Shoulder Arthroplasty

SECOND EDITION

T. Bradley Edwards, MD
Attending Shoulder Surgeon
Fondren Orthopedic Group
Texas Orthopedic Hospital
Houston, Texas

Brent J. Morris, MD
Attending Shoulder and Elbow Surgeon
Fondren Orthopedic Group
Texas Orthopedic Hospital
Houston, Texas

ELSEVIER

ELSEVIER

1600 John F. Kennedy Blvd.
Ste 1800
Philadelphia, PA 19103-2899

SHOULDER ARTHROPLASTY, SECOND EDITION   ISBN: 978-0-323-52940-2

Copyright © 2019 by Elsevier, Inc. All rights reserved.

No part of this publication may be reproduced or transmitted in any form or by any means, electronic or mechanical, including photocopying, recording, or any information storage and retrieval system, without permission in writing from the publisher. Details on how to seek permission, further information about the Publisher's permissions policies and our arrangements with organizations such as the Copyright Clearance Center and the Copyright Licensing Agency, can be found at our website: www.elsevier.com/permissions.

This book and the individual contributions contained in it are protected under copyright by the Publisher (other than as may be noted herein).

Notices

Knowledge and best practice in this field are constantly changing. As new research and experience broaden our understanding, changes in research methods, professional practices, or medical treatment may become necessary.

Practitioners and researchers must always rely on their own experience and knowledge in evaluating and using any information, methods, compounds, or experiments described herein. In using such information or methods they should be mindful of their own safety and the safety of others, including parties for whom they have a professional responsibility.

With respect to any drug or pharmaceutical products identified, readers are advised to check the most current information provided (i) on procedures featured or (ii) by the manufacturer of each product to be administered, to verify the recommended dose or formula, the method and duration of administration, and contraindications. It is the responsibility of practitioners, relying on their own experience and knowledge of their patients, to make diagnoses, to determine dosages and the best treatment for each individual patient, and to take all appropriate safety precautions.

To the fullest extent of the law, neither the Publisher nor the authors, contributors, or editors, assume any liability for any injury and/or damage to persons or property as a matter of products liability, negligence or otherwise, or from any use or operation of any methods, products, instructions, or ideas contained in the material herein.

Previous editions copyright © 2008.

Library of Congress Cataloging-in-Publication Data

Names: Edwards, T. Bradley, author. | Morris, Brent J., author. | Preceded by (work): Gartsman, Gary M. Shoulder arthroplasty.
Title: Shoulder arthroplasty / T. Bradley Edwards, Brent J. Morris.
Description: Second edition. | Philadelphia, PA : Elsevier, [2019] | Preceded by Shoulder arthroplasty / Gary M. Gartsman, T. Bradley Edwards. c2008. | Includes bibliographical references and index.
Identifiers: LCCN 2017056976 | ISBN 9780323529402 (hardcover : alk. paper)
Subjects: | MESH: Shoulder Joint–surgery | Arthroplasty–methods
Classification: LCC RD557.5 | NLM WE 810 | DDC 617.5/72059–dc23 LC record available at https://lccn.loc.gov/2017056976

Senior Content Strategist: Kristine Jones
Content Development Specialist: Mary Hegeler
Publishing Services Manager: Catherine Jackson
Project Manager: Kate Mannix
Design Direction: Paula Catalano
Illustrations Manager: Karen Giacomucci

Printed in China

Last digit is the print number: 9 8 7 6 5 4 3 2 1

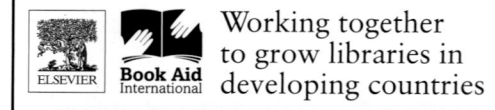

I would be remiss if I did not dedicate the second edition of Shoulder Arthroplasty to my mentor and friend, Gilles Walch. Gilles truly changed my career path 20 years ago when he offered a naïve orthopedic resident who had never been out of North America a chance to study with him in Lyon, France. Gilles, my friend, you taught me not only about shoulder surgery but also about life.

TBE

I owe a tremendous debt of gratitude to Brad Edwards for his friendship and mentoring, and for providing me the opportunity to work on this second edition together. A special thanks to my parents, Lonnie and Cathy, for their love and guidance to direct me along the way. Most importantly, the endless love and support of my wife, Corrie, and children, Miriam and Ben, make it all possible. I am so blessed—you are the joy of my life.

BJM

Preface

Shoulder Arthroplasty was a successful endeavour of Drs. T. Bradley Edwards and Gary Gartsman. Many exciting updates in shoulder arthroplasty have occurred since the publication of the first edition. Dr. Gilles Walch and others have carried forward the pioneering work of Drs. Charles Neer and Paul Grammont in shoulder arthroplasty.

At the time of writing the first edition, reverse shoulder arthroplasty was still a fairly new surgical technique in the United States. The indications for reverse shoulder arthroplasty were limited at that time, and now the indications are rapidly evolving. *Shoulder Arthroplasty*, Second Edition focuses on new applications for reverse shoulder arthroplasty and provides updates with longer-term results following our early experience with reverse shoulder arthroplasty in the United States.

There have been many other important advances in shoulder arthroplasty. Formerly, reverse shoulder arthroplasty and even some anatomic total shoulder arthroplasty humeral stems were long stems and cemented. Now humeral stems are nearly universally press-fit stems and are often shorter stems or even stemless. Furthermore, humeral stems are now convertible to allow for easier conversion from anatomic total shoulder to reverse total shoulder. Additionally, new preoperative surgical planning tools have helped us to better understand the three-dimensional pathology and perform virtual surgery in anatomic and reverse cases.

With these evolving technologies and techniques comes a responsibility to employ these powerful tools wisely. As the number of shoulder arthroplasties performed worldwide continues to grow, surgeons will require more education in shoulder arthroplasty.

Shoulder Arthroplasty, Second Edition shows in detail how we approach all aspects of shoulder replacement in our practice. Our goal was to put these ideas into a simple, user-friendly format to allow practical application by the shoulder surgeon.

T. Bradley Edwards, MD
Brent J. Morris, MD

Contents

SECTION I
The Basics

1. Evolution of Shoulder Arthroplasty — 1
2. Becoming a Shoulder Arthroplasty Surgeon — 8
3. Operating Room Setup — 16
4. Anesthesia, Patient Positioning, and Patient Preparation — 29
5. Long Head of the Biceps Tendon — 35

SECTION II
Unconstrained Shoulder Arthroplasty for Chronic Disease

6. Indications and Contraindications — 39
7. Preoperative Planning and Imaging — 53
8. Surgical Approach — 66
9. Subscapularis — 73
10. Glenoid Exposure — 86
11. Humeral Component — 89
12. Glenoid Component — 106
13. Soft Tissue Balancing — 118
14. Subscapularis and Rotator Interval Repair — 123
15. Wound Closure and Postoperative Orthosis — 130
16. Results and Complications — 134

SECTION III
Reverse Shoulder Arthroplasty

17. Indications and Contraindications — 147
18. Preoperative Planning and Imaging — 160
19. Surgical Approach — 169
20. Glenoid Exposure — 175
21. Humeral Component — 178
22. Glenoid Component — 189
23. Reduction and Deltoid Tensioning — 209
24. Wound Closure and Postoperative Orthosis — 220
25. Results and Complications — 224

SECTION IV
Shoulder Arthroplasty for Fracture

26. Indications and Contraindications — 237
27. Preoperative Planning and Imaging — 242
28. Surgical Approach and Handling of the Tuberosities — 249
29. Humeral Prosthetic Positioning — 254
30. Tuberosity Reduction and Fixation — 268
31. Wound Closure and Postoperative Orthosis — 283
32. Results and Complications — 286

SECTION V
Alternatives to Conventional Shoulder Arthroplasty

33. Stemless Shoulder Arthroplasty — 293
34. Biologic Alternatives to Shoulder Arthroplasty — 308

SECTION VI
Revision Shoulder Arthroplasty

35. Indications and Contraindications — 323
36. Preoperative Planning, Imaging, and Special Tests — 337
37. Surgical Approach — 346
38. Humeral Stem Removal and Glenoid Exposure — 360
39. Humeral Component — 380
40. Glenoid Component — 413
41. Wound Closure and Postoperative Orthosis — 448
42. Results and Complications — 450

SECTION VII
Postoperative Rehabilitation

43. Rehabilitation after Shoulder Arthroplasty — 461

SECTION VIII
The Future

44. Future Directions in Shoulder Arthroplasty — 465

Index — 470

Video Contents

SECTION II

Unconstrained Shoulder Arthroplasty for Chronic Disease

Surgical Approach
Chapter 8, Video 8.1

Unconstrained Total Shoulder Arthroplasty—Humeral Preparation and Humeral Component Placement
Chapter 11, Video 11.1

Unconstrained Total Shoulder Arthroplasty—Glenoid Preparation and Finned, Cementless Central Pegged Glenoid Component Placement
Chapter 12, Video 12.1

Unconstrained Total Shoulder Arthroplasty—Keeled Glenoid Component
Chapter 12, Video 12.2

SECTION III

Reverse Shoulder Arthroplasty

Reverse Shoulder Arthroplasty—Humeral Preparation and Humeral Component Placement
Chapter 21, Video 21.1

Reverse Shoulder Arthroplasty—Glenoid Preparation and Glenoid Component Placement
Chapter 22, Video 22.1

Bony Increased-Offset Reversed Shoulder Arthroplasty (BIO-RSA) Technique—Humeral and Glenoid Preparation and Component Placement
Chapter 22, Video 22.2

SECTION IV

Shoulder Arthroplasty for Fracture

Reverse Shoulder Arthroplasty for Fracture
Chapter 28, Video 28.1

SECTION VI

Revision Shoulder Arthroplasty

Conversion of Anatomic Total Shoulder Arthroplasty to Reverse Shoulder Arthroplasty—Humeral and Glenoid Component Conversion
Chapter 39, Video 39.1—T. Bradley Edwards and Brent J. Morris

ELSEVIER

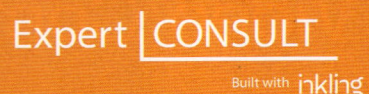

Together, these companion volumes offer comprehensive coverage and trusted guidance on important aspects of shoulder surgery.

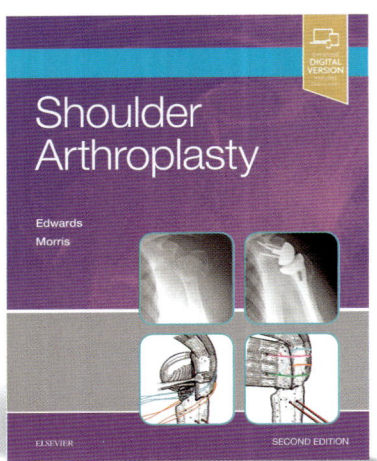

Shoulder Arthroplasty, 2nd Edition

T. Bradley Edwards, MD and Brent J. Morris, MD
2018 • 978-0-323-52940-2

FREE DIGITAL VERSION included with print purchase

- Covers **all key aspects of shoulder replacement surgery** by highlighting new techniques, devices, and implants and providing the latest outcome data for specific conditions and procedures
- Includes indications and contraindications, preoperative planning and imaging, results and complications and more
- **New chapter** on stemless shoulder arthroplasty and new discussions of convertible implants, preoperative planning software, press-fit implants and glenoid reconstructions techniques

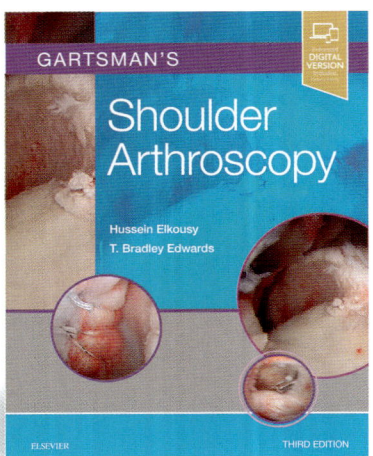

Gartsman's Shoulder Arthroscopy, 3rd Edition

Hussein Elkousy, MD and T. Bradley Edwards, MD
2018 • 978-0-323-52901-3

FREE DIGITAL VERSION included with print purchase

- Covers the **full spectrum of operative shoulder arthroscopy**, including both routine and complex shoulder procedures
- Provides a uniform, consistent approach to walk you through each step of these challenging surgeries
- Features a review of anatomy, indications and contraindications, nonoperative options, preoperative assessment and imaging and much more

Order your copies today | Visit us.elsevierhealth.com

THE BASICS

SECTION 1

Evolution of shoulder arthroplasty

CHAPTER 1

FIRST SHOULDER ARTHROPLASTY

Although Jules Emile Péan is credited with performing the first shoulder arthroplasty, it was probably Themistocles Gluck who first recognized prosthetic replacement as a potential treatment option in the shoulder.[1] Gluck, a Romanian who studied in Germany in the second half of the 19th century, pioneered joint replacement for the treatment of tuberculosis infection. Gluck reported on his design of an ivory shoulder replacement but never documented its use in a living human subject.

The first recorded shoulder arthroplasty was performed in 1893 by Péan, a Parisian surgeon who replaced the shoulder of a patient suffering from tuberculous arthropathy who had refused amputation.[2] Péan implanted a shoulder prosthesis designed and constructed by J. Porter Michaels, a Parisian dentist; the prosthesis consisted of a rubber humeral head that had been boiled in paraffin to harden it and was attached to a platinum shaft via a metal wire. A second metal wire attached the implant to the glenoid. The patient initially "did well" after the surgery before ultimately requiring removal of the prosthesis for recurrence of infection 2 years later.

FIRST-GENERATION SHOULDER ARTHROPLASTY

The first shoulder arthroplasty using a prosthesis with an anatomic design was performed in 1950 by Frederick Krueger.[3] Krueger used a Vitallium implant created by molding proximal humeri obtained from cadavers. He successfully implanted this prosthesis in a young patient with osteonecrosis of the humeral head. The modern era of shoulder arthroplasty, however, was pioneered by Dr. Charles Neer. Neer originally performed hemiarthroplasty to treat complex proximal humeral fractures starting in 1953.[4] Nearly 20 years later, he would report on the use of shoulder replacement for the treatment of glenohumeral arthritis.[5] Neer originally used a monoblock implant; however, variations in humeral head size among patients led to the concept of modularity, which allowed the use of variable humeral head diameters in shoulder arthroplasty. Monoblock implants are now commonly referred to as first-generation shoulder arthroplasty.

SECOND-GENERATION SHOULDER ARTHROPLASTY

The introduction of modular humeral head arthroplasty with variable diameter gave rise to the second generation of shoulder arthroplasty. Although these designs appeared to be an improvement over the earlier monoblock designs, they did not seem to optimally fit all patients. Additionally, not all patients had the good and excellent clinical results reported by Neer after shoulder arthroplasty with first- and second-generation designs.

THIRD-GENERATION SHOULDER ARTHROPLASTY

In the late 1980s, Boileau and Walch hypothesized that variations in anatomy prevented current first- and second-generation shoulder arthroplasty stems from achieving optimal fit within the proximal humerus.[6] They undertook an anatomic study of the proximal humerus that yielded some important conclusions. They discovered that the proximal humerus could be modeled by using a sphere and cylinder. A portion of the sphere represents the articular surface of the proximal humerus. The diameter of the humeral head articular surface was found to be highly variable, as was the thickness of the humeral head. Thickness and diameter were found to have a fixed relationship and correlated with one another linearly. They further found the inclination of the anatomic neck of the humerus relative to the humeral diaphysis to be highly variable. Humeral retroversion, defined by the relationship of the humeral anatomic neck to the transepicondylar axis of the elbow, was found to vary by more than 50 degrees. Finally, the sphere (humeral head) was discovered to be offset, usually posteriorly and medially, from the cylinder (humeral diaphysis). These relationships are summarized in Table 1.1.

The anatomic studies of Boileau and Walch gave rise to the third generation of shoulder arthroplasty: the anatomic (adaptable) prosthesis. The concept behind third-generation implants is to adapt the prosthesis to the individual patient's anatomy instead of trying to force the anatomy to adapt to the prosthesis. Anatomic shoulder arthroplasty stems rely on an anatomic neck cut to replicate the patient's normal humeral retroversion. Multiple humeral head diameters are available. The prosthetic stem has a variable neck shaft (inclination) angle, and the head can be placed in varying degrees of posterior and medial offset, thereby allowing nearly perfect replication of the patient's native anatomy.

Several laboratory studies have demonstrated the clinical relevance of advances in design imposed by third-generation humeral implants. Harryman and colleagues demonstrated that the placement of too thick a humeral component had detrimental effects on glenohumeral motion,[7] whereas Jobe and Iannotti found a decrease in the arc of available glenohumeral motion when too thin a humeral head component was implanted.[8] In an eloquent computer model, Pearl and Kurutz demonstrated the necessity of being able to vary the diameter of the humeral head, offset of the humeral head, and angle of neck inclination of a humeral prosthesis to replicate the patient's native anatomy (Fig. 1.1).[9]

SHORT-STEM AND STEMLESS SHOULDER ARTHROPLASTY

Although the third-generation implants introduced initially in Europe were designed for implantation using cement, the North American market, following trends in hip arthroplasty, demanded implants that could be fixated without the use of cement. As experience grew with the use of press-fit humeral stems, many surgeons noted that the initial fixation occurred at the proximal portion or metaphyseal portion of the implant. This observation, combined with some concerns over medial calcar bone loss possibly related to proximal stress shielding (Fig. 1.2), led to the development of humeral implants with shorter stems designed to exploit this proximal metaphyseal fixation (Fig. 1.3). These short-stem implants retained all the advantages of anatomic restoration of the third-generation implants without the necessity of extending the humeral stem into the diaphysis.

Following the successful implementation of short-stem humeral components, stemless anatomic shoulder arthroplasty was introduced, initially in Europe and subsequently in North America. These stemless devices employ fixation relegated to the metaphyseal portion of the proximal humerus (Fig. 1.4). Experience with these anatomic stemless devices is relatively limited, but early results are encouraging.[10]

GLENOID RESURFACING

Neer first reported on the use of a glenoid component in unconstrained shoulder arthroplasty for the treatment of

TABLE 1.1	Anatomic Variability of the Proximal Humerus	
Dimension	Mean	Range
Humeral head diameter	46.2 mm	37.1 to 56.9 mm
Articular surface diameter	43.3 mm	36.5 to 51.7 mm
Articular surface thickness	15.2 mm	12.1 to 18.2 mm
Inclination	129.6 degrees	123.2 to 135.8 degrees
Retroversion	17.9 degrees	−6.7 to 47.5 degrees
Posterior offset	2.6 mm	−0.8 to 6.1 mm
Medial offset	6.9 mm	2.9 to 10.8 mm

From Boileau P, Walch G: Anatomical study of the proximal humerus: surgical technique consideration and prosthetic design rationale. In Walch G, Boileau P, editors: *Shoulder arthroplasty*, Berlin, 1999, Springer, pp 69–82.

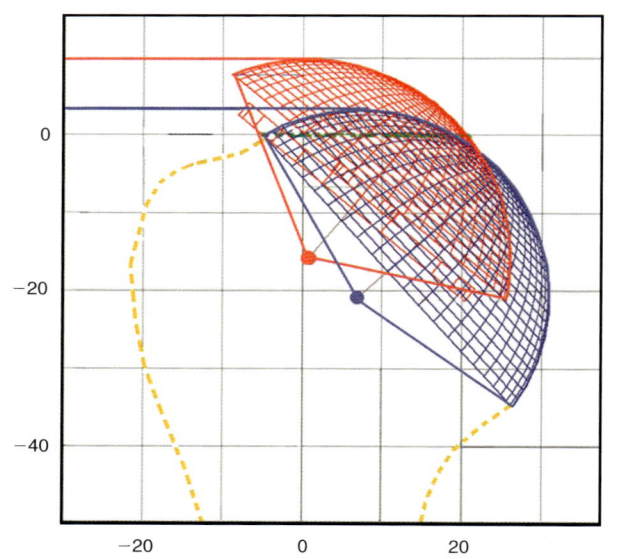
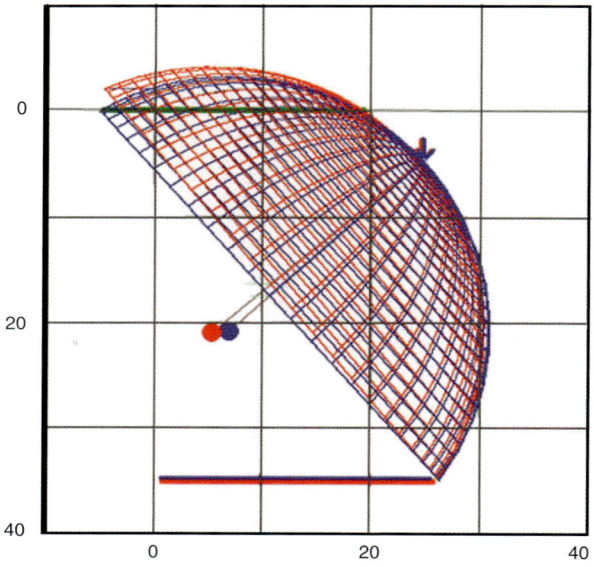

FIGURE 1.1 (A) Inability to reproduce the native anatomy with a prosthesis that has a fixed inclination angle. The native anatomy is depicted in blue, and the closest prosthetic fit is depicted in red. (B) Nearly perfect replication of the native anatomy after variable inclination is introduced into the prosthetic system. (From Pearl ML, Kurutz S: Geometric analysis of commonly used prosthetic systems for proximal humeral replacement, *J Bone Joint Surg Am* 81:660–671, 1999.)

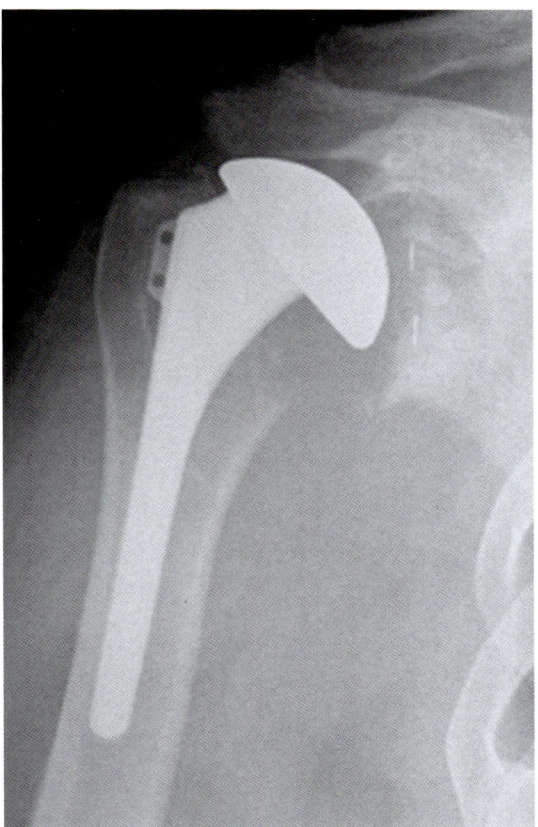

FIGURE 1.2 Medial calcar bone loss occurring with a press-fit third-generation stem.

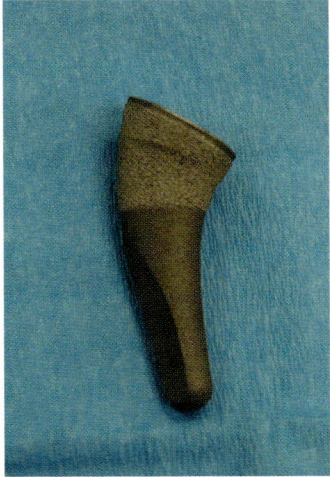

FIGURE 1.3 Short-stem humeral implant designed for metaphyseal press-fit fixation.

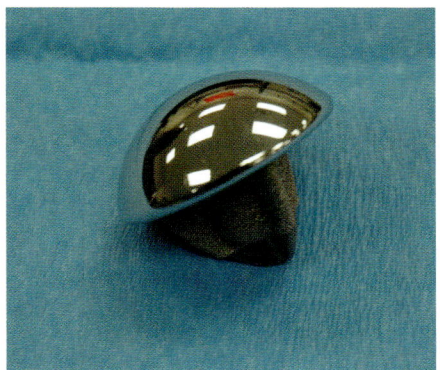

FIGURE 1.4 Stemless humeral implant.

glenohumeral arthritis in 1974.[5] Neer's original implant was a keeled cemented rectangular component (the same anteroposterior diameter superiorly and inferiorly) with a radius of curvature matching the humeral head component.

Advances in glenoid resurfacing have occurred in component design and implantation techniques. Different component designs commonly used include cemented polyethylene keeled convex-back designs, cemented polyethylene keeled flat-back designs, cemented polyethylene pegged convex-back designs, metal-backed designs, and more recently pegged designs employing minimal cement and a cementless central peg. Convex-back designs have been shown experimentally to resist sheer forces better than flat-back designs do, and this has translated into fewer radiolucent lines around the glenoid component in the clinical scenario.[11-13] A larger debate exists over whether to use a keeled or a pegged component. Laboratory studies have demonstrated less micromotion with pegged implants.[14] Clinical studies, however, have reported the superiority of both pegs and keels.[15,16] Because radiographic comparison of these two types of implant is difficult, this debate remains unsolved at present, although trends in North America definitely favor pegged designs. The original metal-backed designs consisted of a metal base plate secured with a screw-type mechanism and a modular polyethylene liner. The thickness of the metal often required that the polyethylene insert be very thin to avoid placing excessive tension on the glenohumeral soft tissues. This thinness resulted in poor wear characteristics of the polyethylene and caused implant failure.[17] Many early metal-backed designs have been abandoned; however, implantation of a glenoid component without the use of cement is still appealing, especially in revision surgery, which may involve compromised glenoid bone stock. Research is ongoing in the development of new and improved metal-backed glenoid designs.

An important advance in the design of glenoid components was recognition of the significance of glenohumeral prosthetic mismatch. Mismatch is defined as the difference in radius of curvature between the humeral head and the glenoid component. Congruent articulations (mismatch = 0) allow optimal surface contact, minimize the risk of surface wear of the glenoid component, and contribute to increased joint stability. However, with these advantages comes a lack of obligate translation (translation between the articular surfaces that normally occurs with shoulder mobility and is absorbed by elastic deformation of the articular cartilage and the glenoid labrum). Lack of obligate translation may lead to loosening of the glenoid component by increasing the stress developed at the implant fixation site. Alternatively, noncongruent articulations (larger glenoid than humeral radius of curvature) allow obligate translation between the humeral head and the glenoid, thereby potentially decreasing the stress observed at the glenoid implant fixation site. Glenoid component wear and joint stability remain a concern in noncongruent articulations. Laboratory investigations have yielded some insight into appropriate mismatch in shoulder arthroplasty, including studies demonstrating that a 4-mm mismatch is necessary to best replicate normal shoulder mobility. Other studies have shown that mismatch in excess of 10 mm risks fracture of the polyethylene component.[18,19] The clinical relevance of these laboratory studies was not clear, however, until Walch and coworkers reported on the influence of glenohumeral prosthetic mismatch on radiolucent lines occurring around the glenoid component.[20] This study found that fewer radiolucent lines occurred at minimum 2-year follow-up when a radial mismatch of at least 6 mm was used during the performance of total shoulder arthroplasty. An upper limit of mismatch was not established, however, thus prompting ongoing studies to discover the ideal glenohumeral prosthetic mismatch.

Another aspect of glenoid resurfacing that has evolved is the implantation technique of glenoid components. Neer originally recommended preparation of a keel slot with a curette to remove a large amount of bone and create a large cement mantle.[5] Gazielly and colleagues alternatively introduced the bone compaction technique for implantation of keeled glenoid components.[21] Radiolucent lines around glenoid components appear on the initial postoperative radiographs in many cases and have been attributed to technical deficiencies.[22] The compaction technique of bone preparation addresses radiolucent lines in three ways. First, compaction of cancellous bone in the glenoid provides a more stable base for the glenoid component than does bone removal via curettage. Second, a compacted bone slot that has the same dimensions as the component keel allows a primary "press fit" fixation, which should help prevent micromotion of the component as the cement polymerizes. Third, the compaction technique uses a smaller amount of cement, which may decrease thermal necrosis of the adjacent glenoid bone. Clinically, a comparison of the curettage technique with the compaction technique has shown superiority of the compaction technique in minimizing radiolucent lines on immediate and 2-year postoperative radiographs.[23]

More recently, preservation of subchondral bone during glenoid preparation has proved important in avoiding glenoid component failure.[24] Consequently a new generation of glenoid implants have been developed that minimize glenoid bone removal during preparation. These adaptable glenoid implants allow the component to match the existing radius of curvature of the native glenoid (Fig. 1.5).

ARTHROPLASTY FOR FRACTURE

Neer's original indication for shoulder arthroplasty—complex fractures of the proximal humerus—remains the most difficult diagnosis for which shoulder arthroplasty is used. Performance of shoulder arthroplasty for fracture is fraught with potential complications and often results in disappointing outcomes. The majority of these poor outcomes are related to nonunion or malunion of the greater and lesser tuberosities after arthroplasty. Boileau and associates have identified four potential causes of tuberosity complications after shoulder arthroplasty for fracture.[25] First, improper positioning of the prosthesis may lead to nonunion of the tuberosities by placing

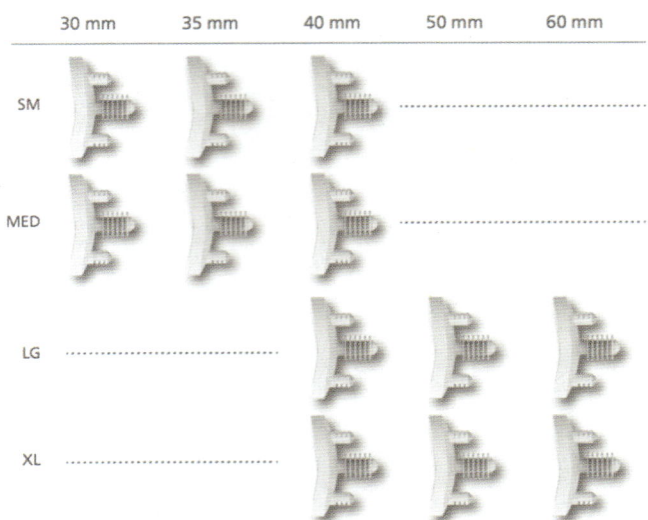

FIGURE 1.5 Adaptable glenoid implants with variable backside radii of curvature. SM, small; MED, medium; LG, large; XL, extra large.

undue tension on the rotator cuff, specifically if the prosthesis is implanted proud or in excessive retroversion (Fig. 1.6). Second, the osteopenic nature of the tuberosities in this patient population makes healing of the tuberosities difficult to achieve. Third, fixation of the tuberosities around the prosthesis is difficult and often results in migration of the tuberosities.[26] Fourth, the large amount of proximal metal used in conventional humeral arthroplasties may act as a hindrance to healing of the tuberosities.

Arthroplasty for fracture has evolved specifically to address these issues of tuberosity complications. First, ancillary instrumentation was developed to allow more reliable placement and testing of the humeral implant before definitive cementation (Fig. 1.7). This intimidating early instrumentation eventually gave way to easier techniques allowing for simpler replication of native anatomy.[27] Second, the interface between the greater and lesser tuberosities and the interface between the tuberosities and the native humerus is now routinely bone-grafted with autogenous bone from the fractured humeral head. Third, a reproducible, biomechanically stable tuberosity fixation technique has been developed. Fourth, fracture-specific implants with less metallic bulk proximally and metaphyseal fenestrations to promote healing of the tuberosities are now available for use in fracture cases (Fig. 1.8). Boileau and colleagues reported on the clinical implications of the use of an arthroplasty system designed for the treatment of proximal humeral fractures and found that tuberosity complications decreased from 49% in procedures involving conventional hemiarthroplasty to 25% in procedures that used a hemiarthroplasty designed for fracture cases.[25]

Despite the advances made in implants, instrumentation, and surgical techniques in unconstrained shoulder arthroplasty for fracture, outcomes may still be disappointing compared with the outcomes obtained for unconstrained arthroplasty in chronic conditions, especially in elderly patients with compromised bone quality. Largely because of these suboptimal results, constrained (reverse) shoulder arthroplasty is now widely used as the primary treatment

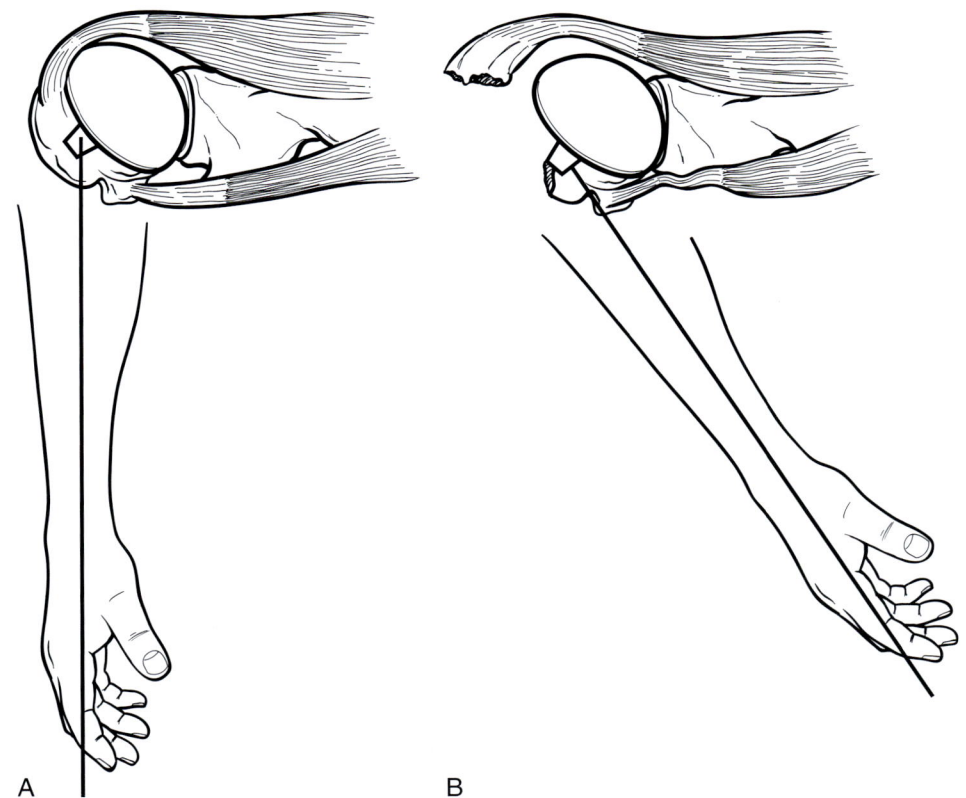

FIGURE 1.6 (A and B) Illustration showing how excessive humeral retroversion can cause migration of the tuberosity.

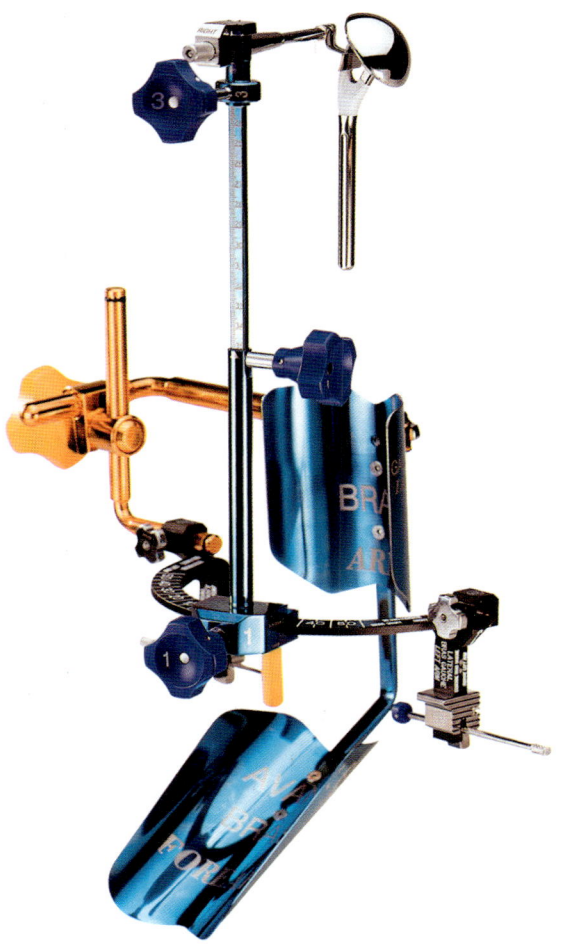

FIGURE 1.7 Early ancillary instrumentation for approximating correct prosthetic height and version.

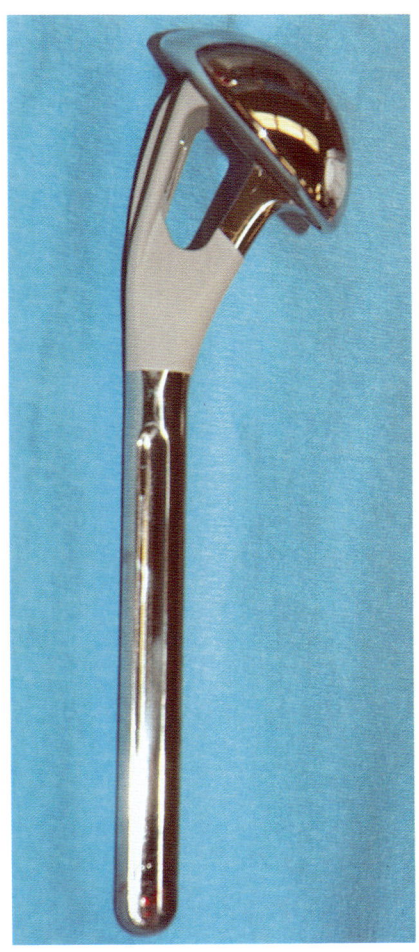

FIGURE 1.8 Humeral stem specifically designed for use in fracture cases. Note the lower profile proximally and the fenestration to allow bone grafting and promotion of tuberosity healing.

in these difficult cases, relegating unconstrained arthroplasty use to fracture cases in young patients with good bone quality and an otherwise unreconstructible scenario.

CONSTRAINED AND SEMICONSTRAINED SHOULDER ARTHROPLASTY

Constrained and semiconstrained arthroplasty was initially introduced in the 1960s to treat patients with glenohumeral arthritis and massive rotator cuff tears. The concept of these devices is to resolve upward migration of the humeral head and thereby restore the normal deltoid moment arm and allow active elevation of the arm powered by the deltoid. Reverse designs, with a sphere fixated to the glenoid and a cup secured to the proximal humerus, were introduced in the past to accomplish this goal. The problem with these early designs was early loosening of the glenoid caused by deltoid forces acting on the laterally offset center of glenohumeral rotation (Fig. 1.9). Such failures eventually resulted in abandonment of these early prosthetic designs.

In 1987, Paul Grammont introduced a new reverse-design prosthesis in an effort to overcome the failures that had plagued earlier attempts. This new prosthesis uses a "glenosphere" component fixated over the scapular neck and places the center of glenohumeral rotation within the bone of the glenoid instead of lateral to it (Fig. 1.10).[28] This prosthesis now has up to 30 years' follow-up in Europe, and glenoid failure rates have not exceeded those of unconstrained total shoulder prostheses in patients with a competent rotator cuff.[29,30] Additionally, although pain relief has been equivalent to that seen with humeral head replacement, postoperative active shoulder elevation has far exceeded the elevation that can be expected after hemiarthroplasty.

Following approval by the U.S. Food and Drug Administration in the United States in 2004, implantation of reverse shoulder prostheses has increased exponentially. Indications for reverse shoulder arthroplasty are now manifold, and reverse shoulder arthroplasty has now become the procedure of choice for many diagnoses previously treated with unconstrained shoulder arthroplasty, such as comminuted proximal humeral fractures in elderly patients. Additionally, the vast majority of revision shoulder arthroplasties are now performed with semiconstrained devices.

As indications for reverse shoulder arthroplasty have expanded, designs of these implants have evolved. Newer reverse shoulder arthroplasty designs employ varying amounts of lateral offset in the humeral and/or glenoid components. Humeral cut depth and inclination angles vary among implant systems. Early results with many of these design variations are encouraging, but one "best" design is yet to be found.

CONVERTIBLE SHOULDER ARTHROPLASTY

As the number of shoulder arthroplasty cases has continued to increase, the number of cases requiring revision surgery has followed suit. Often, removal of the previously placed humeral stem is technically difficult, as many of these stems are well fixed. Revision of unconstrained shoulder

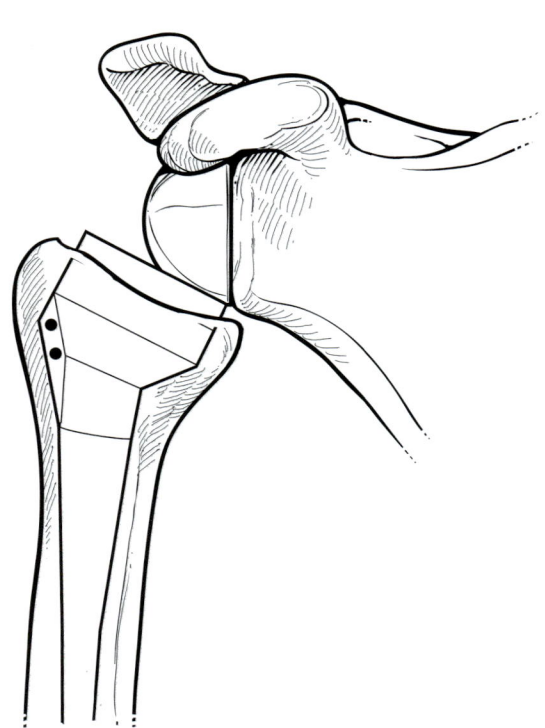

FIGURE 1.9 The laterally located center of rotation of early reverse-design prostheses caused early loosening.

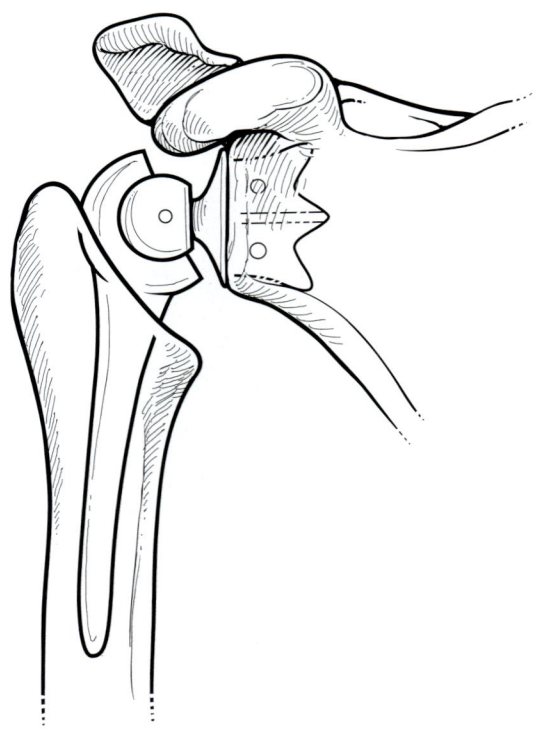

FIGURE 1.10 The center of rotation of the Grammont prosthesis is within the scapular bone, thus theoretically decreasing the potential for loosening.

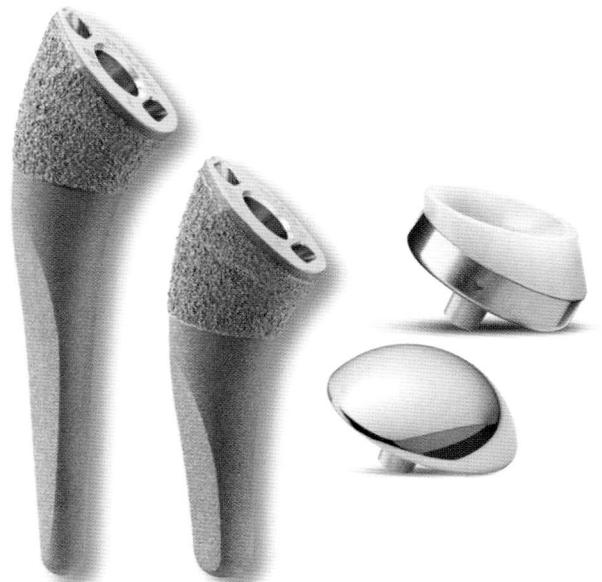

FIGURE 1.11 Convertible implant system that allows revision of an unconstrained shoulder arthroplasty to a semiconstrained shoulder arthroplasty without removal of the humeral stem.

arthroplasty is often performed using a reverse arthroplasty device. Because of these factors, convertible shoulder implants have been developed to allow retention of the humeral stem when an unconstrained shoulder arthroplasty is being revised to a semiconstrained arthroplasty. Additionally, these convertible systems allow a single platform to be used in the primary arthroplasty, whether anatomic or reverse (Fig. 1.11).

REFERENCES

1. Gluck T: Referat über die Durch das moderne chirurgishe Experiment gewonnenen positiven Resultate betreffend die Nacht und den Ersatz von defecten hoherer Gewebe sowie über die Verwertung resorbirbarer und lebendiger Tamons in der Chirurgie, *Arch Klin Chir* 41:187–239, 1891.
2. Lugli T: Artificial shoulder joint by Péan (1893). The facts of an exceptional intervention and the prosthetic method, *Clin Orthop* 133:215–218, 1978.
3. Krueger FJ: A Vitallium replica arthroplasty on the shoulder: a case report of aseptic necrosis of the proximal end of the humerus, *Surgery* 30:1005–1011, 1951.
4. Neer CS: Articular replacement for the humeral head, *J Bone Joint Surg Am* 37:215–228, 1955.
5. Neer CS: Replacement arthroplasty for glenohumeral osteoarthritis, *J Bone Joint Surg Am* 56:1–13, 1974.
6. Boileau P, Walch G: Anatomical study of the proximal humerus: surgical technique consideration and prosthetic design rationale. In Walch G, Boileau P, editors: *Shoulder arthroplasty*, Berlin, 1999, Springer, pp 69–82.
7. Harryman DT, Sidles JA, Harris SL, et al: The effect of articular conformity and the size of the humeral head component on laxity and motion after glenohumeral arthroplasty: a study in cadavera, *J Bone Joint Surg Am* 77:555–563, 1995.
8. Jobe CM, Iannotti JP: Limits imposed on glenohumeral motion by joint geometry, *J Shoulder Elbow Surg* 4:281–285, 1995.
9. Pearl ML, Kurutz S: Geometric analysis of commonly used prosthetic systems for proximal humeral replacement, *J Bone Joint Surg Am* 81:660–671, 1999.
10. Churchill RS, Chuinard C, Wiater JM, et al: Clinical and radiographic outcomes of the Simpliciti canal-sparing shoulder arthroplasty system: a prospective two-year multicenter study, *J Bone Joint Surg Am* 98:552–560, 2016.
11. Anglin C, Wyss UP, Pichora DR: Mechanical testing of shoulder prostheses and recommendations for glenoid design, *J Shoulder Elbow Surg* 9:323–331, 2000.
12. Lacaze F, Kempf JF, Bonnomet F, et al: Primary fixation of glenoid implants: an in vitro study. In Walch G, Boileau P, editors: *Shoulder arthroplasty*, Berlin, 1999, Springer, pp 141–146.
13. Szabo I, Buscayret F, Walch G, et al: Radiographic comparison of flat back and convex back polyethylene glenoid components in total shoulder arthroplasty. Paper presented at the 16th Annual Meeting of the Société Européenne de Chirurgie de l'Epaule et du Coude, September 2002, Budapest.
14. Anglin C, Wyss UP, Nyffeler RW, et al: Loosening performance of cemented glenoid prosthesis design pairs, *Clin Biomech (Bristol, Avon)* 16:144–150, 2001.
15. Gartsman GM, Elkousy HA, Warnock KM, et al: Radiographic comparison of pegged and keeled glenoid components, *J Shoulder Elbow Surg* 14:252–257, 2005.
16. Gazielly D, El-Abiad R: Comparative results of three types of polyethylene cemented glenoid components. In Walch G, Boileau P, Molé D, editors: *2000 Prosthèses d'Epaule…Recul de 2 à 10 Ans*, Paris, 2001, Sauramps Medical, pp 483–488.
17. Boileau P, Avidor C, Krishnan SG, et al: Cemented polyethylene versus uncemented metal-backed glenoid components in total shoulder arthroplasty: a prospective, double-blind, randomized study, *J Shoulder Elbow Surg* 11:351–359, 2002.
18. Karduna AR, Williams GR, Williams JL, et al: Joint stability after total shoulder arthroplasty in a cadaver model, *J Shoulder Elbow Surg* 6:506–511, 1997.
19. Friedman RJ, An YH, Draughn RA: Glenohumeral congruence in total shoulder arthroplasty, *Orthop Trans* 21:17, 1997.
20. Walch G, Edwards TB, Boulahia A, et al: The influence of glenohumeral prosthetic mismatch on glenoid radiolucent lines: results of a multicentric study, *J Bone Joint Surg Am* 84:2186–2191, 2002.
21. Gazielly DF, Allende C, Pamelin E: Results of cancellous compaction technique for glenoid resurfacing. Paper presented at the 9th International Congress on Surgery of the Shoulder, May 2004, Washington, DC.
22. Brems J: The glenoid component in total shoulder arthroplasty, *J Shoulder Elbow Surg* 2:47–54, 1993.
23. Szabo I, Buscayret F, Edwards TB, et al: Radiographic comparison of two different glenoid preparation techniques in total shoulder arthroplasty, *Clin Orthop Relat Res* 431:104–110, 2005.
24. Walch G, Young AA, Boileau P, et al: Patterns of loosening of polyethylene keeled glenoid components after shoulder arthroplasty for primary osteoarthritis: results of a multicenter study with more than five years of follow-up, *J Bone Joint Surg Am* 94:145–150, 2012.
25. Boileau P, Coste JS, Ahrens PM, et al: Prosthetic shoulder replacement for fracture: Results of the multicentre study. In Walch G, Boileau P, Molé D, editors: *2000 Prosthèses d'Epaule…Recul de 2 à 10 Ans*, Paris, 2001, Sauramps Medical, pp 561–578.
26. Gerber C, Wahlström P, Nyffeler R: Suture failure caused by suboptimal prosthetic design may cause secondary tuberosity displacement. Paper presented at the 8th International Congress on Surgery of the Shoulder, April 2001, Cape Town, South Africa.
27. Krishnan SG, Bennion PW, Reineck JR, et al: Hemiarthroplasty for proximal humeral fracture: restoration of the Gothic arch, *Orthop Clin North Am* 39:441–450, 2008.
28. Grammont PM, Baulot E: Delta shoulder prosthesis for rotator cuff rupture, *Orthopedics* 16:65–68, 1993.
29. Favard L, Nové-Josserand L, Levigne C, et al: Anatomical arthroplasty versus reverse arthroplasty in treatment of cuff tear arthropathy. Paper presented at the 14th Annual Meeting of the Société Européenne de Chirurgie de l'Epaule et du Coude, September 2000, Lisbon, Portugal.
30. Bouttens D, Nérot C: Cuff tear arthropathy: Mid term results with the delta prosthesis. Paper presented at the 14th Annual Meeting of the Société Européenne de Chirurgie de l'Epaule et du Coude, September 2000, Lisbon, Portugal.

CHAPTER 2

Becoming a shoulder arthroplasty surgeon

Shoulder arthroplasty is much less frequently performed than hip and knee arthroplasty; it accounts for only 7.5% of inpatient joint replacements in the United States,[1] largely because hip and knee arthrosis is much more common than glenohumeral arthrosis. Additionally, patients with glenohumeral arthrosis tolerate the symptoms better than those with hip and knee arthrosis because they do not rely on their shoulders for locomotion. Consequently a busy general orthopedic surgeon may easily perform more than 100 hip and knee replacements in a given year and yet see fewer than five patients who are candidates for shoulder replacement during that same period. Moreover, most orthopedic residencies offer the same lower extremity–focused arthroplasty experience. This has been confirmed by our shoulder fellows, most of whom have seen fewer than five total shoulder arthroplasties during a 4-year orthopedic residency.

The desire and need to perform shoulder arthroplasty have evolved from advances made in the field of shoulder surgery over the last three decades. Shoulder arthroscopy has developed from a solely diagnostic procedure to a part of the surgical armamentarium that allows treatment of nearly every shoulder problem formerly treated by open surgery. As a result, many orthopedists, largely through technique-driven courses, have become proficient at arthroscopic shoulder procedures, including but not limited to rotator cuff and labral repair. As these same surgeons develop practices in which an increasing number of patients with shoulder problems are treated, it becomes inevitable that they will encounter diagnoses not amenable to arthroscopic treatment, specifically diagnoses best treated by shoulder arthroplasty. An aging population that is living longer and remaining more active has contributed to the increasing number of shoulder arthroplasties performed annually as well. In the United States alone, approximately 105,700 shoulder arthroplasties were performed in 2015, a 6.2% increase over the previous year.[1] This chapter reviews some basic concepts that must be understood when an orthopedic surgeon decides to become a shoulder arthroplasty surgeon.

ANATOMY

An exhaustive review of shoulder anatomy is beyond the scope of this textbook; however, an understanding of open shoulder anatomy is imperative for performing shoulder arthroplasty. Most shoulder arthroplasties are performed through a deltopectoral approach. This section reviews the surgically important anatomic features of this approach.

Cutaneous

The palpable coracoid process marks the proximal extent of the skin incision for the deltopectoral approach. In thin patients, the deltopectoral interval may be palpable, thus helping to direct the skin incision (Fig. 2.1). In revision cases, the skin incision may be extended distally along the lateral aspect of the biceps brachii muscle, which is also palpable (Fig. 2.2).

Subcutaneous

The deltopectoral interval is marked by the cephalic vein. This vein has many small branches, most of which enter the deltoid muscle (Fig. 2.3). The deltoid has attachments at the acromion and the deltoid tuberosity of the humerus (Fig. 2.4). The pectoralis major has attachments at the clavicle, the sternum, and the humerus just lateral to the long head of the biceps brachii tendon.

Coracoid/Conjoined Tendon

Immediately deep to the deltoid and pectoralis major muscles is the conjoined tendon of the coracobrachialis and the short head of the biceps brachii (Fig. 2.5). This structure passes from the tip of the coracoid process (the proximal extent of dissection) to the anterior humeral shaft. The coracoid process also serves as the point of attachment of the coracoacromial ligament laterally and the pectoralis minor tendon medially (Fig. 2.6).

Neurovascular Structures

As the conjoined tendon is retracted medially, the anterior humeral circumflex vessels can be seen passing along the inferior border of the subscapularis tendon (Fig. 2.7). The axillary nerve may be visualized inferior to the anterior humeral circumflex vessels during dissection with the arm held in a forward-flexed and slightly internally rotated position (Fig. 2.8). The musculocutaneous nerve may be visualized as it enters the coracobrachialis and the short head of the biceps brachii, although it is not routinely exposed during shoulder arthroplasty (Fig. 2.9).

Text continued on p. 13

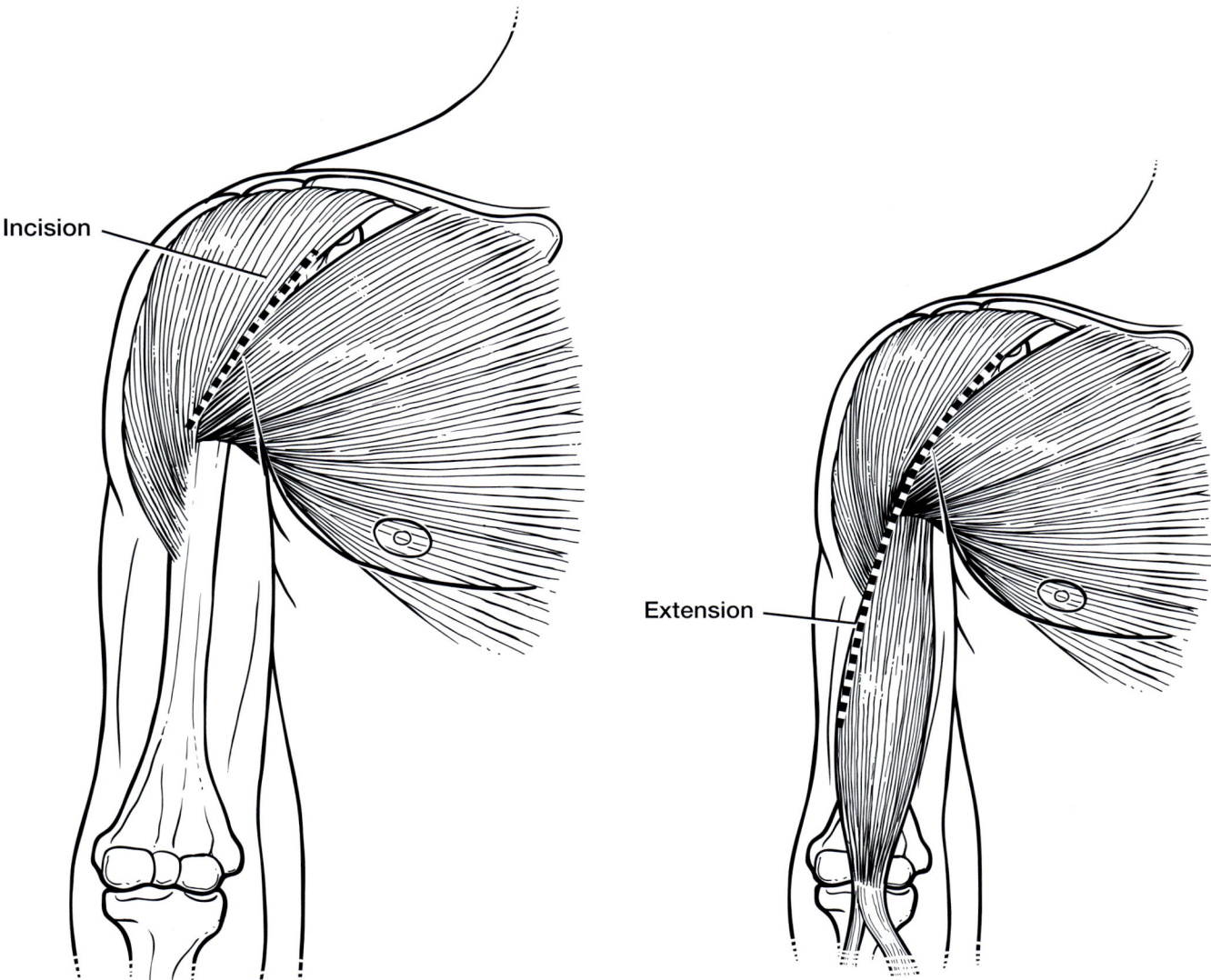

FIGURE 2.1 Skin incision for the deltopectoral approach to the shoulder.

FIGURE 2.2 Extension of the deltopectoral skin incision into an anterolateral approach to the humeral shaft.

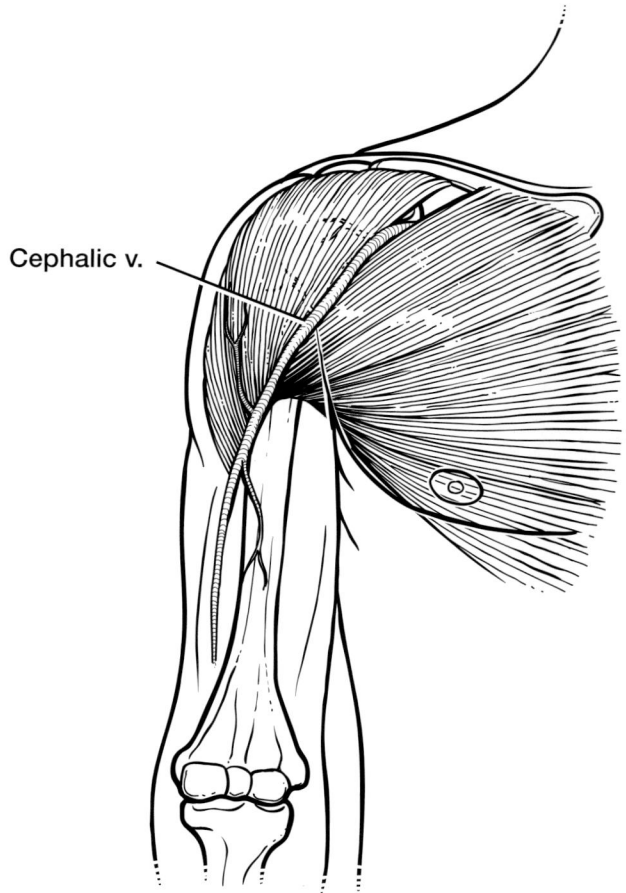

FIGURE 2.3 Cephalic vein marking the deltopectoral interval.

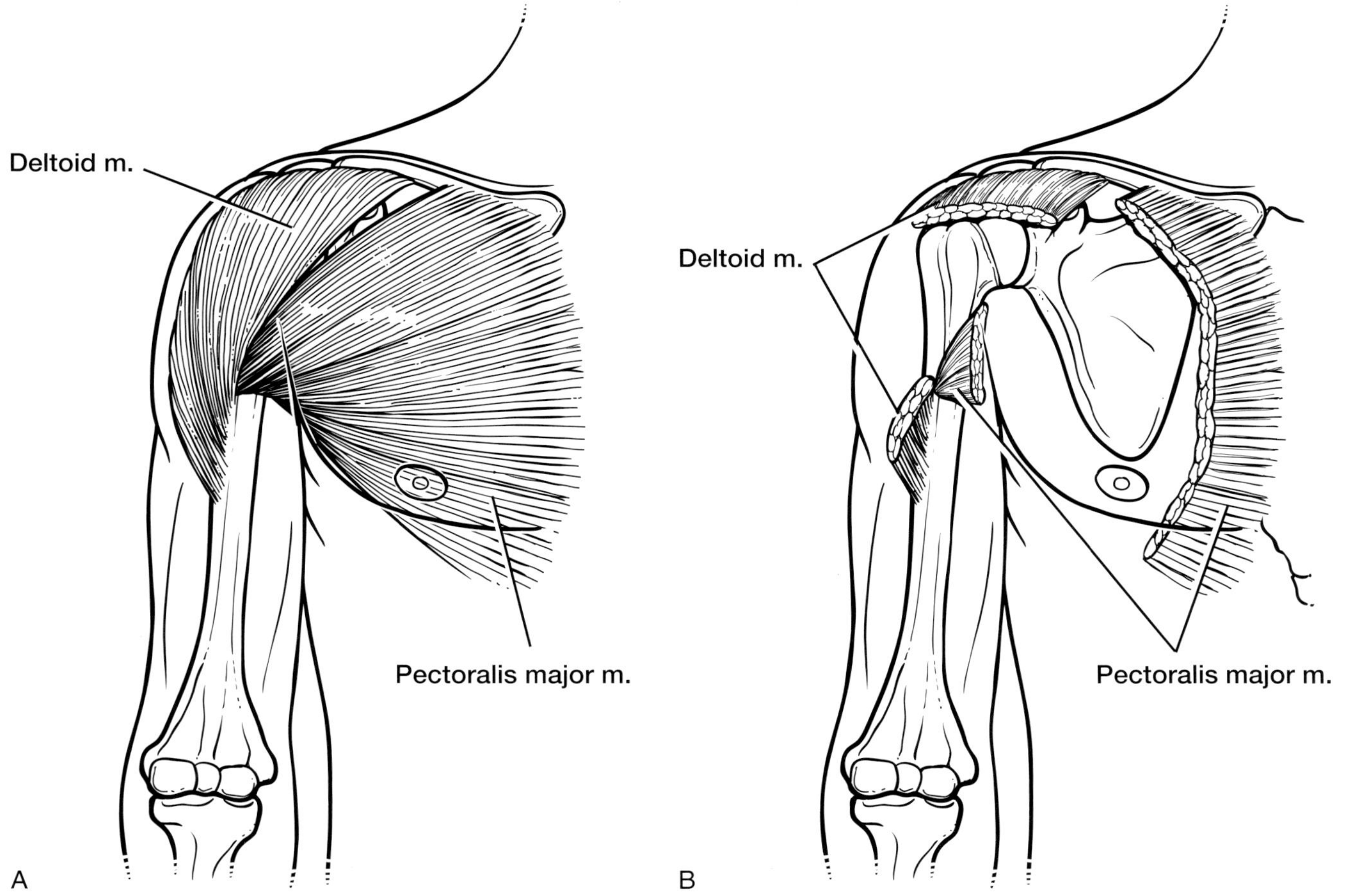

FIGURE 2.4 (A and B) Anatomy of the deltoid and pectoralis major muscles.

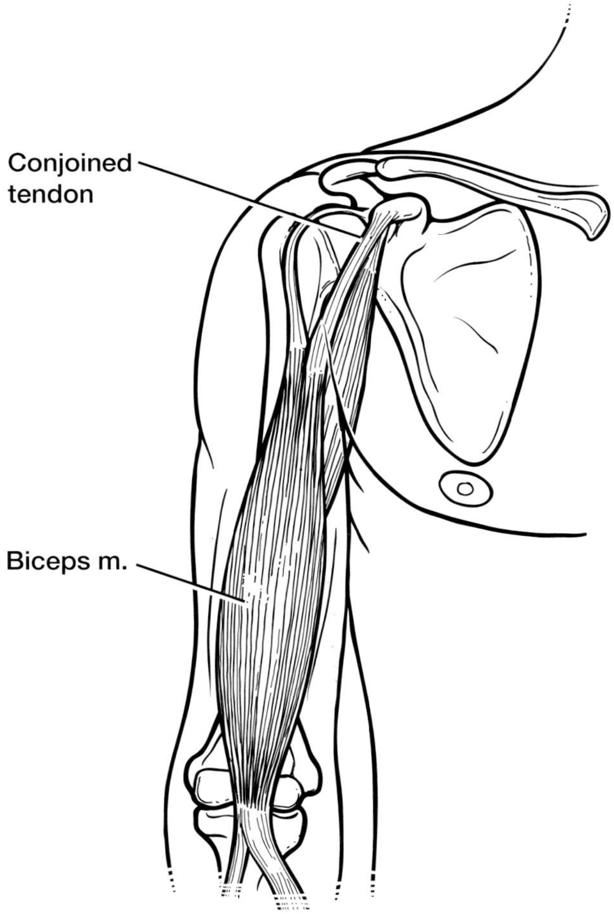

FIGURE 2.5 Anatomy of the conjoined tendon.

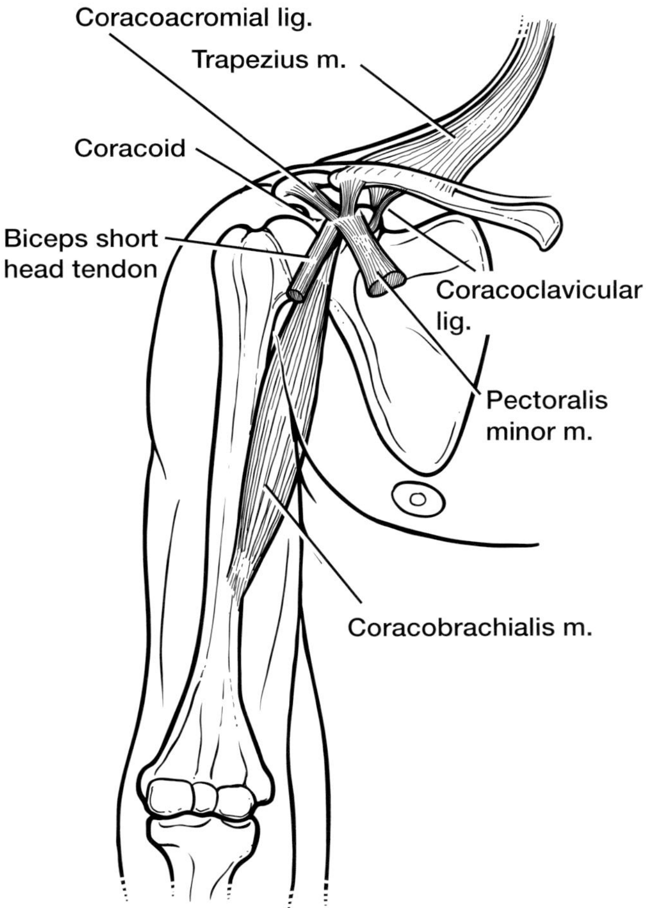

FIGURE 2.6 Structures attaching to the coracoid process.

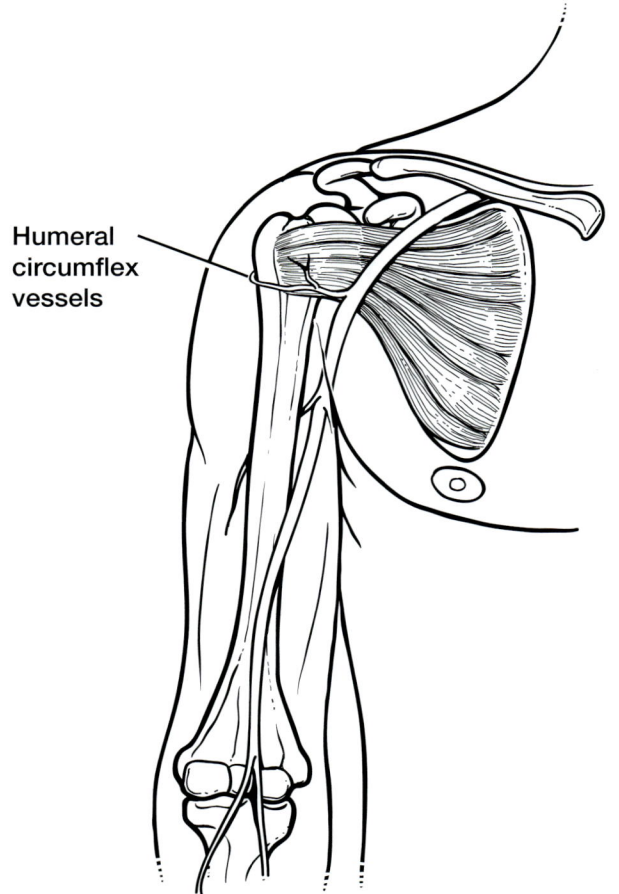

FIGURE 2.7 Anterior humeral circumflex vessels passing over the inferior aspect of the subscapularis.

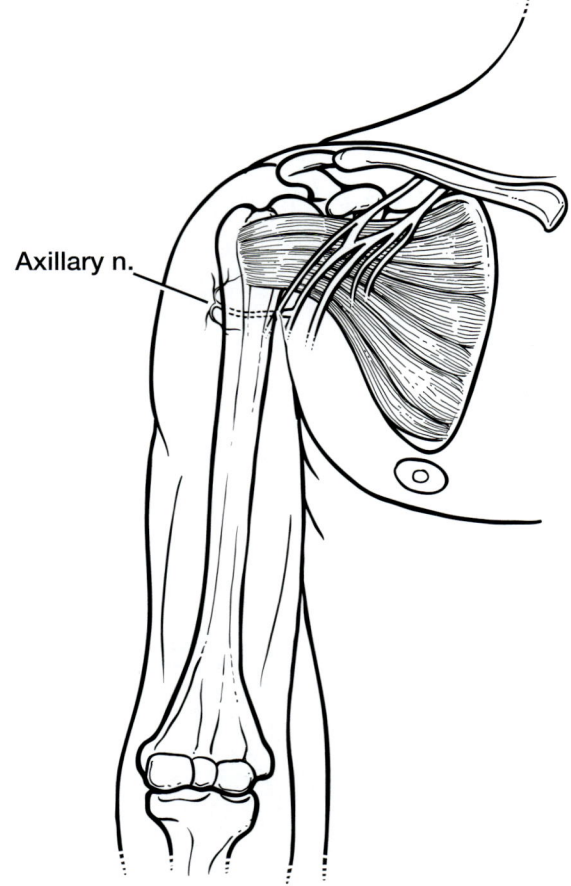

FIGURE 2.8 The axillary nerve.

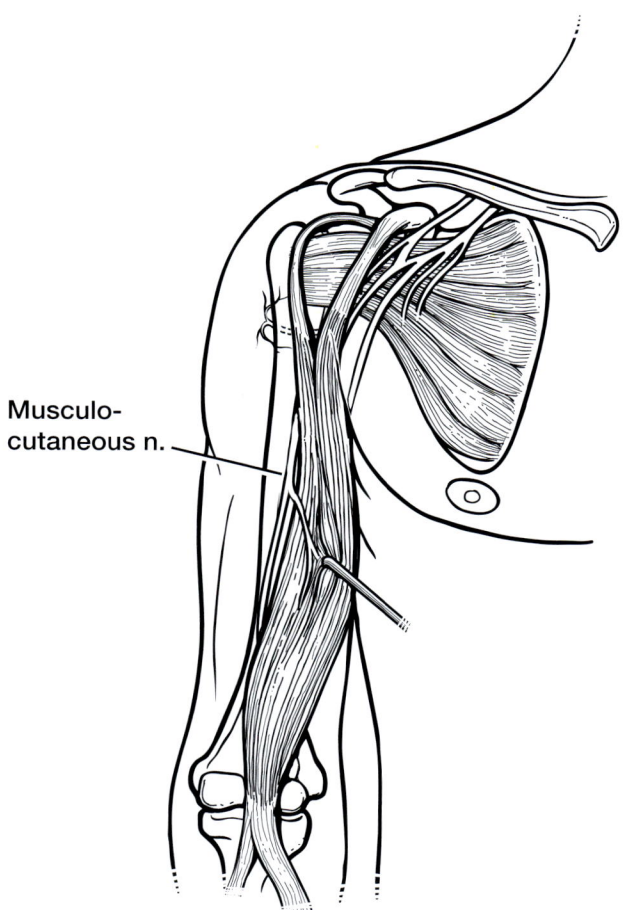

FIGURE 2.9 The musculocutaneous nerve.

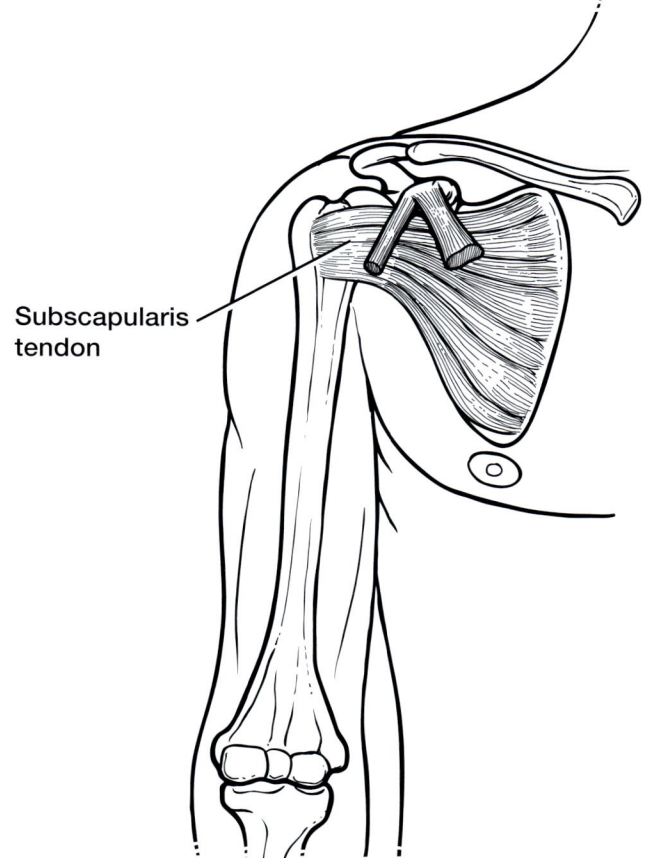

FIGURE 2.10 The subscapularis tendon.

Subscapularis, Rotator Interval, and Biceps

The subscapularis tendon is readily visible just deep to the conjoined tendon as it inserts into the lesser tuberosity of the humerus (Fig. 2.10). The rotator interval is palpable just superior to the subscapularis tendon and is the site of the initial arthrotomy during shoulder arthroplasty (Fig. 2.11). The long head of the biceps brachii exits the bicipital groove of the humerus, traverses the rotator interval, and inserts on the superior glenoid labrum and supraglenoid tubercle.

Glenohumeral Ligaments and Capsule

After a subscapularis tenotomy, the superior, middle, and inferior glenohumeral ligaments may be visualized, as well as the inferior joint capsule (Fig. 2.12). The posterior joint capsule is more readily visualized after the humeral head is resected (Fig. 2.13).

Rotator Cuff

After dislocation of the humeral head, the articular surface of the posterior superior rotator cuff is visible. The "bare area" of the humeral head marks the insertion of the infraspinatus, with the supraspinatus inserting superior and anterior to the bare area. The teres minor inserts immediately inferior to the infraspinatus and is not readily distinguishable as a distinct tendon separate from the infraspinatus (Fig. 2.14).

Osseous Structures

Relevant osseous anatomy consists of the proximal humerus and glenoid. The native anatomy of both these structures can be distorted by arthritic changes or fractures (Fig. 2.15).

IMPLANTS AND TECHNIQUES

In performing shoulder arthroplasty, it is important to realize that "the shoulder is not the hip." Although some of the implant research and development pertaining to hip arthroplasty is applicable to the shoulder, much of it is not. Similarly, technical points of paramount importance during hip arthroplasty are inconsequential in shoulder arthroplasty. Although large forces cross the shoulder during activity, the fact that the shoulder is not a weight-bearing joint accounts for many of these differences.

In total hip arthroplasty, femoral stem loosening has been a problem. Innovations in implants and in insertion techniques have minimized many of these problems. Conversely, the rate of humeral stem loosening is exceptionally low. This

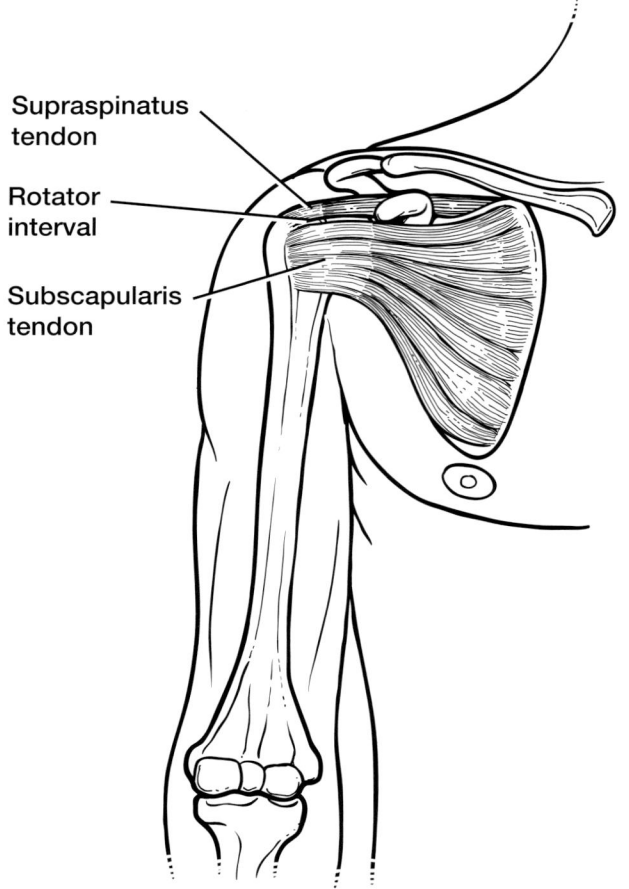

FIGURE 2.11 The rotator interval.

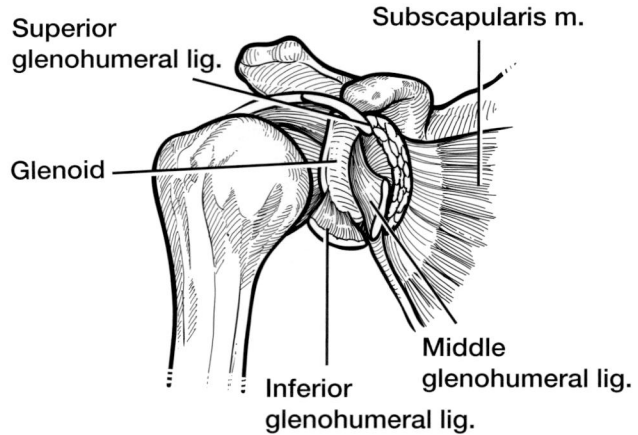

FIGURE 2.12 Glenohumeral ligaments and joint capsule as visualized through the deltopectoral approach.

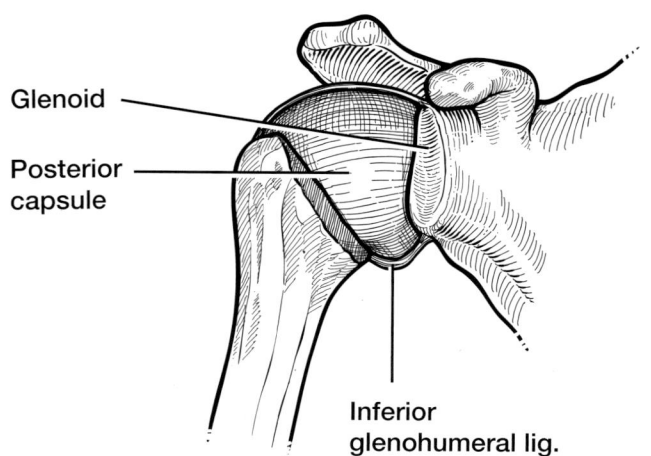

FIGURE 2.13 The posterior joint capsule is readily visualized after resection of the humeral head.

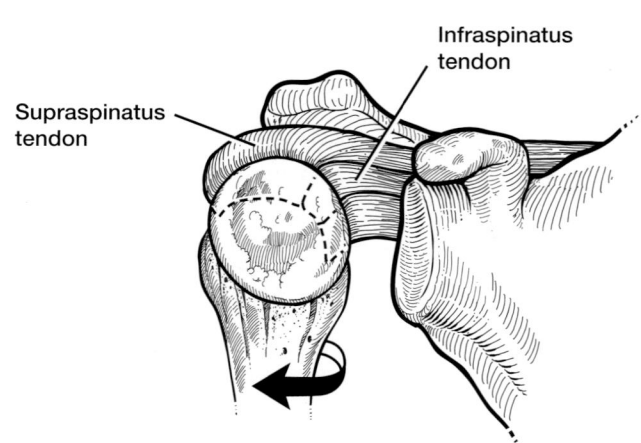

FIGURE 2.14 The posterosuperior rotator cuff.

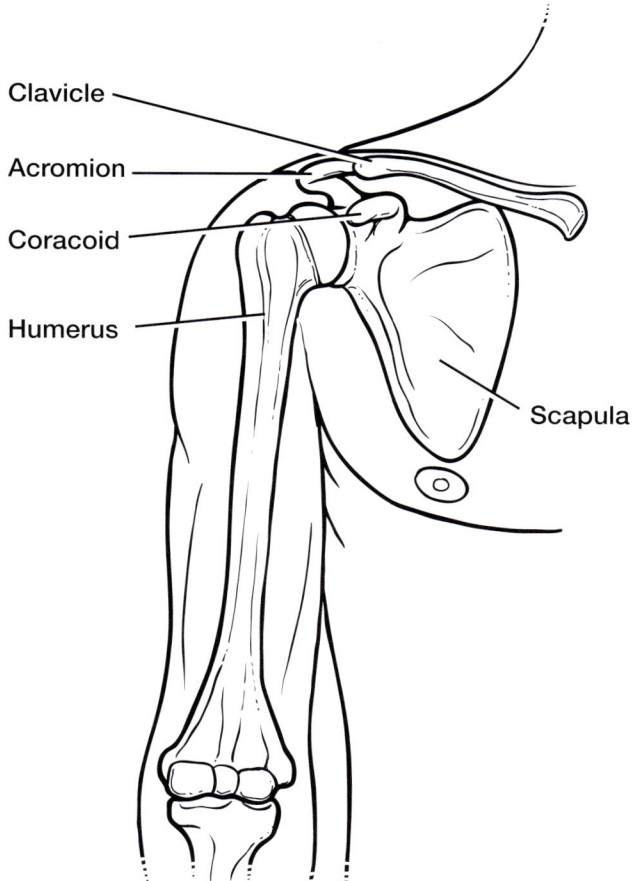

FIGURE 2.15 Osseous anatomy of the shoulder girdle.

low rate of failure has been observed with both cemented and press-fit stems. No single stem type, regardless of fixation or finish type, has proved superior to other types with respect to prosthetic loosening. Additionally, although modernized cementing techniques have proved efficacious in hip arthroplasty, humeral stem loosening is no more prevalent with "finger packing" of cement than with instrumented pressurization.

In contrast to hip arthroplasty, the "socket side" of shoulder arthroplasty has most commonly been the site of failure. Although metal-backed acetabular components in hip arthroplasty have been considered an advance, most metal-backed glenoid components have been disappointing in unconstrained total shoulder arthroplasty.

Overall, it is important for the shoulder arthroplasty surgeon to recognize that the shoulder is a unique joint and that techniques and implants for shoulder arthroplasty are specific to this procedure and not merely extrapolated from those used for lower extremity arthroplasty.

RESOURCES FOR BECOMING A SHOULDER ARTHROPLASTY SURGEON

Many resources are available that attempt to teach shoulder arthroplasty, including courses, instructional videos, textbooks, and Internet resources. Educational courses that aim to teach shoulder arthroplasty, both diverse and specific, are frequently offered by organizations such as the American Academy of Orthopaedic Surgeons (AAOS) and the American Shoulder and Elbow Surgeons (ASES). Additionally, many of the implant manufacturers offer periodic courses on the use of their implants. Many of these courses provide instruction through lecture and laboratory sessions. Most of these courses give the surgeon opportunities to perform shoulder arthroplasty on a cadaver forequarter or on synthetic bones.

Many instructional videos on shoulder arthroplasty are exhibited each year at the annual meeting of the AAOS. These videos demonstrate a variety of shoulder arthroplasty techniques and are available for purchase through the AAOS. Technical videos demonstrating our preferred techniques are provided with this textbook on a DVD.

Many textbooks contain sections on shoulder arthroplasty, including multiple-volume general orthopedic textbooks, textbooks focusing on the shoulder, and those limited to shoulder arthroplasty. This textbook, modeled after *Shoulder Arthroscopy* by Gartsman, was born out of the practical needs we observed while teaching a course in shoulder arthroplasty. This textbook eliminates much of the theoretical discussion of shoulder arthroplasty in favor of providing practical information that actually assists the surgeon in the technical part of the procedure and in postoperative care.

REFERENCE

1. Mendenhall Associates, Inc: A 2016 extremity update. *Orthopedic News Network* 27:1, 2016.

CHAPTER 3

Operating room setup

This chapter outlines the organization of the operating room used for shoulder arthroplasty. Organization of the arthroplasty surgical suite focuses on the correct position of equipment, staff, and lights. In addition, all necessary surgical instrumentation must be available.

OPERATING ROOM LAYOUT

A large operating room is preferable when shoulder arthroplasty is being performed. Larger operating rooms allow a complete set of implants to be stored in the room on a mobile shelving unit to minimize traffic in and out of the operating suite. Our operating suite has two doors: one main door from the hall through which the patient is transported, and a second door going into the substerile area. After the patient is placed on the operating table, the main door is locked to further minimize traffic. A view box is used to display radiographs and secondary imaging studies during the procedure so that they can be referenced quickly if necessary (Fig. 3.1). Additionally, a computer is available for intraoperative review of digital imaging (Fig. 3.2).

An overview of the operating room layout is shown in Fig. 3.3. The operating table is placed directly under the operating lights and is not angled within the room. Anesthesia equipment is located at the head of the operating table. The electrocautery unit is placed on a mobile cart at the foot of the operating table. A Mayo stand is positioned over the patient's lower extremities and comes in from the nonoperative side. Two back tables of equipment are placed on the nonoperative side. The cord for the electrocautery handpiece and the tubing for suction are passed off the foot of the operating table. Mobile shelving units containing a full set of implants are placed against a wall of the operating room.

STAFF POSITIONING

Fig. 3.3 shows the location of each member of the operative team. The operating surgeon stands facing the patient's axilla. The first assistant stands just behind the operative shoulder, facing the surgeon. If available, a second assistant stands on the opposite side of the operating table from the surgeon. The position of the second assistant serves dual purposes: first, it allows the assistant to perform retraction without crowding the surgeon; second, if any observers are present, this allows them to have an unhindered view of the procedure. The surgical technician stands on the nonoperative side of the patient between the back tables and the operating table. If needed in the absence of a second assistant, the surgical technician can use one hand to hold a retractor during selected portions of the procedure.

OVERHEAD LIGHTING

Lighting is critical in performing shoulder arthroplasty. Although some surgeons use accessory lighting (i.e., headlamps) for open shoulder surgery, we have found that proper positioning of the overhead lights precludes the need for such devices. Fig. 3.4 demonstrates proper light positioning during shoulder arthroplasty performed by a right hand–dominant surgeon. The main operating room light is positioned just above the surgeon's left shoulder to prevent the surgeon's operating hand from interfering with the light path. The secondary light is positioned on the surgeon's right side, more cephalic than the main light. These relationships are reversed for a left hand–dominant surgeon.

SURGICAL INSTRUMENTATION

Fig. 3.5 shows the arrangement of instruments placed on the Mayo stand during shoulder arthroplasty. Figs. 3.6 and 3.7 show the arrangement of instruments on the back tables. Table 3.1 lists all instruments in our shoulder arthroplasty set along with their use during the procedure. Table 3.2 lists the sutures and disposable instruments that we have available during shoulder arthroplasty. Table 3.3 lists the specific product sets that we use during shoulder arthroplasty.

CHAPTER 3 ■ Operating Room Setup

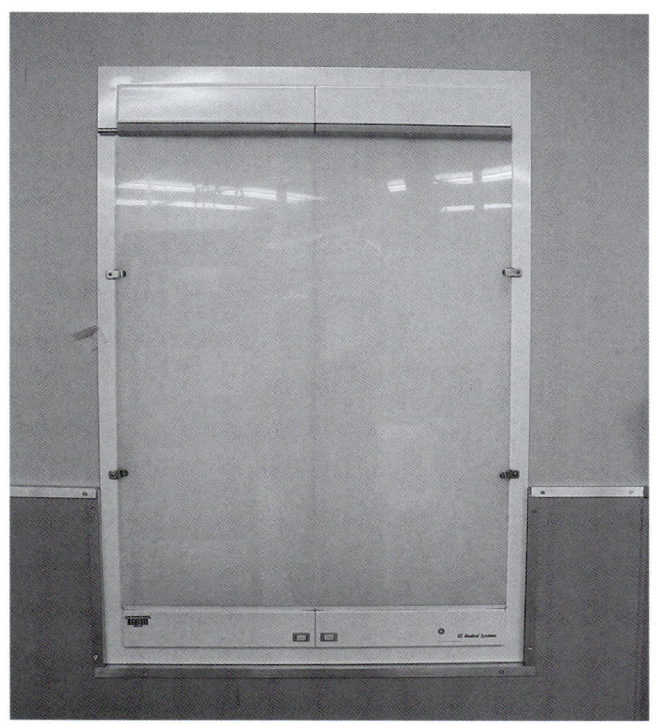

FIGURE 3.1 Typical radiographic view box available in the operating suite.

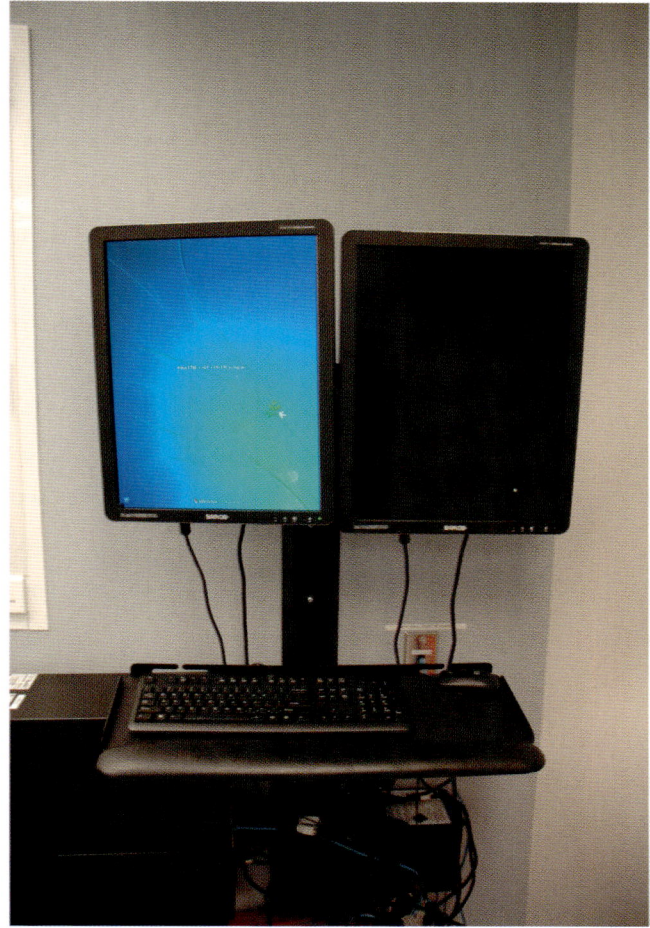

FIGURE 3.2 Computer located in the operating suite used to review secondary imaging studies.

FIGURE 3.3 Overview of the operating room layout.

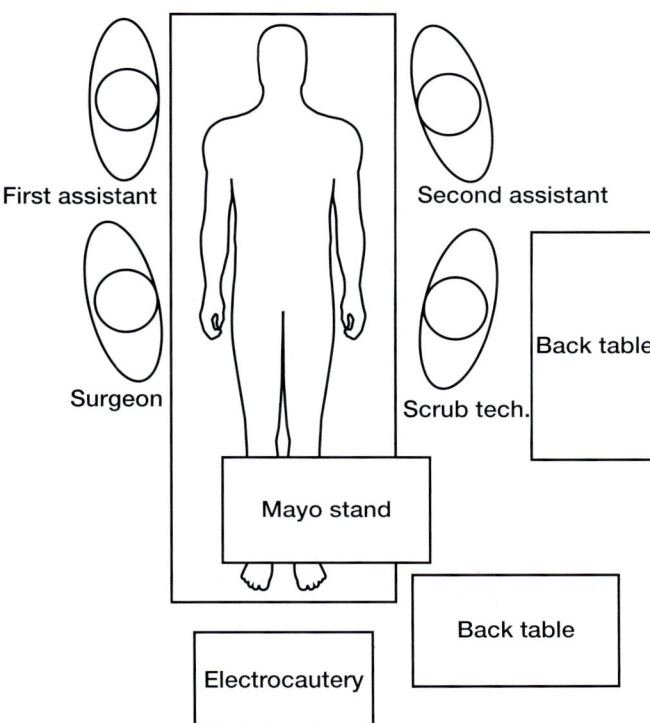

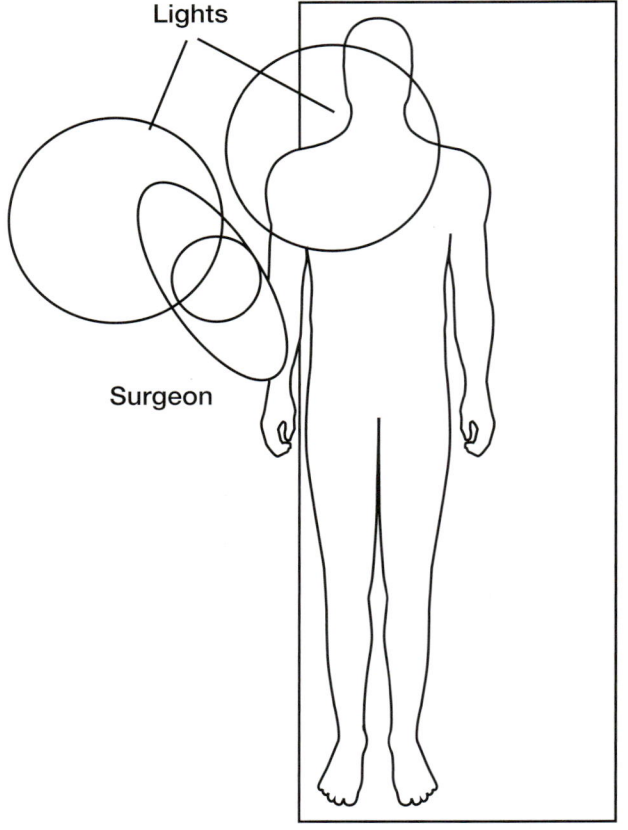

FIGURE 3.4 Position of the overhead lighting for a right hand–dominant surgeon.

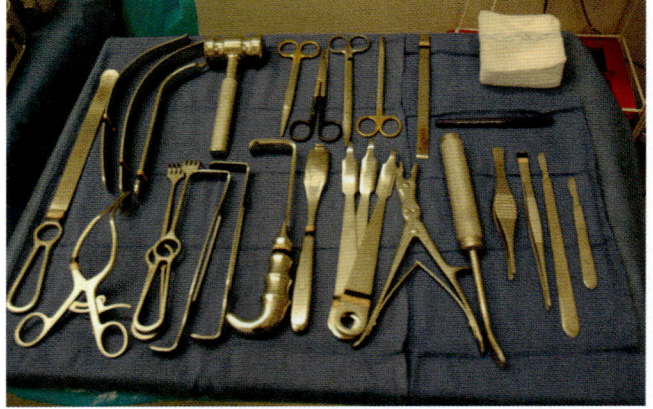

FIGURE 3.5 Arrangement of instruments placed on the Mayo stand during surgery.

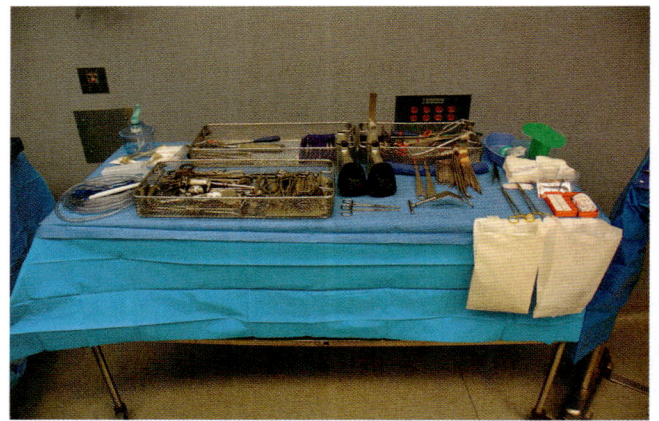

FIGURE 3.6 Arrangement of instruments on one of the back tables.

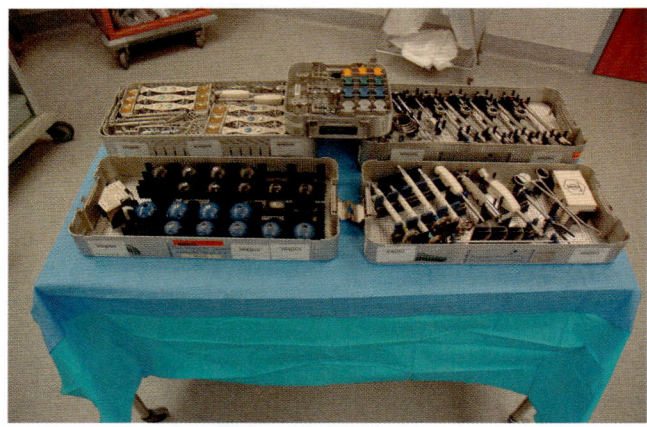

FIGURE 3.7 Arrangement of instruments on the other back table.

TABLE 3.1 Instruments Used During Shoulder Arthroplasty

Instrument	Quantity	Use	Figure
Forceps			
Vascular forceps	2	Dissection	3.8
Ferris-Smith forceps	2	Dissection	3.9
Adson forceps with teeth	1	Skin closure	3.10
Scissors			
Long curved Metzenbaum scissors	1	Dissection, subscapularis release	3.11
Long curved Mayo scissors	1	Dissection	3.12
Straight Mayo scissors	1	Cutting suture	3.13
Bandage scissors	1	Removal of draping	3.14
Retractors			
Medium skin rake	2	Skin retraction	3.15
Army–Navy retractor	2	Deltopectoral retraction	3.16
Cerebellar retractor	2	Deltopectoral retraction	3.17
Hohmann retractor	4	Proximal retraction, humeral retraction, glenoid retraction	3.18
Narrow Richardson retractor	1	Conjoined tendon retraction	3.19
Small glenoid rim retractor	1	Anterior glenoid retraction	3.20B
Trillat humeral head retractor	1	Humeral retraction during glenoid exposure	3.21
Fukuda humeral head retractor	1	Humeral retraction during glenoid exposure	3.22
Long Darrach humeral head retractor	1	Humeral retraction during glenoid exposure	3.23
Large glenoid rim retractor	1	Humeral retraction during glenoid exposure	3.20A
Special Hohmann retractor	1	Inferior medial humeral retraction during humeral preparation	3.24
Double-pointed Hohmann retractor	1	Inferior glenoid retraction	3.25
Clamps			
Kocher hemostat	2	Sponge removal	3.26A
Kelly hemostat	2	Tagging stay sutures	3.26B
Standard hemostat	6	Tagging stay sutures	3.26C
Mosquito hemostat	2	Tagging stay sutures	3.26D
Lahey clamp	1	Handling of tuberosities during fracture cases	3.27
Towel clips	2	Creation of bone tunnels through hard bone (lesser tuberosity)	3.28
Power equipment			
Battery-powered sagittal saw	1	Humeral head osteotomy, humeral shaft osteotomy in revision	3.29
Battery-powered drill/reamer	1	Glenoid preparation	3.30
Miscellaneous			
Long no. 3 knife handle	2	Skin incision, subscapularis tenotomy, biceps tenotomy	3.31
8-inch Mayo needle holder	2	Suture passage	3.32
Cobb elevator	1	Inferior capsular retraction during inferior capsular release	3.33
½-inch straight osteotome	1	Removal of humeral osteophytes	3.34
Mallet	1	Removal of humeral osteophytes, insertion of implants	3.35
1-inch straight osteotome	1	Iliac crest bone graft harvest for glenoid revision	3.36
Freer elevator	1	Removal of excess cement	3.37
¾-inch curved osteotome	1	Iliac crest bone graft harvest for glenoid revision	3.38
Small bone tamp	1	Impaction of bone graft	3.39 *top*
Large bone tamp	1	Impaction of bone graft	3.39 *bottom*
Bone hook	1	Dislocation of proximal humerus after glenoid preparation	3.40
Lamina spreader	1	Distraction between humerus and glenoid for posterior capsule exposure	3.41
Large rongeur	1	Osteophyte removal	3.42A
Small rongeur	1	Osteophyte removal	3.42B
Heavy needle holder	1	Suture passage through hard bone (lesser tuberosity)	3.43
Vise-grip pliers with slap hammer	1	Prosthetic removal during revision	3.44
Large Cobb elevator	1	Prosthetic removal during revision	3.45

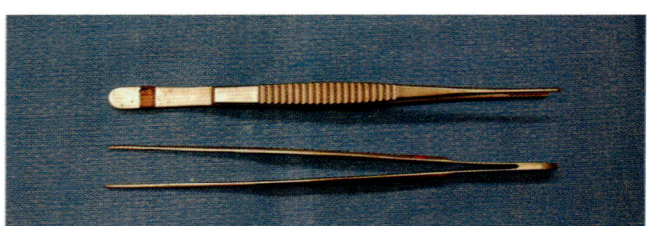

FIGURE 3.8 Vascular forceps.

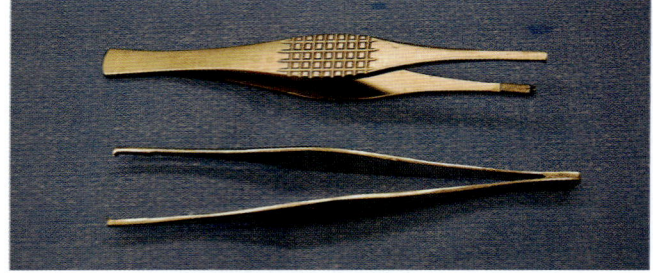

FIGURE 3.9 Ferris–Smith forceps.

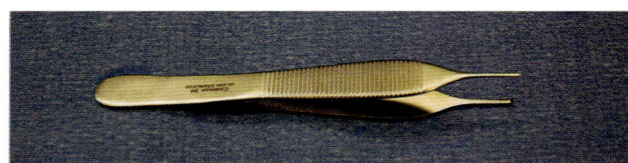

FIGURE 3.10 Adson forceps with teeth.

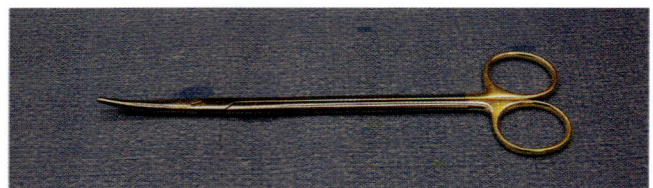

FIGURE 3.11 Long curved Metzenbaum scissors.

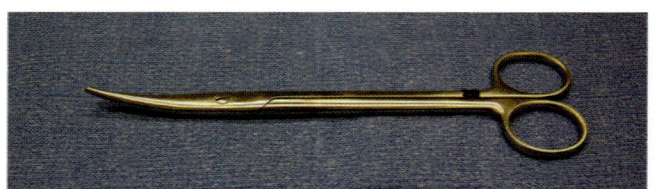

FIGURE 3.12 Long curved Mayo scissors.

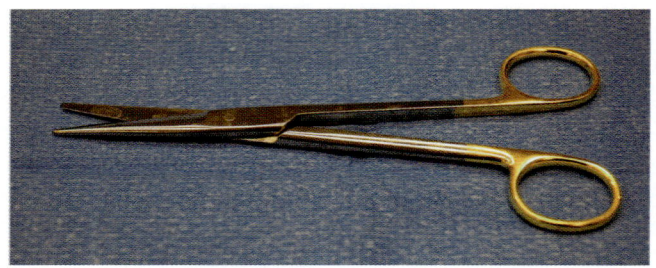

FIGURE 3.13 Straight Mayo scissors.

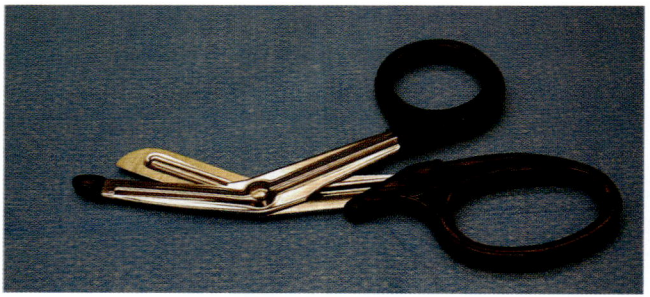

FIGURE 3.14 Bandage scissors.

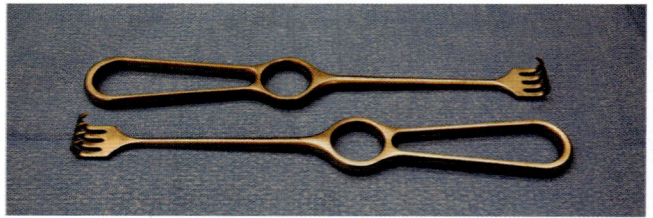

FIGURE 3.15 Medium skin rake.

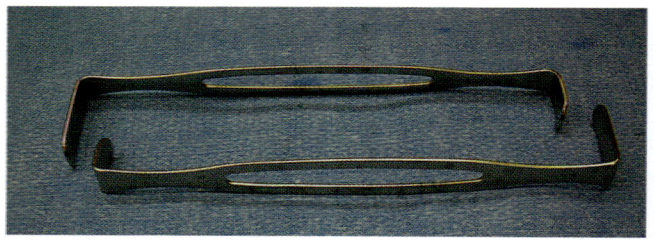

FIGURE 3.16 Army–Navy retractor.

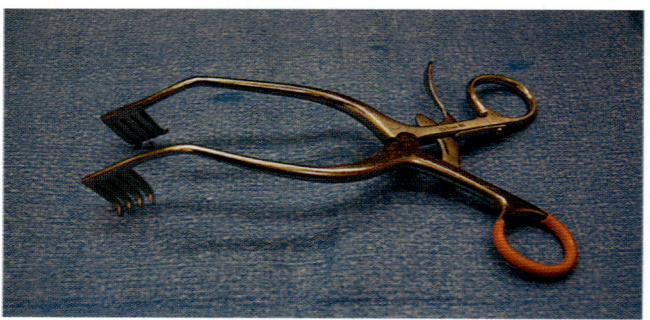

FIGURE 3.17 Cerebellar retractor.

CHAPTER 3 ■ Operating Room Setup

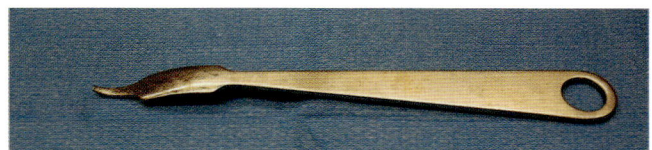

FIGURE 3.18 Hohmann retractor.

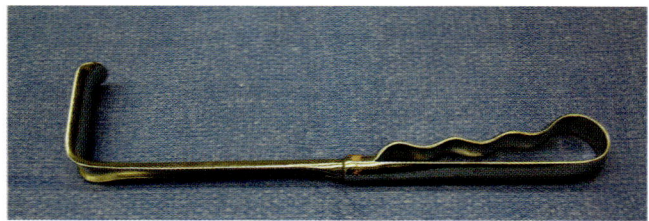

FIGURE 3.19 Narrow Richardson retractor.

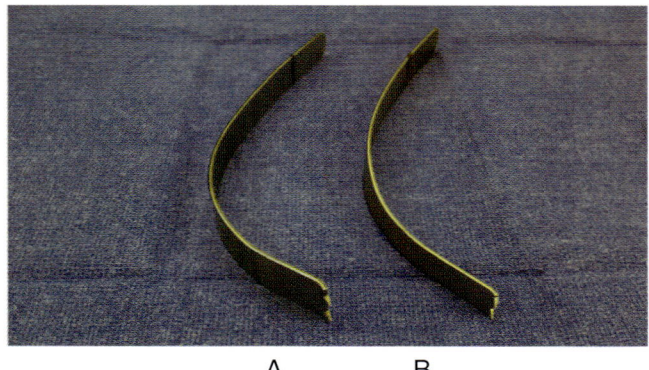

FIGURE 3.20 Large glenoid rim retractor (A) and small glenoid rim retractor (B).

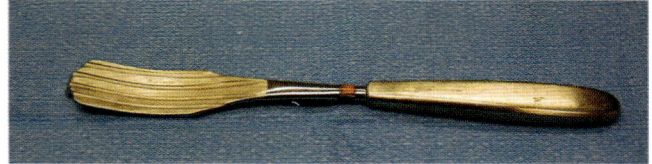

FIGURE 3.21 Trillat humeral head retractor.

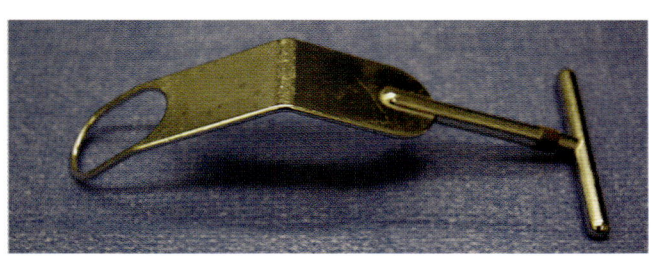

FIGURE 3.22 Fukuda humeral head retractor.

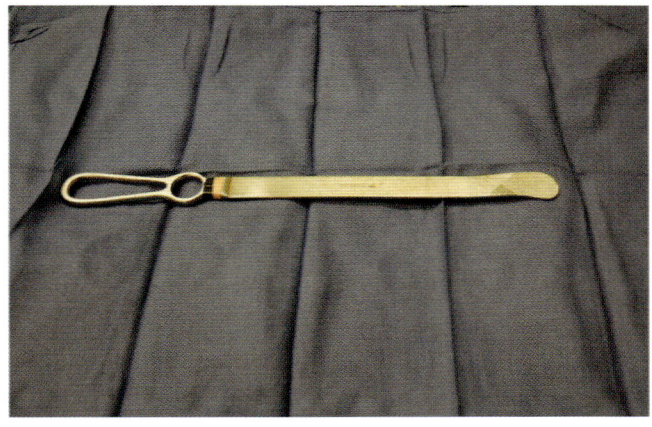

FIGURE 3.23 Long Darrach humeral head retractor.

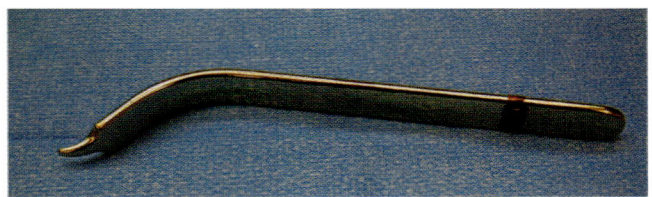

FIGURE 3.24 Special Hohmann retractor.

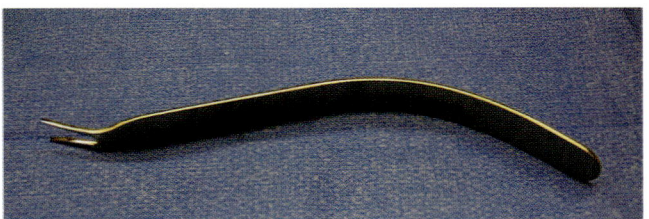

FIGURE 3.25 Double-pointed Hohmann retractor.

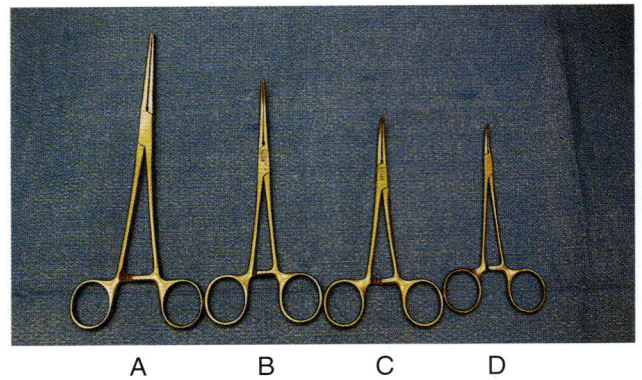

FIGURE 3.26 (A) Kocher hemostat. (B) Kelly hemostat. (C) Standard hemostat. (D) Mosquito hemostat.

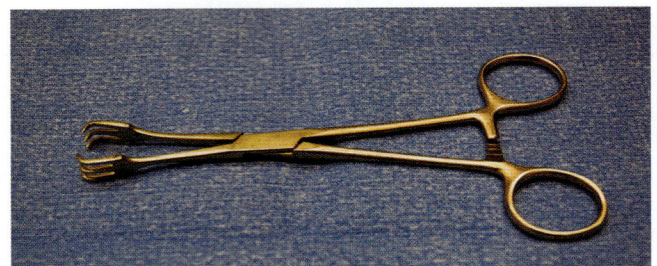

FIGURE 3.27 Lahey clamp.

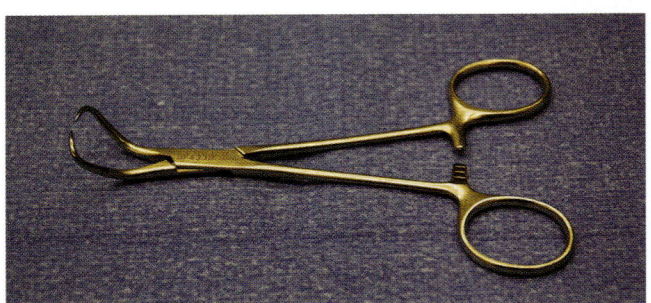

FIGURE 3.28 Towel clips.

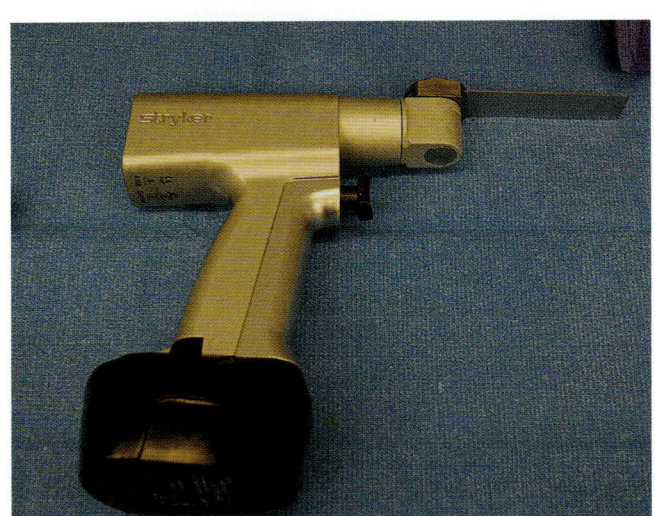

FIGURE 3.29 Battery-powered sagittal saw.

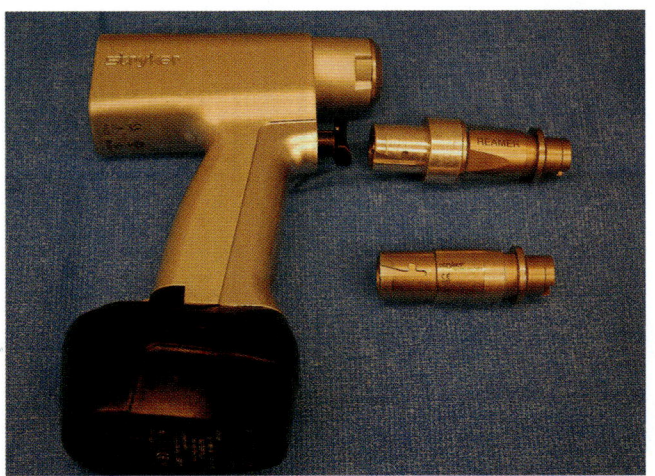

FIGURE 3.30 Battery-powered drill/reamer.

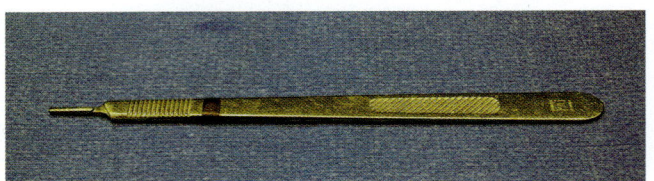

FIGURE 3.31 Long no. 3 knife handle.

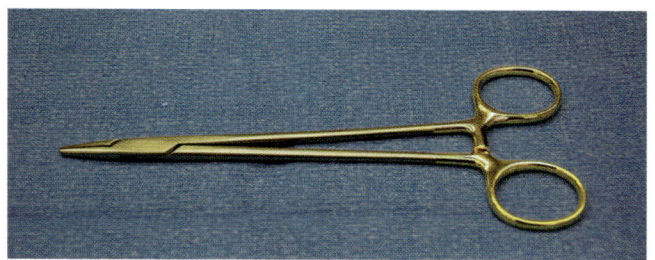

FIGURE 3.32 Eight-inch Mayo needle holder.

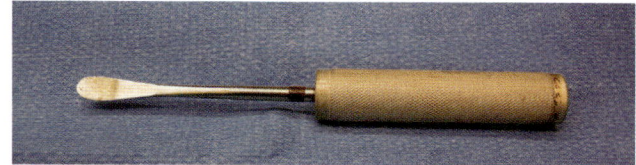

FIGURE 3.33 Cobb elevator.

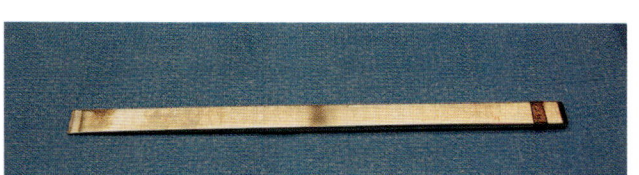

FIGURE 3.34 Half-inch straight osteotome.

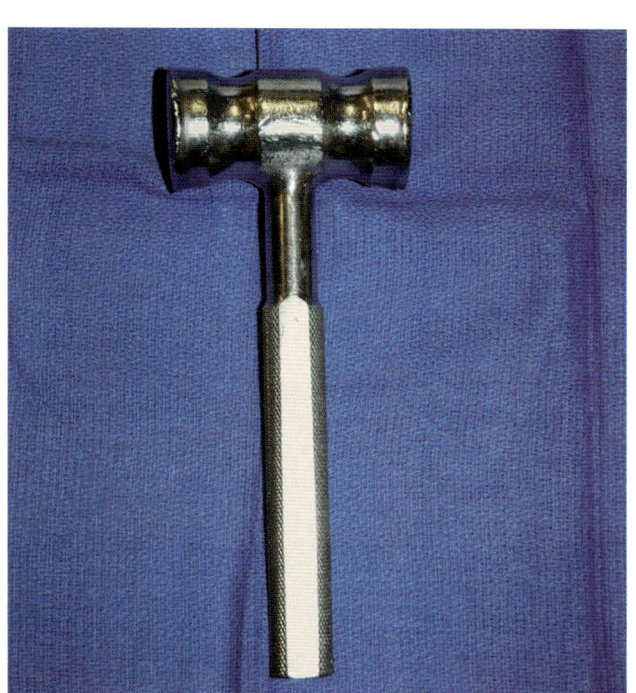

FIGURE 3.35 Mallet.

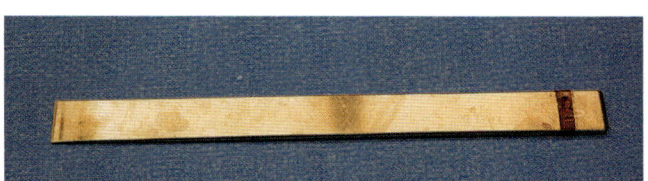

FIGURE 3.36 One-inch straight osteotome.

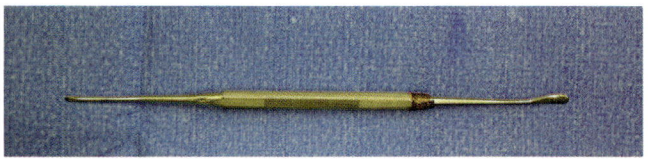

FIGURE 3.37 Freer elevator.

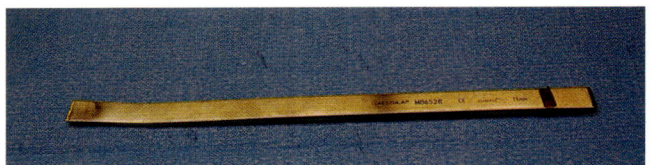

FIGURE 3.38 Three-quarter-inch curved osteotome.

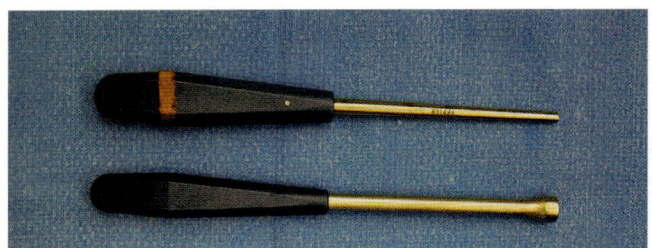

FIGURE 3.39 Small bone tamp *(top)* and large bone tamp *(bottom)*.

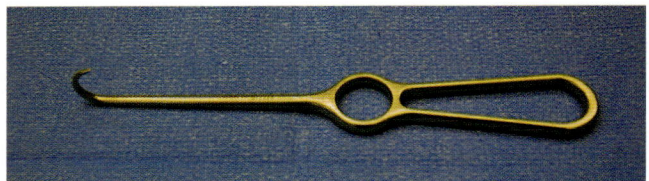

FIGURE 3.40 Bone hook.

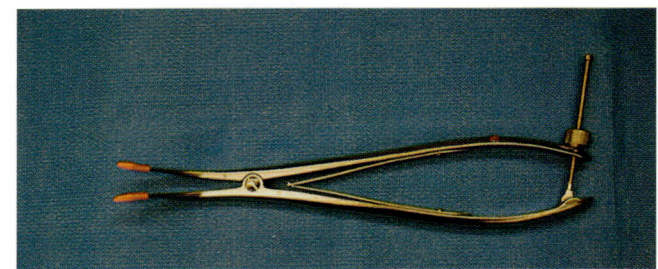

FIGURE 3.41 Lamina spreader.

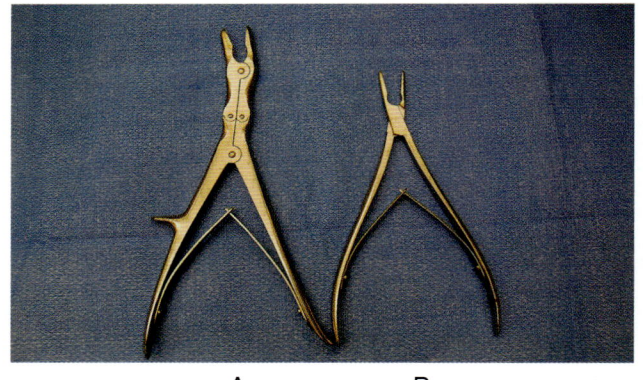

FIGURE 3.42 Large rongeur (A) and small rongeur (B).

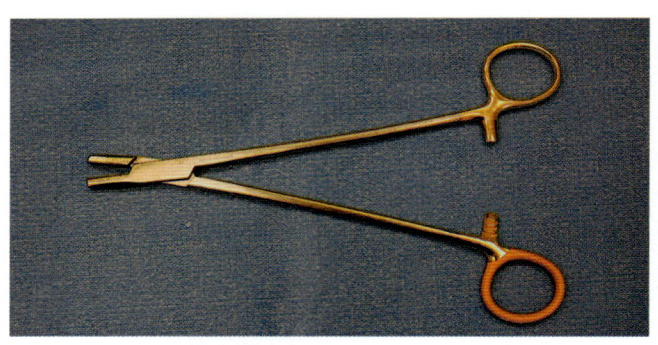

FIGURE 3.43 Heavy needle holder.

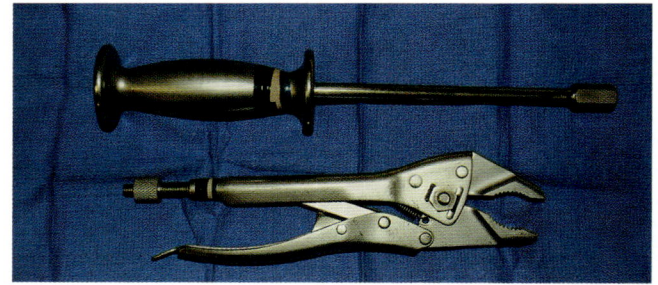

FIGURE 3.44 Vise-grip pliers with slap hammer.

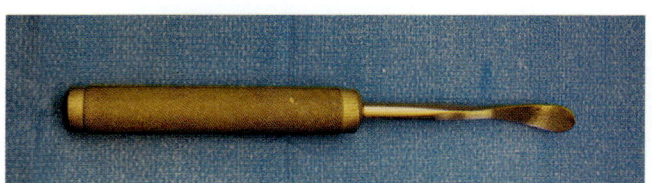

FIGURE 3.45 Large Cobb elevator.

TABLE 3.2   Disposable Instruments and Suture Used During Shoulder Arthroplasty

Instrument	Quantity	Use	Figure
Suture			
No. 0 Vicryl (taper needle)	3	Hemostasis, wound closure	3.46
No. 2 Ethibond (taper needle)	1	Subscapularis stay suture, fixation of biologic glenoid resurfacing	3.46
No. 2 Fiberwire (taper needle)	3	Subscapularis closure, tuberosity fixation	3.46
No. 1 Vicryl (taper needle)	1	Subscapularis closure, posterior capsulorrhaphy	3.46
2-0 Vicryl	1	Wound closure	3.46
3-0 Polydioxanone suture	1	Wound closure	3.46
Skin stapler	1	Wound closure (revision cases)	3.47
Miscellaneous			
Saw blade	1	Humeral head osteotomy	3.48
Electrocautery with needle tip	1	Hemostasis, dissection	3.49
Suction tip with tubing	1	Visualization	3.50
Bulb syringe	1	Irrigation	3.51
Catheter tip 60-mL syringe	1	Cement application	3.52

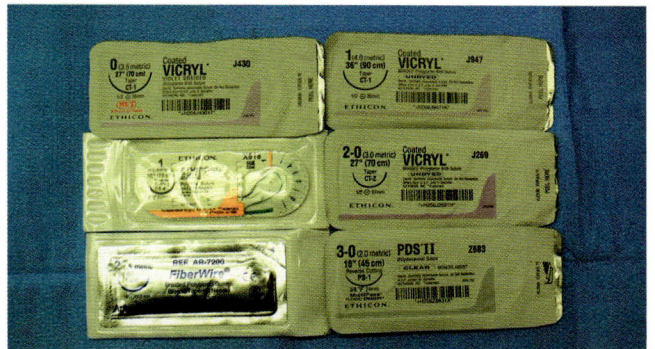

FIGURE 3.46   Suture packages.

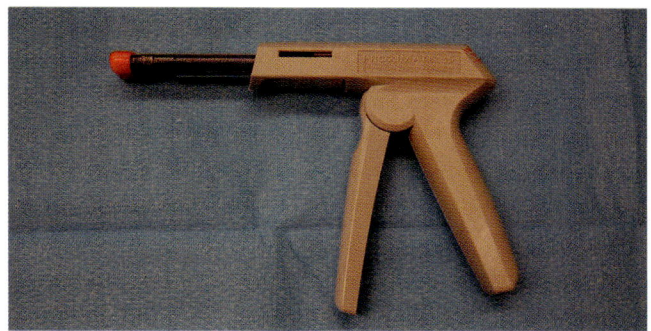

FIGURE 3.47   Skin stapler.

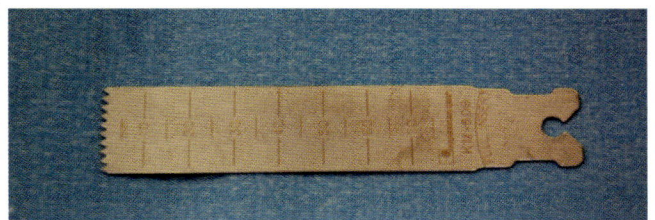

FIGURE 3.48   Saw blade.

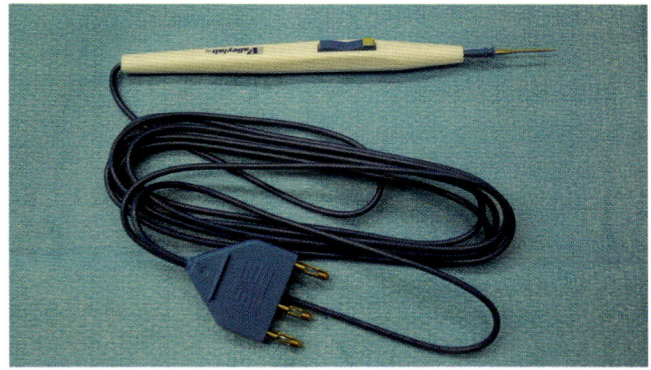

FIGURE 3.49   Electrocautery with needle tip.

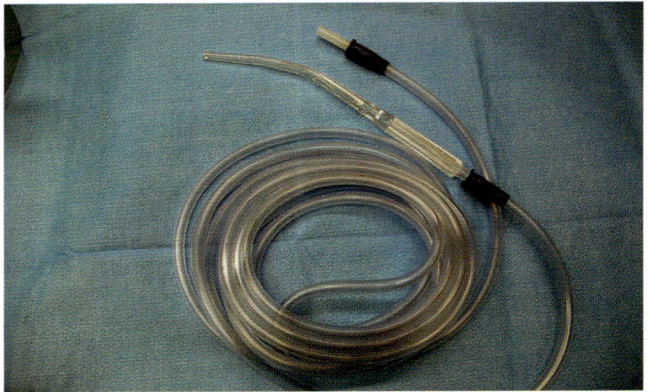

FIGURE 3.50 Suction tip with tubing.

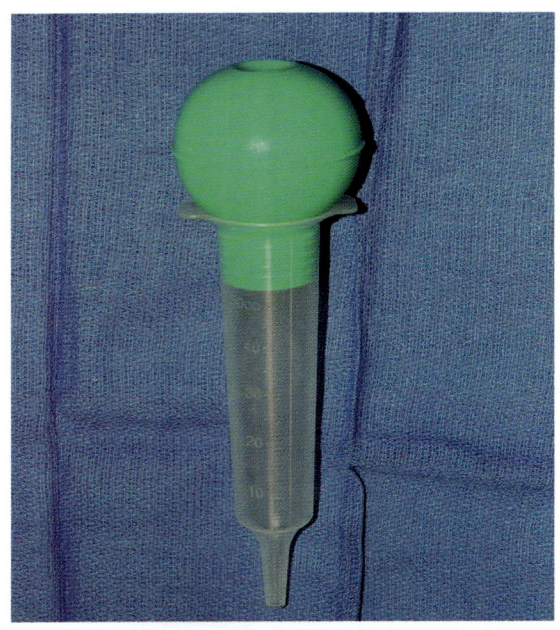

FIGURE 3.51 Bulb syringe.

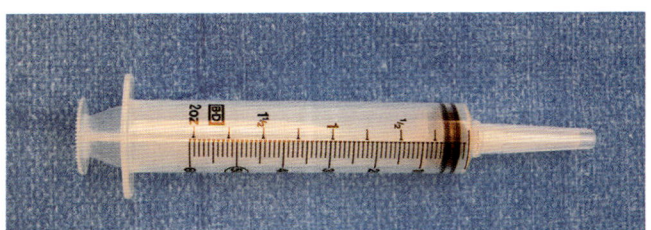

FIGURE 3.52 Catheter-tipped 60-mL syringe.

TABLE 3.3	Specific Instrument Sets Available During Shoulder Arthroplasty		
Set	Manufacturer	Use	Figure
Press-fit convertible humeral stem set	Tornier	Unconstrained and reverse shoulder arthroplasty	3.53
Keel/peg glenoid set	Tornier	Unconstrained shoulder arthroplasty	3.54
Reverse shoulder arthroplasty glenoid set	Tornier	Semiconstrained shoulder arthroplasty	3.55
Fracture arthroplasty set	Tornier	Unconstrained shoulder arthroplasty for fracture	3.56
Long-stem fracture arthroplasty set	Tornier	Unconstrained revision shoulder arthroplasty	3.57
Long-stem reverse shoulder arthroplasty set	Tornier	Semiconstrained cemented revision shoulder arthroplasty	3.58
Adjustable press-fit reverse shoulder arthroplasty set	Tornier	Semiconstrained uncemented revision shoulder arthroplasty	3.59
Cerclage cable set	Kinamed	Fixation of humeral osteotomy during revision	3.60
4.0-mm cannulated screw set	Synthes	Fixation of bone graft in uncontained glenoid defect	3.61
SmartPin bioabsorbable pin set	Linvatec	Fixation of bone graft in uncontained glenoid defect	3.62

CHAPTER 3 ■ Operating Room Setup 27

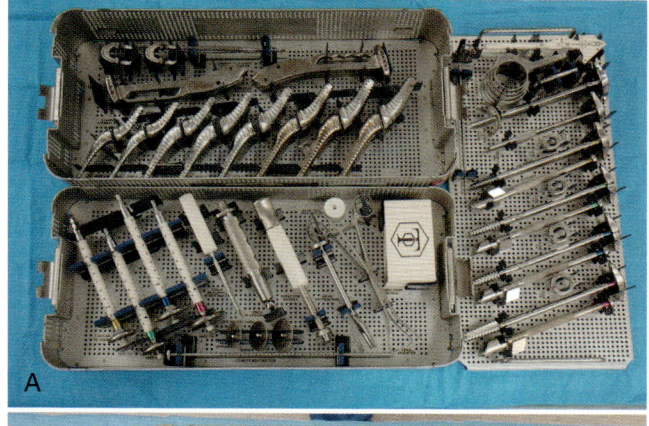

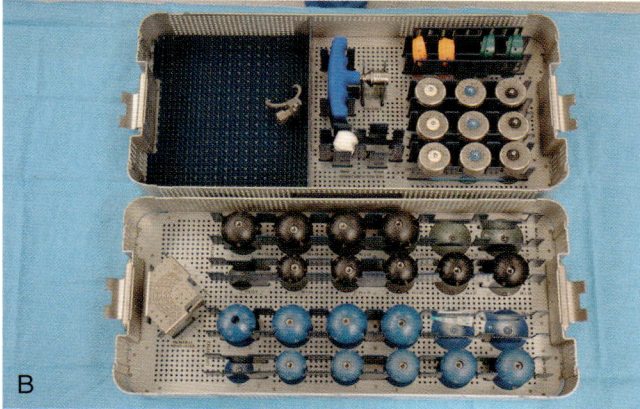

FIGURE 3.53 (A and B) Unconstrained/reverse humeral arthroplasty set.

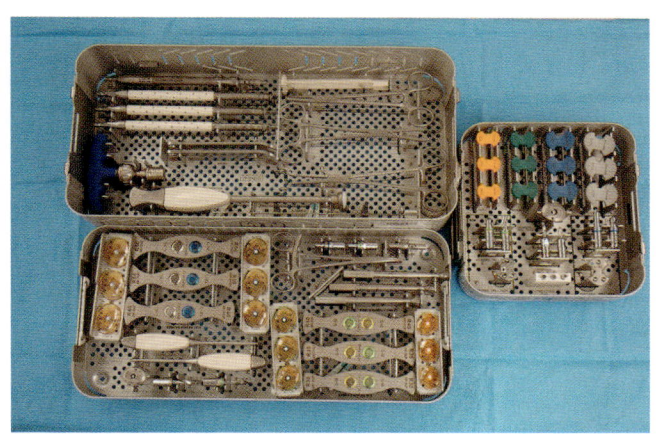

FIGURE 3.54 Unconstrained glenoid set.

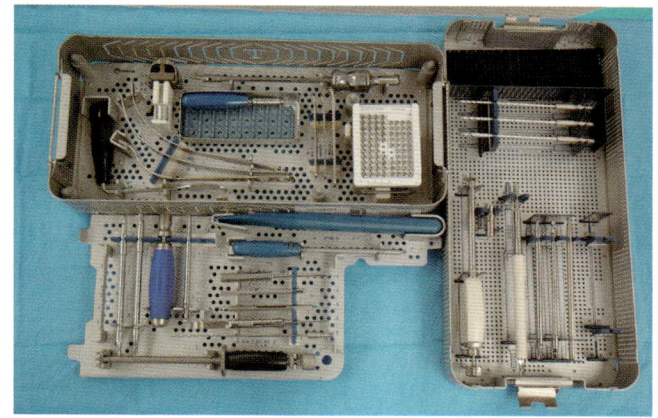

FIGURE 3.55 Reverse glenoid set.

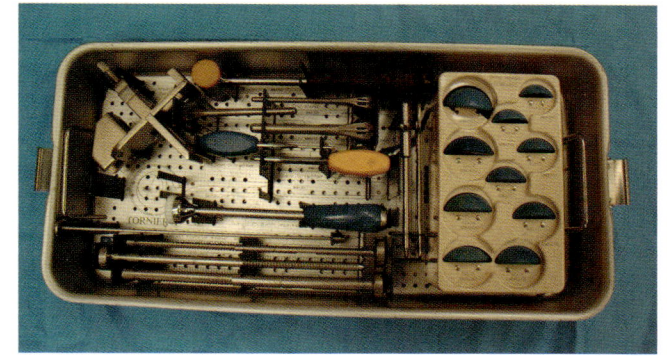

FIGURE 3.56 Fracture arthroplasty set.

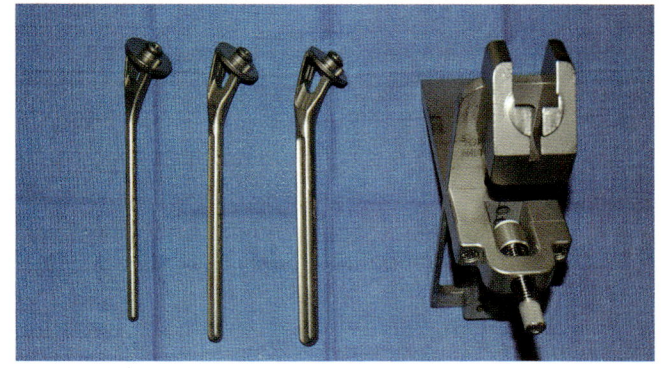

FIGURE 3.57 Long-stem fracture arthroplasty set.

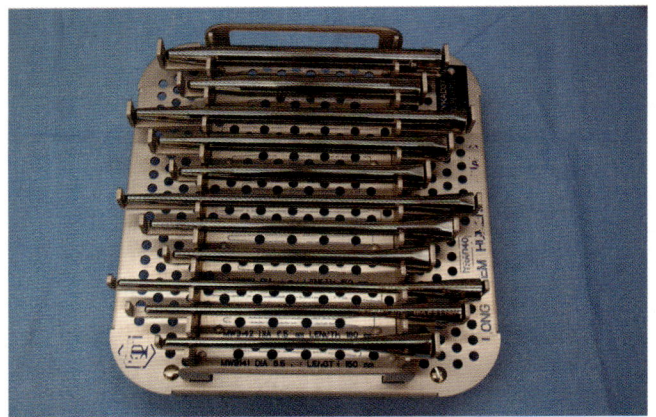

FIGURE 3.58　Long-stem reverse shoulder arthroplasty set.

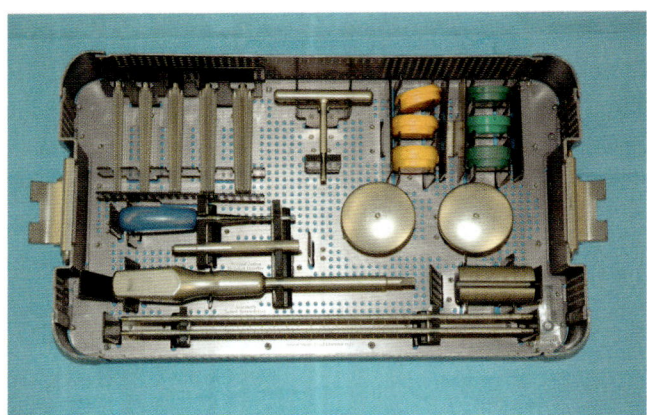

FIGURE 3.59　Adjustable press-fit reverse shoulder arthroplasty set.

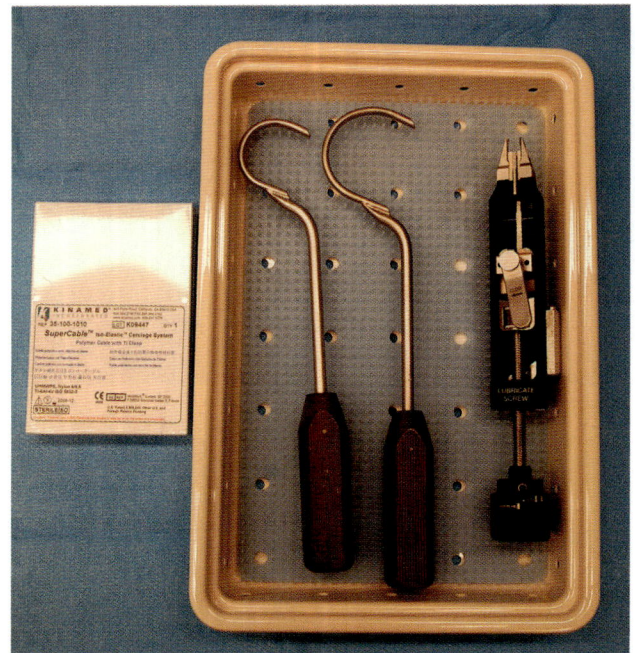

FIGURE 3.60　Cerclage cable set.

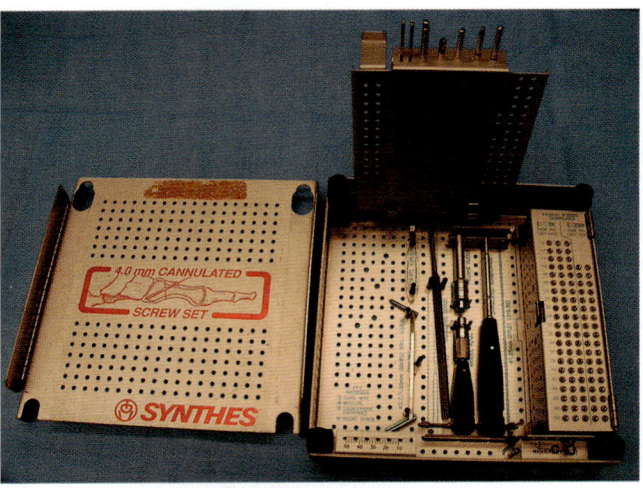

FIGURE 3.61　Four-millimeter cannulated screw set.

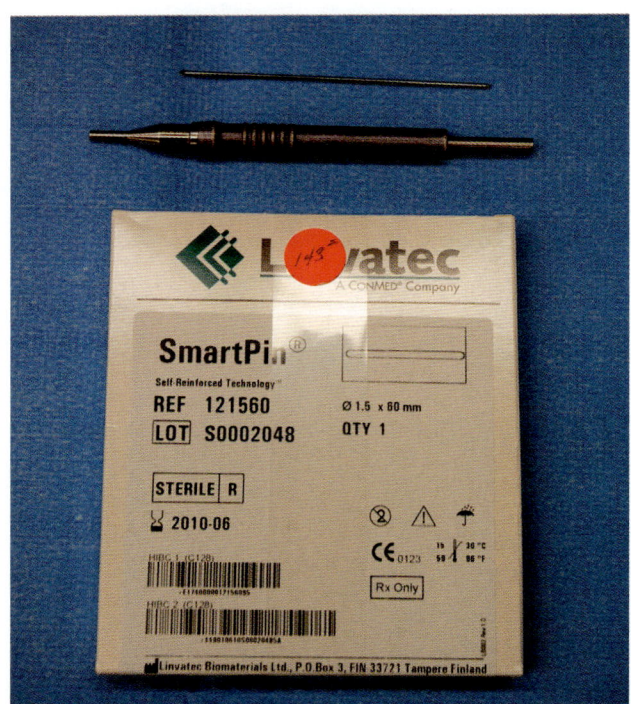

FIGURE 3.62　SmartPin bioabsorbable pin set.

Anesthesia, patient positioning, and patient preparation

CHAPTER 4

This chapter reviews the anesthesia used for shoulder replacement surgery. Additionally, proper patient positioning and surgical preparation and draping are described.

ANESTHESIA

Provided that no contraindication exists, all of our shoulder arthroplasty patients undergo a preoperative interscalene block administered in the preoperative holding area by an anesthesiologist. The interscalene block serves two purposes. First, use of the block minimizes the amount of general anesthetic needed during surgery; second, it aids in postoperative pain management. Our anesthesiologists perform a single shot interscalene block under ultrasound guidance. The single shot block generally lasts 12–18 hours. General anesthesia and neuromuscular paralytic agents are then administered to all patients. Neuromuscular paralysis greatly facilitates exposure during glenoid resurfacing and can be discontinued after implantation of the glenoid component.

PATIENT POSITIONING

Proper patient positioning is crucial during shoulder arthroplasty. We use a standard operating table with the patient positioned sufficiently to the operative side to allow extension of the arm (Fig. 4.1). A rolled sheet is placed between the scapulae to slightly elevate the shoulder off the operating table and allow proper surgical preparation of the posterior aspect of the shoulder (Fig. 4.2). The use of certain types of operating tables developed for shoulder arthroscopy, in which the portion of the table posterior to the scapula is removed, is discouraged because these tables inhibit control of the scapula and thus make glenoid exposure difficult.

The patient is placed in the modified beach-chair position. To obtain the proper position, the operating table is first reflexed (Fig. 4.3) and the patient's knees are flexed (Fig. 4.4). The patient is then placed in a slight Trendelenburg position to prevent him or her from sliding inferiorly on the operating table (Fig. 4.5). Finally, the back of the operating table is elevated approximately 45 to 60 degrees relative to the floor (Fig. 4.6). The position of the patient's head and neck is checked to ensure neutral alignment. Occasionally it is necessary to slightly flex the head portion of the operating table to eliminate cervical extension. Once cervical alignment and the head position are acceptable, the forehead and chin are secured with 1-inch silk adhesive tape as shown in Fig. 4.7. In patients with fragile skin, a dry gauze pad is used to minimize tape contact and prevent skin tears. Care should be taken to pad and protect bony prominences and sites of subcutaneous vulnerable nerves near the elbow (ulnar) and knee (peroneal). Fig. 4.8 shows the final position of the patient before skin preparation.

SURGICAL PREPARATION AND DRAPING

Skin preparation begins the day before surgery. We advise the patient to shave the affected shoulder girdle and axilla; it is not necessary to shave the arm below the elbow. Shaving the surgical area a day in advance allows any skin irritation caused by shaving to subside. Patients are also advised to bathe with an antibacterial soap the morning of surgery before coming to the hospital. Once the patient is in the operating room, the skin of the affected upper extremity and shoulder girdle is cleaned with isopropyl alcohol. A povidone-iodine (Betadine) scrub is then performed. The surgical area is dried with towels and painted with a Betadine solution (Fig. 4.9). In patients with allergy or hypersensitivity to Betadine, a scrub with 4% chlorhexidine gluconate solution (Betasept) is performed (Fig. 4.10). The scrub solution is removed with sterile water and an isopropyl alcohol preparation is applied. The area included in the surgical preparation extends medially to the midline, distally to the level of the nipple, and proximally to the level of the mandible; it also encompasses the entire upper extremity, including the hand (Fig. 4.11).

Draping is initiated when the assistant drapes the patient's hand with an impermeable stockinet (Fig. 4.12). A reinforced disposable paper drape is placed from the inferior aspect of the surgical field and extended over the torso and lower extremities to prevent contamination of the operative team during the remainder of the draping. The stockinet is rolled proximally, past the elbow in most cases, and covered and secured with disposable elastic wrap (Fig. 4.13). In cases where an extensile surgical approach is anticipated, as in revision surgery, the stockinet covers only the hand and forearm. A towel is used to dry an area circumferentially around the shoulder to allow the ensuing "U" drapes to adhere to the skin (Fig. 4.14). A disposable impermeable "U" drape is placed inferiorly to superiorly, with the two limbs of the drape meeting superiorly (Fig. 4.15). A large disposable reinforced paper "U" drape is applied inferiorly to superiorly (Fig. 4.16). A smaller disposable paper "U" drape is placed superiorly to inferiorly (Fig. 4.17). The remaining exposed skin in the surgical field, including the axillary skin, is dried with a towel. In patients with previous

Text continued on p. 34

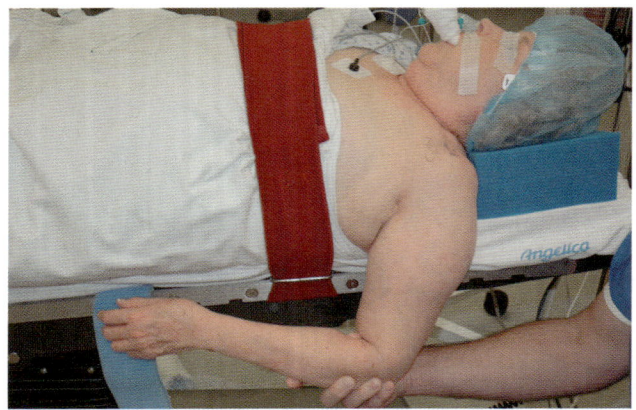

FIGURE 4.1 The patient is positioned sufficiently laterally on the operating table to allow full arm extension.

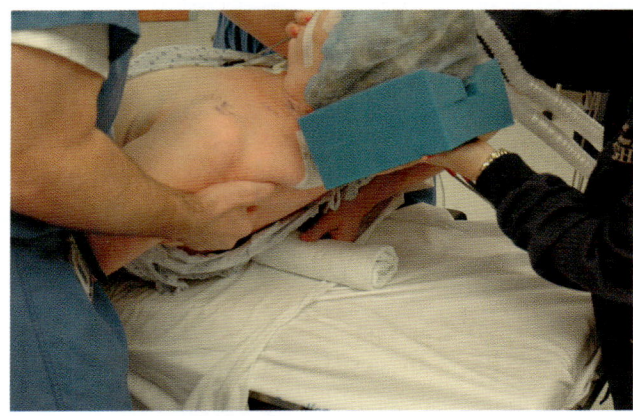

FIGURE 4.2 A rolled sheet is placed between the scapulae.

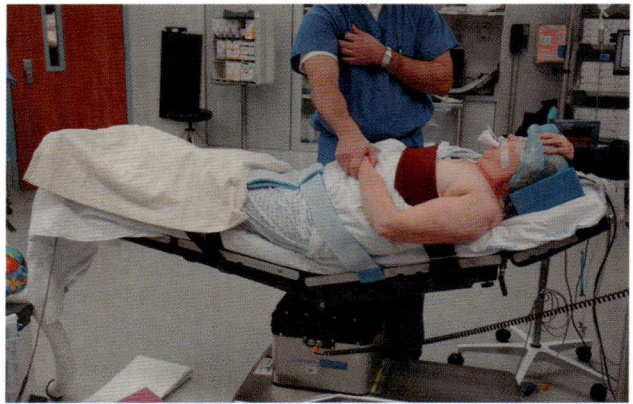

FIGURE 4.3 The operating table is first reflexed.

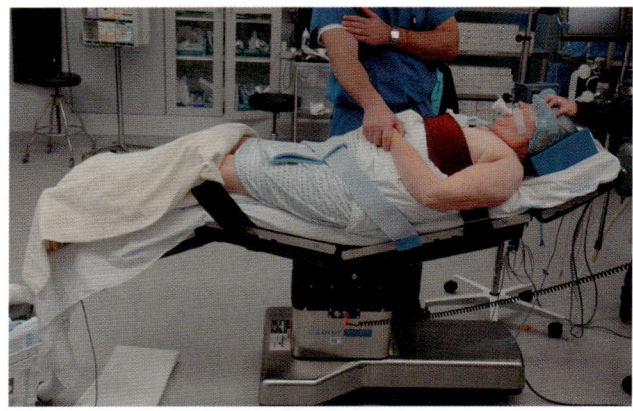

FIGURE 4.4 The patient's knees are flexed.

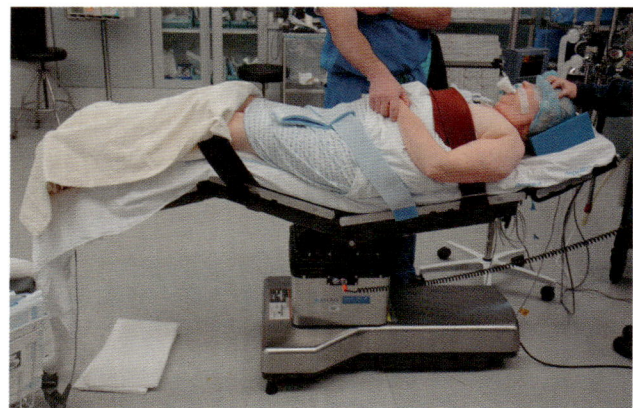

FIGURE 4.5 The patient is then placed in a slight Trendelenburg position to prevent him or her from sliding inferiorly on the operating table.

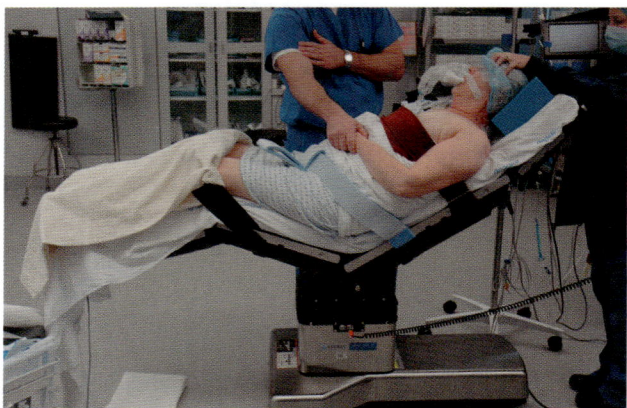

FIGURE 4.6 The back of the operating table is elevated approximately 45 to 60 degrees with respect to the floor.

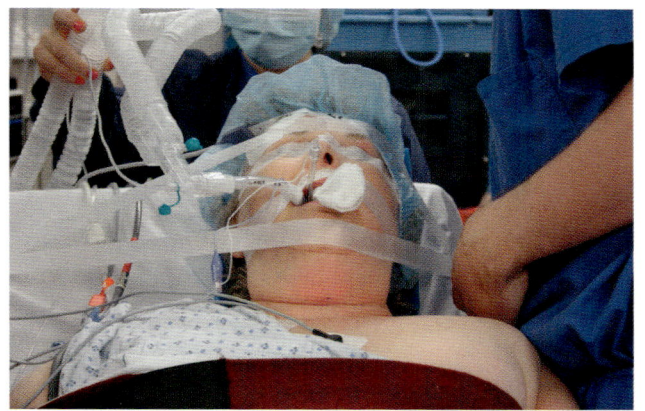

FIGURE 4.7 The forehead and chin are secured with 1-inch silk adhesive tape.

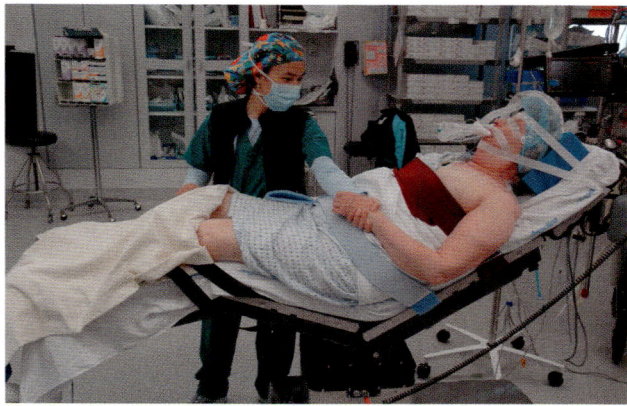

FIGURE 4.8 Final patient position before skin preparation.

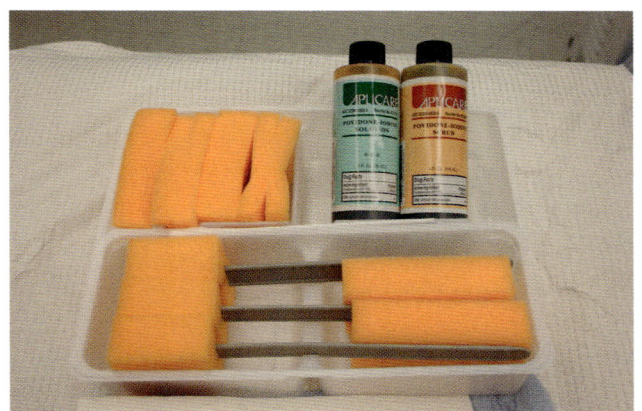

FIGURE 4.9 Povidone-iodine (Betadine) scrub and skin preparation.

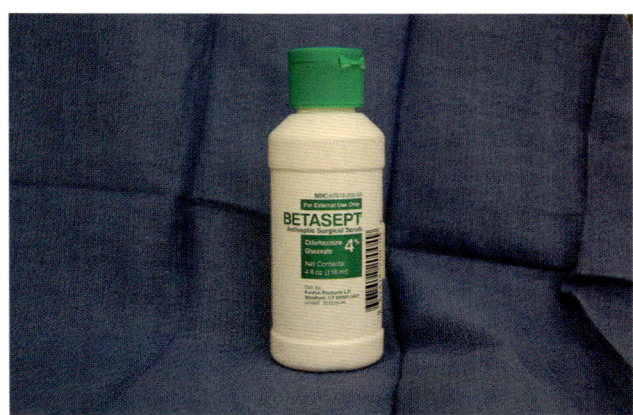

FIGURE 4.10 Chlorhexidine gluconate (Betasept) solution used for surgical scrub in patients with an allergy or hypersensitivity to Betadine.

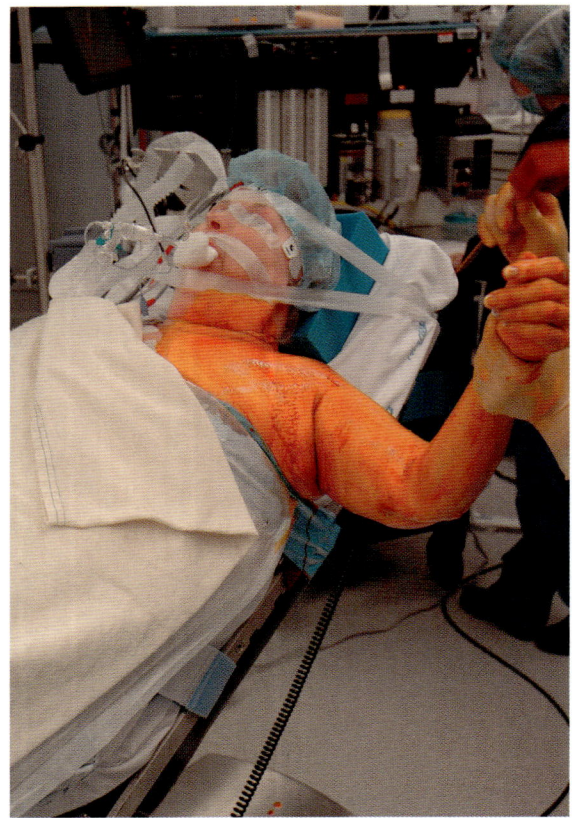

FIGURE 4.11 Completed skin preparation extending medially to the midline, distally to the level of the nipple, proximally to the level of the mandible, and including the entire upper extremity.

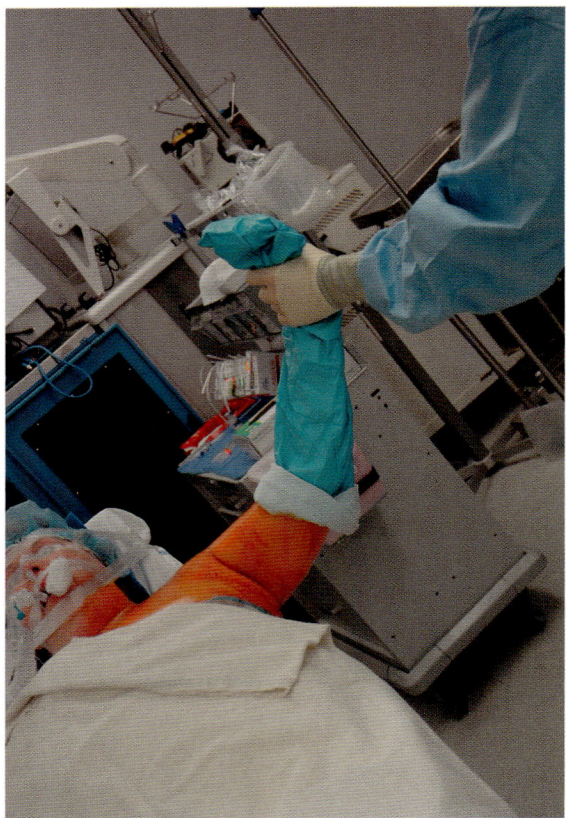

FIGURE 4.12 Placement of an impermeable stockinet.

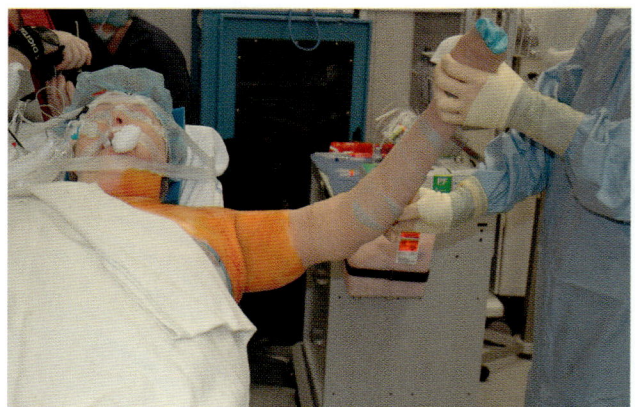

FIGURE 4.13 The stockinet is secured with a disposable elastic wrap.

CHAPTER 4 ■ Anesthesia, Patient Positioning, and Patient Preparation 33

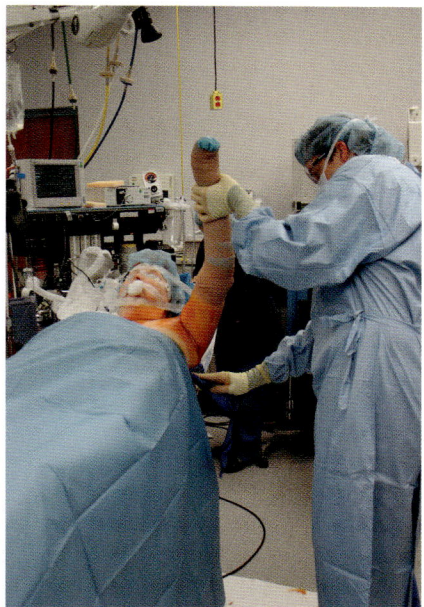

FIGURE 4.14 The area around the shoulder is dried to allow adhesion of the operative drapes.

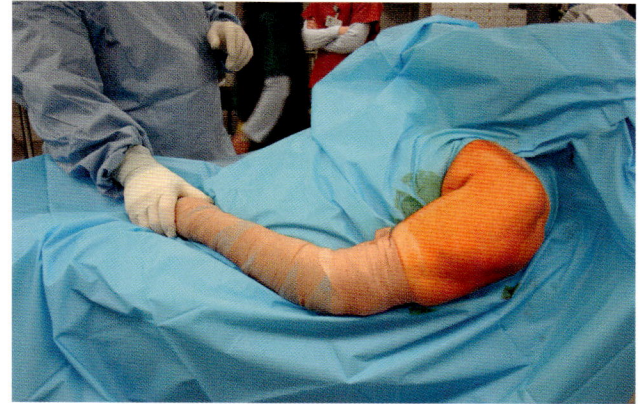

FIGURE 4.15 A disposable impermeable "U" drape is placed inferiorly to superiorly with the two limbs of the drape meeting superiorly.

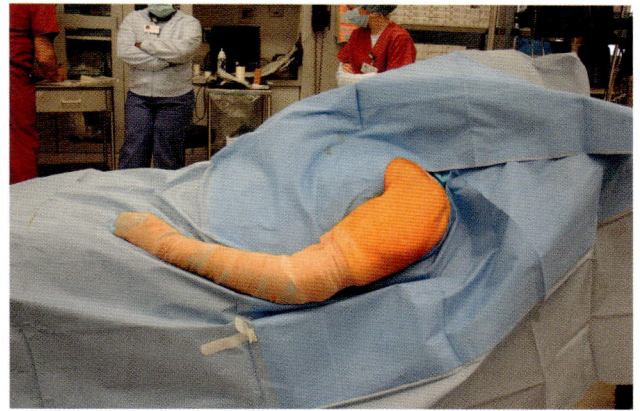

FIGURE 4.16 A large disposable reinforced paper "U" drape is applied inferiorly to superiorly.

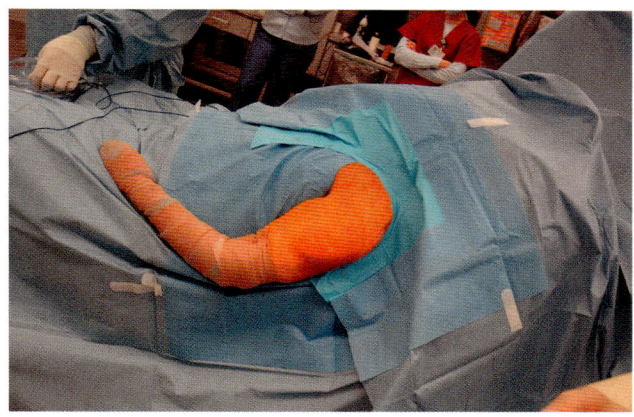

FIGURE 4.17 A smaller disposable paper "U" drape is placed superiorly to inferiorly.

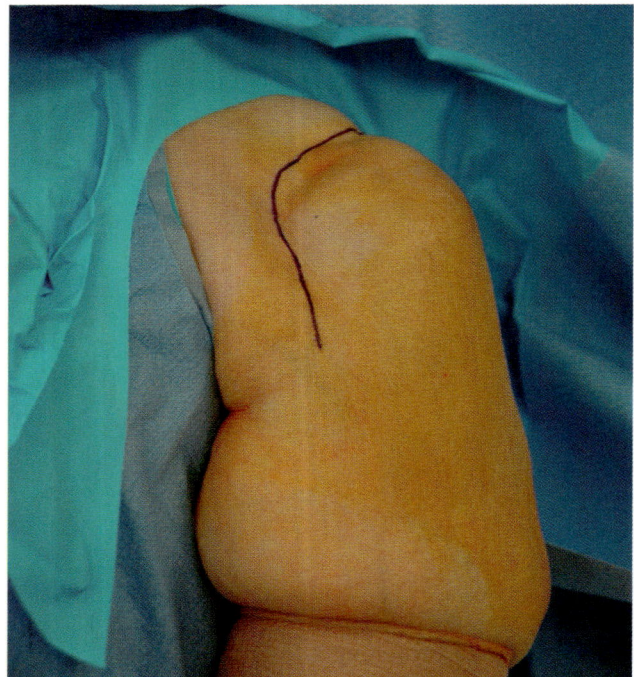

FIGURE 4.18 Previous incisions are marked with a sterile marking pen.

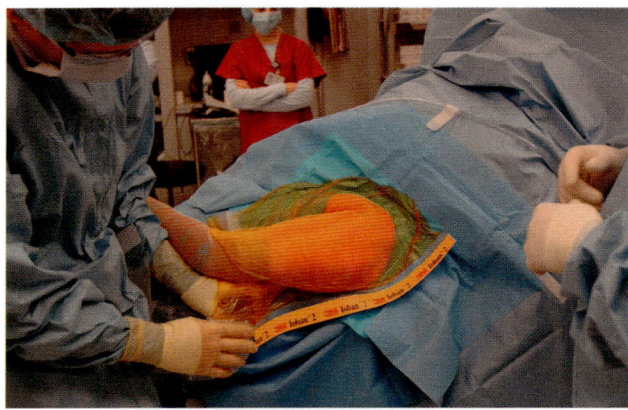

FIGURE 4.19 Placement of an occlusive adhesive drape with the arm abducted to allow isolation of the axilla from the operative field.

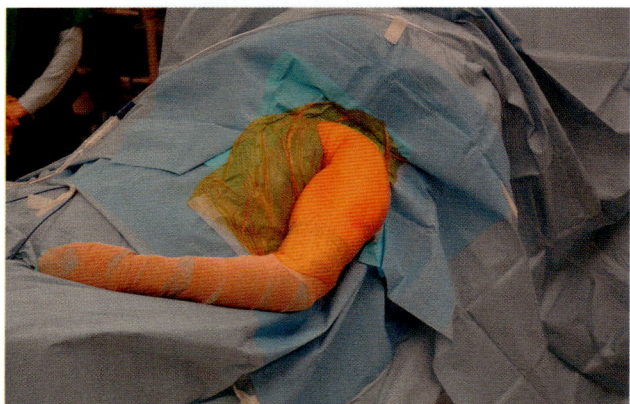

FIGURE 4.20 Final draping.

surgical incisions, skin scars are marked with a skin-marking pen (Fig. 4.18). An occlusive adhesive drape is applied to the shoulder to effectively remove the axilla from the surgical field. We prefer an iodine-impregnated occlusive drape; however, in patients with an iodine allergy or hypersensitivity, we use a non-iodine–impregnated version of the same drape. The occlusive drape is applied by first securing the drape to the posterior aspect of the shoulder. The arm is then abducted and externally rotated as the occlusive drape is placed anteriorly initially and then around the arm to cover the axilla (Fig. 4.19). Final patient positioning and draping are shown in Fig. 4.20.

ACKNOWLEDGMENTS

The authors would like to acknowledge and thank Gurunath Sigireddi, MD, and Steve T. Boozalis, MD, of Greater Houston Anesthesiology and the Department of Anesthesiology at Texas Orthopedic Hospital for their assistance with the anesthesia section of this chapter.

Long head of the biceps tendon

CHAPTER 5

Historically, the functional role of the long head of the biceps tendon has been controversial. Viewpoints have ranged from the biceps being a critical structural restraint to superior migration of the humeral head to being a vestigial structure that has little if any functional role in the shoulder. More recently, the long head of the biceps tendon has been implicated as a source of pain in patients with rotator cuff tears and in those with continued pain after shoulder arthroplasty performed for a proximal humeral fracture.[1,2]

In our patients undergoing shoulder arthroplasty, we have noted gross abnormalities of the long head of the biceps tendon in 60% of the patients. Table 5.1 details bicipital abnormalities observed at the time of shoulder arthroplasty by diagnosis.

Handling of the long head of the biceps tendon during shoulder arthroplasty has ranged from systematic preservation to systematic tenotomy or tenodesis regardless of its condition. In a series of 688 shoulder arthroplasties performed for primary osteoarthritis, concomitant biceps tenodesis or tenotomy was shown to improve outcomes. In this series, 121 shoulders underwent biceps tenodesis or tenotomy at the time of shoulder arthroplasty independent of the condition of the biceps. These patients demonstrated a significantly higher postoperative mean activity score, mean mobility score, mean total Constant score, mean active anterior elevation, and mean active external rotation as well as better subjective results than did patients not undergoing concomitant biceps surgery.[3] Fewer radiolucencies were reported around the glenoid component in shoulders that had undergone biceps tenotomy or tenodesis. Importantly, the incidence of complications was not affected by cutting the long head of the biceps tendon.

Based largely on the findings of the aforementioned study, our preference is to systematically remove the intra-articular portion of the biceps tendon at the time of shoulder arthroplasty in all cases. We do not recognize the long head of the biceps tendon as being essential to normal shoulder function after arthroplasty. We view cutting the biceps at the time of shoulder arthroplasty as akin to a general surgeon's performance of appendectomy during another abdominal procedure; even if the structure appears normal, it serves no critical function and could eventually cause a problem, so it is removed.

In our practice, the decision to perform tenodesis or tenotomy of the long head of the biceps is based on the patient's age, body habitus, and cosmetic concerns. We have anecdotally observed no differences in pain relief or function between tenodesis and tenotomy. In younger patients, thin patients, and those concerned about the appearance of the arm, we opt for biceps tenodesis. In patients not fitting these criteria, biceps tenotomy is sufficient and takes less operative time.

TECHNIQUE FOR HANDLING THE LONG HEAD OF THE BICEPS TENDON

The long head of the biceps tendon may be addressed any time it is visualized during shoulder arthroplasty. In most cases, we remove the intra-articular portion of the biceps just after preparation of the humerus and immediately before preparation of the glenoid because it is easily visualized at this juncture of the procedure. Additionally, in some cases the long head of the biceps tendon may be contracted or found to lack normal excursion. This could potentially hinder glenoid exposure, so the tendon is released before glenoid preparation. However, in fracture cases treated by hemiarthroplasty, the long head of the biceps tendon is left intact as an anatomic point of reference until just before fixation of the tuberosities.

After humeral head resection and proximal humeral preparation, large curved Mayo scissors are placed superior and posterior to the long head of the biceps tendon to allow visualization of the tendon as it enters the bicipital groove (Fig. 5.1). A scalpel is used to transect the tendon at the entrance of the bicipital groove (Fig. 5.2). If tenodesis is to be performed, the tendon is pulled out of the bicipital groove inferiorly and sutured to the pectoralis major tendon with a figure-of-eight no. 1 nonabsorbable braided suture (Fig. 5.3). Residual tendon is sharply removed to complete the tenodesis (Fig. 5.4). When the humeral head is retracted posteriorly for glenoid exposure, the remaining intra-articular stump of the long head of the biceps tendon is removed with Mayo scissors (Fig. 5.5). In cases of obvious tenosynovitis, any remaining bicipital sheath is removed as well.

In fracture cases, the long head of the biceps tendon is released from its insertion at the supraglenoid tubercle with curved Mayo scissors just before tuberosity fixation; it then undergoes tenodesis, if applicable, by the same technique described earlier.

TABLE 5.1	Condition of the Long Head of the Biceps Tendon in Cases of Shoulder Arthroplasty Performed at Texas Orthopedic Hospital From 2003 to 2014			
	Condition of the Long Head of the Biceps Tendon			
Diagnosis	Normal	Rupture	Partial Tear/Synovitis	Spontaneous Tenodesis
Primary osteoarthritis	455	267	39	5
Acute fracture	53	42	9	0
Rotator cuff tear arthropathy	17	87	166	7
Atraumatic osteonecrosis	28	7	5	4
Instability arthropathy	38	29	12	2
Rheumatoid arthritis	6	13	27	2
Posttraumatic arthropathy	32	27	34	13
Revision arthroplasty	19	23	111	10
Miscellaneous diagnoses	6	6	10	5
Total	654	501	413	48

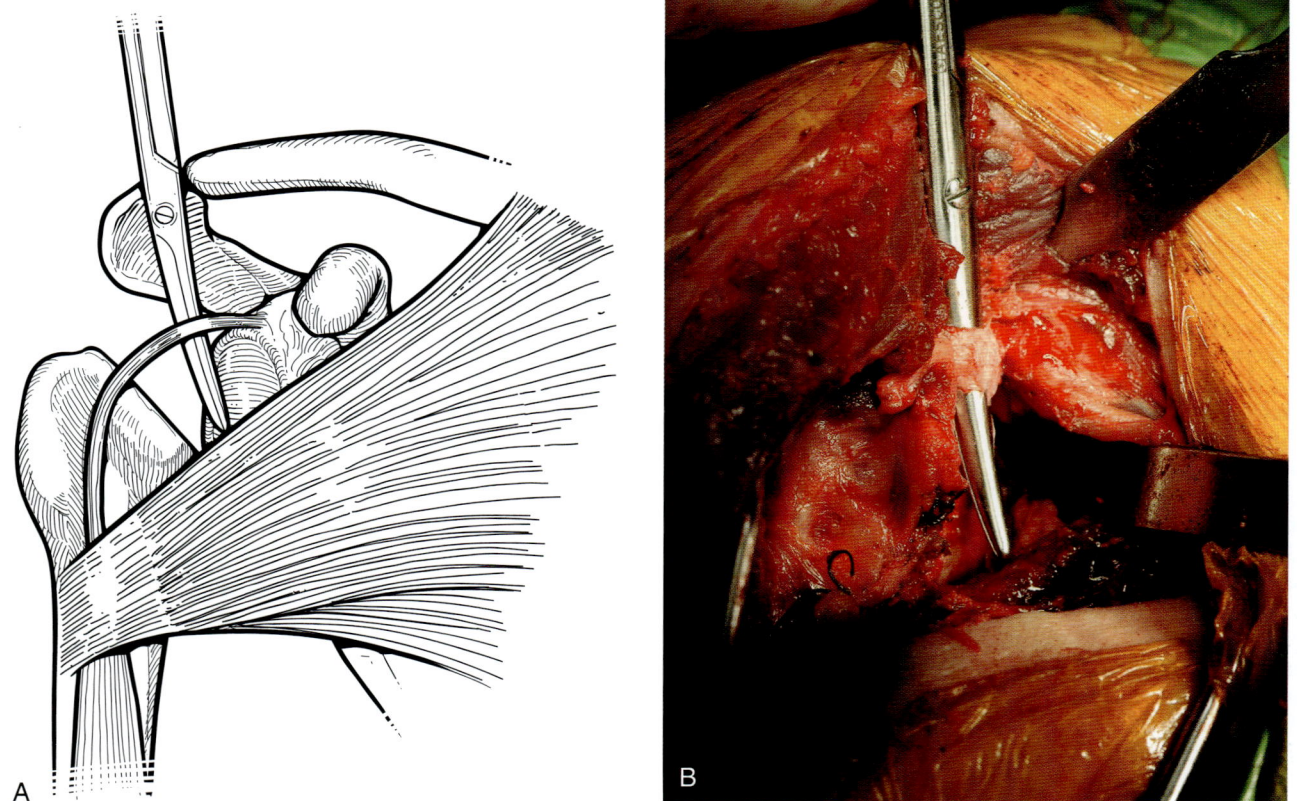

FIGURE 5.1 (A and B) Large curved Mayo scissors are placed superior and posterior to the long head of the biceps tendon to allow visualization of the tendon as it enters the bicipital groove.

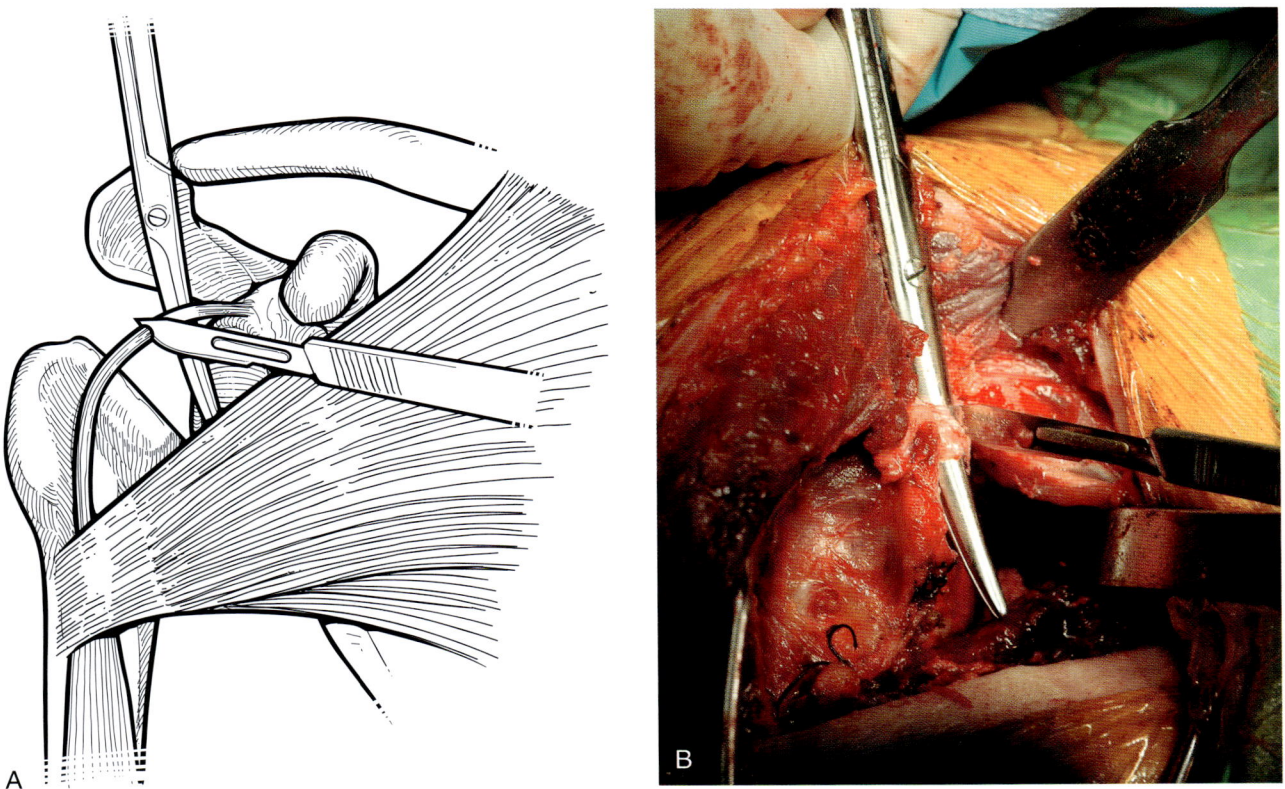

FIGURE 5.2 (A and B) A scalpel is used to transect the tendon at the entrance of the bicipital groove.

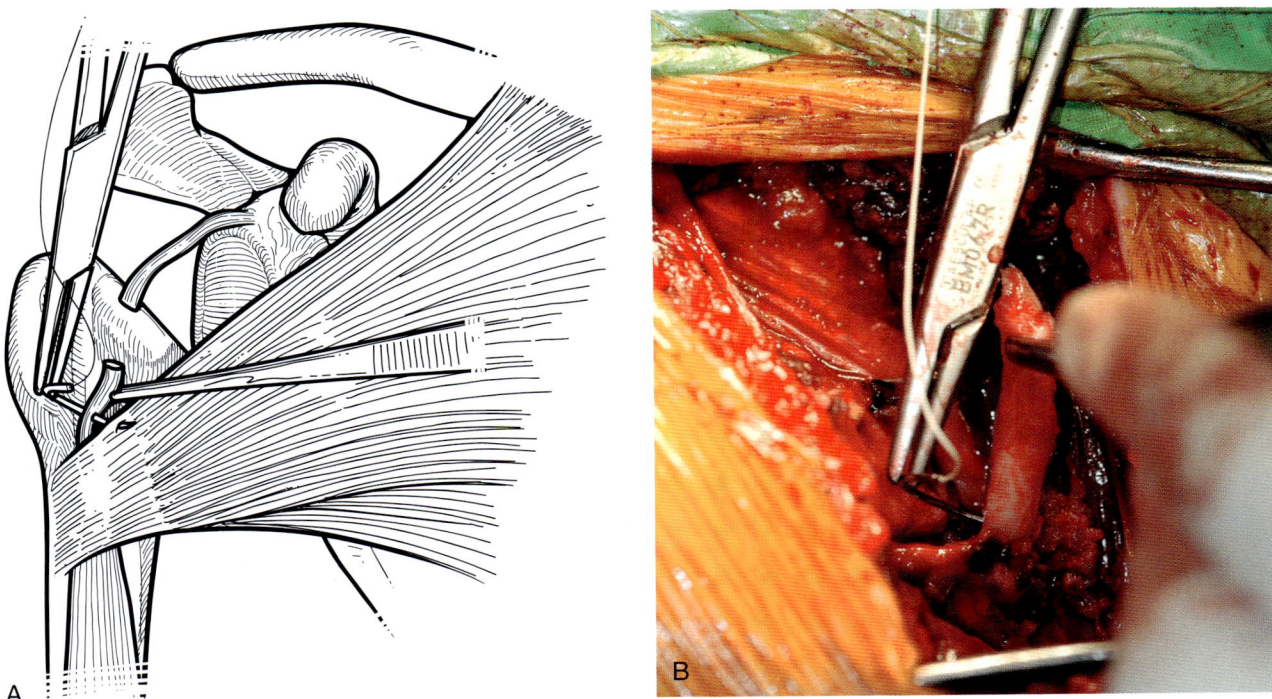

FIGURE 5.3 (A and B) The long head of the biceps tendon is pulled out of the bicipital groove inferiorly and sutured to the pectoralis major tendon with a figure-of-eight no. 1 nonabsorbable braided suture.

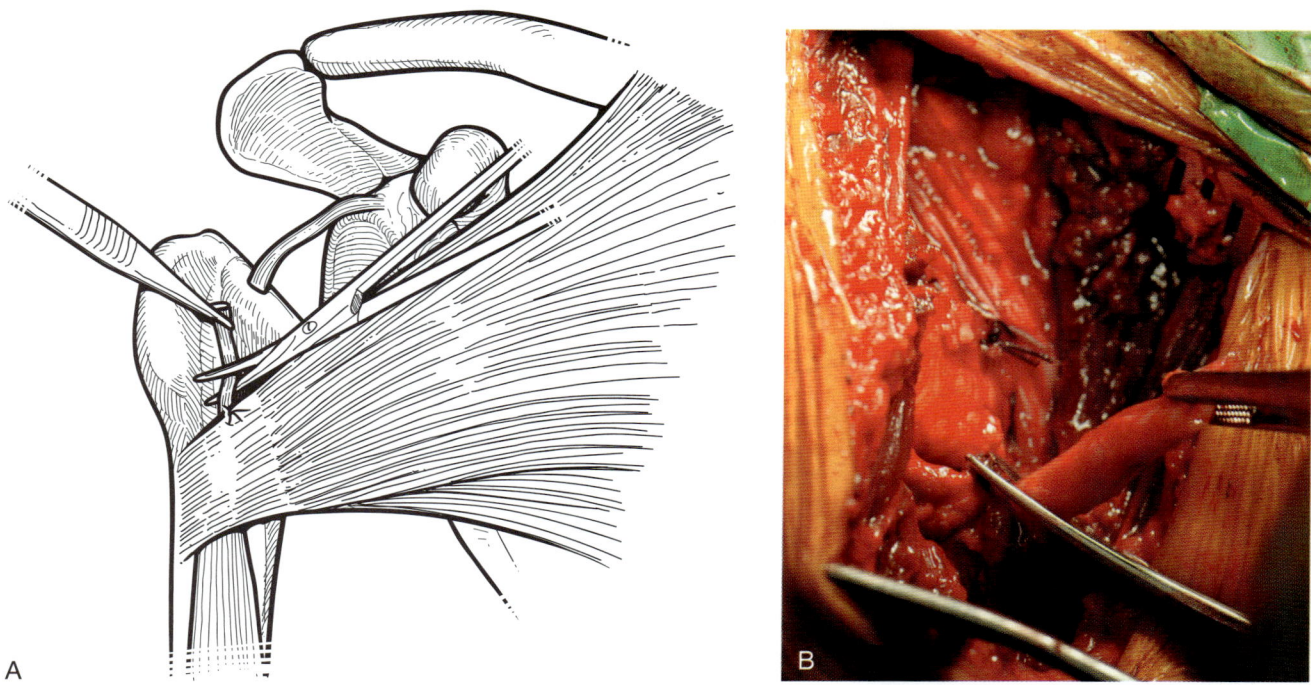

FIGURE 5.4 (A and B) Residual tendon is sharply removed to complete the tenodesis.

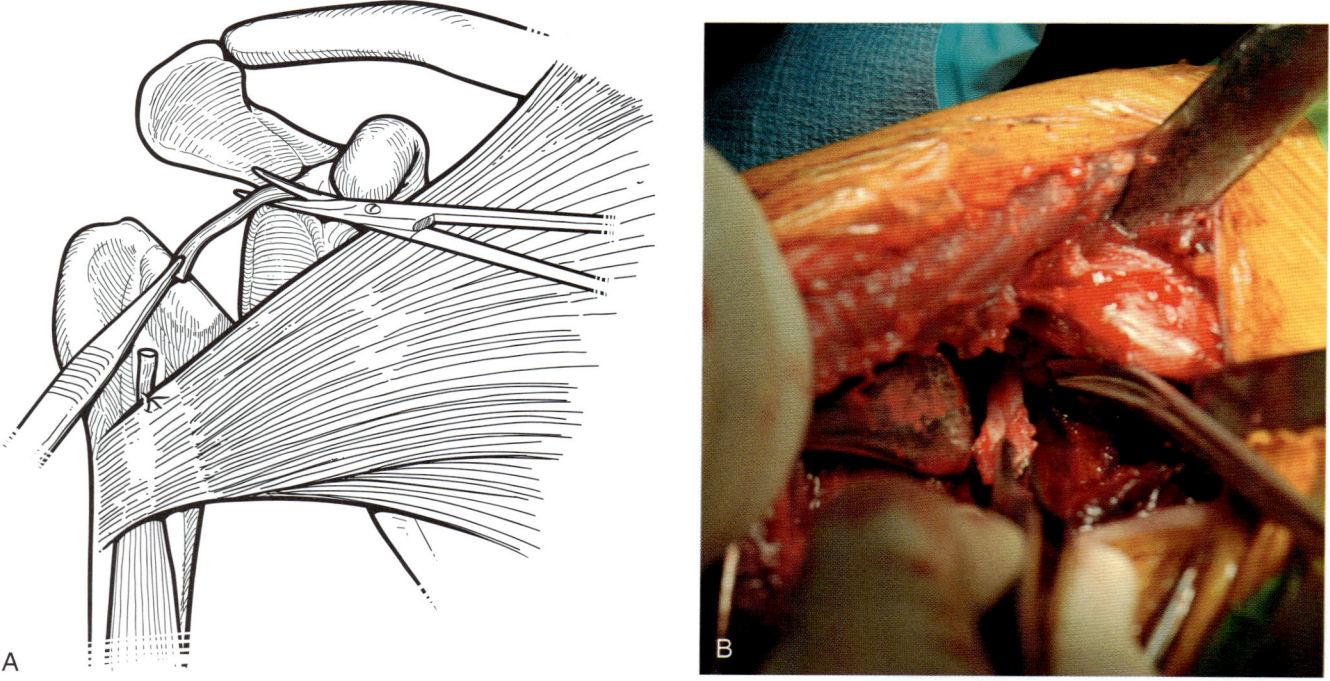

FIGURE 5.5 (A and B) With the humeral head retracted posteriorly for glenoid exposure, the remaining intra-articular stump of the long head of the biceps tendon is removed with Mayo scissors.

REFERENCES

1. Walch G, Edwards TB, Nové-Josserand L, et al: Arthroscopic tenotomy of the long head of the biceps in the treatment of rotator cuff tears: clinical and radiographic results of 307 cases, *J Shoulder Elbow Surg* 14:238–246, 2005.
2. Dines D, Hersch J: Long head of the biceps lesions after shoulder arthroplasty. Paper presented at the 8th International Congress on Surgery of the Shoulder, April 2001, Cape Town, South Africa.
3. Fama G, Edwards TB, Boulahia A, et al: The role of concomitant biceps tenodesis in shoulder arthroplasty for primary osteoarthritis: results of a multicentric study, *Orthopedics* 27:401–405, 2004.

SECTION II

UNCONSTRAINED SHOULDER ARTHROPLASTY FOR CHRONIC DISEASE

CHAPTER 6

Indications and contraindications

Indications for unconstrained shoulder arthroplasty can be divided into arthroplasty performed for acute fracture and arthroplasty performed for chronic shoulder disease. This chapter focuses on indications for unconstrained shoulder arthroplasty in patients with chronic shoulder disease. Indications for unconstrained shoulder arthroplasty in patients with an acute fracture are covered in Chapter 26.

Multiple chronic indications for unconstrained shoulder arthroplasty include, but are not limited to, primary osteoarthritis, inflammatory arthropathies, humeral head osteonecrosis, instability arthropathy, posttraumatic arthritis, fixed glenohumeral dislocation, rotator cuff tear arthropathy (glenohumeral arthritis with a massive rotator cuff tear), postinfectious arthropathy, glenohumeral chondrolysis, proximal humeral fracture nonunion, glenohumeral arthritis associated with neurologic pathology, glenohumeral arthritis associated with previous radiation therapy, glenohumeral arthritis associated with skeletal dysplasia, and tumor. This chapter looks at unique characteristics and special considerations for each of these indications. In addition, indications for total shoulder arthroplasty versus hemiarthroplasty are discussed, and contraindications to unconstrained shoulder arthroplasty are detailed.

HEMIARTHROPLASTY VERSUS TOTAL SHOULDER ARTHROPLASTY: INDICATIONS FOR GLENOID RESURFACING

Indications for glenoid resurfacing in unconstrained shoulder arthroplasty are a much debated topic. We currently favor total shoulder arthroplasty because the results are superior and the complication rate is equal to or lower than that seen in hemiarthroplasty. Our decision on when to perform glenoid resurfacing is detailed according to diagnosis in the following sections.

Two major requirements exist for performance of glenoid resurfacing in unconstrained shoulder arthroplasty: the glenoid bone must be sufficient to allow implantation of components (judged by preoperative imaging studies; see Chapter 7), and the anterior and posterior rotator cuff must be functioning (judged by clinical examination and preoperative imaging studies; see Chapter 7).[1] Lack of either of these requirements represents an absolute contraindication to glenoid resurfacing. A relative contraindication to glenoid resurfacing is young patient age. A "safe" age at which to implant a polyethylene glenoid component has not been established. Concerns of polyethylene wear are heightened in younger patients because of their residual life expectancy.

PRIMARY OSTEOARTHRITIS

Primary osteoarthritis was initially described by Neer and is the most common single indication for shoulder arthroplasty in our practice.[2] In a large multicenter study, primary osteoarthritis was the underlying cause in half of the primary shoulder arthroplasties performed.[3]

Clinical Findings

Clinical findings in patients with primary osteoarthritis include glenohumeral crepitus and stiffness. Rotator cuff testing may be normal or compromised by pain.

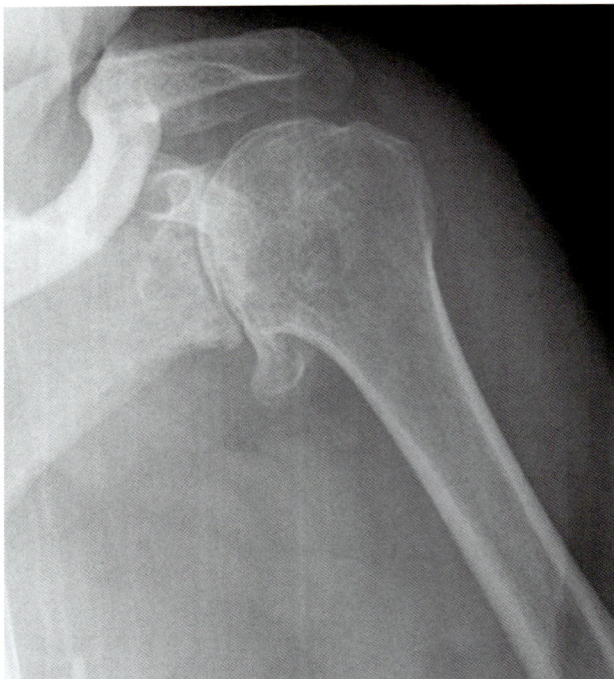

FIGURE 6.1 Radiograph of primary osteoarthritis showing the typical loss of the glenohumeral joint space and the presence of large humeral osteophytes.

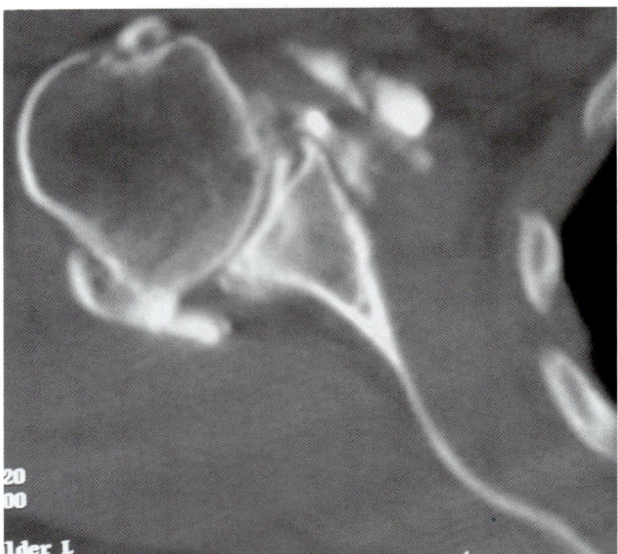

FIGURE 6.3 Computed tomography demonstrating the "classic" biconcave glenoid seen in primary osteoarthritis.

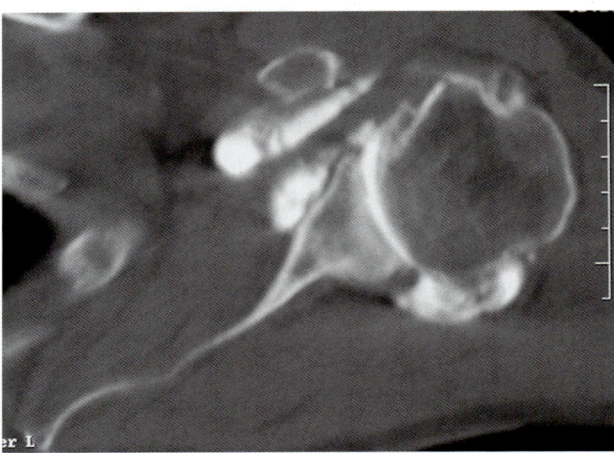

FIGURE 6.4 Computed tomography showing the more common posterior humeral head subluxation without the osseous glenoid erosion seen in primary osteoarthritis.

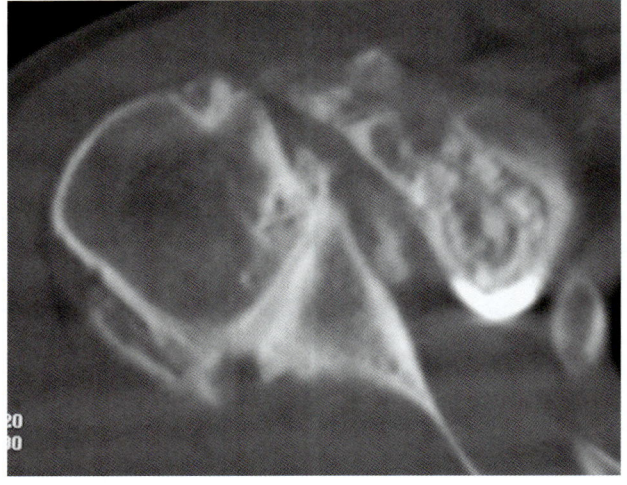

FIGURE 6.2 Large loose body in the subscapularis fossa in a patient with primary osteoarthritis.

Imaging Findings

Plain radiography demonstrates loss of the normal glenohumeral joint space. Humeral head osteophytes are usually present and may be large (Fig. 6.1). Loose bodies may be apparent on plain radiography, especially in the subscapularis recess (Fig. 6.2).

Secondary imaging studies (computed tomography arthrography, magnetic resonance imaging) will show the "classic" posterior glenoid erosion with biconcavity in only 20% of cases (Fig. 6.3).[3] Approximately half of patients with primary osteoarthritis will have the humeral head centered within the glenoid, and another 25% will demonstrate posterior subluxation without osseous erosion (Fig. 6.4).[3] Less than 5% of patients with primary osteoarthritis will demonstrate a dysplastic-appearing glenoid morphology (Fig. 6.5).[3]

Seven percent of patients with primary osteoarthritis have a full-thickness rotator cuff tear limited to the supraspinatus, and an additional 7% have a partial-thickness rotator cuff tear.[4] Moreover, moderate to severe fatty infiltration of the infraspinatus or subscapularis (or both) occurs in approximately 20% of patients with primary osteoarthritis.[4]

Special Considerations

We perform total shoulder arthroplasty in nearly all cases of primary osteoarthritis because it has been shown to be superior to hemiarthroplasty without an increased risk of

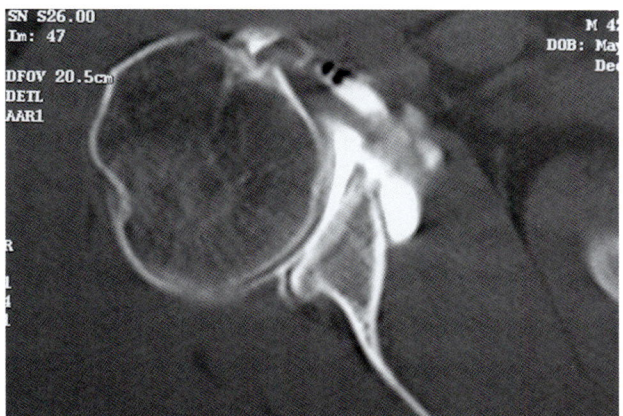

FIGURE 6.5 Dysplastic glenoid morphology seen rarely in primary osteoarthritis. Note the excessive glenoid retroversion present with a relatively well centered humeral head.

complications or reoperations.[5,6] The only patients with primary osteoarthritis in whom we perform hemiarthroplasty are those with insufficient glenoid bone. In patients with anterior or posterior rotator cuff insufficiency, we opt for a reverse-design prosthesis instead of a total shoulder arthroplasty or hemiarthroplasty (see Section III).

RHEUMATOID ARTHRITIS

Rheumatoid arthritis is the most common inflammatory joint disease. Shoulder manifestations develop in 60% to 90% of patients as their disease progresses. In a large multicenter study, rheumatoid arthritis was the underlying cause in 12% of the primary shoulder arthroplasties performed.[7]

Clinical Findings

Clinical findings in patients with rheumatoid arthritis include glenohumeral crepitus and stiffness. Rotator cuff testing may be normal, compromised by pain, or compromised by a rotator cuff tear as rotator cuff tears are more common in patients with rheumatoid arthritis compared with primary osteoarthritis.

Imaging Findings

Plain radiography demonstrates loss of the normal glenohumeral joint space. Humeral head osteophytes are rarely present (Fig. 6.6). The humeral head may be centered or statically migrated, depending on the condition of the rotator cuff.

Secondary imaging studies (computed tomography arthrography, magnetic resonance imaging) may show protrusio-type glenoid morphology (Fig. 6.7). Eight percent of patients with rheumatoid arthritis have a full-thickness rotator cuff tear limited to the supraspinatus, and an additional 9% have a partial-thickness supraspinatus tear.[8] Twelve percent of patients with rheumatoid arthritis have massive rotator cuff tears involving the supraspinatus and infraspinatus tendons.[8] In addition, moderate to severe fatty infiltration of the infraspinatus or the subscapularis (or both)

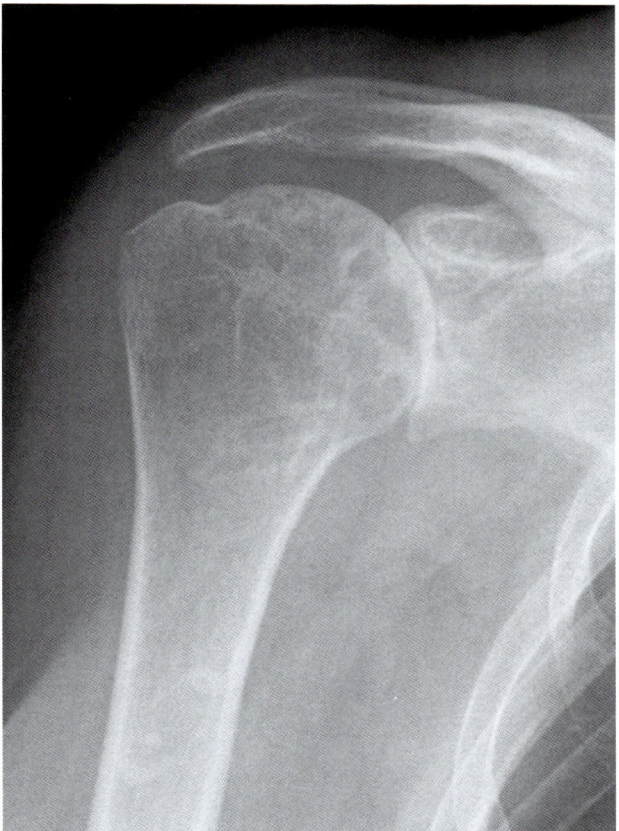

FIGURE 6.6 Radiograph of rheumatoid arthritis showing the typical loss of the glenohumeral joint space and a paucity of humeral osteophytes.

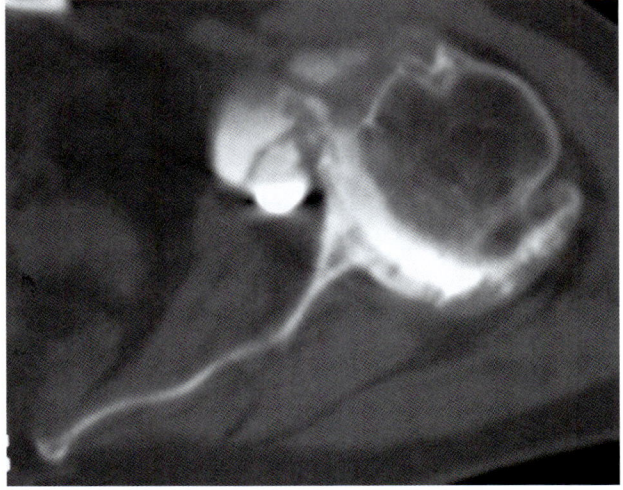

FIGURE 6.7 Computed tomography demonstrating a protrusio-type glenoid morphology seen in rheumatoid arthritis.

occurs in approximately 45% of patients with rheumatoid arthritis.[8]

Special Considerations

We perform total shoulder arthroplasty in nearly all cases of rheumatoid arthritis because it has been shown to be superior to hemiarthroplasty.[9] The only patients with rheumatoid arthritis in whom we perform hemiarthroplasty are those with insufficient glenoid bone. In patients with anterior or posterior rotator cuff insufficiency, we opt for a reverse-design prosthesis (see Section III).

A rare subtype of rheumatoid arthritis that rarely requires shoulder arthroplasty but merits special consideration is juvenile-onset rheumatoid arthritis. In our limited experience, these patients tend to have severe preoperative stiffness that may require more soft tissue releases than normal, including release of the entire pectoralis major. In addition, the humerus and glenoid may be exceptionally small and thus necessitate the use of custom-manufactured implants.

OTHER INFLAMMATORY ARTHROPATHIES

Other inflammatory arthropathies affecting the glenohumeral joint sufficiently to require shoulder arthroplasty are rare and include Paget's disease, ankylosing spondylitis, psoriatic arthritis, systemic lupus erythematosus, scleroderma, and polymyalgia rheumatica. Unfortunately, because of the relative rarity of these conditions, little information is available regarding special considerations for these diseases. When any of these conditions evolve to complete loss of articular cartilage and fail reasonable nonoperative treatment, shoulder arthroplasty may be considered. Provided that the rotator cuff is competent and sufficient glenoid bone stock exists, we opt to resurface the glenoid in these patients.

HUMERAL HEAD OSTEONECROSIS

Although humeral head osteonecrosis is rare, it is the most common nontraumatic indication for shoulder hemiarthroplasty in our practice. In a large multicenter study, osteonecrosis was the underlying cause in only 5% of the primary shoulder arthroplasties performed.[10] Many factors have been implicated as contributing to atraumatic osteonecrosis, including corticosteroid use, alcohol abuse, and hematologic disorders. Despite the influence of these factors, most cases of humeral head osteonecrosis are idiopathic.

Clinical Findings

Clinical findings in patients with atraumatic osteonecrosis range from solely subjective complaints of pain to glenohumeral crepitus and stiffness, such as seen in primary osteoarthritis. Rotator cuff testing is usually normal but may be compromised by pain, especially in the later stages.

Imaging Findings

Radiographic classification of humeral head osteonecrosis has evolved from that described for the femoral head.[11,12] Stage I is a preradiographic stage that requires diagnosis by magnetic resonance imaging or scintigraphy. Stage II is characterized by a zone of osteopenia surrounding a zone of relatively increased osseous density with the sphericity of the humeral head preserved (Fig. 6.8). Stage III is characterized by the presence of a subchondral fracture (the "crescent sign");

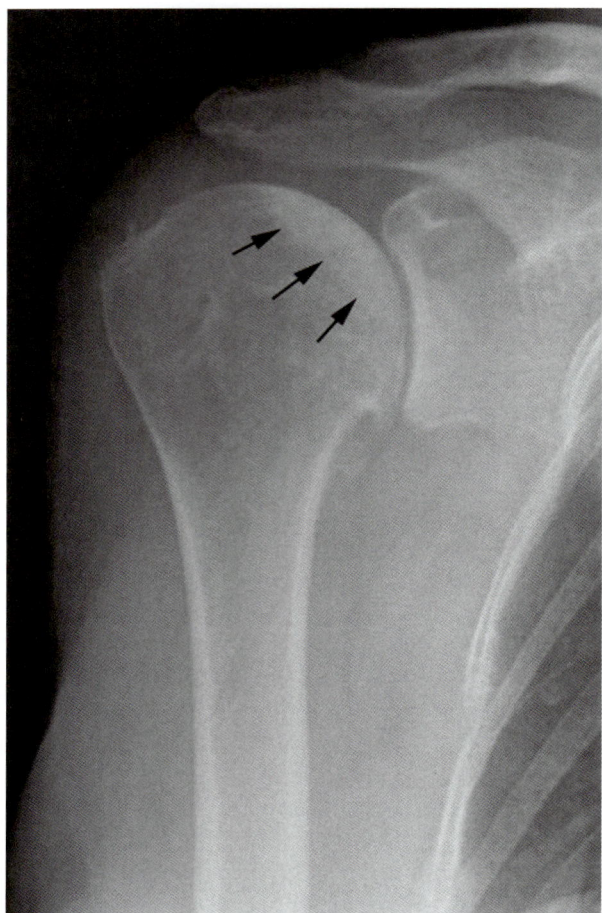

FIGURE 6.8 Stage II osteonecrosis is characterized by a zone of osteopenia surrounding a zone of relatively increased osseous density *(arrows)*, with the sphericity of the humeral head preserved.

sphericity of the humeral head is preserved (Fig. 6.9). Stage IV corresponds to loss of sphericity of the humeral head as a result of collapse of the necrotic segment (Fig. 6.10). Stage V is characterized by loss of glenoid articular cartilage with secondary osteoarthritis (Fig. 6.11). Stage VI is characterized by osseous collapse of the humeral head with medialization of the humerus relative to the glenoid (Fig. 6.12).

Magnetic resonance imaging will reliably show the area of osteonecrosis in all except the earliest cases (what has been described as stage 0 in the hip and characterized by increased intraosseous pressure without imaging abnormalities), as shown in Fig. 6.13. Secondary imaging studies (computed tomography arthrography, magnetic resonance imaging) almost always show a concentric glenoid.

The incidence of rotator cuff tears in patients with atraumatic osteonecrosis is similar to that observed in primary osteoarthritis. Conversely, moderate to severe fatty infiltration of the infraspinatus or subscapularis (or both) occurs less frequently than with primary osteoarthritis.[10]

Special Considerations

We perform hemiarthroplasty for stage I, II, III, and IV osteonecrosis because the results have been shown to be equal to those of total shoulder arthroplasty.[12] In patients with

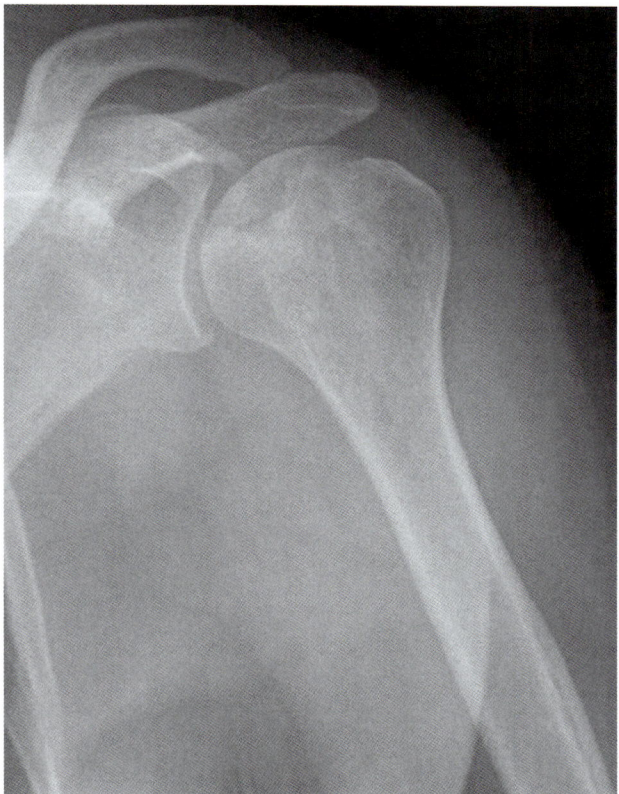

FIGURE 6.9 Stage III osteonecrosis is characterized by the presence of a subchondral fracture (the "crescent sign"); the sphericity of the humeral head is preserved.

stage V and VI osteonecrosis, we perform total shoulder arthroplasty if no contraindications to glenoid resurfacing exist.

INSTABILITY ARTHROPATHY

Instability arthropathy of the shoulder necessitating shoulder arthroplasty is a rare entity; it is seen in less than 5% of unconstrained primary shoulder arthroplasties in our practice. Patients with previous shoulder dislocations treated operatively and nonoperatively are included in this category. Patients usually fall into a bimodal distribution with regard to age at the time of initial dislocation. The first group of patients dislocate their shoulder when they are relatively young, and progressive arthropathy develops over a period of several years. The second group of patients are older (>60 years) at the time of initial dislocation and are prone to a rapidly developing glenohumeral arthritis that may result in a complete loss of articular cartilage within months of the initial dislocation. We have not been able to distinguish between what has previously been termed "capsulorrhaphy arthropathy" and "instability arthropathy" and consequently include these patients in a single entity under the diagnosis of instability arthropathy.[13]

Clinical Findings

Clinical findings in patients with instability arthropathy include glenohumeral crepitus and stiffness. Rotator cuff

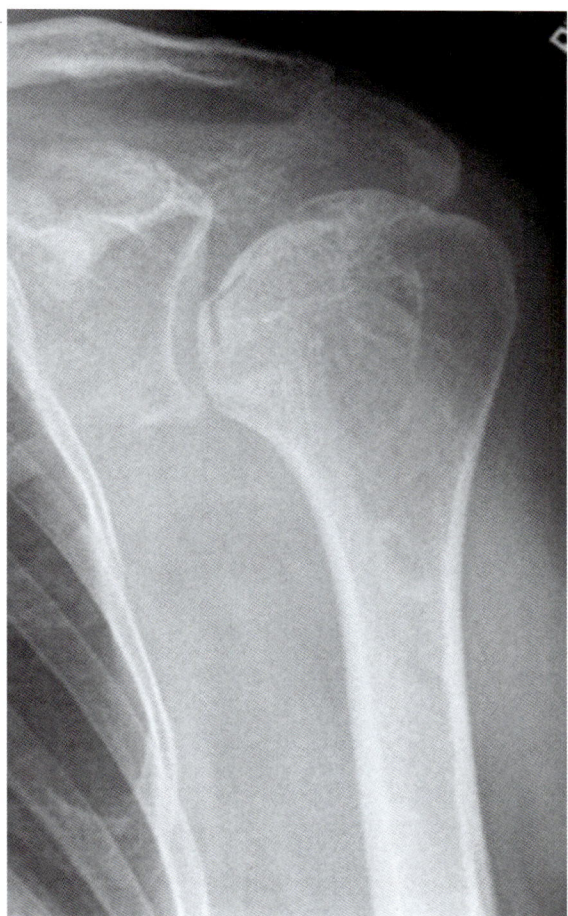

FIGURE 6.10 Stage IV osteonecrosis corresponds to loss of sphericity of the humeral head caused by collapse of the necrotic segment.

testing may be normal or compromised by pain or rotator cuff tearing.

Imaging Findings

Plain radiography demonstrates loss of the normal glenohumeral joint space. In patients with slowly progressing arthropathy, the radiographic changes are very similar to those of primary osteoarthritis and consist of humeral head osteophytes with or without loose bodies (Fig. 6.14). In older patients with rapidly appearing instability arthropathy, loss of the glenohumeral joint space with a paucity of osteophytes is apparent (Fig. 6.15).

Secondary imaging studies (computed tomography arthrography, magnetic resonance imaging) show posterior subluxation with or without glenoid erosion with biconcavity in 20% of cases, and this finding occurs in both patients who have previously undergone stabilization surgery and those who have not.[13] Twenty percent of patients with instability arthropathy have a full-thickness rotator cuff tear, with most being limited to the supraspinatus tendon.[13]

Special Considerations

We perform total shoulder arthroplasty in nearly all cases of instability arthropathy because it has been shown to be

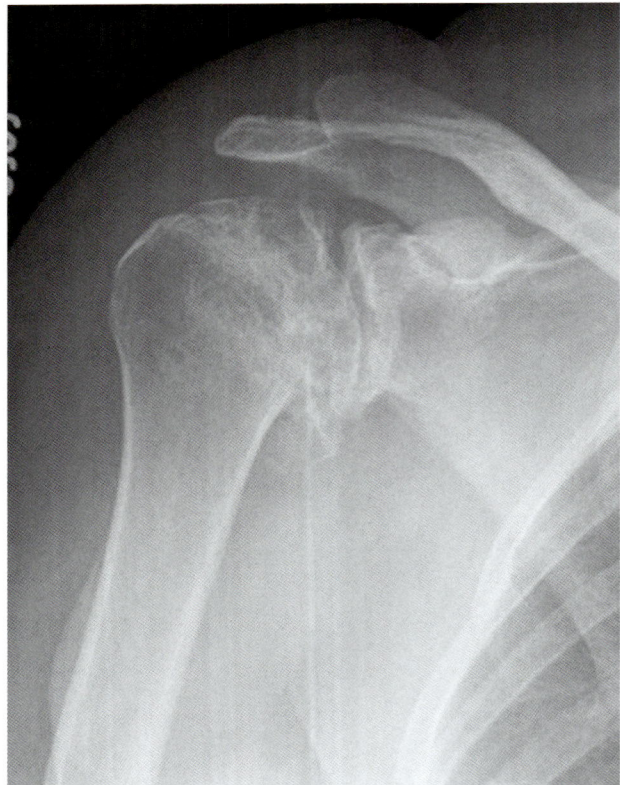

FIGURE 6.11 Stage V osteonecrosis is characterized by loss of glenoid articular cartilage with secondary osteoarthritis.

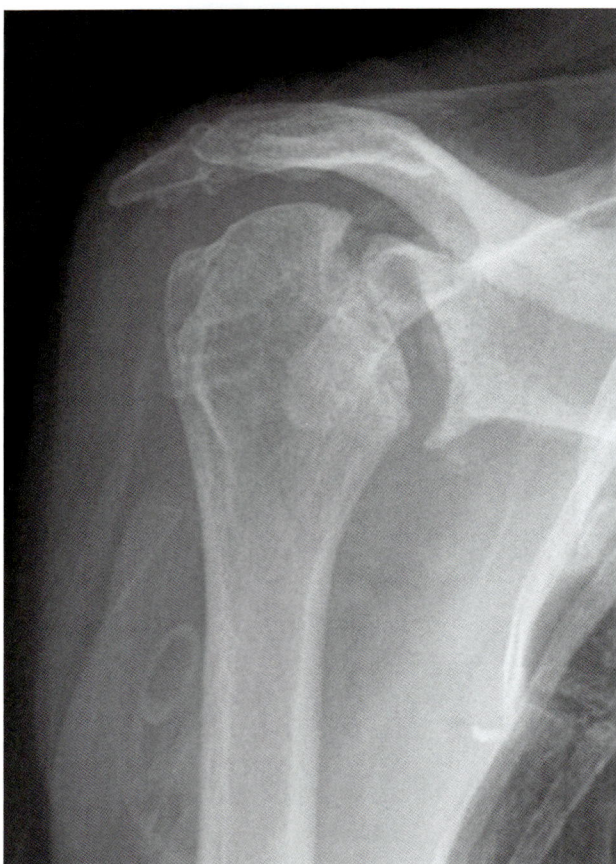

FIGURE 6.12 Stage VI osteonecrosis is characterized by osseous collapse of the humeral head with medialization of the humerus relative to the glenoid.

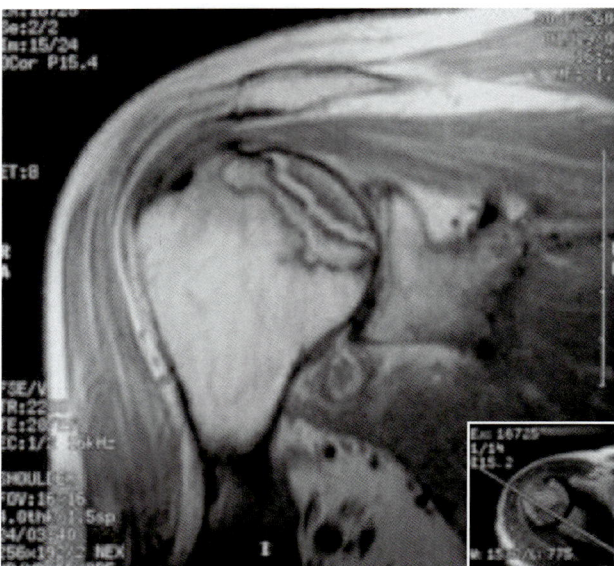

FIGURE 6.13 Magnetic resonance imaging showing an area of osteonecrosis of the humeral head.

superior to hemiarthroplasty and is not associated with an increased risk of complications or reoperations.[13] The only patients with instability arthropathy in whom we perform hemiarthroplasty are those with insufficient glenoid bone. In patients with anterior or posterior rotator cuff insufficiency, we opt for a reverse-design prosthesis instead of total shoulder arthroplasty or hemiarthroplasty (see Section III).

POSTTRAUMATIC ARTHRITIS

Posttraumatic glenohumeral arthritis covers a large spectrum of causes, including chondral damage secondary to blunt trauma and malunion and nonunion of the proximal humerus after fracture. This diagnosis can be relatively uncomplicated to treat when little glenohumeral osseous deformity is present (Fig. 6.16) or extremely difficult to treat in the case of severe proximal humeral malunion (Fig. 6.17). The integrity of the rotator cuff and the position of the tuberosities are very important when considering a patient for shoulder arthroplasty. If the rotator cuff is largely intact and the tuberosities are acceptably positioned to allow nearly normal rotator cuff function, unconstrained shoulder arthroplasty is our treatment of choice. In situations in which rotator cuff or tuberosity compromise (nonunion, severe malunion) is severe and would require a greater tuberosity osteotomy, we opt for a reverse-design prosthesis (see Section III).

Rarely, posttraumatic arthritis will develop after a glenoid fracture (Fig. 6.18). In these cases, it is of paramount

CHAPTER 6 ■ Indications and Contraindications 45

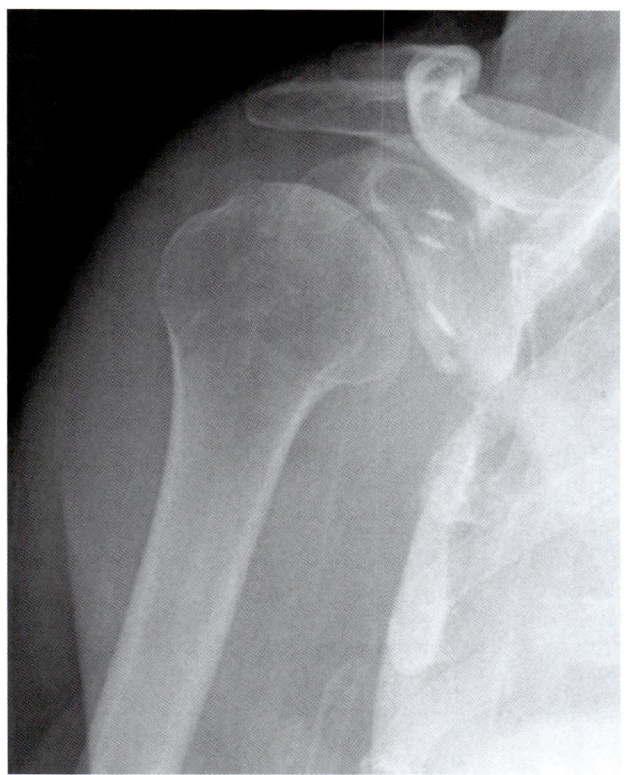

FIGURE 6.14 Slowly progressing instability arthropathy.

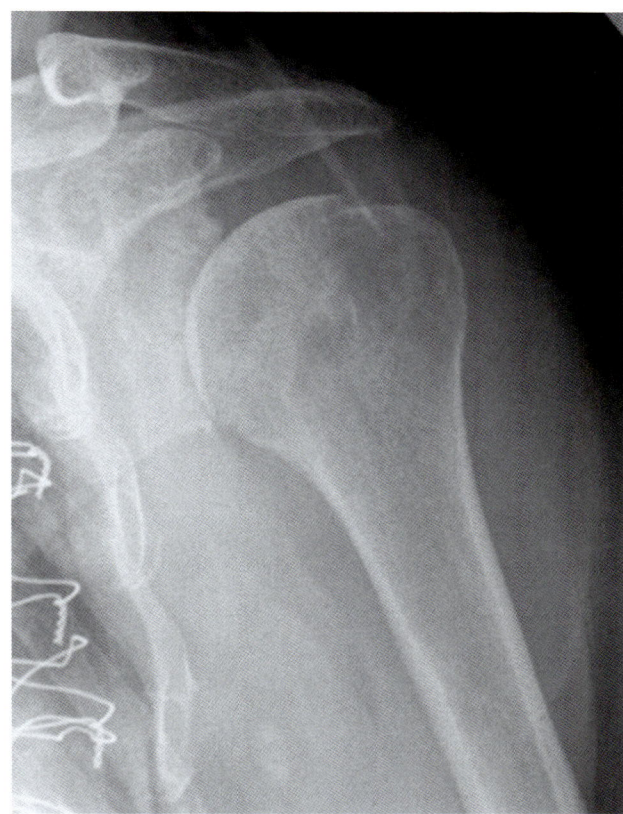

FIGURE 6.15 Rapidly appearing instability arthropathy in an older patient.

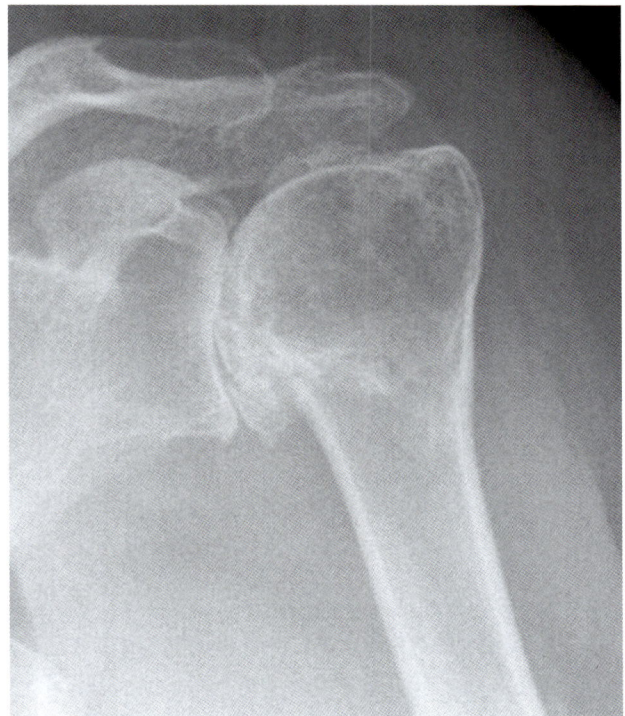

FIGURE 6.16 Posttraumatic arthritis with minimal residual deformity.

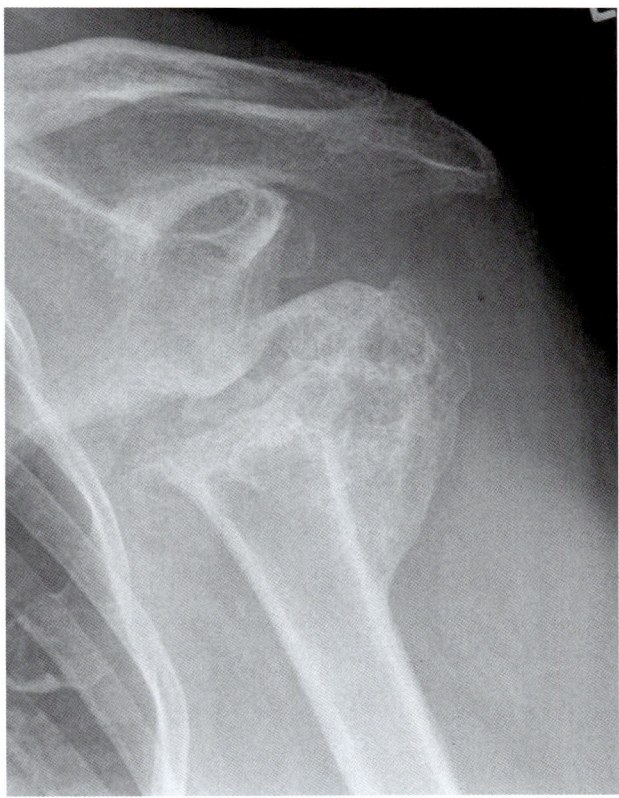

FIGURE 6.17 Posttraumatic arthritis with severe proximal humeral malunion.

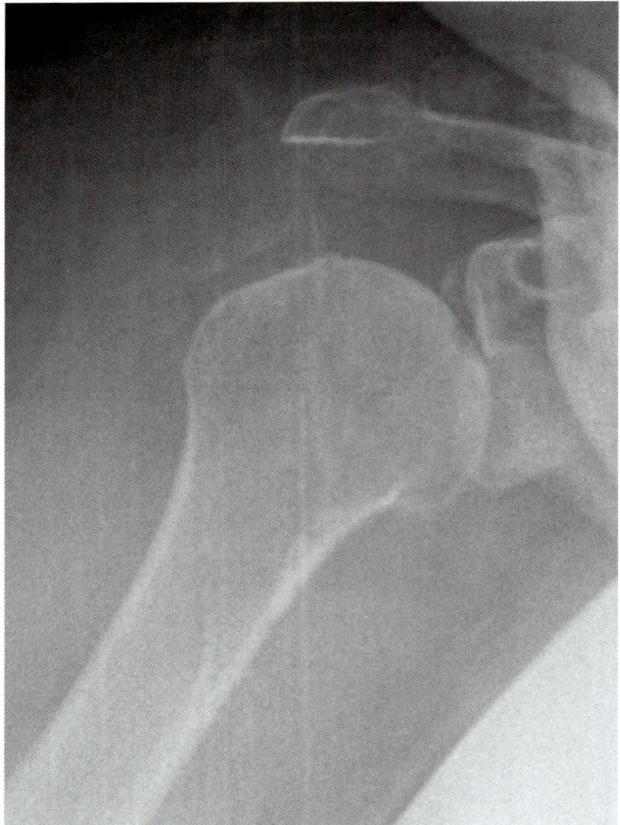

FIGURE 6.18 Posttraumatic arthritis after fracture of the glenoid.

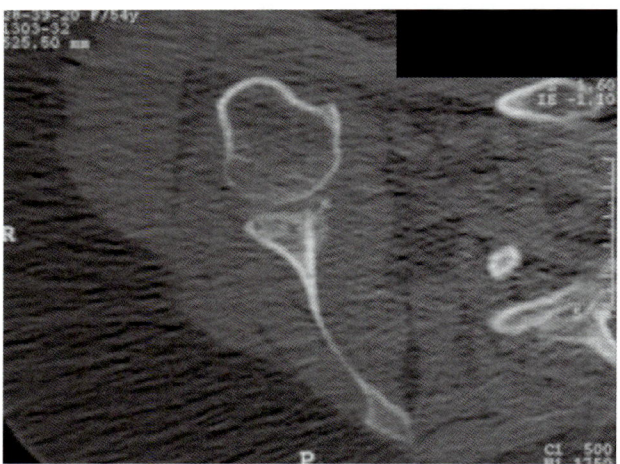

FIGURE 6.19 Computed tomography of a patient with posttraumatic arthritis after a glenoid fracture.

importance to ensure that the osseous glenoid is sufficient to allow placement of a glenoid component (Fig. 6.19). We prefer computed tomography arthrography rather than magnetic resonance imaging.

Clinical Findings

Clinical findings in patients with posttraumatic arthritis are variable. Findings in patients with relatively well-preserved proximal humeral anatomy are similar to those of primary osteoarthritis with its requisite glenohumeral crepitus and stiffness. In patients with distortion of proximal humeral anatomy as a result of malunion, shoulder stiffness may be exceptionally severe and attributable to mechanical impingement, subdeltoid contracture, and subacromial contracture, in addition to the glenohumeral incongruity and capsular contracture seen in primary osteoarthritis. Rotator cuff testing may be normal or compromised by pain or rotator cuff tearing.

Imaging Findings

Plain radiography demonstrates loss of the normal glenohumeral joint space. Other radiographic findings are variable, as previously mentioned, and depend on the source of the posttraumatic arthritis (chondral injury, malunion, etc.)

Secondary imaging studies (computed tomography arthrography, magnetic resonance imaging), like plain radiography, show variable findings, depending on the deformity present. We much prefer the use of computed tomography arthrography over magnetic resonance imaging in this diagnosis for the osseous detail provided.

Special Considerations

We perform total shoulder arthroplasty in nearly all cases of posttraumatic arthritis because it has been shown to be superior to hemiarthroplasty without an increased risk of complications or reoperations.[14] The only patients with posttraumatic arthritis in whom we perform hemiarthroplasty are those with insufficient glenoid bone. In patients with anterior or posterior rotator cuff insufficiency or in those who would require a greater tuberosity osteotomy to perform humeral arthroplasty, we opt for a reverse-design prosthesis instead of total shoulder arthroplasty or hemiarthroplasty (see Section III).

FIXED GLENOHUMERAL DISLOCATION

A distinct subset of patients with glenohumeral instability are those with fixed (chronic) glenohumeral dislocations (Fig. 6.20). These dislocations can be anterior or posterior. Long-standing dislocations can result in severe glenohumeral arthritis with complete loss of proximal humeral articular cartilage, especially in older patients. Our results using unconstrained shoulder arthroplasty in this subset of patients have been disappointing.[15] We now use a reverse-design prosthesis in this patient subset (see Section III).

ROTATOR CUFF TEAR ARTHROPATHY (GLENOHUMERAL OSTEOARTHRITIS WITH A MASSIVE ROTATOR CUFF TEAR)

Historically, hemiarthroplasty was the operative treatment of choice in patients with osteoarthritis combined with a massive irreparable rotator cuff tear (Fig. 6.21). Unconstrained total shoulder arthroplasty is contraindicated because of the

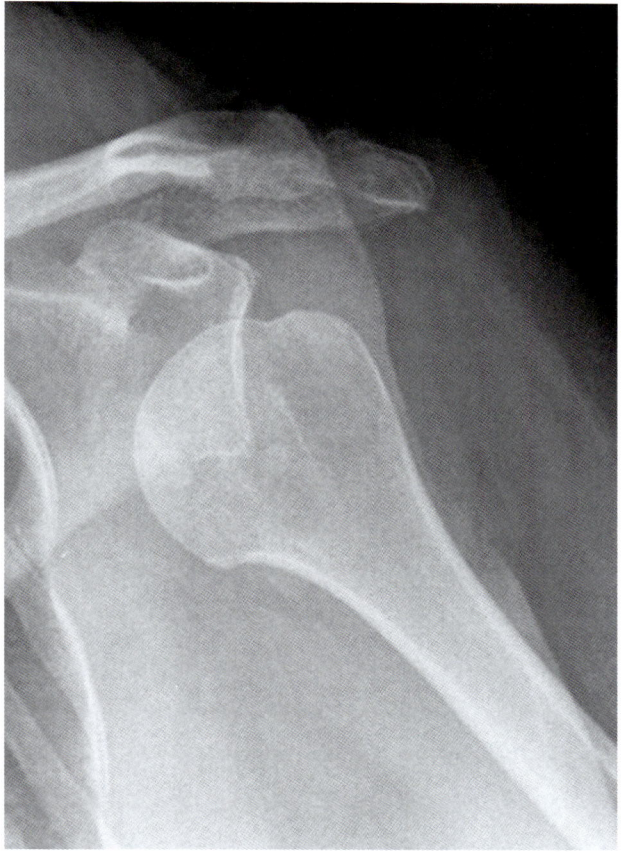

FIGURE 6.20 Chronic dislocation of the glenohumeral joint.

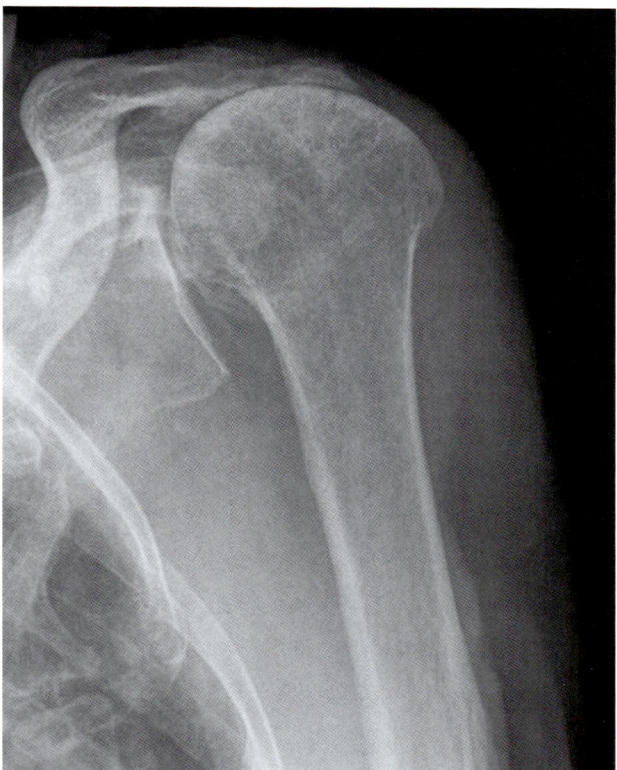

FIGURE 6.21 Glenohumeral arthritis combined with a massive rotator cuff tear.

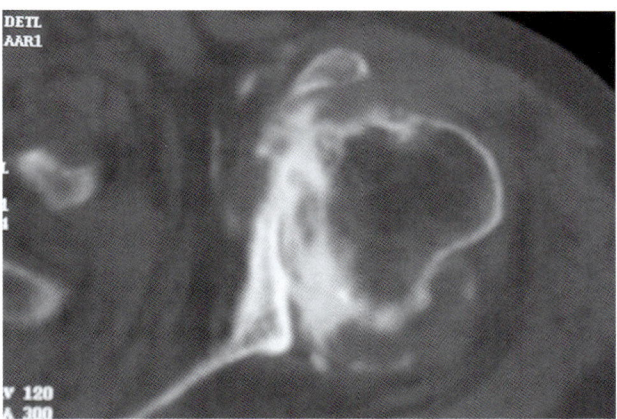

FIGURE 6.22 Computed tomography of a patient with rotator cuff tear arthropathy and insufficient glenoid bone stock to allow implantation of a reverse-prosthesis glenoid component.

risk of loosening of the glenoid component by eccentric loading of the glenoid component.[1] However, the results of hemiarthroplasty for this diagnosis have been disappointing, with most patients achieving only modest improvement postoperatively.[16]

Since its introduction in the United States and because of its superior results, we have used the reverse prosthesis in nearly all cases of osteoarthritis with massive irreparable rotator cuff tears that we have treated operatively.[16] We still consider the use of unconstrained hemiarthroplasty in patients with insufficient glenoid bone stock to support the reverse-prosthesis glenoid component and in elderly patients with severe osteopenia who would seemingly be at increased risk for glenoid failure after the implantation of a reverse-design prosthesis (Fig. 6.22).

POSTINFECTIOUS ARTHROPATHY

Postinfectious arthropathy is a rare and somewhat controversial indication for shoulder arthroplasty. Successful shoulder arthroplasty in these patients depends on complete eradication of the infection before shoulder arthroplasty is undertaken. We use a systematic approach in our work-up of these patients preoperatively (see Chapter 7). We first confirm through review of previous medical records the type of infection (hematogenous versus postoperative, type of organism). We also ensure that the infection was properly and adequately treated. Consultation with an infectious disease specialist is obtained and continued throughout the preoperative work-up and the shoulder arthroplasty. Unfortunately, postinfectious arthropathy often involves damage to the rotator cuff, necessitating implantation of a reverse-design prosthesis. An unconstrained total shoulder arthroplasty is indicated in the rare setting of postinfectious arthropathy with an intact rotator cuff.

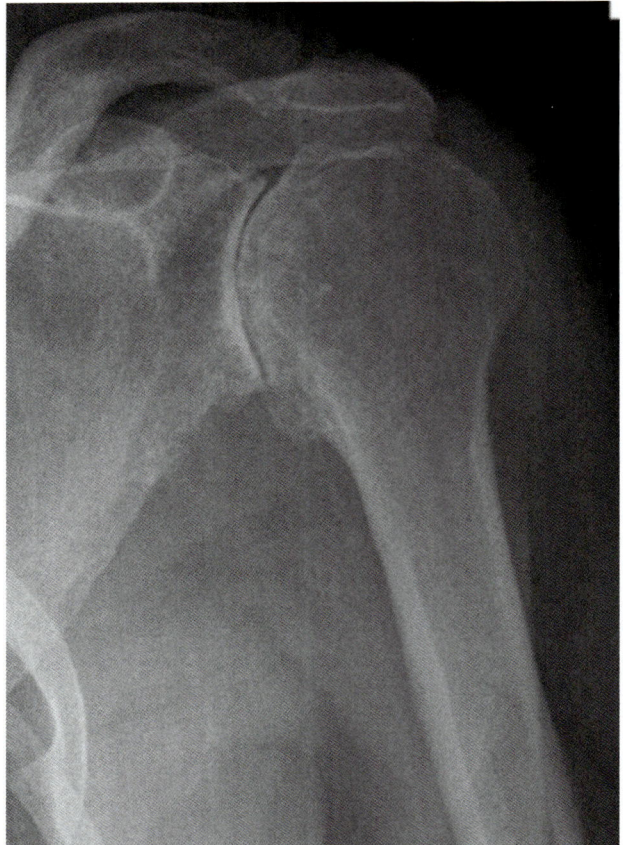

FIGURE 6.23 Radiograph of a patient with postinfectious arthropathy.

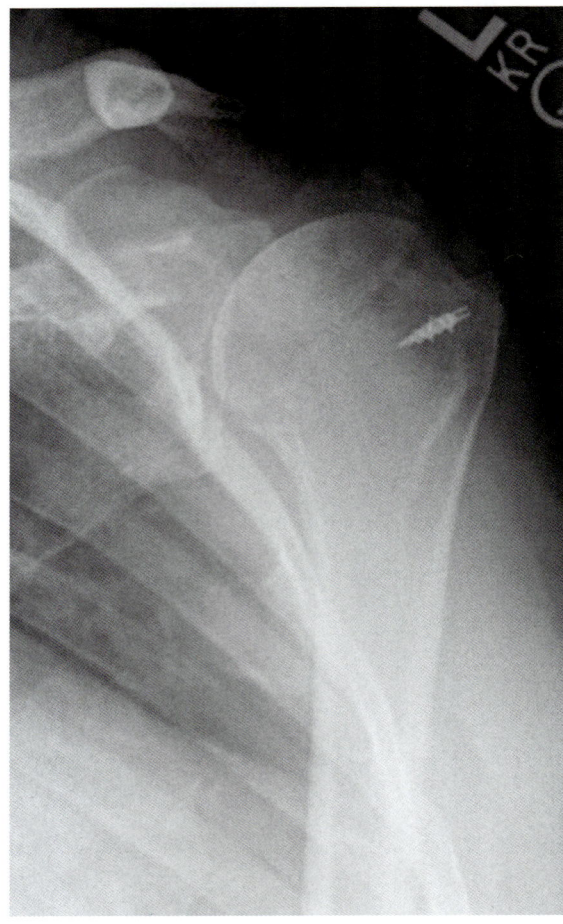

FIGURE 6.24 Static superior migration of the humeral head in a patient with postinfectious arthropathy after an attempt at rotator cuff repair that became infected.

Clinical Findings

Clinical findings in patients with postinfectious arthropathy are variable. Most patients demonstrate glenohumeral crepitus and severe stiffness. Rotator cuff testing may be normal but is often compromised because many of these cases are caused by postoperative infections emanating from an attempt at rotator cuff repair.

Imaging Findings

Plain radiography demonstrates loss of the normal glenohumeral joint space in nearly all cases (Fig. 6.23). Humeral head osteophytes may be present if the condition has been long-standing and has progressed over many years. The humeral head may be statically subluxated superiorly or anterosuperiorly in cases of massive rotator cuff tearing (Fig. 6.24).

Secondary imaging studies (computed tomography arthrography, magnetic resonance imaging) show various findings. The osseous humeral head and glenoid are usually well preserved, although in patients with previous osteomyelitis, substantial bony deficiency may be present as a result of either the infection or subsequent osseous débridement. The condition of the rotator cuff is variable in postinfectious arthropathy, with patients who have undergone a previous attempt at rotator cuff repair more likely to demonstrate rotator cuff compromise.

Special Considerations

In all patients with postinfectious arthropathy, we follow our published algorithm to rule out ongoing infection.[17] We begin with serum studies including a complete blood count with differential, a sedimentation rate, and C-reactive protein. Fluoroscopically guided aspiration of the glenohumeral joint is performed after the patient has been off all antibiotics for at least 2 weeks (even antibiotics used for other conditions such as respiratory infections). The aspirate is cultured for 21 days for aerobic bacteria, anaerobic bacteria, mycobacteria, and fungi. Holding the cultures for 21 days allows for detection of *Propionibacterium acnes* and *Staphylococcus epidermidis,* which have longer incubation periods.[17] The aspirate is also sent for alpha defensin (Synovasure Alpha Defensin Test, Zimmer, Inc., Warsaw, IN). At the time of fluoroscopically guided aspiration, patients undergo computed tomography arthrography or magnetic resonance imaging (if they are allergic to radiographic contrast material).

The patient is considered actively infected if aspirate cultures are positive and is treated as such, with the

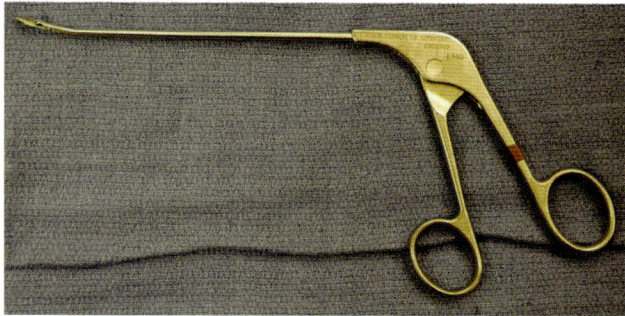

FIGURE 6.25 Arthroscopic punch used to obtain a synovial biopsy specimen in patients with a previous shoulder infection.

arthroplasty being delayed indefinitely. If the aspirate demonstrates moderate to many white blood cells or serum testing is highly suggestive of infection (increased white blood cells, increased C-reactive protein), infection is considered possible even in the absence of a positive culture. Isolated elevation of the sedimentation rate is not considered by us a reliable indicator of infection in this patient population.

In all patients with postinfectious arthropathy and negative aspirate cultures, arthroscopic synovial biopsy is performed before arthroplasty. An arthroscopic punch is used to obtain more than 10 synovial specimens from multiple sites within the joint before the administration of perioperative antibiotics (Fig. 6.25); after obtaining the synovial specimens, standard perioperative intravenous antibiotics are administered immediately. These specimens are sent for microscopic analysis by a pathologist and cultured for aerobic bacteria, anaerobic bacteria, mycobacteria, and fungi and again held for 21 days. If these cultures are positive or if findings of the frozen section are indicative of infection (more than five polymorphonuclear leukocytes per high-power field on five consecutive fields), the patient is considered actively infected and treated as such, and the arthroplasty is delayed indefinitely.[18] If this work-up is negative for infection, the patient is a candidate for total shoulder arthroplasty. With these criteria, our infection rate has been no higher for this indication than for primary osteoarthritis.

We perform total shoulder arthroplasty in nearly all cases of postinfectious arthropathy when the rotator cuff is intact. The only patients with postinfectious arthropathy in whom we perform hemiarthroplasty are those with insufficient glenoid bone. In patients with anterior or posterior rotator cuff insufficiency, we opt for a reverse-design prosthesis (see Section III).

GLENOHUMERAL CHONDROLYSIS

A rare but disturbing disease process that we are seeing with increasing frequency is glenohumeral chondrolysis.[19] We have observed this diagnosis in patients in the early portion of their third decade. Nearly all patients have a history of an arthroscopic shoulder stabilization procedure, with or without the use of thermal energy.[19] We have even observed a patient with glenohumeral chondrolysis at age 21 after a single dislocation with no surgery performed.

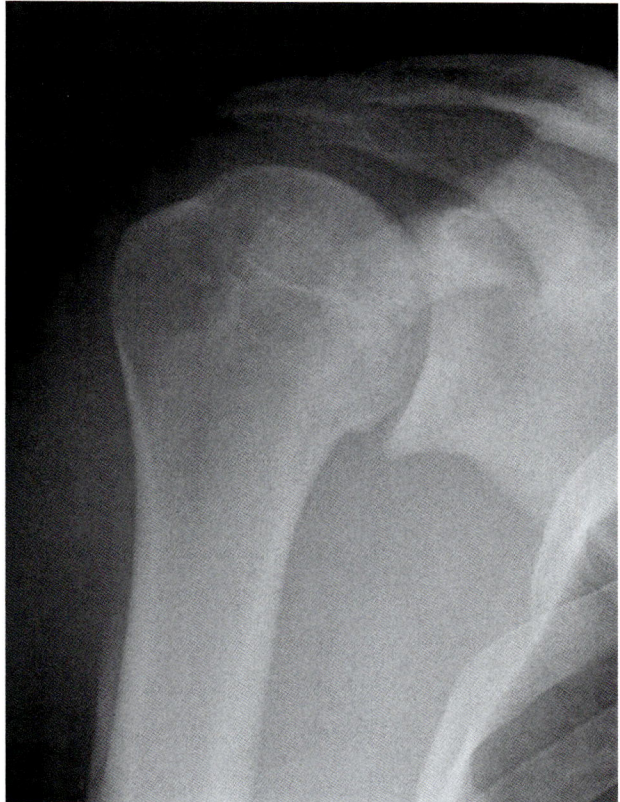

FIGURE 6.26 Radiograph of a 20-year-old patient with complete glenohumeral chondrolysis after arthroscopic surgery for instability.

The chondrolysis that occurs is diffuse and affects both the humeral head and glenoid.

Clinical Findings

Clinical findings in patients with glenohumeral chondrolysis include glenohumeral crepitus and stiffness. Rotator cuff testing is usually normal but may be compromised by pain.

Imaging Findings

Plain radiography demonstrates loss of the normal glenohumeral joint space. Humeral head osteophytes are absent (Fig. 6.26).

Secondary imaging studies show concentric loss of glenohumeral articular cartilage. The rotator cuff is generally intact, and any osseous wear is minimal and centrally oriented.

Special Considerations

A major challenge in dealing with cases of glenohumeral chondrolysis is young patient age. Because the disease occurs on both the humeral head and the glenoid, we are compelled to address the glenoid pathology and not simply perform a hemiarthroplasty. We have been disappointed with results of biologic resurfacing and hemiarthroplasty in these patients,

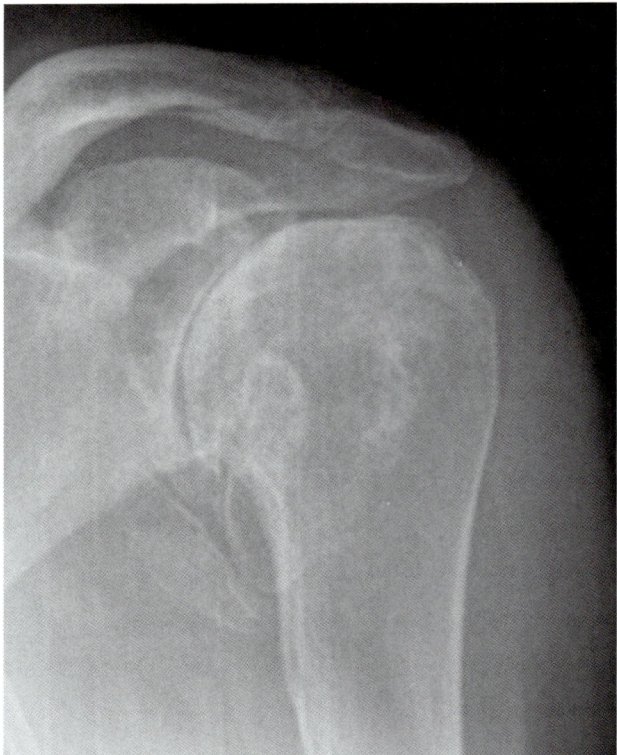

FIGURE 6.27 Radiograph of a patient with Parkinson's disease and glenohumeral arthritis.

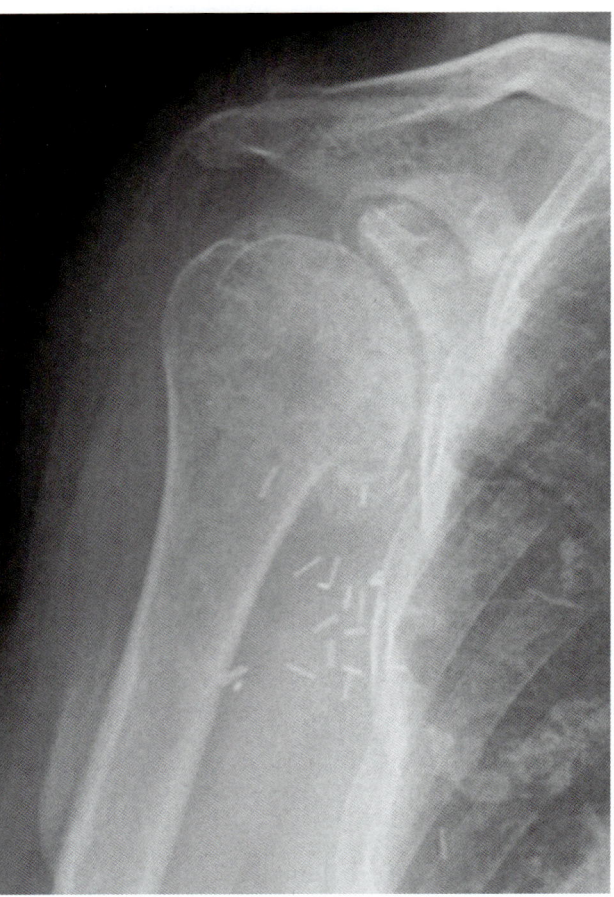

FIGURE 6.28 Radiograph of a patient with glenohumeral arthritis associated with previous radiation therapy.

and despite young patient age we elect to perform unconstrained total shoulder arthroplasty. Our results with arthrodesis in this population have been disappointing, and hence we avoid this procedure in nearly all cases.

GLENOHUMERAL ARTHRITIS ASSOCIATED WITH NEUROLOGIC PATHOLOGY

Infrequently, we encounter patients with glenohumeral osteoarthritis combined with a systemic neurologic disorder. The most common neurologic disorder in patients with glenohumeral arthritis is Parkinson's disease.[20] Clinically, these patients may be functioning at a lower level than patients with primary osteoarthritis. Radiographically and on secondary imaging studies, these patients resemble those with primary osteoarthritis (Fig. 6.27).

GLENOHUMERAL ARTHRITIS ASSOCIATED WITH PREVIOUS RADIATION THERAPY

An indication for shoulder arthroplasty that we are seeing less frequently is glenohumeral arthritis after radiation therapy (Fig. 6.28).[21] Most patients in this diagnostic group have undergone radiation therapy for the treatment of breast cancer or lymphoma. Radiographically, some cases resemble aseptic osteonecrosis and other cases resemble inflammatory arthropathy. This indication is becoming less common as radiotherapy technology improves and becomes less toxic.

GLENOHUMERAL ARTHRITIS ASSOCIATED WITH SKELETAL DYSPLASIA

An exceedingly rare indication for unconstrained shoulder arthroplasty is glenohumeral arthritis associated with skeletal dysplasia. Little is known about this entity. Our limited experience with this indication has led us to treat it like primary osteoarthritis (i.e., perform total shoulder arthroplasty), provided that the anterior and posterior rotator cuff is intact and the osseous glenoid is sufficient. Many of these patients require custom-manufactured implants because of their small size and osseous distortion (Fig. 6.29).

TUMOR

Tumors about the shoulder girdle are an exceptionally rare indication for unconstrained shoulder arthroplasty. In our practice, we infrequently assist in reconstruction

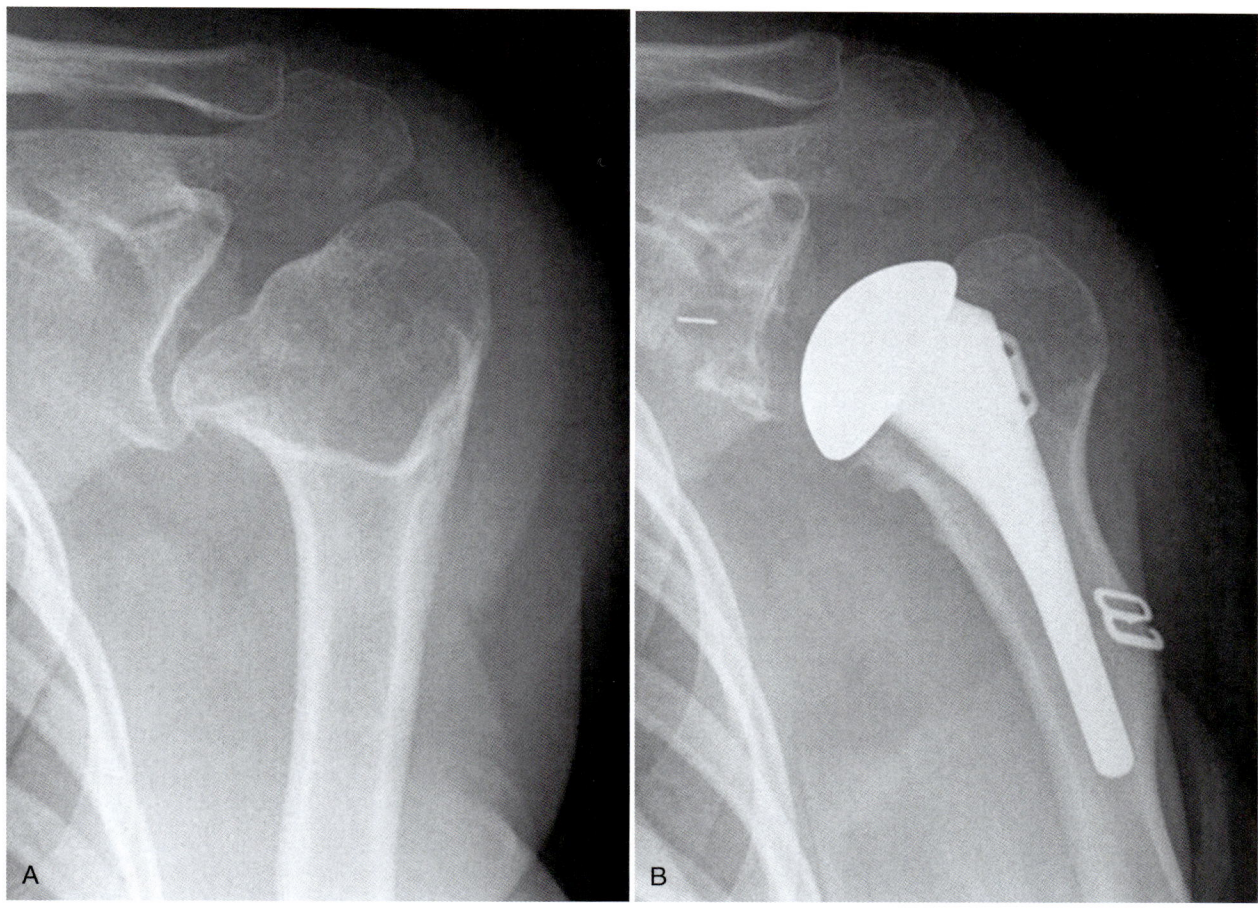

FIGURE 6.29 (A) Radiograph of a patient with glenohumeral arthritis and achondroplasia. (B) A custom-manufactured humeral stem of shorter length was required.

TABLE 6.1 Contraindications to Unconstrained Shoulder Arthroplasty

Contraindication	Absolute or Relative	Comments
Poor generalized health	Relative	Appropriate perioperative medical treatment required
Active infection	Absolute	
Axillary nerve palsy	Relative	Probably better suited for resection arthroplasty or arthrodesis
Suprascapular nerve palsy	Relative	Glenoid component contraindicated; better suited for a reverse prosthesis
Massive rotator cuff tear	Relative	Glenoid component contraindicated; better suited for a reverse prosthesis
Insufficient humeral bone stock	Absolute	
Insufficient glenoid bone stock	Relative	Glenoid component contraindicated; better suited for hemiarthroplasty
Ankylosed shoulder	Absolute	
Previous shoulder arthrodesis	Absolute	
Upper motor neuron lesion	Relative	Absolute contraindication if the patient has uncontrolled shoulder spasticity
Poor patient motivation	Absolute	

of the shoulder after tumor resection by an orthopedic oncologic surgeon. If the resection leaves the rotator cuff and tuberosities intact and attached to the humeral diaphysis, an unconstrained prosthesis can be considered and would usually consist of a hemiarthroplasty. However, in nearly all cases of shoulder girdle tumor, the rotator cuff is substantially compromised by the resection. In our practice, we opt for use of a reverse-design prosthesis (see Section III).

CONTRAINDICATIONS TO UNCONSTRAINED SHOULDER ARTHROPLASTY

Contraindications to unconstrained shoulder arthroplasty are listed in Table 6.1. Some of these contraindications are absolute and others are relative. In addition, some situations are contraindications to glenoid resurfacing with an unconstrained implant but not to unconstrained hemiarthroplasty.

REFERENCES

1. Franklin JL, Barrett WP, Jackins SE, et al: Glenoid loosening in total shoulder arthroplasty: association with rotator cuff deficiency, *J Arthroplasty* 3:39–46, 1988.
2. Neer CS, 2nd: Replacement arthroplasty for glenohumeral osteoarthritis, *J Bone Joint Surg Am* 56:1–13, 1974.
3. Edwards TB: Primary glenohumeral osteoarthritis: epidemiological, clinical, and radiographic findings in patients undergoing shoulder arthroplasty. In Walch G, Boileau P, Molé D, editors: *2000 Prosthèses d'Epaule ... Recul de 2 à 10 Ans*, Paris, 2001, Sauramps Medical, pp 65–72.
4. Edwards TB, Boulahia A, Kempf JF, et al: The influence of the rotator cuff on the results of shoulder arthroplasty for primary osteoarthritis: results of a multicenter study, *J Bone Joint Surg Am* 84:2240–2248, 2002.
5. Edwards TB, Kadakia NR, Boulahia A, et al: A comparison of hemiarthroplasty and total shoulder arthroplasty in the treatment of primary glenohumeral osteoarthritis: results of a multicenter study, *J Shoulder Elbow Surg* 12:207–213, 2003.
6. Gartsman GM, Roddey TS, Hammerman SM: Shoulder arthroplasty with or without resurfacing of the glenoid in patients who have osteoarthritis, *J Bone Joint Surg Am* 82:26–34, 2000.
7. Aswad R, Franceschi JP, Levigne C: Rheumatoid arthritis: epidemiology and preoperative radiographic assessment. In Walch G, Boileau P, Molé D, editors: *2000 Prosthèses d'Epaule ... Recul de 2 à 10 Ans*, Paris, 2001, Sauramps Medical, pp 159–162.
8. Vandermaren C, Docquier P: Shoulder arthroplasty in rheumatoid arthritis: influence of the rotator cuff on the results. In Walch G, Boileau P, Molé D, editors: *2000 Prosthèses d'Epaule ... Recul de 2 à 10 Ans*, Paris, 2001, Sauramps Medical, pp 177–182.
9. Loehr J, Levigne C: Shoulder arthroplasty in rheumatoid arthritis: Influence of the glenoid on the results. In Walch G, Boileau P, Molé D, editors: *2000 Prosthèses d'Epaule ... Recul de 2 à 10 Ans*, Paris, 2001, Sauramps Medical, pp 171–176.
10. Willems WJ: Atraumatic avascular osteonecrosis of the humeral head: Epidemiology and radiology. In Walch G, Boileau P, Molé D, editors: *2000 Prosthèses d'Epaule ... Recul de 2 à 10 Ans*, Paris, 2001, Sauramps Medical, pp 121–126.
11. Cruess RL: Steroid-induced avascular necrosis of the head of the humerus, *J Bone Joint Surg Br* 58:313–317, 1976.
12. Nové-Josserand L, Basso M: Prosthèses d'épaule sur ostéonécroses avasculaires: Facteurs pronostiques. In Walch G, Boileau P, Molé D, editors: *2000 Prosthèses d'Epaule ... Recul de 2 à 10 Ans*, Paris, 2001, Sauramps Medical, pp 135–142.
13. Matsoukis J, Tabib W, Guiffault P, et al: Shoulder arthroplasty in patients with a prior anterior shoulder dislocation: results of a multicenter study, *J Bone Joint Surg Am* 85:1417–1424, 2003.
14. Duparc F, Trojani C, Boileau P: Results of shoulder arthroplasty in cephalic collapse or necrosis following proximal humerus fractures (type 1 fracture sequelae). In Walch G, Boileau P, Molé D, editors: *2000 Prosthèses d'Epaule ... Recul de 2 à 10 Ans*, Paris, 2001, Sauramps Medical, pp 279–289.
15. Matsoukis J, Tabib W, Guiffault P, et al: Primary unconstrained shoulder arthroplasty in patients with a fixed anterior glenohumeral dislocation: results of a multicenter study, *J Bone Joint Surg Am* 88:547–552, 2006.
16. Favard L, Lautmann S, Sirveaux F, et al: Hemiarthroplasty versus reverse shoulder arthroplasty in the treatment of osteoarthritis with massive rotator cuff tear. In Walch G, Boileau P, Molé D, editors: *2000 Prosthèses d'Epaule ... Recul de 2 à 10 Ans*, Paris, 2001, Sauramps Medical, pp 261–268.
17. Morris BJ, Waggenspack WN, Laughlin MS, et al: Reverse shoulder arthroplasty for management of postinfectious arthropathy with rotator cuff deficiency, *Orthopedics* 38(8):e701–e707, 2015.
18. Feldman DS, Lonner JH, Desai P, et al: The role of intraoperative frozen sections in revision total joint arthroplasty, *J Bone Joint Surg Am* 77:1807–1813, 1995.
19. Larsen MW, Higgins LD, Basamania CJ: Severe glenohumeral chondrolysis following shoulder arthroscopy: A series of 6 cases treated with hemiarthroplasty. Paper presented at the 22nd Open Meeting of the American Shoulder and Elbow Surgeons, March 2006, Chicago.
20. Garreau de Loubresse C: Prothèse d'épaule et affections neurologiques. In Walch G, Boileau P, Molé D, editors: *2000 Prosthèses d'Epaule ... Recul de 2 à 10 Ans*, Paris, 2001, Sauramps Medical, pp 195–203.
21. Godenèche A: Shoulder arthroplasty and previous radiotherapy. In Walch G, Boileau P, Molé D, editors: *2000 Prosthèses d'Epaule ... Recul de 2 à 10 Ans*, Paris, 2001, Sauramps Medical, pp 143–148.

Preoperative planning and imaging

CHAPTER 7

Although the majority of cases of unconstrained shoulder arthroplasty are routine, certain patients have unique characteristics that merit special consideration. Preoperative planning identifies patients who may require deviation from routine unconstrained shoulder arthroplasty. Preoperative planning should be done well in advance of the surgical procedure and not be an afterthought the morning of surgery. The surgeon should review the patient's clinical history and physical examination, radiographs, and any secondary imaging studies. This chapter presents our approach to preoperative planning for unconstrained shoulder arthroplasty.

CLINICAL HISTORY AND EXAMINATION

Although a description of a detailed shoulder history and examination are beyond the scope of this textbook, certain aspects of the history and physical examination are important in preoperative planning for unconstrained shoulder arthroplasty. The shoulder-specific complaints of the patient are reviewed, such as the type of symptoms (pain, stiffness, weakness), duration of symptoms (weeks, months, years), and previous treatment (activity modification, nonsteroidal antiinflammatory medications, corticosteroid injections, viscosupplementary injections, previous surgery). These shoulder-specific complaints help the surgeon decide which patients are candidates for shoulder replacement surgery. A patient with complaints of only mild pain, mild weakness, or mild stiffness (or any combination of these complaints) may initially best be treated with nonoperative (or nonarthroplasty) modalities, even if radiographs demonstrate end-stage glenohumeral arthritis. Similarly, a patient with a sudden onset of symptoms of short duration to date may be experiencing a transient acute rotator cuff tendinitis concomitantly with chronic glenohumeral arthritis that has been well tolerated. In this situation, a period of nonoperative treatment would certainly be indicated. Special attention is given to factors that could make the operative procedure more difficult. Chronic use of nonsteroidal antiinflammatory medications can result in excessive operative blood loss, so such drugs should be discontinued the week before surgery.

Any previous surgery merits special consideration. The type of surgery should be noted. Although previous arthroscopic procedures are usually inconsequential to the performance of shoulder arthroplasty, previous open procedures may introduce difficulties. Specifically, previous instability surgery may have resulted in severe stiffness, especially in external rotation, and may have caused excessive scar tissue that will make the surgical approach more difficult. The type of surgical procedure should be elucidated whenever possible. Procedures that alter normal anatomic relationships, such as tendon transfers (subscapularis transfers—i.e., the Magnuson-Stack procedure or Putti-Platt procedure) and coracoid transfers (Latarjet or Bristow procedure) are especially important in considering the surgical approach. Previous rotator cuff surgery may focus attention on determining preoperative rotator cuff integrity.

Any symptoms of infection, especially in patients who have previously undergone surgery or injections, should be investigated further. If a patient has a history of infection after shoulder surgery or has had symptoms suggestive of infection (systemic fever, shoulder warmth or redness), a preoperative infection workup—including hematologic evaluation with a complete blood cell count and differential, sedimentation rate, and C-reactive protein—is indicated. Additionally, a fluoroscopically guided shoulder aspirate is obtained and the specimen submitted for aerobic, anaerobic, fungal, and mycobacterial culture; these cultures are held for 21 days to allow for the detection of *Propionibacterium acnes* and *Staphylococcus epidermidis*. The aspirate is also sent for alpha defensin (Synovasure Alpha Defensin Test [Zimmer, Inc., Warsaw, IN]), which is used to detect infection. If the findings are suggestive or diagnostic of infection, shoulder arthroplasty is postponed or canceled until infectious disease consultation is obtained and the infection is appropriately treated. In all patients with postinfectious arthropathy and negative aspirate cultures, arthroscopic synovial biopsy is performed as an additional precaution to rule out infection before arthroplasty (Table 7.1).

Any medical history of systemic illness (diabetes mellitus, cardiac problems, etc.) should be considered in the preoperative planning. Although these factors may not affect the actual surgical procedure, they may necessitate special considerations in the patient's postoperative care. Appropriate medical consultations should be obtained well in advance of the surgery date. The availability of appropriate care, including consultants for these systemic illnesses, should be confirmed before surgery.

All our patients undergo a thorough shoulder examination. Motion and rotator cuff strength are of critical importance. Both active and passive mobility is recorded. Mobility parameters recorded are elevation in the plane of the scapula (Fig. 7.1), abduction (Fig. 7.2), external rotation with the arm at the side (Fig. 7.3), external rotation with the arm abducted 90 degrees (when possible; Fig. 7.4), and internal rotation as determined by the vertebral level reached with an outstretched thumb (Fig. 7.5). Any incongruity of the glenohumeral joint as indicated by the presence of glenohumeral crepitus with motion is noted, as is any discrepancy in active and passive mobility.

TABLE 7.1	Workup for Infection Before Unconstrained Shoulder Arthroplasty
Test	If Abnormal
White blood cell count with differential	Increase suspicion for infection; consider arthroscopic biopsy
Sedimentation rate	Increase suspicion for infection if combined with an abnormal white blood cell count or C-reactive protein; consider arthroscopic biopsy
C-reactive protein	Increase suspicion for infection; consider arthroscopic biopsy
Fluoroscopically guided aspiration	Consider the shoulder as actively infected and treat as such; arthroscopic biopsy is unnecessary
Arthroscopic biopsy	Consider the shoulder as actively infected and treat as such

Rotator cuff examination consists of testing each tendon of the rotator cuff by isolating it as much as possible. Jobe's test is used to test supraspinatus integrity (Fig. 7.6).[1] The external rotation lag sign and evaluation of external rotation strength with the arm at the side are used to test the infraspinatus (Figs. 7.7 and 7.8).[2] The teres minor is tested via the horn blower's sign (Fig. 7.9).[3] The subscapularis is tested with the belly press test and, when mobility allows, the lift-off test (Figs. 7.10 and 7.11).[4]

The results of the clinical history and physical examination are documented in the patient's chart and reviewed well in advance of surgery as part of preoperative planning.

RADIOGRAPHY

Radiographs are obtained in all patients who are candidates for shoulder arthroplasty. We prefer an anteroposterior view of the glenohumeral joint with the arm in neutral rotation (Fig. 7.12), an axillary view (Fig. 7.13), and a scapular outlet view (Fig. 7.14). The anteroposterior radiograph is used to evaluate the glenohumeral joint space, the presence of humeral and glenoid osteophytes, the size of the humeral canal (Fig. 7.15), the presence of any loose bodies (Fig. 7.16), and the presence of any deformity of the humeral shaft (Fig. 7.17) because these factors may all have an impact

Text continued on p. 59

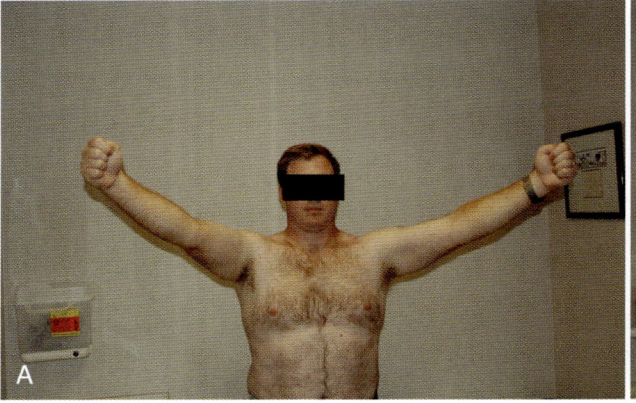 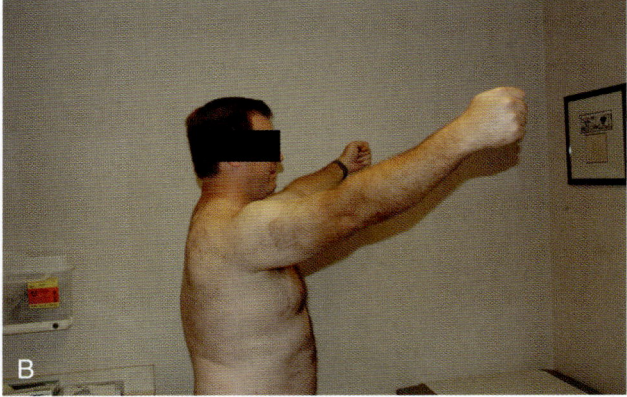

FIGURE 7.1 (A and B) Elevation in the plane of the scapula.

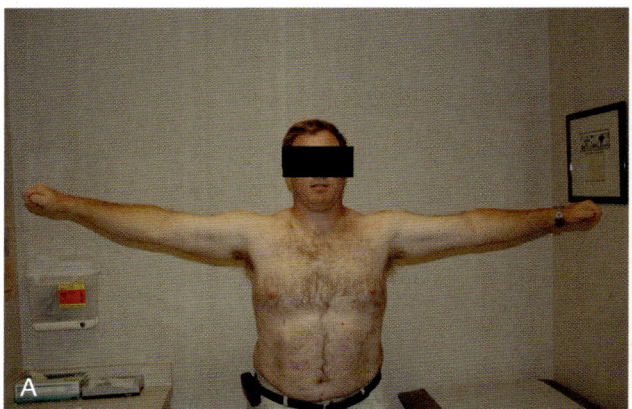 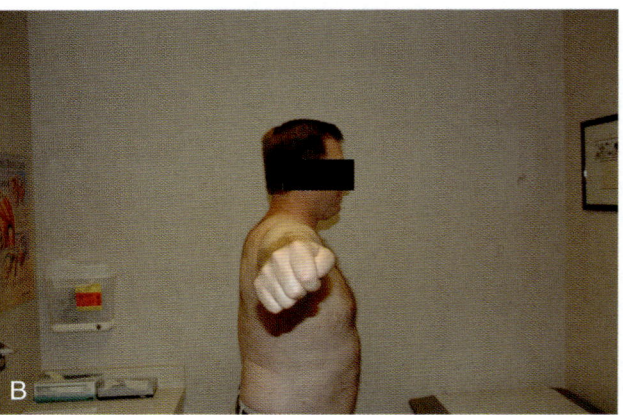

FIGURE 7.2 (A and B) Abduction. The arm is kept in the coronal plane.

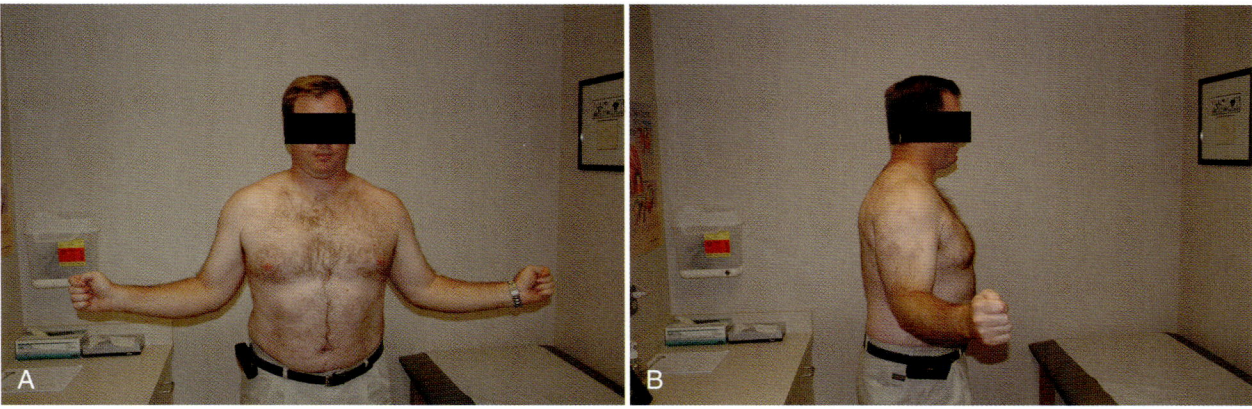

FIGURE 7.3 (A and B) External rotation with the arm at the side.

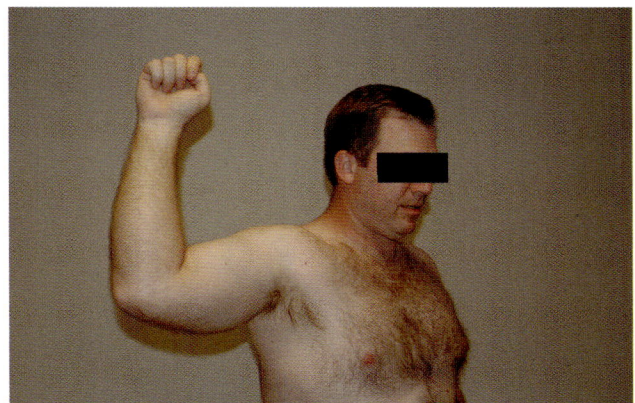

FIGURE 7.4 External rotation with the arm abducted 90 degrees. Measurement of this mobility parameter is not possible in all patients because of limited mobility in severe cases.

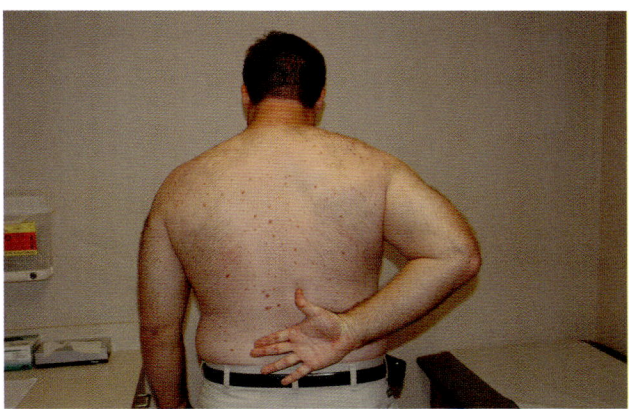

FIGURE 7.5 Internal rotation as measured by the vertebral level reached with an outstretched thumb.

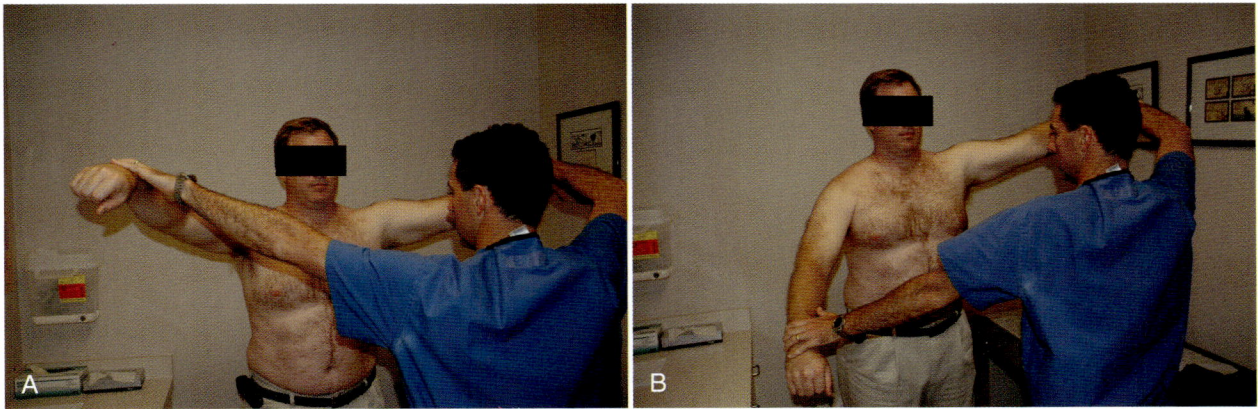

FIGURE 7.6 (A and B) Jobe's test for supraspinatus integrity. The patient elevates the pronated arm in the plane of the scapula and resists the downward force of the examiner.

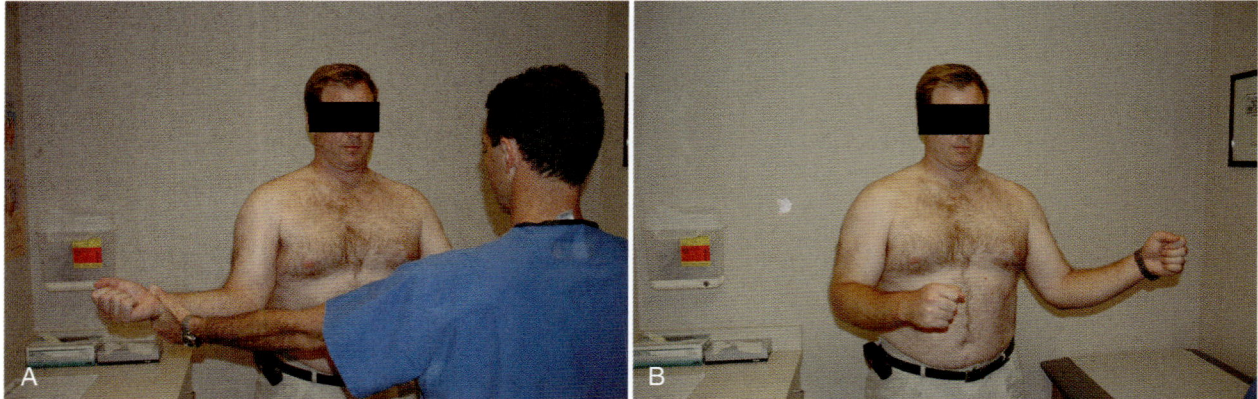

FIGURE 7.7 (A and B) External rotation lag sign for infraspinatus integrity. The examiner maximally rotates the arm externally at the side and asks the patient to maintain this position. If the patient is unable to maintain this position, the test is considered positive for infraspinatus insufficiency.

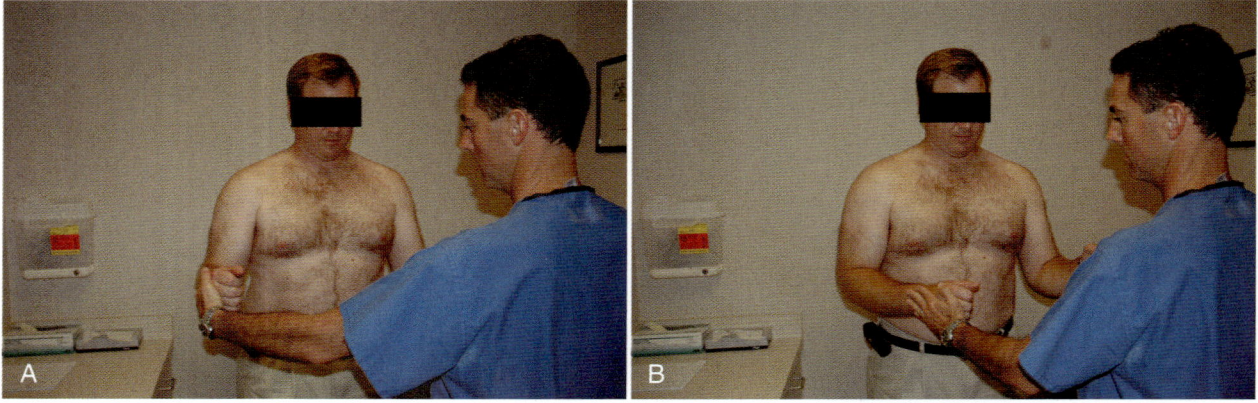

FIGURE 7.8 (A and B) Evaluation of external rotation strength with the arm at the side. The patient resists the examiner's internally directed force. Weakness in this position may indicate infraspinatus insufficiency.

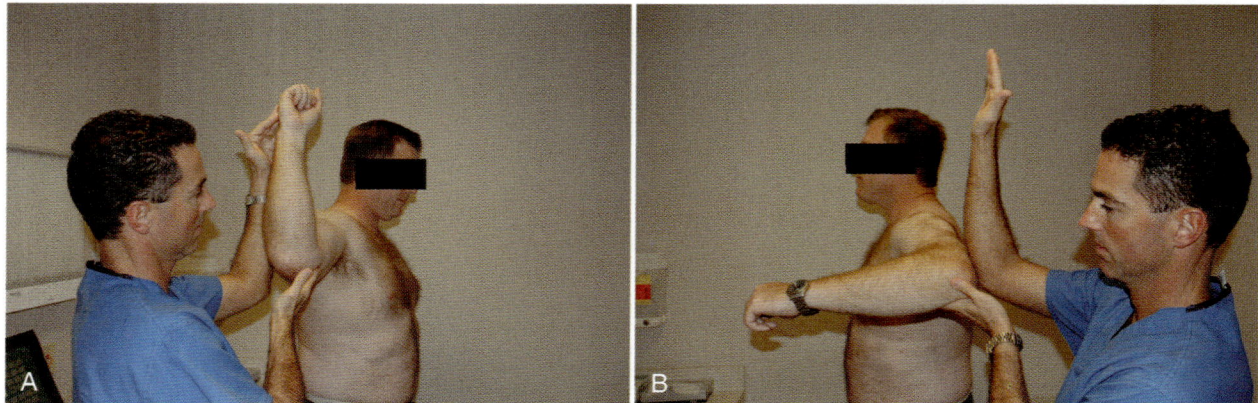

FIGURE 7.9 (A and B) The horn blower's sign for evaluation of the teres minor. The patient is asked to actively rotate the 90-degree abducted arm externally. Inability to perform this maneuver may indicate teres minor insufficiency.

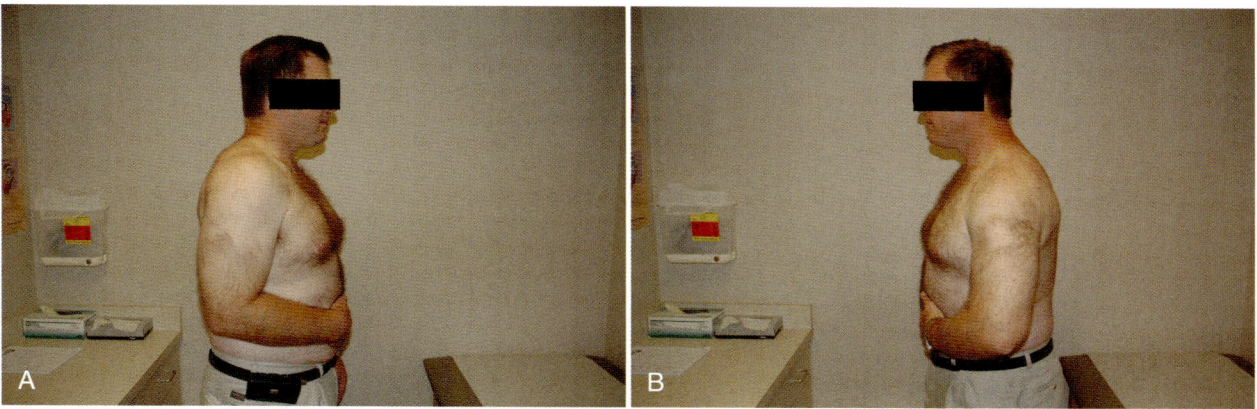

FIGURE 7.10 Belly press test for subscapularis insufficiency. The test is considered positive if the patient must flex the wrist and extend the arm to press on the abdomen. (A) Positive test. (B) Negative test.

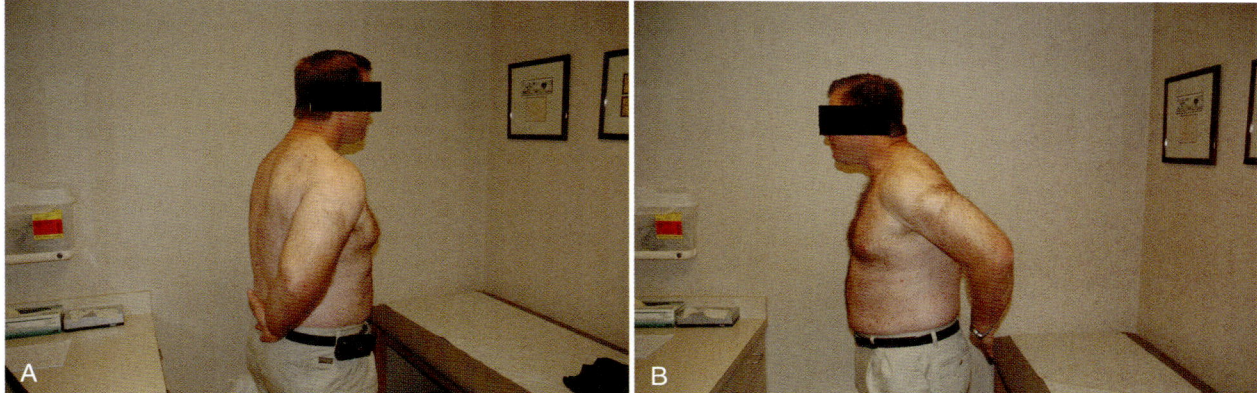

FIGURE 7.11 The lift-off test for subscapularis insufficiency. The test is considered positive if the patient is unable to lift the hand off the back. (A) Positive test. (B) Negative test.

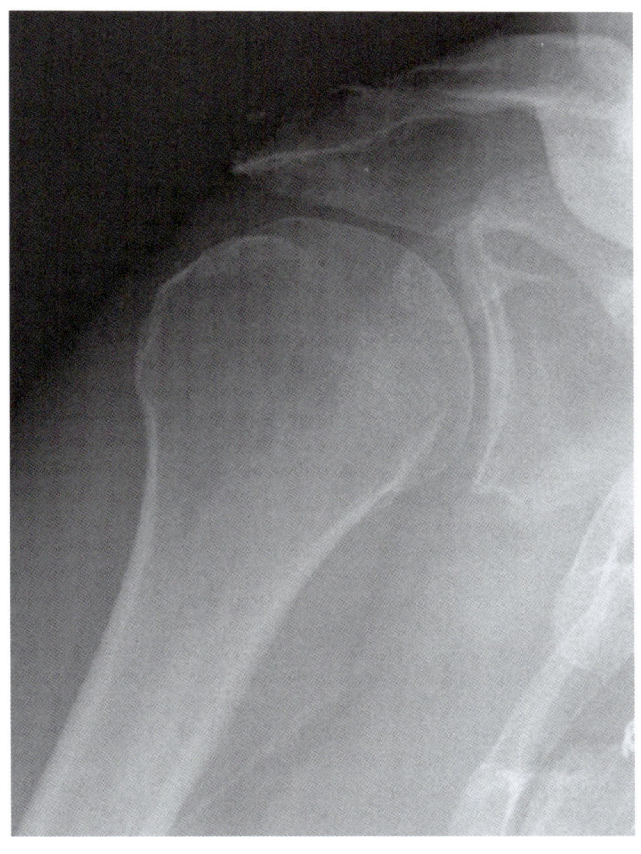

FIGURE 7.12 Anteroposterior radiograph of the glenohumeral joint with the arm in neutral rotation.

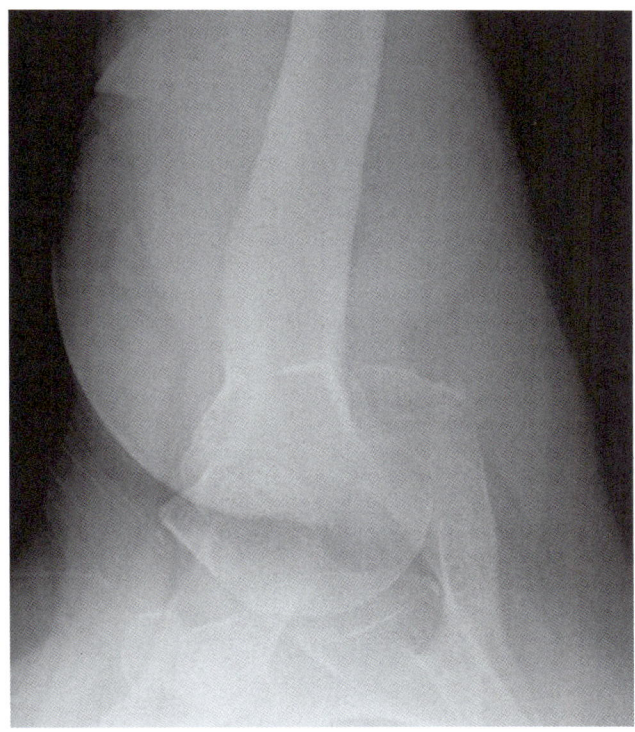

FIGURE 7.13 Axillary radiograph.

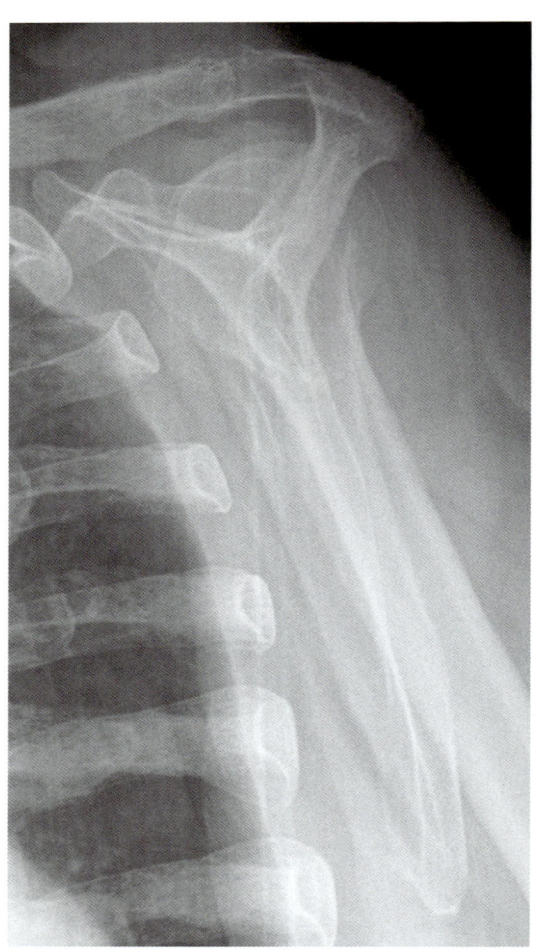

FIGURE 7.14 Scapular outlet radiograph.

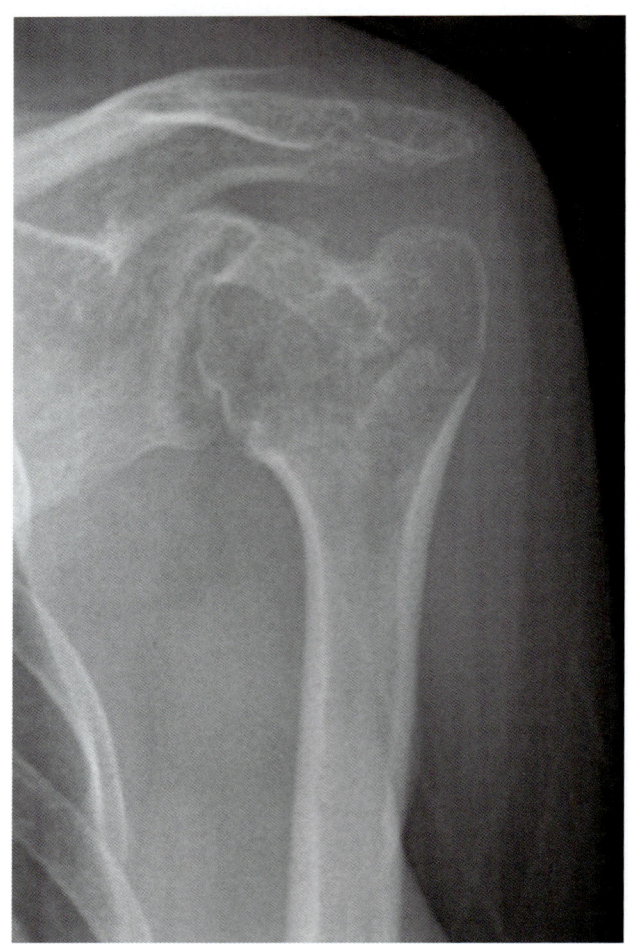

FIGURE 7.15 Anteroposterior radiograph of a patient with juvenile rheumatoid arthritis and an exceptionally small humeral intramedullary canal. A standard humeral component is too large for this patient, so a custom-manufactured stem is required.

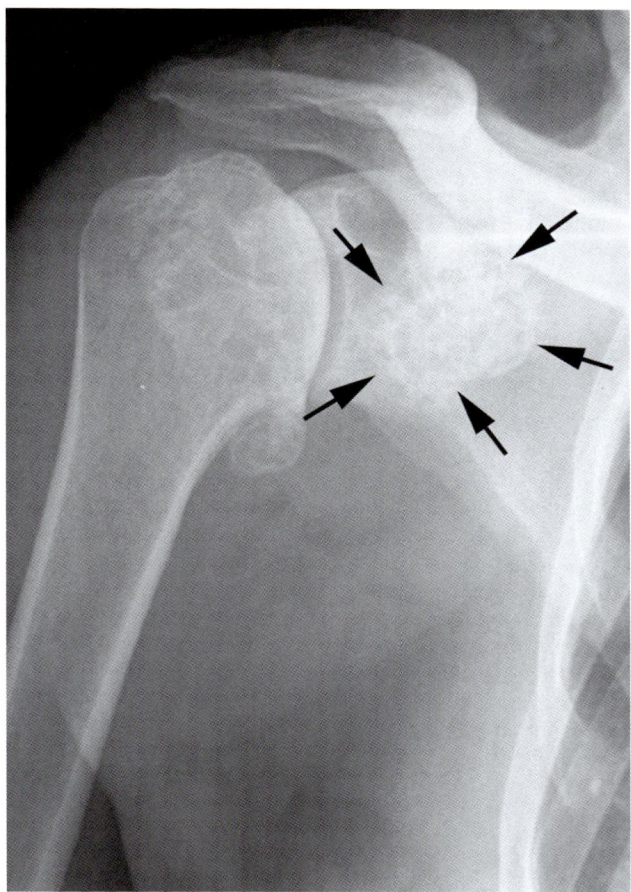

FIGURE 7.16 Large loose body *(arrows)* in the subscapularis recess identified on an anteroposterior radiograph. It should be removed at the time of arthroplasty.

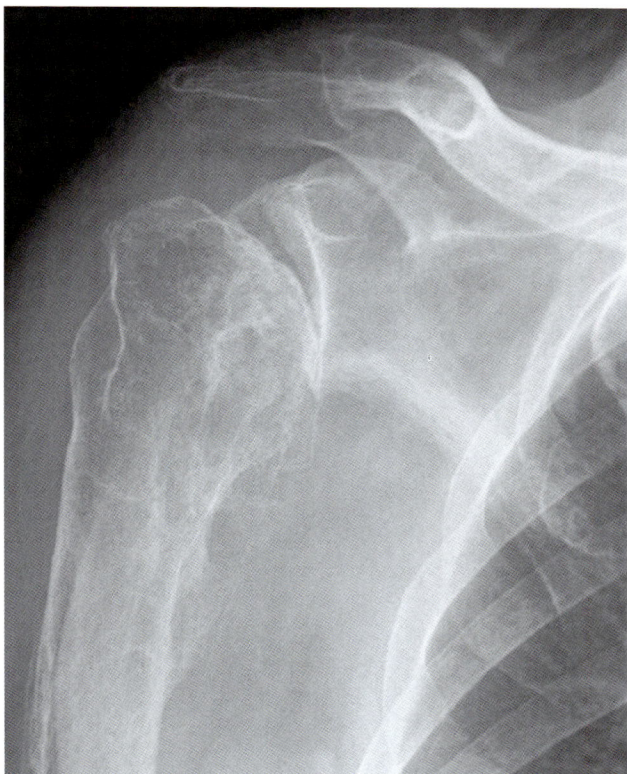

FIGURE 7.17 Proximal humeral diaphyseal malunion in a patient with glenohumeral arthritis.

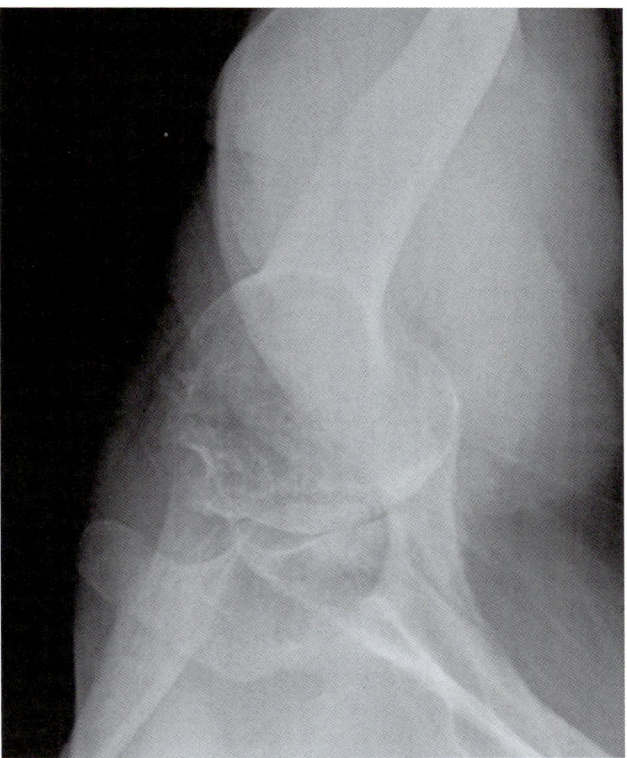

FIGURE 7.18 Posterior glenoid wear with posterior humeral head subluxation identified on an axillary radiograph.

on the planned procedure. The axillary radiograph is used to evaluate the glenohumeral joint space, the presence of anterior or posterior humeral head subluxation, and the presence of osseous glenoid wear and dysplasia (Fig. 7.18). The scapular outlet radiograph is used to evaluate for the presence of anterior or posterior humeral head subluxation (Fig. 7.19), loose bodies in the subscapularis recess, and any deformity of the humeral shaft. Findings on these radiographs help the surgeon to predict the need for a smaller humeral stem or possibly even a custom implant (proximal humeral deformity), predict the need to remove large loose bodies in the subscapularis recess that may not be visible at the time of surgery, and note cases in which the glenoid portion of the procedure may be exceptionally difficult.

Ideally, these radiographs are taken with magnification under fluoroscopic control to allow accurate assessment of the glenohumeral joint space and an accurate measure of the acromiohumeral interval, an important predictor of static humeral subluxation resulting from rotator cuff insufficiency. Some patients arrive at our clinic with radiographs taken by a referring physician. If these radiographs are judged to be of sufficient quality, are less than 6 months old, and no unusual circumstances (e.g., an excessively small humeral intramedullary canal) exist, radiographs are not repeated. In all other cases, radiographs are repeated with magnification and fluoroscopically controlled techniques.

Most shoulder arthroplasty prosthetic systems have radiographic templates available for preoperative planning (Fig. 7.20). However, most shoulder arthroplasty systems are transitioning away from manual radiographic templates to a digital format, which also provides the option of creating patient-specific instrumentation. Furthermore, the use of modern adaptable anatomic prosthetic systems minimizes the need for radiographic templates in most cases because humeral stem size, humeral head size and position, and glenoid size will be determined intraoperatively. In select cases, such as those of patients with substantial deformity of the proximal humerus (Fig. 7.21) or an excessively small humeral canal, use of radiographic templates preoperatively is mandatory. We use these templates to determine whether existing prefabricated implants are sufficient or a custom-manufactured implant is required.

SECONDARY IMAGING

A secondary imaging study is obtained in all patients before unconstrained shoulder arthroplasty to evaluate the rotator cuff and, more importantly, glenoid morphology. Our preferred secondary imaging modality is computed tomography arthrography. We find that it provides the greatest osseous detail and allows concomitant evaluation of the rotator cuff tendons and musculature. Some patients come to our clinic with a magnetic resonance imaging scan. If the scan allows sufficient evaluation of the osseous structures and rotator cuff and is less than 6 months old, we will not order additional secondary imaging.

Glenoid morphology is classified by computed tomography (or magnetic resonance imaging) according to the system of Walch and colleagues (Fig. 7.22).[5,6] In type A, or concentric glenoid morphology, the humeral head is centered and loads are equally distributed on the glenoid. Glenoid osseous erosion may be minor, type A1, or major, type A2. Type B, or nonconcentric glenoid morphology, is characterized by a posteriorly subluxated humeral head and asymmetric loads across the glenoid. Type B1 shows narrowing of the posterior joint space, subchondral sclerosis, and osteophytes, and type B2 demonstrates a biconcave glenoid resulting from posterior osseous erosion. Type C or the dysplastic glenoid is defined by glenoid retroversion greater than 25 degrees and a centered or only slightly subluxated humeral head. New three-dimensional computed tomography reconstructions help to further classify glenoid morphology based on degrees of retroversion and percentage of subluxation. A newly described type is type B3.[6] Walch and colleagues describe the

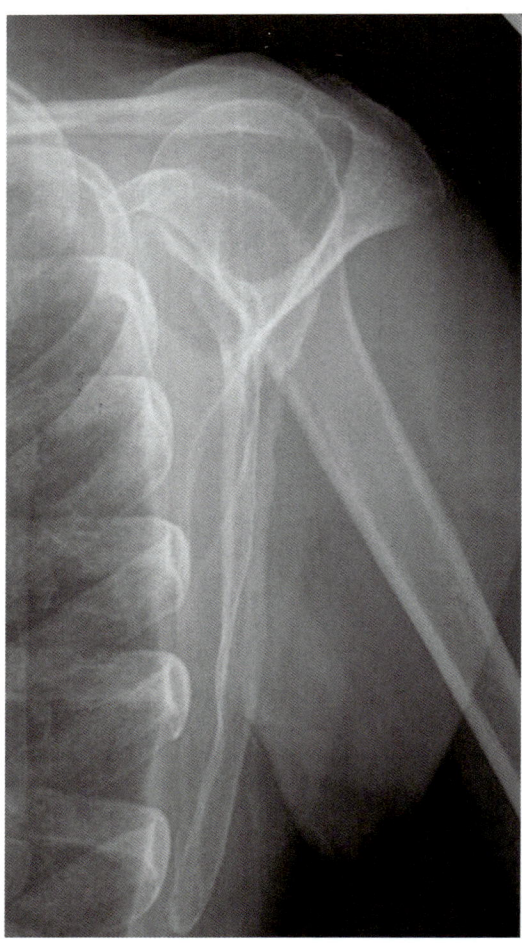

FIGURE 7.19 Anterosuperior humeral head subluxation with coracohumeral impingement identified on a scapular outlet radiograph.

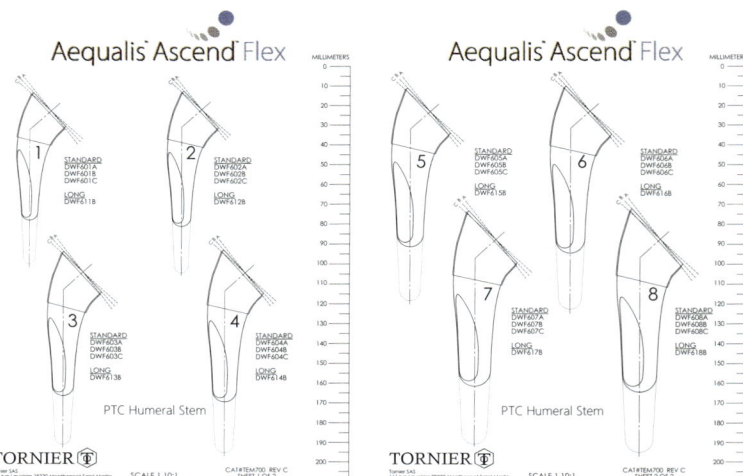

FIGURE 7.20 (A and B) Radiographic templates for preoperative planning for unconstrained shoulder arthroplasty.

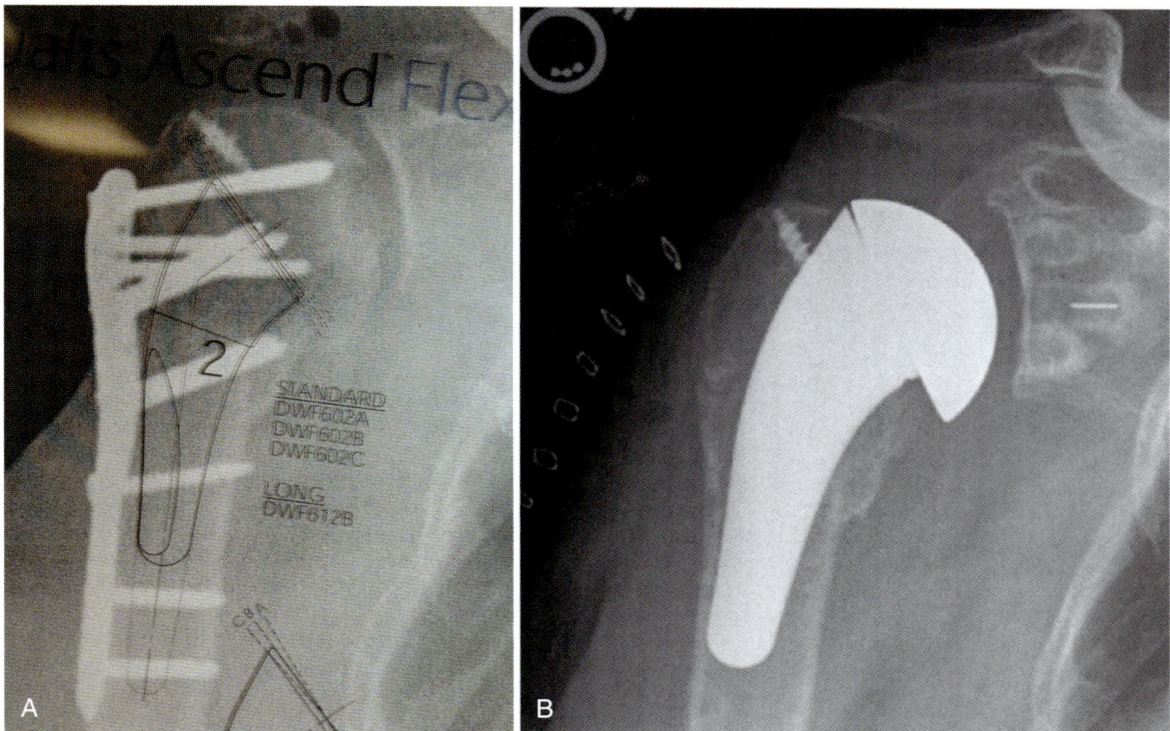

FIGURE 7.21 (A) Preoperative radiographic templating in a patient with a proximal humeral diaphyseal malunion. (B) In this case, a short humeral stem was selected and successfully implanted.

B3 glenoid as monoconcave (rather than biconcave in B2) with posterior bone wear and severe pathologic retroversion (at least 15 degrees) or posterior humeral head subluxation (of at least 70%), or both. Classification of glenoid morphology is critical in two scenarios when unconstrained shoulder arthroplasty is being performed. First, in a patient with severe glenoid erosion (A2, B2, or B3) or severe dysplasia (C), insufficient glenoid bone stock may prohibit implantation of a standard glenoid component (Fig. 7.23). In cases of insufficient glenoid bone stock, the surgeon may opt for hemiarthroplasty, choose to alter the glenoid component (i.e., shorten the keel or pegs), consider a posteriorly augmented glenoid component, or possibly in extreme circumstances consider a reverse-design prosthesis. Second, in cases of posterior humeral head subluxation and a biconcave glenoid (B2), posterior capsulorrhaphy may be required at the time of shoulder arthroplasty. When these cases are identified by preoperative secondary imaging, an additional step of testing glenohumeral stability with the trial components is included as part of the surgical technique (Chapter 13).

The rotator cuff is next evaluated with secondary imaging modalities, including assessment of tendon integrity and evaluation of muscle quality (fatty infiltration). In addition, the condition of the long head of the biceps tendon is noted, particularly its position (centered, subluxated, dislocated, ruptured) to help identify it at the time of surgery. Although full-thickness rotator cuff tears limited to the supraspinatus tendon may not change the operative plan, tears of the supraspinatus combined with either posterior (infraspinatus) or anterior (subscapularis) rotator cuff tears are contraindications to glenoid resurfacing and may best be treated with a reverse-design prosthesis (Fig. 7.24).[7] The degree of fatty infiltration of the supraspinatus and infraspinatus musculature has been shown to influence the results of unconstrained shoulder arthroplasty in patients with primary osteoarthritis.[7] Although we do not necessarily change our operative plan based on fatty infiltration, we routinely classify the degree of fatty infiltration of these muscles by using a three-tiered modification of the Goutallier classification to help determine the patient's postoperative prognosis.[8] The soft tissue axial sections of a computed tomography scan or the T1-weighted axial sections of magnetic resonance imaging are used to classify fatty infiltration (Fig. 7.25).

PREOPERATIVE PLANNING SOFTWARE AND PATIENT-SPECIFIC INSTRUMENTATION

Preoperative planning software has been introduced to enable surgeons to plan the anticipated surgery virtually, including humeral and glenoid implantation. Most shoulder arthroplasty companies have a software tool for preoperative planning. The software is typically formatted off nonarthrogram computed tomography scans to create three-dimensional reconstructions allowing evaluation of glenoid morphology including degrees of retroversion and percentage of humeral head subluxation (Fig. 7.26). Currently, if one is opting to use one of these preoperative planning systems, it is necessary to obtain a computed tomography scan without intraarticular contrast using specific protocols established by the software company. The surgeon can implant the glenoid component virtually to determine the appropriate size of the glenoid component, backside radius of curvature, and desired location

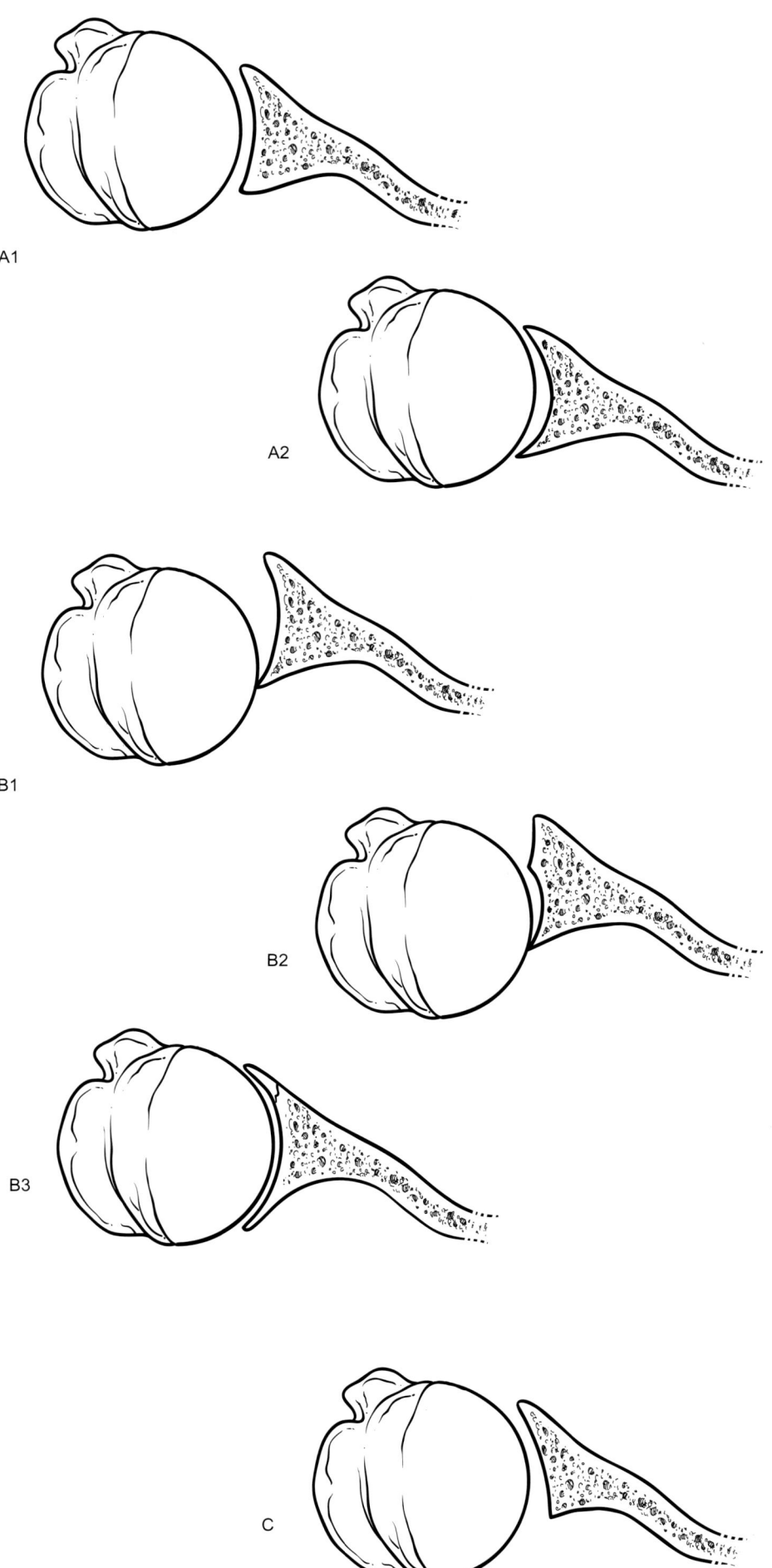

FIGURE 7.22 Schematic of glenoid morphology as described by Walch and colleagues. (A) Type A1 glenoid with concentric loading. (B) Type A2 glenoid with concentric loading and excessive central wear. (C) Type B1 glenoid with eccentric loading causing posterior subluxation of the humeral head. (D) Type B2 glenoid with eccentric loading, posterior subluxation of the humeral head, and excessive posterior glenoid wear (biconcave glenoid). (E) Type B3 glenoid representing severe posterior glenoid wear and excessive retroversion that is monoconcave. (F) Type C glenoid representing glenoid dysplasia.

to ensure appropriate version, seating, and depth of reaming as well as to minimize glenoid perforation (Figs. 7.27 and 7.28A). The three-dimensional plan can be used with or without a patient-specific guide (see Fig. 7.28). The patient-specific guide is created to provide reproducibility of guide-pin placement for instrumentation of the glenoid. Multiple preoperative planning software programs and patient-specific guides have been shown to improve the reproducibility of guide-pin placement for glenoid instrumentation.[9-11] Clinical data have not been presented to date to show an advantage in glenoid component survival or patient outcomes with or without a patient-specific guide.

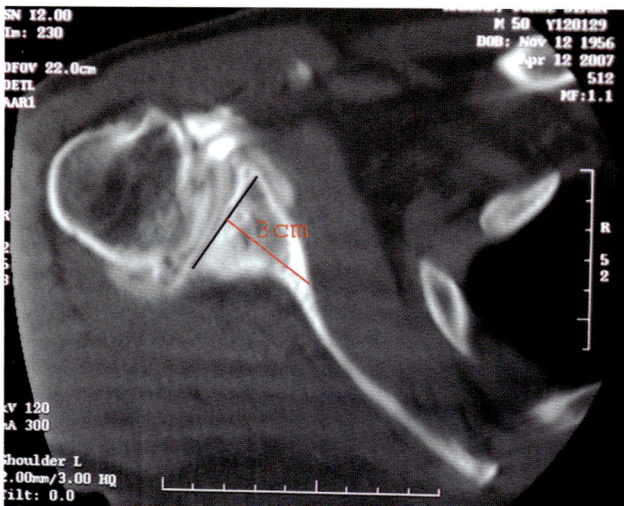

FIGURE 7.23 Measurement of the depth of the glenoid vault with a computed tomography scan preoperatively to determine whether a standard glenoid implant may be used.

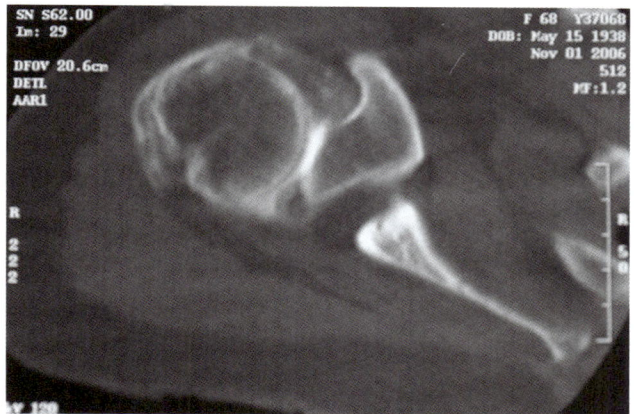

FIGURE 7.24 Computed tomography arthrography demonstrating a large tear of the rotator cuff involving the supraspinatus and infraspinatus, for which unconstrained total shoulder arthroplasty is contraindicated. In this case either a semiconstrained reverse-design prosthesis (preferable) or hemiarthroplasty should be used.

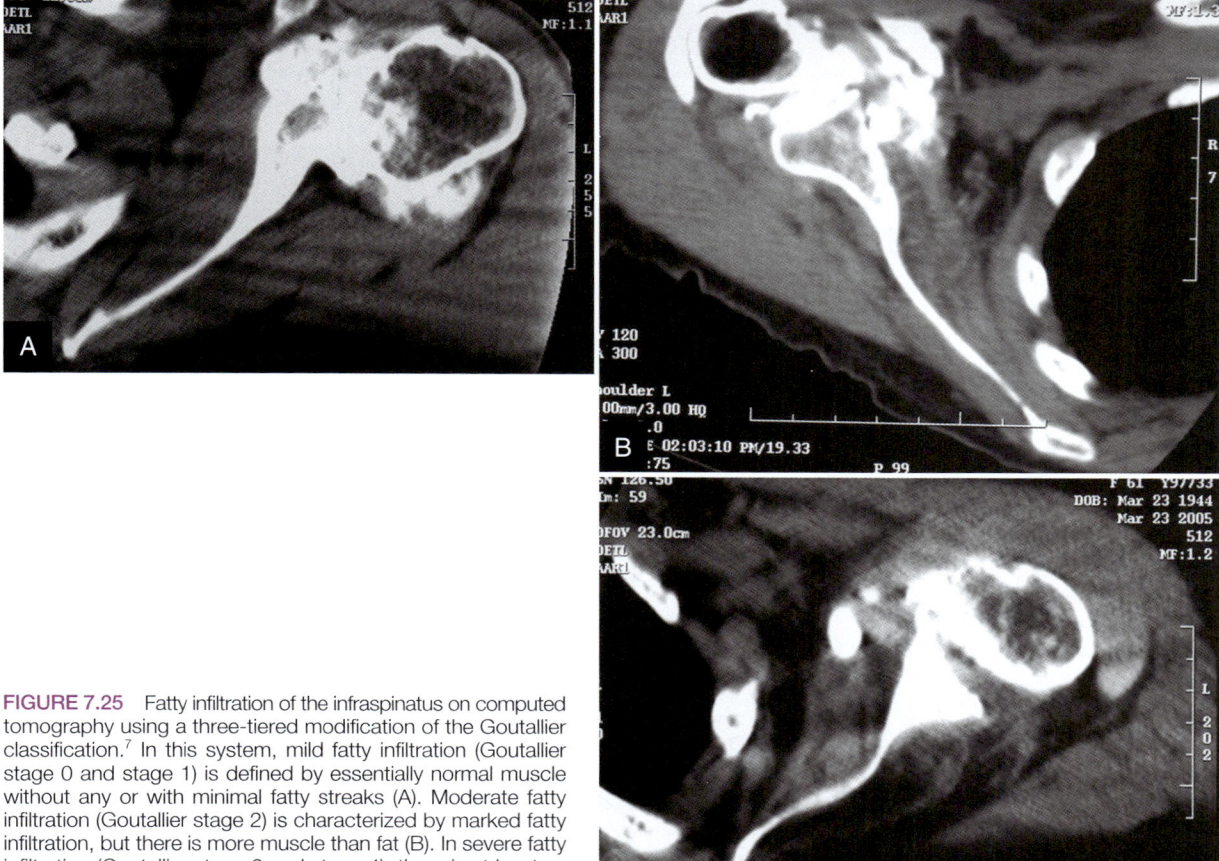

FIGURE 7.25 Fatty infiltration of the infraspinatus on computed tomography using a three-tiered modification of the Goutallier classification.[7] In this system, mild fatty infiltration (Goutallier stage 0 and stage 1) is defined by essentially normal muscle without any or with minimal fatty streaks (A). Moderate fatty infiltration (Goutallier stage 2) is characterized by marked fatty infiltration, but there is more muscle than fat (B). In severe fatty infiltration (Goutallier stage 3 and stage 4), there is at least as much fat as muscle (C). The same classification system is used for the subscapularis.

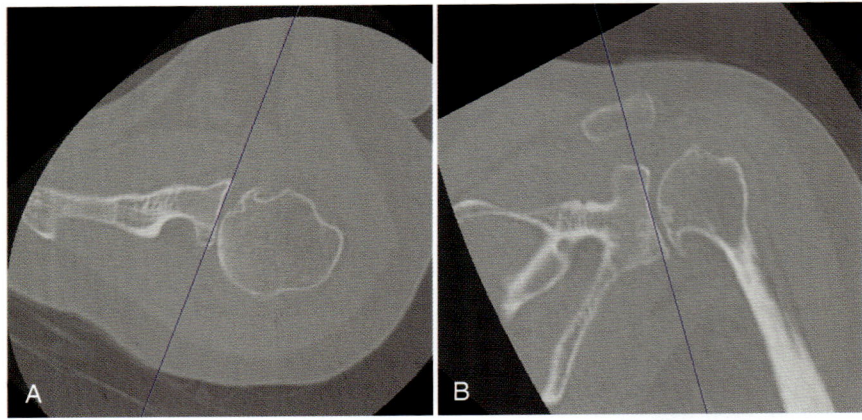

FIGURE 7.26 Preoperative planning software using computed tomography to determine retroversion (18 degrees) (A) and superior inclination (12 degrees) (B).

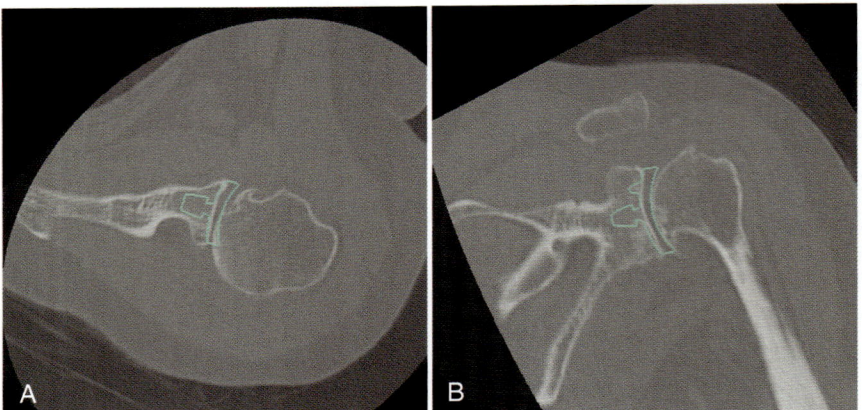

FIGURE 7.27 Preoperative planning software using computed tomography to determine axial (A) and coronal (B) virtual glenoid component placement. The green highlighted glenoid component implies that there is no glenoid perforation, which would alternatively display as red with any glenoid perforation with the peg(s) or keel.

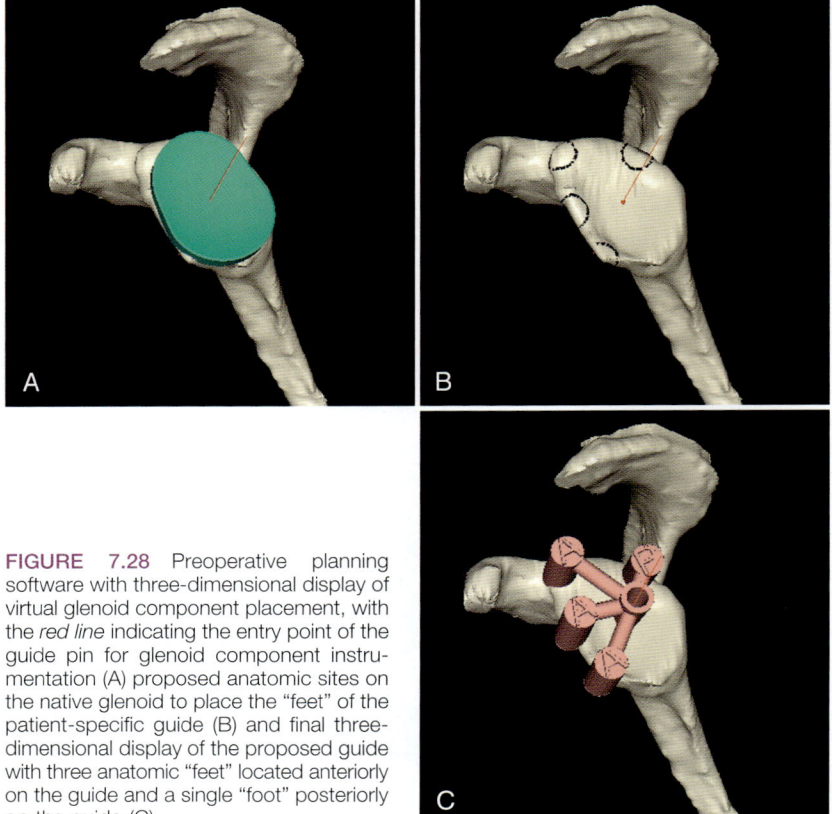

FIGURE 7.28 Preoperative planning software with three-dimensional display of virtual glenoid component placement, with the *red line* indicating the entry point of the guide pin for glenoid component instrumentation (A) proposed anatomic sites on the native glenoid to place the "feet" of the patient-specific guide (B) and final three-dimensional display of the proposed guide with three anatomic "feet" located anteriorly on the guide and a single "foot" posteriorly on the guide (C).

REFERENCES

1. Jobe FW, Jobe C: Painful athletic injuries of the shoulder, *Clin Orthop Relat Res* 173:117–124, 1983.
2. Hertel R, Ballmer FT, Lambert SM, et al: Lag signs in the diagnosis of rotator cuff rupture, *J Shoulder Elbow Surg* 5:307–313, 1996.
3. Gerber C, Vinh TS, Hertel R, et al: Latissimus dorsi transfer for the treatment of massive tears of the rotator cuff: a preliminary report, *Clin Orthop Relat Res* 232:51–61, 1988.
4. Gerber C, Krushell RJ: Isolated rupture of the tendon of the subscapularis muscle: clinical features in 16 cases, *J Bone Joint Surg Br* 73:389–394, 1991.
5. Walch G, Badet R, Boulahia A, et al: Morphologic study of the glenoid in primary glenohumeral osteoarthritis, *J Arthroplasty* 14:756–760, 1999.
6. Bercik MJ, Kruse K, 2nd, Yalizis M, et al: A modification to the Walch classification of the glenoid in primary glenohumeral osteoarthritis using three-dimensional imaging, *J Shoulder Elbow Surg* 25(10):1601–1606, 2016, doi:10.1016/j.jse.2016.03.010. [Epub 2016 Jun 6].
7. Edwards TB, Boulahia A, Kempf JF, et al: The influence of the rotator cuff on the results of shoulder arthroplasty for primary osteoarthritis: results of a multicenter study, *J Bone Joint Surg Am* 84:2240–2248, 2002.
8. Goutallier D, Postel JM, Bernageau J, et al: Fatty muscle degeneration in cuff rupture, *Clin Orthop Relat Res* 304:78–83, 1994.
9. Hendel MD, Bryan JA, Barsoum WK, et al: Comparison of patient-specific instruments with standard surgical instruments in determining glenoid component position: a randomized prospective clinical trial, *J Bone Joint Surg Am* 94:2167–2175, 2012.
10. Throckmorton TW, Gulotta LV, Bonnarens FO, et al: Patient-specific targeting guides compared with traditional instrumentation for glenoid component placement in shoulder arthroplasty: a multi-surgeon study in 70 arthritic cadaver specimens, *J Shoulder Elbow Surg* 24(6):965–971, 2015, doi:10.1016/j.jse.2014.10.013. [Epub 2014 Dec 19].
11. Walch G, Vezeridis PS, Boileau P, et al: Three-dimensional planning and use of patient-specific guides improve glenoid component position: an in vitro study, *J Shoulder Elbow Surg* 24:302–309, 2015.

CHAPTER 8

Surgical approach

For primary unconstrained shoulder arthroplasty we use a deltopectoral approach in all cases. This chapter details this commonly used surgical approach to the glenohumeral joint (Video 8.1).

The surgical approach begins with identification of the topographic anatomy (Fig. 8.1). The coracoid process is readily palpable in all but the most obese patients and those who have previously undergone a surgical procedure involving the coracoid process. In thin patients, the deltopectoral interval may be palpable and is useful in guiding orientation of the skin incision. The skin incision, made with a no. 10 scalpel blade, is extended distally and laterally along the anticipated location of the deltopectoral interval from the tip of the coracoid process for 10 to 15 cm, depending on the size of the patient (Fig. 8.2). To minimize hemorrhage, we use a needle-tip electrocautery for subcutaneous dissection and for most of the deep dissection throughout the procedure. Medium-size skin rakes are used for retraction during this portion of the approach. The cephalic vein is located to identify the interval between the deltoid and the pectoralis major. In many cases, the cephalic vein is covered with a layer of fatty tissue, and identification of this tissue aids in locating the vein (Fig. 8.3). If difficulty is encountered in locating the cephalic vein (congenitally small or absent vein), the deltopectoral interval can be readily detected proximally by identifying a small triangular area devoid of muscle tissue between the proximal portions of the deltoid and pectoralis major muscles (Fig. 8.4). Once located, the cephalic vein is dissected free of the pectoralis major muscle with Metzenbaum scissors. We prefer to retract the cephalic vein laterally with the deltoid because most of the branches of the cephalic vein are based on the deltoid. Medial retraction of the cephalic vein with the pectoralis major disrupts these deltoid branches and introduces unwanted hemorrhage.

After the deltopectoral interval has been identified and developed, Army–Navy retractors are used to maintain the interval. The humeral insertion of the pectoralis major tendon is identified. Division of the superior centimeter of the pectoralis major tendon enhances exposure of the inferior aspect of the subscapularis, the anterior humeral circumflex vessels, and the axillary nerve (Fig. 8.5). A self-retaining deltopectoral retractor—we prefer a cerebellar-type retractor—is inserted to maintain exposure. Next, the conjoined tendon is identified and traced proximally to its insertion on the coracoid process. Large curved Mayo scissors are used to create a space superior to the coracoid process by placing the scissors just over the top of the coracoid and spreading the blades. The creation of this space allows the surgeon to place the tip of a Hohmann-type retractor behind the base of the coracoid process to provide proximal retraction (Fig. 8.6).

The arm is placed in an abducted and externally rotated position, and the apex that is formed by the insertions of the coracoacromial ligament and conjoined tendon to the coracoid process is identified (Fig. 8.7). This apex is developed with the needle-tip electrocautery to release the clavipectoral fascia. The lateral aspect of the conjoined tendon is released with the electrocautery, and the conjoined tendon is relaxed by forward flexing the arm; the tendon is then retracted medially with a narrow Richardson retractor to expose the subscapularis tendon and anterior humeral circumflex vessels (the "three sisters") (Fig. 8.8). We prefer to use a narrow Richardson retractor for the conjoined tendon instead of a self-retaining type of retractor because we believe that it minimizes the possibility of prolonged compression and damage to the musculocutaneous nerve.

With the arm externally rotated, the anterior humeral circumflex vessels are suture-ligated at the inferior border of the subscapularis with no. 0 dyed absorbable braided suture. The proper site of ligation approximates the location of the anatomic neck of the humerus, with the vessels being ligated on each side of the anatomic neck. The suture limbs are cut approximately 15 mm long. This, combined with the dyed suture, allows easier identification of the ligation site during subsequent subscapularis tenotomy (Fig. 8.9).

The axillary nerve can be identified by direct visualization at this point if desired. We do not routinely identify the axillary nerve, but it is important to be intimately familiar with its location. Familiarity with the location of the axillary nerve ensures its protection throughout the procedure (Fig. 8.10). In primary surgery, this vital nerve is almost always in its normal location, but in revision surgery that is rarely the case. The experience gained by dissecting the nerve in primary surgery or in a cadaveric lab dissection pays great dividends when the surgeon must find the nerve in the scar tissue associated with revision operations. In order to expose the axillary nerve, the narrow Richardson retractor is moved slightly inferiorly along the conjoined tendon to just below the location of the anterior humeral circumflex vessels. The arm is flexed forward in neutral rotation, and blunt dissection is undertaken by spreading the tips of Metzenbaum scissors in the axillary fat inferior and deep to the humeral circumflex vessels. Table 8.1 lists the steps in the deltopectoral approach for easy reference.

CHAPTER 8 ■ Surgical Approach

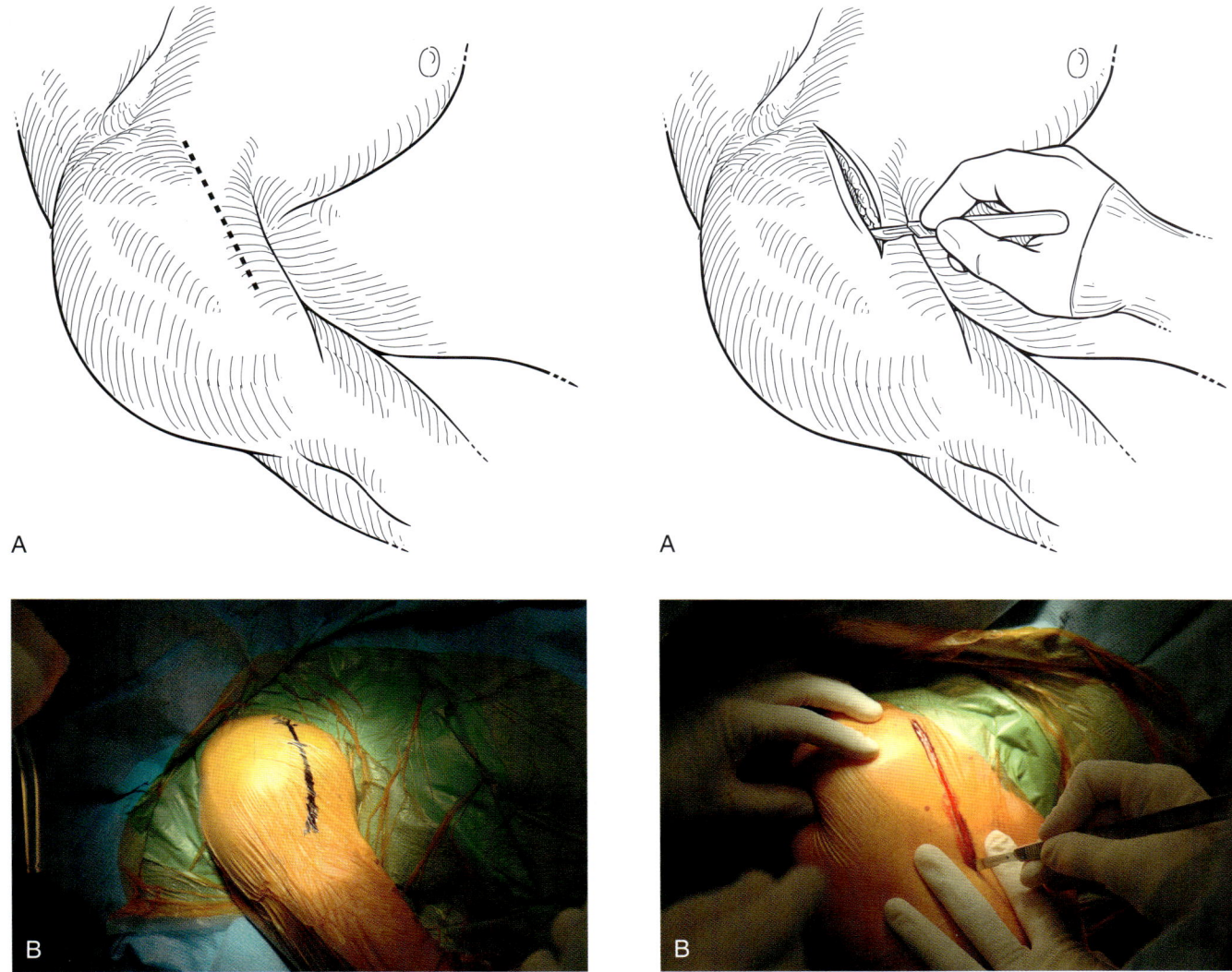

FIGURE 8.1 (A and B) Topographic anatomy of the shoulder delineated for use in the deltopectoral approach.

FIGURE 8.2 (A and B) Skin incision for the deltopectoral approach.

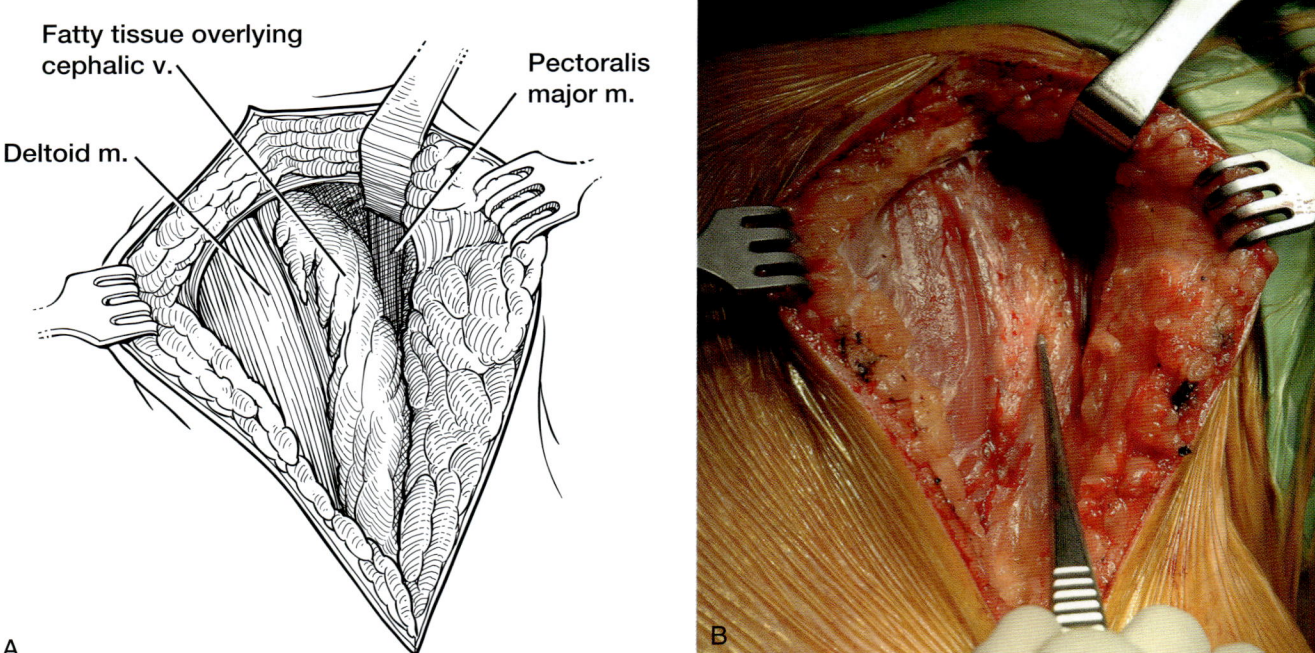

FIGURE 8.3 (A and B) Fatty tissue overlying the cephalic vein aids in its detection and the subsequent identification of the deltopectoral interval.

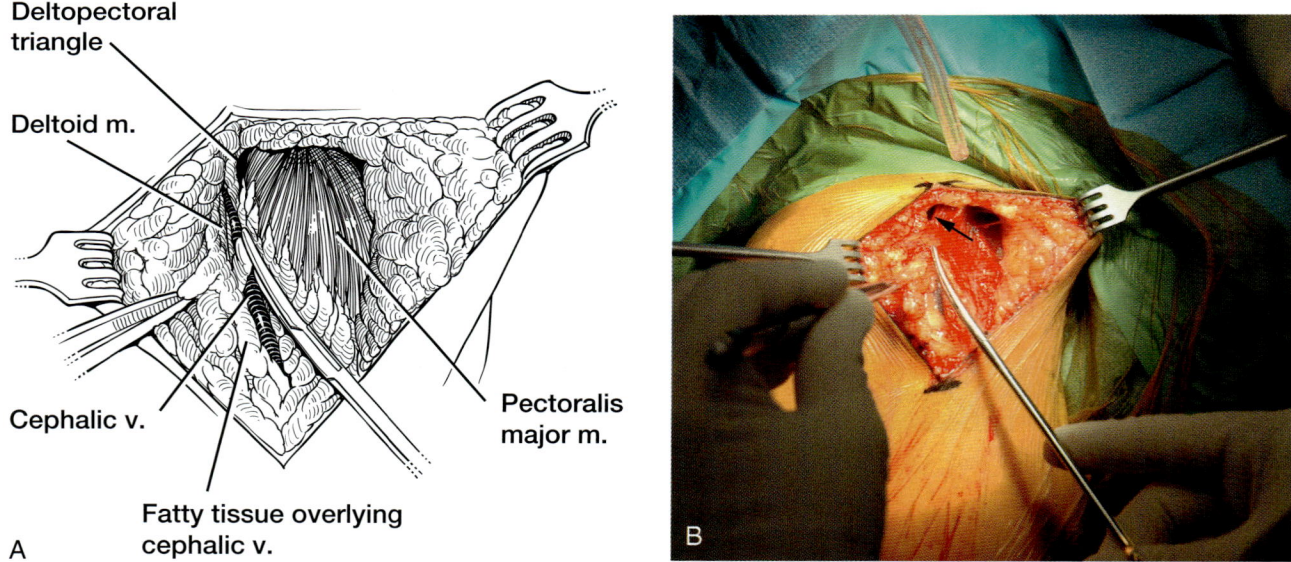

FIGURE 8.4 (A and B) Proximal deltopectoral interval. Note the triangular area devoid of muscle tissue (*arrow* in B), which aids in identifying this interval.

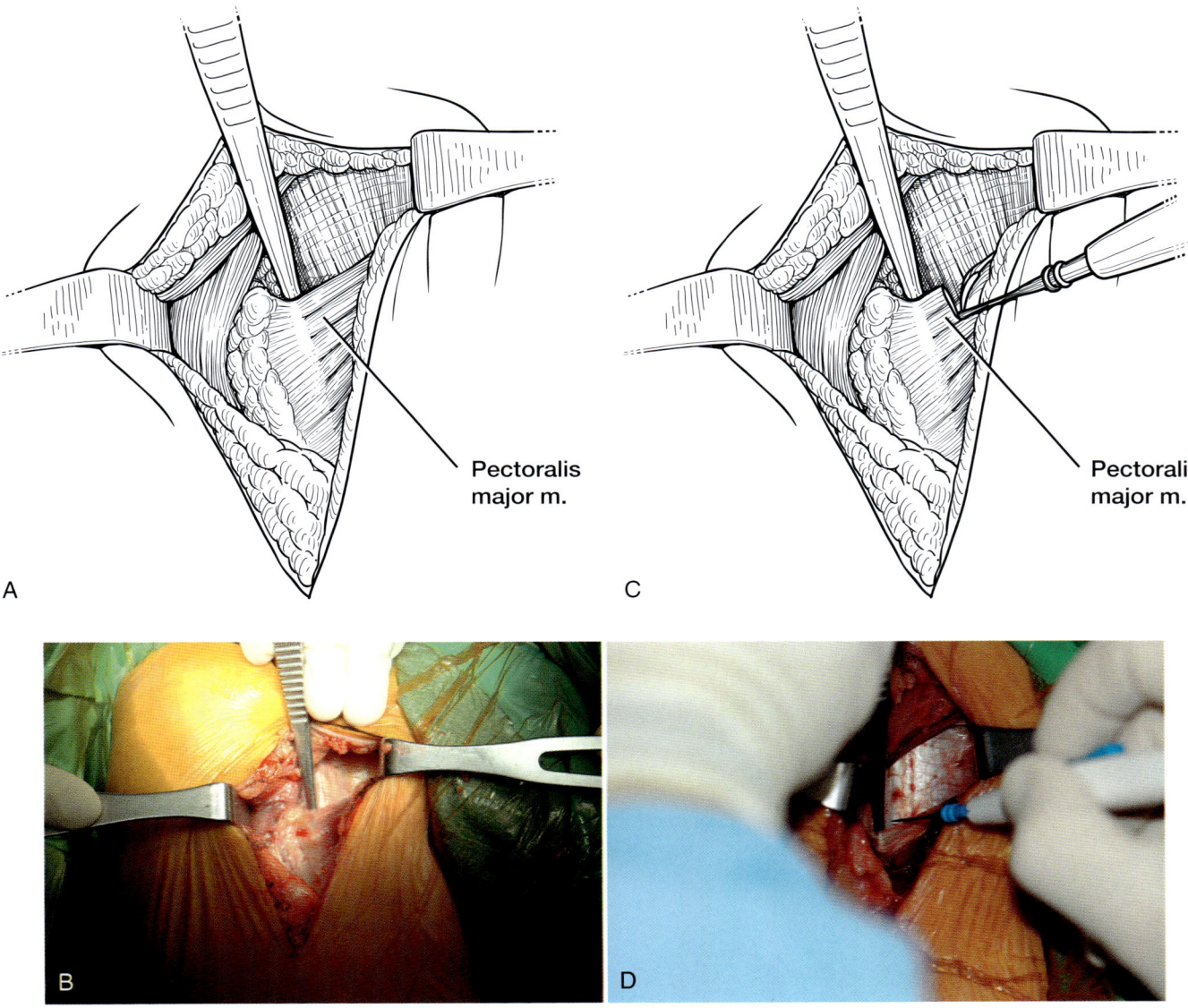

FIGURE 8.5 (A to D) Identification and release of the superior aspect of the pectoralis major tendon.

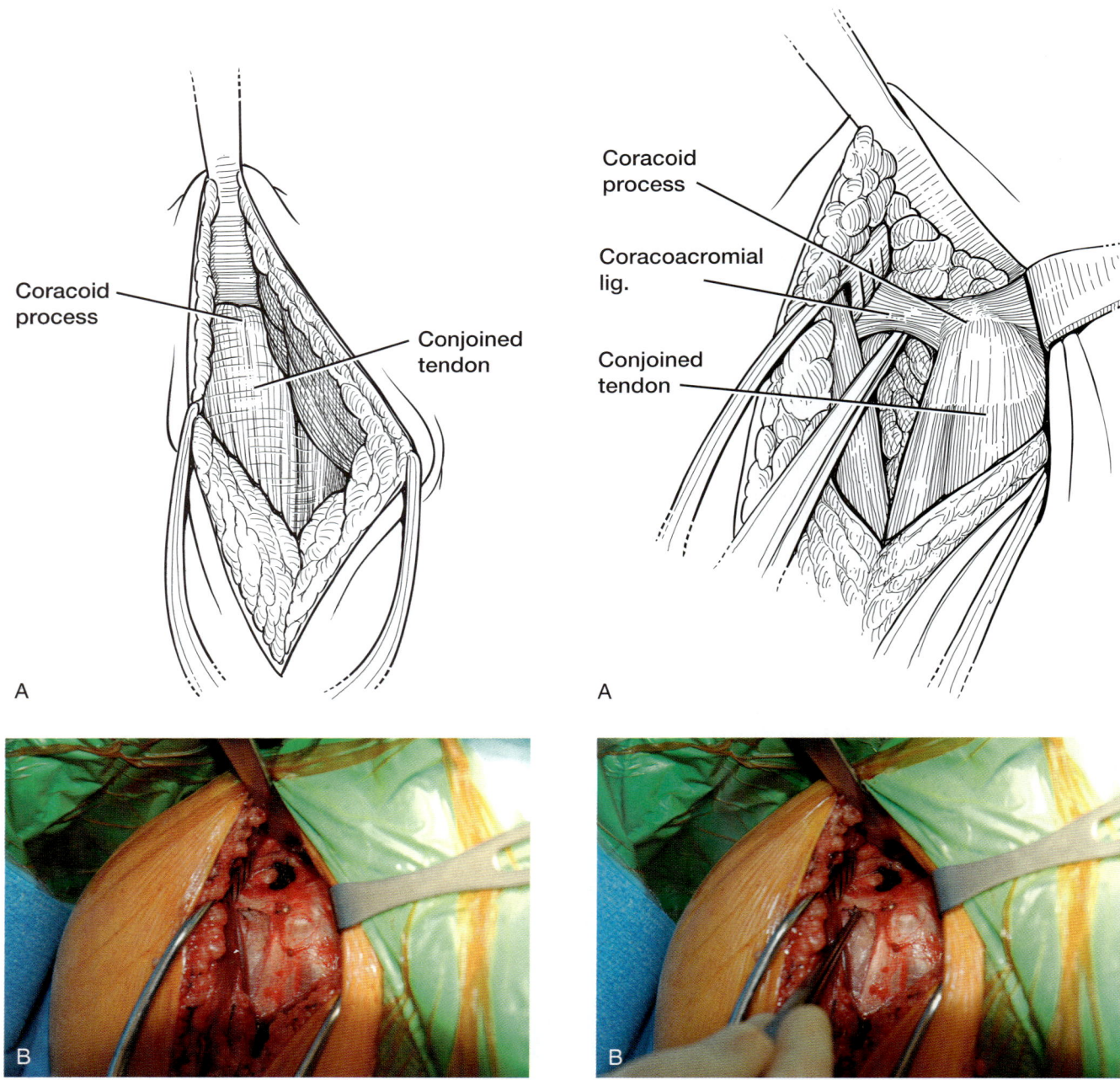

FIGURE 8.6 (A and B) Completed retractor placement for the deltopectoral approach.

FIGURE 8.7 (A and B) Identification of the coracoacromial ligament and lateral aspect of the conjoined tendon.

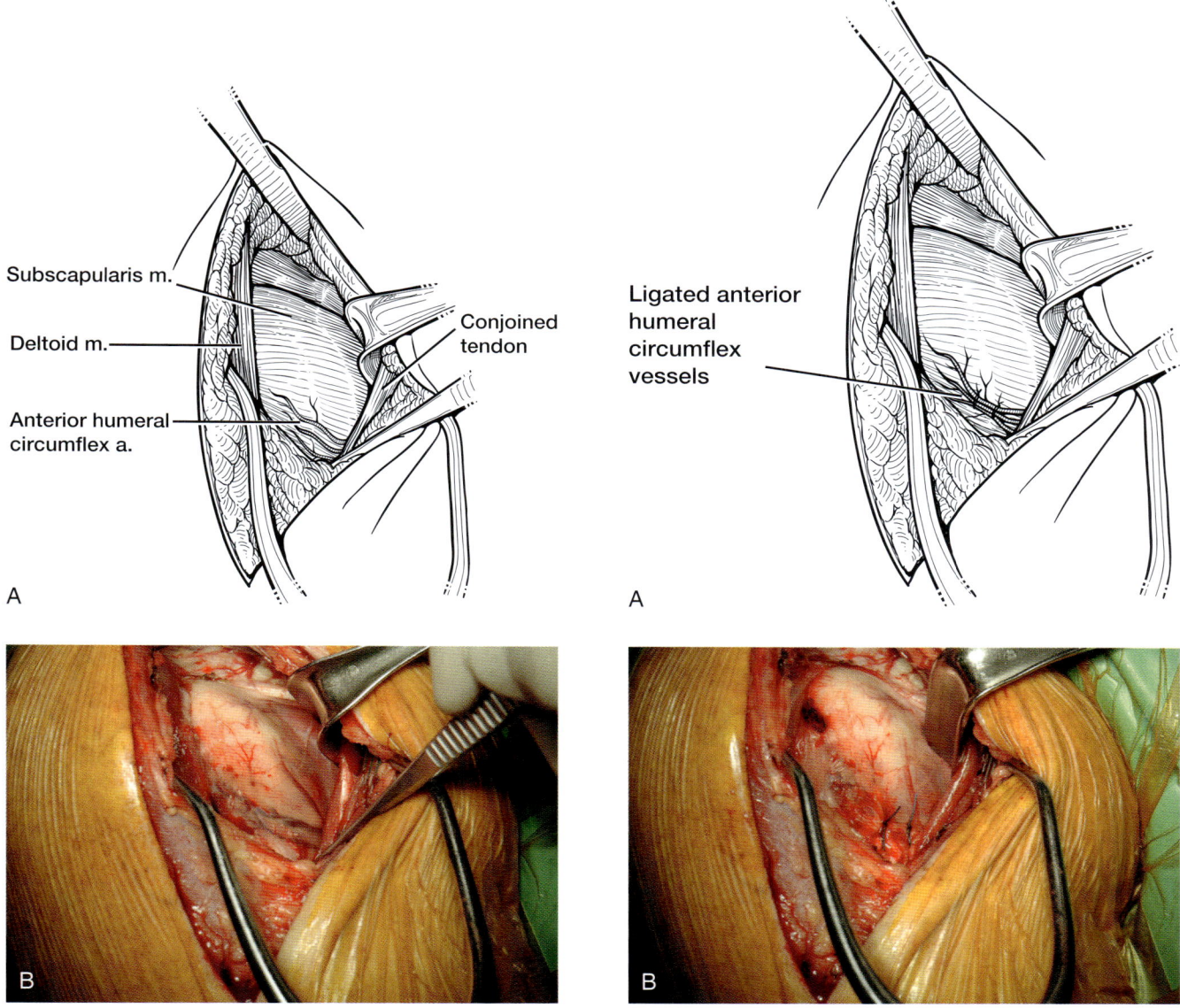

FIGURE 8.8 (A and B) Medial retraction of the conjoined tendon allows visualization of the subscapularis muscle and anterior humeral circumflex vessels.

FIGURE 8.9 (A and B) Ligation of the anterior humeral circumflex vessels on each side of the anatomic neck of the humerus. The suture is of the dyed variety, and the suture limbs are cut long to allow easier identification of this site during subsequent subscapularis tenotomy.

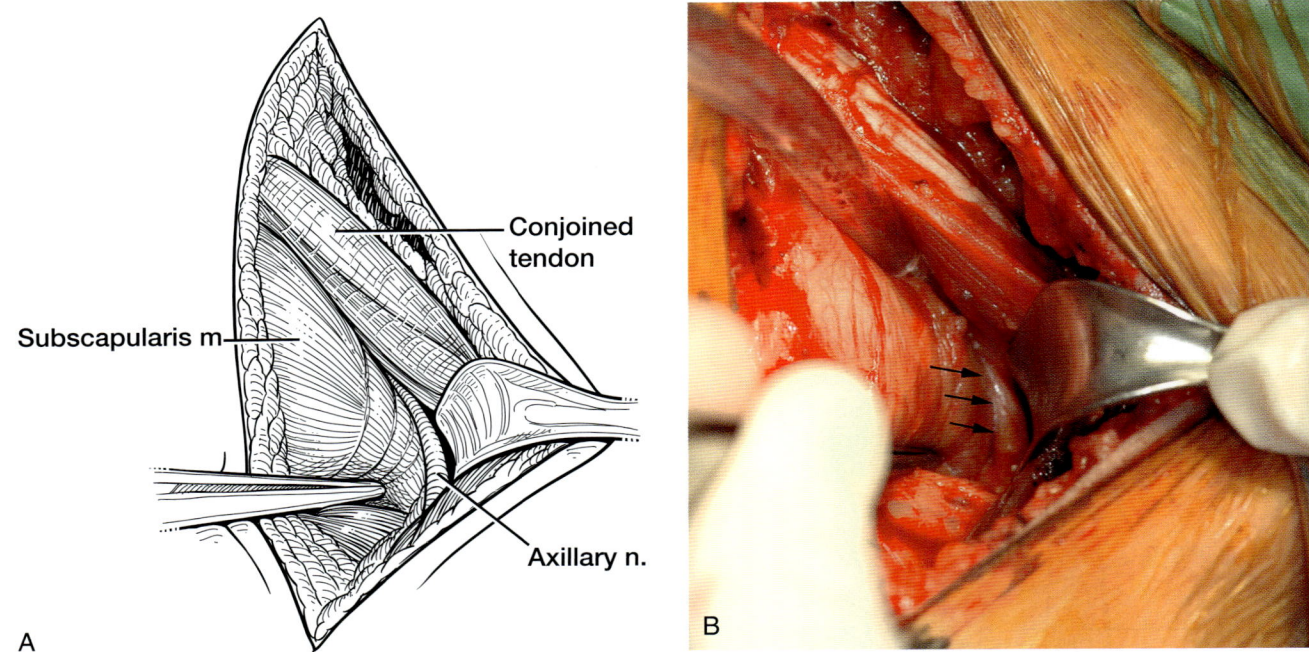

FIGURE 8.10 (A and B) Identification of the axillary nerve (*arrows* in B) through direct visualization.

TABLE 8.1	Steps in the Deltopectoral Approach
Step	Procedure
1	Palpate the coracoid process
2	Perform skin incision of the tip of the coracoid process 15 cm along the deltopectoral interval
3	Perform subcutaneous dissection with needle-tip electrocautery
4	Dissect and retract the cephalic vein laterally with the deltoid
5	Identify the insertion of the pectoralis major tendon on the humerus and divide the superior 1 cm
6	Apply self-retaining retractor to the deltopectoral interval
7	Identify the conjoined tendon and trace it to the coracoid process
8	Place a Hohmann retractor superior to the coracoid process
9	Abduct and externally rotate the arm
10	Identify the lateral aspect of the conjoined tendon
11	Release the lateral aspect of the conjoined tendon
12	Retract the conjoined tendon medially with a narrow Richardson retractor
13	Expose the subscapularis and anterior humeral circumflex vessels
14	Suture-ligate the anterior humeral circumflex vessels with dyed no. 0 braided suture
15	Move the Richardson retractor slightly inferiorly along the conjoined tendon
16	Flex the arm forward in neutral rotation
17	When desired, identify the axillary nerve in fat inferior and deep to the circumflex vessels

Subscapularis

CHAPTER 9

After the deltopectoral surgical approach is completed, the next step in performing unconstrained shoulder arthroplasty is management of the subscapularis musculotendinous unit. Various techniques for obtaining anterior access to the glenohumeral joint during shoulder arthroplasty have been described, including complete and partial subscapularis tenotomy, lesser tuberosity osteotomy, and access to the joint solely through the rotator interval. In many patients in whom shoulder arthroplasty is performed, the subscapularis lacks normal excursion, thereby creating loss of external rotation. In such cases, surgical techniques must address this soft tissue contracture to allow sufficient postoperative external rotation and minimize the incidence of postoperative dehiscence of the subscapularis. This chapter details our preferred technique for handling the subscapularis, including accessing the glenohumeral joint and addressing loss of external rotation caused by subscapularis contracture.

TECHNIQUE FOR HANDLING THE SUBSCAPULARIS

After the conjoined tendon is retracted medially with a narrow Richardson retractor, the subscapularis is readily visualized. In some cases a hypertrophic subscapularis bursa may be present, and a bursectomy is necessary to allow adequate visualization of the subscapularis tendon. To minimize hemorrhage, we perform bursectomy with the needle-tip electrocautery. Once the subscapularis tendon is adequately visualized, two stay sutures of no. 1 nonabsorbable braided suture are double-passed through the tendon approximately 15 mm lateral to the musculotendinous junction, one in the superior half and one in the inferior half of the tendon (Fig. 9.1). Adduction and external rotation of the surgical arm allows improved visualization of the subscapularis tendon for placement of the stay sutures.

The glenohumeral joint is opened initially through the rotator interval. The tips of large curved Mayo scissors are passed tangential and just superior to the subscapularis tendon and used to puncture the rotator interval tissue for access to the glenohumeral joint. Once the glenohumeral joint is entered, the scissors are spread to enlarge the arthrotomy (Fig. 9.2). Usually, after the Mayo scissors are spread, synovial fluid egresses from the joint.

The next step involves elevation of the subscapularis from its humeral insertion to allow further access to the glenohumeral joint. We prefer performing a complete subscapularis tenotomy because it allows unhindered access to the glenohumeral joint and sufficient release of subscapularis contracture. Additionally, tenotomy does not risk disruption of the existing proximal humeral osseous anatomy, as may occur with lesser tuberosity osteotomy. The location of the tenotomy is critical to allow adequate repair after insertion of the prosthesis is completed. We perform the tenotomy along the anatomic neck of the humerus while leaving a small amount of tendon on the lesser tuberosity to use in later subscapularis closure. The shoulder is placed in neutral to slight external rotation during this portion of the procedure. To identify the anatomic neck of the humerus, a no. 10 scalpel blade on a long handle is used to further open the rotator interval from the initial arthrotomy site extending laterally along the superior border of the subscapularis tendon (Fig. 9.3). Once the anatomic neck of the humerus is identified by observing the lateral extent of the articular surface, the scalpel blade is directed inferiorly to transect the superior two-thirds of the subscapularis tendon along the anatomic neck of the humerus (Fig. 9.4A and B). At the inferior third of the subscapularis, we switch to the needle-tip electrocautery and complete the tenotomy. The needle tip passes between the previously placed anterior humeral circumflex ligation sutures and cauterizes these vessels (Fig. 9.4C and D). As the subscapularis tenotomy is completed, the shoulder is progressively externally rotated to allow visualization of the inferior humeral capsular attachment. This capsule is released from the humerus with the needle-tip electrocautery while keeping the electrocautery in contact with the humerus (Fig. 9.5). Release of the capsular attachments on the humeral side is important as it improves humeral mobilization and ultimately aids in glenoid exposure.

A humeral head retractor (we prefer the modified Trillat type of retractor) is placed in the glenohumeral joint, and the humeral head is retracted posteriorly. To facilitate insertion of this retractor, the shoulder is initially externally rotated and moved into internal rotation as the retractor is pushed posteriorly between the humeral head and the glenoid. With the humeral head retracted posteriorly and traction applied to stay sutures in the subscapularis tendon, the glenohumeral ligaments are readily visualized (Fig. 9.6). To increase subscapularis excursion, circumferential release of the subscapularis tendon is performed. The superior glenohumeral ligament is first released with large curved Mayo scissors along the superior aspect of the subscapularis tendon (Fig. 9.7). The middle glenohumeral ligament, which

Text continued on p. 82

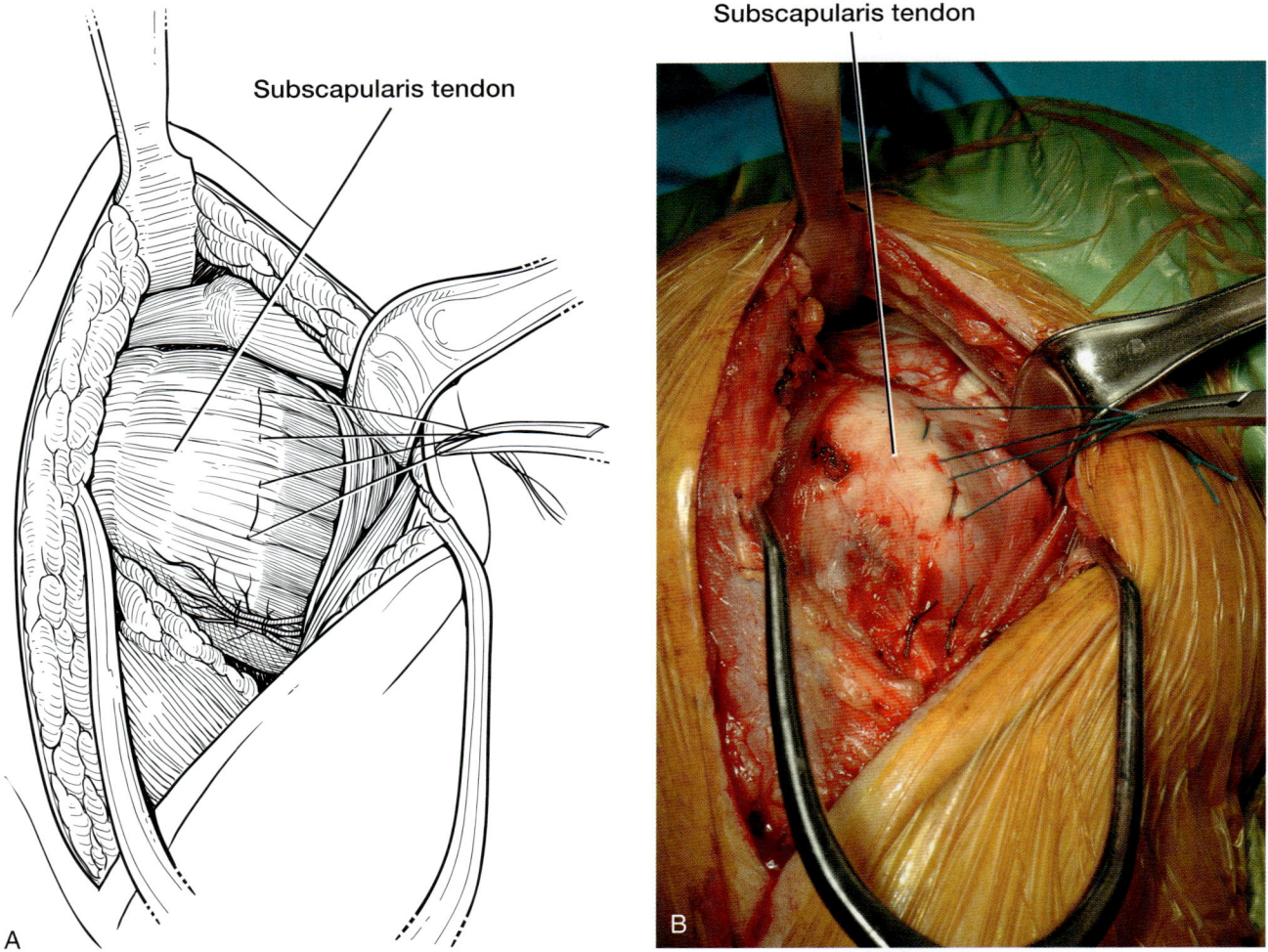

FIGURE 9.1 (A and B) Stay sutures placed in the subscapularis tendon before subscapularis tenotomy.

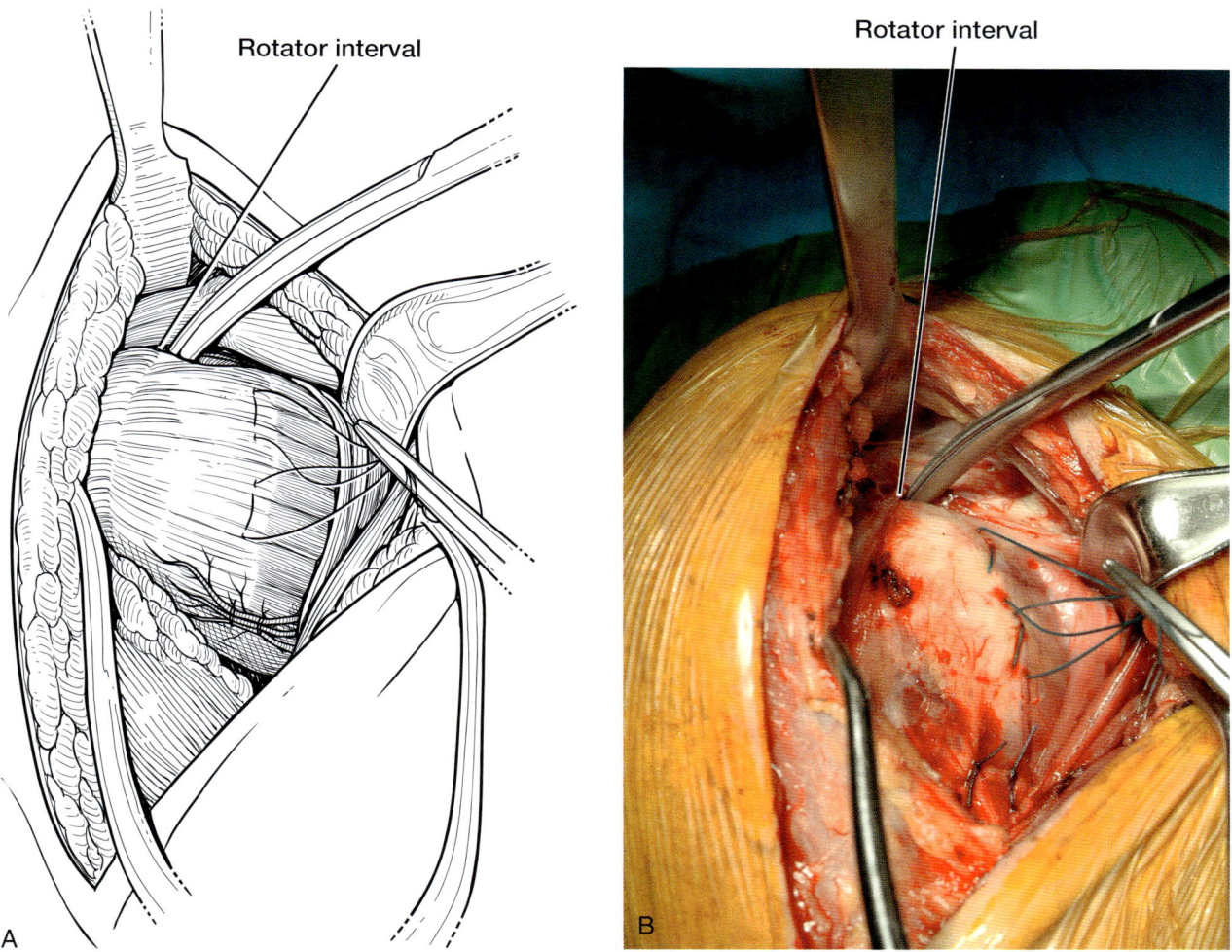

FIGURE 9.2 (A and B) Arthrotomy of the glenohumeral joint through the rotator interval with large Mayo scissors.

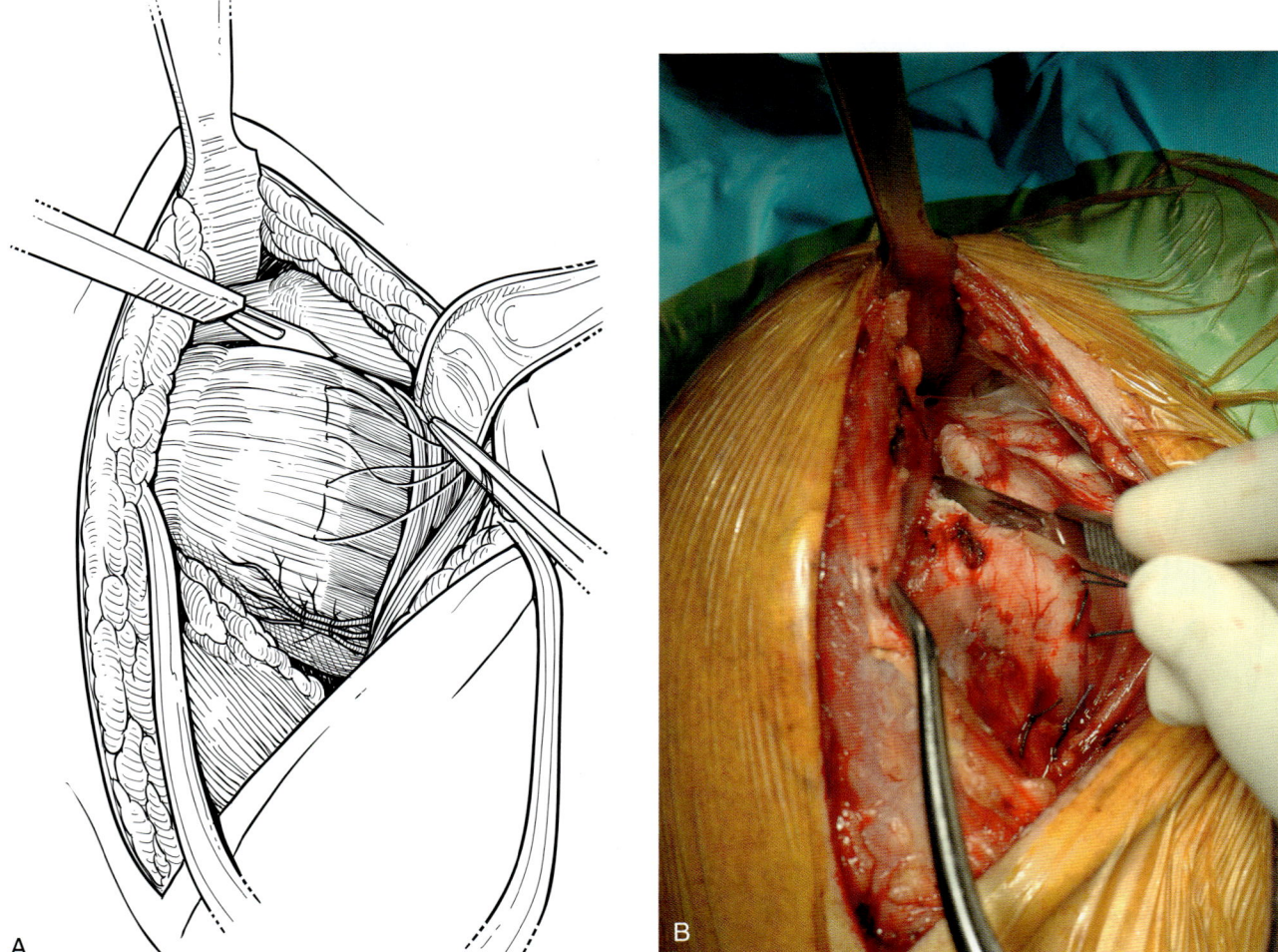

FIGURE 9.3 (A and B) Extension of the rotator interval arthrotomy laterally to the anatomic neck in preparation for subscapularis tenotomy.

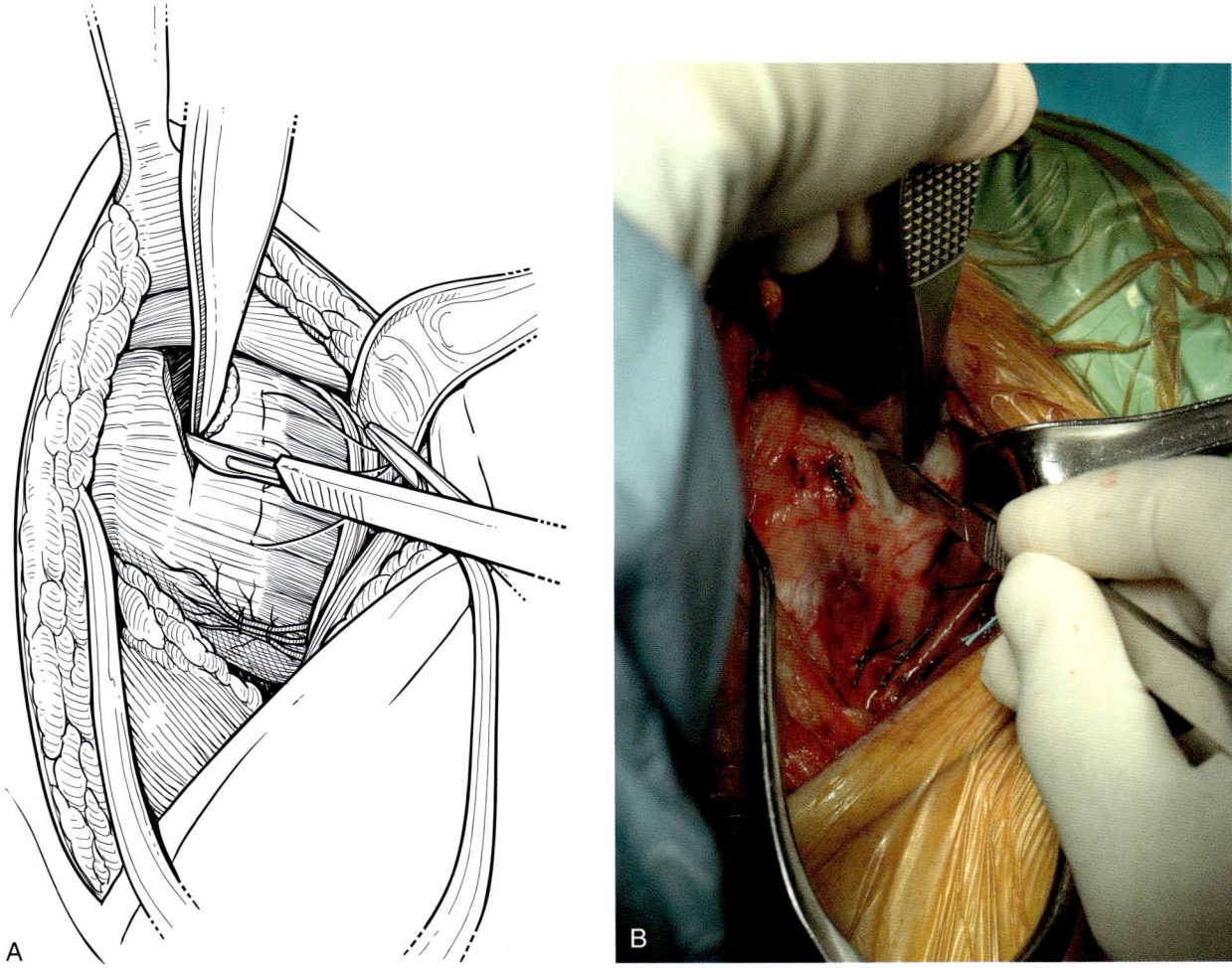

FIGURE 9.4 Performance of subscapularis tenotomy. (A and B) The superior two-thirds of the tendon is transected with the scalpel.

Continued

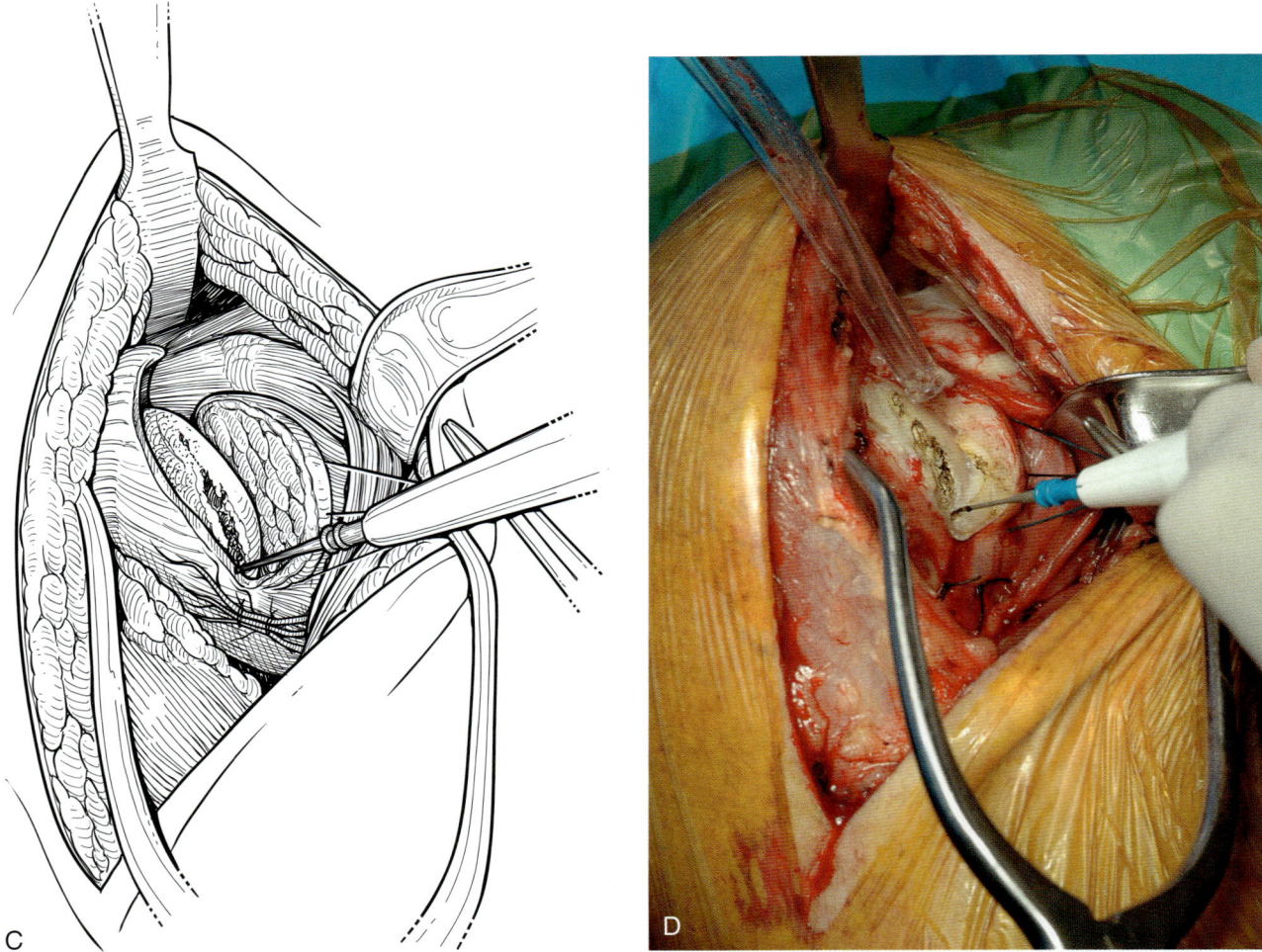

FIGURE 9.4, cont'd (C and D) The inferior third of the tendon is transected by passing the needle-tip electrocautery between the ligation sutures previously placed around the anterior humeral circumflex vessels during the surgical approach.

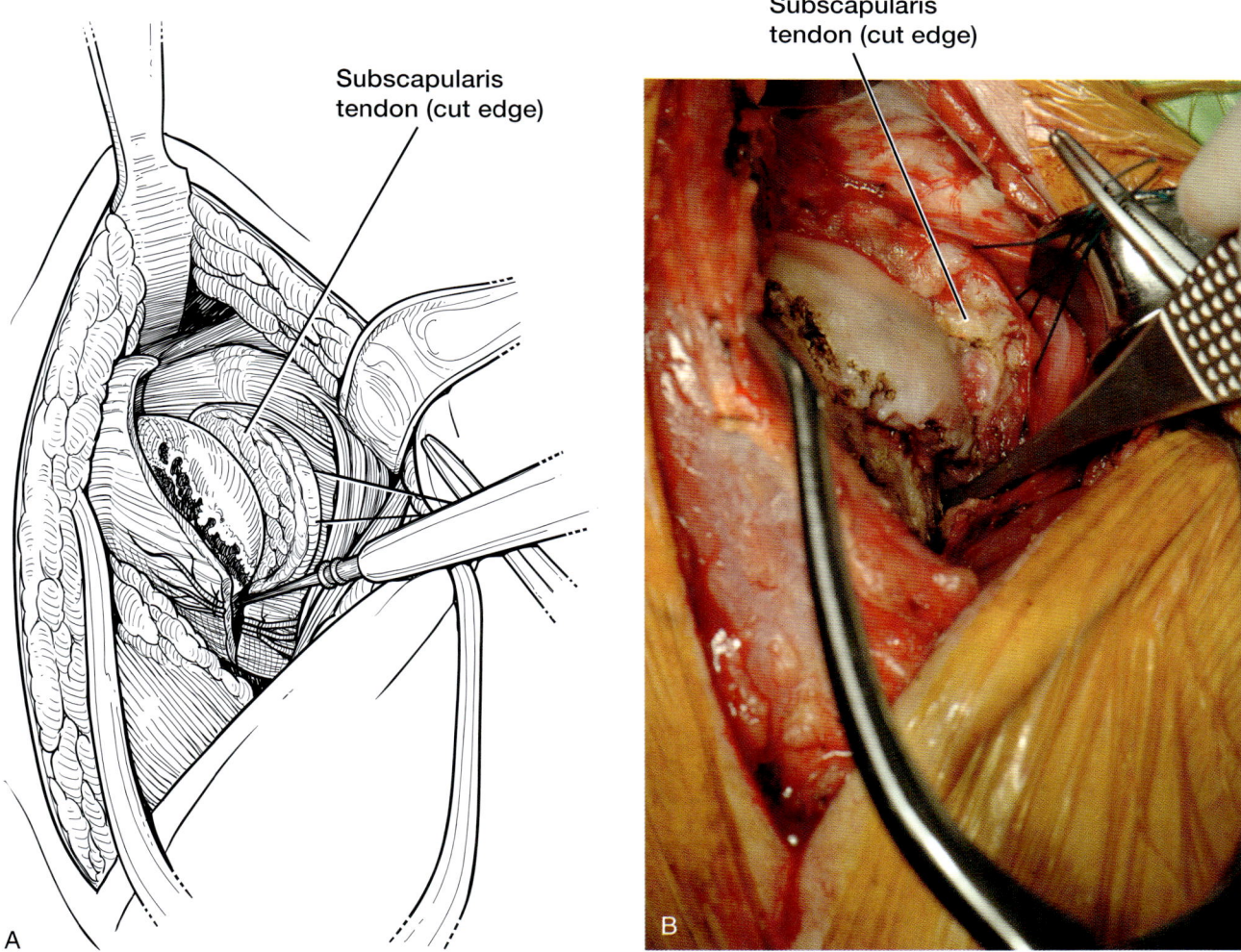

FIGURE 9.5 (A and B) Release of the medial joint capsule from the humerus with the needle-tip electrocautery.

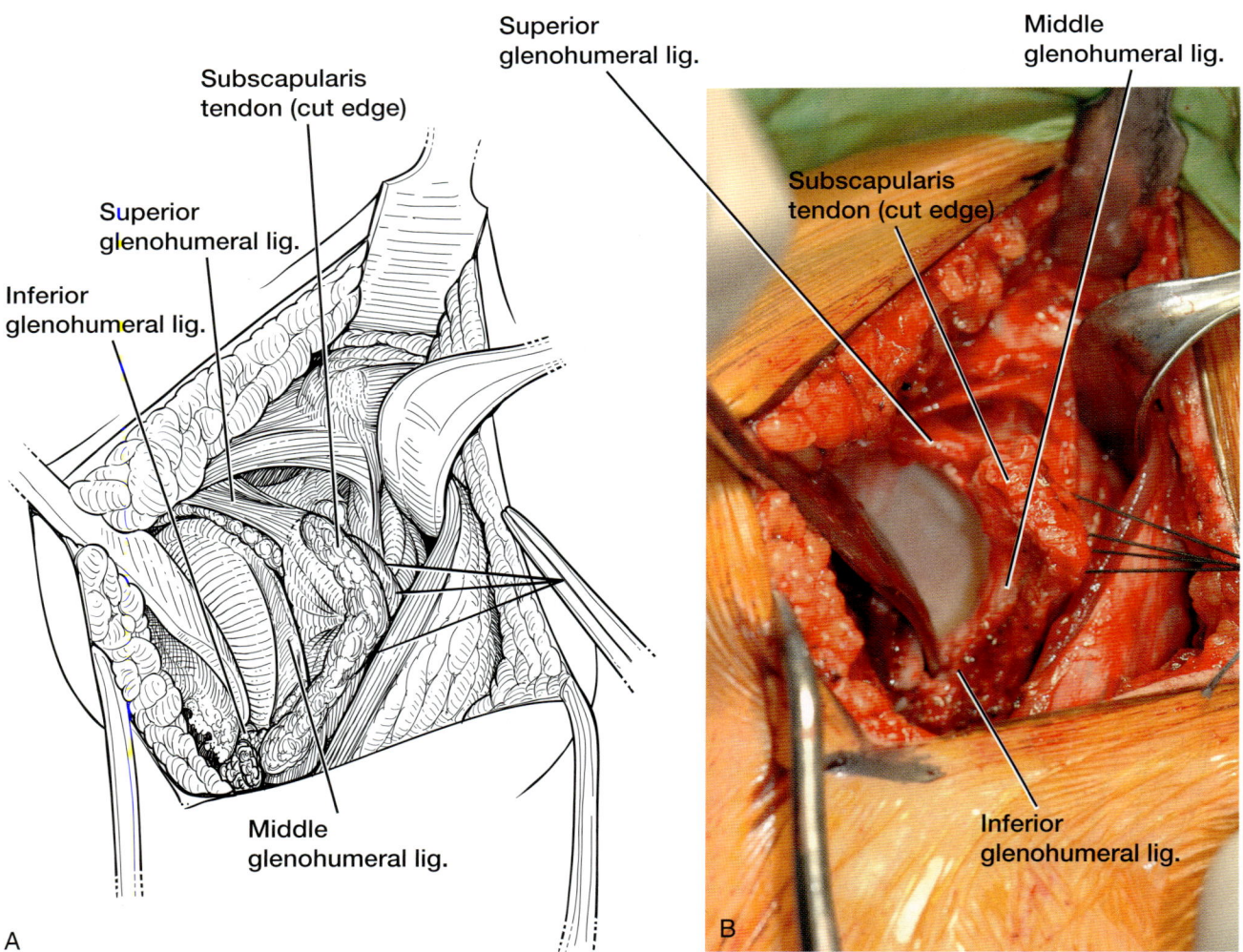

FIGURE 9.6 (A and B) Visualization of the superior, middle, and inferior glenohumeral ligaments after subscapularis tenotomy.

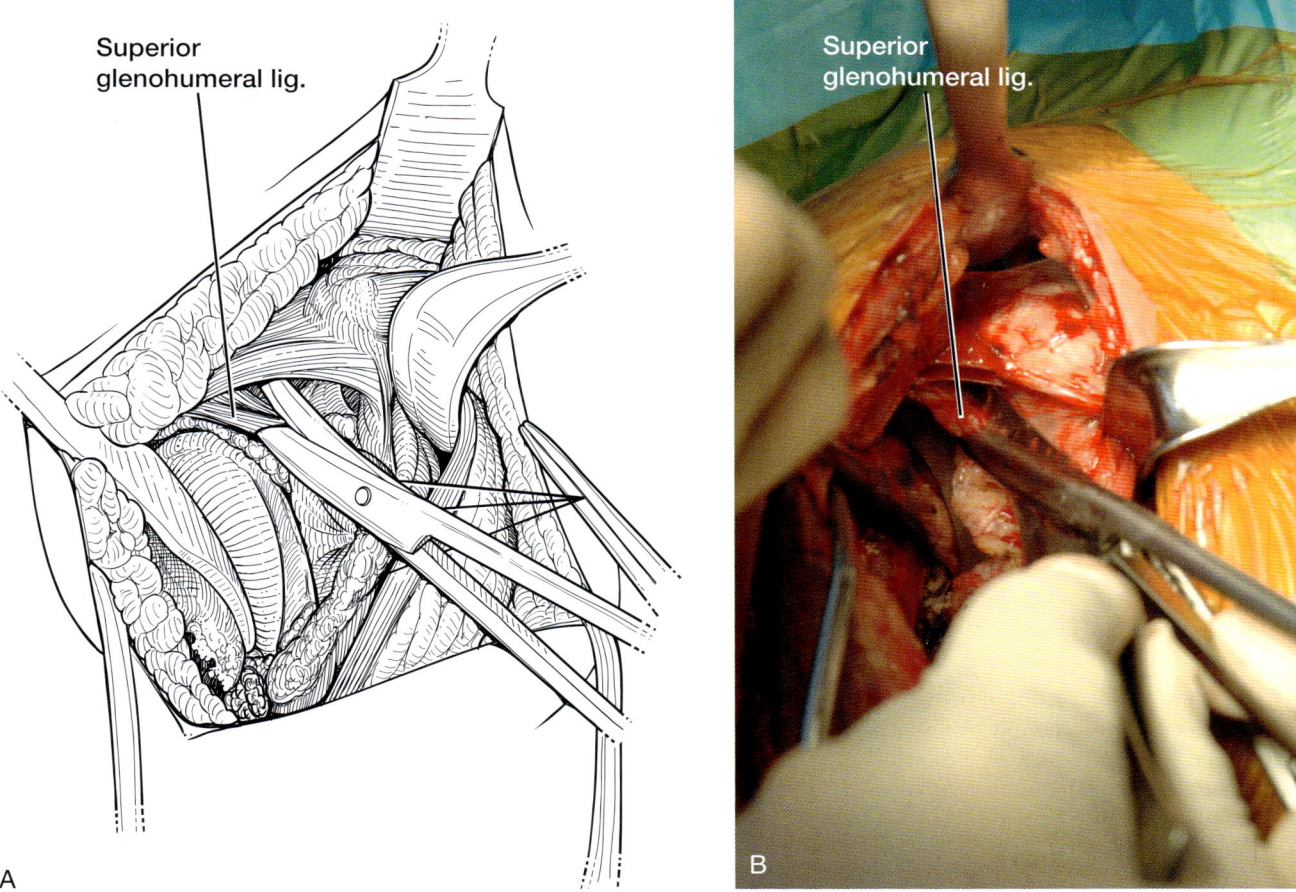

FIGURE 9.7 (A and B) Transection of the superior glenohumeral ligament during release of the subscapularis tendon.

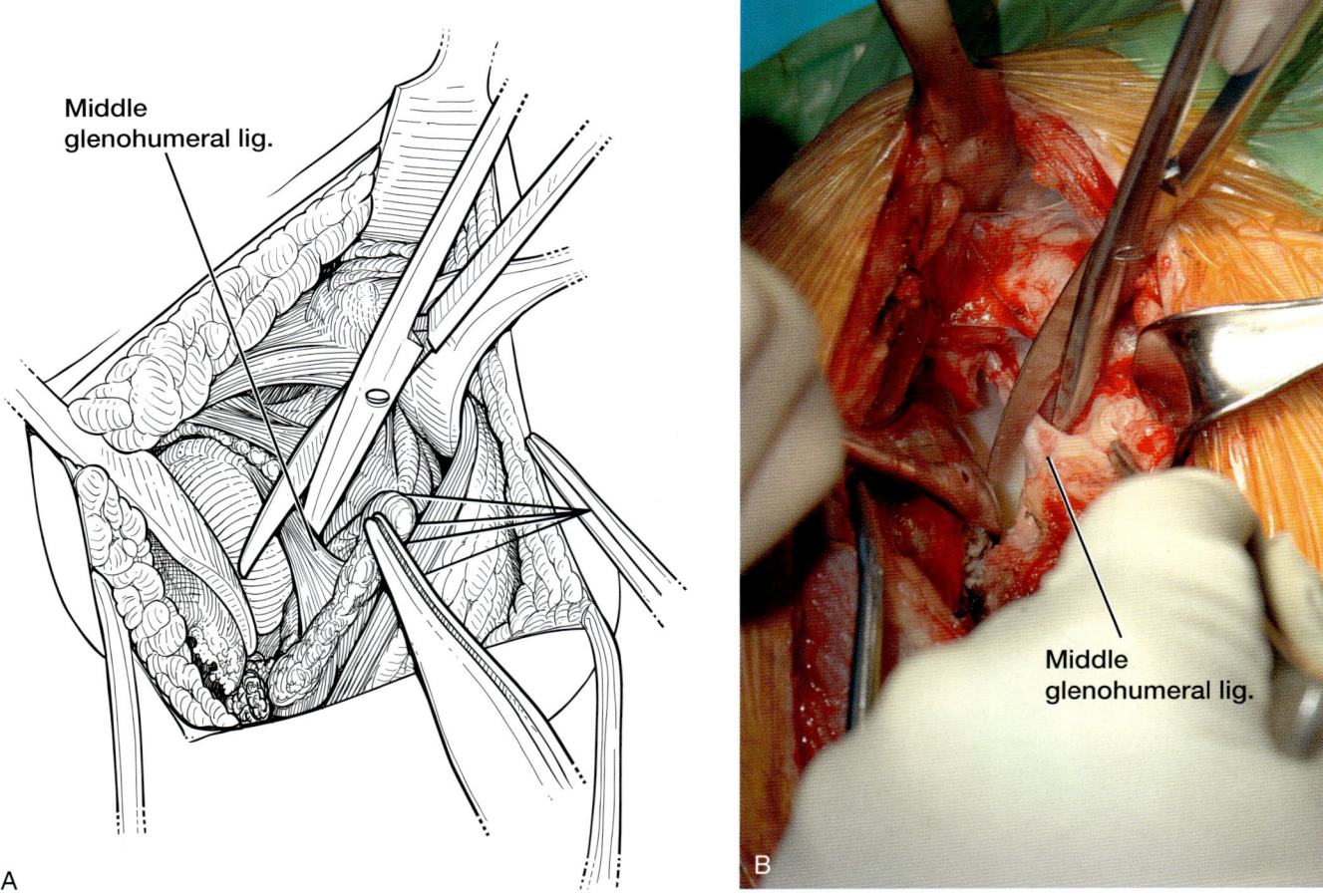

FIGURE 9.8 (A and B) Transection of the middle glenohumeral ligament during release of the subscapularis tendon.

may be absent in up to one-third of patients, is released parallel to the anterior glenoid rim with large curved Mayo scissors (Fig. 9.8). Anteriorly and inferiorly the tissue plane between the capsuloligamentous structures and the primarily muscular inferior portion of the subscapularis is identified and established with large curved Mayo scissors. Once this plane is established, the inferior glenohumeral ligament is divided with the scissors. Risk of injury to the axillary nerve is avoided because the muscular portion of the subscapularis isolates it from the path of the scissors (Fig. 9.9). After release of the glenohumeral ligaments, the intraarticularly located subscapularis recess is readily accessible. This recess should be routinely inspected for loose bodies. We remove all loose bodies (Fig. 9.10). In most cases, these loose bodies are osseous and may be anticipated by identification on preoperative imaging studies. Finally, blunt dissection with a Cobb elevator is used to release any adhesions that remain anterior to the subscapularis (Fig. 9.11). After release of the subscapularis, which effectively lengthens the contracted tendon, increased excursion should be possible. A sponge is used to tuck the subscapularis into the subscapularis fossa; it is held with a small anterior glenoid rim retractor (Fig. 9.12).

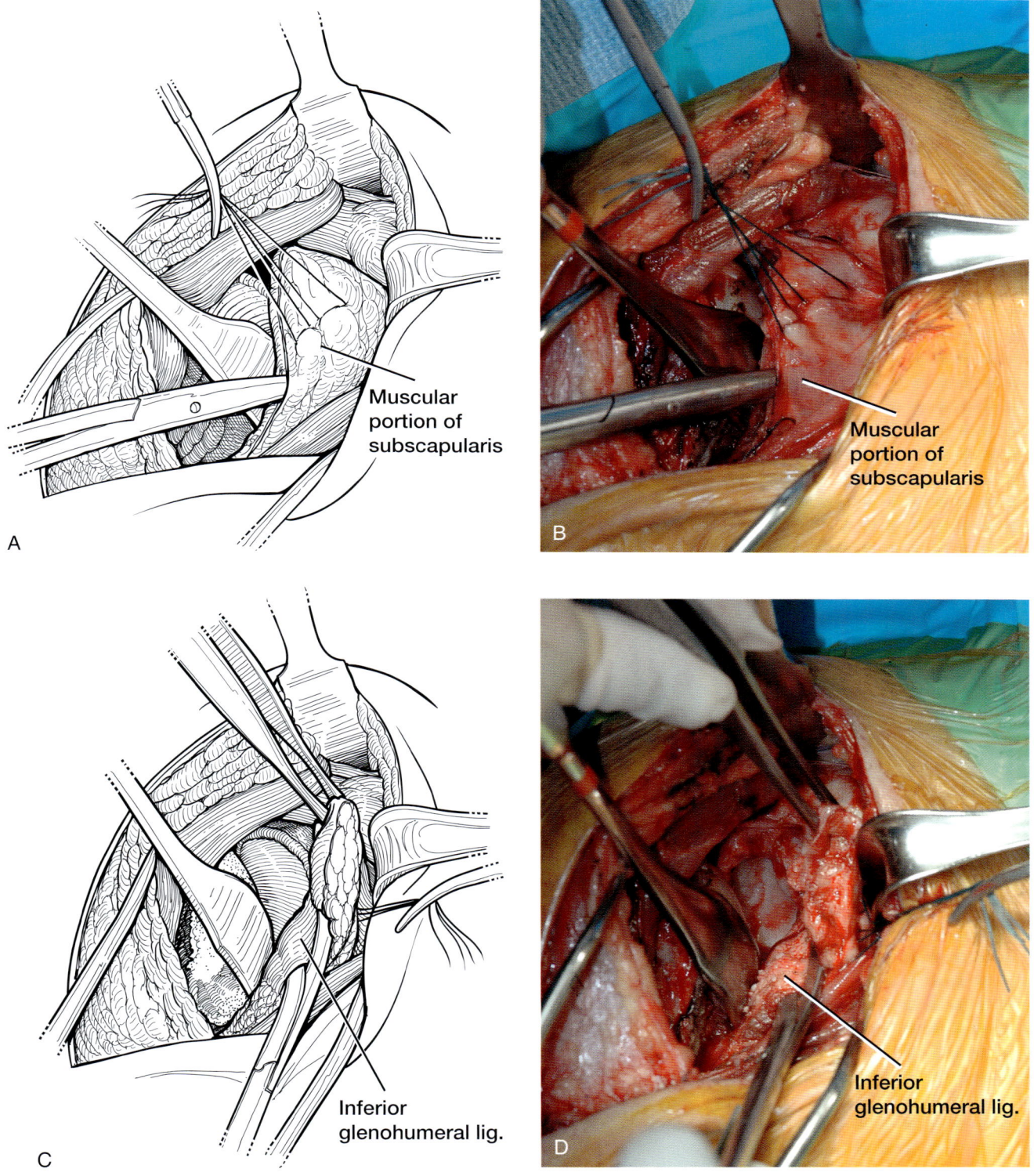

FIGURE 9.9 (A to D) Transection of the inferior glenohumeral ligament during release of the subscapularis. The muscular portion of the subscapularis inferiorly protects the axillary nerve during release.

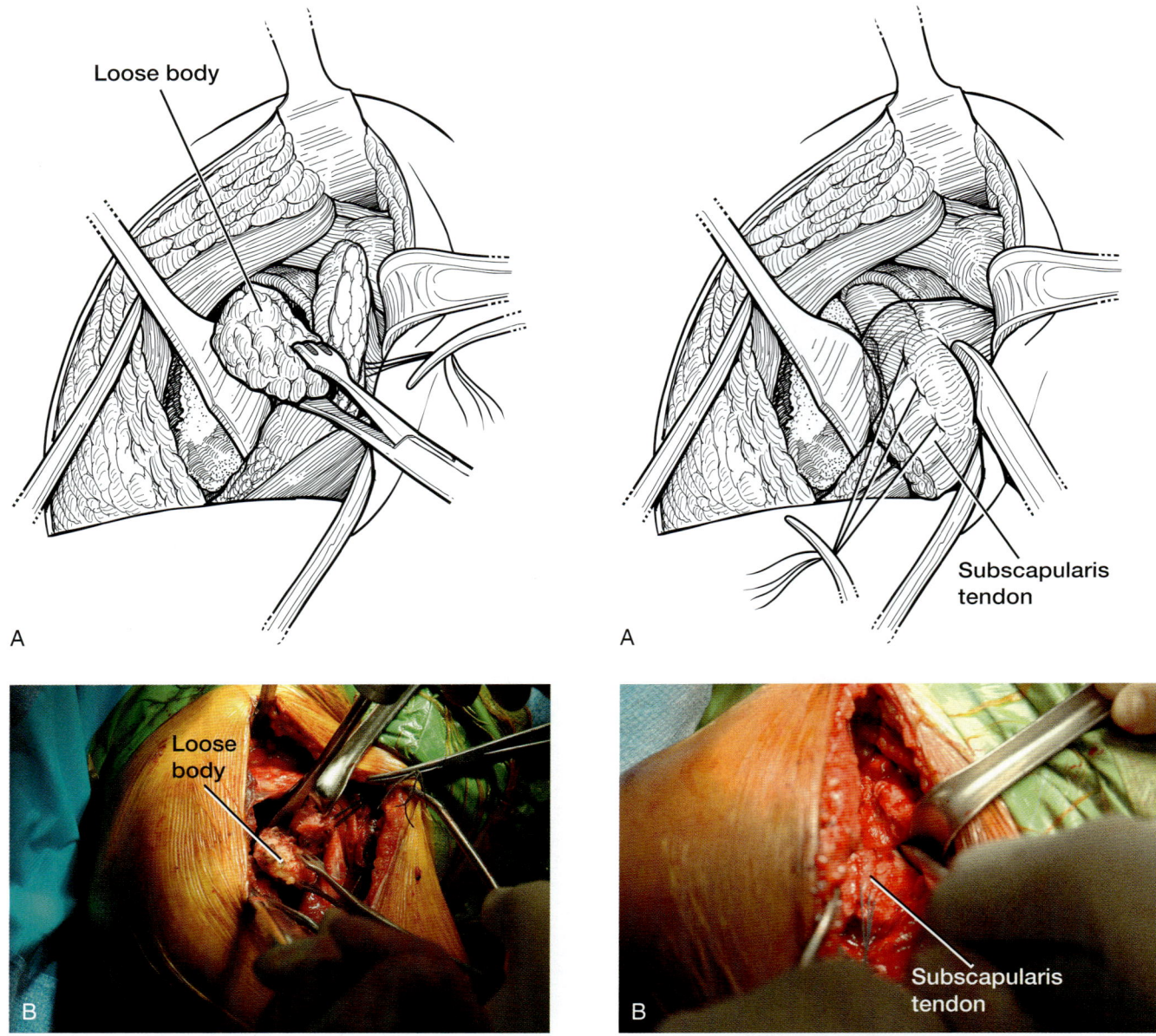

FIGURE 9.10 (A and B) A loose body identified in the subscapularis recess after release of the glenohumeral ligaments.

FIGURE 9.11 (A and B) Release of extraarticular adhesions anterior to the subscapularis with a Cobb elevator.

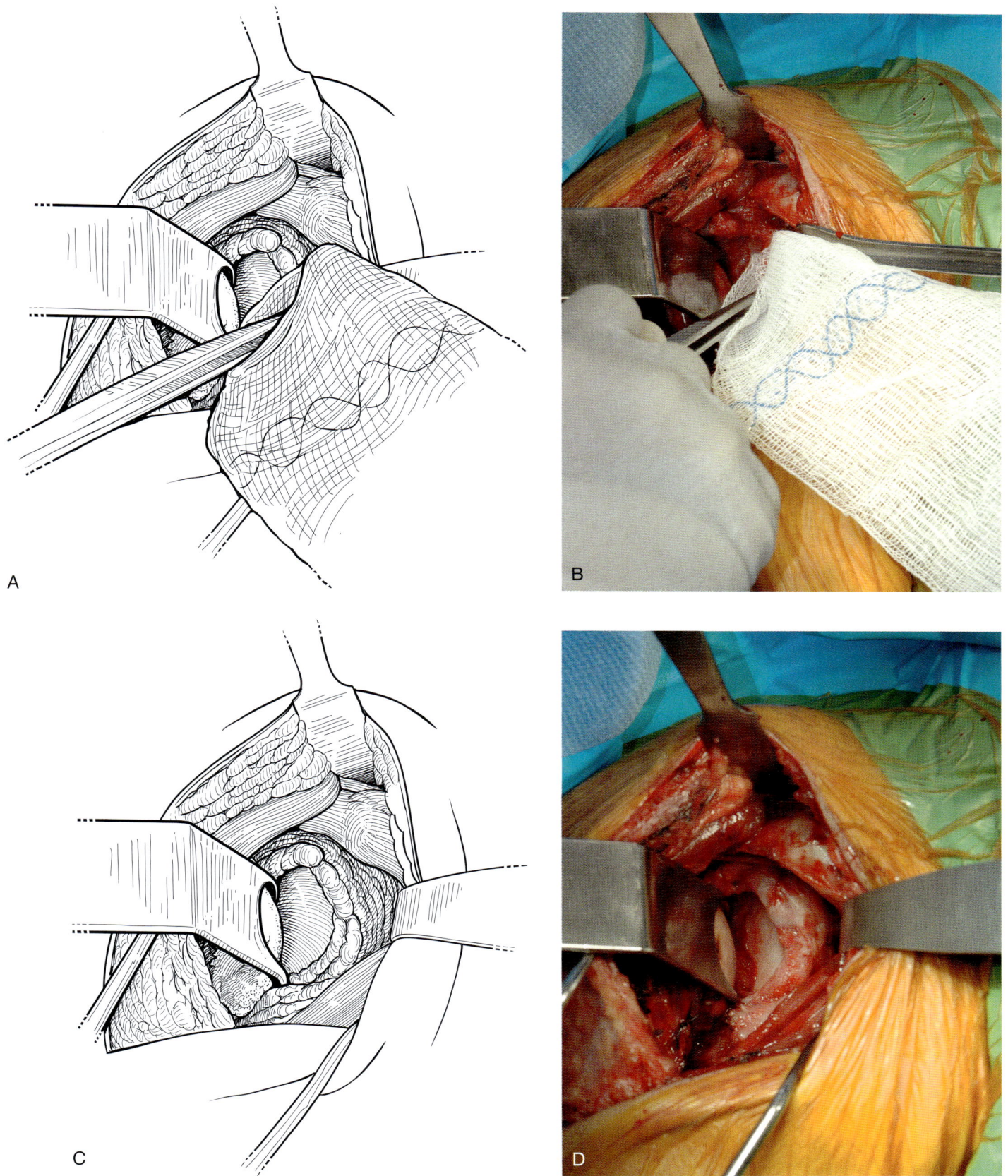

FIGURE 9.12 A sponge is used to tuck the subscapularis into the subscapularis fossa (A and B); it is held with a small glenoid rim retractor (C and D).

Glenoid exposure

Whenever we have questioned surgeons who routinely perform hemiarthroplasty instead of total shoulder arthroplasty for conditions such as primary osteoarthritis about why they chose not to resurface the glenoid, by far the most common response is that they encounter problems with glenoid exposure. When questioned further, it is evident that most of these surgeons simply lack the information necessary to correctly and reliably provide visualization of the osseous glenoid. Glenoid exposure can be simplified by following a sequence of surgical steps. This chapter outlines our systematic technique of capsular release, which provides sufficient visualization for glenoid resurfacing.

TECHNIQUE FOR GLENOID EXPOSURE

Anterior Release

After the subscapularis is retracted medially with a sponge and small anterior glenoid rim retractor, attention is turned to glenoid exposure. A needle-tip electrocautery is used to excise any remaining labrum beginning at the base of the coracoid process and extending inferiorly to the 5 o'clock position in a right shoulder (7 o'clock in a left shoulder). This allows identification of the osseous anterior margin of the glenoid (Fig. 10.1).

Inferior Release

In nearly all cases, implantation of a glenoid component requires release of the inferior capsule to obtain adequate exposure. The tip of the electrocautery is used to release the inferior capsule directly off the rim of the glenoid bone (Fig. 10.2). To avoid damaging the axillary nerve, the tip of the electrocautery must be kept in contact with glenoid bone. This release is extended sufficiently medially toward the axillary border of the scapula to completely transect the capsule and expose the muscular fibers of the long head of the triceps inserting on the inferior osseous glenoid. Visualization of the muscular fibers of the triceps or the axillary border of the scapula indicates that dissection of the capsule is sufficient.

Posterior Release

The amount of posterior subluxation present on preoperative secondary imaging studies (computed tomography, magnetic resonance imaging) determines the posterior extent of release. In shoulders without posterior subluxation, the release continues posteriorly to the 8 o'clock position for right shoulders (4 o'clock position for left shoulders). In shoulders that have preexisting posterior subluxation, either with or without posterior glenoid erosion, the release continues initially to only the 6 o'clock position. These patients often have a distended posterior capsule; therefore, to avoid further compromising these posterior structures, no more release is performed than is absolutely necessary. If release to only the 6 o'clock position proves inadequate later during glenoid reaming, the release can be extended at that time. A Cobb elevator can be used to check the release for completeness (Fig. 10.3). Fig. 10.4 shows the completed release.

CHAPTER 10 ■ Glenoid Exposure 87

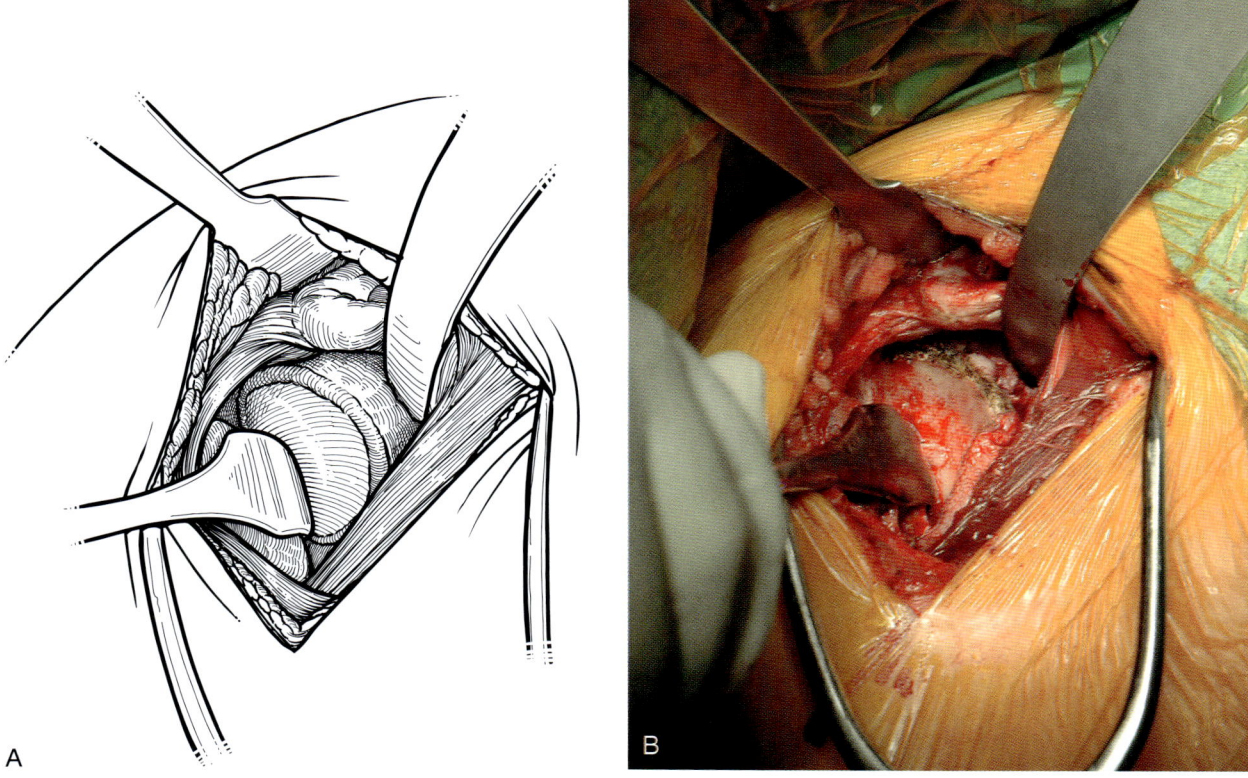

FIGURE 10.1 (A and B) Identification of the anterior osseous margin of the glenoid after excision of the anterior glenoid labrum.

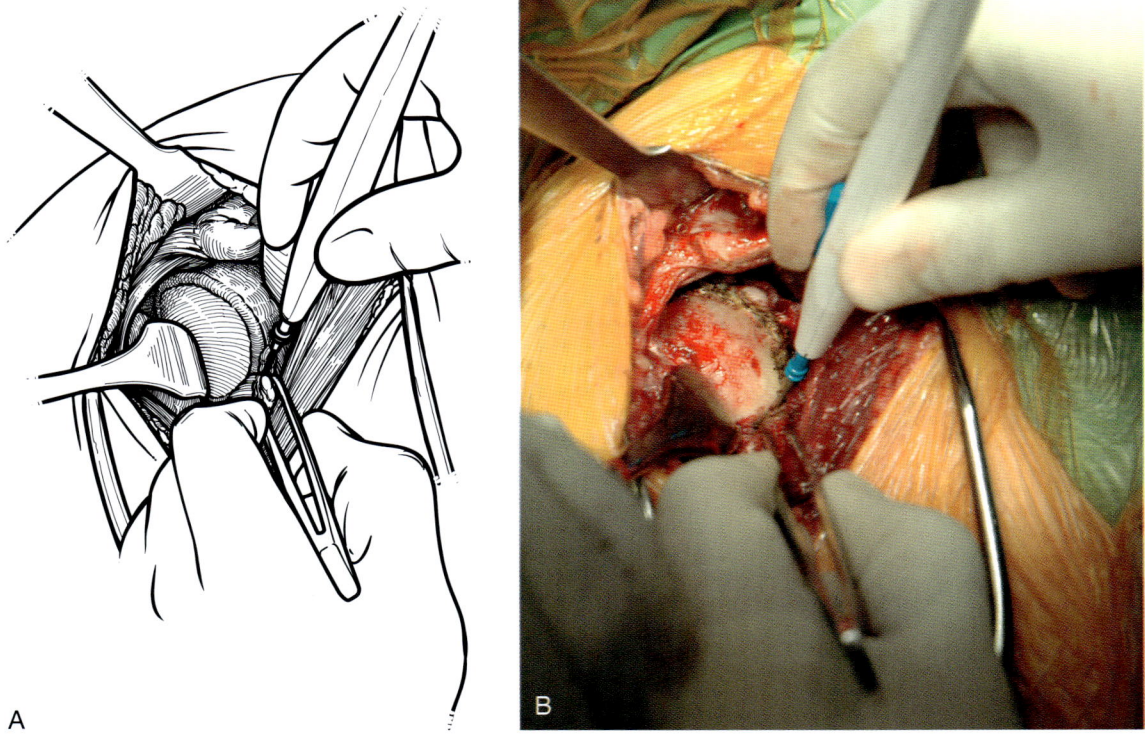

FIGURE 10.2 (A and B) Release the inferior capsule directly off the rim of the glenoid with the electrocautery.

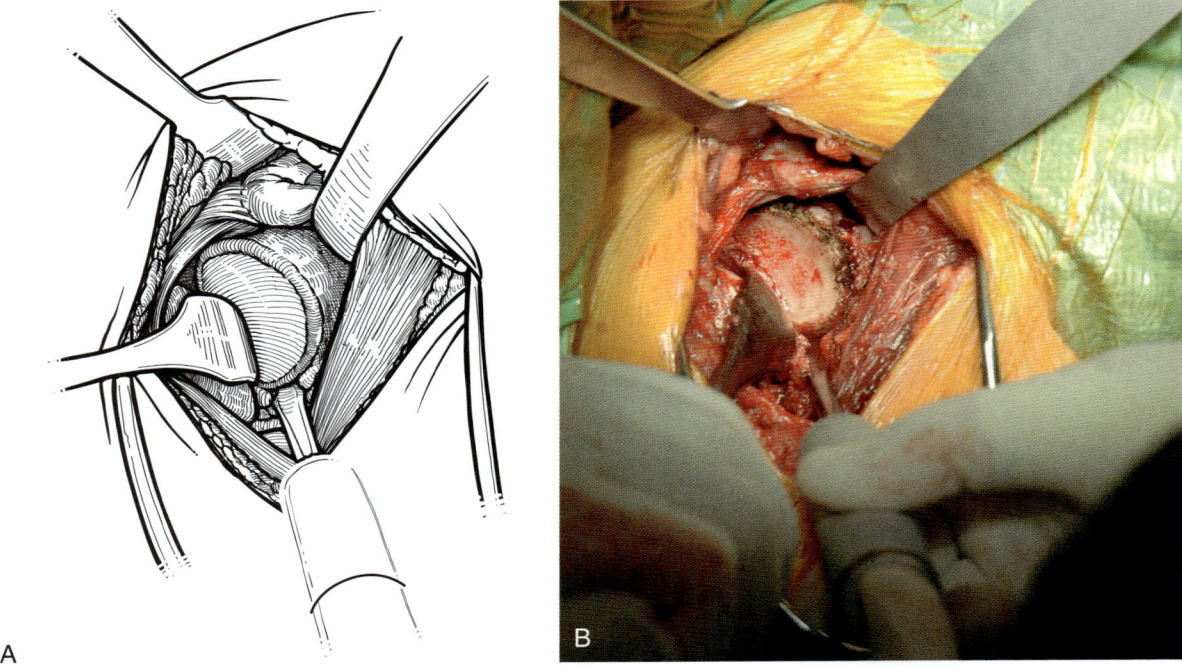

FIGURE 10.3 (A and B) A Cobb elevator is used to check the adequacy of the inferior capsular release.

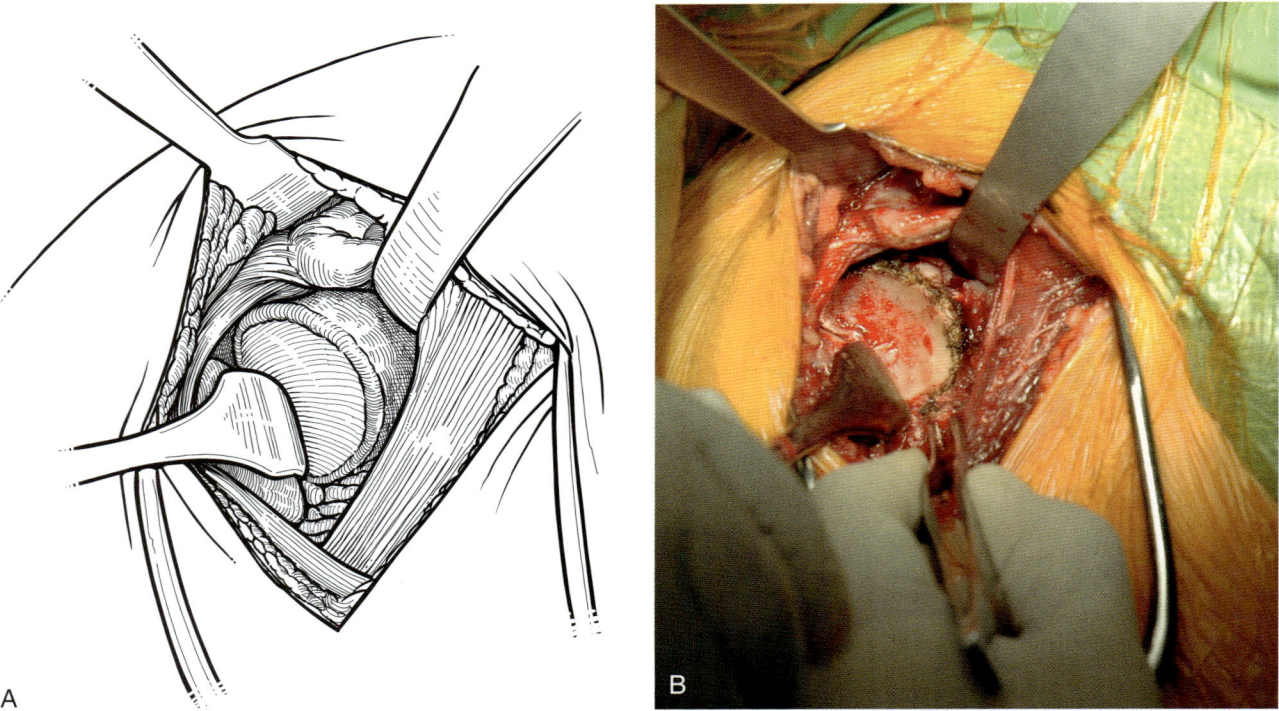

FIGURE 10.4 (A and B) Completed glenoid exposure. Note how much of the glenoid is visible even before humeral head resection.

Humeral component

CHAPTER 11

For unconstrained shoulder arthroplasty, both cemented and uncemented humeral stemmed components are available (Figs. 11.1 and 11.2). The incidence of aseptic loosening of cemented humeral stems is less than 2%.[1] Similarly, the incidence of aseptic loosening of uncemented textured humeral stems is negligible.[2] Implantation of smooth, polished humeral components without cement has led to a 55% incidence of humeral loosening and should be avoided.[1] In most cases of unconstrained shoulder arthroplasty, the choice of cemented or uncemented humeral stems is based on surgeon preference. In our practice, we prefer the use of uncemented humeral stems in most cases. Use of uncemented humeral stems eliminates the time required for cement preparation and insertion. Our indication for use of a cemented humeral stem is preexisting deformity of the proximal humerus or severe proximal humeral osteopenia precluding initial fixation of an uncemented humeral stem. Many different prosthetic systems are available for unconstrained shoulder arthroplasty, and it is beyond the scope of this textbook to describe the specific techniques used for each of these systems. This chapter describes the technique for preparation of the proximal humerus with the prosthetic system we used at the time of printing of this textbook. Most of the steps are applicable regardless of the system used.

TECHNIQUE FOR INSERTION OF AN UNCEMENTED HUMERAL COMPONENT

Once the inferior capsule is released from the neck of the glenoid, as described in Chapter 10, humeral preparation begins (Video 11.1). The humeral head retractor is removed, and the humeral head is dislocated by externally rotating and extending the arm (Fig. 11.3). A Hohmann retractor positioned superior to the coracoid process is moved to the margin of the bare area of the humeral head articular surface (junction of the supraspinatus and infraspinatus) and a modified Hohmann retractor (see Chapter 3) is placed inferiorly and medially at the surgical neck of the humerus. This completes the proximal humeral exposure (Fig. 11.4). The presence and extent of humeral head osteophytes will vary with the underlying diagnosis. Whereas conditions such as primary osteoarthritis typically include large osteophytes, other conditions such as rheumatoid arthritis have a paucity of osteophytes. The anteroposterior radiograph is helpful in determining the presence and extent of humeral osteophytes. To identify the true anatomic neck of the humerus, the osteophytes are removed with a half-inch straight osteotome (Fig. 11.5). Typically a layer of adipose tissue is present between the osteophytes and the native humerus and aids in identifying the normal margin of the humeral head articular surface (Fig. 11.6). The insertion of the infraspinatus tendon should be readily visible on the posterior aspect of the humerus (Fig. 11.7). It is critical to visualize the infraspinatus to prevent damage to the posterior rotator cuff during humeral head resection. Additionally, in using a prosthesis with an anatomic design, the location of the posterior rotator cuff (infraspinatus) defines humeral version (which varies from 7 degrees of anteversion to 48 degrees of retroversion) and, consequently, version of the humeral head cut.[3] After the insertion of the infraspinatus is identified, the humeral head is removed at the anatomic neck of the humerus with an oscillating saw (Fig. 11.8). We prefer to make a freehand anatomic humeral head cut, but various implant-specific intramedullary or extramedullary cut guides are available if desired. The key is to avoid damage to the posterior rotator cuff regardless of the humeral head resection technique. We believe it acceptable to leave the bare area of the humeral head because this allows a margin of error for protection of the posterior rotator cuff during humeral head resection. Proper head resection at the anatomic neck correctly replicates humeral version. Fig. 11.9 depicts the relationship between humeral version and insertion of the rotator cuff.

We use a convertible anatomic prosthetic system (Aequalis Ascend Flex, Tornier, Inc., Bloomington, Minnesota) with the goal of reproducing the normal anatomy of each patient. This system permits specification of humeral stem diameter, humeral head diameter, anatomic neck inclination, humeral head offset, and convertibility to reverse total shoulder arthroplasty. The stem primarily achieves press fit in the metaphyseal portion of the humerus. With this system, the humeral canal is identified and entered with an awl; the entry point is typically on the anterolateral aspect of the cut surface because of the normal posterior and medial offset of the humeral head with respect to the humeral diaphysis (Fig. 11.10). A sequential series of humeral sounders are inserted to determine the diaphyseal size of the humerus (Fig. 11.11). The size and shape of the sounders correspond to the size and shape of the matching humeral components. Each sounder corresponds to two sizes depending on how far the sounder is advanced distally in the humerus. After determining the appropriately sized sounder, the sounder

Text continued on p. 94

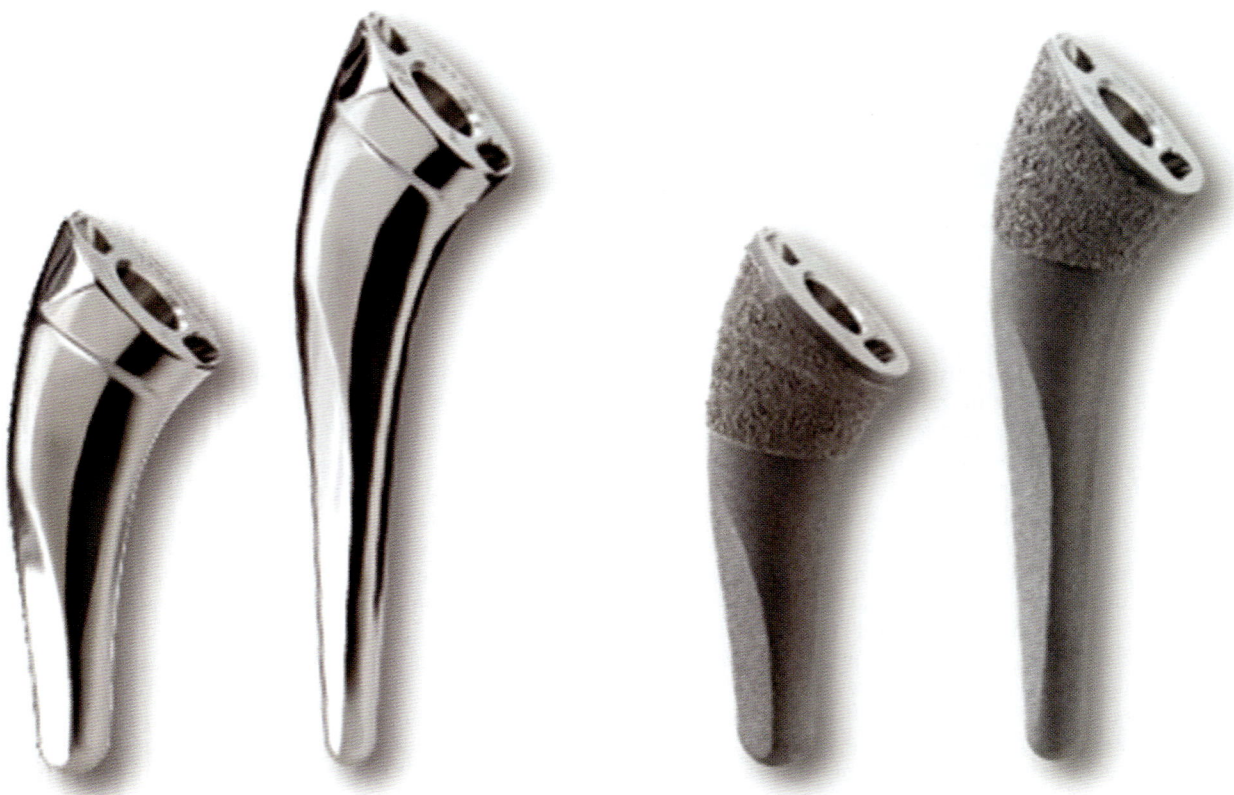

FIGURE 11.1 Cemented humeral stem. Note the smooth, polished stem design.

FIGURE 11.2 Uncemented humeral stem. Note the textured proximal finish.

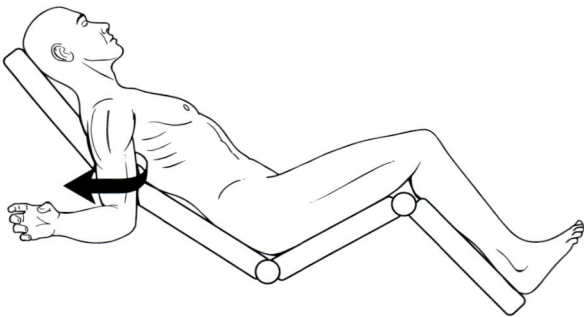

FIGURE 11.3 Maneuver (external rotation and extension) for dislocation of the humeral head.

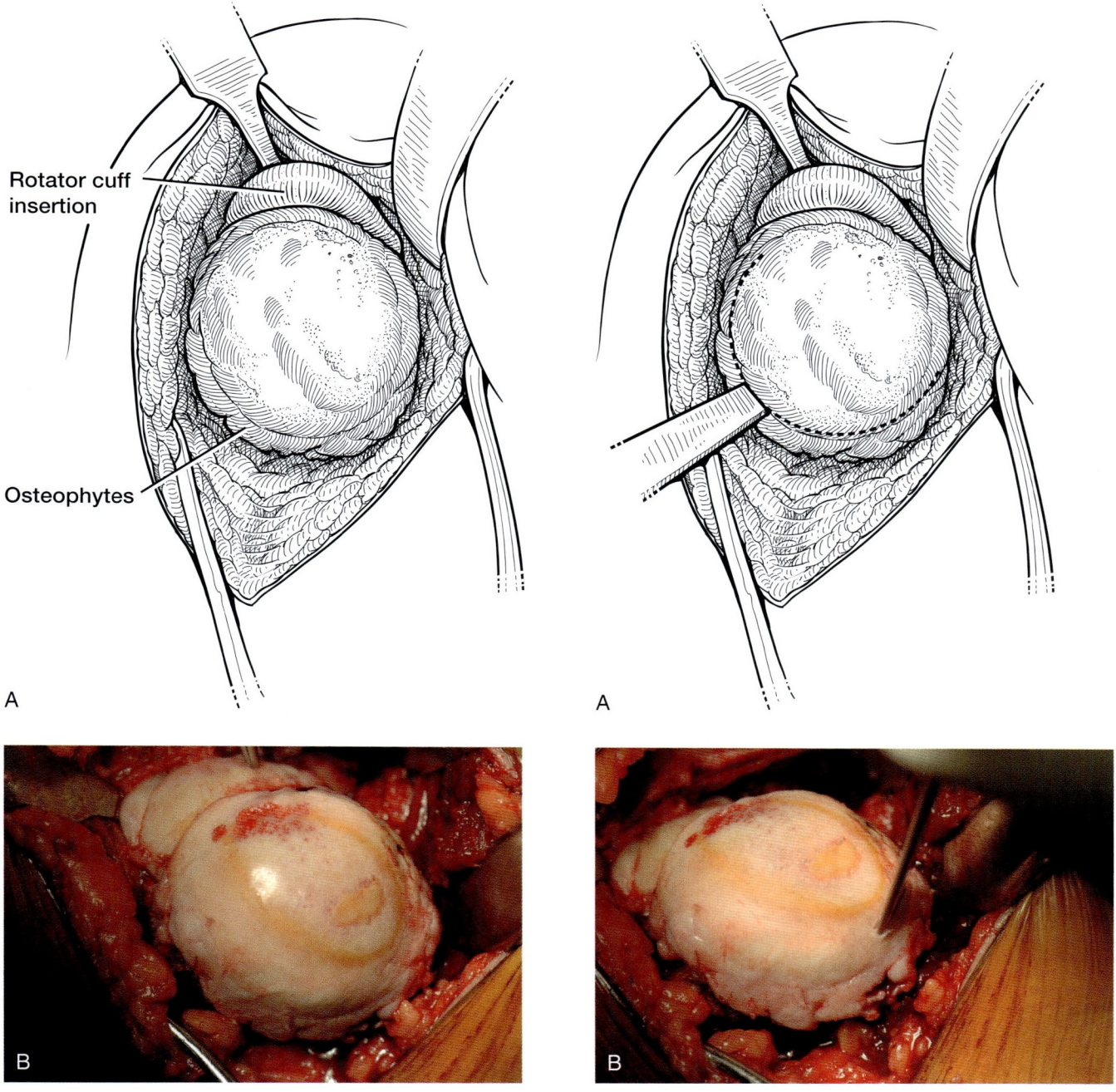

FIGURE 11.4 (A and B) The dislocated proximal humerus reveals peripheral osteophytes.

FIGURE 11.5 (A and B) Peripheral humeral osteophytes are removed with an osteotome to expose the anatomic neck of the humerus.

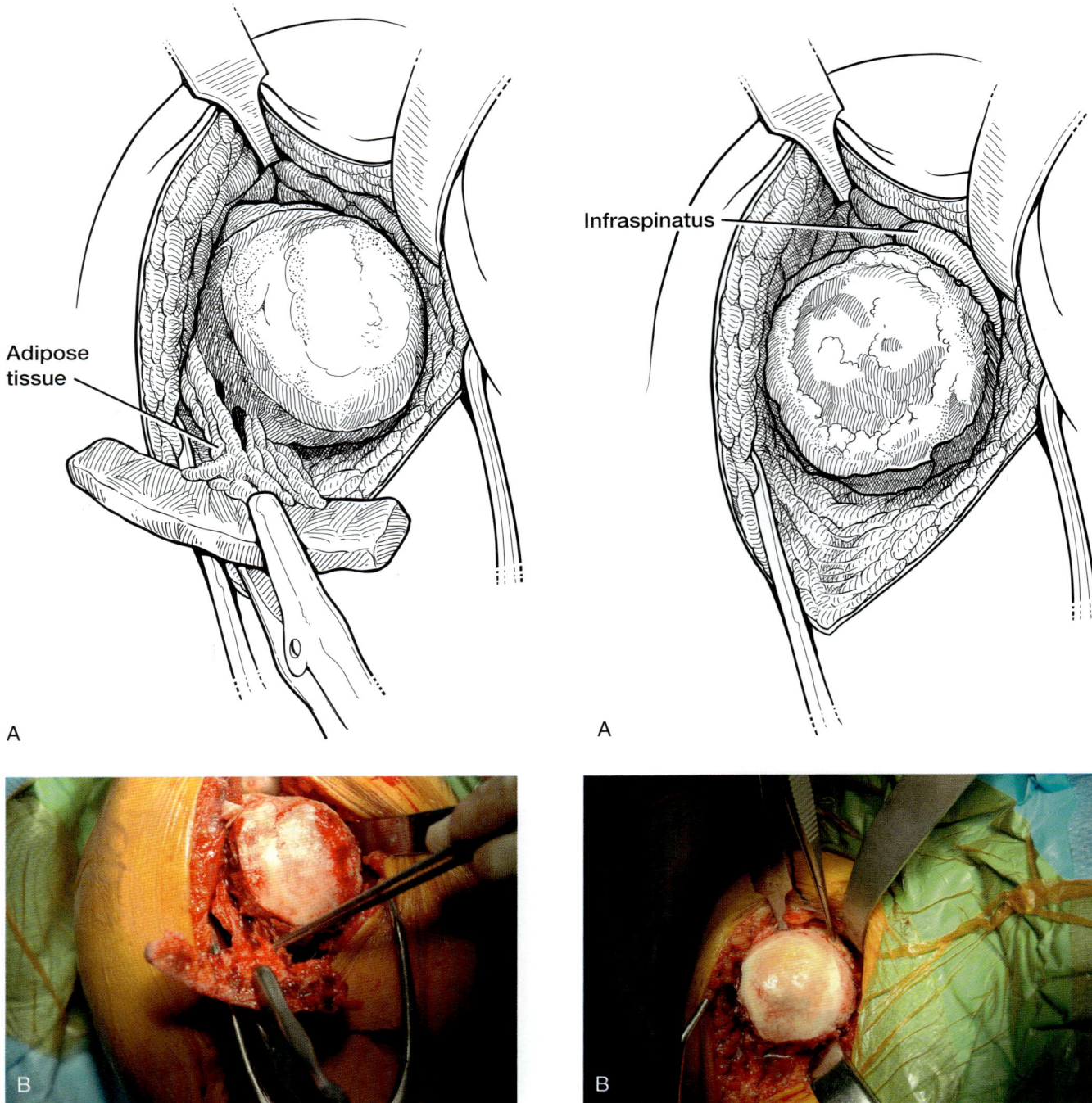

FIGURE 11.6 (A and B) A layer of adipose tissue interposed between the osteophytes and the native humerus.

FIGURE 11.7 (A and B) Identification of the infraspinatus insertion on the greater tuberosity at the posterior aspect of the humerus.

CHAPTER 11 ■ Humeral Component

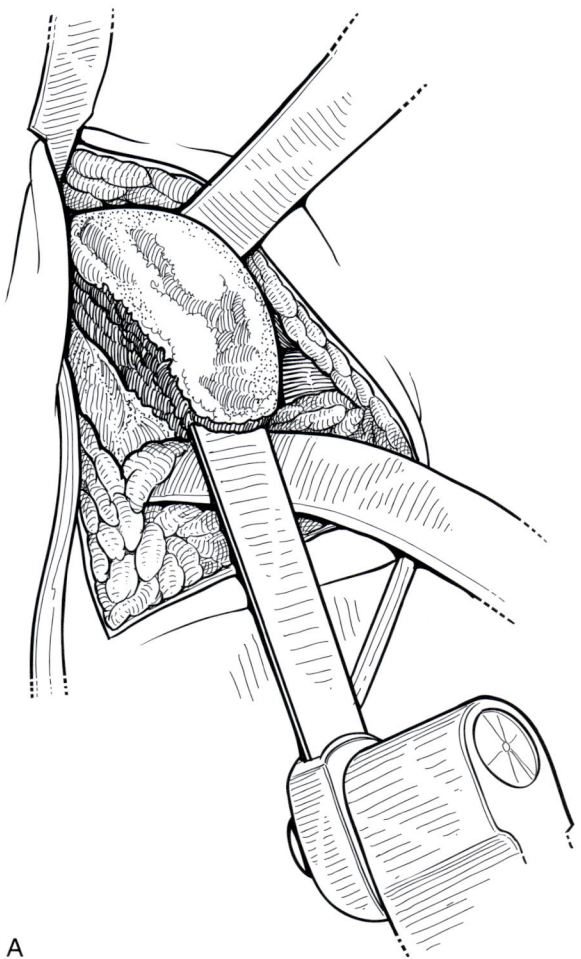

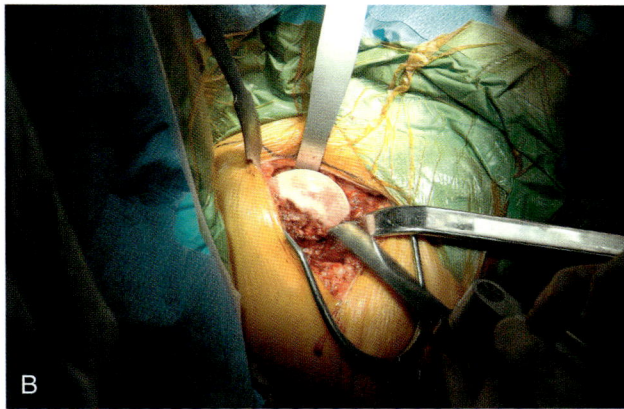

FIGURE 11.8 (A and B) Resection of the humeral head with an oscillating saw.

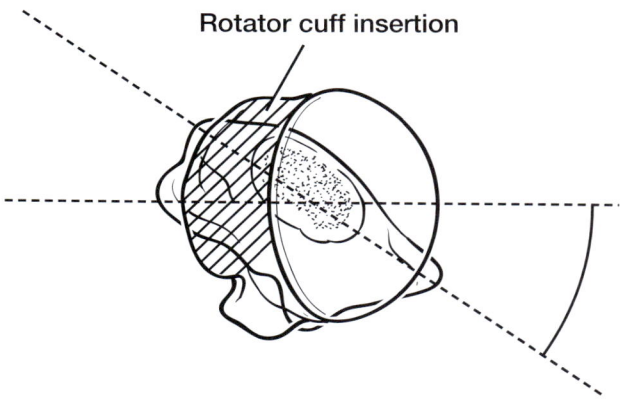

FIGURE 11.9 Depiction of the relationship between the insertion of the posterior rotator cuff (infraspinatus) and humeral version.

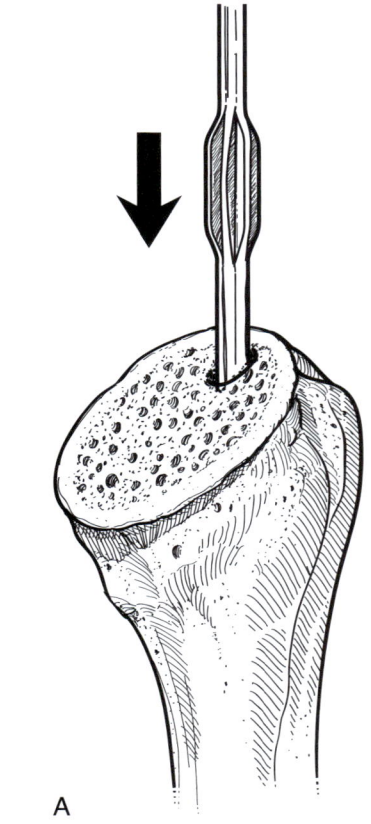

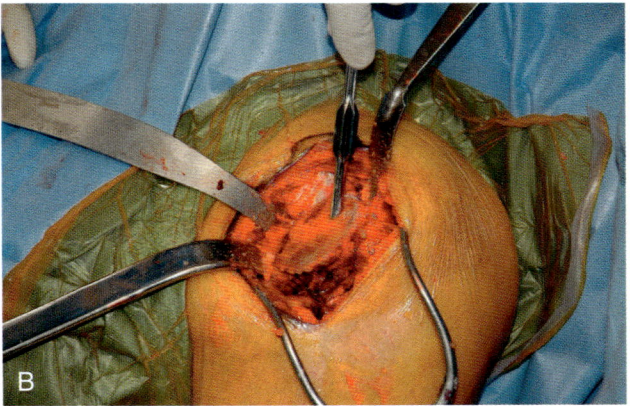

FIGURE 11.10 (A and B) An awl is used to locate and open the humeral canal. The entry point is generally located on the anterolateral aspect of the cut surface because of the normal posterior and medial offset of the humeral head with respect to the humeral diaphysis.

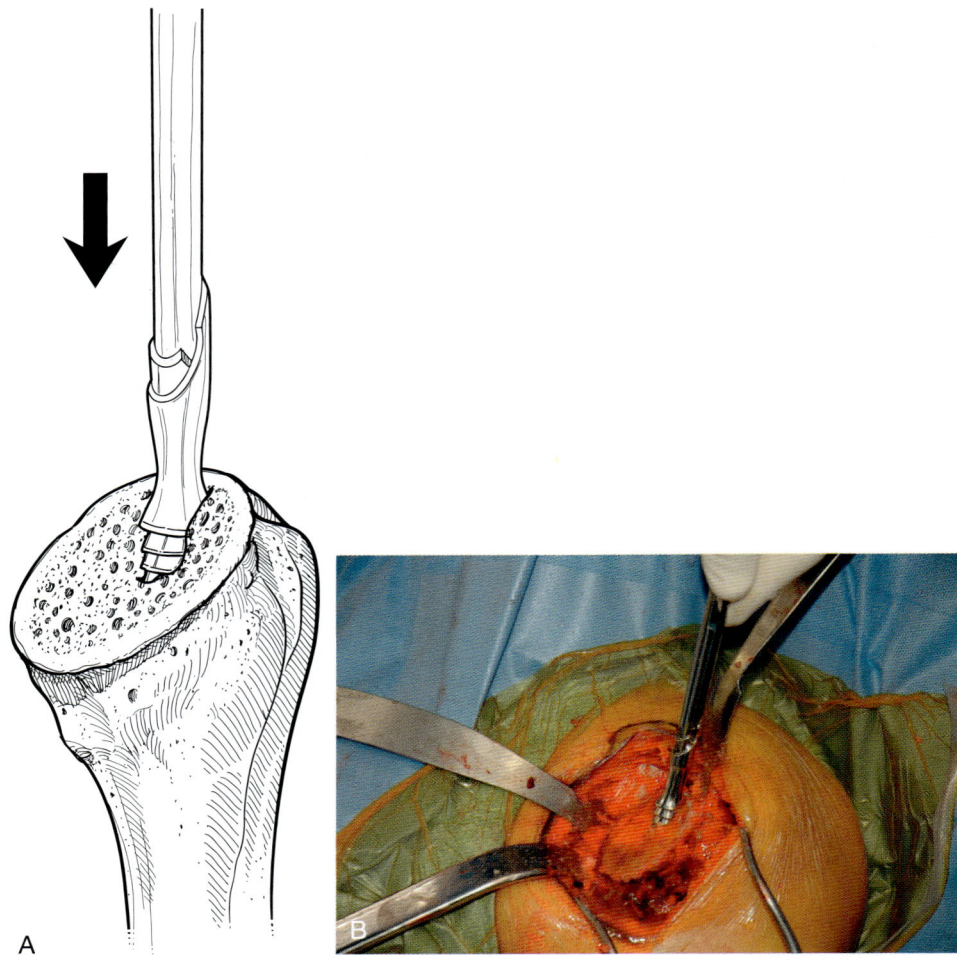

FIGURE 11.11 (A and B) Sounding of the proximal humerus.

is left in the intramedullary canal and the corresponding punch template attached (Fig. 11.12). The punch removes a small portion of bone medially to prepare for humeral compactor placement. The punch and sounder are removed. A sequential series of humeral compactors are placed next (Fig. 11.13). The sounders and humeral compactors are designed to compact bone rather than to cut or remove bone, which is common with reaming or broaching. We routinely start with the compactor that is at least three sizes below the final sounder size so as to prevent humeral fracture. For example, if the sounder was size 5, then we would start with a size 3 humeral compactor and work our way up to a size 5 compactor. The humeral compactors are sequentially inserted and impacted until the depth-stop contacts the resected edge (Fig. 11.14). The humeral compactors have a variable inclination angle, and the pivoting neck is locked into place with a screwdriver once the final compactor is in place and the depth-stop is flush with the resected edge (Fig. 11.15). The impactor handle used to insert the humeral compactor also accepts a version rod to determine the degrees of retroversion of the humeral component if needed in the case of altered proximal humeral anatomy (Fig. 11.16). The version is gauged off the version rod relative to the forearm. The size and press fit of the trial component can be tested with a "twist test," where the impactor handle is twisted to determine the press fit of the trial component (Fig. 11.17). The impactor handle is removed after the size of the trial humeral compactor and degree of version are determined (Fig. 11.18). If needed, a calcar planer or saw can be used to match the cut surface of the humerus to the compactor surface (Fig. 11.19).

A trial prosthetic humeral head is selected to match the size of the resected humeral head (Fig. 11.20). Most humeral heads are slightly elliptical; if this is the case, the smaller diameter is selected. Additionally, if the resected humeral head is between the sizes available in the prosthetic system, the smaller size is initially selected to avoid "overstuffing" the glenohumeral joint. The trial head is then placed on the trial compactor stem. The system we use incorporates variable medial and posterior head offsets, allowing the surgeon to position the head at the appropriate indexed positions. Additionally, two different offsets (high and low) are available for each head diameter (Fig. 11.21). Rotation of the head provides nearly limitless offset options. Graduated markings on the trial heads allow the selected offset position to be replicated with the final implant by aligning the marker on the head with the lateral aspect of the stem. The position that provides the best coverage of the cut humeral surface is selected (Fig. 11.22). Care is taken to avoid overhang of

Text continued on p. 99

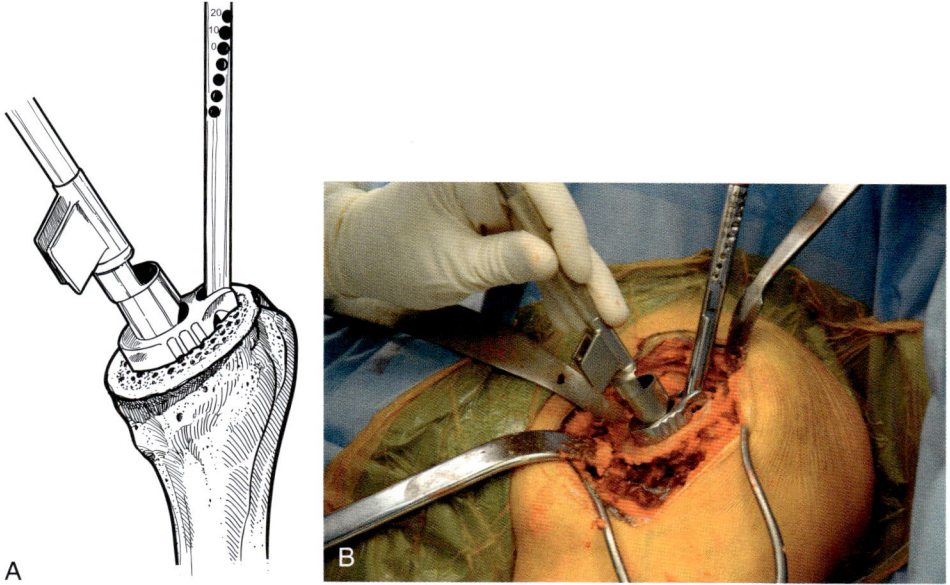

FIGURE 11.12 (A and B) A punch is used to remove a small amount of metaphyseal bone so as to permit progressive broaching.

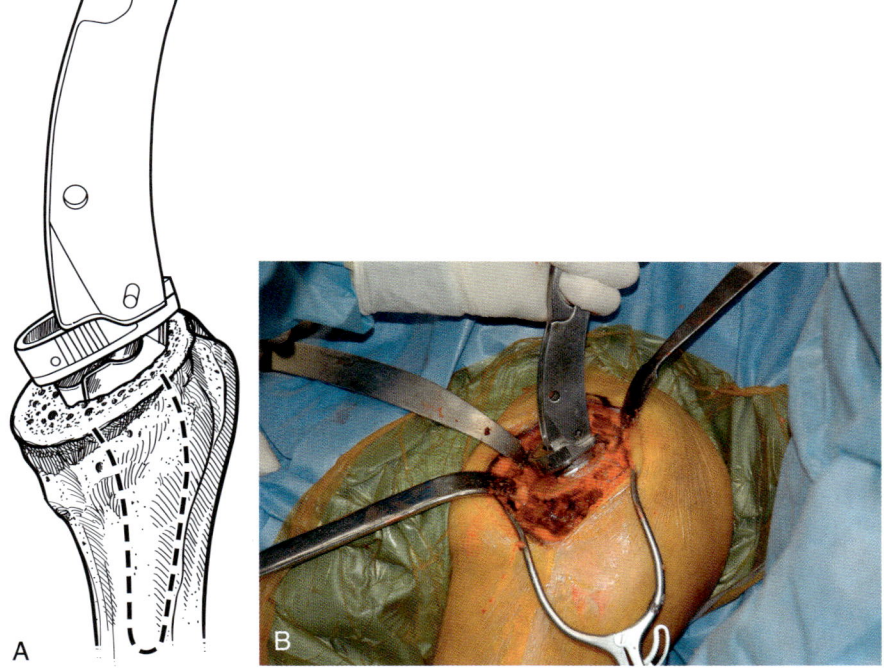

FIGURE 11.13 (A and B) Progressive metaphyseal broaching is performed.

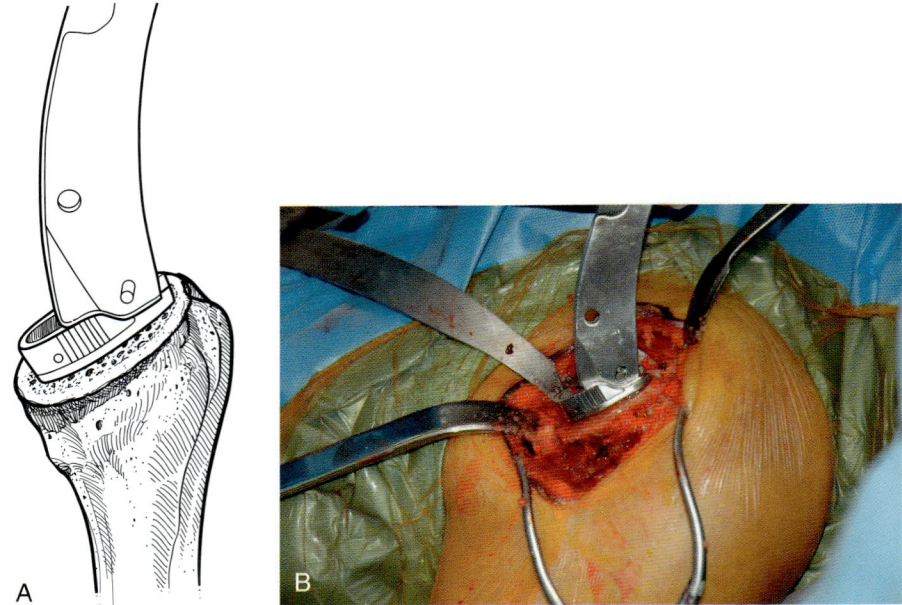

FIGURE 11.14 (A and B) The humeral compactors are sequentially inserted and impacted until the depth stop contacts the resected edge.

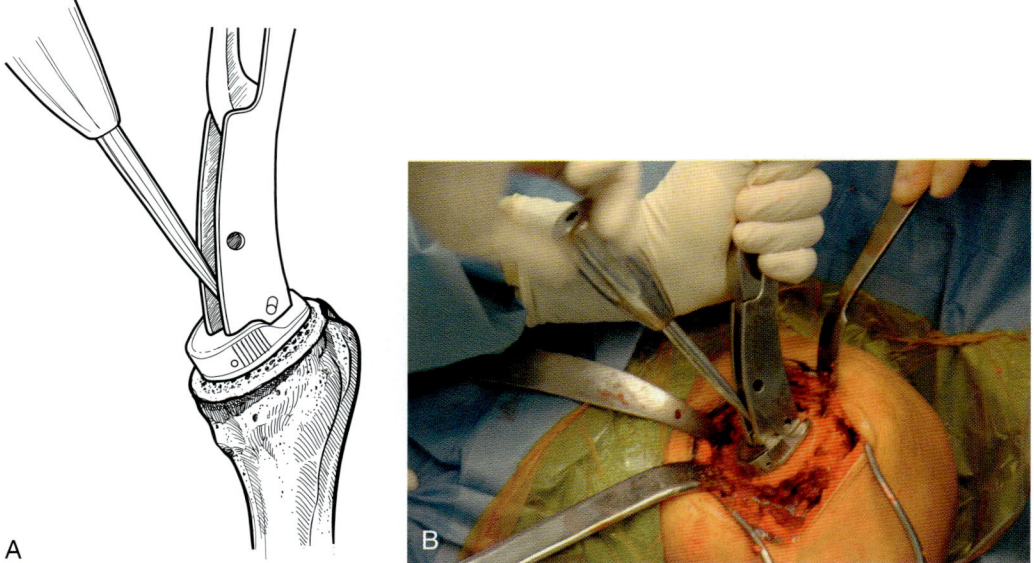

FIGURE 11.15 (A and B) The pivoting neck is locked into place with a screwdriver once the final compactor is in place and the depth stop is flush with the resected edge.

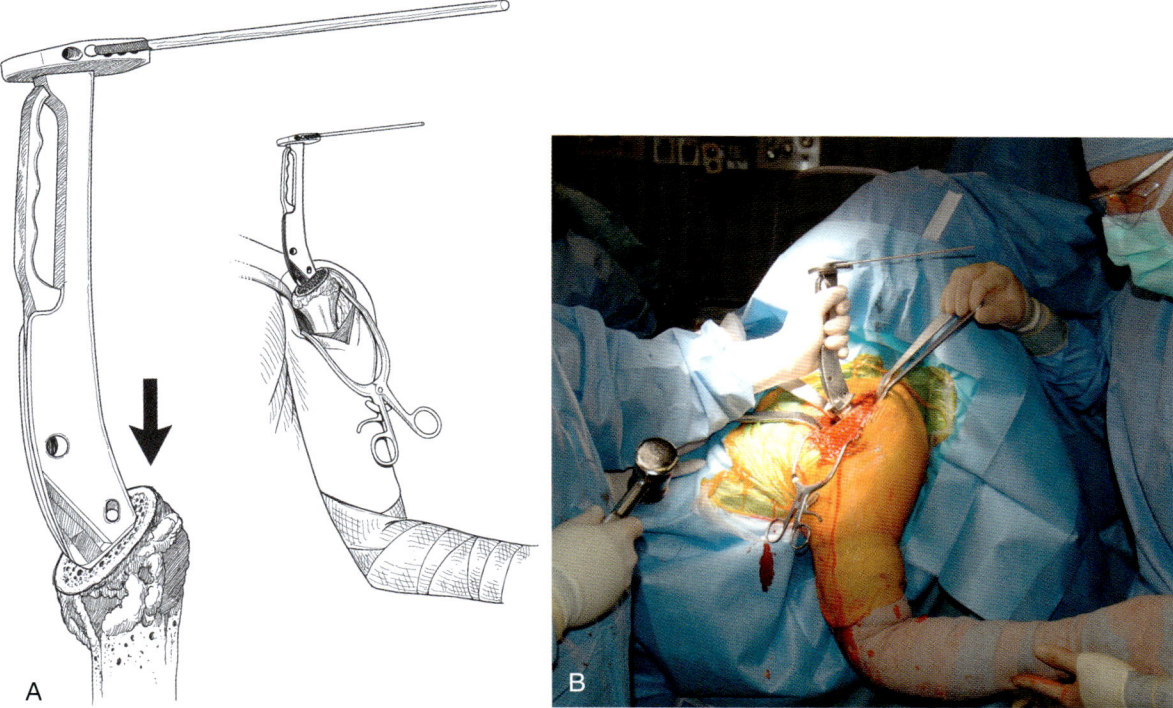

FIGURE 11.16 (A and B) Version guide, which aligns parallel to the forearm, can be used on the compactor handle. It is necessary to use this guide only in the case of altered humeral anatomy that affects the version (i.e., a rotational malunion).

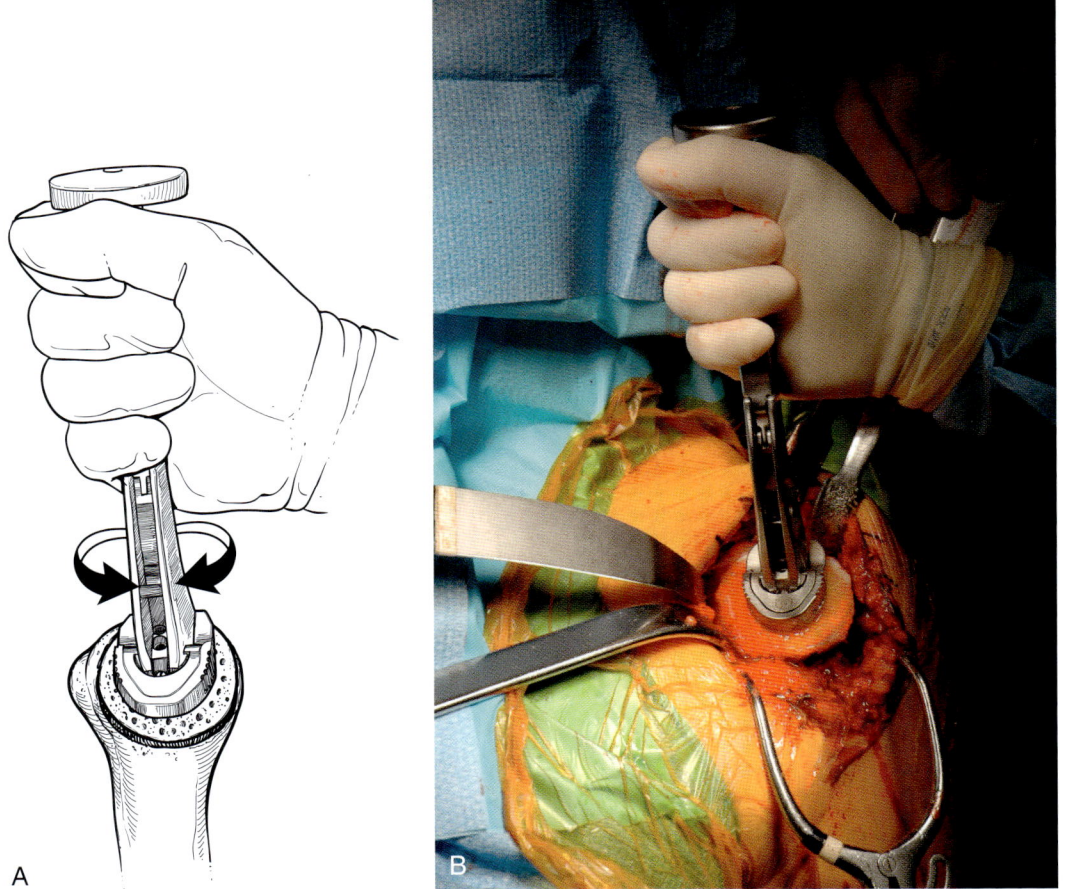

FIGURE 11.17 (A and B) The twist test to evaluate the rotational stability of an uncemented humeral component. If torsional stress applied to the compactor handle yields no gross motion and rotates the arm, there is adequate rotational stability.

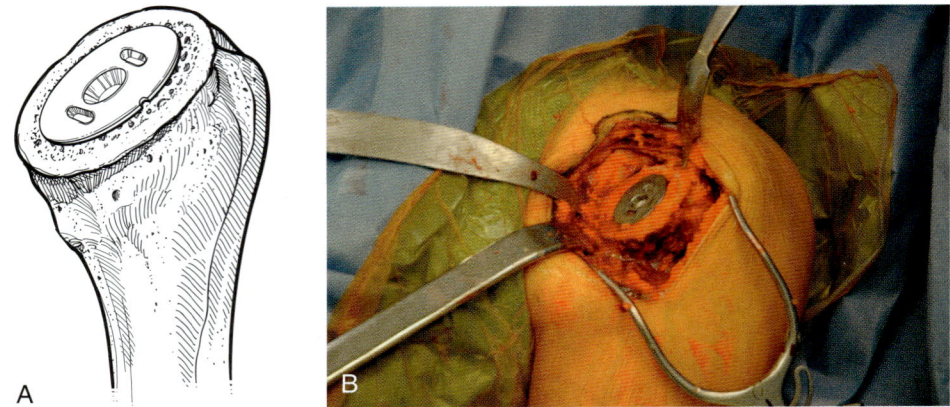

FIGURE 11.18 (A and B) Cut humeral surface with trial stem (compactor) in place.

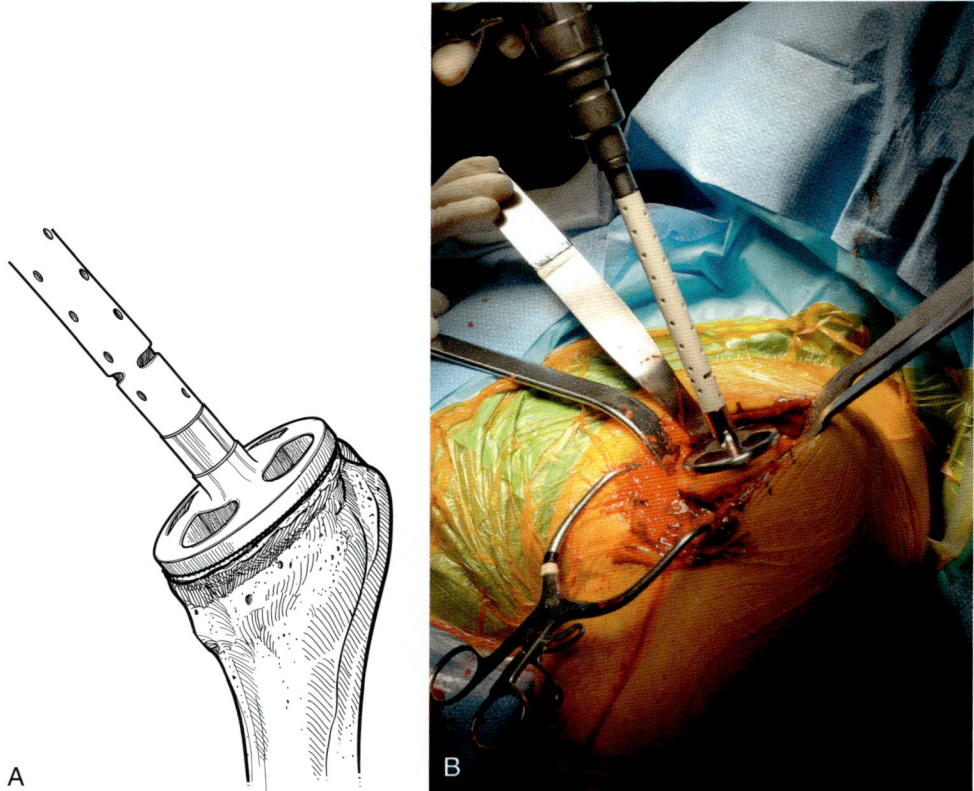

FIGURE 11.19 (A and B) A planer can be used to slightly correct inclination should the cut inclination differ slightly from the preset inclination angles available for the prosthetic system.

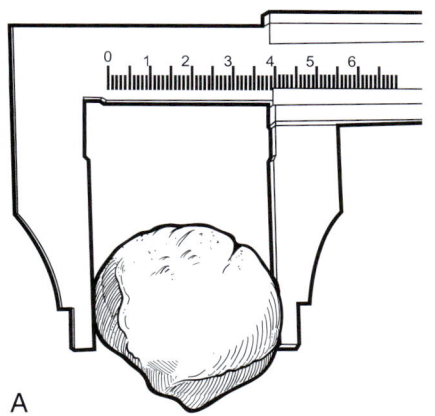
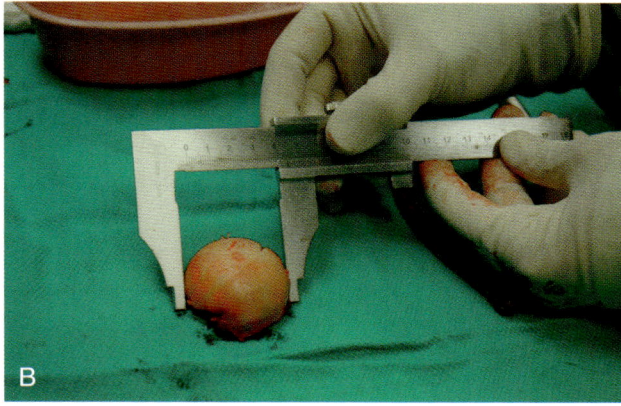

FIGURE 11.20 The resected humeral head can be measured with calipers or compared in size with the trial humeral heads available.

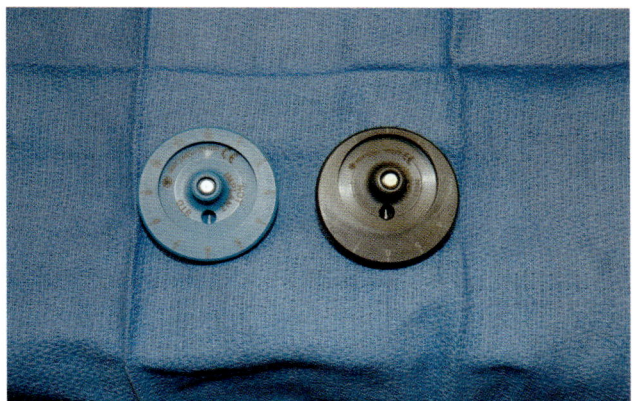

FIGURE 11.21 High- and low-offset heads available. The low-offset heads are 1.5 mm offset from the center and the high-offset heads range from 3.5 to 4.0 mm offset from the center, depending on the size chosen.

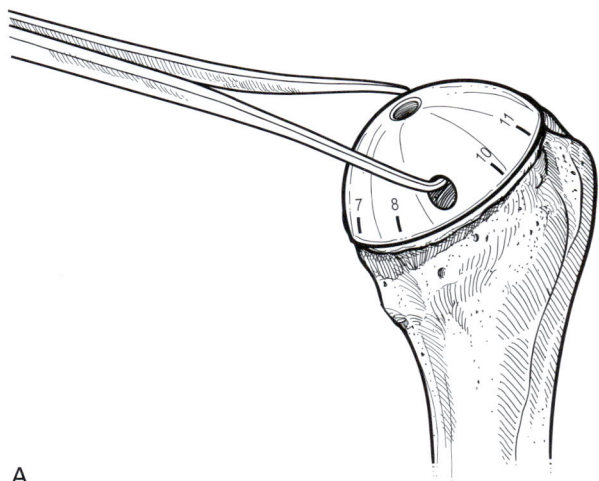
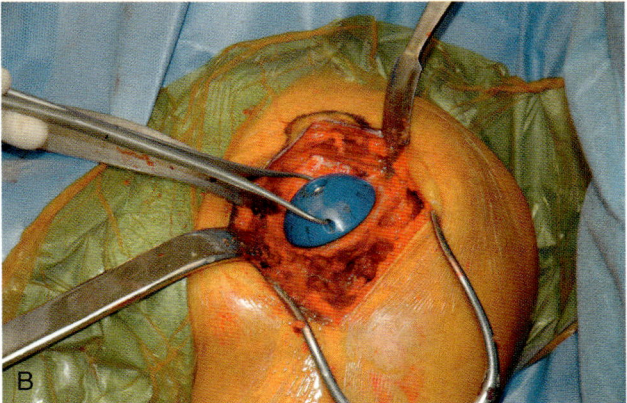

FIGURE 11.22 (A and B) Placement of the trial humeral head. The trial head is rotated until the indexed position providing the best coverage of the cut humeral surface is discovered.

the prosthetic head anteriorly, superiorly, and posteriorly so as to prevent impingement of the rotator cuff. Inferior overhang, though not ideal, is acceptable. If a large amount of overhang is observed at any index, the selected head is probably too large. In areas in which the prosthetic head does not quite cover the cut humeral surface, a rongeur can be used to trim the cut surface and create a better fit. If a glenoid component is to be inserted, the trial head is removed and the cut humeral surface is covered with a humeral cut protector to prevent deformation of the humeral cut surface during glenoid preparation and implantation (Fig. 11.23). Care is taken to note the humeral head offset index before disassembling the trial humeral component so that the final humeral implant may be properly assembled.

After the cut protector has been inserted, tenotomy or tenodesis of the biceps tendon is performed (as described in Chapter 5), the glenoid is addressed (as described in Chapter 12), and soft tissue balancing is completed (as described in Chapter 13) in cases of total shoulder arthroplasty. The humeral trial (compactor) is removed and the proper inclination confirmed (Fig. 11.24). The final humeral implant is assembled on the back table by an assistant (Fig. 11.25). Before insertion of the final humeral implant, three no. 2 nonabsorbable braided sutures are placed through the humeral stump of the subscapularis tendon, into the lesser tuberosity, and out through the intramedullary canal of the humerus to be used in later reattachment of the subscapularis (Fig. 11.26). These sutures are tagged with three different types of hemostats to identify the sutures as superior, middle,

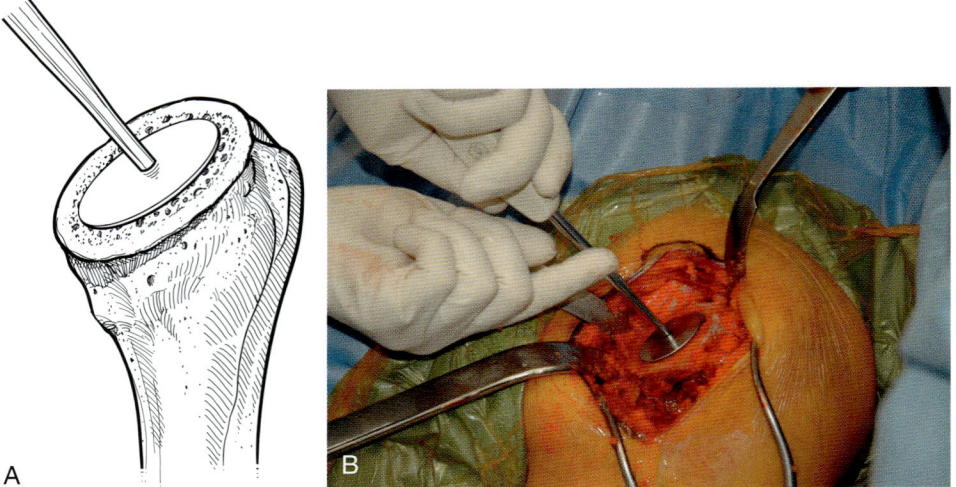

FIGURE 11.23 (A and B) A humeral cut protector is placed after removal of the trial humeral component and before glenoid preparation.

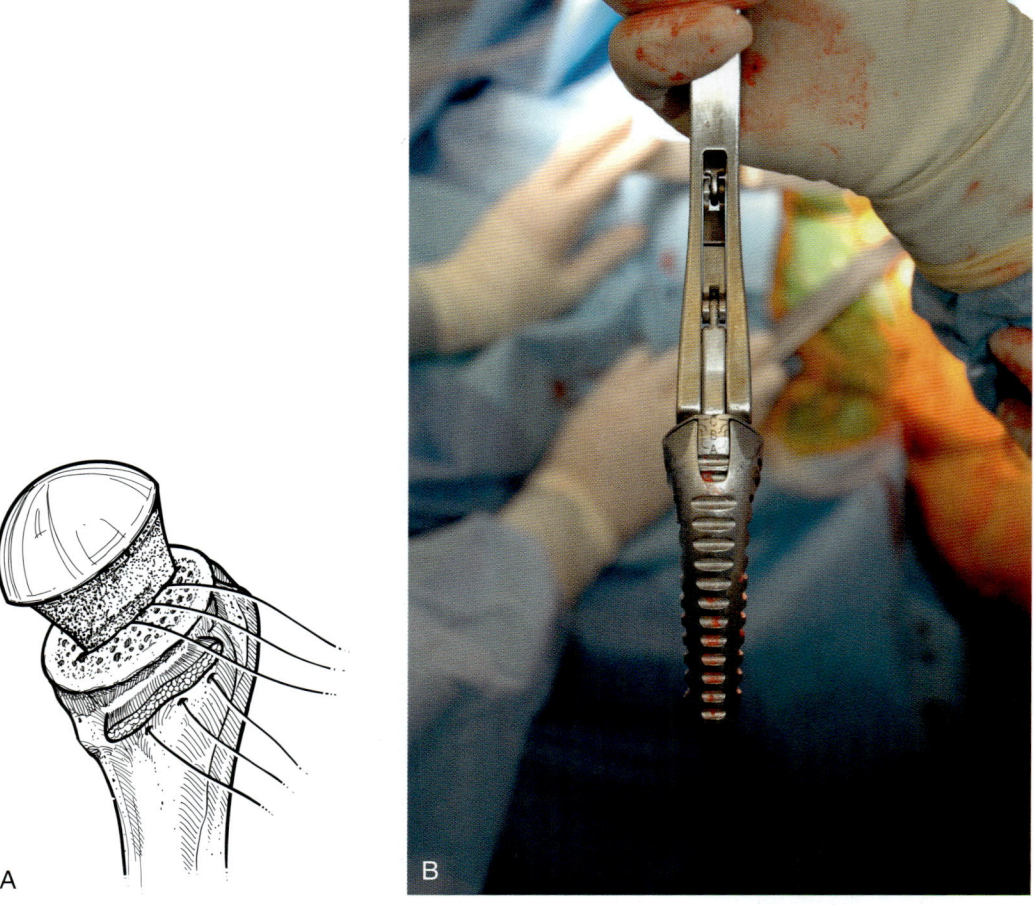

FIGURE 11.24 (A and B) The humeral trial (compactor) is removed and the proper inclination confirmed.

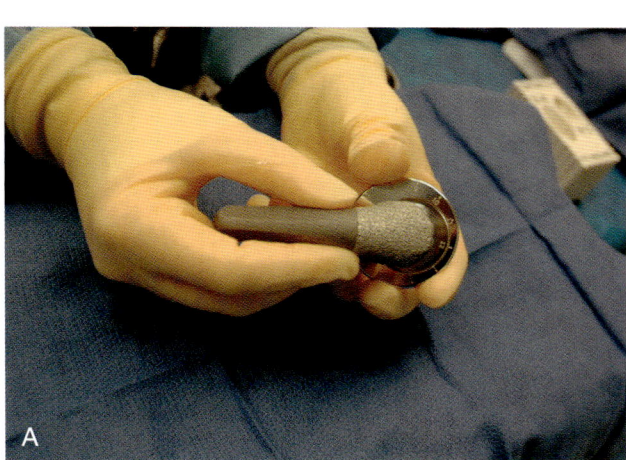
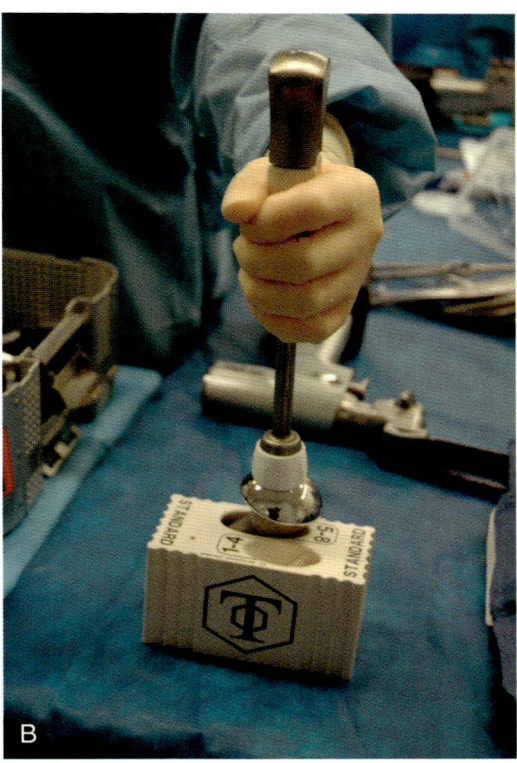

FIGURE 11.25 (A and B) Assembly of the humeral implant. The humeral head is impacted onto the humeral stem at the selected posteromedial offset index.

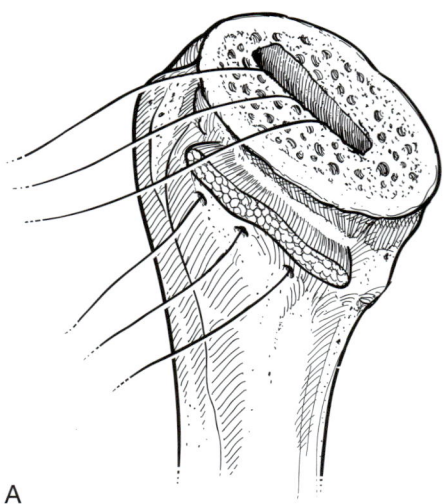

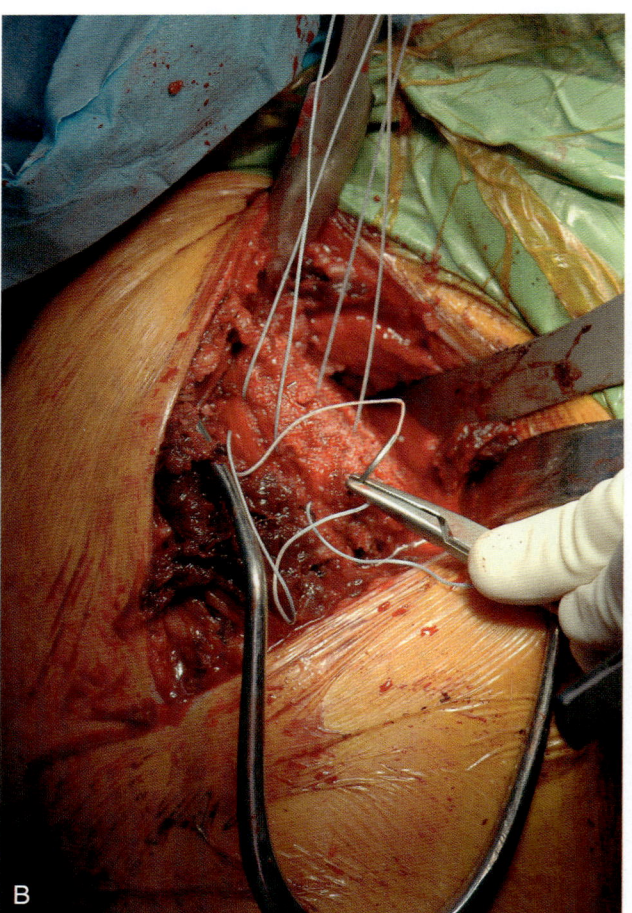

FIGURE 11.26 (A and B) Placement of transosseous sutures for later reattachment of the subscapularis.

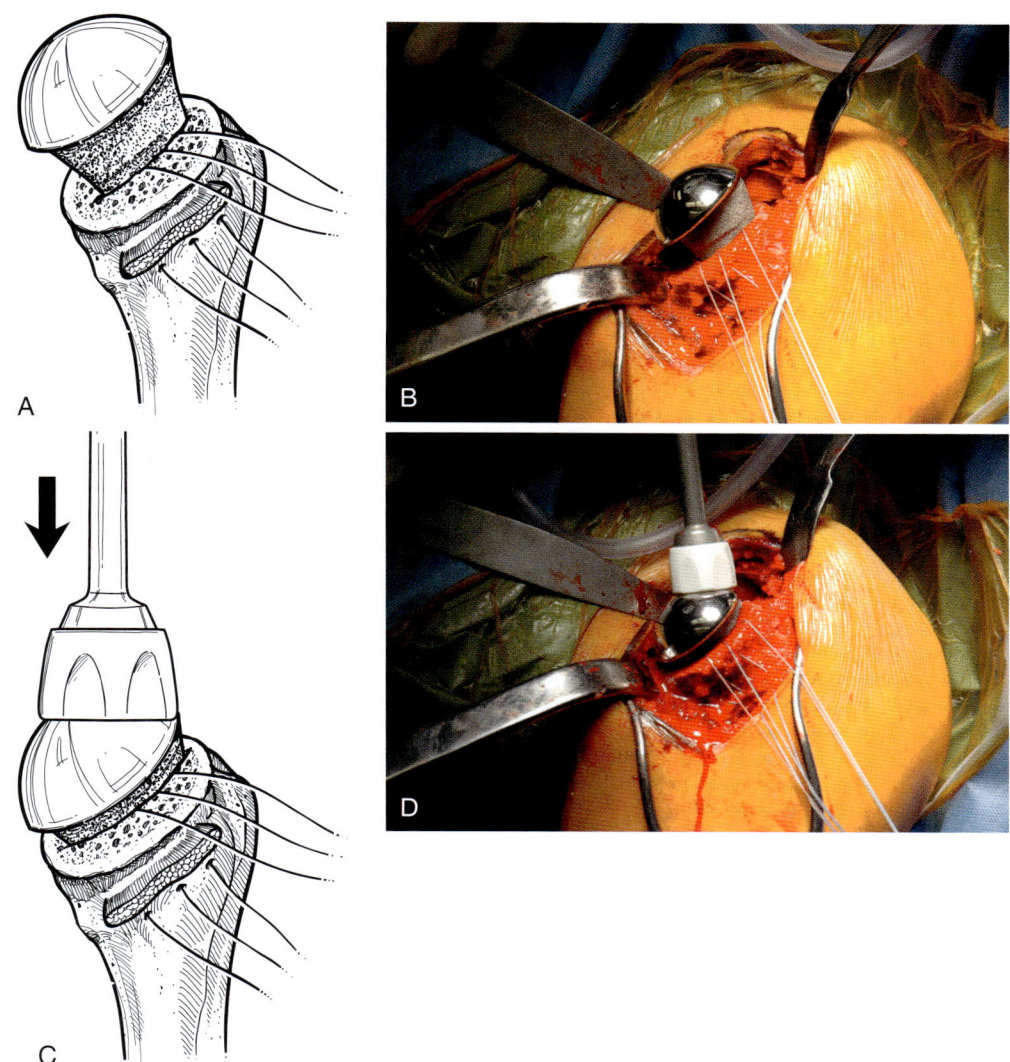

FIGURE 11.27 (A to D) Insertion of the humeral implant.

and inferior (we use a curved Kelly hemostat superiorly, a mosquito hemostat on the middle suture, and a regular hemostat inferiorly). The humeral implant is then impacted into place while making sure to avoid inadvertent rotation of the component during insertion (Fig. 11.27).

TECHNIQUE FOR INSERTION OF A CEMENTED HUMERAL COMPONENT

The technique for insertion of a cemented humeral stem is not too dissimilar from the technique described for insertion of an uncemented humeral stem. Humeral exposure, osteotomy, and humeral sided preparation are performed in the same way as for an uncemented humeral stem. Insertion of the trial stem and selection of the trial humeral head and its posterior medial offset index are identical to that for an uncemented humeral stem, as are humeral head trial removal and insertion of a cut protector. Preparation of the glenoid and soft tissue balancing are carried out as described in Chapters 12 and 13.

Before insertion of the humeral stem, an insertion device is used to place a cement restrictor 1 cm distal to the distalmost extent of the stem (Fig. 11.28). Sutures for reattachment of the subscapularis are placed as described earlier. The humeral canal is irrigated with sterile saline and dried with suction and gauze sponges. Bone cement (we prefer to use DePuy CMW 2 [DePuy, Inc., Warsaw, Indiana] because of its accelerated curing time of <8 minutes) is introduced with a catheter-tip syringe (Fig. 11.29). The canal is filled with cement and the assembled humeral stem is inserted and then seated with an impactor (Fig. 11.30). It is not necessary to pressurize the cement. Excess cement is removed with a Freer elevator. It is not necessary to allow the cement to cure before reducing the glenohumeral joint unless the humeral metaphysis is compromised (tuberosity fracture), in which case the cement should be allowed to cure before the glenohumeral joint is reduced.

104 SECTION II ■ Unconstrained Shoulder Arthroplasty for Chronic Disease

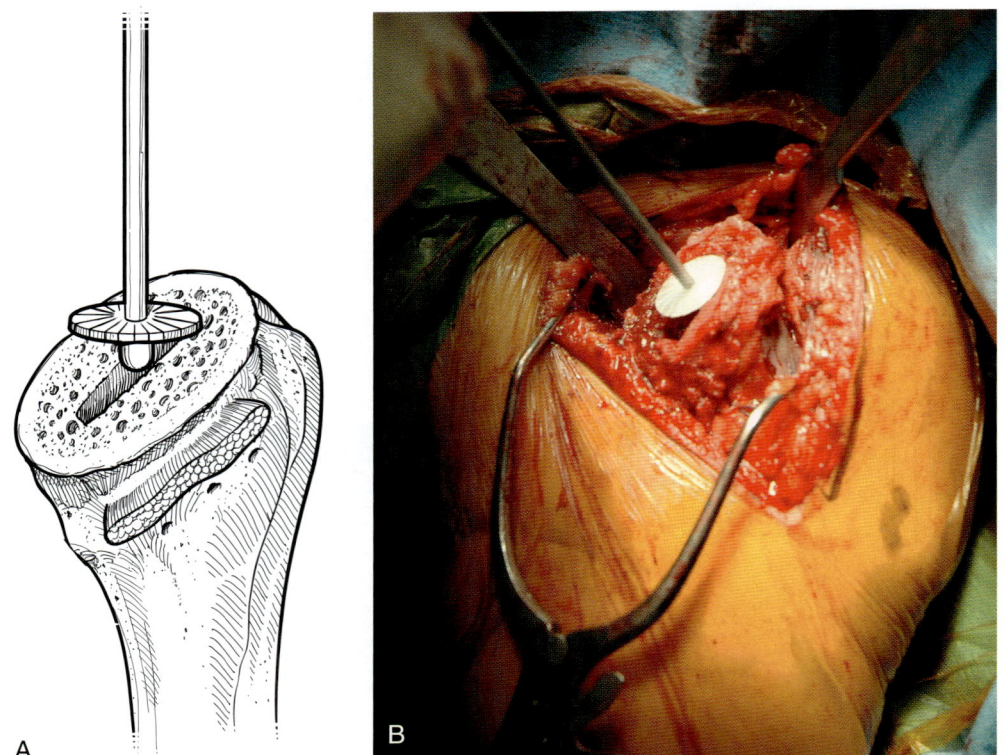

FIGURE 11.28 (A and B) Insertion of a cement restrictor before insertion of a cemented humeral stem. The cement restrictor allows 1 cm of cement distal to the tip of the humeral stem.

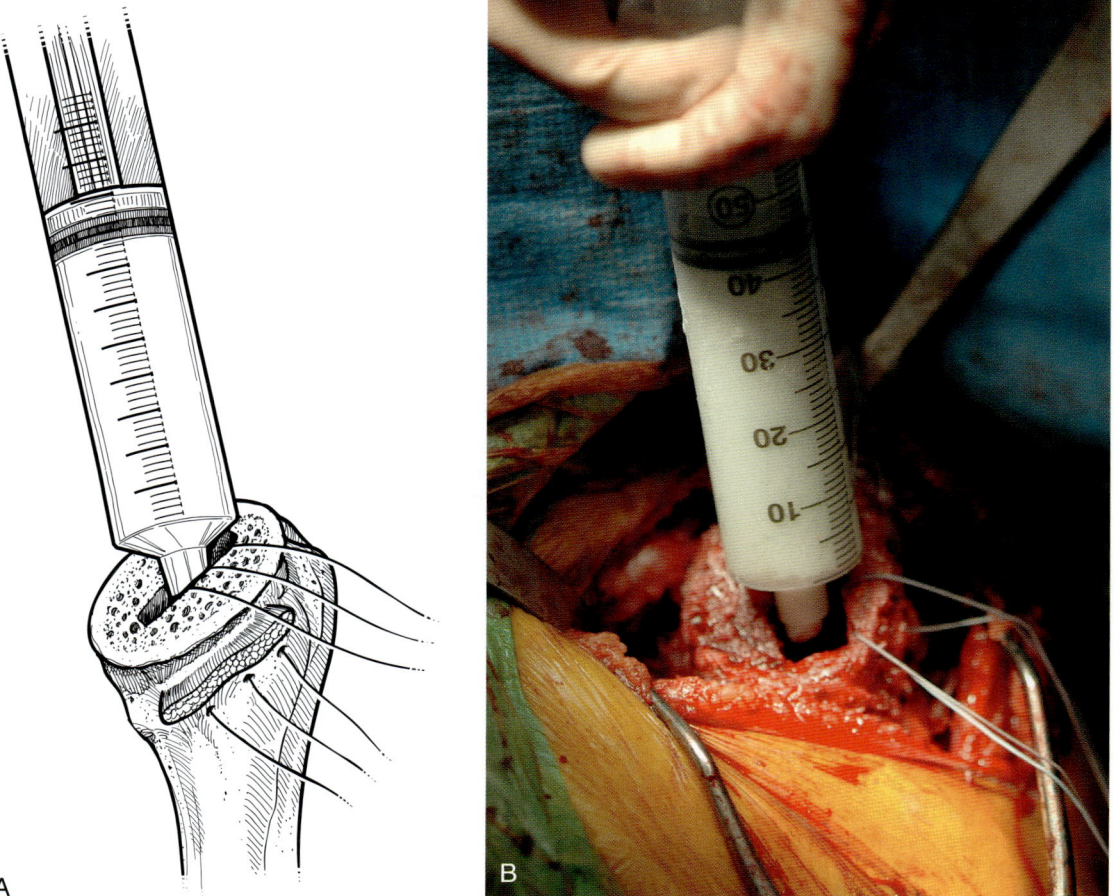

FIGURE 11.29 (A and B) Cement is inserted into the humeral canal with a catheter-tip syringe.

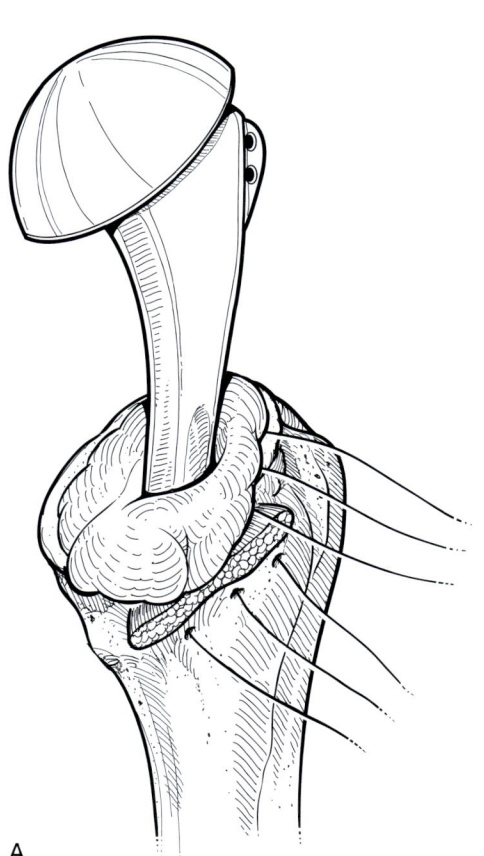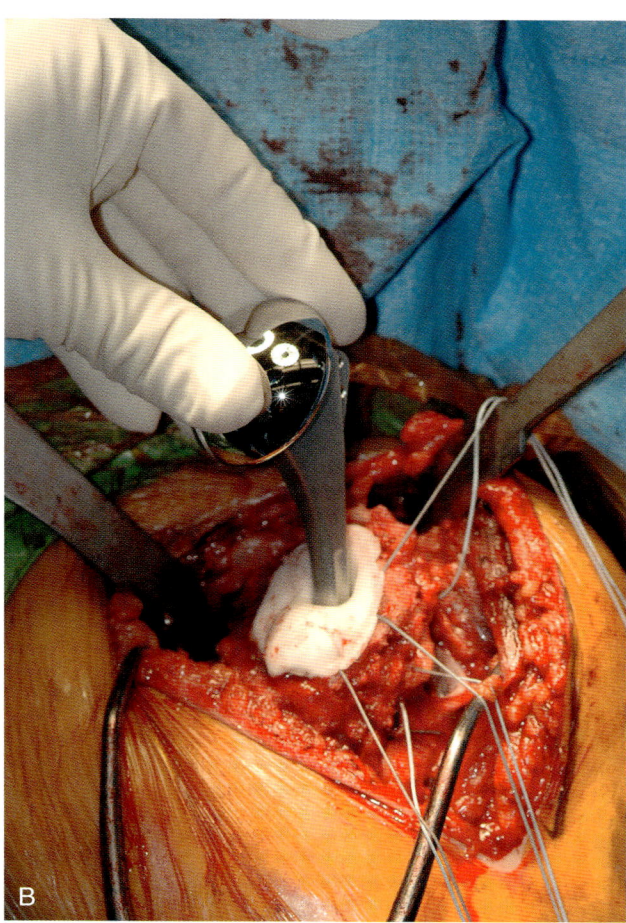

FIGURE 11.30 (A and B) Insertion of a cemented humeral stem.

REFERENCES

1. Trojani C, Boileau P, Coste JS, et al: Aseptic loosening in Aequalis shoulder arthroplasty. In Walch G, Boileau P, Molé D, editors: *2000 Prosthèses d'Epaule…Recul de 2 à 10 Ans*, Paris, 2001, Sauramps Medical, pp 437–441.
2. Matsen FA, III, Iannotti JP, Rockwood CA, Jr: Humeral fixation by press-fitting of a tapered metaphyseal stem: a prospective radiographic study, *J Bone Joint Surg Am* 85:304–308, 2003.
3. Boileau P, Walch G: Anatomical study of the proximal humerus: surgical technique consideration and prosthetic design rationale. In Walch G, Boileau P, editors: *Shoulder arthroplasty*, Berlin, 1999, Springer, pp 69–82.

CHAPTER 12

Glenoid component

Historically, the glenoid component has been the "weak link" of shoulder replacement. In addition to being the most difficult part of the surgical procedure, the glenoid component is the most likely site of component failure, which has led many surgeons to avoid glenoid resurfacing in nearly all cases. Fortunately, glenoid component materials and designs have improved greatly, as have techniques for implantation of glenoid components. Problems with the glenoid component are becoming less common, perhaps leading more surgeons to consider glenoid resurfacing in more cases. As detailed in Chapter 6, we prefer to implant a glenoid component in most nonfracture indications for unconstrained shoulder arthroplasty because of results superior to those of hemiarthroplasty in most diagnoses. The main contraindication to glenoid resurfacing in patients with a competent rotator cuff is insufficient glenoid bone to support implantation of a glenoid component. Such cases are readily identifiable with preoperative imaging studies (Fig. 12.1).

The steps involved in implantation of the glenoid component include obtaining glenoid exposure (detailed in Chapter 10), reaming the glenoid surface, selecting the size of glenoid component to be implanted, selecting the type of glenoid component to be implanted, preparing the native glenoid bone for implantation of the glenoid component (Videos 12.1 and 12.2), and final implantation of the glenoid component. Each facet of this process is detailed in this chapter.

REAMING THE GLENOID SURFACE

Reaming the glenoid surface serves two purposes: first, it provides a congruent surface that matches the apposing surface of the implant by removing any remaining cartilage and smoothing the osseous surface, and second, it corrects any deformity caused by bony wear, as identified on preoperative imaging (Fig. 12.2). If no deformity is present, "light" reaming is performed. However, in patients with posterior glenoid wear, the anterior portion of the glenoid should be preferentially reamed to correct the deformity. Recent research by Walch et al. has shown that preservation of glenoid subchondral bone is important to help resist compressive and eccentric forces and is important for longevity of the glenoid component.[1] Some newer glenoid components allow matching the backside radius of curvature of the glenoid component and glenoid reamer to the radius of curvature of the native glenoid to help preserve subchondral bone.

After humeral preparation and insertion of the humeral cut protector (see Chapter 11), the humeral head retractor is replaced to retract the proximal humerus posteriorly and expose the glenoid (Fig. 12.3). It is helpful to mark the center point of the glenoid with an electrocautery. It is also important to realize that with severe deformity or biconcavity, the center point will change (the new center point is posterior to the original center point after "reaming away" a portion of the anterior glenoid) by preferentially reaming the anterior glenoid, and this should be considered when identifying the center point. The system that we commonly use has glenoid components with variable backside radius of curvature options to match the native glenoid anatomy. The native glenoid radius of curvature is measured at this point using radius of curvature gauges (Fig. 12.4). A guide with a stop can be used when drilling a pilot hole through the center point of the glenoid (Fig. 12.5). The tip of a reamer of the appropriate glenoid size (see the next section) is introduced into the pilot hole (Fig. 12.6). Introduction of the reamer is usually the most difficult part of glenoid resurfacing. A few techniques are helpful when performing this portion of the procedure in exceptionally stiff shoulders. We first confirm with the anesthesiologist that the patient is adequately relaxed with paralytic agents. We then determine which posterior glenoid retractor yields the best exposure. We start with the large Darrach retractor or the modified Trillat humeral head retractor. If this proves inadequate, we will also try a Fukuada humeral head retractor, a large glenoid rim retractor, or one or more Hohmann retractors (these retractors are shown in Chapter 3). Many times it is necessary for the assistant retracting the humeral head to perform a maneuver with the humeral head retractor to facilitate insertion of the reamer. This is done by first forcefully retracting posteriorly and then relaxing the retractor to allow clearance of the posterior aspect of the reamer. The retractor can be left in place in a relaxed position during the actual reaming. This technique is illustrated in Fig. 12.7. Rarely, despite the use of these techniques for exposure of the glenoid and insertion of the reamer, it may not be possible to insert the reamer tip into the pilot hole. In this scenario, we remove the humeral head retractor completely and insert a laminar spreader between the glenoid and humerus. One limb of the laminar spreader is placed at the most superior aspect of the glenoid surface, and the other limb is placed on the cut surface of the proximal humerus. The laminar spreader is opened to distract the glenohumeral joint and retract the humerus laterally.

Text continued on p. 110

CHAPTER 12 ■ Glenoid Component

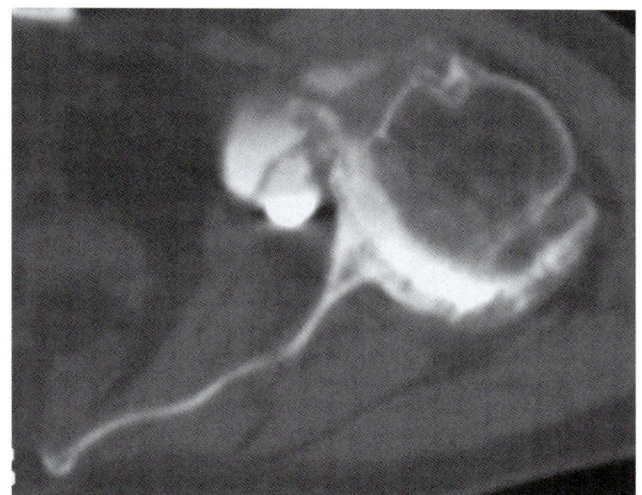

FIGURE 12.1 Case involving insufficient glenoid bone stock to allow implantation of a glenoid component.

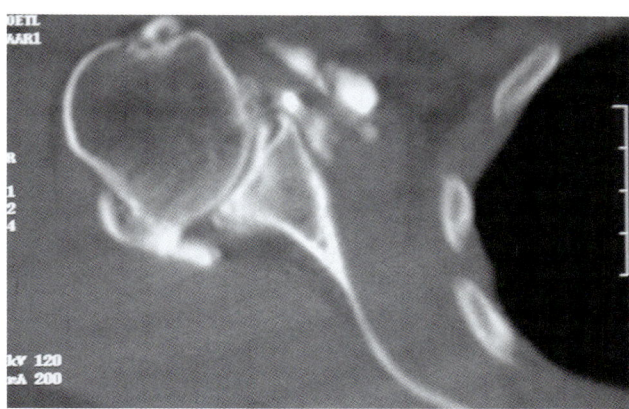

FIGURE 12.2 Example of identification of a biconcave glenoid deformity identified on preoperative imaging studies. This deformity should be corrected by eccentric reaming during the surgical procedure.

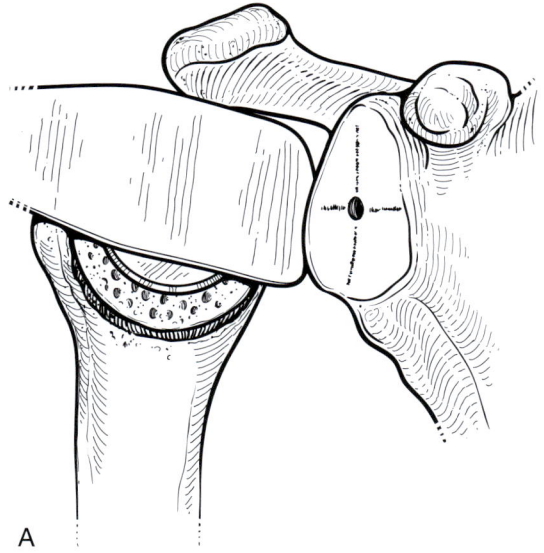
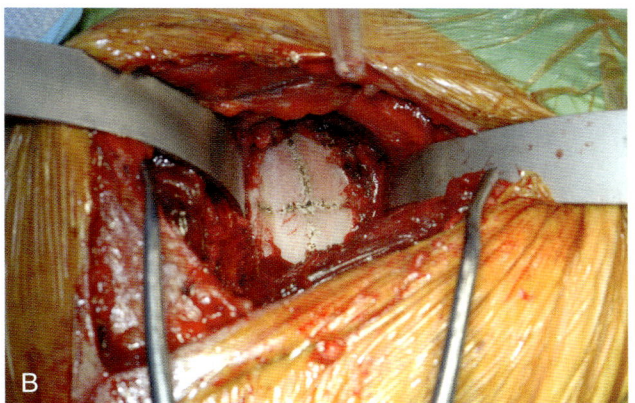

FIGURE 12.3 (A and B) Glenoid exposure. The center point of the glenoid has been marked with the electrocautery.

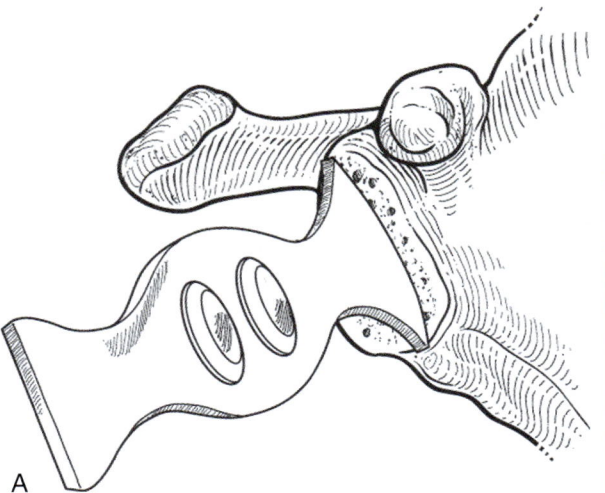
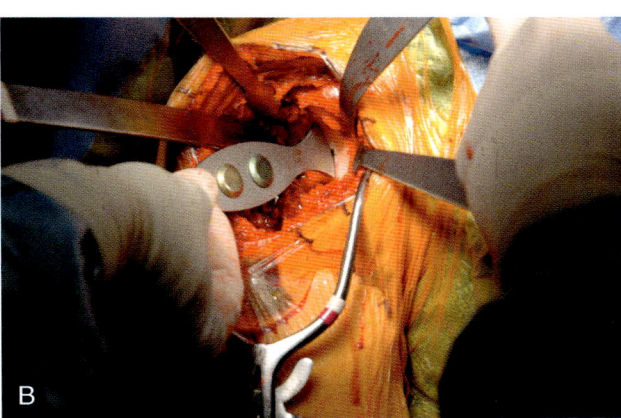

FIGURE 12.4 (A and B) Measurement of the radius of curvature of the native glenoid.

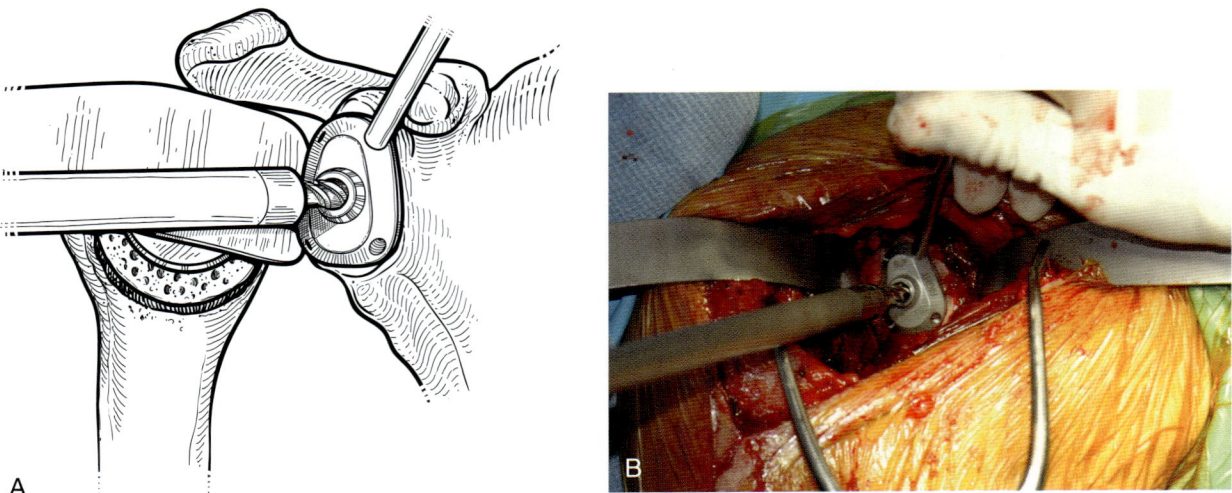

FIGURE 12.5 (A and B) Drilling of the central pilot hole in the glenoid.

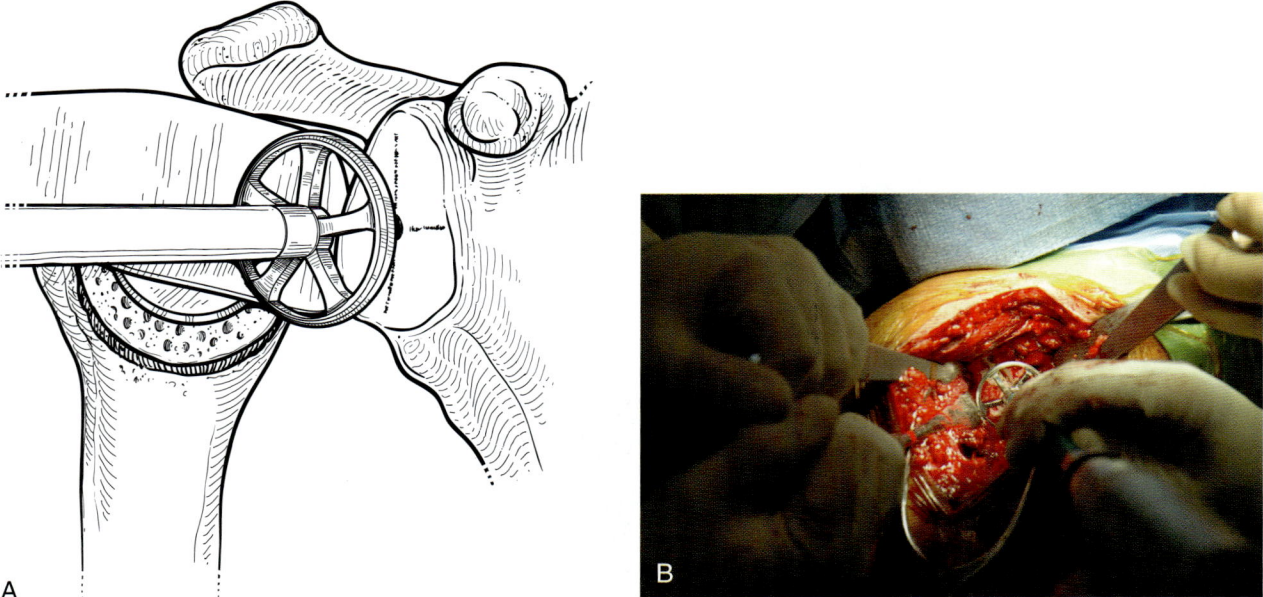

FIGURE 12.6 (A and B) Introduction of the reamer tip into the central pilot hole.

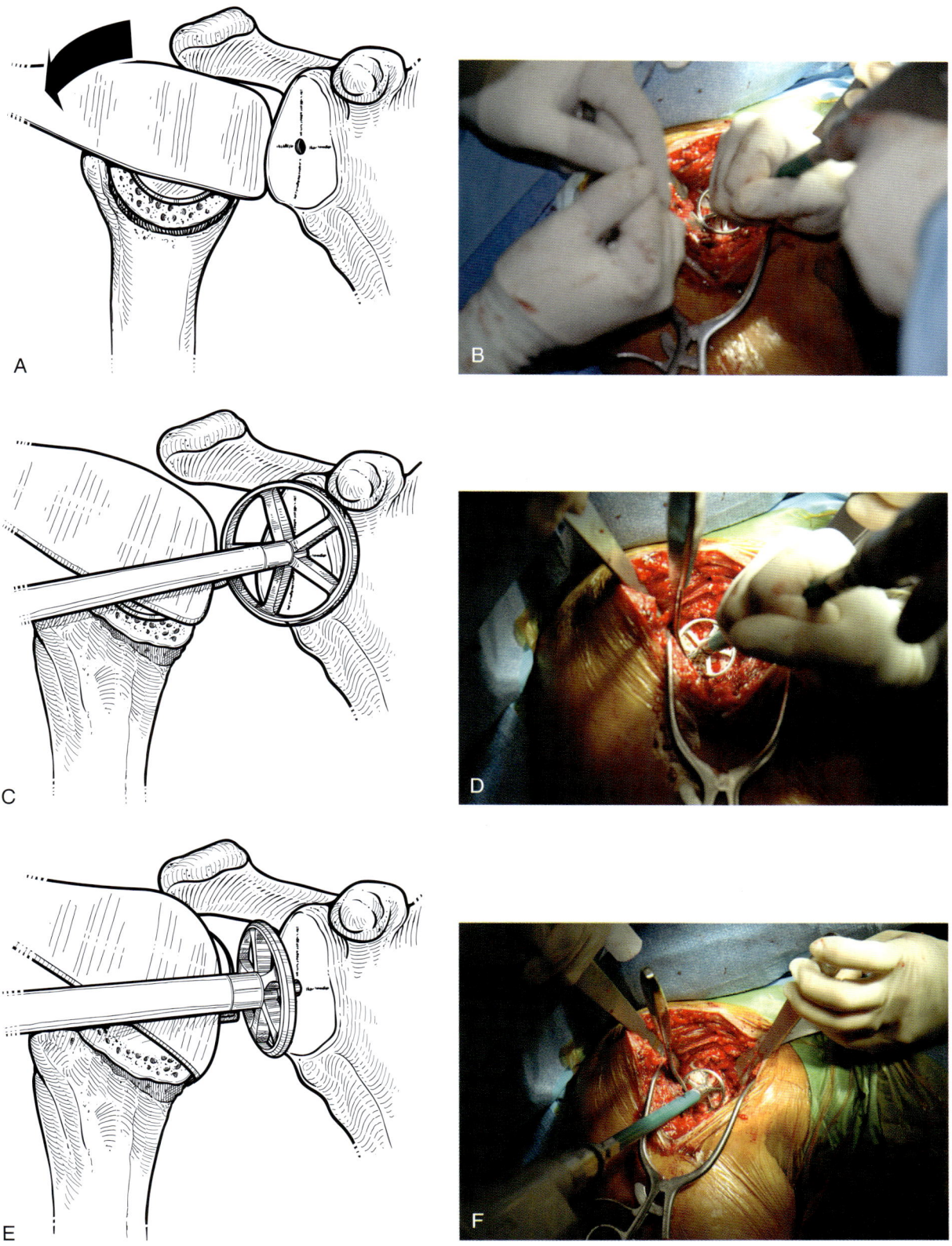

FIGURE 12.7 (A to F) Maneuver for insertion of the reamer in a stiff shoulder.

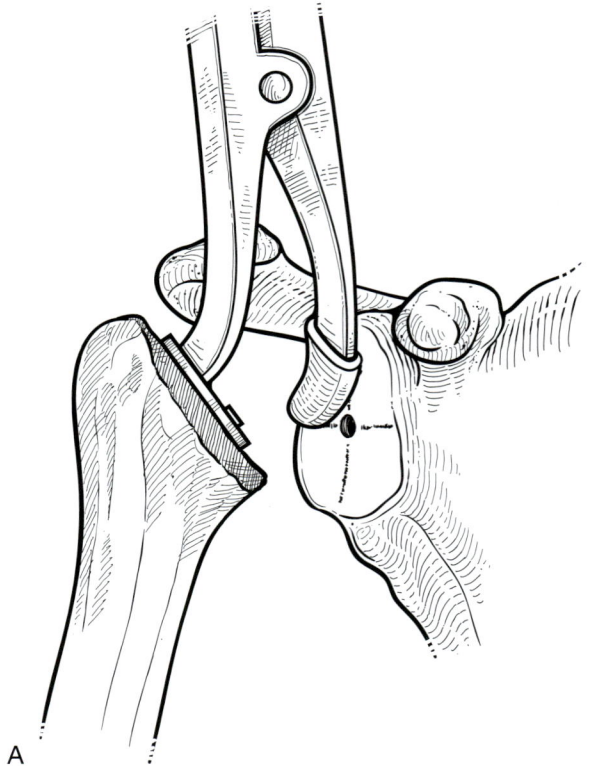

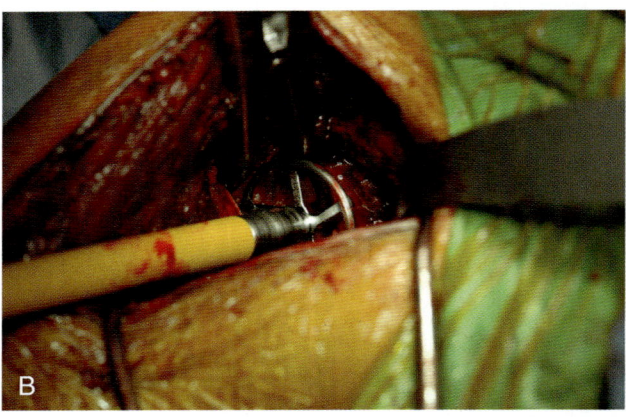

FIGURE 12.8 (A and B) Technique for using a laminar spreader to facilitate insertion of the glenoid reamer in an excessively stiff shoulder.

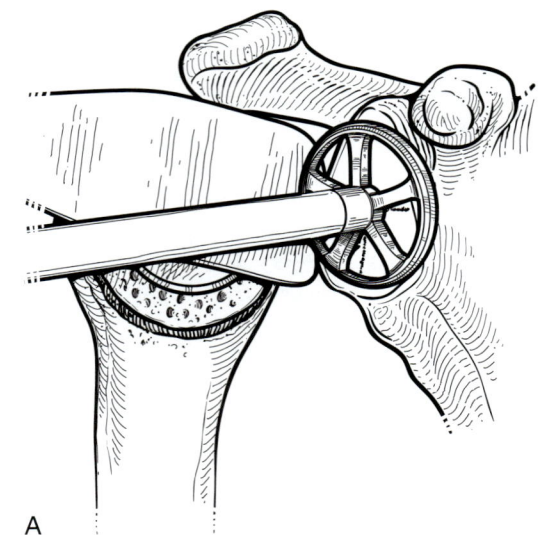

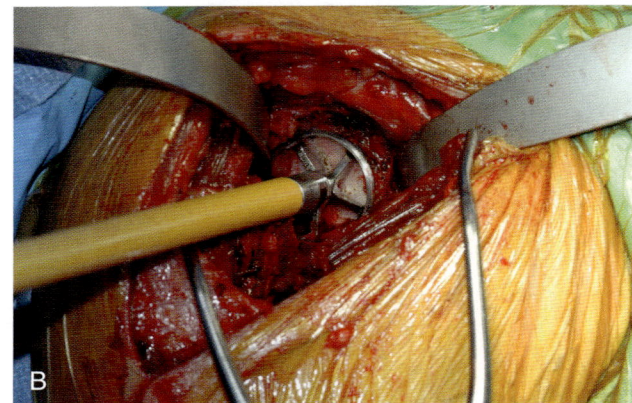

FIGURE 12.9 (A and B) Reaming of the glenoid surface.

This technique allows insertion of the glenoid reamer by eliminating obstruction of the reamer by the posterior humeral head retractor (Fig. 12.8). By using these techniques sequentially, we have yet to perform a shoulder arthroplasty in which we were unable to resurface the glenoid because of inadequate exposure.

After the tip of the reamer is inserted into the pilot hole, the cutting surface of the reamer is slightly distracted away from the glenoid surface as the reamer is started. This helps avoid glenoid fracture by preventing the reamer from suddenly engaging any prominent areas on the glenoid. The drill for the reamer is placed on the "ream" function rather than "drill" function to also help avoid glenoid fracture. The reamer is advanced medially to engage the glenoid bone (Fig. 12.9). In patients with a concentric glenoid (identified on preoperative computed tomography (CT) or magnetic resonance imaging; Chapter 7), reaming is performed only until a surface matching the radius of curvature of the reamer (same radius of curvature as on the back side of the glenoid component) is obtained. Any remaining glenoid cartilage should be removed; however, it is unnecessary to ream past the subchondral bone to cancellous bone.

Cases of asymmetric glenoid wear represent a challenging problem. Asymmetric glenoid wear is almost always posterior in primary osteoarthritis and creates a biconcave glenoid with the humeral head articulating with the posterior concavity or "neoglenoid"(Fig. 12.10). This biconcavity may not be grossly apparent during surgical visualization, hence the need for adequate preoperative imaging studies (Chapter 7). In addition to providing a concentric surface for the glenoid component, an additional goal of reaming in this scenario is to eliminate the biconcave glenoid morphology and restore the glenoid to a single-concavity morphology with appropriate version (2 to 8 degrees of retroversion). Preoperative planning with CT or magnetic resonance imaging helps determine the amount of correction necessary (Fig. 12.11; see Chapter 7 for more details). When reaming a biconcave glenoid, the anterior glenoid is preferentially reamed until a single concavity is achieved and the glenoid surface has been reoriented into correct version. As reaming

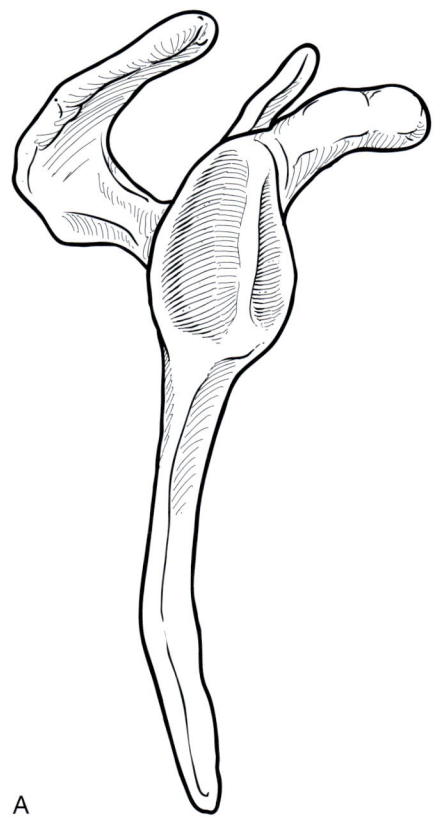

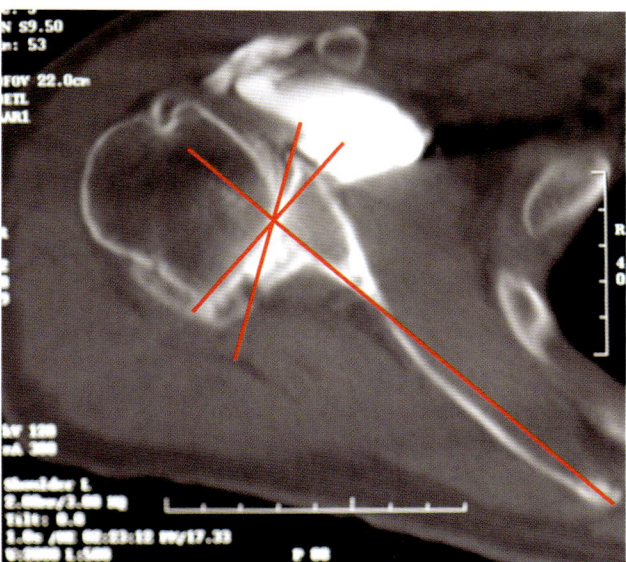

FIGURE 12.11 Determination of the correction needed in a case of primary osteoarthritis with glenoid biconcavity.

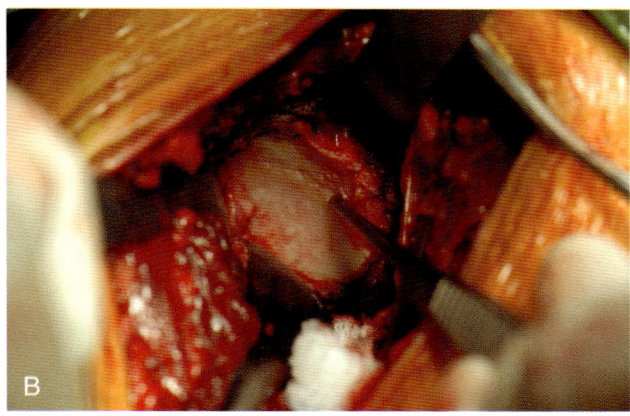

FIGURE 12.10 (A and B) Glenoid biconcavity in primary osteoarthritis identified on preoperative computed tomography.

progresses, the reamer should be periodically removed and the glenoid surface checked. A ridge on the glenoid surface demarcating the two concavities of the glenoid surface should move progressively posteriorly until it is no longer visible (Fig. 12.12).

SELECTING THE SIZE OF THE GLENOID COMPONENT

Selection of glenoid component size is based on coverage of the glenoid surface and, more importantly, on glenohumeral component mismatch. Glenohumeral prosthetic mismatch is defined as the difference in radius of curvature between the humeral head and glenoid components. Mismatch of at least 5.5 mm has been associated with fewer postoperative radiolucent lines.[2] Mismatch of greater than 10 mm has been shown biomechanically to risk fracture of the polyethylene glenoid component.[3] In the prosthetic system that we use, the preferred mismatch is obtained by combining a given humeral head size with a given glenoid component size (Table 12.1). The size of the humeral head is first selected as described in Chapter 11. The corresponding glenoid size is selected so that glenohumeral prosthetic mismatch is optimized. Occasionally, the native glenoid surface area is larger than the surface of the selected glenoid component. In this case a larger glenoid component is selected to provide better surface coverage and increased glenohumeral prosthetic mismatch. In the rare scenario in which the selected glenoid component is larger than the native glenoid surface, the preferentially selected glenoid component is used while some peripheral overhanging of the glenoid component is accepted to respect a mismatch of at least 5.5 mm.

SELECTING THE TYPE OF GLENOID COMPONENT

After the glenoid has been reamed and the size of glenoid component selected, the type of glenoid to be implanted is determined, typically pegged, keeled (Video 12.2), or a newer finned, cementless central pegged component (see Video 12.1). All three of the components are all-polyethylene convex-back components inserted with cement (Figs. 12.13 to 12.15). We prefer the new pegged component with a cementless finned central peg. Radiographic studies have shown superior early results with pegged components, including a randomized prospective study.[4,5] Laboratory biomechanical studies have also favored fixation of pegged components.[6] Clinical outcomes have been equivocal or shown slightly

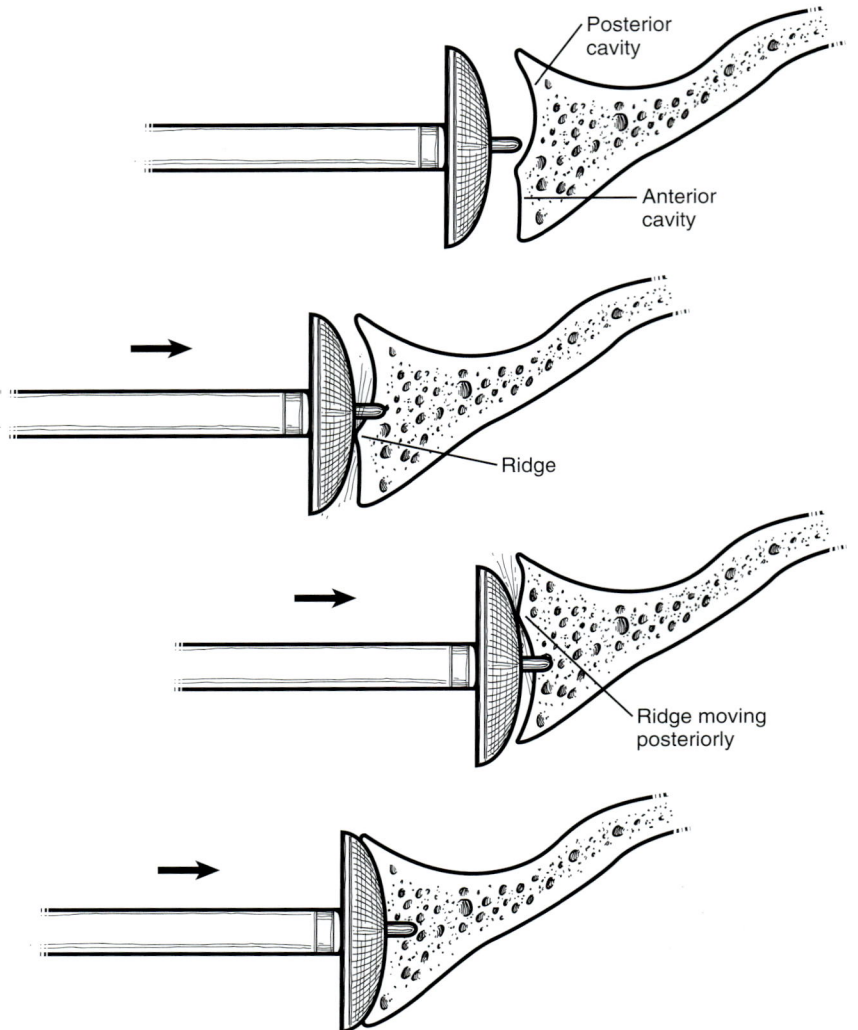

FIGURE 12.12 The ridge of bone demarcating the two glenoid concavities moves progressively posteriorly during eccentric glenoid reaming.

TABLE 12.1	Glenohumeral Prosthetic Mismatch Values and Recommendations[a] for the Aequalis Ascend Flex/Perform Shoulder Arthroplasty System[b]											
Size	Heads	37 × 13.5	39 × 14	41 × 15	43 × 16	46 × 17	48 × 18	50 × 16	50 × 19	52 × 19	52 × 23	54 × 23	54 × 27
Glenoid	Radius of Curvature	19.5	20.6	21.5	22.5	24	25	27.5	26	27.3	26.2	27.35	27
Small	27.7	8.2	7.1	6.2	5.2	3.7	2.7	0.2	1.7	0.4	1.5	0.35	0.7
Medium	59.6	10.3	9.2	8.3	7.3	5.8	4.8	2.3	3.8	2.5	3.6	2.45	2.8
Large	31.8	12.3	11.2	10.3	9.3	7.8	6.8	4.3	5.8	4.5	5.6	4.45	4.8
XL	33.9	14.4	13.3	12.4	11.4	9.9	8.9	6.4	7.9	6.6	7.7	6.55	6.9

[a]Shaded boxes represent recommendations.
[b]Wright Medical, Inc., Memphis, Tennessee.
XL, Extra large.

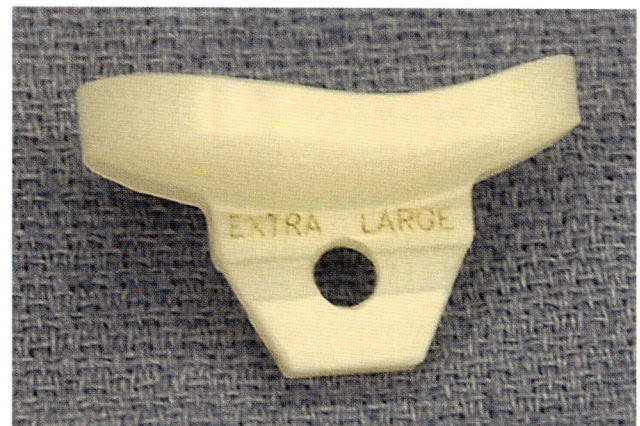

FIGURE 12.13 Keeled, all-polyethylene convex-back glenoid component.

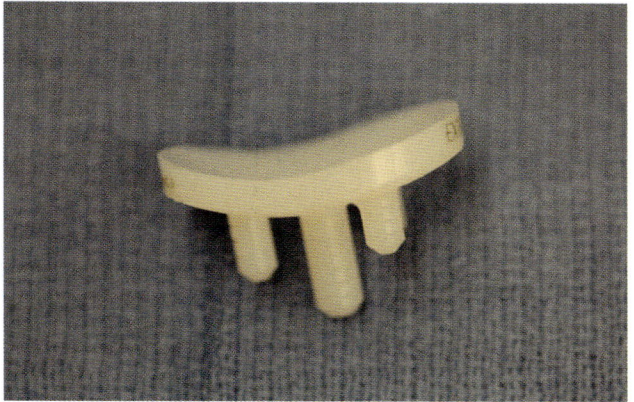

FIGURE 12.14 Pegged, all-polyethylene convex-back glenoid component.

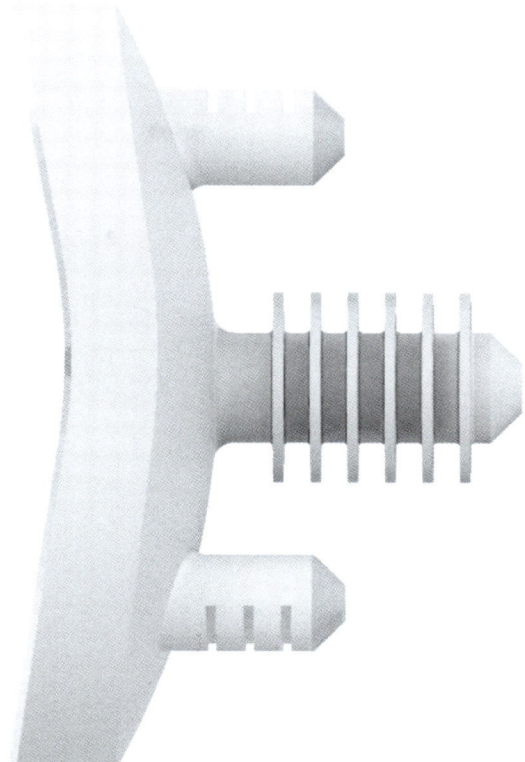

FIGURE 12.15 Pegged, all-polyethylene convex-back glenoid component with cementless central peg.

better results with keeled components.[7] Finned, central cementless pegged components have shown the existence of bony interdigitation using CT analysis.[8] Early results with the finned, central cementless pegged components at 2-year and 5-year follow-up are promising.[8,9]

In most scenarios, we believe that selection of a keeled or pegged glenoid component is based largely on surgeon preference. New preoperative surgical planning software may help to determine if a specific component may fit the patient's anatomy the best, especially for a shallow glenoid vault (Chapter 7).

PREPARING THE GLENOID BONE

When using a pegged glenoid component, a template is used to drill the peg holes (Fig. 12.16). A trial glenoid component is inserted to ensure full seating of the component (Fig. 12.17). The peg holes are then irrigated with sterile saline and dried with a sponge, an inexpensive technique shown to be as effective as the use of hemostatic agents and compressed carbon dioxide.[10]

The technique used for preparing the native glenoid bone has been shown to influence the radiographic results when a keeled glenoid component has been selected.[11] When implanting a keeled glenoid component, we prefer using the bony compaction technique pioneered by Gazielly.[12] Holes are drilled superior and inferior to the original pilot hole with use of a template device, and any remaining bony bridge is broken with a rongeur (Fig. 12.18). A keel punch that is the same size as the keel of the glenoid component is impacted into the native glenoid to finish preparation of the keel slot (Fig. 12.19). A trial glenoid component is inserted to ensure full seating of the component. The trial component is removed, and the keel slot is irrigated with sterile saline and dried in the same manner as with a pegged component.

FINAL IMPLANTATION OF THE GLENOID COMPONENT

The final component is cemented in place with polymethylmethacrylate (we prefer to use DePuy CMW 2 bone cement [DePuy, Inc., Warsaw, Indiana] because of its accelerated curing time of less than 8 minutes) in the keel slot/peg holes only (Fig. 12.20). An impactor impacts and holds the component in place while the cement cures.

When using our preferred finned cementless central pegged component and our preferred fast-setting cement, cement is introduced only into the peripheral peg holes. With this component, primary stability is obtained by the finned central peg, making it unnecessary to wait for the cement to polymerize prior to continuing the procedure.

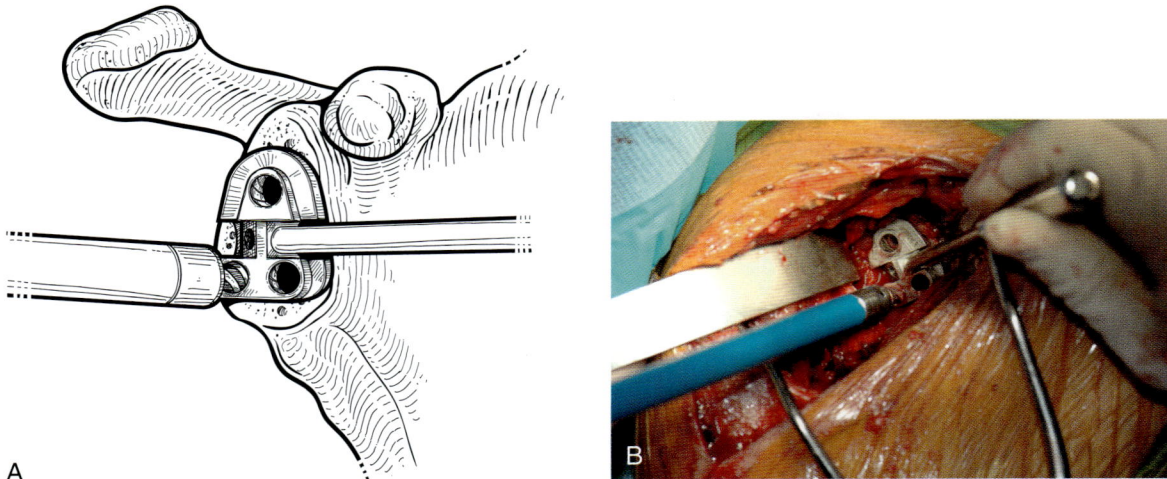

FIGURE 12.16 (A and B) Preparation of the glenoid for a pegged glenoid component.

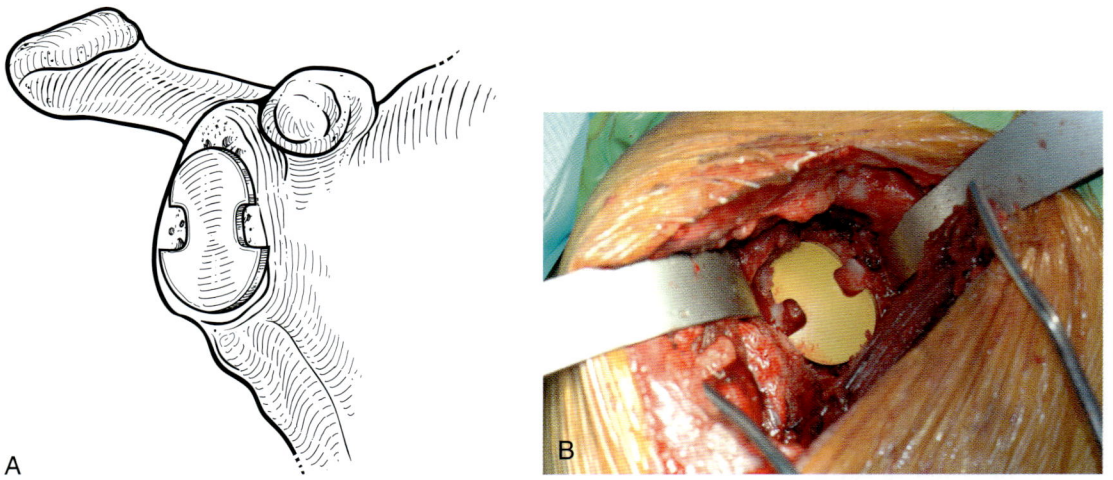

FIGURE 12.17 (A and B) Placement of the trial glenoid component to ensure that the component fully seats.

CHAPTER 12 ■ Glenoid Component 115

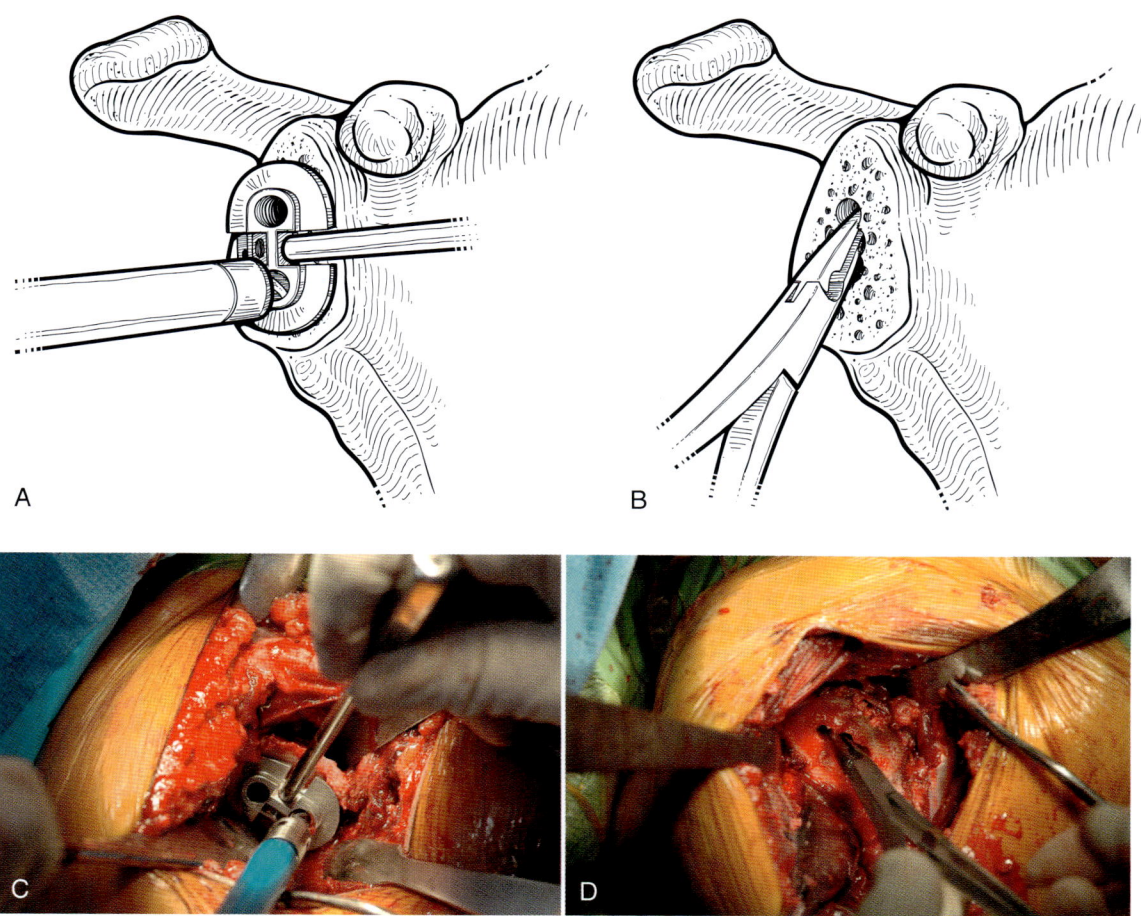

FIGURE 12.18 (A to D) Creation of the keel slot by first drilling holes superior and inferior to the original pilot hole via a template. The bony bridges between these holes are removed with a small rongeur.

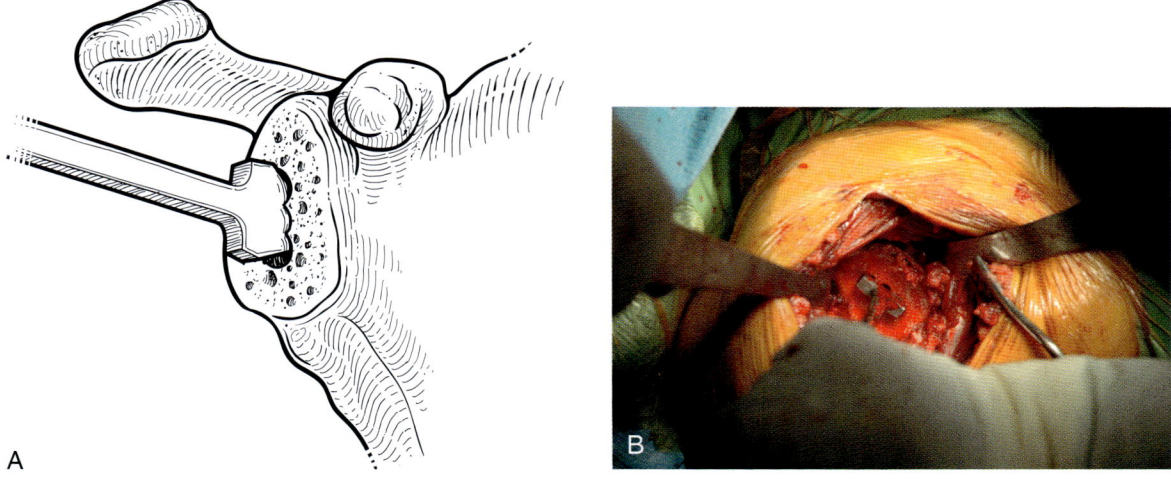

FIGURE 12.19 (A and B) Compaction of the glenoid vault to complete creation of the keel slot.

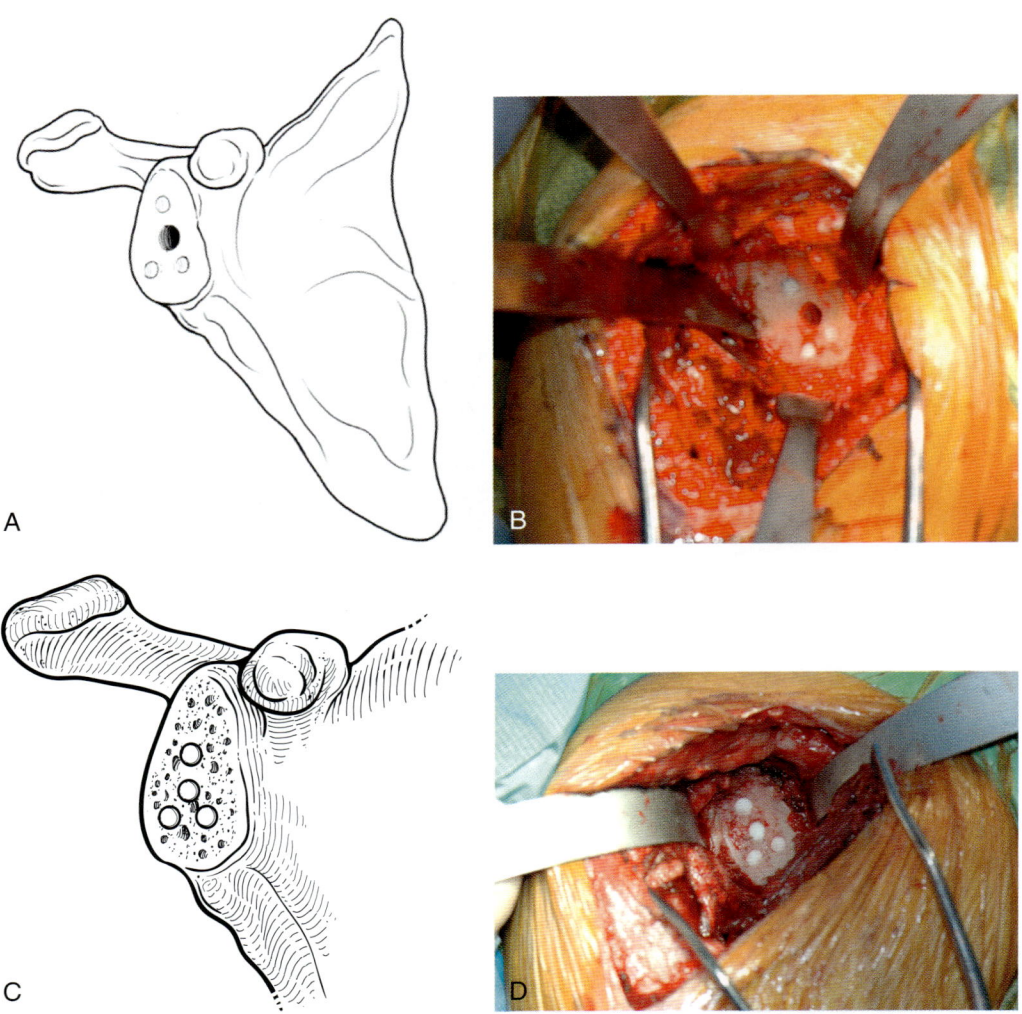

FIGURE 12.20 (A to H) Cementing the final glenoid component. (A and B) Finned cementless central pegged component. (C and D) Pegged component.

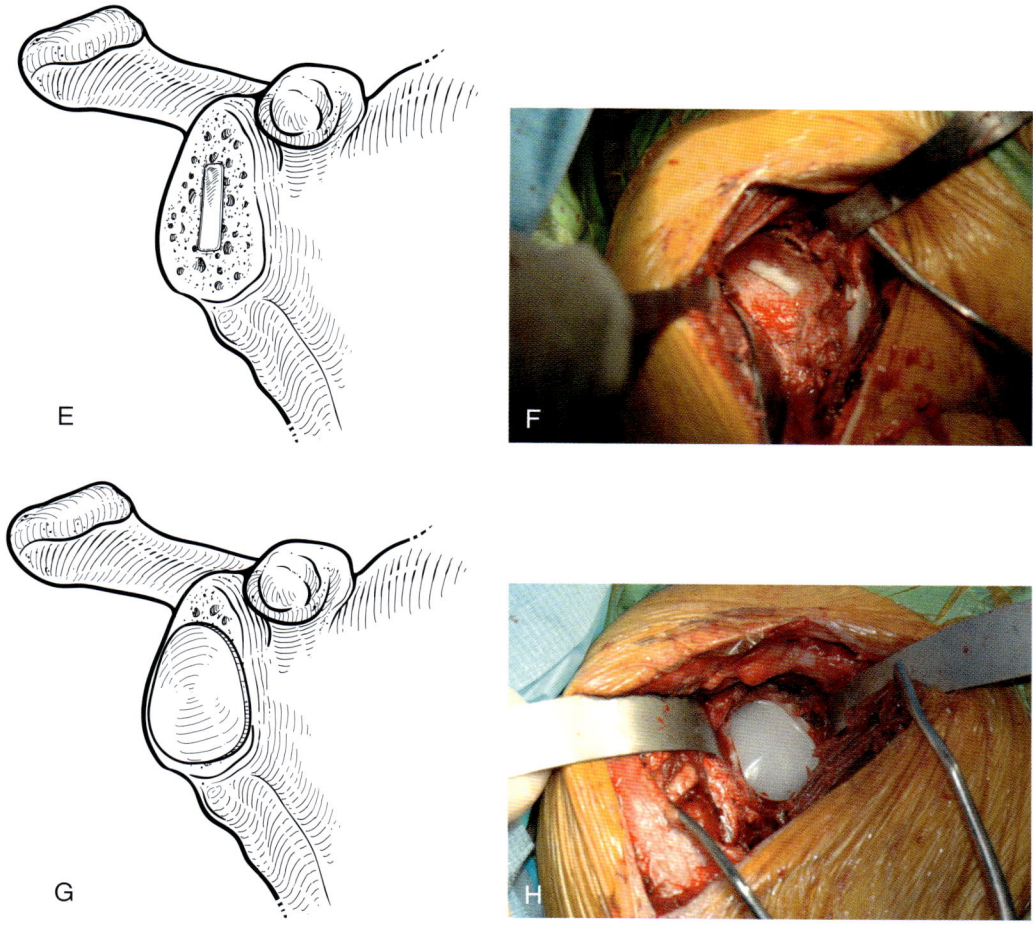

FIGURE 12.20, cont'd (E and F) Keeled component. (G and H) Final component in place.

REFERENCES

1. Walch G, Young AA, Boileau P, et al: Patterns of loosening of polyethylene keeled glenoid components after shoulder arthroplasty for primary osteoarthritis: results of a multicenter study with more than five years of follow-up, *J Bone Joint Surg Am* 94:145–150, 2012.
2. Walch G, Edwards TB, Boulahia A, et al: The influence of glenohumeral prosthetic mismatch on glenoid radiolucent lines: Results of a multicentric study, *J Bone Joint Surg Am* 84:2186–2191, 2002.
3. Friedman RJ, An YH, Draughn RA: Glenohumeral congruence in total shoulder arthroplasty, *Orthop Trans* 21:17, 1997.
4. Gartsman GM, Elkousy HA, Warnock KM, et al: Radiographic comparison of pegged and keeled glenoid components, *J Shoulder Elbow Surg* 14:252–257, 2005.
5. Anglin C, Wyss UP, Nyffeler RW, et al: Loosening performance of cemented glenoid prosthesis design pairs, *Clin Biomech (Bristol, Avon)* 16:144–150, 2001.
6. Edwards TB, Labriola JE, Stanley RJ, et al: Radiographic comparison of pegged and keeled glenoid components using modern cementing techniques: a prospective randomized study, *J Shoulder Elbow Surg* 19:251–257, 2010.
7. Gazielly D, El-Abiad R: Comparative results of three types of polyethylene cemented glenoid components. In Walch G, Boileau P, Molé D, editors: *2000 Prosthèses d'Epaule … Recul de 2 à 10 Ans*, Paris, 2001, Sauramps Medical, pp 483–488.
8. Arnold RM, High RR, Grosshans KT, et al: Bone presence between the central peg's radial fins of a partially cemented pegged all poly glenoid component suggest few radiolucencies, *J Shoulder Elbow Surg* 20:315–321, 2011.
9. Churchill RS: Trends in glenoid component design in unconstrained shoulder arthroplasty, *J Shoulder Elbow Surg* 20:S41–S46, 2011.
10. Edwards TB, Sabonghy EP, Elkousy HA, et al: Glenoid component insertion in total shoulder arthroplasty: comparison of three techniques for drying the glenoid prior to cementation, *J Shoulder Elbow Surg* 16(3 Suppl):S107–S110, 2007.
11. Szabo I, Buscayret F, Edwards TB, et al: Radiographic comparison of two different glenoid preparation techniques in total shoulder arthroplasty, *Clin Orthop Relat Res* 431:104–110, 2005.
12. Gazielly DF, Allende C, Pamelin E: Results of cancellous compaction technique for glenoid resurfacing. Paper presented at the 9th International Congress on Surgery of the Shoulder, May 2004, Washington, DC.

CHAPTER 13

Soft tissue balancing

The use of a prosthetic system that adapts to the patient's anatomy decreases the need for soft tissue balancing. In most cases, little additional soft tissue balancing is necessary after the steps of the procedure have been followed as described in this textbook. Two notable exceptions exist. The first is in an individual, usually with a diagnosis of primary osteoarthritis or instability arthropathy, who has marked posterior glenoid wear and posterior glenohumeral subluxation on preoperative computed tomography or magnetic resonance imaging. The second is in an individual with an exceptionally tight posterior capsule, most commonly seen in our practice in patients with juvenile-onset inflammatory arthropathy.

EVALUATING THE NEED FOR SOFT TISSUE BALANCING

In patients with posterior glenoid wear (type B2 glenoid morphology; see Chapter 7), the sequence of surgical steps is altered. After the glenoid component is implanted, we insert the trial humeral prosthesis instead of the final humeral implant. This is helpful in judging prosthetic stability. After the trial humeral component is reinserted, the glenohumeral joint is reduced. With the arm externally rotated 30 degrees, force is applied in a posterior direction to the proximal humerus. There are two keys that allow the surgeon to determine whether the soft tissues are properly balanced. First, the prosthetic humeral head should subluxate posteriorly approximately 30% to 50% of its diameter and spontaneously reduce on release of the posteriorly directed force. If spontaneous reduction does not occur, posterior capsulorrhaphy may be necessary. Second, if posterior translation of at least 30% of the diameter of the humeral head is not possible, posterior capsular release may be necessary.

PERFORMING A POSTERIOR CAPSULORRHAPHY

In many patients with posterior glenoid wear and posterior humeral head subluxation, the posterior capsule has become distended and ineffective in maintaining posterior glenohumeral stability, even after the osseous glenoid deformity has been corrected by reaming (Fig. 13.1). In such cases, posterior capsulorrhaphy serves to tighten the posterior capsule and prevent posterior instability. To perform this procedure, the trial humeral implant is removed and a laminar spreader with protective rubber sleeves on the tips is placed between the humerus and glenoid to expose the posterior capsule (Fig. 13.2). Three no. 1 braided absorbable sutures (one superior, one in the middle, and one inferior) are passed through the posterior capsule in a mediolateral direction to imbricate the posterior capsule (Fig. 13.3). The laminar spreader is removed and the sutures are tied sequentially. The excess suture limbs are cut from the superior and middle capsulorrhaphy sutures, but the inferior suture is left uncut (Fig. 13.4). The sutures for subscapularis repair and the final humeral implant are placed (see Chapter 11) after posterior capsulorrhaphy, and stability is reevaluated. Stability is usually greatly improved after posterior capsulorrhaphy. In the rare circumstance in which the glenohumeral joint remains dislocated on stability testing after posterior capsulorrhaphy has been performed, the excess inferior suture limbs can be brought through the glenohumeral joint and rotator interval and sutured to the coracoacromial ligament just lateral to its insertion on the coracoid. This helps to avoid posterior instability in the early postoperative phase (Fig. 13.5). Because these sutures are absorbable, no long-term consequence of passing the sutures through the glenohumeral joint have been observed when they have been necessary.

PERFORMING A POSTERIOR CAPSULAR RELEASE

Rarely, posterior translation of at least 30% of the diameter of the humeral head will be impossible during stability testing. We have observed this scenario most commonly in patients with inflammatory arthropathy as the underlying condition for which they are undergoing shoulder arthroplasty. When this occurs, we perform a posterior capsular release in which the final humeral implant is left in place and a laminar spreader with protective rubber sleeves on the tips is placed between the humeral and glenoid components to expose the posterior capsule (Fig. 13.6). The posterior capsule is then released under direct visualization just adjacent to the glenoid component with a no. 10 scalpel blade on a long handle from the 12 o'clock to the 6 o'clock positions (Fig. 13.7). After posterior capsular release, stability is reevaluated. In the rare scenario where the posterior capsule remains too tight after posterior capsular release, consideration is given to decreasing the size of the prosthetic head.

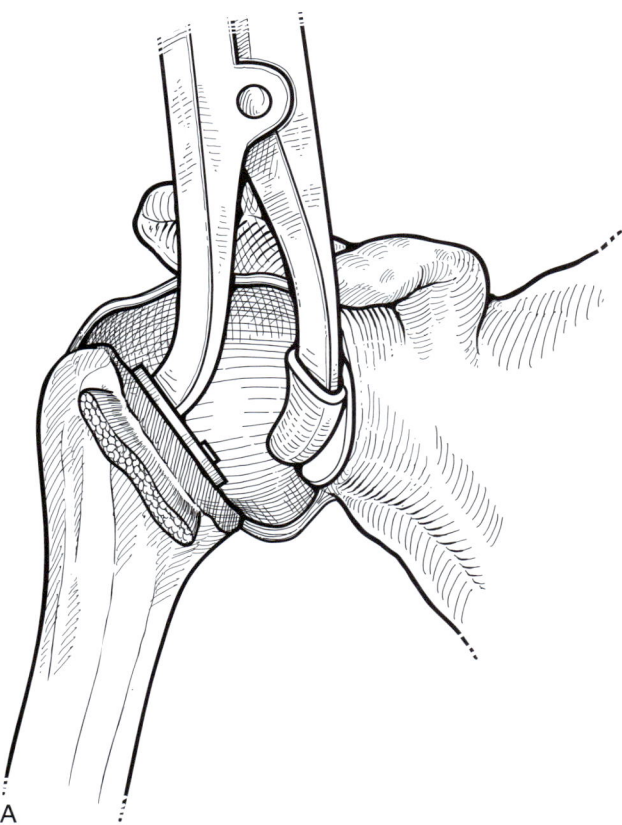

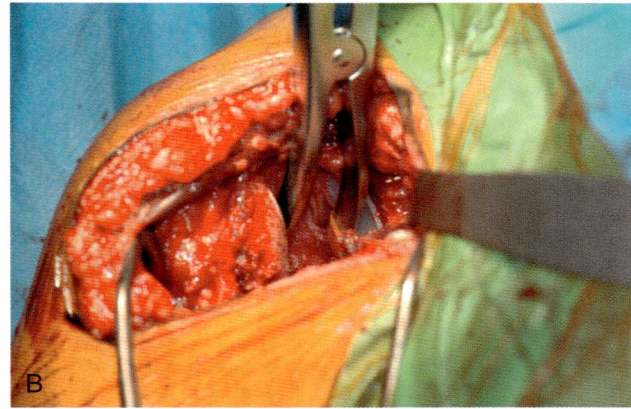

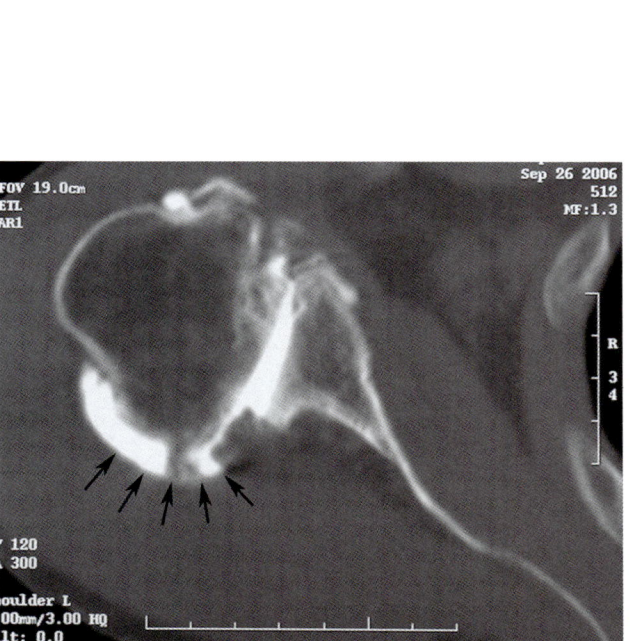

FIGURE 13.1 Computed tomography showing posterior glenoid wear. The posterior glenoid capsule has been enhanced to show its marked distention *(arrows)*.

FIGURE 13.2 (A and B) Laminar spreader placed between the humerus and glenoid to expose the posterior capsule.

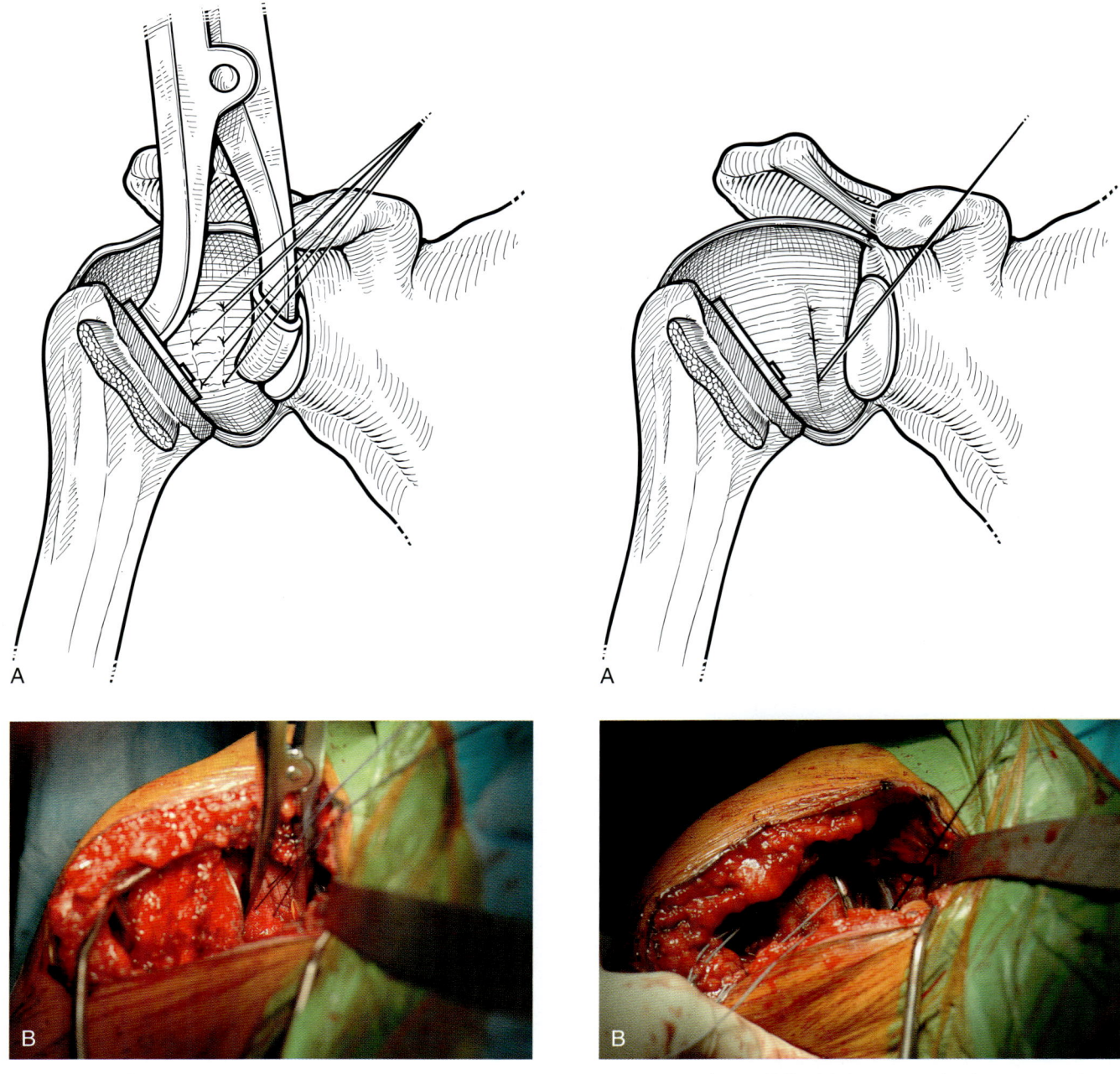

FIGURE 13.3 (A and B) Imbrication sutures placed in the posterior capsule.

FIGURE 13.4 (A and B) The inferior capsulorrhaphy suture is left uncut until stability has been retested.

CHAPTER 13 ■ Soft Tissue Balancing

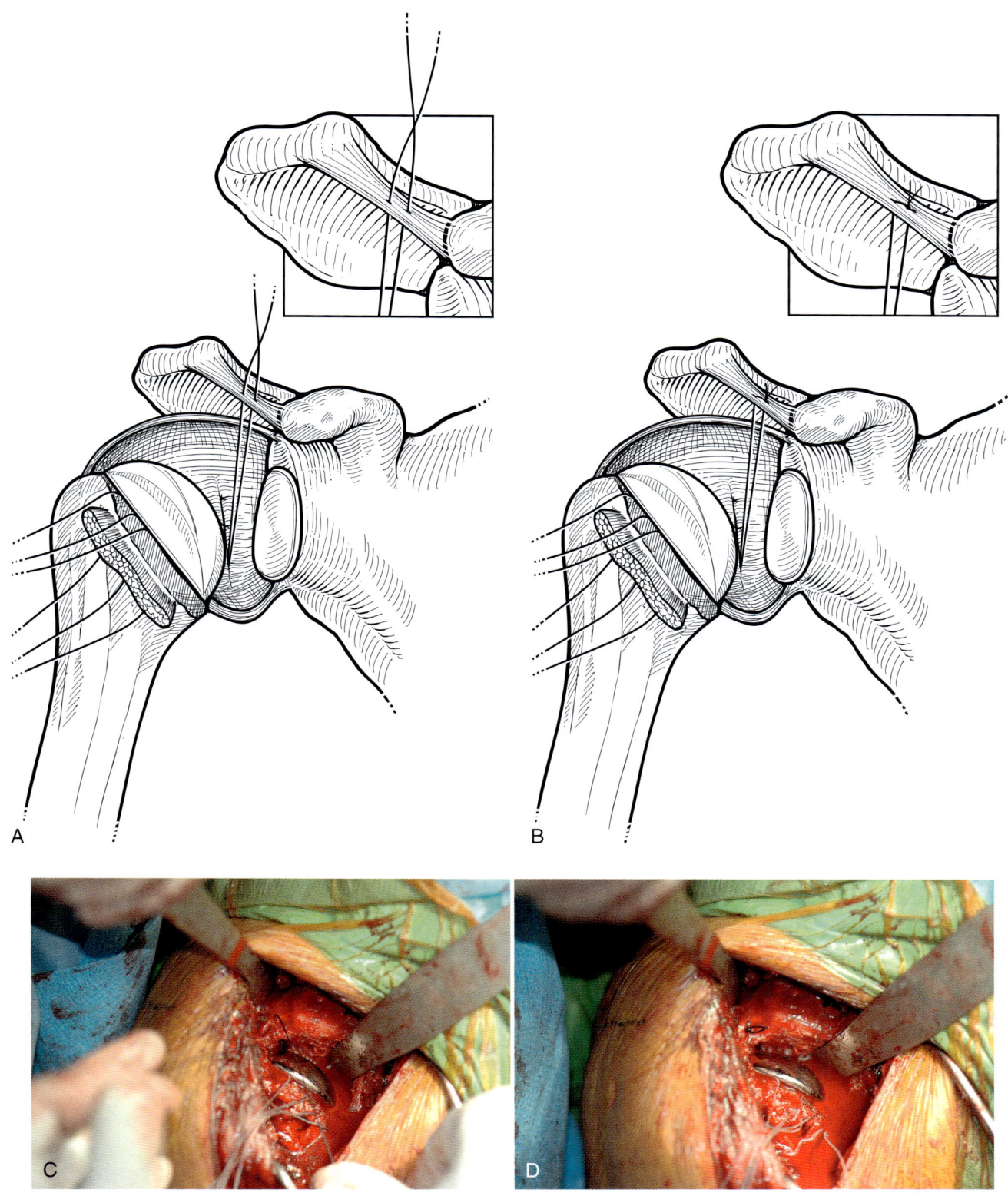

FIGURE 13.5 (A to D) Suturing the inferior capsulorrhaphy suture to the coracoacromial ligament in cases of residual posterior instability after posterior capsulorrhaphy.

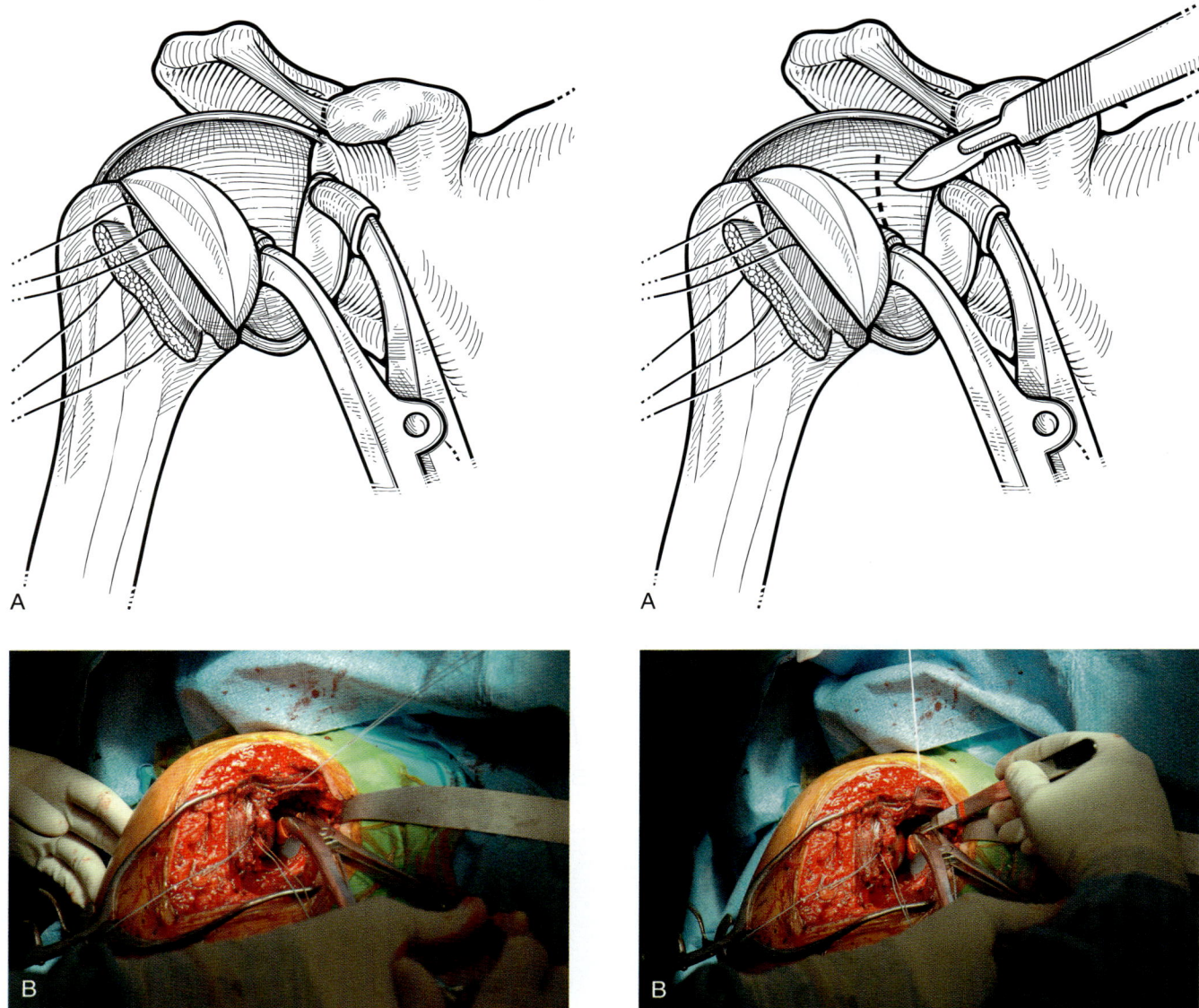

FIGURE 13.6 (A and B) Exposure of a tight posterior capsule with the laminar spreader.

FIGURE 13.7 (A and B) Release of a tight posterior capsule with a scalpel.

Subscapularis and rotator interval repair

CHAPTER 14

Failure of subscapularis repair occurs in 2% of patients after shoulder arthroplasty for primary osteoarthritis.[1] Prognostic factors for the development of symptoms after subscapularis failure are unclear. Many patients will be asymptomatic after failure of subscapularis repair, with subscapularis weakness detected only on postoperative examination. However, symptoms of weakness or anterior instability (or both) will develop in some patients. Additionally, even in patients who are asymptomatic, there is concern over the failure of the subscapularis, which causes eccentric anterior loading and subsequent loosening of the glenoid component. For these reasons, every effort should be made to perform a secure subscapularis repair. We prefer a repair that incorporates both transosseous and transtendinous components. In addition to subscapularis repair, we also routinely close the rotator interval to further decrease the risk for postoperative glenohumeral instability. Rotator interval closure in an anatomic shoulder arthroplasty cadaveric model improved load to failure of the subscapularis tenotomy repair and decreased gap formation of the repair under cyclic load.[2]

TECHNIQUE FOR REPAIR OF THE SUBSCAPULARIS AND ROTATOR INTERVAL

After the completion of soft tissue balancing, final preparations are made for implantation of the humeral component and subsequent subscapularis repair. Three no. 2 nonabsorbable braided sutures are placed through the lesser tuberosity and the humeral stump of the subscapularis tendon, as detailed in Chapter 11, to be used for reattachment of the subscapularis (Fig. 14.1). These sutures are placed just before insertion of the final humeral implant. The final humeral implant is then impacted into place and its stability checked (Chapters 11 and 13).

The small anterior glenoid rim retractor is removed and replaced with a narrow Richardson retractor, which is used to retract the conjoined tendon medially. The previously placed sponge is visualized and removed from the subscapularis fossa with a Kocher clamp (Fig. 14.2). Removal of this sponge reveals the stay sutures placed in the subscapularis tendon during the surgical approach. The Kocher clamp is placed on these stay sutures to obtain control of the subscapularis (Fig. 14.3). The limb of the superior suture exiting the medullary canal is passed from deep to superficial through the superior portion of the subscapularis tendon not more than 1 cm medial to its terminus. The same limb is then passed through the humeral stump of the subscapularis and back through the superior portion of the subscapularis tendon, as before (Fig. 14.4). This suture is tied with a square surgeon's knot using five throws. The subscapularis stay sutures are removed, and the suture passing and tying procedure is repeated for the middle suture and then the inferior suture. This technique yields a transosseous and transtendinous repair (Fig. 14.5). No effort is made to imbricate the subscapularis or to medialize its insertion; the repair should be as anatomic as possible.

The rotator interval is closed with a single figure-of-eight stitch with the residual no. 2 braided nonabsorbable suture from the subscapularis repair (Fig. 14.6). The repaired tissue should consist of the rotator interval capsule. Direct suturing of the subscapularis tendon to the supraspinatus tendon should be avoided because this could substantially limit external rotation postoperatively. Additionally, care is required to avoid imbricating the rotator interval, which could also lead to postoperative limitation of external rotation. The rotator interval and subscapularis repair are then reinforced with a no. 1 braided absorbable suture on a taper needle in a running nonlocking technique. The final repair is shown in Fig. 14.7. After the subscapularis and rotator interval are closed, passive external rotation with the arm at the patient's side is documented to assist in directing postoperative rehabilitation (Fig. 14.8). Ideally, we like to observe at least 30 degrees of external rotation with the arm at the side after repair of the subscapularis and rotator interval. If we are unable to obtain this, we remove the rotator interval suture. If external rotation remains less than 30 degrees (as may be the case in patients with severe preoperative stiffness), we accept whatever external rotation is obtained after removal of the rotator interval suture. We do not recommend heroic attempts, such as Z-plasty tendon lengthening of the subscapularis, to obtain more external rotation because such attempts can seriously compromise the integrity of the subscapularis tendon.

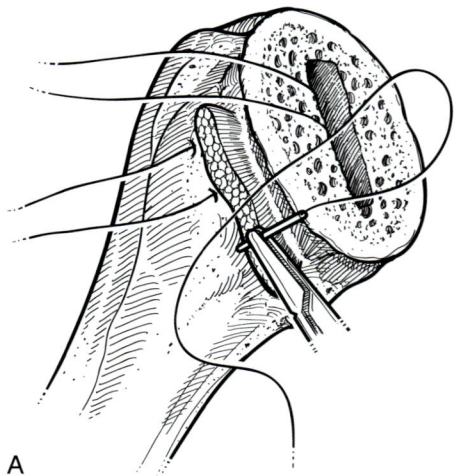

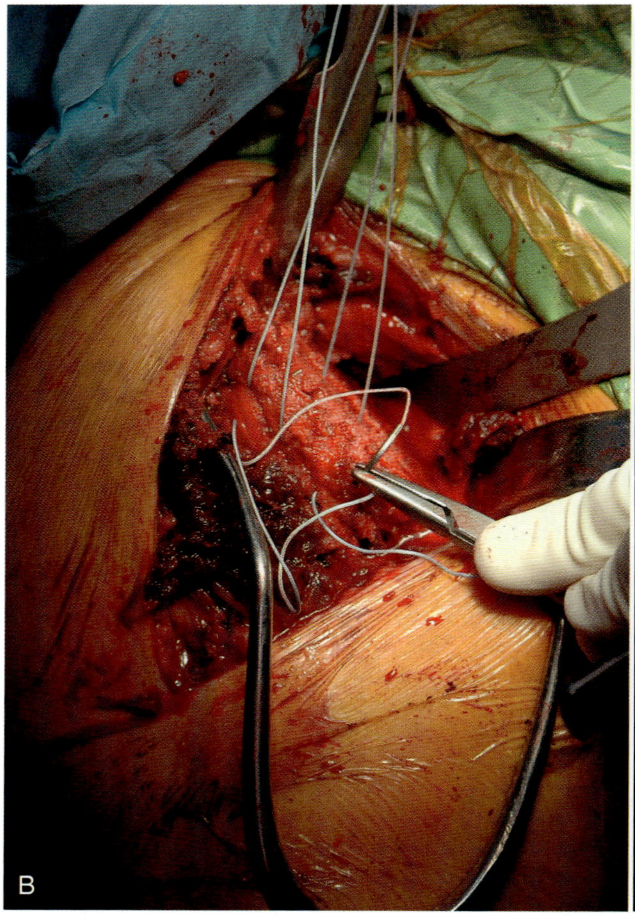

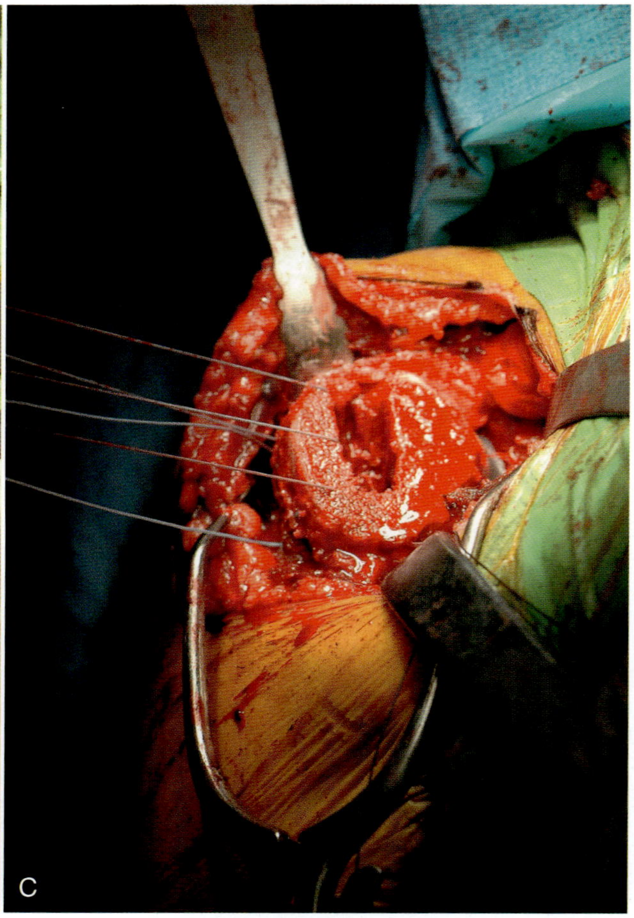

FIGURE 14.1 (A to C) Placement of transosseous sutures for later subscapularis repair.

CHAPTER 14 ■ Subscapularis and Rotator Interval Repair 125

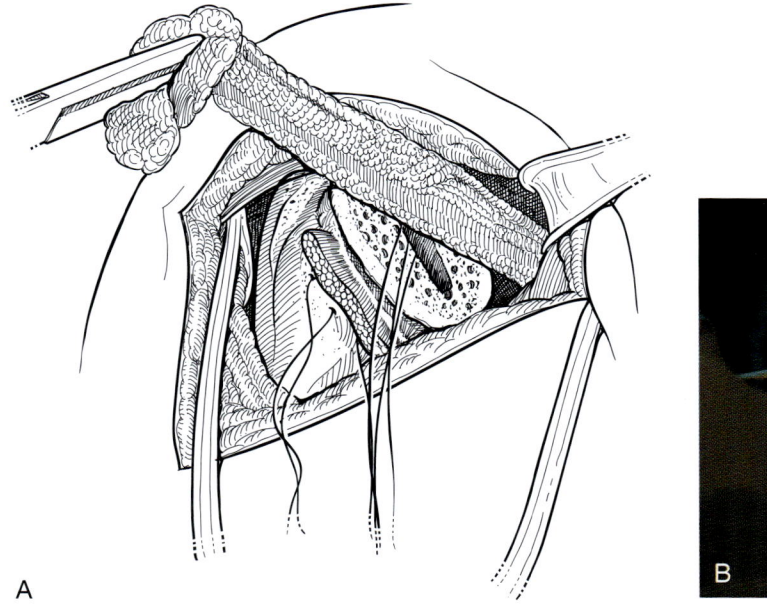
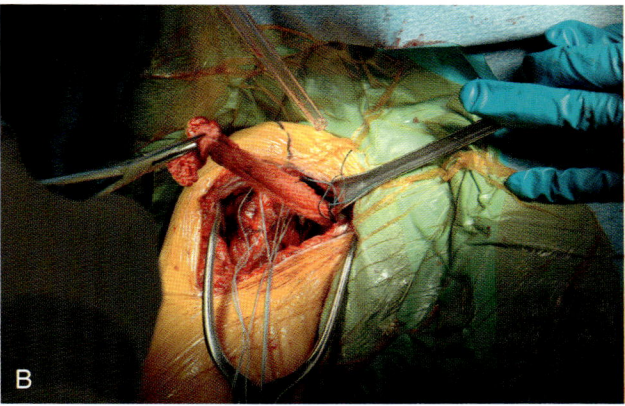

FIGURE 14.2 (A and B) Removal of the previously placed sponge to expose the subscapularis.

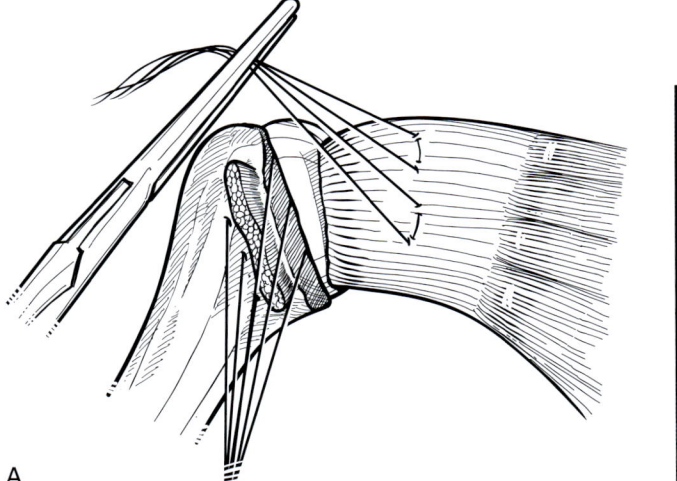
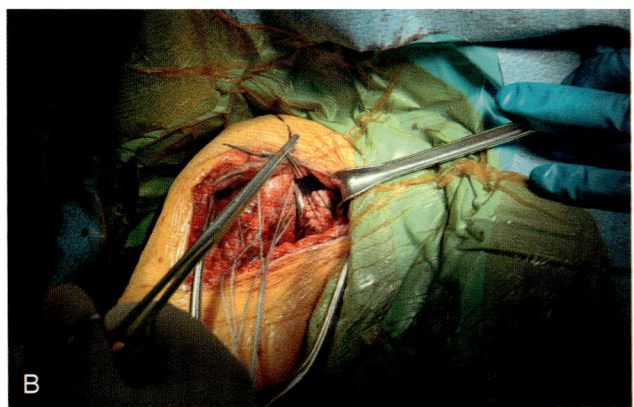

FIGURE 14.3 (A and B) Obtaining control of the subscapularis with stay sutures.

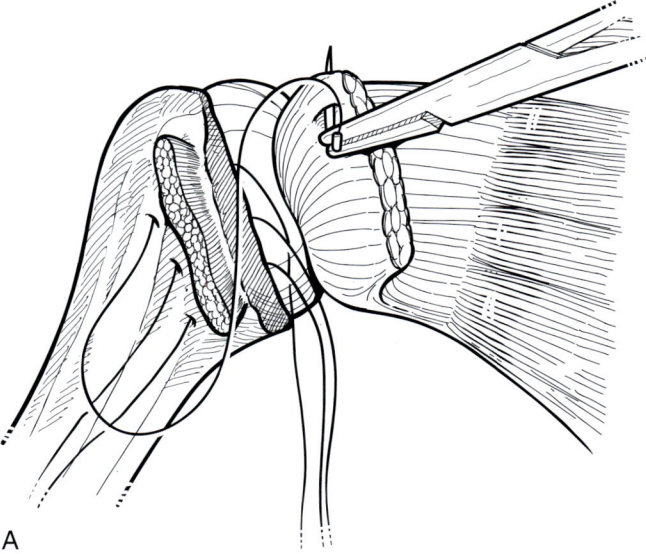
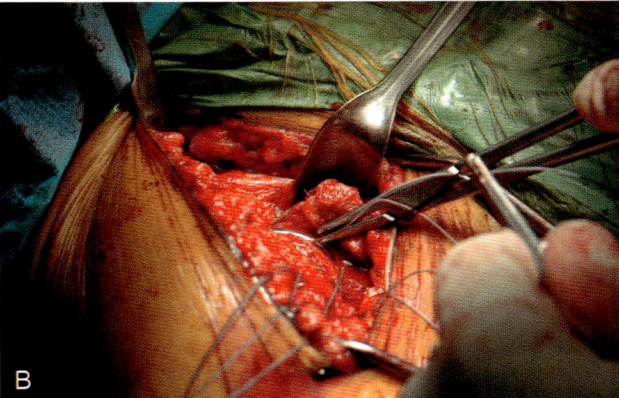

FIGURE 14.4 (A and B) Technique of passing suture through the subscapularis during repair.

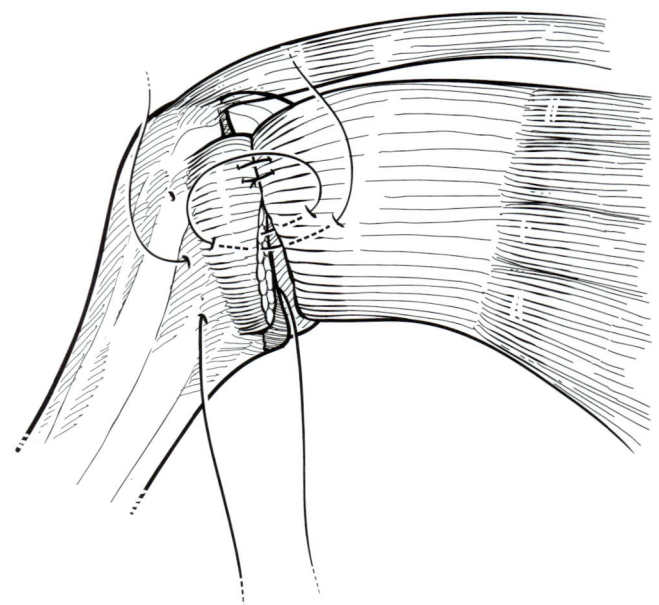

FIGURE 14.5 This technique yields a transosseous and transtendinous repair.

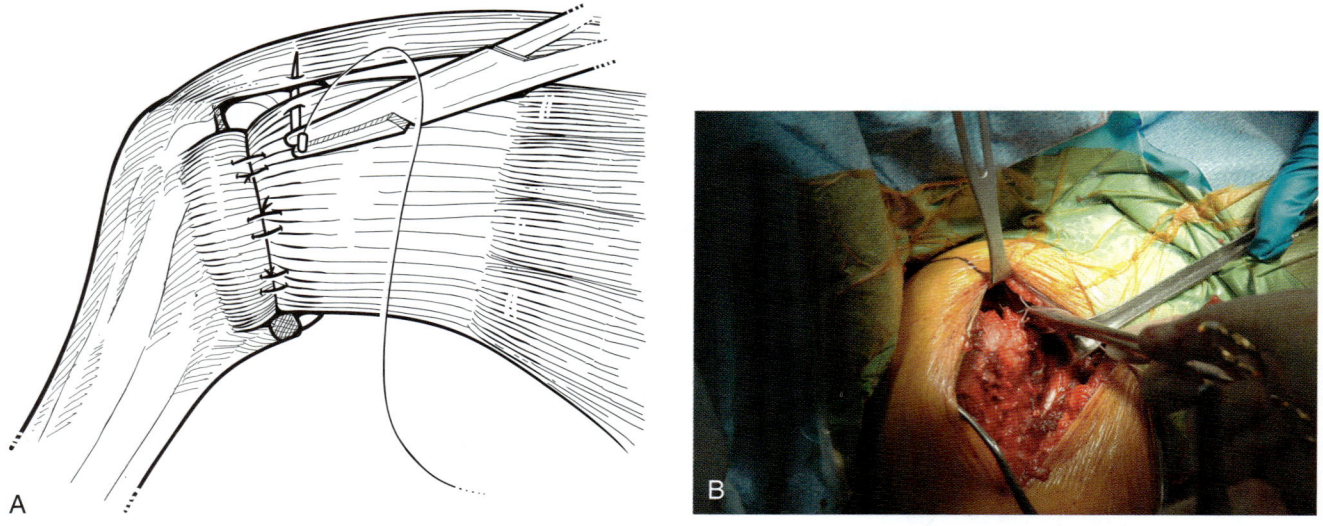

FIGURE 14.6 (A and B) Repair of the rotator interval.

CHAPTER 14 ■ Subscapularis and Rotator Interval Repair

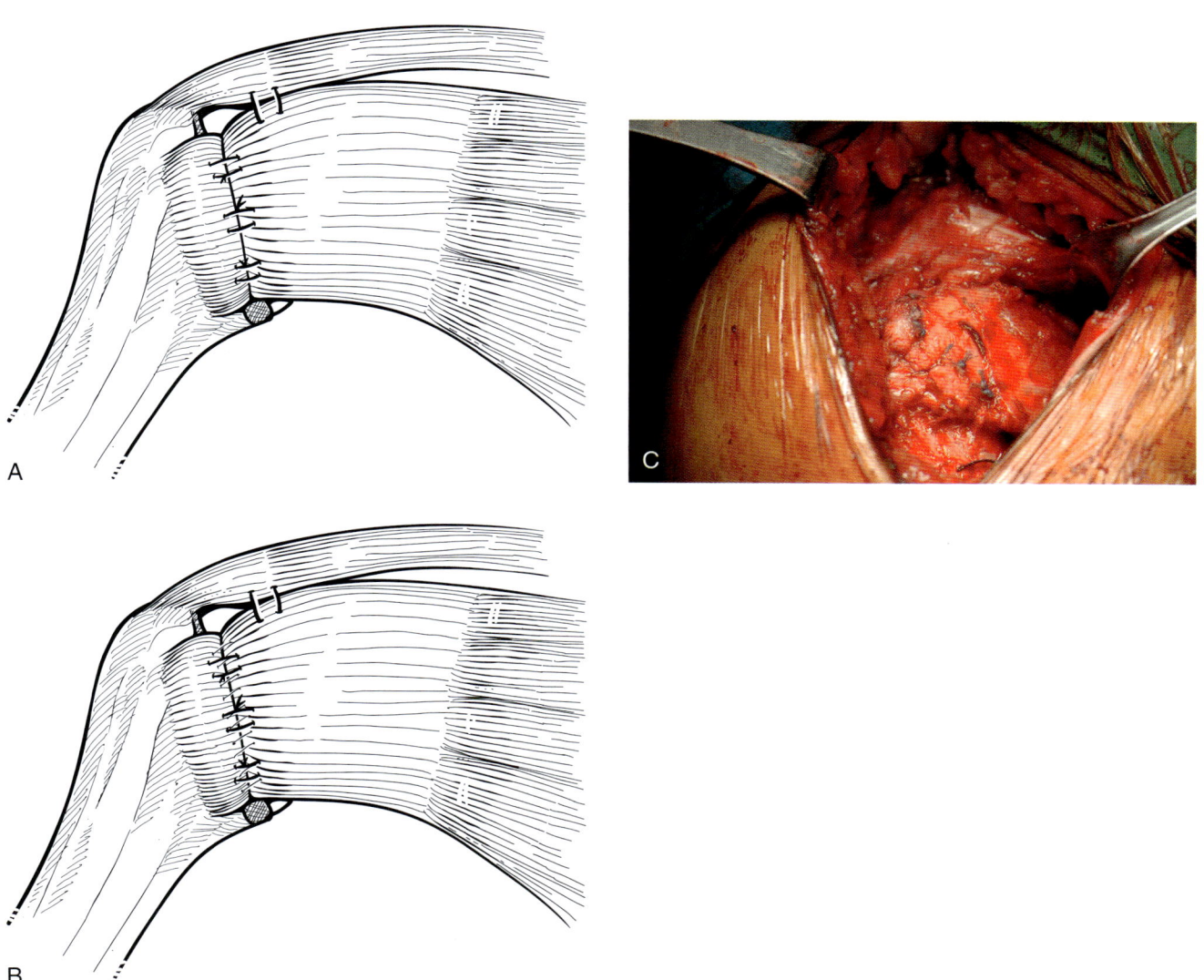

FIGURE 14.7 (A to C) Completed repair of the subscapularis and rotator interval.

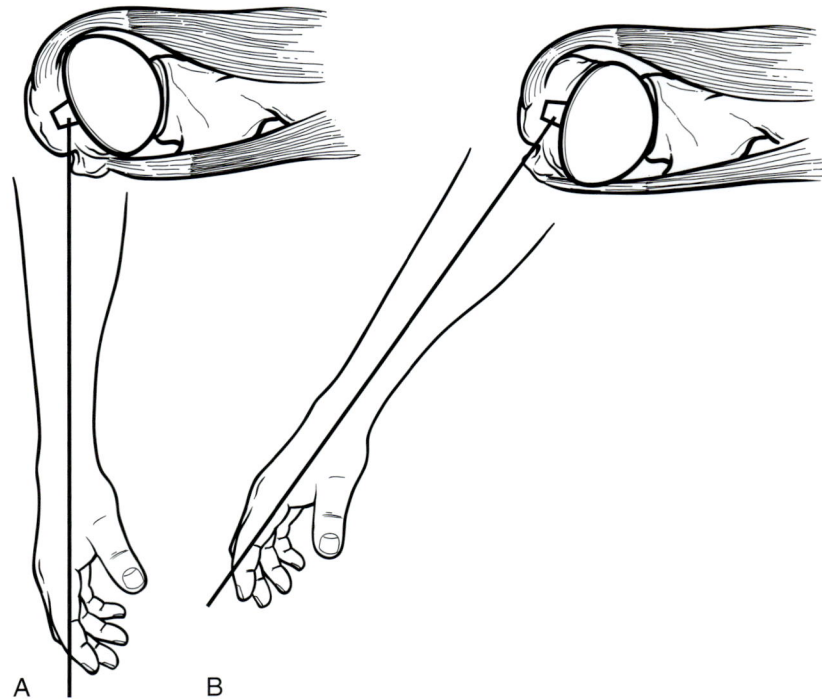
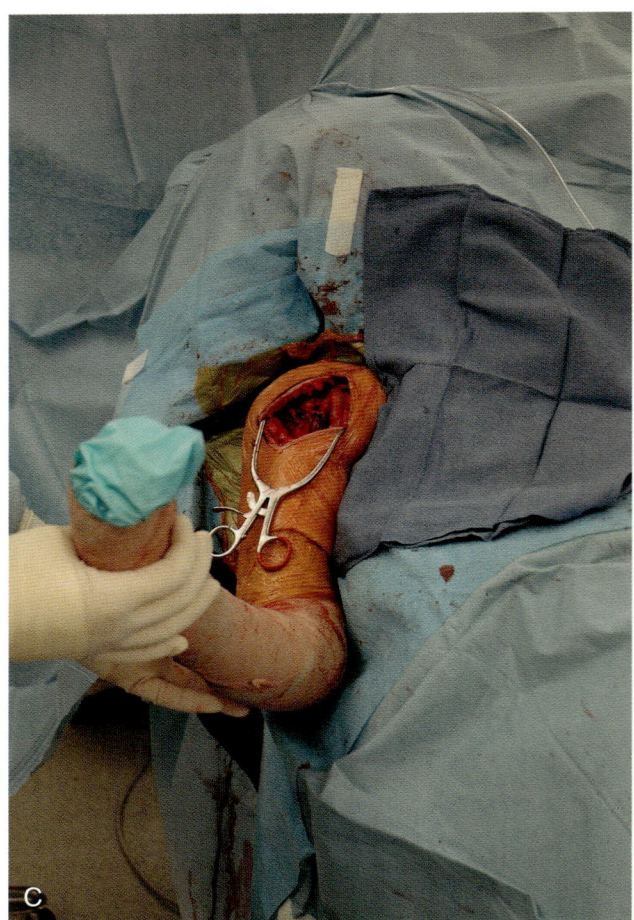

FIGURE 14.8 (A to C) Assessment of passive external rotation after subscapularis repair.

REFERENCES

1. Lafosse L, Kempf JF: Omarthrose primitive: resultats cliniques et radiologiques. In Walch G, Boileau P, Molé D, editors: *2000 Prosthèses d'Epaule ... Recul de 2 à 10 Ans*, Paris, 2001, Sauramps Medical, pp 73–85.
2. Daly CA, Hutton WC, Jarrett CD: Biomechanical effects of rotator interval closure in shoulder arthroplasty, *J Shoulder Elbow Surg* 25(7):1094–1099, 2016, doi:10.1016/j.jse.2015.12.003. Epub 2016 Feb 17.

CHAPTER 15
Wound closure and postoperative orthosis

The final steps of the operative procedure are wound closure and placement of the postoperative orthosis. These steps are relatively elementary but no less important than other aspects of the procedure.

TECHNIQUE FOR WOUND CLOSURE

After closure of the subscapularis and rotator interval, the wound is irrigated with 800 mL of antibiotic-impregnated sterile saline (50,000 units bacitracin per liter sterile normal saline) via a bulb syringe. The wound is checked to ensure that adequate hemostasis has been achieved. The electrocautery is used as necessary to minimize any residual hemorrhage. No drain is used because it has been shown to be unnecessary during unconstrained shoulder arthroplasty.[1] We do not close the deltopectoral interval but initiate our closure with the overlying fascial layer. This layer is reapproximated with no. 0 braided absorbable suture via an interrupted figure-of-eight technique (Fig. 15.1). The subcutaneous fascia is reapproximated with 2-0 braided absorbable suture via an interrupted figure-of-eight technique (Fig. 15.2). The skin is reapproximated with 3-0 undyed absorbable monofilament suture in a subcuticular running closure (Fig. 15.3).

The occlusive draping is removed adjacent to the incision, and the skin is cleansed of blood with a saline-soaked sponge and then dried. Half-inch Steri-Strips are placed over the incision (Fig. 15.4). Sterile gauze is placed over the incision and a sterile absorbent pad is placed over the gauze (Fig. 15.5). The dressing is secured with 3-inch foam tape (Fig. 15.6). The remaining surgical drapes are then removed.

The dressing is maintained in place until postoperative day 3, at which time it is removed and not replaced. After removal of the dressing, the patient is allowed to shower, but submerging the incision in a bathtub is prohibited until 2 weeks postoperatively. The patient removes the Steri-Strips progressively as they lose their adhesion to the skin, typically after 10 to 14 days.

POSTOPERATIVE ORTHOSIS

The postoperative orthosis is placed in the operating room immediately after the dressing is applied. The type of orthosis used is determined by the procedure performed. We use two types of postoperative orthoses. For unconstrained shoulder arthroplasty without an associated posterior capsulorrhaphy, we use a simple sling (Fig. 15.7). This is used for the patient's comfort and protection and is discontinued whenever the patient decides that it is no longer required, usually between 2 and 4 weeks postoperatively. We ask patients to avoid externally rotating beyond neutral for 4 weeks (6 weeks for inflammatory arthropathy) and to avoid pushing or pulling their body weight with the operated extremity for 8 weeks to protect the subscapularis repair.

In patients who have undergone an associated posterior capsulorrhaphy, we use a neutral-rotation sling (Fig. 15.8). This sling is maintained for 4 weeks to protect the posterior capsulorrhaphy. Patients are allowed to remove the sling only for hygiene and rehabilitative exercises. Additionally, patients who have undergone posterior capsulorrhaphy are cautioned against cross-body adduction and internal rotation behind the back for the first 4 postoperative weeks.

CHAPTER 15 ■ Wound Closure and Postoperative Orthosis

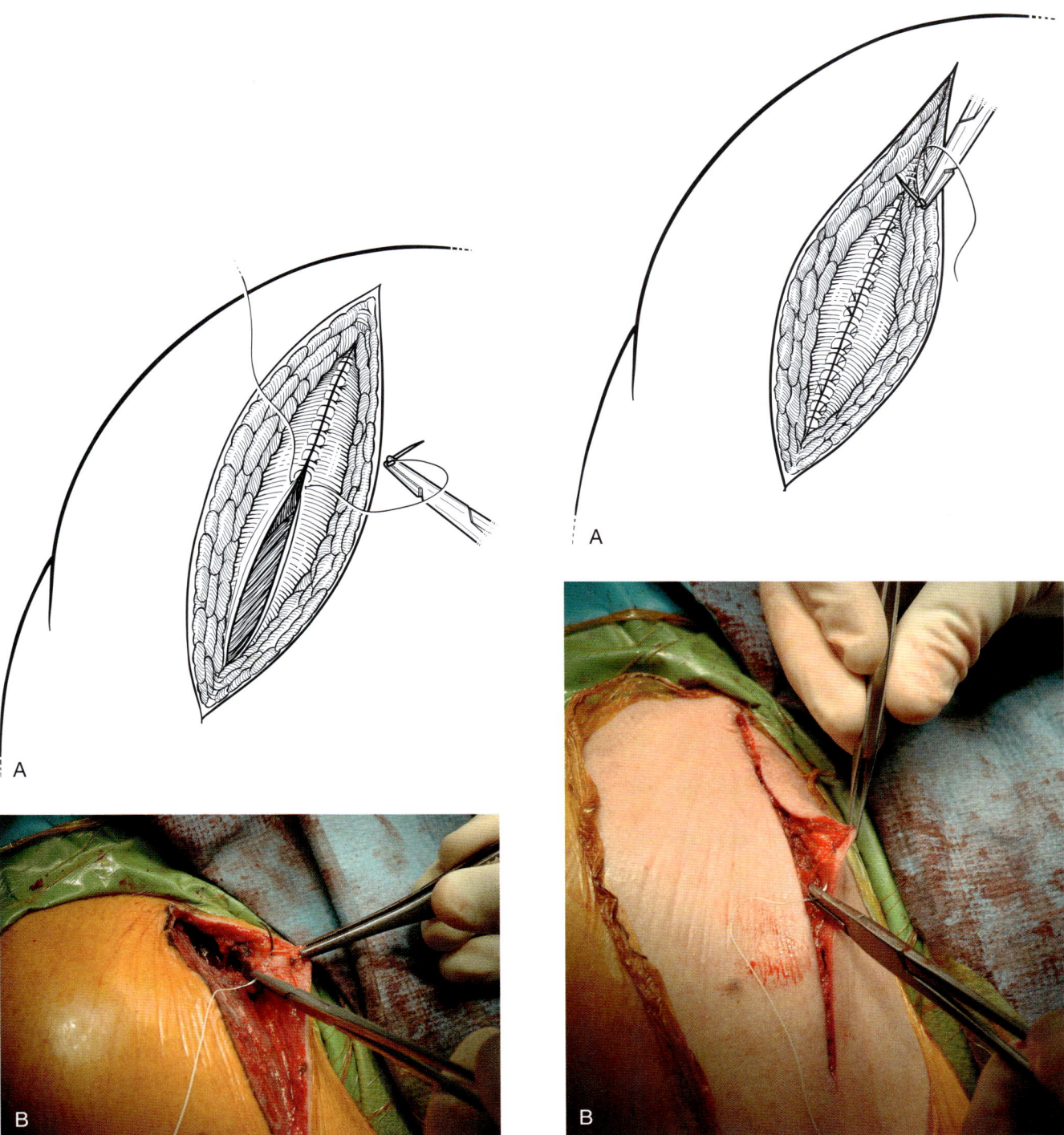

FIGURE 15.1 (A and B) Closure of the deep fascial layer.

FIGURE 15.2 (A and B) Closure of the subcutaneous fascia.

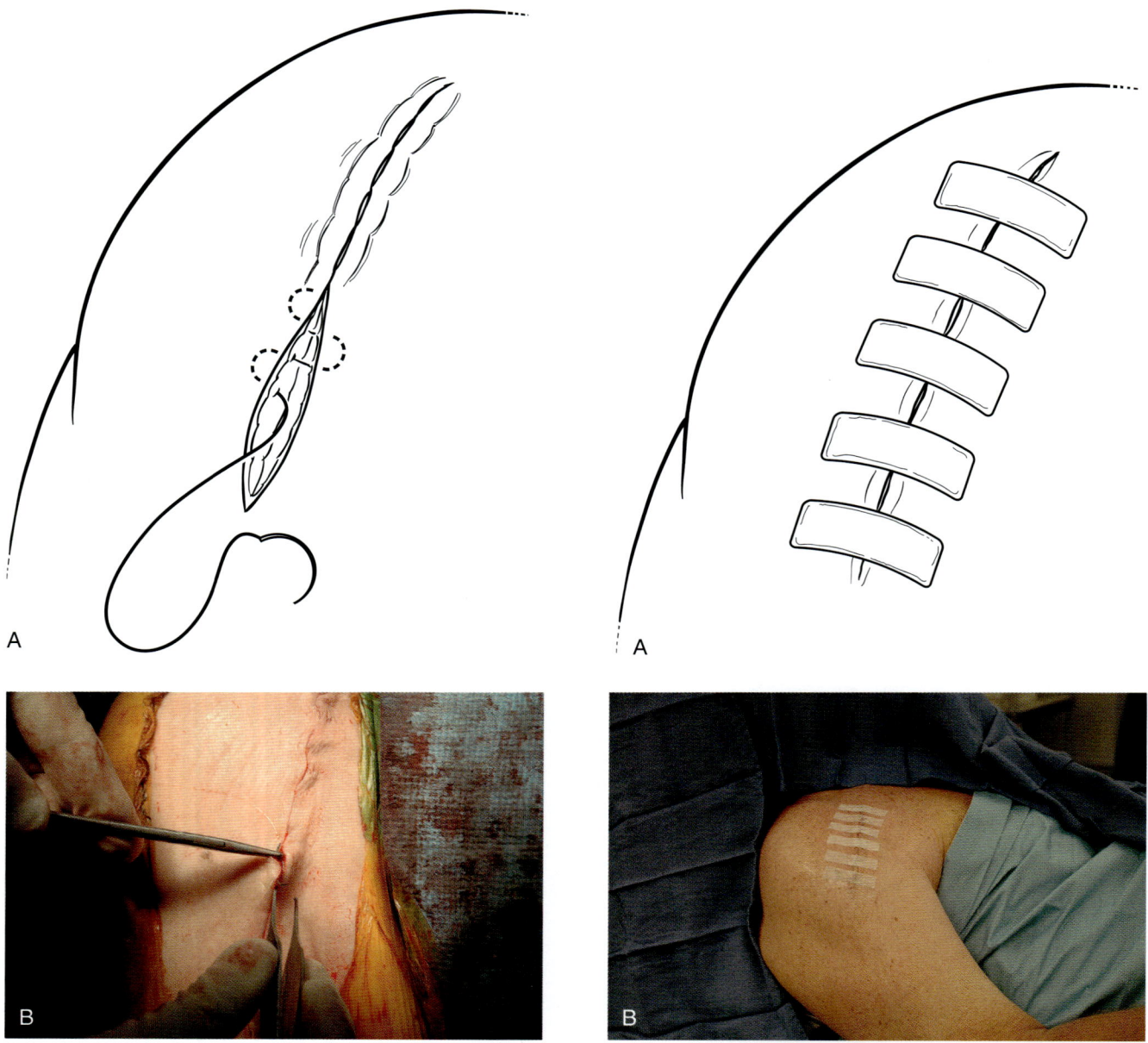

FIGURE 15.3 (A and B) Subcuticular skin closure.

FIGURE 15.4 (A and B) Steri-Strips covering the incision.

CHAPTER 15 ■ Wound Closure and Postoperative Orthosis

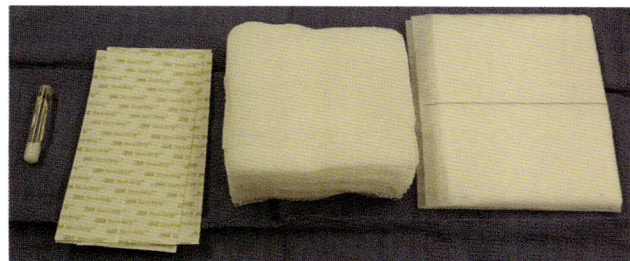

FIGURE 15.5 Sterile dressings used after shoulder arthroplasty.

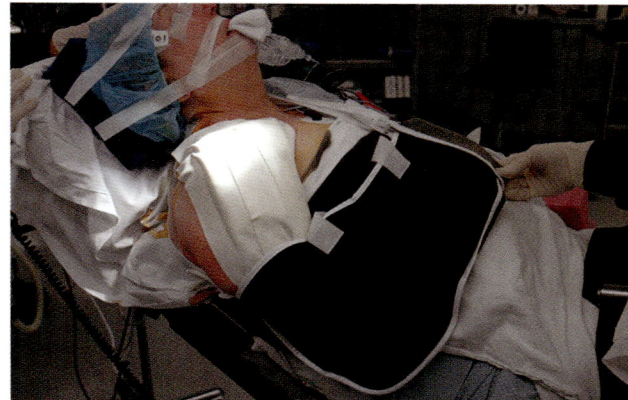

FIGURE 15.7 Simple sling used in most cases of unconstrained shoulder arthroplasty.

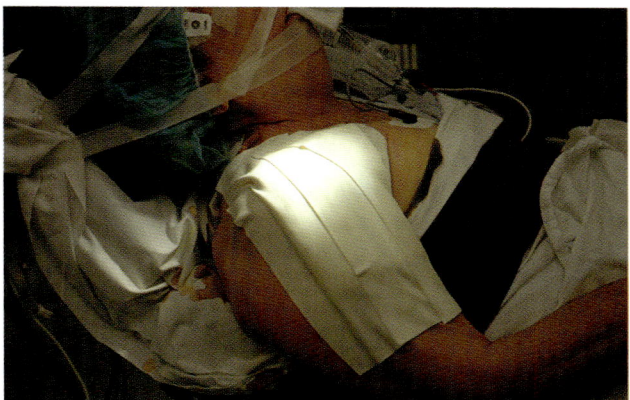

FIGURE 15.6 Completed postoperative dressing.

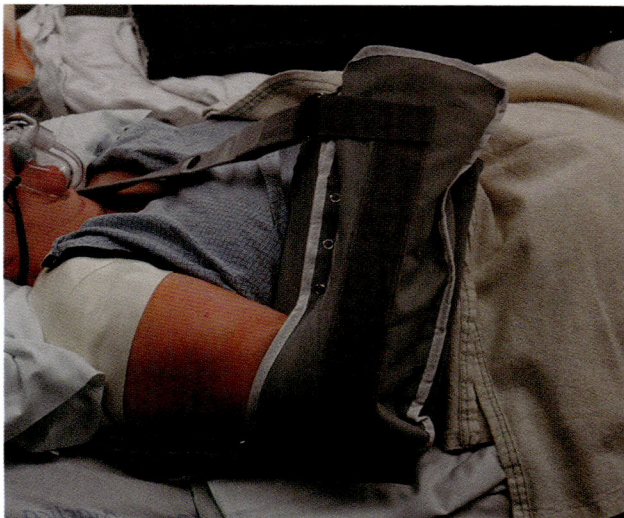

FIGURE 15.8 Application of a neutral rotation sling in patients who have undergone an associated posterior capsulorrhaphy.

REFERENCE

1. Gartsman GM, Milne JC, Russell JA: Closed wound drainage in shoulder surgery, *J Shoulder Elbow Surg* 6:288–290, 1997.

CHAPTER 16

Results and complications

The results of unconstrained shoulder arthroplasty have been reported by multiple investigators. These results vary predominantly according to the underlying indication for which the arthroplasty was performed. To our knowledge, the largest reported database of results of unconstrained shoulder arthroplasty was presented in Nice, France, in 2001.[1] Because of the large number of patients enrolled, this multicenter study has allowed meaningful conclusions to be drawn about the outcomes and complications of unconstrained shoulder arthroplasty. Our results have largely mirrored those reported in the Nice study. This chapter reports the results of unconstrained shoulder arthroplasty for the treatment of nonfracture conditions by drawing from information in the Nice database and our arthroplasty database, which was prospectively established in 2003. Additionally, the most frequent complications and their treatment are outlined.

RESULTS

The results of unconstrained shoulder arthroplasty vary mainly with the cause for which the arthroplasty is performed. The best results are obtained in the treatment of primary osteoarthritis and osteonecrosis, whereas results are least satisfactory for posttraumatic arthritis and rotator cuff tear arthropathy. Tables 16.1 and 16.2 detail the results of unconstrained shoulder arthroplasty for the most common indications.[2-8] These tables express the results in terms of active mobility; patient satisfaction; the Constant score, a shoulder-specific outcomes device incorporating pain, mobility, activity, and strength; and the age- and gender-adjusted Constant score.[9,10]

INTRAOPERATIVE COMPLICATIONS

Intraoperative complications are uncommon during shoulder arthroplasty and may be divided into complications involving the humerus, glenoid, musculotendinous soft tissues (rotator cuff), and neurovascular structures.

Humerus

Intraoperative complications involving the humerus are rare. The most common humeral complication is iatrogenic fracture, which usually results from performing an overly aggressive dislocation maneuver without previous adequate soft tissue release. Patients with osteopenia (i.e., inflammatory arthropathy) and those with severe preoperative stiffness (i.e., posttraumatic arthritis) are at most risk for this complication. These fractures may occur at the humeral diaphysis or proximally and involve the tuberosities. Fractures involving the humeral diaphysis should be reduced and a long-stem humeral implant placed. Allograft struts and cerclage cables may be added in patients with severe osteopenia (Fig. 16.1).

Intraoperative fractures involving the greater or lesser tuberosities (or both) are usually nondisplaced. Many of these fractures are stable or become stable once the humeral implant has been placed (Fig. 16.2). If a tuberosity fracture is not satisfactorily stable, suture fixation of the tuberosity is performed and the postoperative rehabilitation adjusted accordingly to allow healing of the tuberosity.

Glenoid

Intraoperative glenoid fractures are more common than humeral injury. These fractures almost always occur during preparation (reaming) of the glenoid. Patients with osteopenia are most at risk. Fractures may involve only the peripheral glenoid rim or may extend significantly into the articular surface. Adequate capsular release helps minimize the risk of glenoid fracture. Additionally, a motorized reamer (not a drill) should be used to prepare the glenoid surface. The reamer should be started before the surgeon applies force to engage the reamer onto the glenoid face. This avoids having the reamer "catch" an edge of the glenoid, which may cause a fracture.

Fractures that involve only a small portion of the peripheral rim usually require no treatment, and the glenoid component can be inserted as planned. Glenoid fractures that extend into the central portion of the glenoid (keel slot or peg holes) should be bone-grafted with the humeral head and placement of a glenoid component should be avoided. Placement of a glenoid component in a patient with a fracture involving the central portion of the glenoid can result in early glenoid failure (Fig. 16.3).

Rotator Cuff

With proper glenoid exposure, intraoperative injury to the rotator cuff is rare. The key to avoiding rotator cuff injury during unconstrained shoulder arthroplasty is adequate visualization of the rotator cuff before resection of the humeral head (see Chapter 11). If the rotator cuff is adequately

TABLE 16.1 Results of Unconstrained Shoulder Arthroplasty According to Underlying Cause in the Nice Multicenter Study

Etiology	Absolute Constant Score (Points)		Adjusted Constant Score (%)		Active Forward Flexion (Degrees)		Active External Rotation (Degrees)		Excellent/Good Subjective Results (%)
	Preoperative	Postoperative	Preoperative	Postoperative	Preoperative	Postoperative	Preoperative	Postoperative	
Primary osteoarthritis ($n = 689$)[2]	32	71	43	96	92	142	8	41	93
Rheumatoid arthritis ($n = 172$)[3]	26	56	34	73	79	120	15	39	90
Osteonecrosis ($n = 80$)[4]	30	70	37	88	89	142	15	41	90
Post-traumatic arthritis ($n = 203$)[5]	27	57	NA[a]	NA	80	112	2	30	81
Fixed dislocation ($n = 11$)[6]	21	46	28	60	49	90	13	26	73
Cuff tear arthropathy ($n = 66$)[7]	25	46	NA	NA	76	96	10	22	NA
Instability arthropathy ($n = 55$)[8]	301	66	38	80	82	139	4	39	94

[a]Not available. These data were not reported in the referenced article/chapter.
From Walch G, Boileau P: Presentation of the multicentric study. In Walch G, Boileau P, Molé D, editors: *2000 Prothèses d'Epaule … Recul de 2 à 10 Ans*, Paris, Sauramps Medical, 2001, pp 11–20.

TABLE 16.2	Results of Unconstrained Shoulder Arthroplasty According to Underlying Cause in the Authors' Prospective Database From 2003 to 2014								
	Absolute Constant Score (Points)		Adjusted Constant Score (%)		Active Forward Flexion (Degrees)		Active External Rotation (Degrees)		Excellent/Good Subjective Results (%)
Etiology	Preoperative	Postoperative	Preoperative	Postoperative	Preoperative	Postoperative	Preoperative	Postoperative	
Primary osteoarthritis (n = 388)	28	78	36	103	87	160	12	45	90
Rheumatoid arthritis (n = 11)	21	66	30	90	72	142	18	54	91
Atraumatic osteonecrosis (n = 8)	42	74	58	104	106	158	26	48	88
Instability arthropathy (n = 34)	28	81	32	96	89	163	6	44	94

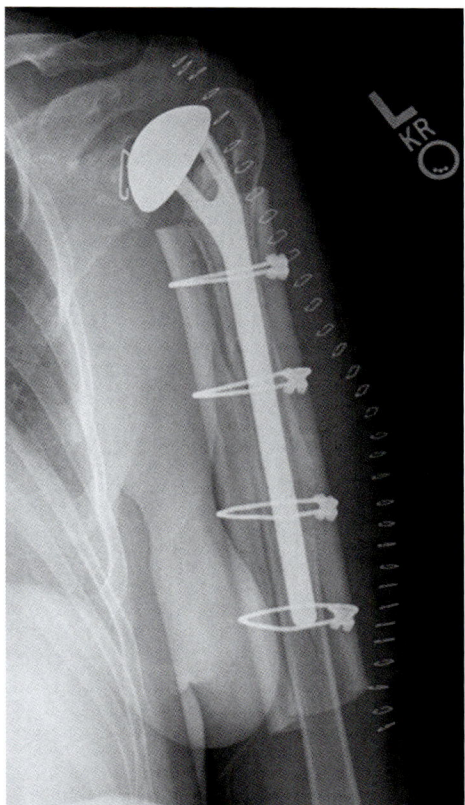

FIGURE 16.1 Fixation of an intraoperative humeral diaphyseal fracture with a long-stem humeral implant, allograft cortical struts, and cerclage cables.

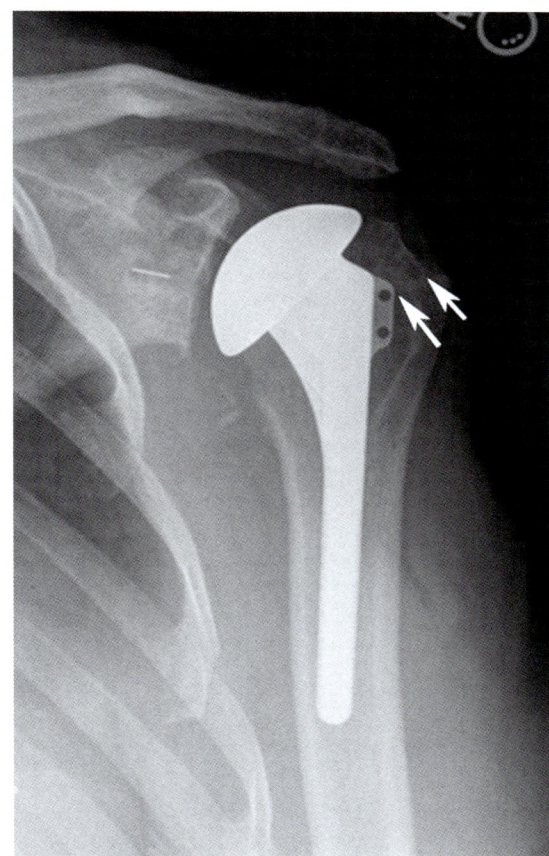

FIGURE 16.2 Nondisplaced fractures of the greater tuberosity *(arrows)* are usually sufficiently stable after placement of the humeral implant.

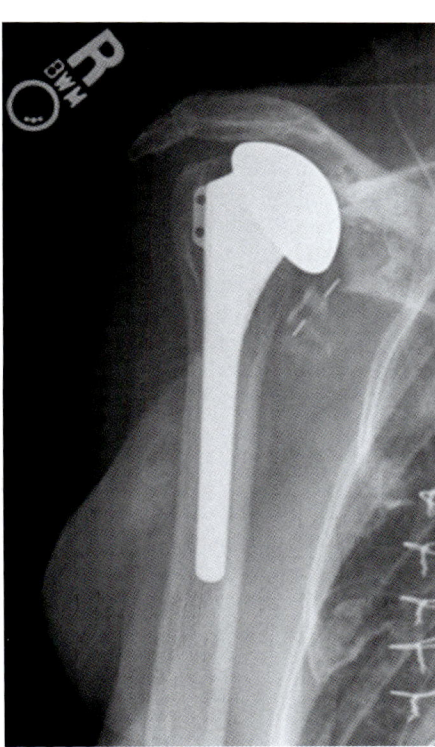

FIGURE 16.3 Early glenoid failure caused by placement of a glenoid component despite the occurrence of an intraoperative glenoid fracture.

visualized, inadvertent damage to the rotator cuff by the saw during humeral head resection can be avoided.

Neurovascular Structures

Catastrophic injury to neurovascular structures around the shoulder is exceedingly rare. Transient neuropraxia involving the axillary nerve, however, is one of the most common complications that we observe in unconstrained shoulder arthroplasty (up to 3% of cases).

The neural structures most at risk during unconstrained shoulder arthroplasty are the axillary and musculocutaneous nerves. During primary arthroplasty, these nerves should not be at risk for transection when an accepted operative technique is being used. Neuropraxic injury caused by stretch most commonly involves the axillary nerve, but any nerves within the brachial plexus can be involved. Care should be taken in positioning the patient to maintain the cervical spine in neutral alignment in order to avoid a stretch injury of the brachial plexus. We have yet to establish risk factors for neuropraxic injury to the axillary nerve. Intraoperative nerve monitoring studies have shown that nerve injury with anatomic shoulder arthroplasty may be increased with extremes of motion during the case and for patients with preoperative decreased passive external rotation, decreased forward flexion, and a history of prior open shoulder surgery.[11,12] These studies were based on intraoperative nerve monitoring and short-term electromyography and cannot definitively establish risk factors for long-term clinical implications. Logic would suggest that patients with the most stiffness, creating difficulty in glenoid exposure, would be at highest risk for this type of complication. Our clinical experience has not borne this out, however, and currently we are unable to predict which patients are most likely to experience this complication. Patient education preoperatively is of paramount importance in dealing with neuropraxia because patients are much more accepting if they have heard about the possibility of this complication before surgery. Axillary nerve (and other nerve) neuropraxia is treated by observation, with most patients recovering by 3 to 4 months postoperatively.

Although tearing of the cephalic vein is common and largely without consequence, significant arterial and venous injuries occurring during primary unconstrained shoulder arthroplasty performed for nonfracture indications are exceptionally rare. Injuries to the major upper extremity vessels are generally due to overzealous medial dissection, which is not needed during shoulder arthroplasty. Should such an injury occur, emergency intraoperative consultation with a vascular surgeon is required after cross-clamping of the injured vessel.

POSTOPERATIVE COMPLICATIONS

Postoperative complications are more common than intraoperative complications and occur in up to 20% of cases of unconstrained shoulder arthroplasty.[1] The most common postoperative complications include wound problems (dehiscence, hematoma), glenoid problems, humeral problems, instability, rotator cuff problems, stiffness, and infection.

Wound Problems

Wound problems occur early after unconstrained shoulder arthroplasty. Hematoma is most easily avoided by extensive use of electrocautery during shoulder arthroplasty. Suture ligation, in addition to electrosurgical cauterization, of the anterior humeral circumflex vessels also minimizes the incidence of postoperative wound hematoma. When a hematoma occurs, it is managed by symptomatic nonoperative treatment (warm compresses, pain medication). Operative drainage is reserved for situations in which drainage persists beyond 1 week or infection is suspected (see later), but it is rarely necessary.

Wound dehiscence occasionally occurs when susceptible patients have a reaction to dissolving subcutaneous sutures. The presence of minimal serous drainage distinguishes this complication from the more serious deep infection. Superficial wound dehiscence is treated by local wound care, including removal of any residual dissolving suture material and chemical cauterization of any granulating tissue with silver nitrate applicators (Fig. 16.4).

Glenoid Problems

Glenoid problems after unconstrained shoulder arthroplasty are the most common complications necessitating revision surgery. Glenoid complications can develop after both total

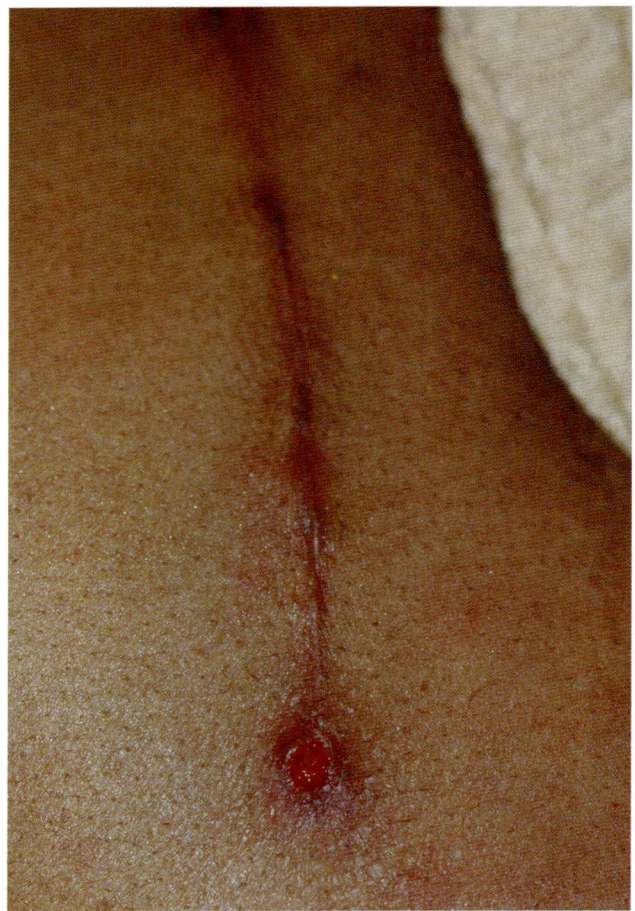

FIGURE 16.4 Superficial wound dehiscence.

shoulder arthroplasty and isolated humeral head replacement (hemiarthroplasty). Glenoid component failure after total shoulder arthroplasty can occur as a result of loosening of the glenoid component from the host bone (Fig. 16.5) or as a result of mechanical breakage of the glenoid implant (Fig. 16.6). Glenoid component problems, when symptomatic, usually require revision surgery (see Section VI).

After hemiarthroplasty, erosion of the remaining glenoid articular cartilage and osseous glenoid can occur. This can take place early or late and is multifactorial in its cause.[13] Successful treatment of glenoid erosion generally requires revision surgery, during which the glenoid is resurfaced (Fig. 16.7).

Humeral Problems

Humeral problems after unconstrained shoulder arthroplasty are rare and can be divided into loosening of the humeral component and periprosthetic humeral fracture. Aseptic loosening of cemented and surface-prepared (grit-blasted, porous-coated, etc.) uncemented unconstrained humeral stems develops in less than 1% of cases. Whenever loosening of a humeral stem occurs, infection must be ruled out (Fig. 16.8; see later). In the rare instance of symptomatic aseptic loosening of the humeral component, treatment is

Text continued on p. 140

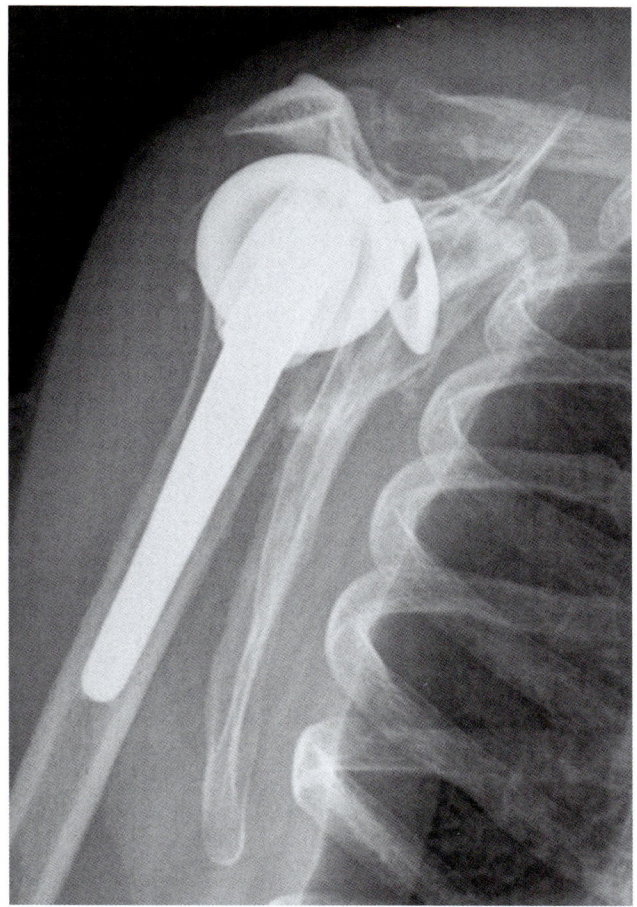

FIGURE 16.5 Aseptic loosening of a glenoid component.

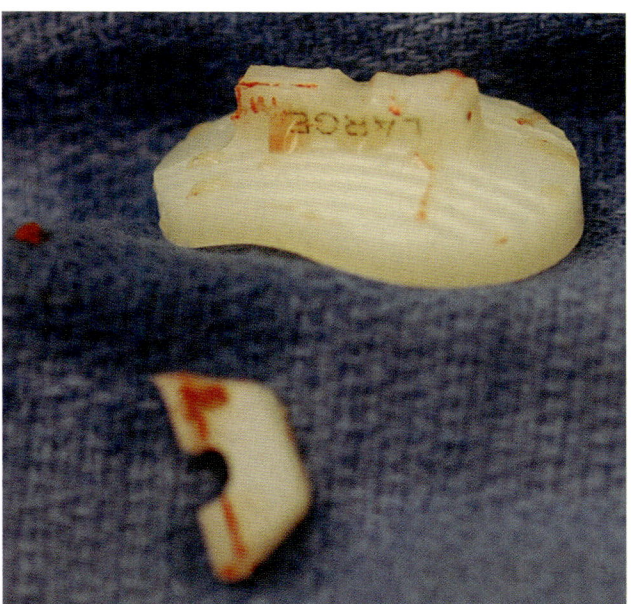

FIGURE 16.6 Fracture of a glenoid component.

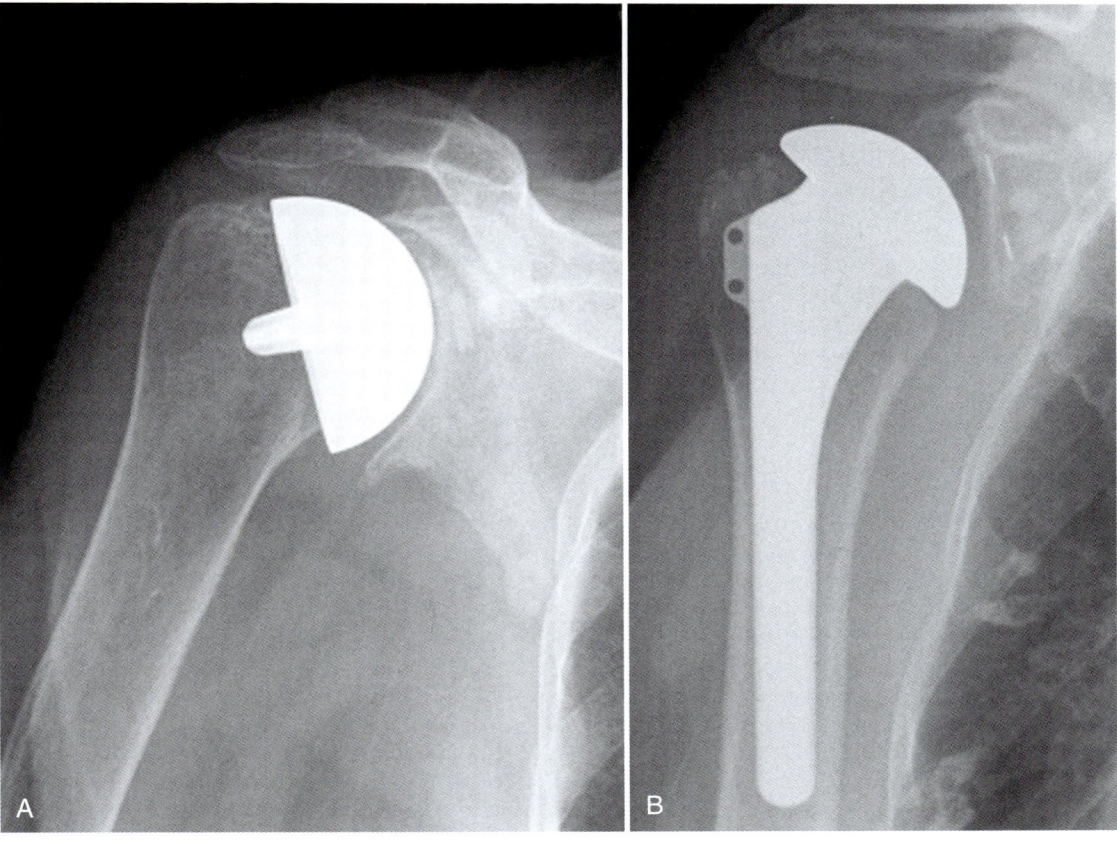

FIGURE 16.7 Symptomatic glenoid erosion (A) necessitating revision surgery for insertion of a glenoid component (B).

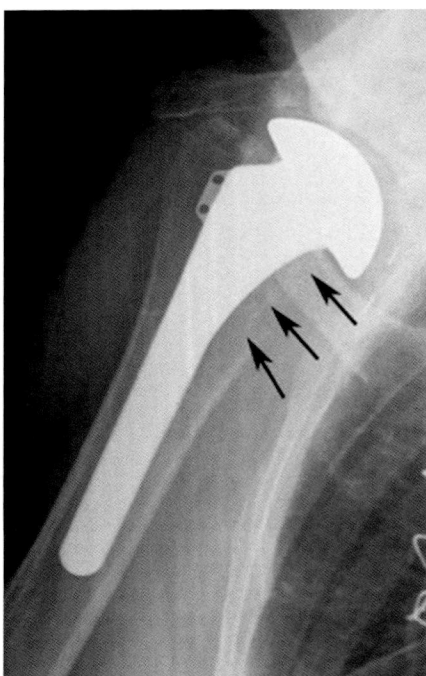

FIGURE 16.8　Septic loosening of a humeral stem *(arrows)*.

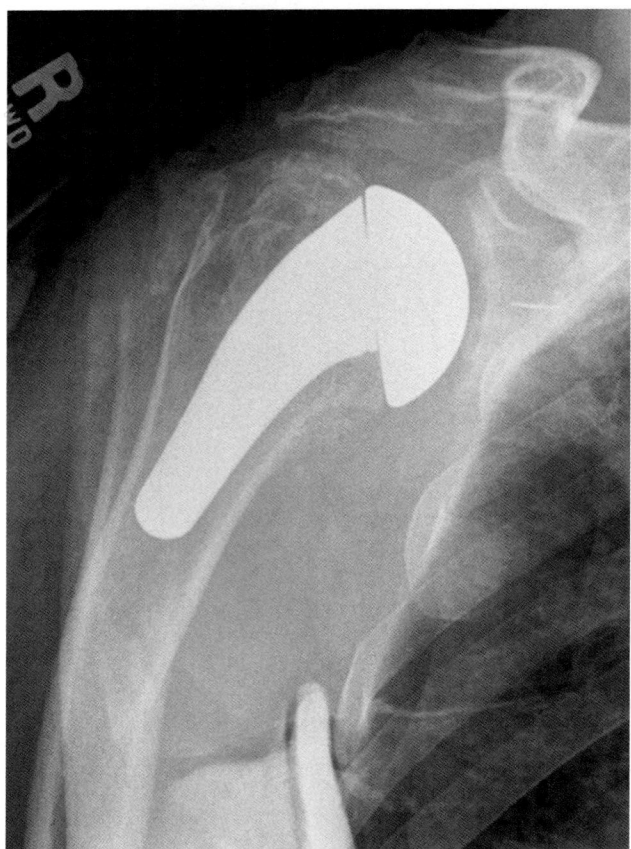

FIGURE 16.9　Periprosthetic humeral diaphyseal fracture resulting from a fall.

revision of the humeral stem, usually with a cemented humeral component (see Section VI).

Periprosthetic humeral fractures are more common than loosening of the humeral component and are almost always the result of a fall or similar low-energy trauma (Fig. 16.9). The majority of these fractures occur just distal to the tip of the humeral stem, and most can be treated nonoperatively. Nonoperative treatment consists of fracture bracing, activity modification, pain medication, and frequent radiographic monitoring. If the fracture has not healed within 3 months, we incorporate the use of an external bone stimulator (OL 1000 Bone Growth Stimulator, Donjoy Orthopedics, Vista, California). Despite these measures, periprosthetic humeral fractures treated nonoperatively may take more than 9 months to heal.[14] Our criteria for recommending operative treatment of periprosthetic fractures (revision surgery; see Section VI) include complete displacement, angulation greater than 30 degrees, loosening of the humeral component, or failure of nonoperative treatment (Fig. 16.10).

Instability

Instability after unconstrained shoulder arthroplasty is usually related to one or more of three factors, including the prosthesis (alignment, size), the capsule, and the rotator cuff. Cases where prosthetic problems have led to dynamic or static shoulder instability require correction to resolve the instability. Prosthetic problems may be related to the humeral side (excessive retroversion, causing posterior instability; excessive anteversion, causing anterior instability; too small a prosthetic head, causing global instability) or the glenoid side (failure to correct posterior glenoid wear, causing posterior instability). Revision arthroplasty (see Section VI) is the treatment of instability related to a prosthetic problem.

Capsular problems leading to instability are generally related to failure to perform posterior capsulorrhaphy at the time of primary arthroplasty in a patient with posterior glenoid wear and a chronically distended posterior capsule, resulting in posterior instability (Fig. 16.11; see Chapter 13). Required treatment consists of revision surgery with performance of posterior capsulorrhaphy (marginally successful) or conversion to a reverse prosthesis (more predictable outcome; Fig. 16.12).

Rotator cuff problems can cause static and dynamic instability. Unconstrained arthroplasty in patients with a compromised rotator cuff often results in static instability (Fig. 16.13). These patients are best treated initially with a reverse-design prosthesis to avoid this potential complication. Rarely, in a patient with a previously intact rotator cuff who has undergone unconstrained shoulder arthroplasty, a massive rotator cuff tear will develop and contribute to static instability (Fig. 16.14). These patients, when symptomatic, are best treated by revision to a reverse-design prosthesis (Fig. 16.15).

Dynamic instability after unconstrained shoulder arthroplasty most commonly occurs as anterior instability secondary to failure of the subscapularis repair. If this is diagnosed early, an attempt at subscapularis repair is warranted. Occasionally, failure of the subscapularis repair may be related to implantation of too large a humeral head component (Fig. 16.16). In this situation, subscapularis repair should be accompanied by exchange of the humeral head component

Text continued on p. 144

CHAPTER 16 ■ Results and Complications 141

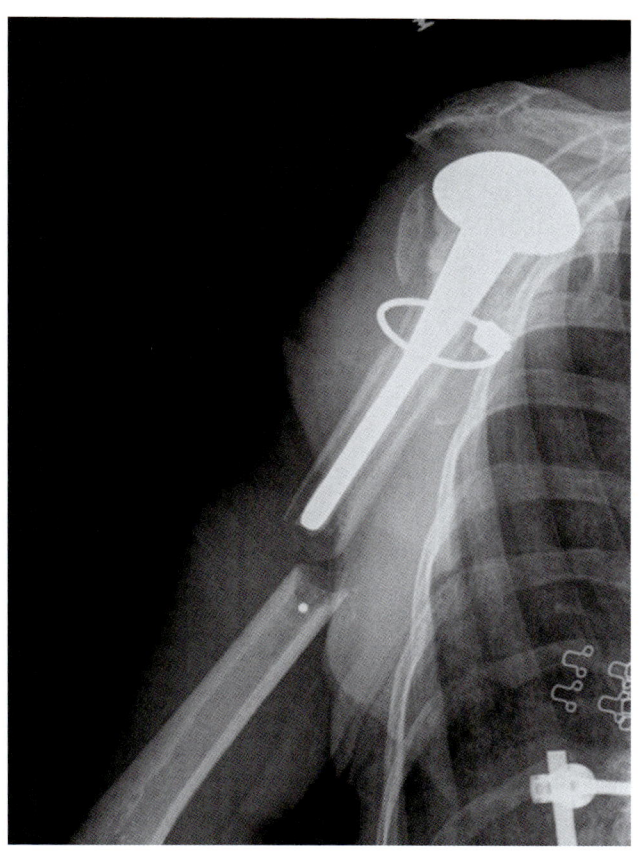

FIGURE 16.10 Periprosthetic humeral diaphyseal fracture failing 9 months of nonoperative treatment, including use of a bone stimulator.

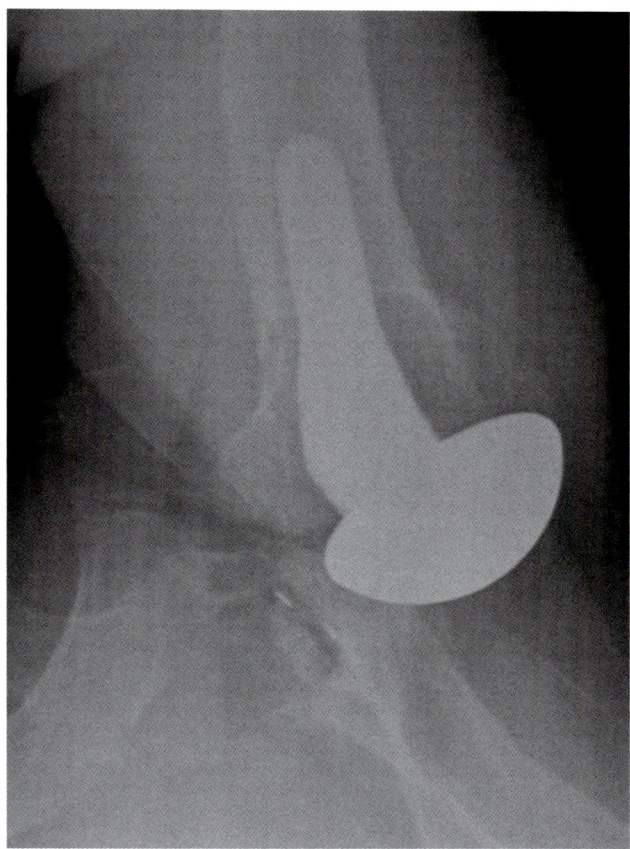

FIGURE 16.11 Posterior instability of an unconstrained shoulder arthroplasty.

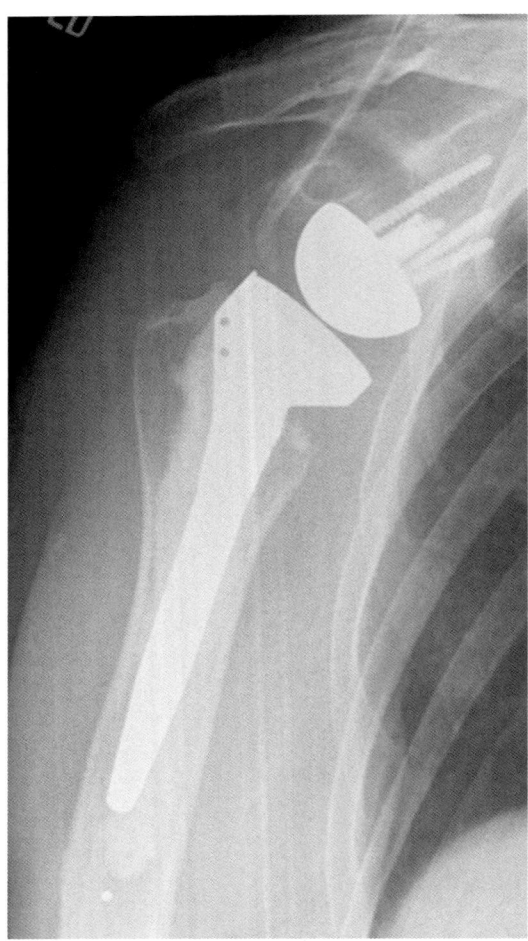

FIGURE 16.12 Revision of an unconstrained shoulder arthroplasty to a reverse arthroplasty for the treatment of postoperative posterior shoulder instability.

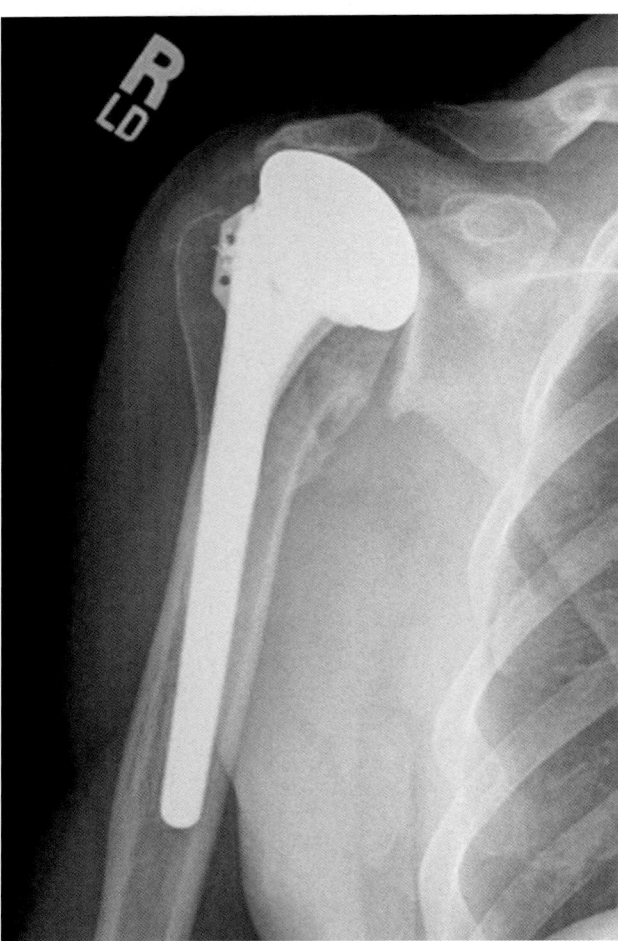

FIGURE 16.13 Anterosuperior escape of a hemiarthroplasty in a patient with a massive rotator cuff tear.

CHAPTER 16 ■ Results and Complications 143

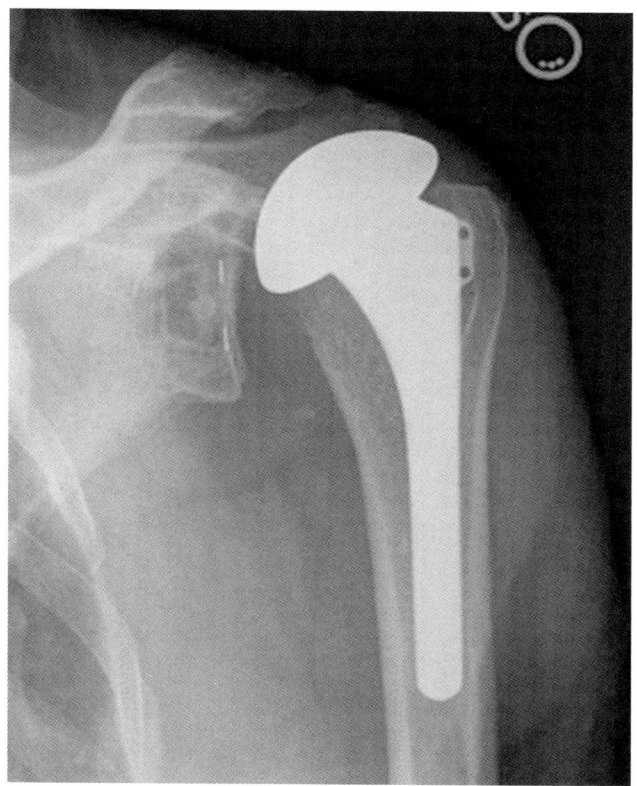

FIGURE 16.14 Radiograph of a patient who had undergone total shoulder arthroplasty for primary osteoarthritis. The patient did well until a massive degenerative rotator cuff tear developed and led to static proximal migration of the humerus some years after the index arthroplasty.

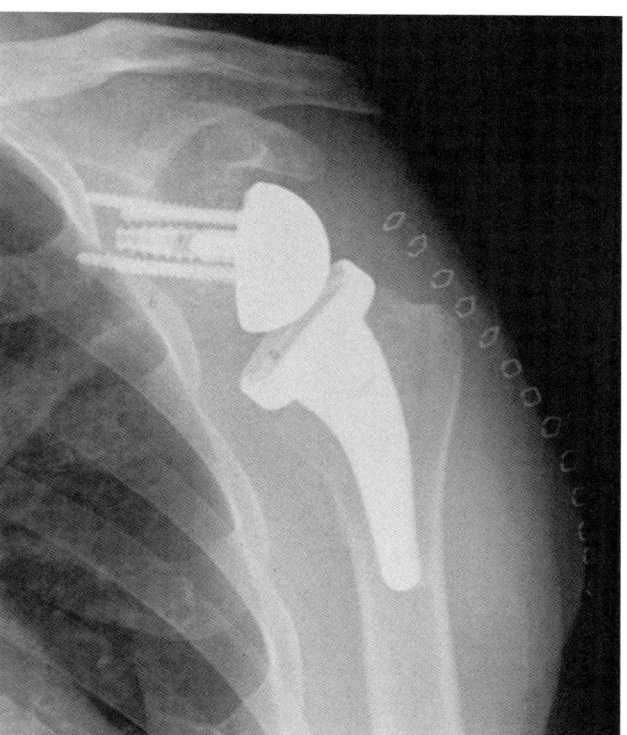

FIGURE 16.15 Revision of an unconstrained arthroplasty with a reverse prosthesis in a patient with static proximal migration of the humerus.

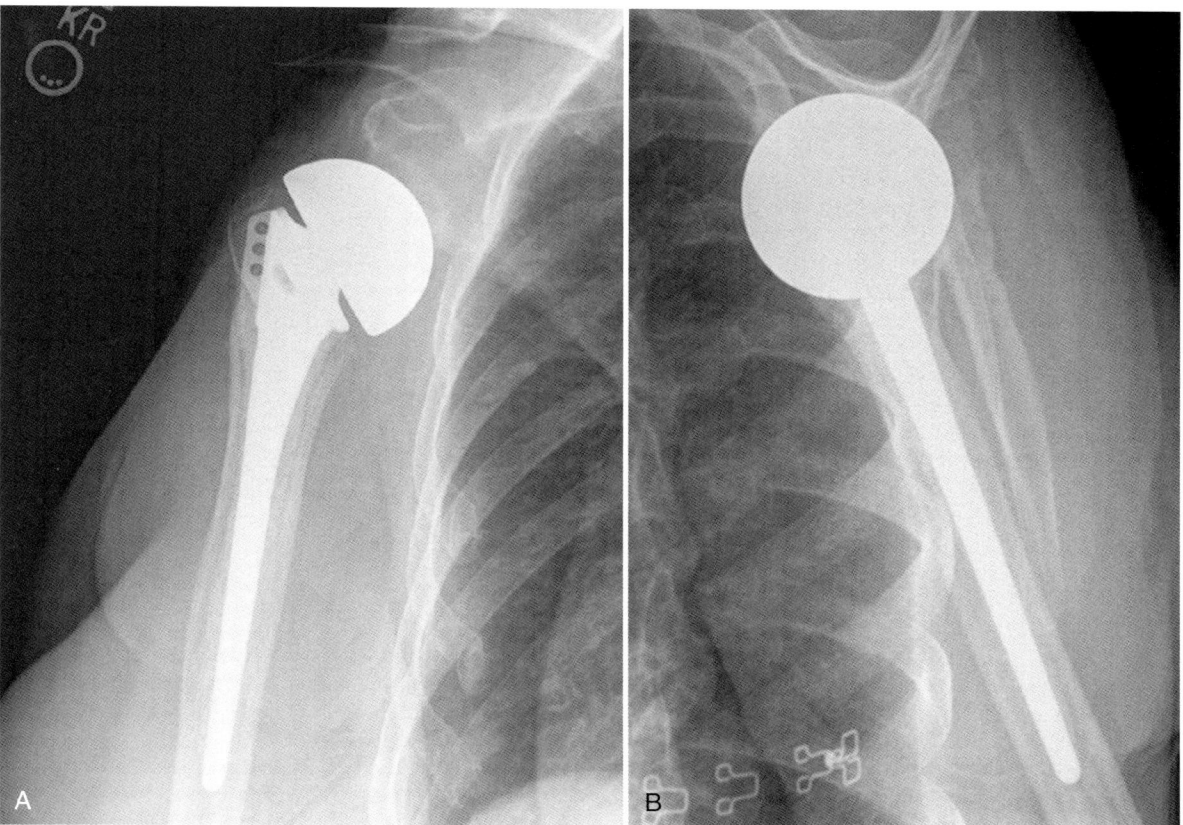

FIGURE 16.16 (A and B) Subscapularis repair failure caused by implantation of too large a humeral head.

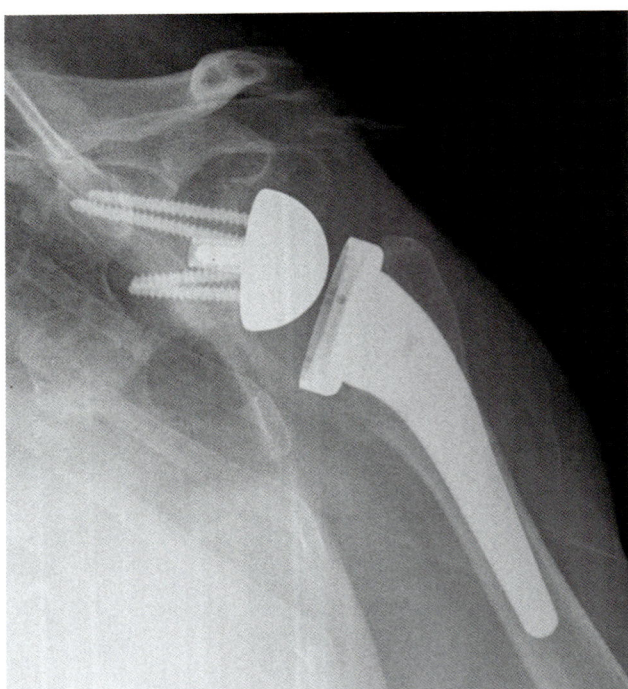

FIGURE 16.17 Revision arthroplasty with a reverse prosthesis in a patient with dynamic anterior shoulder instability secondary to failure of the subscapularis repair.

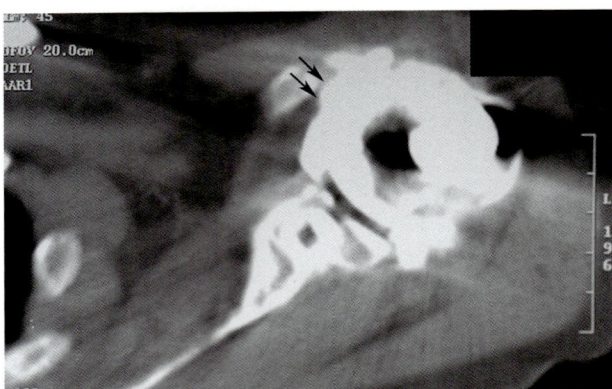

FIGURE 16.18 Computed tomography arthrogram demonstrating disruption of the subscapularis (*arrows*).

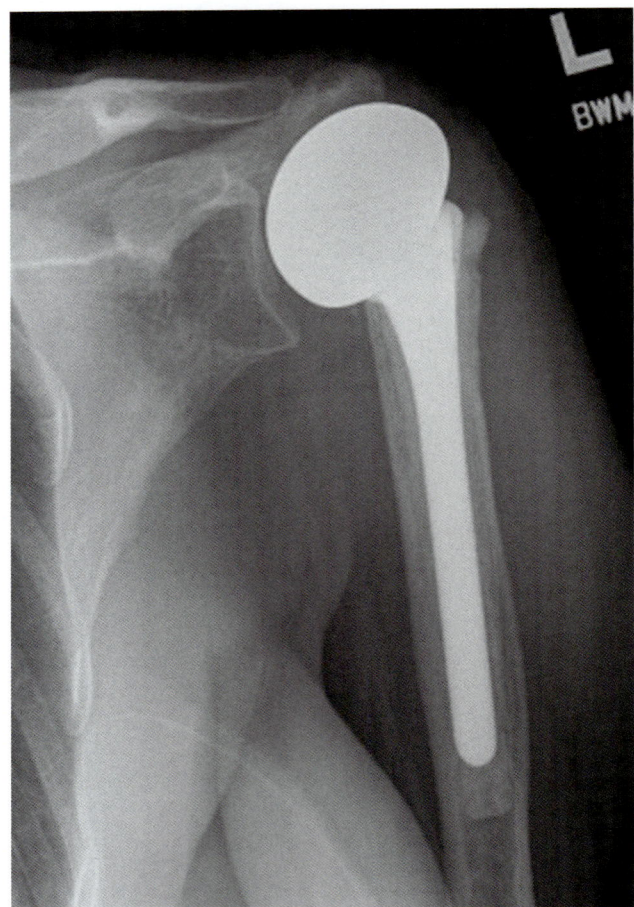

FIGURE 16.19 Postoperative shoulder stiffness caused by insertion of too large a humeral head component.

for one smaller in size. If diagnosed after 4 to 6 weeks postoperatively, subscapularis repair is not usually possible and we opt for revision to a reverse-design prosthesis (Fig. 16.17).

Rotator Cuff Problems

Symptomatic problems of the rotator cuff after unconstrained shoulder arthroplasty often result in instability and are described earlier under "Instability." Failure of the subscapularis repair is the most common postoperative rotator cuff problem that we observe, yet it occurs in less than 3% of cases.[1] When subscapularis failure is minimally symptomatic or asymptomatic, no treatment is indicated. When symptomatic, treatment is indicated as described previously under "Instability."

Isolated internal rotation weakness is not diagnostic of subscapularis failure after unconstrained shoulder arthroplasty. It is common for individuals to lose some internal rotation strength after tenotomy and repair of the subscapularis during shoulder arthroplasty. Subscapularis failure should be documented by computed tomography arthrography before operative treatment of this complication is considered (Fig. 16.18).

Stiffness

Glenohumeral stiffness after unconstrained shoulder arthroplasty is related to capsular contracture or the prosthesis (or to both). Prosthetic problems resulting in stiffness are almost always the result of implantation of too large a humeral component (Fig. 16.19). Rehabilitation with capsular stretching can be attempted in an effort to improve mobility. If this fails (no improvement over a 6-month period), revision surgery consisting of downsizing of the humeral head and open release of any capsular contractures is indicated.

Stiffness related to capsular contracture almost always responds to nonoperative management with aquatic-based rehabilitation (see Chapter 43). If a patient shows no improvement in mobility over a 6-month course of rehabilitation and has no obvious prosthetic problem, we will consider him or her a candidate for arthroscopic capsular contracture release.

Infection

Fortunately, infection after shoulder arthroplasty is much less common than infection after hip or knee arthroplasty; it has occurred in less than 1% of all cases in our practice. Patients most at risk for infection are those with systemic illness (diabetes mellitus), those with compromised soft tissues (radiation-induced osteonecrosis, posttraumatic arthritis), and those with inflammatory arthropathy (rheumatoid arthritis). These infections are most commonly caused by *Staphylococcus aureus* or *Propionibacterium acnes*. Infections after shoulder arthroplasty can be divided into perioperative (within 6 weeks of surgery) and late (hematogenous) infections.

Early perioperative infections are initially treated by multiple (two or three) irrigation and débridement procedures with retention of the components. At the last planned irrigation and débridement procedure, absorbable antibiotic-impregnated beads (Stimulan, Biocomposites, Inc., Staffordshire, England) are placed in the soft tissues around the shoulder. Consultation with an infectious disease specialist is obtained, and a minimum of 6 weeks of intravenous antibiotics tailored to the specific organism causing the infection (or covering the most likely offending organisms if cultures remain negative despite obvious infection) is usually recommended. If this regimen fails, prosthetic removal ensues, as detailed in Section VI.

Late-appearing infections are treated by removal of the prosthesis and intravenous antibiotics as detailed in Section VI. The decision regarding whether to place a revision shoulder arthroplasty or continue with a resection arthroplasty is patient-specific.

REFERENCES

1. Walch G, Boileau P: Presentation of the multicentric study. In Walch G, Boileau P, Molé D, editors: *2000 Prosthèses d'Epaule … Recul de 2 à 10 Ans*, Paris, 2001, Sauramps Medical, pp 11–20.
2. Lafosse L, Kempf JF: Omarthrose primitive: Resultats cliniques et radiologiques. In Walch G, Boileau P, Molé D, editors: *2000 Prosthèses d'Epaule … Recul de 2 à 10 Ans*, Paris, 2001, Sauramps Medical, pp 73–85.
3. Gohlke F: Clinical and radiographic results of shoulder arthroplasty in rheumatoid arthritis. In Walch G, Boileau P, Molé D, editors: *2000 Prosthèses d'Epaule … Recul de 2 à 10 Ans*, Paris, 2001, Sauramps Medical, pp 163–169.
4. Versier G, Marchaland JP: Ostéonécorse avasculaire aseptique de la tête humérale (onath): Résultats cliniques et radiologiques des prostheses d'épaule. In Walch G, Boileau P, Molé D, editors: *2000 Prosthèses d'Epaule … Recul de 2 à 10 Ans*, Paris, 2001, Sauramps Medical, pp 127–134.
5. Trojani C, Boileau P, LeHeuc JC, et al: Sequelae of fractures of the proximal humerus: Surgical classification. In Walch G, Boileau P, Molé D, editors: *2000 Prosthèses d'Epaule … Recul de 2 à 10 Ans*, Paris, 2001, Sauramps Medical, pp 271–277.
6. Matsoukis J, Tabib W, Guiffault P, et al: Primary unconstrained shoulder arthroplasty in patients with a fixed anterior glenohumeral dislocation: results of a multicenter study, *J Bone Joint Surg Am* 88:547–552, 2006.
7. Oudet D, Favard L, Lautmann S, et al: La prosthèse d'épaule aequalis dans les omarthroses avec rupture massive et non réparable de la coiffe. In Walch G, Boileau P, Molé D, editors: *2000 Prosthèses d'Epaule … Recul de 2 à 10 Ans*, Paris, 2001, Sauramps Medical, pp 241–246.
8. Matsoukis J, Tabib W, Guiffault P, et al: Shoulder arthroplasty in patients with a prior anterior shoulder dislocation: results of a multicenter study, *J Bone Joint Surg Am* 85:1417–1424, 2003.
9. Constant CR, Murley AH: A clinical method of functional assessment of the shoulder, *Clin Orthop Relat Res* 214:160–164, 1987.
10. Constant CR: Assessment of shoulder function. In Gazielly D, Gleyze P, Thomas T, editors: *The Cuff*, New York, 1997, Elsevier, pp 39–44.
11. Nagda SH, Rogers KJ, Sestokas AK, et al: Neer Award 2005: peripheral nerve function during shoulder arthroplasty using intraoperative nerve monitoring, *J Shoulder Elbow Surg* 16(3 Suppl):S2–S8, 2007. [Epub 2006 Jul 26].
12. Parisien RL, Yi PH, Hou L, et al: The risk of nerve injury during anatomical and reverse total shoulder arthroplasty: an intraoperative neuromonitoring study, *J Shoulder Elbow Surg* 25(7):1122–1127, 2016.
13. Hertel R, Lehmann O: Glenoid erosion after hemiarthroplasty of the shoulder. In Walch G, Boileau P, Molé D, editors: *2000 Prosthèses d'Epaule … Recul de 2 à 10 Ans*, Paris, 2001, Sauramps Medical, pp 417–423.
14. Kumar S, Sperling JW, Haidukewych GH, et al: Periprosthetic humeral fractures after shoulder arthroplasty, *J Bone Joint Surg Am* 86:680–689, 2004.

REVERSE SHOULDER ARTHROPLASTY

Indications and contraindications

SECTION III

CHAPTER 17

Reintroduction of reverse-design shoulder arthroplasty has added a powerful device to the shoulder surgeon's armamentarium. Reverse ball-and-socket shoulder prostheses were initially introduced in the 1960s to treat patients with glenohumeral arthritis and massive rotator cuff tears. The concept of these and subsequent devices is to resolve upward migration of the humeral head and thereby restore the normal deltoid moment arm. This allows the deltoid to power active elevation of the arm (Fig. 17.1). The problem with the initial designs was early loosening of the glenoid caused by the action of deltoid forces on the laterally offset center of glenohumeral rotation (Fig. 17.2). These failures eventually resulted in abandonment of these early prosthetic designs.

In 1987, Paul Grammont introduced a reverse-design prosthesis that used a "glenosphere" component fixated over the scapular neck. In an effort to overcome the failures that had plagued earlier attempts, Grammont's design placed the center of glenohumeral rotation within the bone of the glenoid instead of lateral to it (Fig. 17.3).[1] Most available reverse prostheses take advantage of Grammont's ingenuity.

The reverse prosthesis was originally introduced to treat rotator cuff tear arthropathy. The reverse prosthesis resurfaces the glenohumeral joint with a total shoulder arthroplasty to treat the arthritis component and restores normal deltoid tension to allow active elevation—goals that are infrequently accomplished with conventional unconstrained hemiarthroplasty. Because the results from this implant were observed to be good and the complication rate low for this select indication, indications were expanded as experience broadened. Currently, a reverse prosthesis is considered in a patient who has severe rotator cuff dysfunction but would otherwise be a candidate for unconstrained shoulder arthroplasty. This chapter details the specific indications for which we use a reverse prosthesis as a primary shoulder arthroplasty. Another application for a reverse prosthesis is revision arthroplasty. We cover that scenario in Section VI.

ROTATOR CUFF TEAR ARTHROPATHY (GLENOHUMERAL OSTEOARTHRITIS WITH MASSIVE ROTATOR CUFF TEAR)

Rotator cuff tear arthropathy was initially described by Neer and consists of a massive irreparable rotator cuff tear combined with glenohumeral arthritis and, in the late stages, humeral head osteonecrosis.[2] This entity has gradually expanded to include all patients with massive rotator cuff tears and glenohumeral arthritis, even in the absence of humeral head osteonecrosis. Although we believe that rotator cuff tear arthropathy as described by Neer and glenohumeral osteoarthritis with a massive rotator cuff tear are two distinct entities, the clinical scenarios are sufficiently similar that we consider them together both in our practice and in this textbook.

Rotator cuff tear arthropathy (glenohumeral osteoarthritis with a massive rotator cuff tear) is the single most common indication for which we perform reverse shoulder arthroplasty. This indication accounts for nearly half of our cases of reverse shoulder arthroplasty.

Clinical Findings

Clinical findings in patients with glenohumeral osteoarthritis and a massive rotator cuff tear are variable and depend on both the degree of arthritis and the specific tendons of the rotator cuff that are torn. Most patients demonstrate some glenohumeral crepitus with stiffness. Additionally, acromiohumeral crepitus may be present.

Testing of the individual rotator cuff tendons will typically demonstrate obvious insufficiency. Rotator cuff insufficiency may involve the posterior superior rotator cuff (supraspinatus, infraspinatus, teres minor), the anterior superior rotator cuff (supraspinatus, subscapularis), or the entire rotator cuff. Additionally, the long head of the biceps tendon is often ruptured, as demonstrated by the characteristic deformity of the upper part of the arm. Chapter 7 details clinical testing of the rotator cuff.

Text continued on p. 149

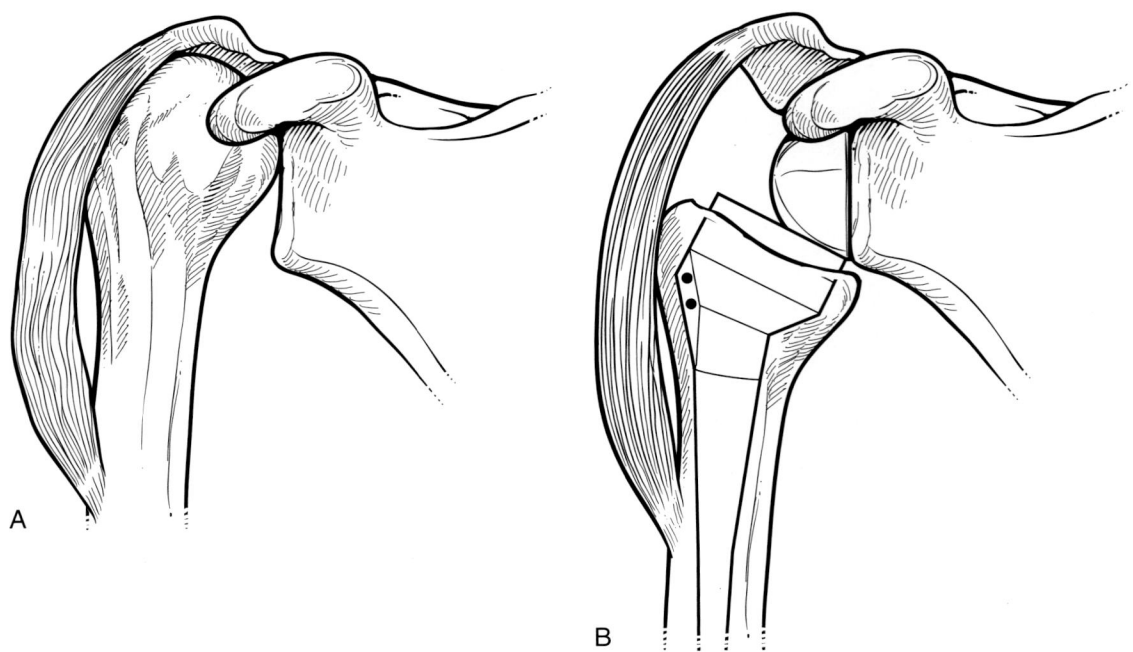

FIGURE 17.1 (A and B) Restoration of deltoid tension with a reverse-design prosthesis.

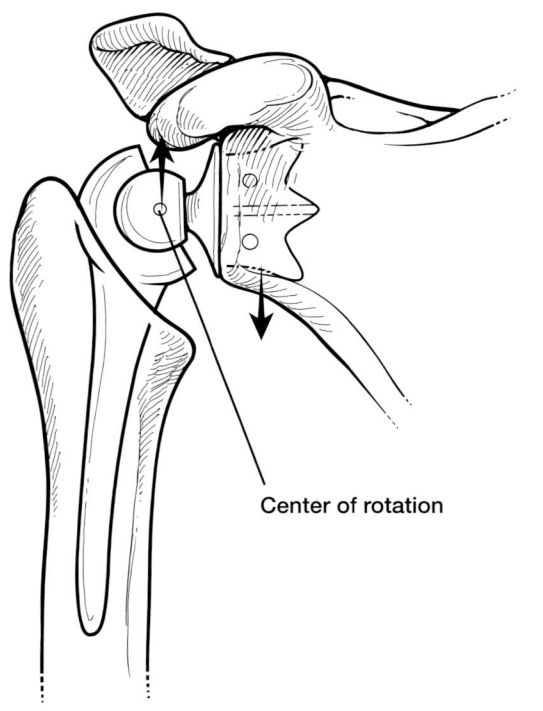

FIGURE 17.2 Forces acting on the glenoid fixation, causing loosening of early reverse prosthetic designs.

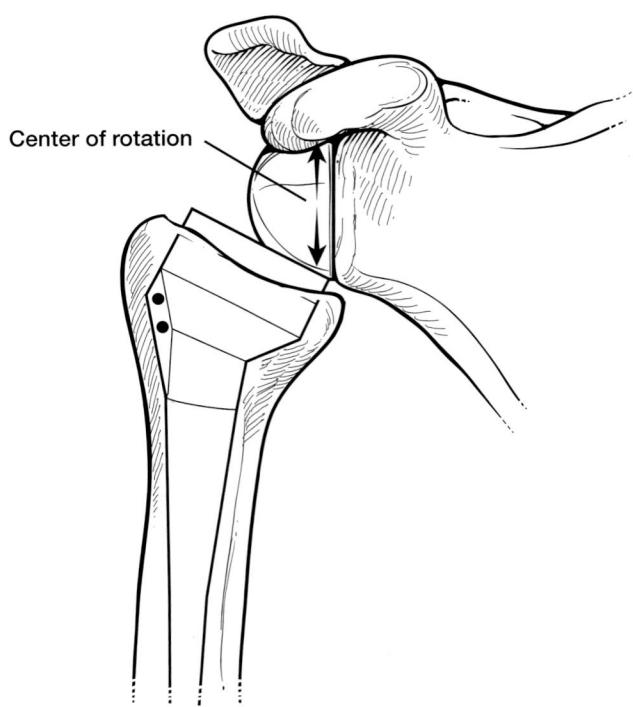

FIGURE 17.3 A "Grammont designed" reverse prosthesis using a medialized center of rotation to decrease the risk of loosening of the glenoid component.

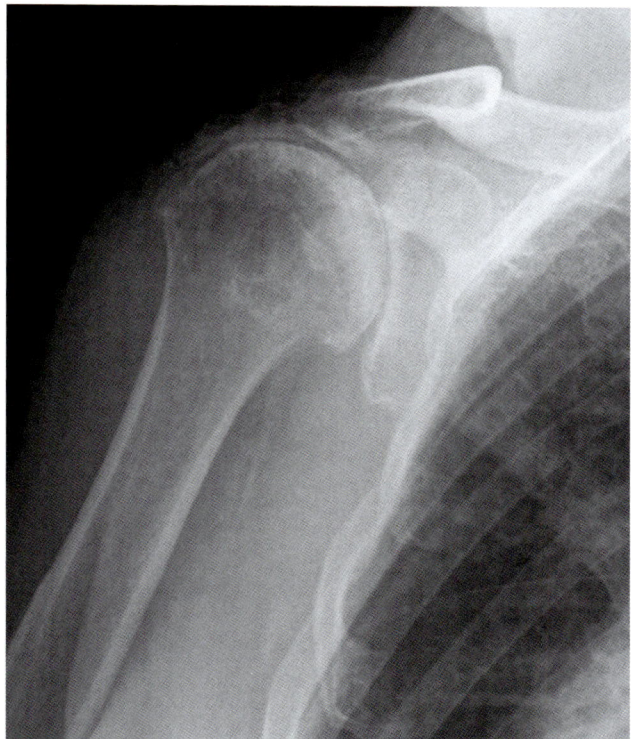

FIGURE 17.4 Radiograph demonstrating superior migration of the humeral head in a patient with osteoarthritis and a massive rotator cuff tear involving the posterior superior rotator cuff.

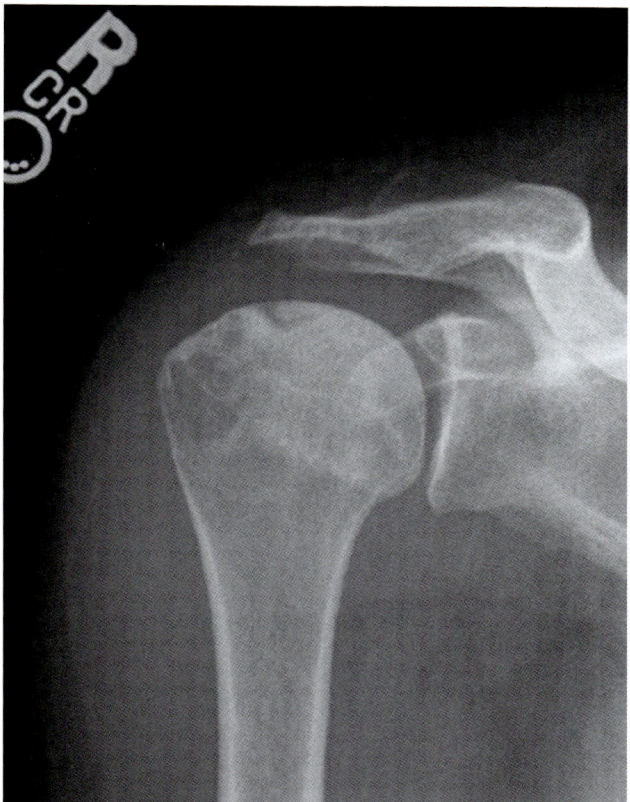

FIGURE 17.6 Acromial changes mirroring the radius of curvature of the humeral head in a patient with chronic rotator cuff insufficiency and only mild chronic humeral head superior migration.

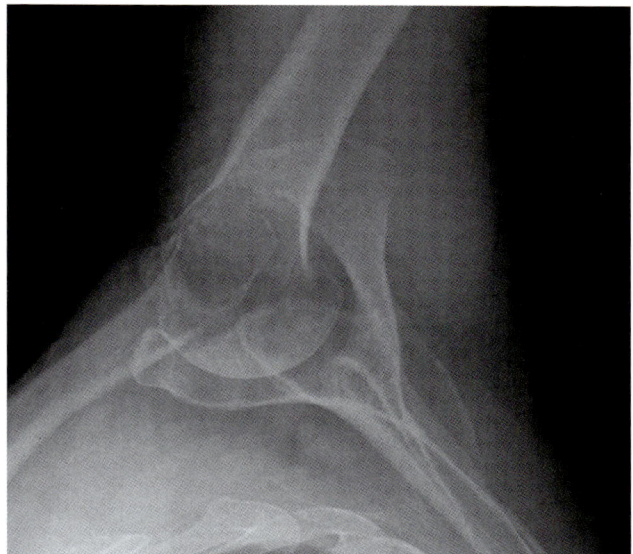

FIGURE 17.5 Axillary radiograph of a patient with static anterior migration of the humeral head caused by chronic anterior superior rotator cuff insufficiency.

Imaging Findings

Plain radiography demonstrates loss of the normal glenohumeral joint space. Humeral head osteophytes may or may not be present. Static migration of the humeral head is almost always present. In patients with insufficiency of the posterior superior rotator cuff, the humeral head migration occurs in a superior direction (Fig. 17.4). In patients with insufficiency of the anterior superior rotator cuff, static anterior migration may be apparent on just the axillary radiograph (Fig. 17.5). Less frequently, the patient may demonstrate only dynamic migration of the humeral head as a result of rotator cuff insufficiency. Acromial changes on radiographs of patients with no apparent static superior humeral head migration may show evidence of this dynamic instability (Fig. 17.6). Patients with osteoarthritis and a massive rotator cuff tear will frequently have osseous wear on the undersurface of the acromion, the superior glenoid, or both (Fig. 17.7). Less frequently, insufficiency fractures of the acromion may be caused by wear (Fig. 17.8). These stress fractures, however, do not contraindicate use of a reverse prosthesis.

Secondary imaging studies (computed tomography arthrography, magnetic resonance imaging) will always show rotator cuff tears involving more than one tendon (Fig. 17.9). The rotator cuff muscle belly of the torn tendons shows fatty infiltration (Fig. 17.10). In cases with long-standing rotator

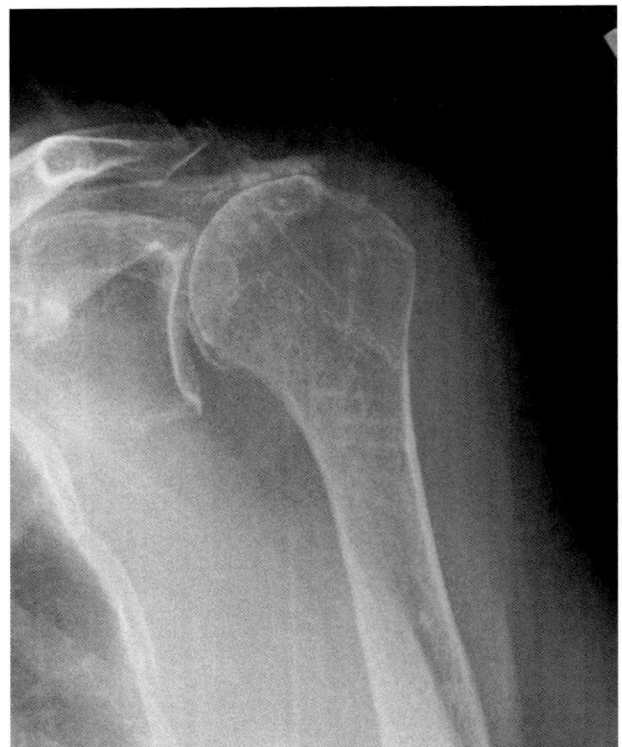

FIGURE 17.7 Acromial wear in a patient with rotator cuff tear arthropathy.

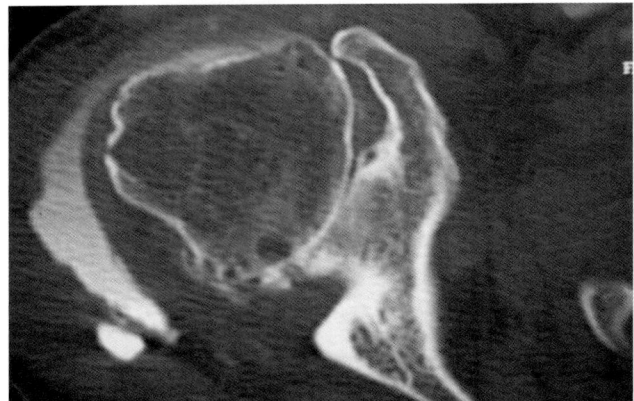

FIGURE 17.9 Computed tomography arthrogram demonstrating a massive rotator cuff tear with glenohumeral arthritis.

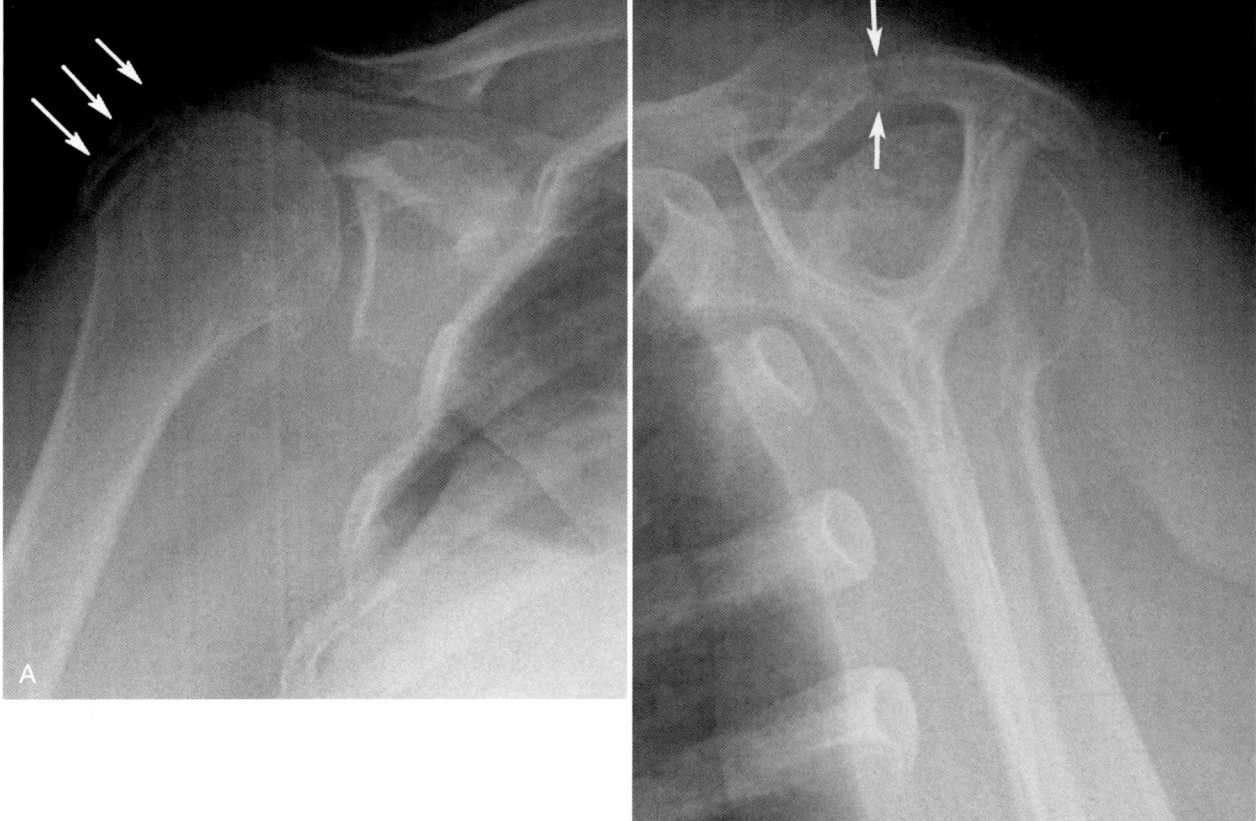

FIGURE 17.8 (A and B) Insufficiency fracture of the acromion *(arrows)* in a patient with rotator cuff tear arthropathy.

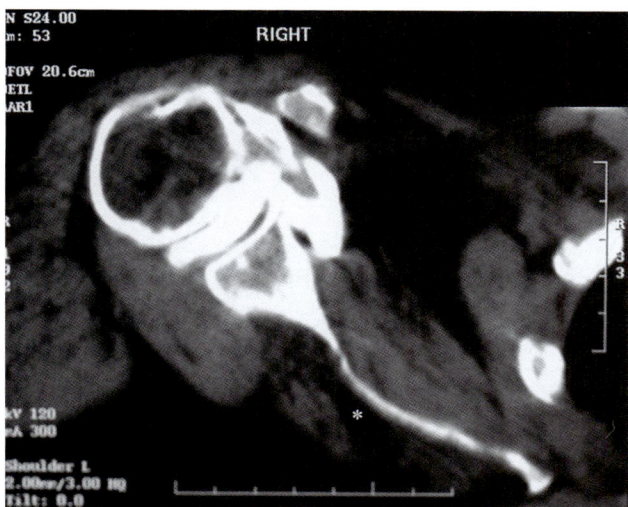

FIGURE 17.10 Computed tomography arthrogram demonstrating severe fatty infiltration of the infraspinatus *(asterisk)*. Compare with the normal subscapularis.

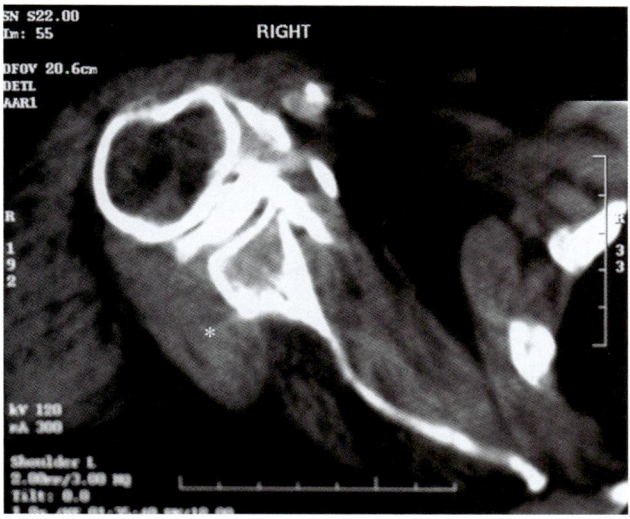

FIGURE 17.11 Computed tomography arthrogram demonstrating hypertrophy of the teres minor in a patient with infraspinatus insufficiency *(asterisk)*.

cuff tears involving the infraspinatus in which the teres minor is intact, the teres minor muscle belly may demonstrate compensatory hypertrophy (Fig. 17.11).

Secondary imaging studies can confirm osseous wear (glenoid, acromion) in patients with glenohumeral osteoarthritis and a massive rotator cuff tear. Coronal sections of computed tomography or magnetic resonance imaging have been used to classify superior glenoid wear (Fig. 17.12).[3]

Special Considerations

We emphasize that this patient group (osteoarthritis with a massive rotator cuff tear/rotator cuff tear arthropathy) consists only of individuals with *glenohumeral* osteoarthritis and massive *irreparable* rotator cuff tears involving *more than one* rotator cuff tendon. Patients with glenohumeral osteoarthritis and rotator cuff tears limited to the supraspinatus tendon do not fit this criterion and are best treated with other options (nonoperative treatment or unconstrained total shoulder arthroplasty). Furthermore, patients with massive irreparable rotator cuff tears *without* glenohumeral arthritis do not fit into this group and are rarely treated with a reverse prosthesis.

RHEUMATOID ARTHRITIS (INFLAMMATORY ARTHROPATHY) WITH MASSIVE ROTATOR CUFF TEAR

More than 10% of patients considered for shoulder arthroplasty with an underlying diagnosis of rheumatoid arthritis have a large tear of the rotator cuff that contraindicates unconstrained total shoulder arthroplasty.[4] These patients are candidates for either reverse shoulder arthroplasty (our preferred treatment) or unconstrained hemiarthroplasty (our preferred treatment only in cases of severe osseous insufficiency).

Clinical Findings

Clinical findings in patients with rheumatoid arthritis and a massive rotator cuff tear include glenohumeral crepitus and stiffness. Acromiohumeral crepitus may be present. Testing of the individual rotator cuff tendons will typically demonstrate obvious insufficiency. The rotator cuff insufficiency may involve the posterior superior rotator cuff (supraspinatus, infraspinatus, teres minor), the anterior superior rotator cuff (supraspinatus, subscapularis), or all of the rotator cuff tendons. Additionally, the long head of the biceps tendon is often ruptured, as demonstrated by the characteristic deformity of the upper part of the arm. Chapter 7 details clinical testing of the rotator cuff.

Imaging Findings

Plain radiography demonstrates loss of the normal glenohumeral joint space. Humeral head osteophytes are rarely seen (Fig. 17.13). Static migration of the humeral head is almost always present. In patients with insufficiency of the posterior superior rotator cuff, the humeral head migration occurs in a superior direction (Fig. 17.14). In patients with insufficiency of the anterior superior rotator cuff, static anterior migration may be apparent only on the axillary radiograph. Patients with rheumatoid arthritis and a massive rotator cuff tear may have severe osseous wear on the undersurface of the acromion, the superior glenoid, or both (Fig. 17.15). Additionally, severe destruction of the humeral head may be present (Fig. 17.16).

As in cases of rotator cuff tear arthropathy, secondary imaging studies (computed tomography arthrography, magnetic resonance imaging) will show rotator cuff tears involving more than one tendon in all cases. The rotator cuff muscle belly of the torn tendons will show fatty infiltration.

Osseous wear/destruction (glenoid, acromion, humeral head) is seen on secondary imaging studies. Severe loss of

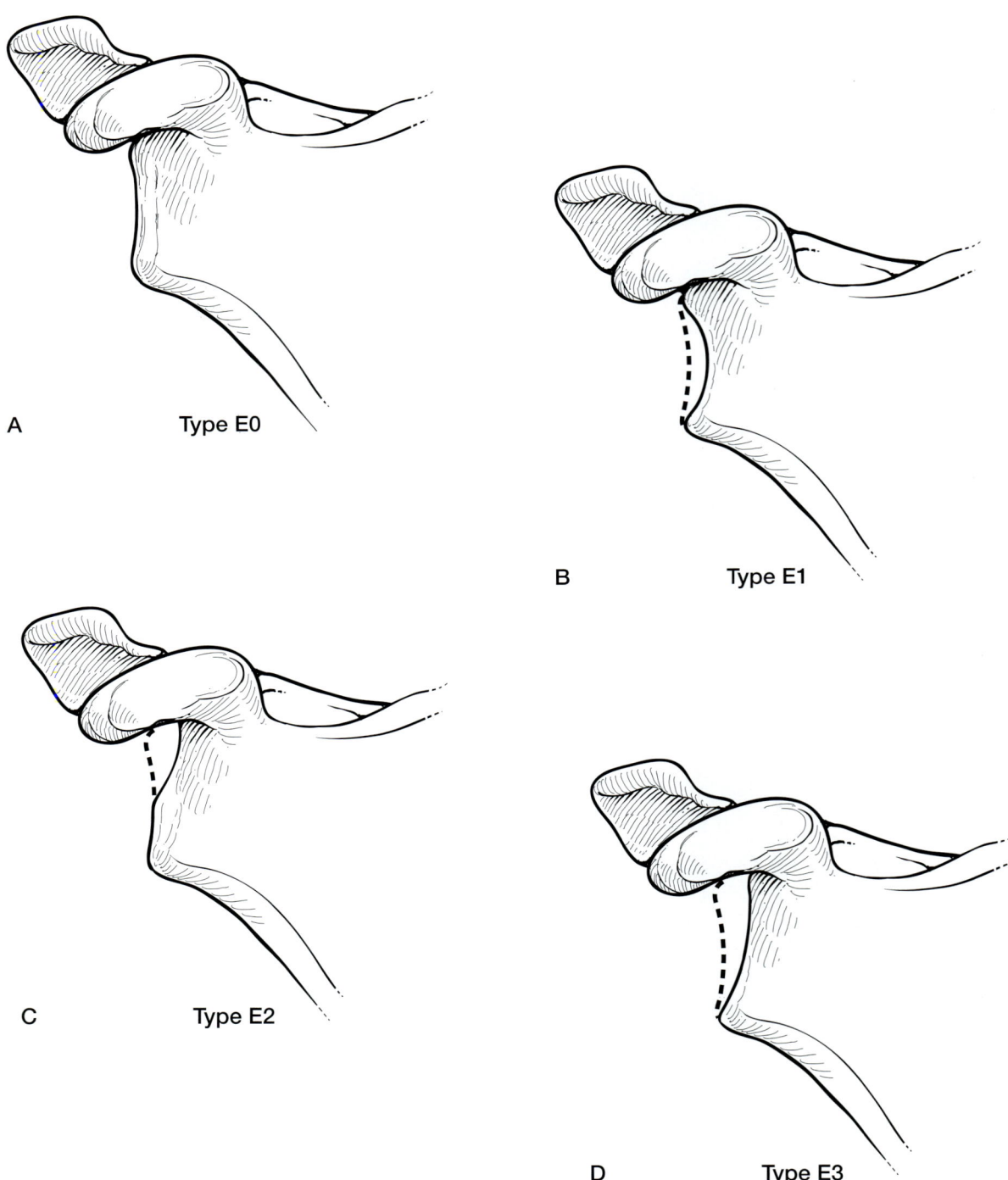

FIGURE 17.12 Classification of superior glenoid wear. (A) E0 represents normal glenoid morphology. (B) E1 represents central glenoid wear. (C) E2 represents superior glenoid wear with superior biconcavity. (D) E3 represents severe superior glenoid wear with a superiorly oriented glenoid morphology. (From Oudet D, Favard L, Lautmann S, et al: La prosthèse d'épaule Aequalis dans les omarthroses avec rupture massive et non réparable de la coiffe. In Walch G, Boileau P, Molé D, editors: *2000 Prosthèses d'Epaule ... Recul de 2 à 10 Ans*. Paris, Sauramps Medical, 2001, pp 241–246.)

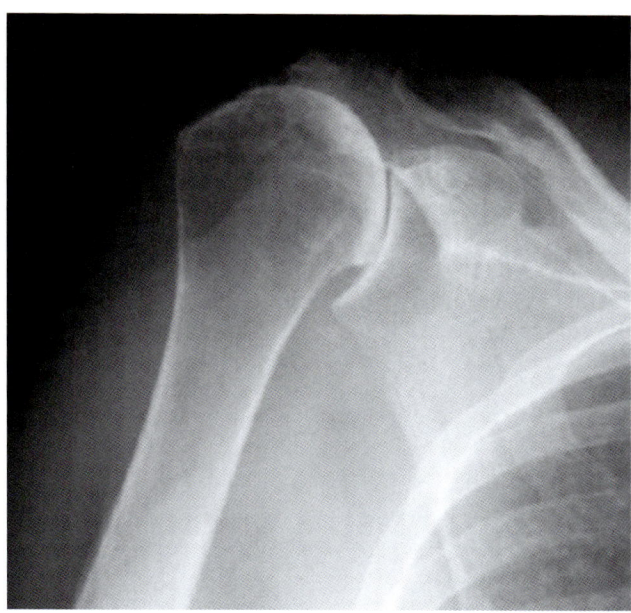

FIGURE 17.13 Radiograph of a patient with rheumatoid arthritis, demonstrating a paucity of osteophytes.

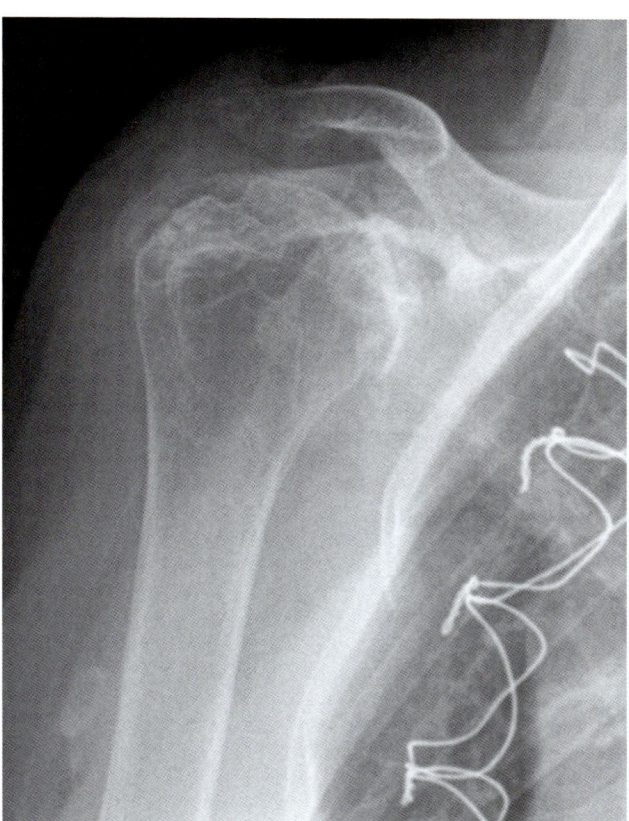

FIGURE 17.15 Severe osseous wear of both the glenoid and acromion occurring in a patient with rheumatoid arthritis and a massive rotator cuff tear.

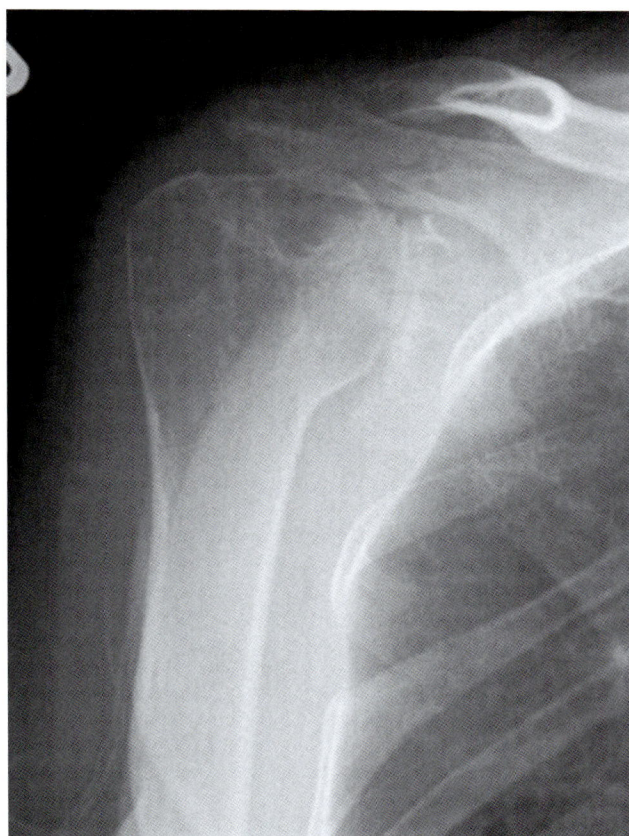

FIGURE 17.14 Radiograph of a patient with rheumatoid arthritis and a massive posterior superior rotator cuff tear, demonstrating superior migration of the humeral head.

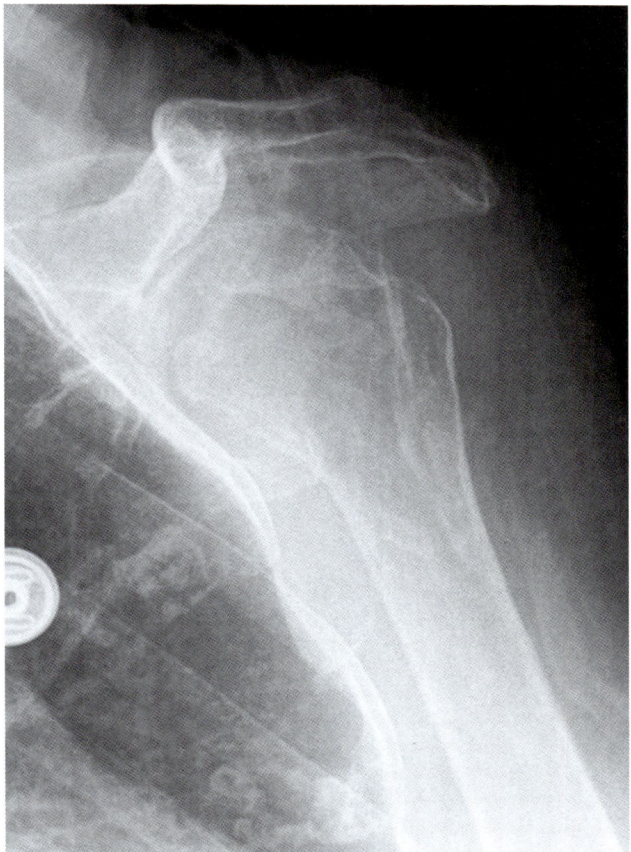

FIGURE 17.16 Rheumatoid arthritis with destruction of the humeral head.

glenoid bone with glenoid "protrusio" morphology may be present (Fig. 17.17).

Special Considerations

As in cases of osteoarthritis with a massive rotator cuff tear/rotator cuff tear arthropathy, we emphasize that use of a reverse prosthesis in rheumatoid arthritis should be reserved for patients with *glenohumeral* osteoarthritis and massive *irreparable* rotator cuff tears involving *more than one* rotator cuff tendon. Patients with inflammatory arthritis and rotator cuff tears limited to the supraspinatus tendon do not fit this criterion and are best treated with other options (nonoperative treatment or unconstrained total shoulder arthroplasty).

PROXIMAL HUMERAL NONUNION

Posttraumatic proximal humeral fracture problems include proximal humeral nonunion and malunion. In certain cases, severe loss of proximal humeral bone prohibits the preferred treatment of proximal humeral nonunion—operative fixation and bone grafting. Proximal humeral bone loss often results from osteopenia, failed attempts at previous operative treatment, or a combination. Previously, no good solution was available in these difficult cases. Because unconstrained shoulder arthroplasty with attempted fixation of the residual tuberosities has largely been unsatisfactory in the treatment of this problem, we now consider this a reasonable indication for use of a reverse prosthesis provided that no other reasonable option can reliably provide pain relief and return of function (Fig. 17.18).

PROXIMAL HUMERAL MALUNION

Many cases of glenohumeral arthritis with proximal humeral malunion are treatable by unconstrained shoulder arthroplasty (see Chapter 6). Certain cases, however, yield unpredictable results with unconstrained arthroplasty, and the use of reverse shoulder arthroplasty may be indicated. Specifically, in cases of severe malunion in which distorted proximal humeral anatomy prohibits insertion of an unconstrained humeral implant without disruption of the rotator cuff (Fig. 17.19) or in cases where the proximal humeral malunion is accompanied by a massive irreparable rotator cuff tear, shoulder

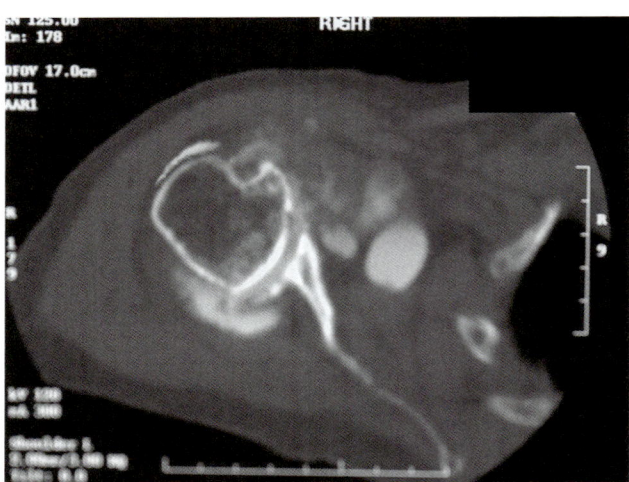

FIGURE 17.17 Computed tomography demonstrating severe glenoid bone loss in a patient with rheumatoid arthritis and a massive rotator cuff tear.

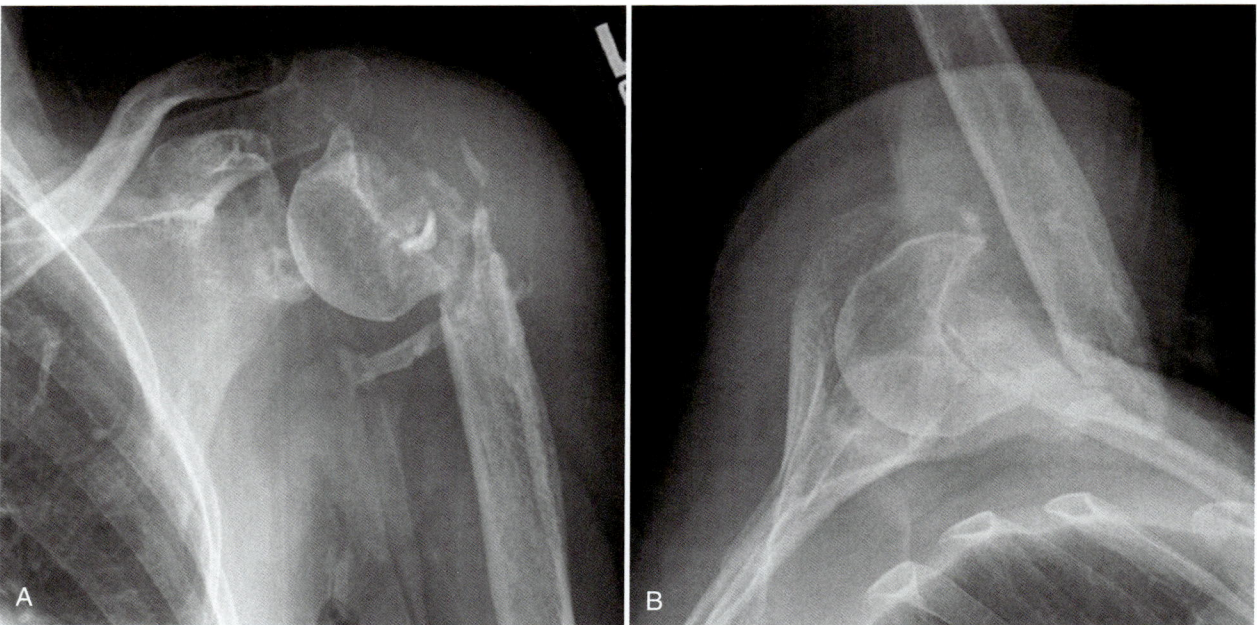

FIGURE 17.18 (A and B) A case of proximal humeral nonunion that has failed multiple attempts at open reduction and internal fixation. The remaining proximal humerus is insufficient to allow successful fixation.

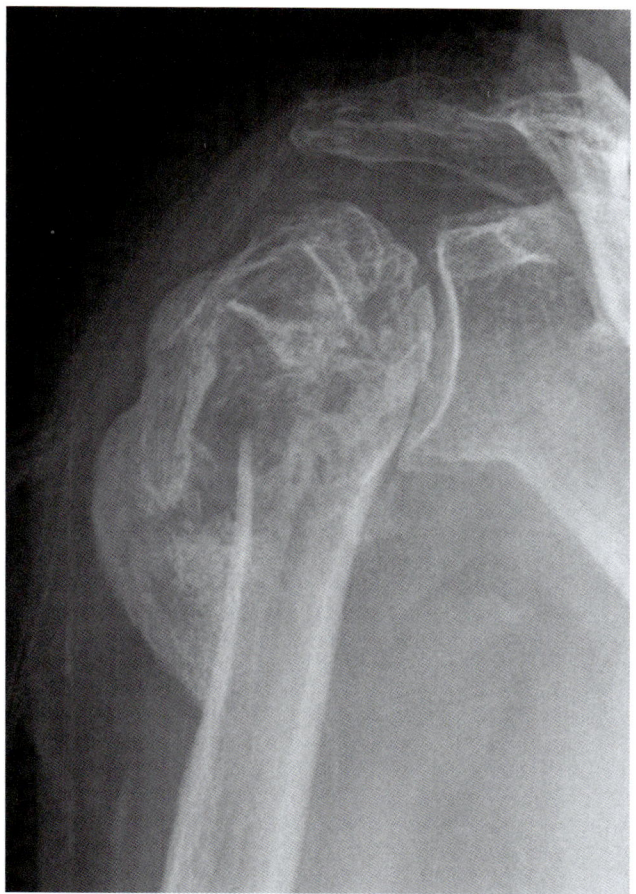

FIGURE 17.19 Posttraumatic arthritis in a patient with severe malunion of the proximal humerus. Use of an unconstrained arthroplasty in this patient would require either violation of the rotator cuff or greater tuberosity osteotomy. We prefer the use of a reverse-design prosthesis in this scenario.

arthroplasty with a reverse prosthesis may be the best operative option.

Clinical Findings

Clinical findings in patients with proximal humeral malunion are variable. In patients with distortion of the proximal humeral anatomy caused by malunion, shoulder stiffness may be exceptionally severe and attributable to mechanical impingement, subdeltoid contracture, and subacromial contracture, in addition to the glenohumeral incongruity and glenohumeral capsular contractures seen in primary osteoarthritis. Rotator cuff testing may be normal or compromised by pain, rotator cuff tearing, or both.

Imaging Findings

Plain radiography demonstrates loss of the normal glenohumeral joint space. Other radiographic findings are variable and depend on the severity of the proximal humeral malunion.

Secondary imaging studies (computed tomography arthrography, magnetic resonance imaging), like plain radiography, show variable findings depending on the deformity present. The rotator cuff may be compromised on secondary imaging studies.

Special Considerations

We perform unconstrained total shoulder arthroplasty in cases of posttraumatic arthritis where the rotator cuff is competent and the proximal humeral anatomy allows insertion of an unconstrained humeral component. In patients with rotator cuff insufficiency or those who would require a greater tuberosity osteotomy to perform humeral arthroplasty, we opt for a reverse-design prosthesis (see Fig. 17.19).

MASSIVE ROTATOR CUFF TEAR WITH CHRONIC PSEUDOPARALYSIS BUT WITHOUT GLENOHUMERAL OSTEOARTHRITIS

A rare and somewhat controversial indication for reverse shoulder arthroplasty is a massive irreparable rotator cuff tear with chronic pseudoparalysis but no glenohumeral arthritis. In such cases, the massive rotator cuff tear leads to inability to counteract the glenohumeral shear forces of the deltoid and prevents active elevation of the arm. Pain may or may not be a complaint in this subset of patients. Neurologic examination and neurodiagnostic testing, if performed, are both normal. Patients have usually failed prolonged (>6 months) attempts at rehabilitation with physical therapy. In these cases, we offer the patient a reverse prosthesis provided that no other reasonable option is available.

Clinical Findings

Patients with chronic pseudoparalysis have a normal neurologic examination. Anterosuperior escape of the humeral head may be palpable on attempts at active arm elevation. Rotator cuff testing will usually indicate which rotator cuff musculotendinous units are compromised. The subscapularis is generally torn in patients with chronic pseudoparalysis and seems to play a major role in the ongoing inability to elevate the arm.

Imaging Findings

Plain radiography demonstrates maintenance of the normal glenohumeral joint space. Static migration of the humeral head is almost always present. In patients with insufficiency of the posterior superior rotator cuff, the humeral head migration occurs in a superior direction (Fig. 17.20). In patients with insufficiency of the anterior superior rotator cuff, static anterior migration may be apparent on the axillary radiograph only. Osseous wear is uncommon in this indication.

As in cases of rotator cuff tear arthropathy, secondary imaging studies (computed tomography arthrography, magnetic resonance imaging) will show rotator cuff tears involving more than one tendon in all cases. The subscapularis is usually involved in the rotator cuff tear. The rotator cuff muscle belly of the torn tendons shows marked fatty infiltration.

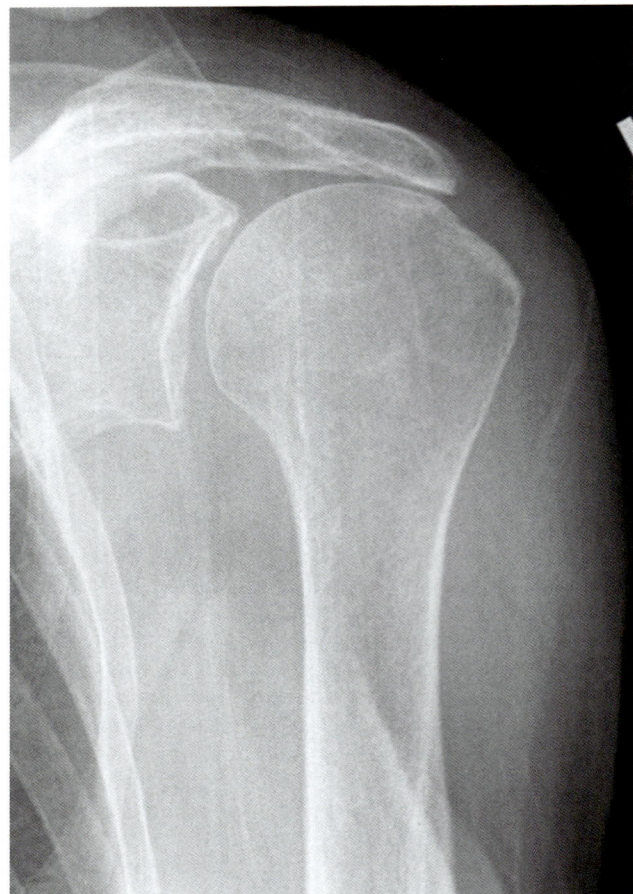

FIGURE 17.20 Proximal migration of the humeral head in a patient with a massive irreparable rotator cuff tear but without glenohumeral arthritis.

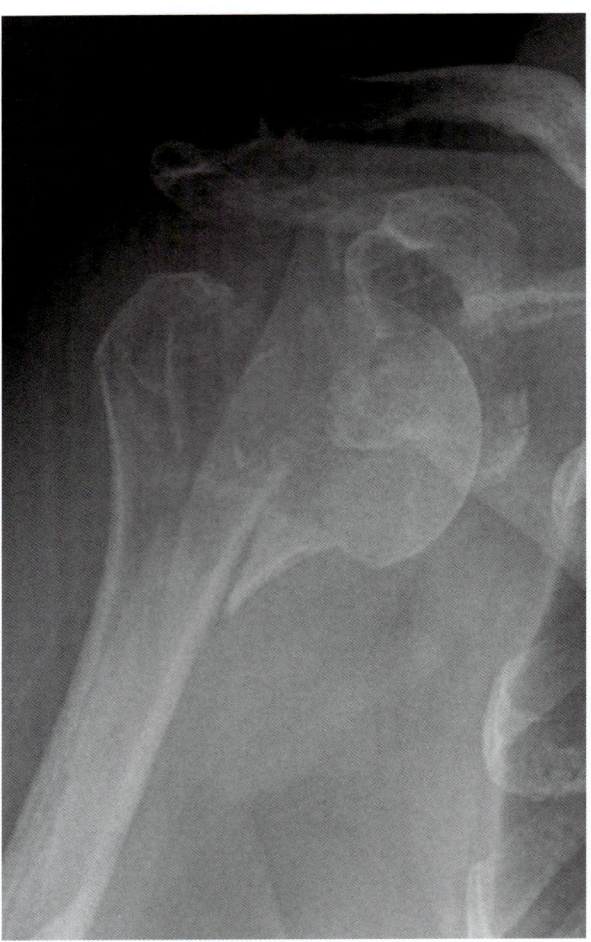

FIGURE 17.21 Radiograph of a 93-year-old active patient with age-related osteopenia and a four-part fracture-dislocation of the proximal humerus. We believe that this patient would be best treated with a reverse prosthesis.

Special Considerations

Most patients with massive irreparable rotator cuff tears and pseudoparalysis can be treated effectively without reverse shoulder replacement. We institute a physical therapy program in all of these patients as well as symptomatic nonoperative treatment (analgesics, modalities, corticosteroid injections). After 6 months, if the patient is still unable to actively elevate the arm, he or she is considered a candidate for reverse shoulder arthroplasty provided that no contraindications exist. If the patient is able to elevate the arm but it remains painful, he or she is considered for other nonarthroplasty interventions, such as arthroscopic débridement with biceps tenotomy or tendon transfer.

ACUTE FRACTURE

Elderly patients with severe osteopenia who have complex proximal humeral fractures—which would normally indicate replacement with a hemiarthroplasty (see Chapter 26)—may be candidates for treatment with a reverse prosthesis (Fig. 17.21). In these difficult cases, even a perfectly performed hemiarthroplasty with fixation of the tuberosities may result in tuberosity nonunion and migration because of impaired healing due to osteopenia and local biology. In these cases, we may opt for a reverse prosthesis combined with fixation of the tuberosities, as described in Chapter 30. In this scenario, in the event that the tuberosities do not heal, the patient still obtains reasonable pain relief and some active elevation; moreover, the need for further surgery is thus minimized.

FIXED GLENOHUMERAL DISLOCATION

Our outcomes using unconstrained shoulder arthroplasty for the treatment of fixed glenohumeral dislocations in elderly patients have been disappointing because we have observed a high rate of recurrent instability.[5] For this reason, we now use a reverse prosthesis as our implant of choice for fixed glenohumeral dislocations in elderly patients.[6]

Clinical Findings

Patients with fixed glenohumeral dislocations have very limited active mobility of the involved shoulder. Findings

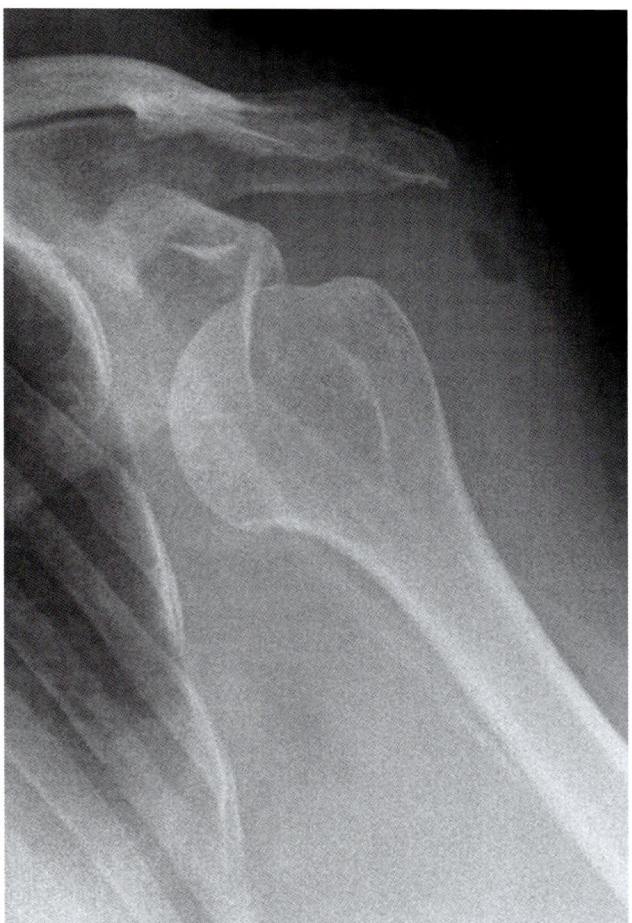

FIGURE 17.22 Fixed anterior dislocation in an elderly patient.

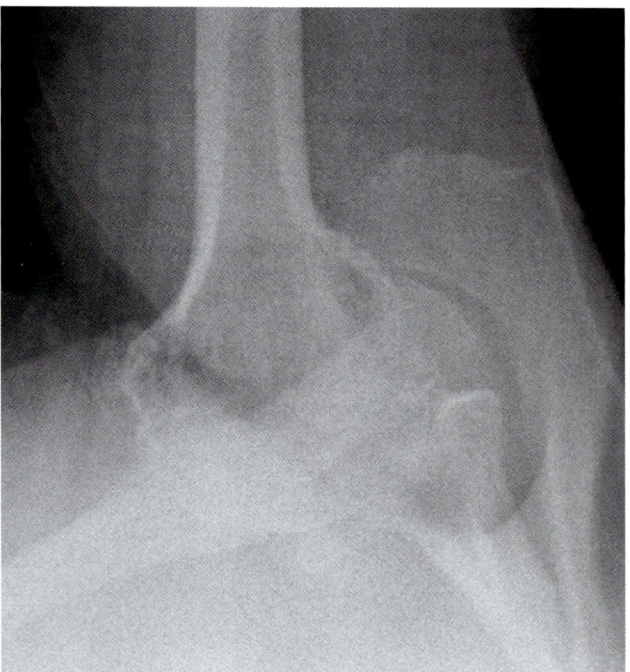

FIGURE 17.23 Axillary radiograph demonstrating a fixed anterior dislocation of the glenohumeral joint with severe loss of the anterior glenoid.

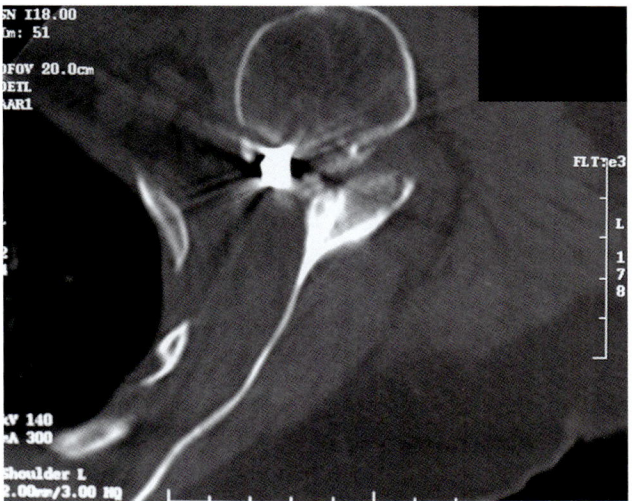

FIGURE 17.24 Computed tomography in a patient with a fixed anterior dislocation and severe anterior glenoid bone erosion.

are invariably consistent with massive rotator cuff tearing. Special attention should be paid to the neurologic examination, specifically axillary nerve function. Glenohumeral crepitus is usually present with shoulder motion.

Imaging Findings

Plain radiography demonstrates dislocation of the glenohumeral joint (Fig. 17.22). Axillary radiography may be difficult to perform because of the dislocation. If obtained, the axillary radiograph may demonstrate substantial wear of the osseous glenoid (Fig. 17.23).

Secondary imaging studies almost always demonstrate a massive rotator cuff tear. Frequently, erosion of the anterior or posterior glenoid occurs as a result of the chronic articulation of the dislocated humeral head (Fig. 17.24). Additionally, the humeral head may be eroded because of this pathologic articulation (Fig. 17.25).

Special Considerations

Implantation of a reverse prosthesis in this subset of patients is technically difficult. Glenoid bone grafting may be required to address anterior or posterior glenoid bone loss.

POSTINFECTIOUS ARTHROPATHY

Postinfectious arthropathy can occur after a rotator cuff repair that subsequently became infected (Fig. 17.26). In this scenario, the rotator cuff repair usually fails and may result in rotator cuff insufficiency, similar to that observed in rotator cuff tear arthropathy. In cases of postinfectious arthropathy coupled with severe rotator cuff dysfunction, a reverse prosthesis is our implant of choice. Just as with postinfectious arthropathy and a competent rotator cuff, successful shoulder

TABLE 17.1	Contraindications to Reverse Shoulder Arthroplasty	
Contraindication	Absolute or Relative	Comments
Poor general health	Relative	Appropriate perioperative medical treatment required
Active infection	Absolute	
Axillary nerve palsy	Absolute	Better suited for resection arthroplasty or arthrodesis
Deltoid insufficiency	Absolute	
Insufficient humeral bone stock	Absolute	
Insufficient glenoid bone stock	Absolute	Glenoid component contraindicated; better suited for hemiarthroplasty
Ankylosed shoulder	Absolute	
Previous shoulder arthrodesis	Absolute	
Upper motor neuron lesion	Relative	Absolute contraindication if the patient has uncontrolled shoulder spasticity
Poor patient motivation	Absolute	

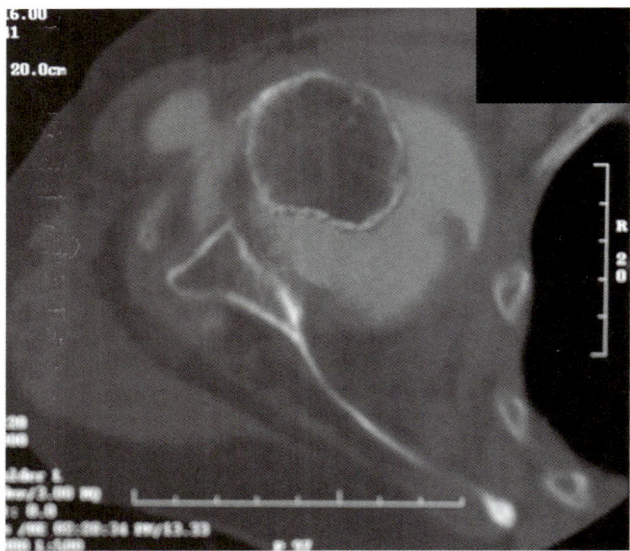

FIGURE 17.25 Computed tomography in a patient with a fixed anterior dislocation and osseous erosion of the humeral head.

arthroplasty in these patients depends on complete eradication of the previous infection before shoulder arthroplasty is undertaken.[7] Our approach for workup of these patients is detailed in the section on postinfectious arthropathy in Chapter 6.

TUMOR

Tumors about the shoulder girdle are an exceptionally rare indication for reverse shoulder arthroplasty. In our practice, we infrequently assist in reconstruction of the shoulder after tumor resection by an orthopedic oncologic surgeon. If resection requires removal of the rotator cuff, tuberosities, or both and leaves the humeral diaphysis and glenoid, a reverse prosthesis can be considered in the reconstruction (Fig. 17.27).[8]

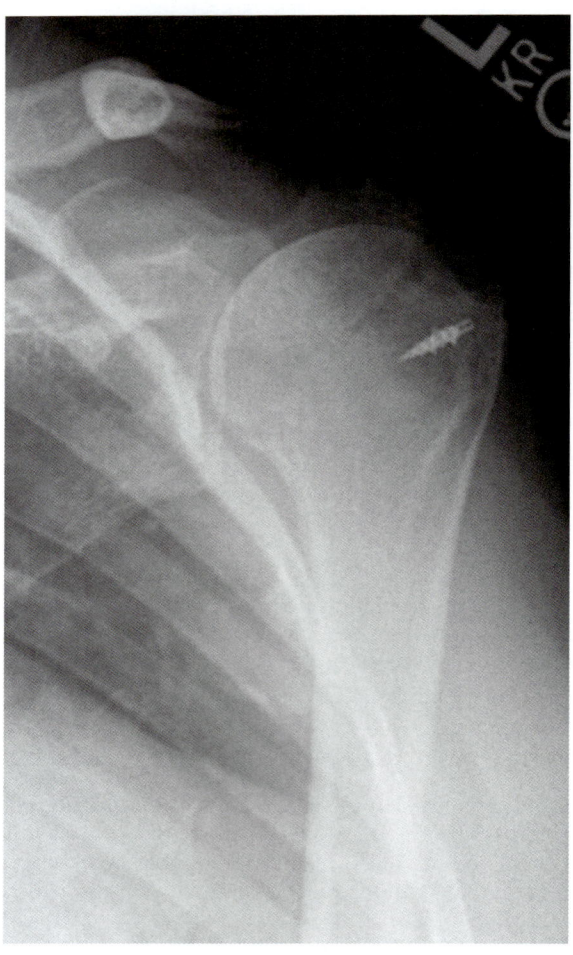

FIGURE 17.26 Radiograph of a patient with postinfectious arthropathy after failed rotator cuff repair.

CONTRAINDICATIONS TO REVERSE SHOULDER ARTHROPLASTY

Contraindications to reverse shoulder arthroplasty are listed in Table 17.1. Some of these contraindications are absolute, whereas others are relative.

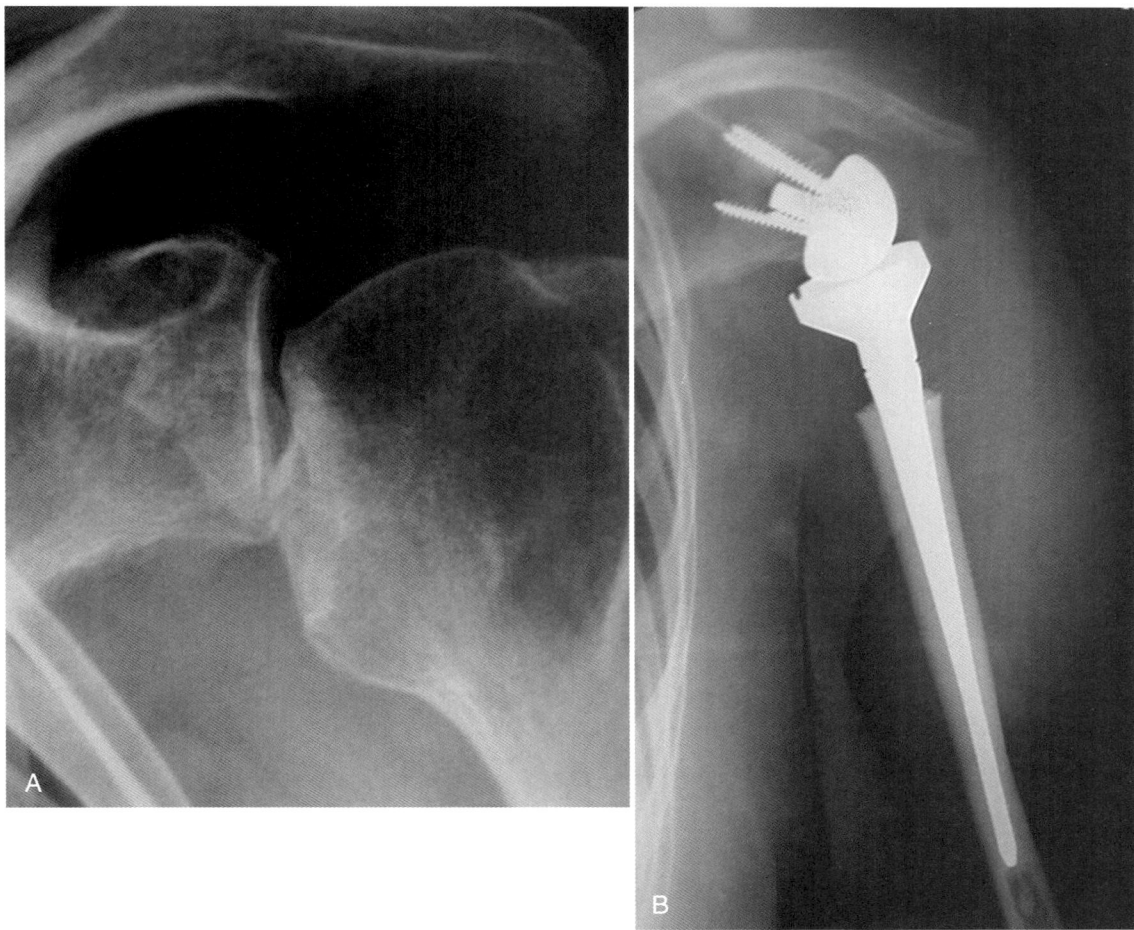

FIGURE 17.27 (A and B) Radiographs of a patient with a desmoid tumor of the shoulder girdle. The patient underwent reconstruction with a reverse prosthesis after tumor resection.

REFERENCES

1. Grammont PM, Baulot E: Delta shoulder prosthesis for rotator cuff rupture, *Orthopedics* 16:65–68, 1993.
2. Neer CS, 2nd, Craig EV, Fukuda H: Cuff tear arthropathy, *J Bone Joint Surg Am* 65:1232–1244, 1983.
3. Oudet D, Favard L, Lautmann S, et al: La prosthèse d'épaule Aequalis dans les omarthroses avec rupture massive et non réparable de la coiffe. In Walch G, Boileau P, Molé D, editors: *2000 Prosthèses d'Epaule ... Recul de 2 à 10 Ans*, Paris, 2001, Sauramps Medical, pp 241–246.
4. Vandermaren C, Docquier P: Shoulder arthroplasty in rheumatoid arthritis: influence of the rotator cuff on the results. In Walch G, Boileau P, Molé D, editors: *2000 Prosthèses d'Epaule ... Recul de 2 à 10 Ans*, Paris, 2001, Sauramps Medical, pp 177–182.
5. Matsoukis J, Tabib W, Guiffault P, et al: Primary unconstrained shoulder arthroplasty in patients with a fixed anterior glenohumeral dislocation: results of a multicenter study, *J Bone Joint Surg Am* 88:547–552, 2006.
6. Cortés ZE, Edwards TB, Elkousy HA, et al: Reverse total shoulder arthroplasty as treatment for fixed anterior shoulder dislocation. Paper presented at a conference titled *Treatment of Complex Shoulder Problems*, January 2005, Tampa, FL.
7. Morris BJ, Waggenspack WN, Laughlin MS, et al: Reverse shoulder arthroplasty for management of postinfectious arthropathy with rotator cuff deficiency, *Orthopedics* 38(8):e701–e707, 2015.
8. Sikka RS, Voran M, Edwards TB, et al: Desmoid tumor of the subscapularis presenting as isolated loss of shoulder external rotation: a report of two cases, *J Bone Joint Surg Am* 86:159–164, 2004.

CHAPTER 18

Preoperative planning and imaging

Reintroduction of the reverse-design prosthesis has allowed surgeons to treat complicated shoulder pathology for which no good solution existed before availability of this implant. The severity and diversity of shoulder pathology treatable with a reverse prosthesis make preoperative planning even more important in these cases than with primary unconstrained shoulder arthroplasty. Candidates for a reverse prosthesis may include patients with substantial proximal humeral or glenoid bone loss or both. Because of the complex nature of many of these cases, preoperative planning should be done well in advance of the surgical procedure and not as an afterthought the morning of surgery. As with unconstrained shoulder arthroplasty, preoperative planning for reverse shoulder arthroplasty requires that the surgeon review the patient's clinical history and physical examination, radiographs, and secondary imaging studies. This chapter outlines our approach to preoperative planning for reverse shoulder arthroplasty.

CLINICAL HISTORY AND EXAMINATION

The same type of clinical history and physical examination is used for candidates for reverse shoulder arthroplasty as for candidates for unconstrained shoulder arthroplasty (see Chapter 7). Because most candidates for reverse shoulder arthroplasty have a compromised rotator cuff, it is important to obtain a detailed history of the patient's complaints (pain only; weakness only; pain and weakness; pain, weakness, and stiffness).

Any previous surgery, especially attempts at rotator cuff repair and fracture surgery, merits special consideration. The type of surgical approach (arthroscopic or open) should be noted. Previous open surgery may compromise deltoid function to a degree that contraindicates use of a reverse prosthesis.

As with unconstrained shoulder arthroplasty, any symptoms of previous infection, especially in patients who have undergone surgery or injections, should be investigated further. If patients have a history of infection after shoulder surgery or have had symptoms suggestive of infection (systemic fevers, shoulder warmth, redness), a preoperative infection workup is indicated. Our approach for workup of these patients is detailed in the postinfectious arthropathy section of Chapter 6. We follow our published algorithm to rule out ongoing infection.[1] We begin with serum studies including a complete blood count with differential, a sedimentation rate, and C-reactive protein. Fluoroscopically guided aspiration of the glenohumeral joint is performed after the patient has been off all antibiotics for at least 2 weeks (even antibiotics used for other conditions, such as respiratory infections). The aspirate is cultured for 21 days for aerobic bacteria, anaerobic bacteria, mycobacteria, and fungi. Holding the cultures for 21 days allows for detection of *Propionibacterium acnes* and *Staphylococcus epidermidis*, which have longer incubation periods.[1] The aspirate is also sent for alpha defensin (Synovasure Alpha Defensin Test [Zimmer, Inc., Warsaw, IN]). If the findings are suggestive or diagnostic of infection, shoulder arthroplasty is postponed or canceled until infectious disease consultation is obtained and the infection is appropriately treated.

Any medical history of systemic illness (diabetes mellitus, cardiac problems) should be considered in the preoperative planning. Although these factors may not affect the actual surgical procedure, they may necessitate special considerations in the patient's postoperative care. The availability of appropriate care of these systemic illnesses, including the availability of consultants, should be confirmed before surgery.

All of our patients undergo a thorough shoulder examination, much of which is detailed in Chapter 7. The visual appearance of the shoulder yields useful information in candidates for reverse shoulder arthroplasty. The presence and location of surgical scars are noted (Fig. 18.1). In thin patients, anterosuperior escape of the humeral head caused by anterosuperior rotator cuff deficiency may be obvious (Fig. 18.2) or may be noted only when the patient attempts arm elevation or abduction. Special attention should be paid to the condition of the deltoid, especially if it has previously been surgically violated (Fig. 18.3). The condition of the deltoid is best evaluated by asking the patient to push against the examiner's hand to observe an isometric contraction. Any areas of deltoid origin that may not have healed to the acromion after a previous operation should be noted. Atrophy of the supraspinatus and infraspinatus should be noted as well (Fig. 18.4).

Both active and passive mobility is recorded, as detailed in Chapter 7. The presence of glenohumeral crepitus with motion is recorded, as is any discrepancy in active and passive mobility. Special attention should be paid to evaluation of the deltoid muscle. If deltoid contractility appears to be compromised, additional evaluation with electromyography and nerve conduction studies should be performed before further consideration for implantation of a reverse prosthesis.

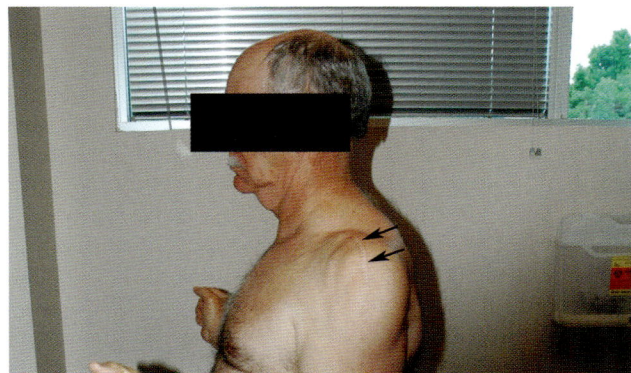

FIGURE 18.1 Scar from a previous open rotator cuff repair *(arrows)* in a candidate for implantation of a reverse prosthesis.

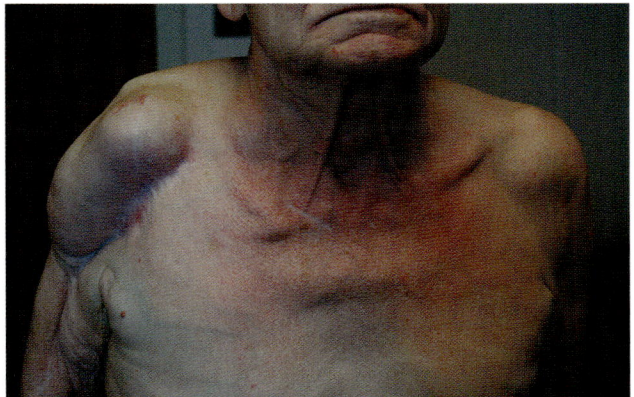

FIGURE 18.2 Obvious anterosuperior escape of the humeral head.

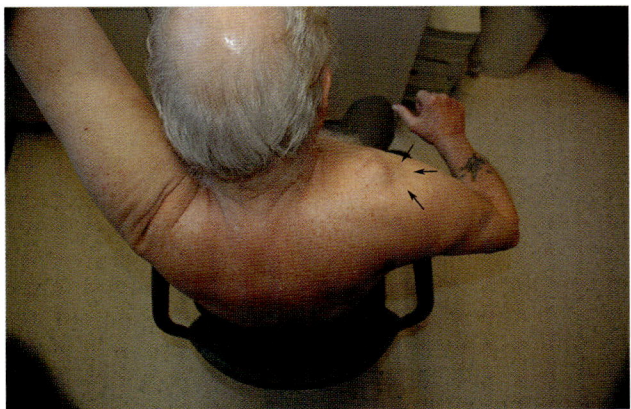

FIGURE 18.3 Patient with previous surgery involving detachment of the deltoid *(arrows)*.

Rotator cuff examination consists of testing each tendon of the rotator cuff by isolating it as much as possible. Jobe's test is used to test supraspinatus integrity.[2] The infraspinatus is tested by the external rotation lag sign and external rotation strength with the arm at the side.[3] The horn blower's sign is used to test the teres minor.[4] The subscapularis is tested with the belly press test and, when mobility allows, the lift-off test.[5] Performance of the various rotator cuff tests is depicted in Chapter 7.

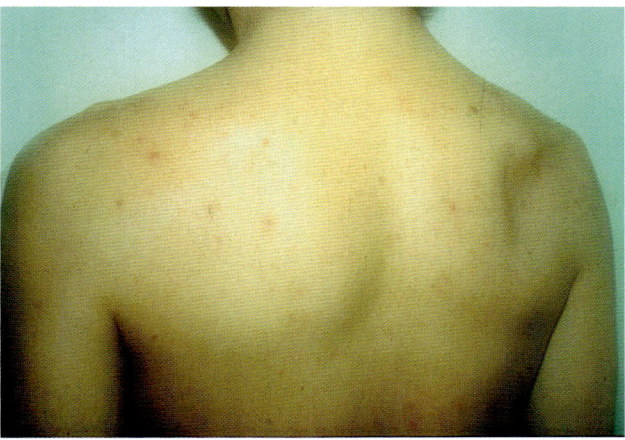

FIGURE 18.4 Patient with supraspinatus and infraspinatus atrophy.

The results of the clinical history and examination are documented in the patient's chart and reviewed well in advance of surgery as part of preoperative planning. Findings are discussed with the patient in terms of postoperative outcome and patient expectations. For example, it is important for patients without posterior rotator cuff function (no infraspinatus or teres minor) to understand that the operation will not restore their ability to actively externally rotate the arm.

RADIOGRAPHY

Radiographs are obtained in all patients who are being considered as candidates for reverse shoulder arthroplasty. An anteroposterior view of the glenohumeral joint with the arm in neutral rotation, an axillary view, and a scapular outlet view are the views that we use for all shoulder arthroplasty patients. The anteroposterior radiograph is used to evaluate the glenohumeral joint space, the presence of humeral and glenoid osteophytes, the size of the humeral canal, the presence of any loose bodies, any deformity of the humeral shaft, any static superior migration of the humeral head (Fig. 18.5), and any superior glenoid wear (Fig. 18.6). The axillary radiograph is used to evaluate the glenohumeral joint space, the presence of anterior or posterior humeral head subluxation, and any osseous glenoid wear and dysplasia. The scapular outlet radiograph is used to evaluate the condition of the acromion (thin, fractured, deficient); it also serves to check for the presence of anterior, posterior, or superior humeral head subluxation (Fig. 18.7), loose bodies in the subscapularis recess, and any deformity of the humeral shaft.

Ideally, these radiographs are taken with magnification and fluoroscopic control. Some patients come to our clinic with radiographs taken by a referring physician. If these radiographs are judged to be of sufficient quality, are less than 6 months old, and do not show any unusual circumstances (e.g., an excessively small humeral intramedullary canal), they are not repeated. In all other cases, radiographs are repeated with magnification and fluoroscopically controlled techniques.

Bilateral full-length magnification-controlled anteroposterior humeral radiographs are obtained in patients demonstrating proximal humeral bone loss from causes such as fracture

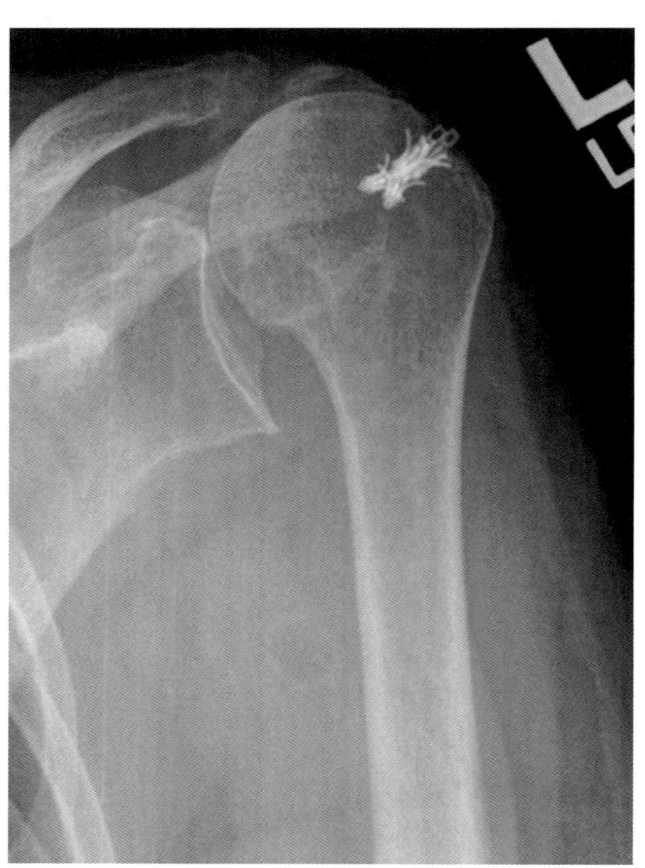

FIGURE 18.5 Static superior migration of the humeral head.

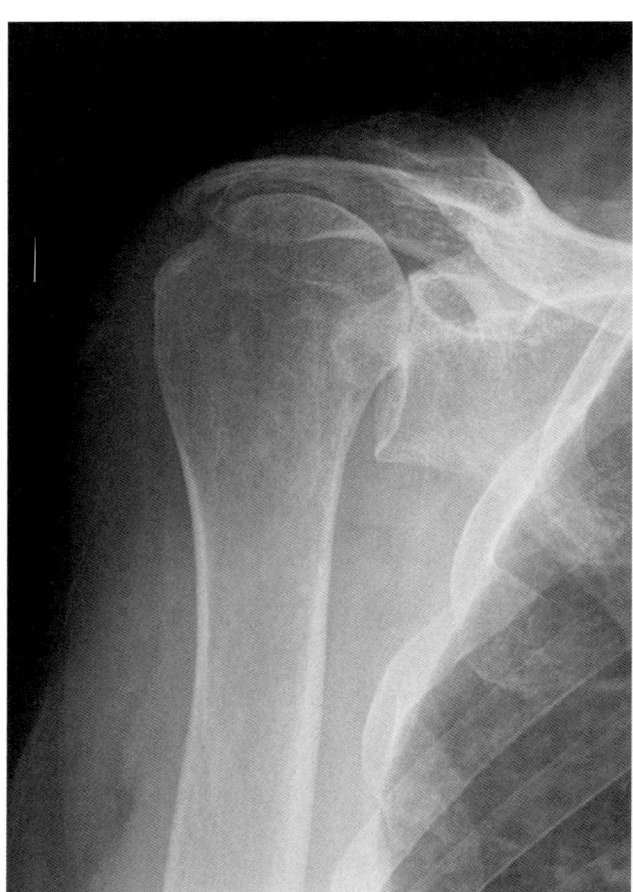

FIGURE 18.6 Superior glenoid wear from static superior humeral head migration.

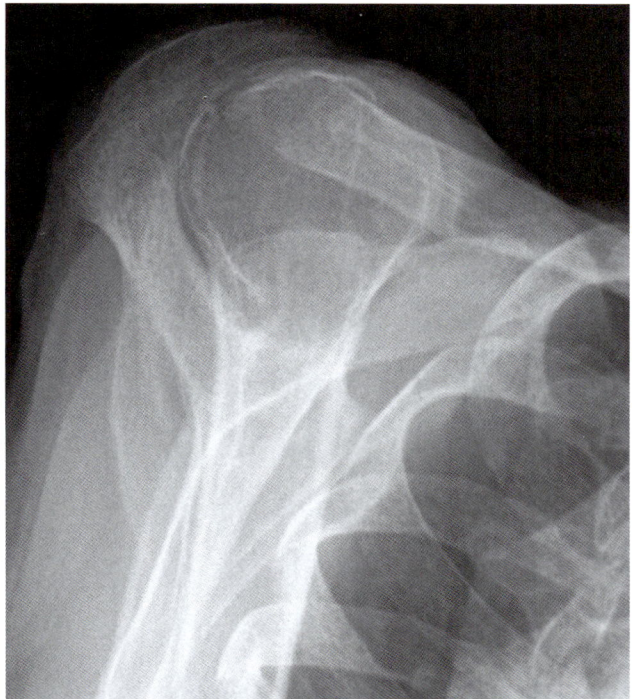

FIGURE 18.7 Superior humeral head migration demonstrated on an outlet radiograph.

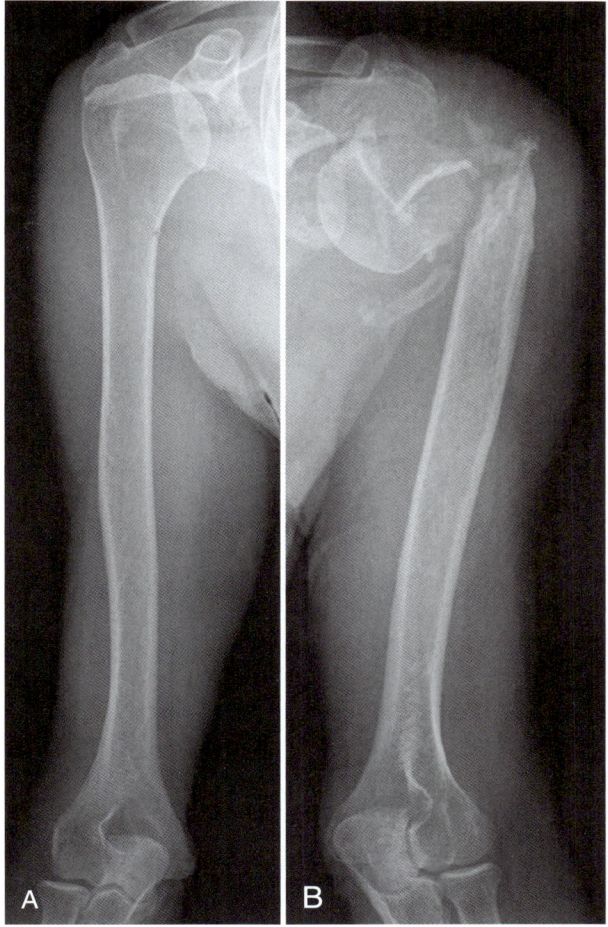

FIGURE 18.8 (A and B) Bilateral humeral radiographs taken to help estimate the level at which the humeral component should be implanted in a patient with severe proximal humeral bone loss.

nonunion (Fig. 18.8). These radiographs are used to help select the height at which to implant the humeral stem.

Most reverse shoulder arthroplasty prosthetic systems have radiographic templates available for preoperative planning. For routine problems such as rotator cuff tear arthropathy, we usually do not use preoperative radiographic templating because we have not found it to be useful. In cases of proximal humeral bone loss, preoperative radiographic templating is done on full-length humeral radiographs. The desired position of the reverse prosthesis is templated on the radiograph of the unaffected humerus and the level of the metaphyseal-diaphyseal junction of the humeral component is marked (Fig. 18.9). The distance from the transepicondylar axis at the elbow to this point is measured (Fig. 18.10). A mark is made at the same distance from the transepicondylar axis on the affected radiograph. A second mark is made at the most proximal extent of the humeral shaft (Fig. 18.11). The distance between the desired prosthetic level at the metaphyseal-diaphyseal junction and the proximal extent of the humeral shaft is measured (Fig. 18.12). A ruler is used during surgery to measure the distance and mark the level on the humeral stem for the desired prosthetic position (Fig. 18.13). This technique of preoperative planning provides only a guideline and may be superseded by intraoperative observations. In general, intraoperative deltoid tension is more important in determining the correct prosthetic position than preoperative radiographic templating. Preoperative planning does, however, provide a starting point for establishing proper prosthetic height.

Rarely, proximal humeral bone loss (previous trauma, tumor, etc.) is sufficiently severe to necessitate use of a custom implant or proximal humeral composite bone graft. Templates are useful to determine whether existing prefabricated implants are sufficient or a custom-manufactured implant is required (Fig. 18.14).

SECONDARY IMAGING

A secondary imaging study is obtained in all patients before reverse shoulder arthroplasty to evaluate the rotator cuff and osseous morphology. As with unconstrained shoulder arthroplasty, our preferred secondary imaging modality in most cases is computed tomography arthrography. Nonarthrogram computed tomography could be utilized to evaluate osseous morphology in cases where the rotator cuff is clearly deficient on the basis of examination and radiographs. If a patient has a previous magnetic resonance imaging scan that allows sufficient evaluation of the osseous structures and rotator cuff and is less than 6 months old, we will not order additional secondary imaging. In the scenario of a patient with possible deltoid muscle detachment from previous open rotator cuff surgery, our imaging modality of choice becomes magnetic resonance imaging, which in our experience more easily shows deltoid pathology.

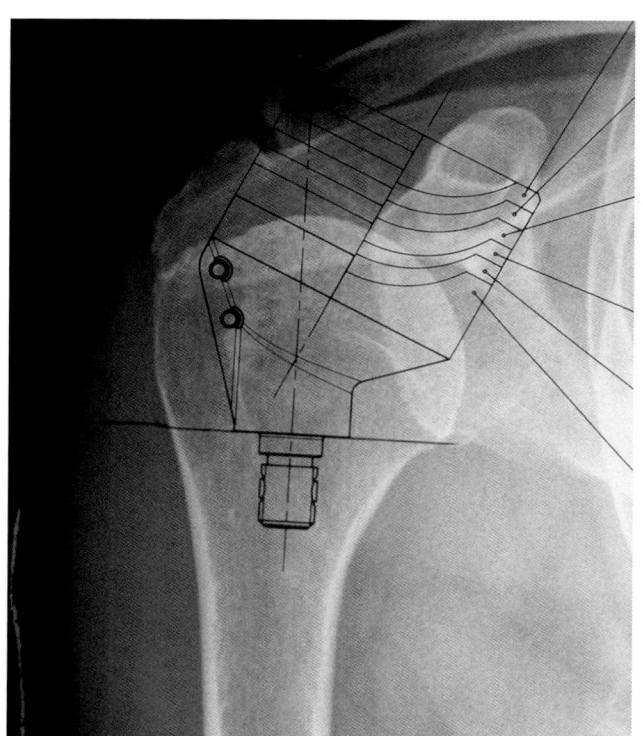

FIGURE 18.9 The desired position of a reverse prosthesis is templated on the unaffected humeral radiograph and the level of the metaphyseal-diaphyseal junction of the humeral component is marked.

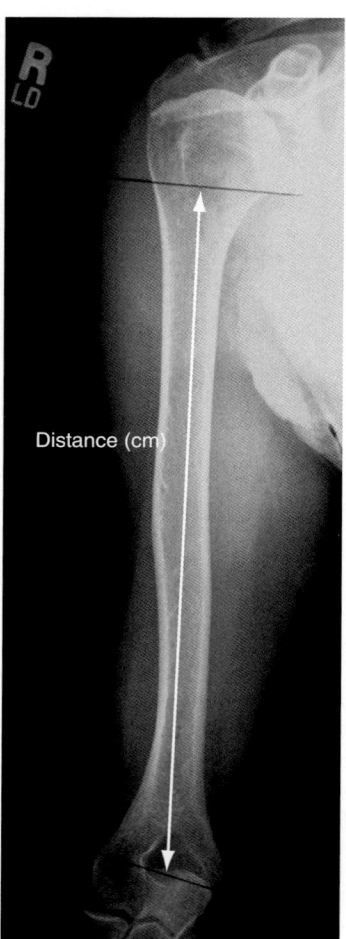

FIGURE 18.10 The distance from the transepicondylar axis at the elbow to the level of the metaphyseal-diaphyseal junction of the humeral component is measured.

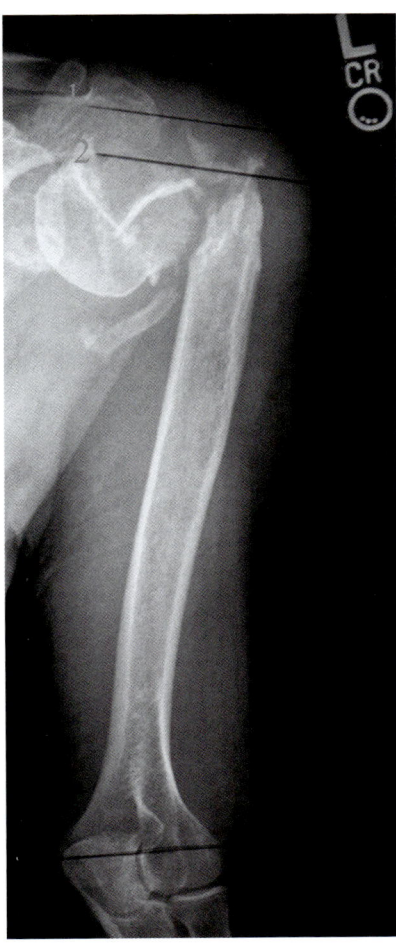

FIGURE 18.11 A mark (1) is made at the same distance from the transepicondylar axis on the affected radiograph. A second mark (2) is made at the most proximal extent of the humeral shaft.

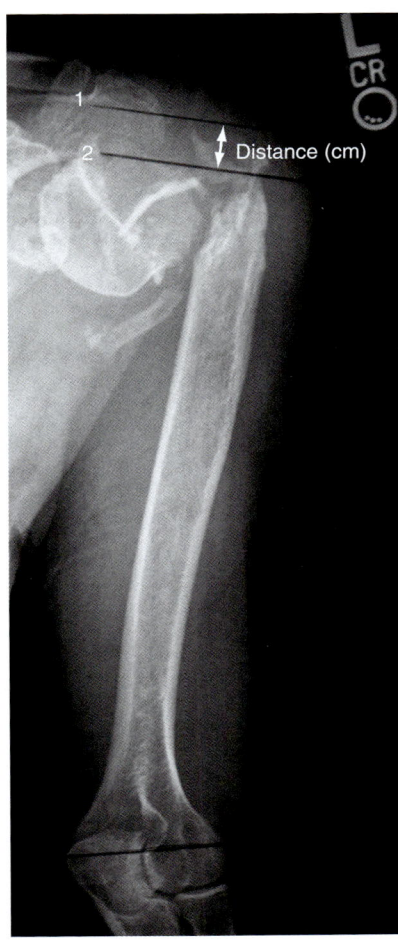

FIGURE 18.12 The distance between the desired prosthetic level at the metaphyseal-diaphyseal junction (1) and the proximal extent of the humeral shaft (2) is measured.

On a computed tomography scan (or magnetic resonance image), axial glenoid morphology is classified according to the system of Walch and colleagues, as described in Chapter 7.[6] New three-dimensional computed tomography reconstructions help to further classify glenoid morphology based on degrees of retroversion and percentage of subluxation.[7] A newly described type is type B3.[7] Walch and colleagues describe the B3 glenoid as monoconcave (rather than biconcave, as in B2) with posterior bony wear and severe pathologic retroversion (at least 15 degrees) or posterior humeral head subluxation (of at least 70%) or both.[7] Preoperative planning and classification of glenoid morphology is critical, especially in patients with severe glenoid erosion and posterior subluxation (B3) or insufficient glenoid bone stock. In these cases, a reverse prosthetic design may be preferred over an unconstrained shoulder arthroplasty even in the setting of an intact rotator cuff. A posterior bone graft may be necessary in the case of a severe B3 glenoid to reorient the glenoid to neutral.

The axial sections of the secondary imaging scan are also used to measure the depth of the glenoid vault in order to determine whether sufficient bone exists to implant the 15-mm peg of the reverse prosthesis base plate (Fig. 18.15).

Additionally, coronal glenoid morphology is classified as described by Sirveaux and associates (Fig. 18.16).[8] In this system, type E0 represents no glenoid wear, type E1 represents central glenoid wear, type E2 represents superior glenoid wear with superior biconcavity, and type E3 represents severe superior glenoid wear extending inferiorly and reorienting the glenoid surface to a superiorly tilted position. A superior bone graft may be necessary to reorient the glenoid to a neutral or inferiorly directed position in cases of severe superior glenoid bone wear (Fig. 18.17).

The rotator cuff is next evaluated with secondary imaging modalities, including assessment of tendinous integrity and evaluation of muscle quality (fatty infiltration). In addition, the condition of the long head of the biceps tendon is noted, particularly its position (centered, subluxated, dislocated, ruptured), to assist in identifying it at the time of surgery. Each tendon of the rotator cuff is individually evaluated with the secondary imaging study. Even though tears or fatty infiltration of the rotator cuff (or both) may not contraindicate use of a reverse prosthesis, knowledge of the status of the rotator cuff helps to determine the postoperative prognosis. Moreover, a completely nonfunctioning posterior rotator cuff may be an indication for use of a latissimus dorsi transfer

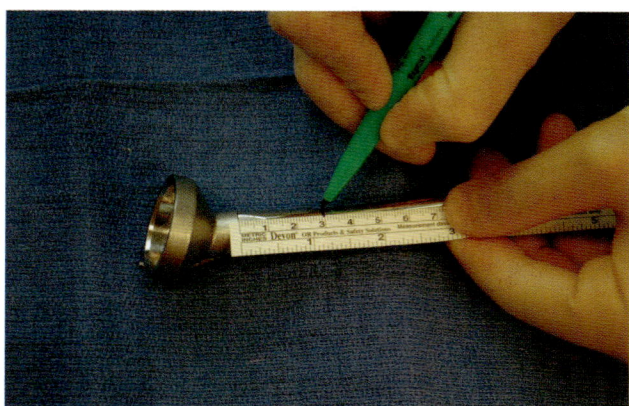

FIGURE 18.13 A ruler is used during surgery to measure the distance and mark on the humeral stem the level for the desired prosthetic position.

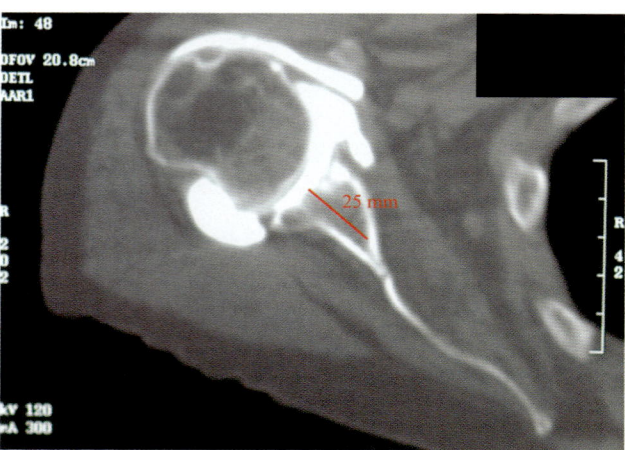

FIGURE 18.15 Measurement of the depth of the glenoid vault with a computed tomography scan taken preoperatively to determine whether the glenoid is sufficient for implantation of the reverse prosthesis base plate.

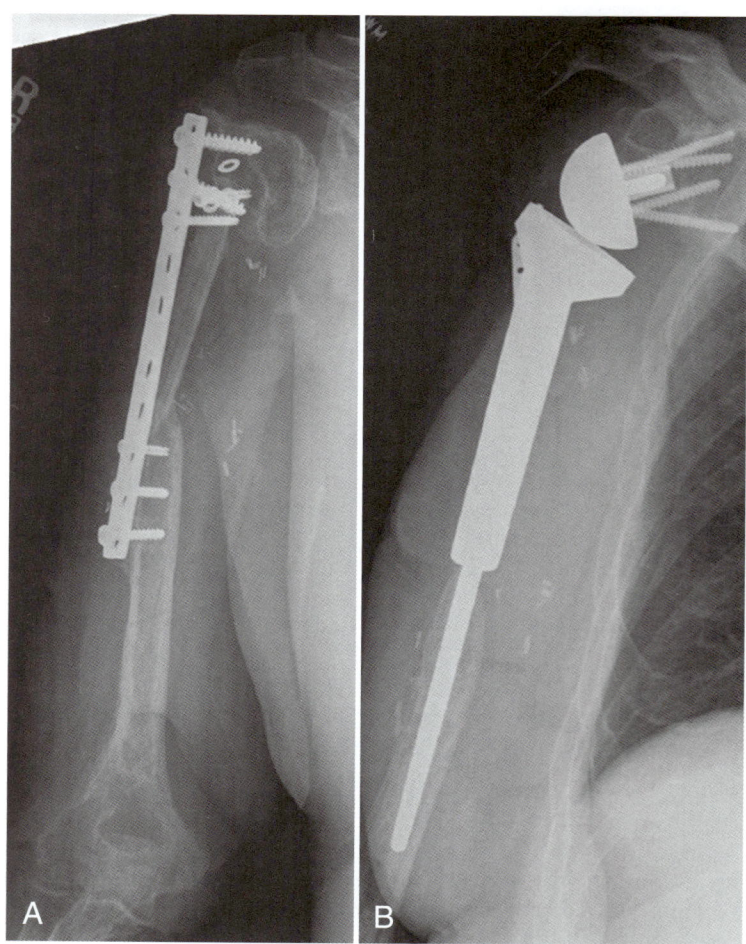

FIGURE 18.14 (A and B) A case in which a custom-manufactured implant was required to accommodate for severe proximal humeral bone loss.

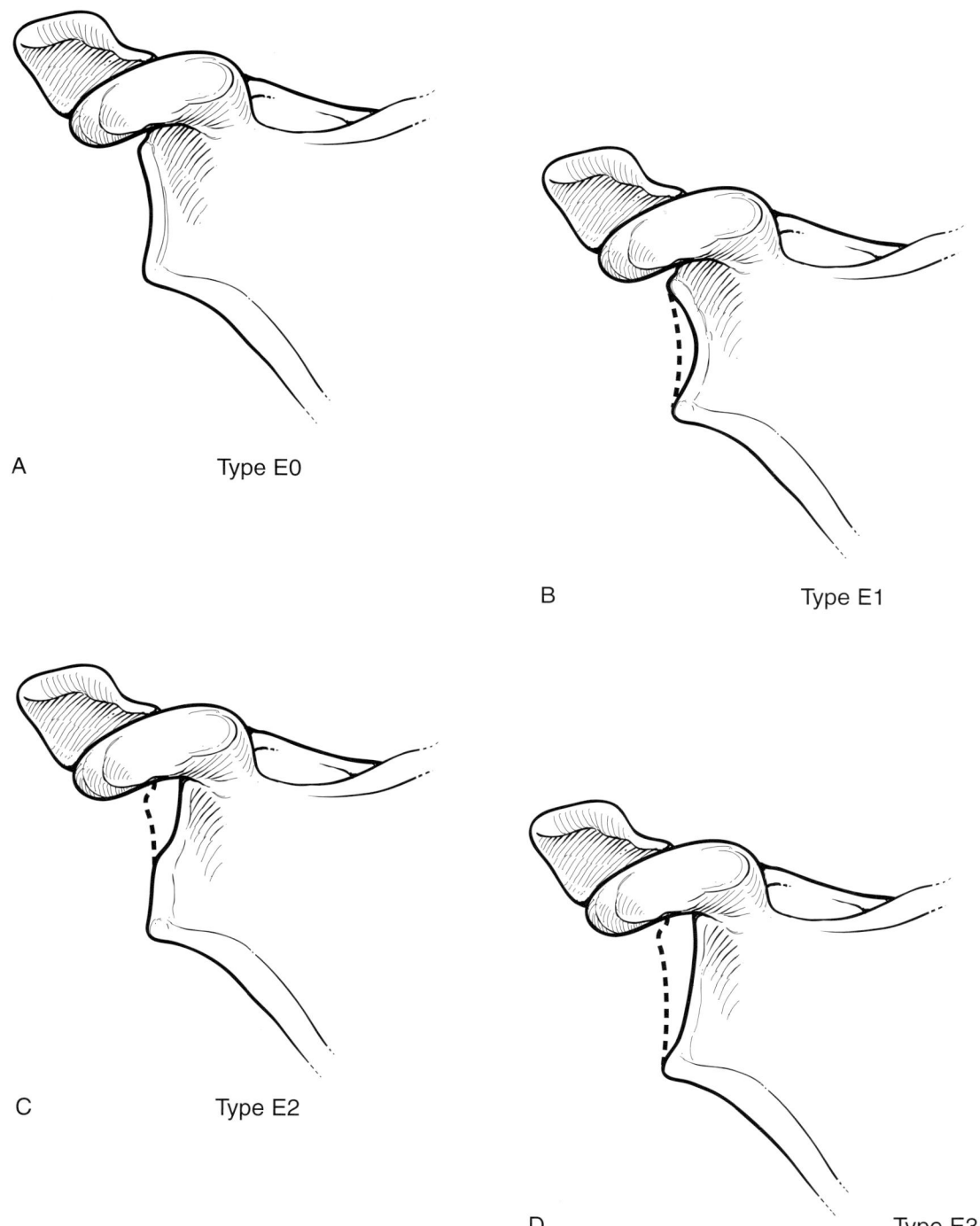

FIGURE 18.16 Classification of coronal glenoid morphology. (A) Type E0 represents no glenoid wear. (B) Type E1 represents central glenoid wear. (C) Type E2 represents superior glenoid wear with superior biconcavity. (D) Type E3 represents severe superior glenoid wear extending inferiorly and reorienting the glenoid surface to a superiorly tilted position.

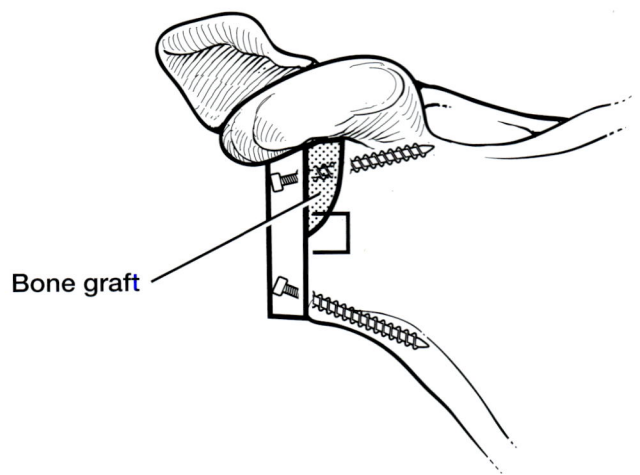

FIGURE 18.17 In cases of severe superior glenoid bony wear, a superior bone graft may be necessary to reorient the glenoid to a neutral or inferiorly directed position.

with the reverse prosthesis to better restore postoperative external rotation, although the usefulness of this adjunctive procedure is not yet well established in this scenario.

PREOPERATIVE PLANNING SOFTWARE AND PATIENT-SPECIFIC INSTRUMENTATION

Preoperative planning software (see Chapter 7) has been introduced to enable surgeons to plan the anticipated surgery virtually, including implantation of the humeral and glenoid components for reverse shoulder arthroplasty. The software is typically formatted off nonarthrogram computed tomography scans to create three-dimensional reconstructions that allow for the evaluation of glenoid morphology, including degrees of retroversion and percentage of humeral head subluxation. The surgeon can virtually implant the glenoid component and determine the appropriate glenosphere size, base-plate size, and desired location on the glenoid to ensure appropriate version, seating, depth of reaming, and appropriate glenoid bone stock. The three-dimensional plan can be used with or without a patient-specific guide. Such a guide is created to provide reproducibility of guide-pin placement for instrumentation of the glenoid.

REFERENCES

1. Morris BJ, Waggenspack WN, Laughlin MS, et al: Reverse shoulder arthroplasty for management of postinfectious arthropathy with rotator cuff deficiency, *Orthopedics* 38(8):e701–e707, 2015.
2. Jobe FW, Jobe C: Painful athletic injuries of the shoulder, *Clin Orthop Relat Res* 173:117–124, 1983.
3. Hertel R, Ballmer FT, Lambert SM, et al: Lag signs in the diagnosis of rotator cuff rupture, *J Shoulder Elbow Surg* 5:307–313, 1996.
4. Gerber C, Vinh TS, Hertel R, et al: Latissimus dorsi transfer for the treatment of massive tears of the rotator cuff: a preliminary report, *Clin Orthop Relat Res* 232:51–61, 1988.
5. Gerber C, Krushell RJ: Isolated rupture of the tendon of the subscapularis muscle: clinical features in 16 cases, *J Bone Joint Surg Br* 73:389–394, 1991.
6. Walch G, Badet R, Boulahia A, et al: Morphologic study of the glenoid in primary glenohumeral osteoarthritis, *J Arthroplasty* 14:756–760, 1999.
7. Bercik MJ, Kruse K, 2nd, Yalizis M, et al: A modification to the Walch classification of the glenoid in primary glenohumeral osteoarthritis using three-dimensional imaging, *J Shoulder Elbow Surg* 25(10):1601–1606, 2016, doi:10.1016/j.jse.2016.03.010. [Epub 2016 Jun 6].
8. Sirveaux F, Favard L, Oudet D, et al: Grammont inverted total shoulder arthroplasty in the treatment of glenohumeral osteoarthritis with massive rupture of the cuff: results of a multicentre study of 80 shoulders, *J Bone Joint Surg Br* 86:388–395, 2004.

Surgical approach

CHAPTER 19

Two surgical approaches have been described for implantation of a reverse prosthesis. The anterior superior approach was initially used because it makes use of the rotator cuff defect. More recently, the deltopectoral approach has been used for insertion of a reverse prosthesis. We insert nearly all reverse prostheses through the deltopectoral approach, which is our preferred approach for five reasons:

1. *Deltoid violation.* A reverse prosthesis relies on the deltoid muscle to power elevation of the arm. The anterior superior approach violates the deltoid muscle, which may be a problem.
2. *Level of humeral resection.* Glenoid exposure in using the anterior superior approach may require more resection of the proximal humerus than when the deltopectoral approach is used. With the anterior superior approach, the humerus is retracted inferiorly to obtain access to the glenoid. If glenoid exposure is inadequate after appropriate soft tissue release, the only solution to enhance glenoid exposure is resection of more of the proximal humerus. More bone resection may make proper deltoid tensioning difficult and lead to weakness in elevation.
3. *Glenoid component positioning.* It is generally agreed that the reverse glenoid component should be placed inferiorly on the glenoid face to help prevent impingement of the humeral component on the scapula and subsequent scapular notching. The need to retract the humerus inferiorly to access the glenoid with the anterior superior approach creates more difficulty in getting the glenoid component aligned with the inferior aspect of the glenoid face. Debate exists on whether inferior tilt should be introduced during glenoid reaming so that the glenoid component is better positioned to avoid scapular notching. However, it is agreed that superior tilt should be avoided. Using the anterior superior approach risks inadvertently placing the glenoid component in a superiorly tilted position, which risks glenoid failure (Fig. 19.1).
4. *Extensile exposure.* The deltopectoral approach can easily be extended into an anterolateral approach to the humerus, whereas the axillary nerve limits distal extension of the anterior superior approach. Review of a consecutive series of 100 reverse prostheses implanted at Texas Orthopedic Hospital demonstrates that the underlying etiology necessitated a more extensile exposure than that which could be obtained with an anterior superior approach in 36 cases (18 nonunion/malunion, 17 revision, 1 fixed dislocation requiring anterior glenoid reconstruction with iliac crest autograft).
5. *Familiarity.* One-third of our shoulder replacements involve the use of a reverse prosthesis. The other two-thirds use an unconstrained device implanted through a deltopectoral approach. We are very comfortable performing unconstrained shoulder arthroplasty through a deltopectoral approach and do not substantially change this approach in implanting a reverse prosthesis.

TECHNIQUE FOR THE DELTOPECTORAL APPROACH

The deltopectoral approach used for implantation of a reverse prosthesis is nearly identical to the deltopectoral approach used for unconstrained shoulder arthroplasty described in Chapter 8. The skin incision, subcutaneous dissection, development of the deltopectoral interval, identification of the conjoined tendon and coracoid process, and retractor placement proceed as detailed in Chapter 8 and shown in Figs. 8.1 through 8.6.

With the arm abducted and externally rotated, the apex formed by the insertion of the coracoacromial ligament and the conjoined tendon onto the coracoid process is identified. The coracoacromial ligament is sectioned just lateral to its insertion on the coracoid with a needle-tip electrocautery to enhance exposure of the superiorly migrated humeral head (Fig. 19.2). This is in contrast to the surgical approach used for unconstrained shoulder arthroplasty, in which the coracoacromial ligament is preserved to act as a static restraint to anterior superior migration. When we use a reverse prosthesis, the prosthetic design eliminates the need for this static restraint.

The conjoined tendon is retracted medially to expose the anterior aspect of the glenohumeral joint. The anterior humeral circumflex vessels (the "three sisters") are suture-ligated together just as in cases of unconstrained shoulder arthroplasty. The arm is then placed in forward flexion and neutral rotation. At this point, if desired, the axillary nerve can be identified by direct visualization after blunt dissection. In cases where the subscapularis is intact, it is handled identically to cases of unconstrained shoulder arthroplasty. Two stay sutures of no. 2 polyester are placed in the subscapularis tendon near the musculotendinous junction. The

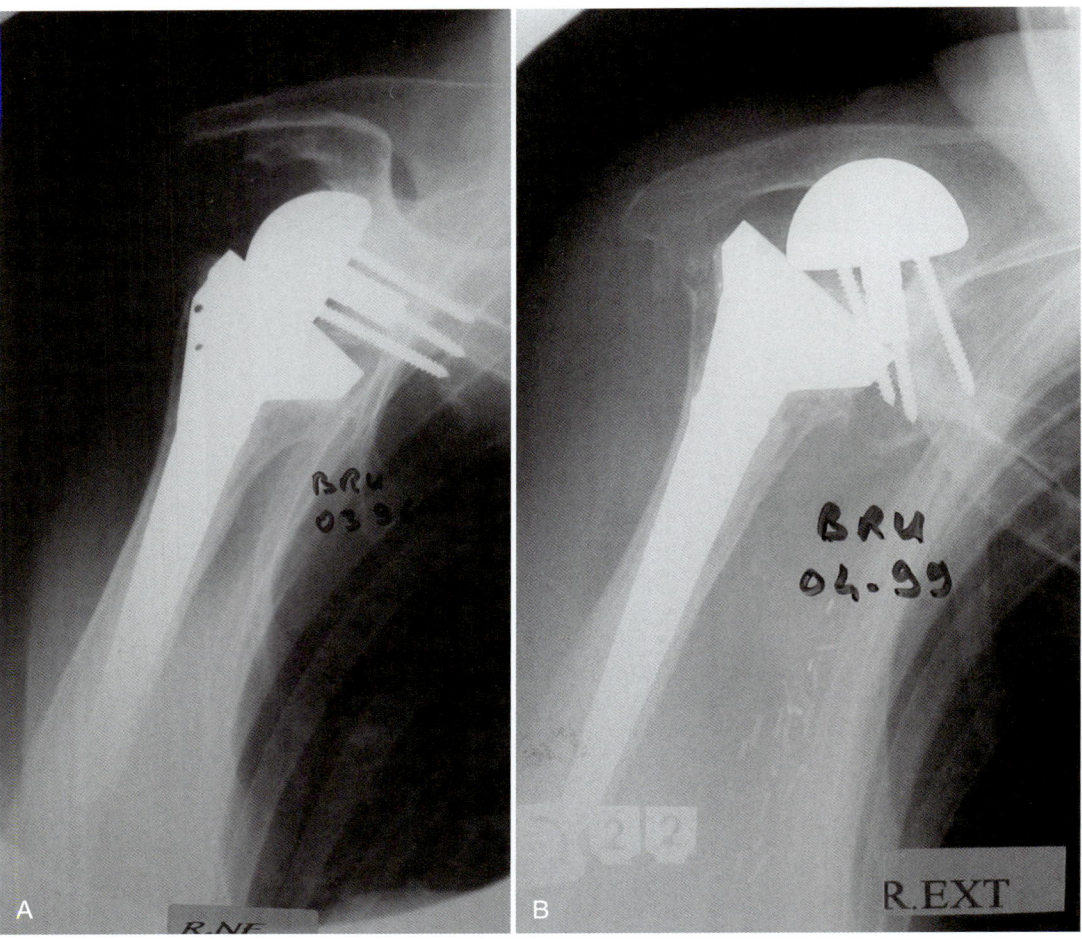

FIGURE 19.1 (A) Radiograph of a reverse prosthesis implanted through an anterior superior approach with the glenoid component inadvertently inserted with a superior tilt. (B) This malpositioned implant eventually failed.

glenohumeral joint is often already accessible through a large rotator cuff tear superiorly (Fig. 19.3). The anatomic neck of the humerus is identified, and a scalpel is used to transect the subscapularis tendon and joint capsule along the anatomic neck of the humerus. The electrocautery replaces the scalpel at the inferior portion of the subscapularis to cauterize the previously ligated anterior humeral circumflex vessels. A humeral head retractor is placed in the glenohumeral joint and is used to retract the humeral head posteriorly. A circumferential release of the subscapularis tendon is performed, with release of the superior, middle, and inferior glenohumeral ligaments just as in unconstrained shoulder arthroplasty. The subscapularis is then tucked into the subscapularis fossa with forceps and held with a glenoid rim retractor. In contrast to cases of unconstrained arthroplasty, no sponge is placed in the subscapularis fossa because insertion of screws for fixation of the glenoid base plate risks entrapment of the sponge with screws as they penetrate the anterior scapular cortex (Fig. 19.4). If the subscapularis tendon is not present, the remaining subscapularis bursa is excised to expose the glenohumeral joint, and the humeral head retractor and glenoid rim retractor are inserted. If the subscapularis tendon is present, the intraarticular portion of the long head of the biceps tendon is handled as described in Chapter 5 (tenotomy or tenodesis).

TECHNIQUE FOR THE ANTERIOR SUPERIOR APPROACH

The anterior superior approach used for implantation of a reverse prosthesis is indicated in our practice for patients with deltoid detachment, which has usually occurred following a prior open rotator cuff repair. The patient setup is the same as for a deltopectoral approach, and the positioning is important to allow proximal subluxation of the humeral head for humeral-sided preparation. Often the prior incision is utilized for the exposure (Fig. 19.5). The incision should extend along the anterolateral edge of the acromion and follow the deltoid muscle fibers. The incision should not extend beyond 5 cm from the edge of the acromion so as to prevent injury to the axillary nerve. In primary cases without a history of deltoid detachment, the anterior deltoid is often removed from the acromial edge and later repaired. In cases with prior deltoid detachment, the anterior deltoid must be repaired as well.

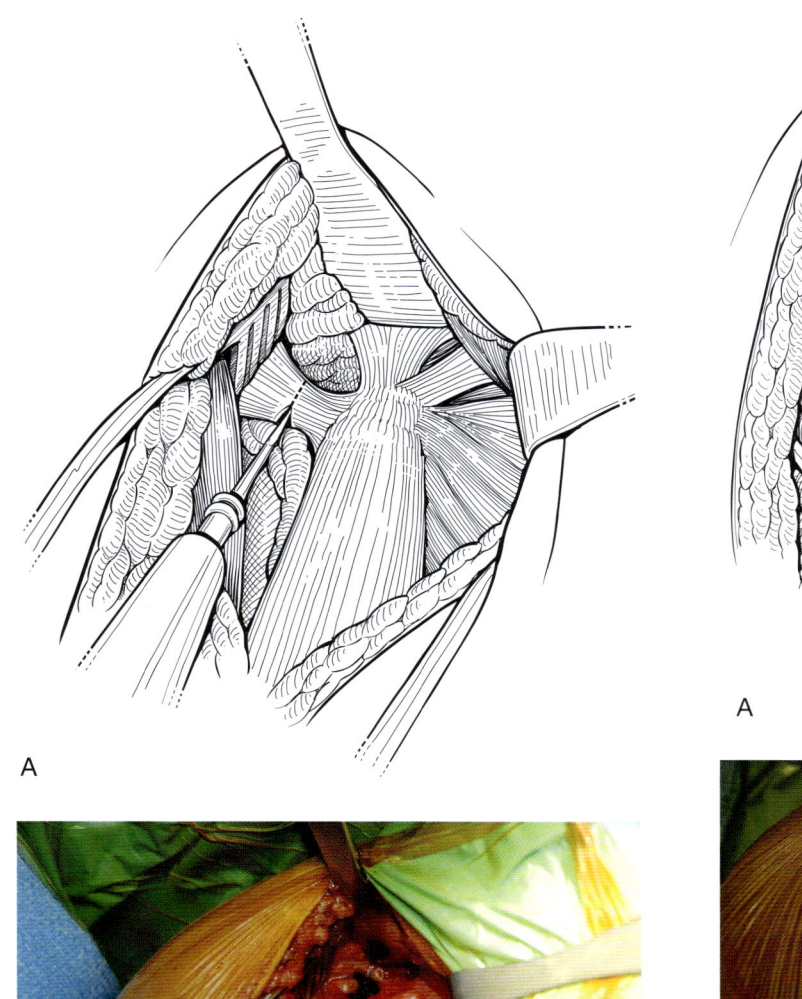

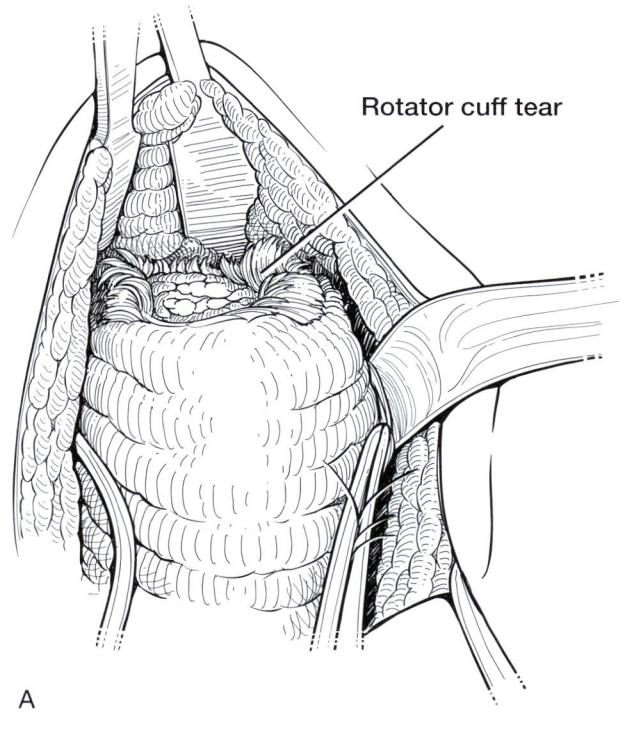

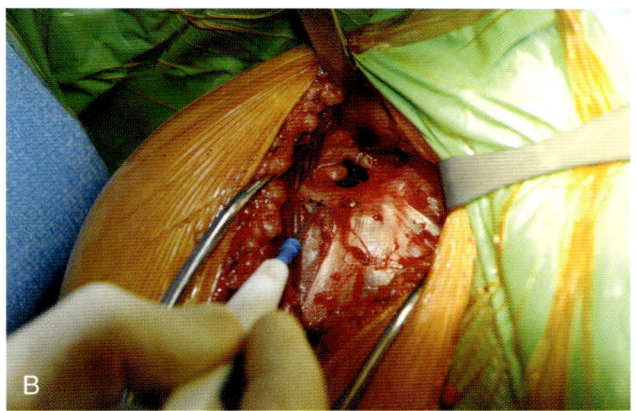

FIGURE 19.2 (A and B) Release of the coracoacromial ligament with the electrocautery.

FIGURE 19.3 (A and B) The glenohumeral joint visualized through a large rotator cuff tear.

After the skin incision, the deltoid muscle fibers are split and the underlying subacromial bursa is identified and resected (Fig. 19.6). The anterior portion of the deltoid is removed (and later repaired) to aid in exposure and the coracoacromial ligament is sectioned. The underlying rotator cuff is identified. In cases where the subscapularis is intact, it is handled identically to cases of unconstrained shoulder arthroplasty.

The assistant applies a superior force under the elbow to provide proximal subluxation of the humeral head for humeral-sided instrumentation (Fig. 19.7). Following humeral-sided preparation, the trial is left in place and a cut protector is placed. Anterior, posterior, and inferior glenoid retractors are placed to provide glenoid exposure (Fig. 19.8). Glenoid preparation and the remainder of the

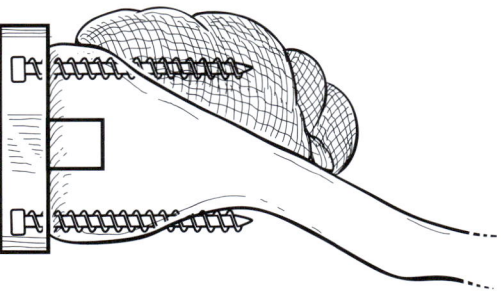

FIGURE 19.4 If a sponge is placed in the subscapularis fossa, screws used for base-plate fixation may engage and incarcerate the sponge. In implanting a reverse prosthesis, a sponge is not used in the subscapularis fossa to avoid this situation.

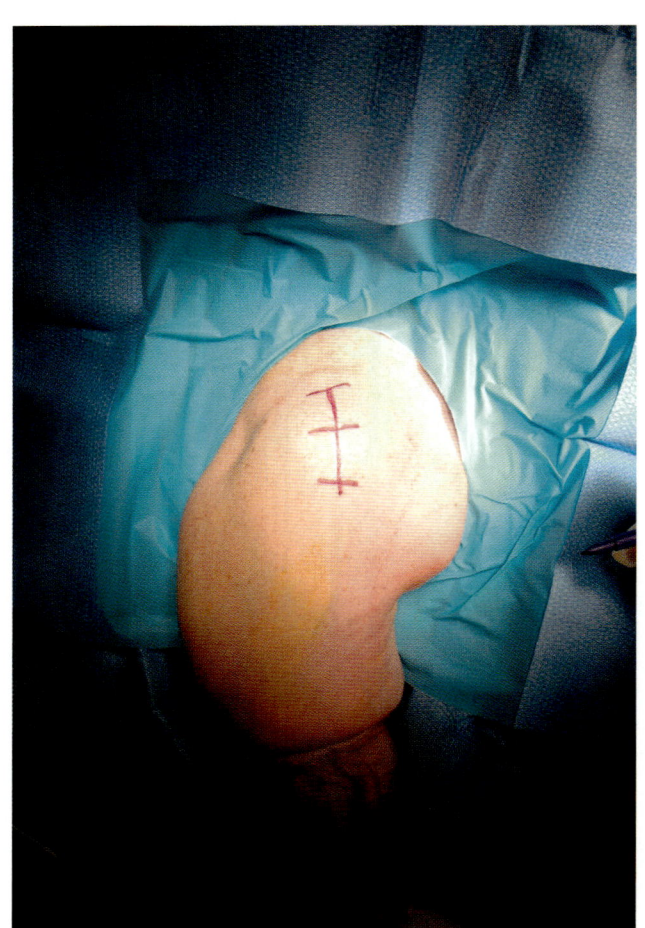

FIGURE 19.5 The prior skin incision is utilized for the anterior superior approach.

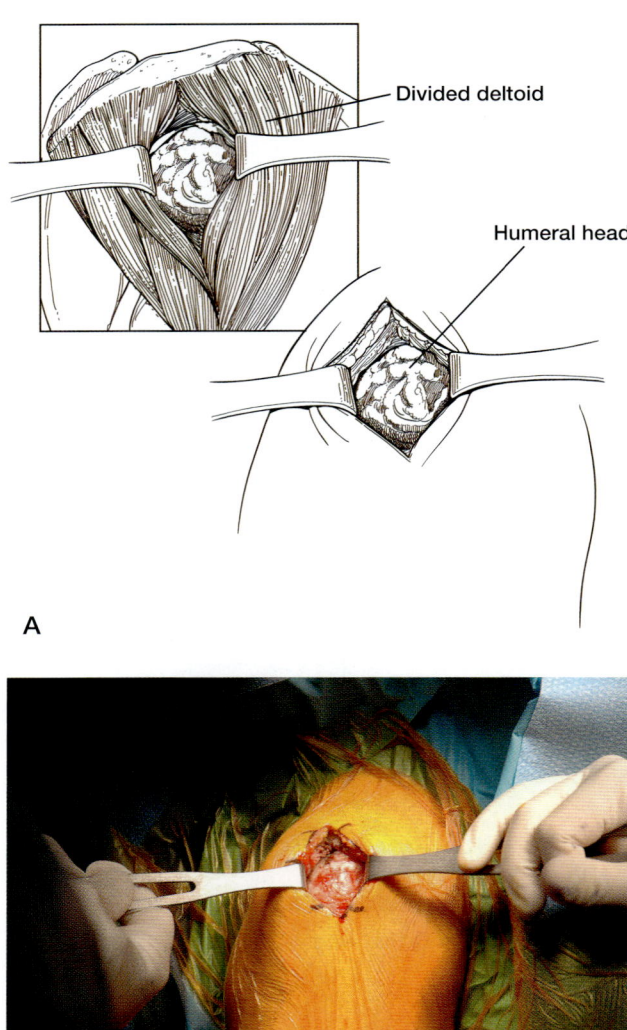

FIGURE 19.6 (A and B) The deltoid muscle fibers are split and the underlying subacromial bursa is identified and resected.

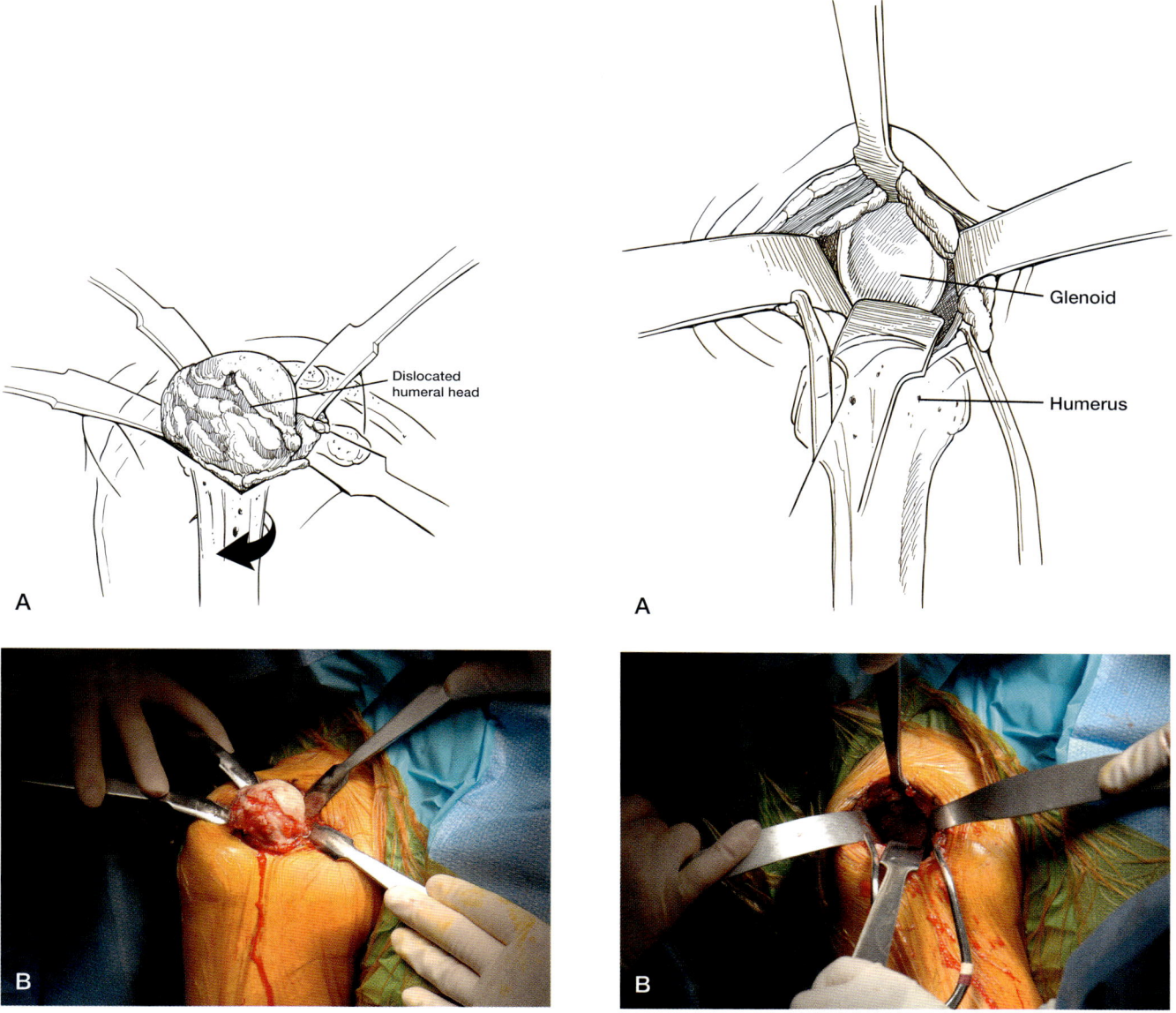

FIGURE 19.7 (A and B) The assistant applies a superior force under the elbow to provide proximal subluxation of the humeral head for humeral-sided instrumentation.

FIGURE 19.8 (A and B) Exposure of the glenoid with the humerus retracted inferiorly using the anterior superior approach.

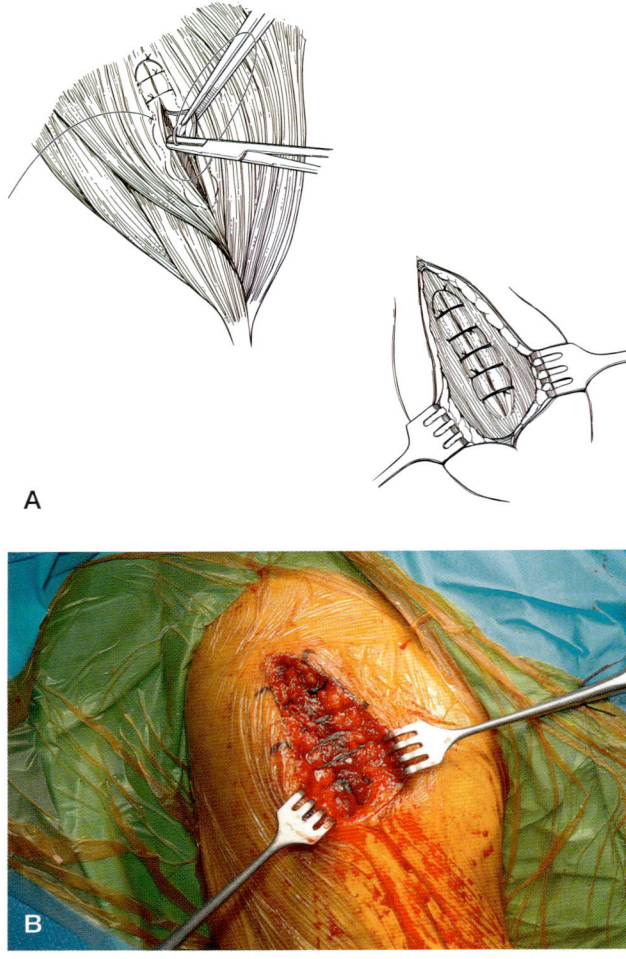

FIGURE 19.9 (A and B) Closure of the defect in the deltoid.

procedure are completed identically to cases of reverse shoulder arthroplasty from a deltopectoral approach with the key exception of deltoid reattachment and repair at the end of the case. The longitudinal split or acquired defect in the deltoid is first addressed by running a no. 5 nonabsorbable braided suture peripherally along the defect to act as a rip stop. Following placement of the rip-stop suture, the longitudinal split is closed with interrupted no. 5 nonabsorbable braided sutures passing behind the rip-stop suture line (Fig. 19.9).

Glenoid exposure

CHAPTER 20

The technique for glenoid exposure is no less important for implantation of a reverse prosthesis than it is in cases of unconstrained total shoulder arthroplasty. In fact, certain aspects of reverse prosthesis cases may make glenoid exposure more difficult than in cases of unconstrained total shoulder arthroplasty. For example, static subluxation of the proximal humerus may increase the difficulty of proximal humeral retraction during glenoid exposure.

The steps and technique of glenoid exposure are essentially identical to those performed for unconstrained total shoulder arthroplasty. Care is taken to avoid releasing more of the glenohumeral joint capsule than necessary to allow adequate glenoid exposure for implantation of the reverse prosthesis while avoiding prosthetic dislocation. In many cases where the reverse prosthesis is indicated, the glenohumeral joint capsule helps to provide stability to the glenohumeral joint. With the rotator cuff absent or severely compromised, stability of the prosthetic joint is provided by a combination of the inherent prosthetic biomechanics, the large muscles crossing the glenohumeral joint (deltoid, biceps), and any residual glenohumeral joint capsule. Because fibers from the large muscles crossing the glenohumeral joint are prone to elongation, which may compromise prosthetic tension and hence prosthetic stability over time, every effort should be made to preserve as much joint capsule as possible to enhance prosthetic stability.

TECHNIQUE FOR GLENOID EXPOSURE

After the subscapularis, if present, is retracted medially with a small glenoid rim retractor, attention is turned to glenoid exposure. Any remaining labrum is excised from the base of the coracoid process; the exposure is then extended inferiorly to the 5 o'clock position in a right shoulder (7 o'clock in a left shoulder) with the needle-tip electrocautery. This allows identification of the osseous anterior margin of the glenoid as well as inspection of the superior aspect of the glenoid for evidence of erosion (Fig. 20.1). The tip of the electrocautery is used to release the inferior capsule directly off the rim of the glenoid bone, stopping initially at the 6 o'clock position (Fig. 20.2). To prevent damage to the axillary nerve, the tip of the electrocautery must be kept in contact with the glenoid bone. This release is extended far enough medially to completely transect the capsule and expose the muscular fibers of the long head of the triceps inserting on the inferior osseous glenoid. Adequacy of glenoid exposure is then evaluated by having an assistant provide maximal retraction on the proximal humerus and verifying complete neuromuscular paralysis with the anesthesiologist or nurse anesthetist (Fig. 20.3). An adequate release is accomplished if the surgeon believes that glenoid reaming and implantation of the reverse glenoid component would be possible after appropriate humeral head resection. If exposure is thought to be adequate, no further capsular release is performed. If the release is thought to be insufficient, capsular transection is continued around to the 7 o'clock position in a right shoulder (5 o'clock position in a left shoulder) and the exposure is reevaluated. The process is repeated until the release is considered adequate. This stepwise progression helps to prevent too large a release, which could potentially lead to prosthetic instability.

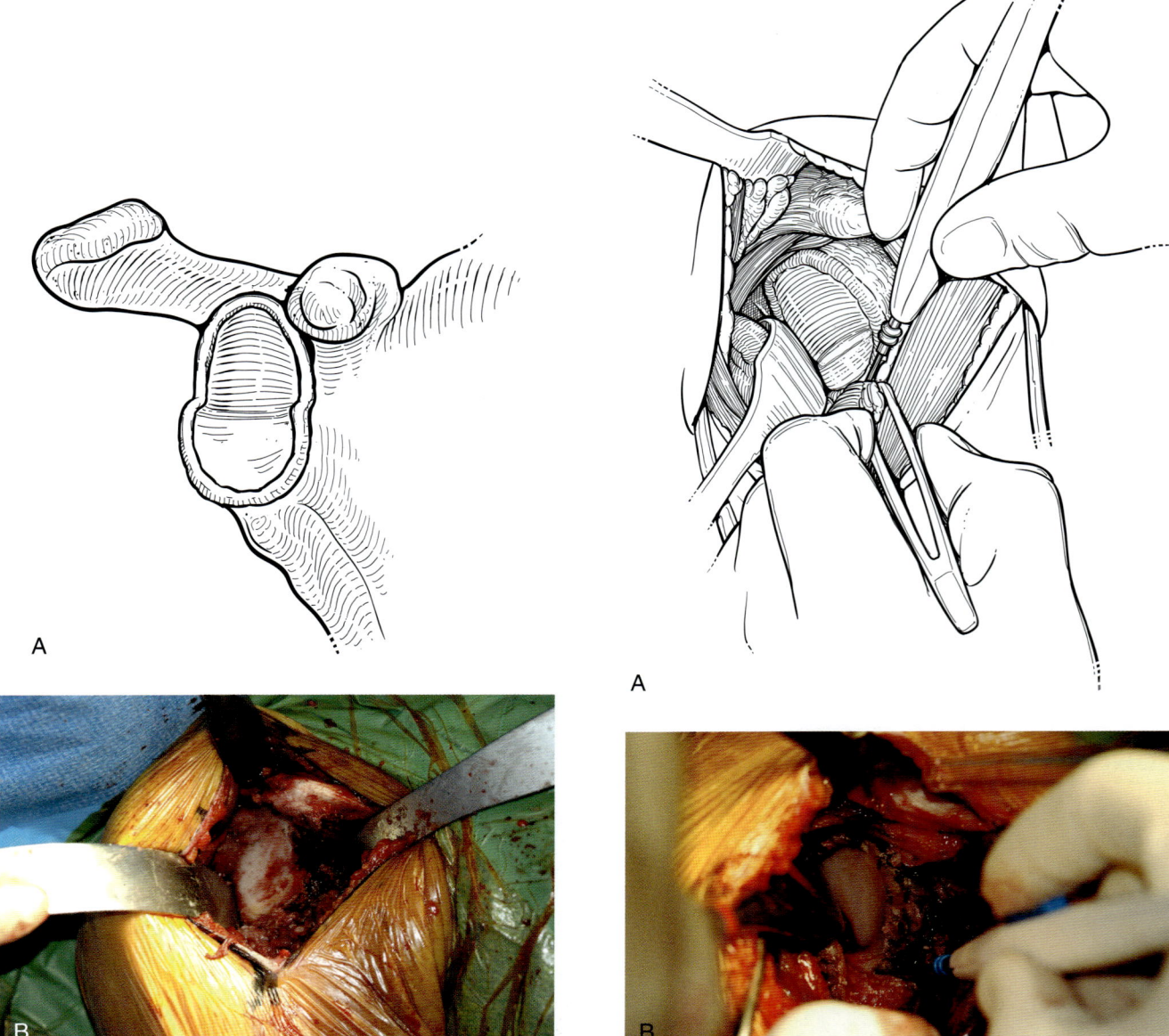

FIGURE 20.1 (A and B) Superior erosion of the glenoid in a case of rotator cuff tear arthropathy.

FIGURE 20.2 (A and B) Release the inferior capsule directly off the rim of the glenoid and extending it initially to the 6 o'clock position with the electrocautery.

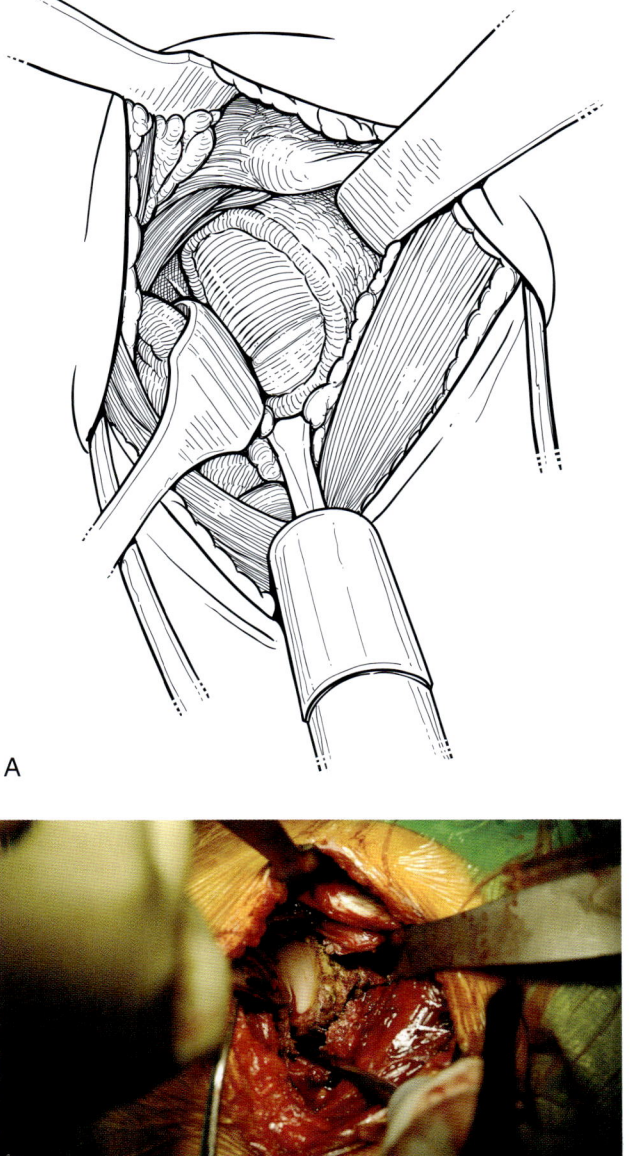

FIGURE 20.3 (A and B) Evaluation of the adequacy of glenohumeral release.

CHAPTER 21

Humeral component

Humeral preparation and implantation of the humeral component of a reverse prosthesis are in some ways easier than with unconstrained arthroplasty. In many cases for which a reverse prosthesis is implanted, the rotator cuff is severely compromised or absent, which facilitates exposure of the proximal humerus.

We implant nearly all reverse-prosthesis humeral components with an uncemented press-fit technique. In the past, we implanted all reverse-prosthesis humeral components with polymethylmethacrylate, but new advances on the humeral side have allowed us to transition to press-fit components. The stem we prefer is a short press-fit stem. The stem shape and length was designed to replicate the internal geometry of the proximal humerus, and it was not simply a shortening of an existing longer stem. The short stem length is our preferred stem, but longer stem options are available if needed. The stem relies on press-fit fixation primarily in the metaphyseal area. Furthermore, the collarless face of the stem is flush with the resection surface and allows humeral convertibility from an unconstrained total shoulder arthroplasty to a reverse shoulder arthroplasty.

Many different implant companies manufacture reverse-design shoulder prostheses. It is beyond the scope of this textbook to describe the specific techniques used for each of these systems. To us, the critical design feature for any reverse-prosthetic system is a modification of the traditional Grammont-designed medialized center of rotation of the glenohumeral articulation. We believe that long-term success can be achieved if the implant system selected adheres to this clinically tested principle. This chapter describes the technique for preparation of the proximal humerus for our preferred prosthetic system. Most of the steps, however, are applicable regardless of the system used.

TECHNIQUE FOR INSERTION OF A REVERSE-PROSTHESIS HUMERAL COMPONENT (Video 21.1)

Once the inferior capsule has been released from the neck of the glenoid, as described in Chapter 20, humeral preparation begins. The humeral head retractor is removed and the humeral head is dislocated by externally rotating and extending the arm. This maneuver is typically easier than in cases of unconstrained arthroplasty because the compromised rotator cuff offers little resistance to proximal humeral dislocation. A Hohmann retractor positioned superior to the coracoid process is moved to the margin of the humeral head, which is often "bald" (devoid of any discernible rotator cuff), and a modified Hohmann retractor is placed inferiorly and medially at the surgical neck of the humerus to complete the proximal humeral exposure (Fig. 21.1).

In most patients being treated with a reverse prosthesis, minimal if any peripheral humeral head osteophytes are present. In the uncommon situation where large humeral osteophytes exist, they are removed with a half-inch osteotome and mallet, just as in cases of unconstrained shoulder arthroplasty (see Chapter 11). Humeral osteophytes are removed to facilitate identification of the anatomic neck of the humerus to guide resection of the humeral head and to avoid mechanical impingement between the osteophytes and the axillary border of the scapula (Fig. 21.2). We used a traditional Grammont design for many years that relied on a minimal humeral head resection. Now we utilize a modification of the traditional Grammont design that permits an anatomic humeral head resection to match that of an anatomic shoulder arthroplasty. The anatomic cut along the humeral head provides consistency in our humeral component technique for both anatomic and reverse shoulder arthroplasty.

The humeral head is resected along the anatomic neck with a saw (Fig. 21.3). If the posterior rotator cuff is completely absent, it may be difficult to identify the anatomic neck. In these cases, the humeral resection is made in approximately 30 degrees of retroversion. This estimate will be adjusted during broaching, as described further on. A starter awl is used to open the humeral canal (Fig. 21.4). A sequential series of humeral sounders are inserted to determine the diaphyseal size of the humerus (Fig. 21.5). The size and shape of the sounders correspond to the distal size and shape of the matching humeral components. After determining the appropriately sized sounder, the sounder is left in the intramedullary canal and the corresponding punch template is attached (Fig. 21.6). The punch removes a small portion of bone medially to prepare for humeral compactor placement (Fig. 21.7). The punch and sounder are then removed (Fig. 21.8). A sequential series of humeral compactors are placed next (Fig. 21.9). For a reverse shoulder arthroplasty, the pivoting necks on the humeral compactors are locked on the "B" setting, or 132.5 degrees for this particular system. We routinely start with the compactor that is at least three sizes below the final sounder size to prevent humeral fracture. For example, if the sounder was the size 5-to-6 sounder, then we would start with a 2 or

Text continued on p. 184

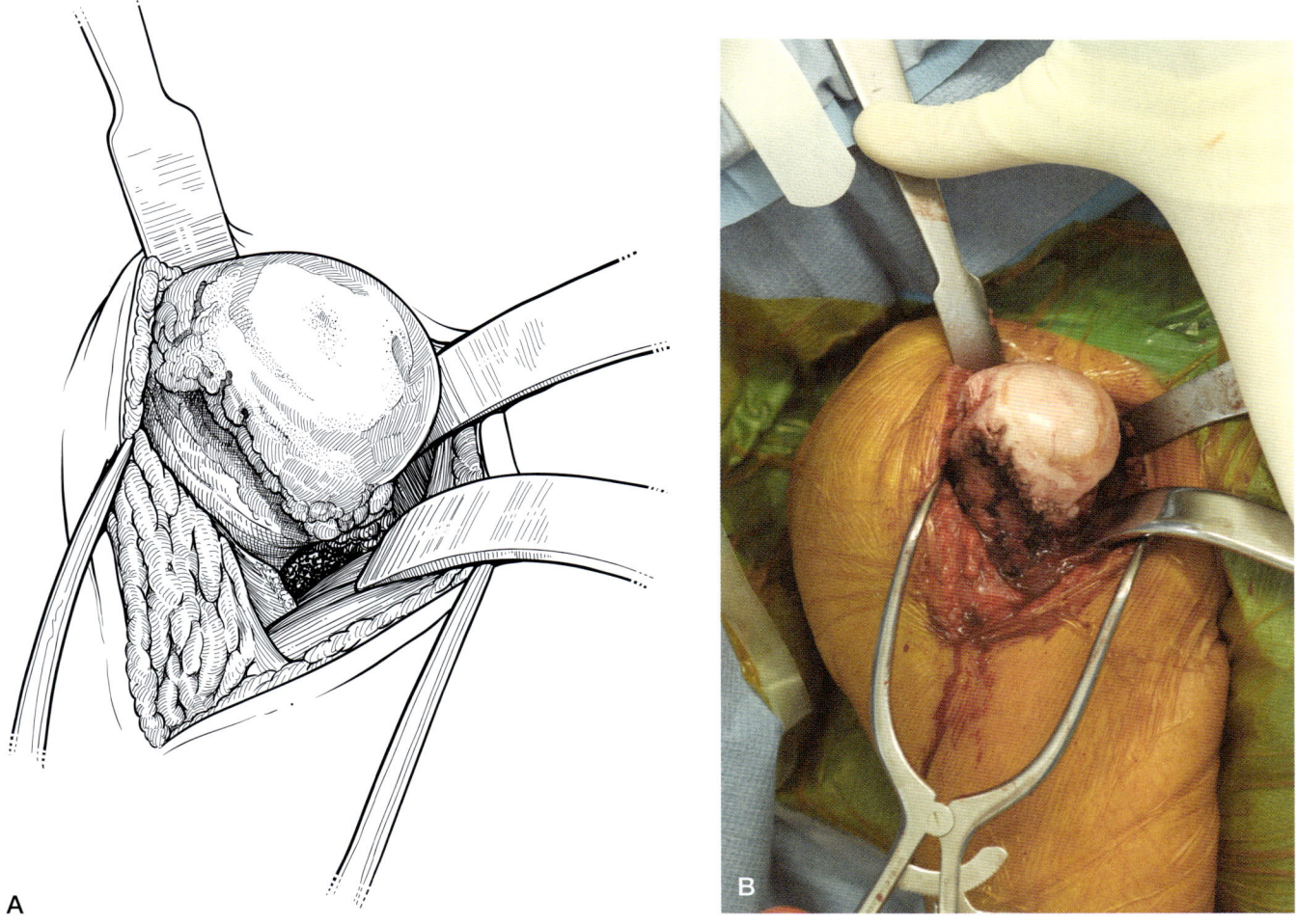

FIGURE 21.1 (A and B) Completed exposure of the proximal humerus in preparation for insertion of a reverse prosthesis.

SECTION III ■ Reverse Shoulder Arthroplasty

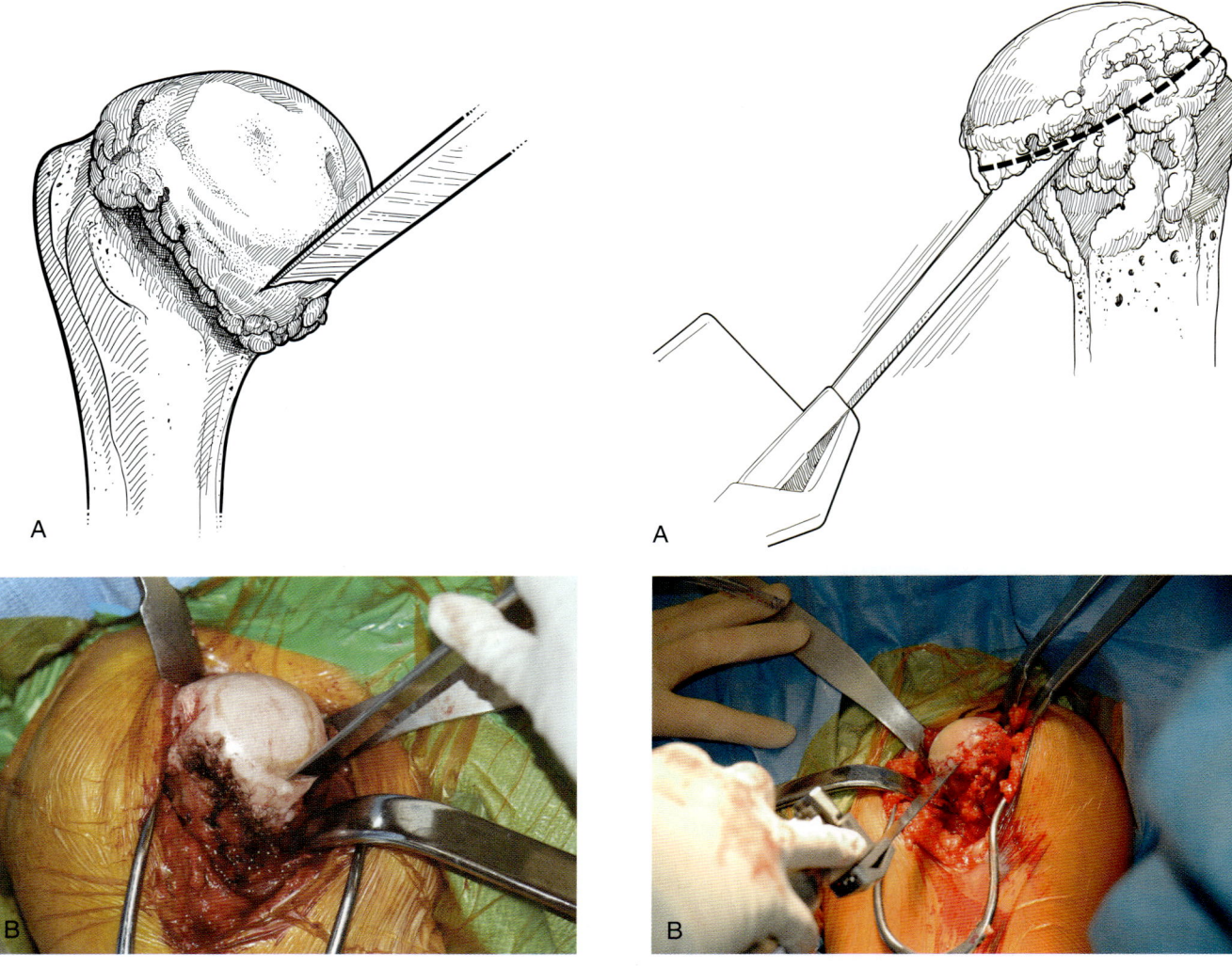

FIGURE 21.2 (A and B) Large proximal humeral osteophytes may cause mechanical impingement after implantation of a reverse prosthesis if not removed.

FIGURE 21.3 (A and B) The humeral head is resected along its anatomical neck.

CHAPTER 21 ■ Humeral Component   181

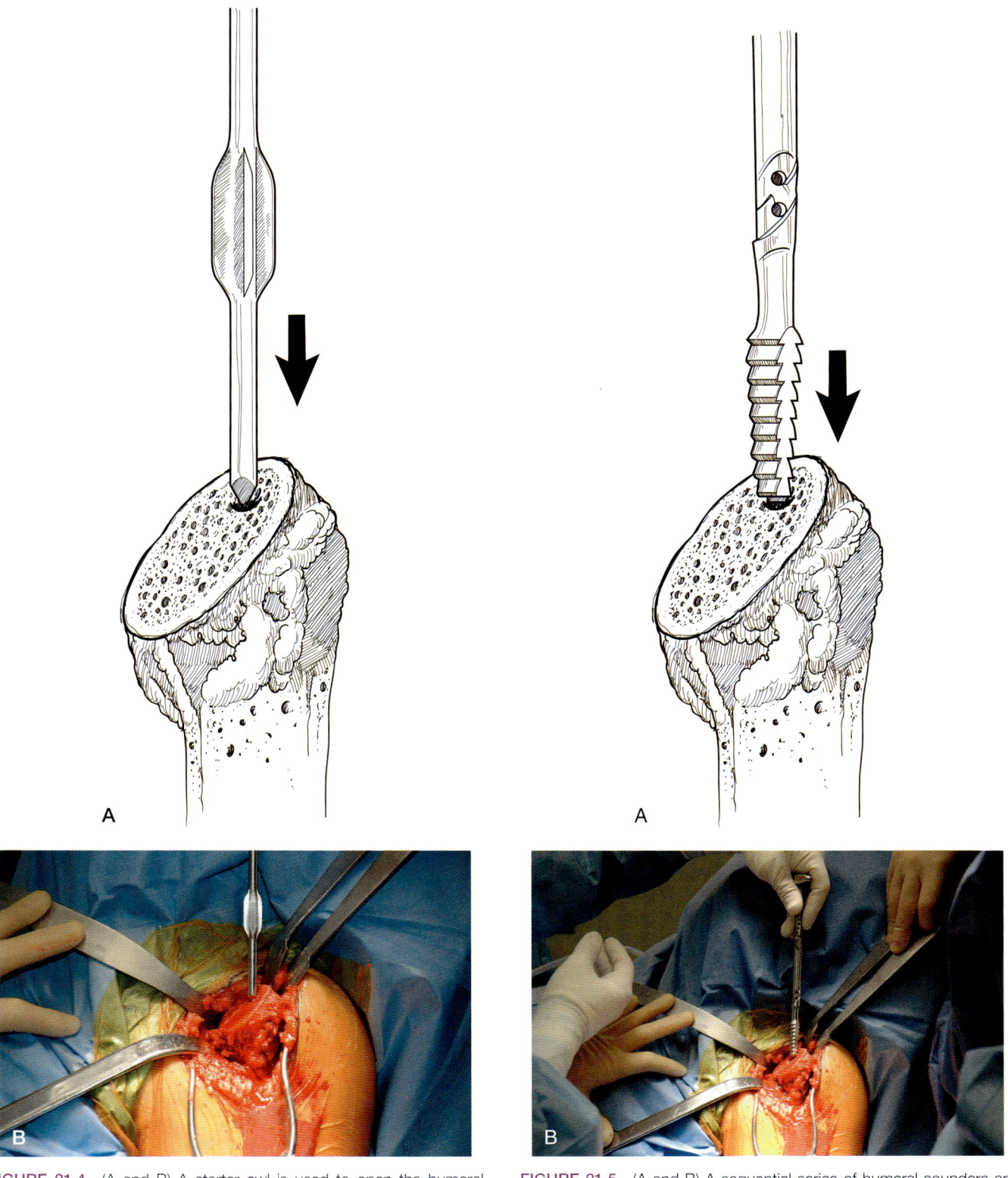

FIGURE 21.4 (A and B) A starter awl is used to open the humeral canal.

FIGURE 21.5 (A and B) A sequential series of humeral sounders are inserted to determine the diaphyseal size of the humerus.

182 SECTION III ■ Reverse Shoulder Arthroplasty

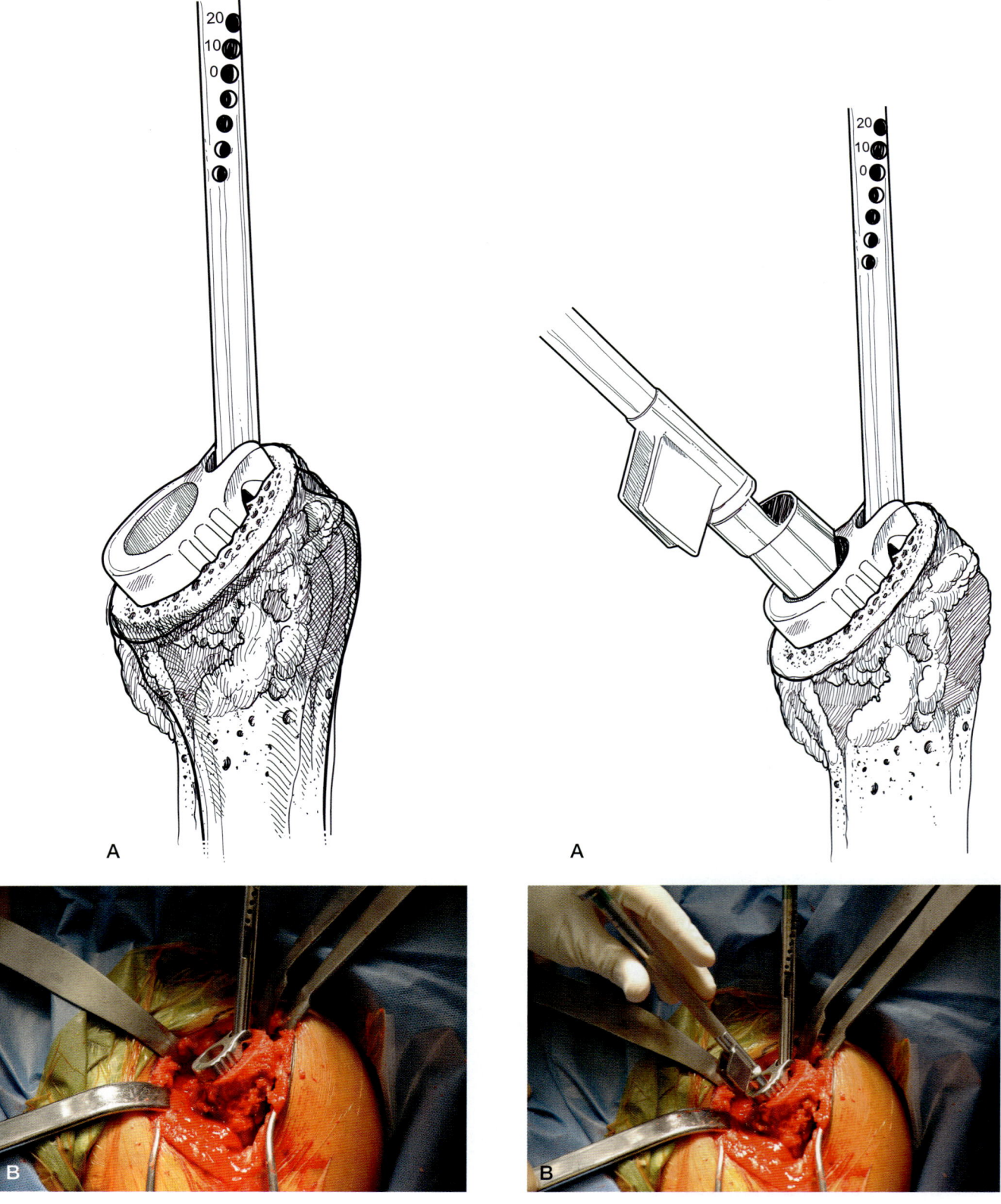

FIGURE 21.6 (A and B) After determining the appropriately sized sounder, the sounder is left in the intramedullary canal and the corresponding punch template is attached.

FIGURE 21.7 (A and B) The punch removes a small portion of bone medially.

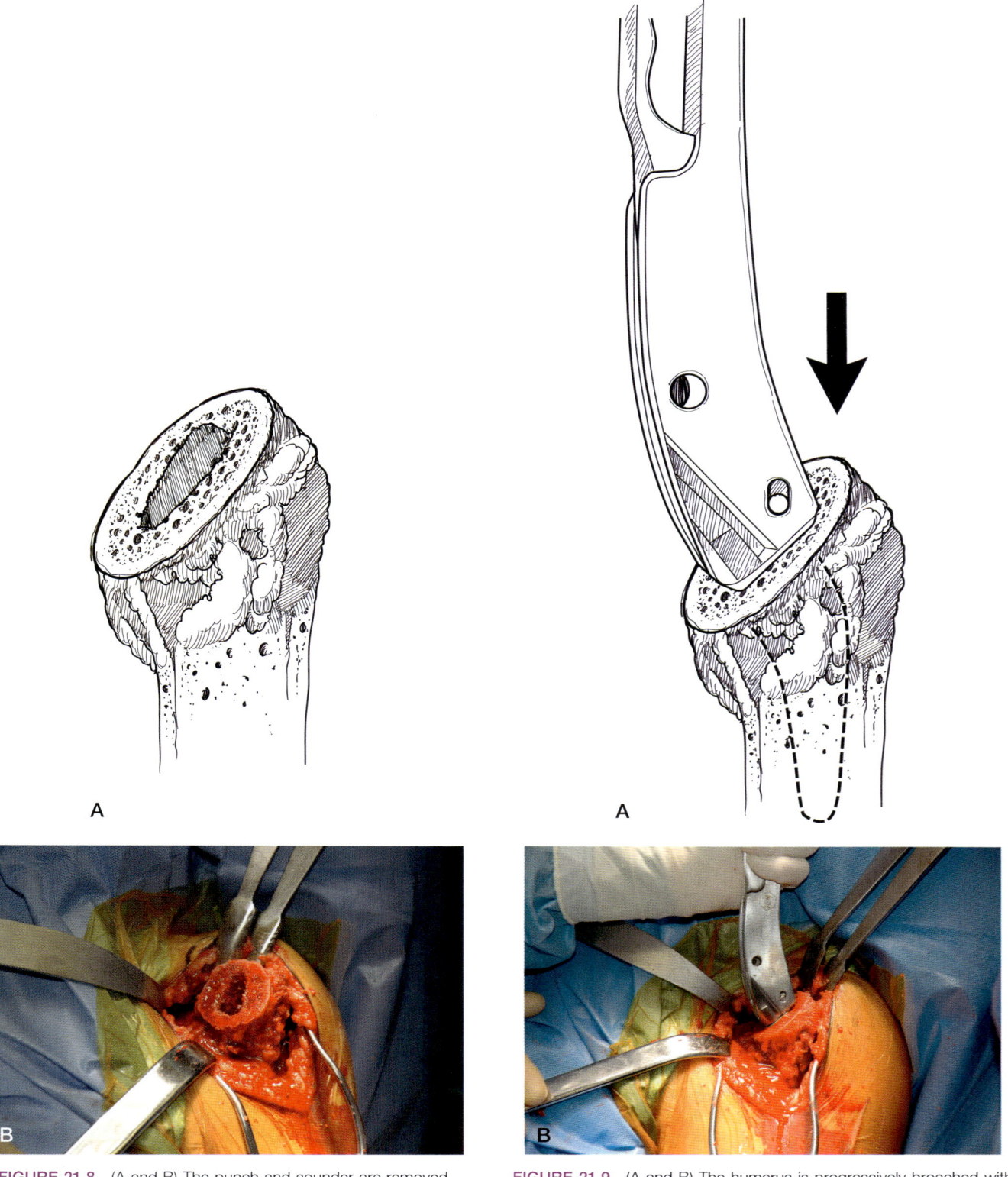

FIGURE 21.8 (A and B) The punch and sounder are removed.

FIGURE 21.9 (A and B) The humerus is progressively broached with the compactors.

3 humeral compactor and work our way up to a size 5 or 6 compactor. The humeral compactors are sequentially inserted until the final compactor has been inserted. The impactor handle used to insert the humeral compactor also accepts a version rod to determine the degrees of retroversion of the humeral component (Fig. 21.10). If the posterior rotator cuff is still present, allowing for identification of the patient's native humeral version, the humeral resection is made respecting this anatomy just as in the case of an unconstrained shoulder arthroplasty (see Chapter 11). In cases where the native humeral version is not easily identified because of lack of the posterior rotator cuff, the version is gauged off the version rod at 30 degrees of retroversion relative to the forearm. The size and press fit of the trial component can be tested with a "twist test," where the impactor handle is twisted to determine the press fit of the trial component (Fig. 21.11). The impactor handle is removed and a calcar planer or saw can be used to match inclination and version of the cut surface of the humerus to the compactor surface if needed (Fig. 21.12).

A cut protector is placed on the trial humeral component, and the glenoid is prepared and implanted as detailed in

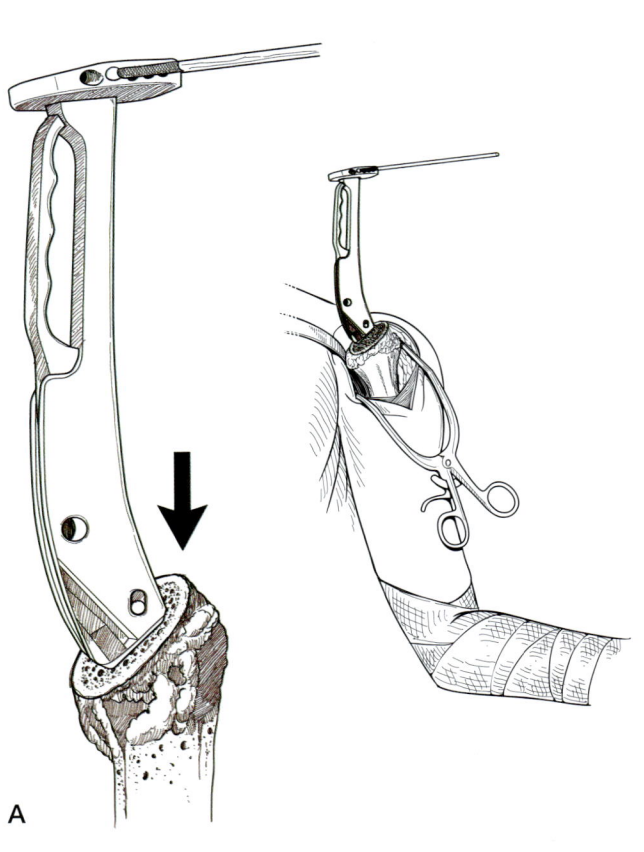
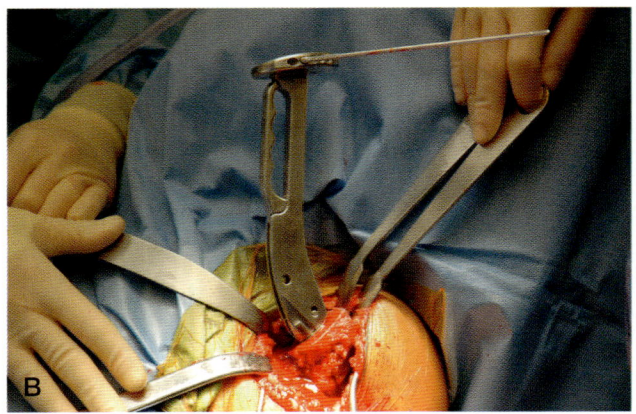

FIGURE 21.10 (A and B) The impactor handle used to insert the humeral compactor also accepts a version rod to determine the degrees of retroversion of the humeral component.

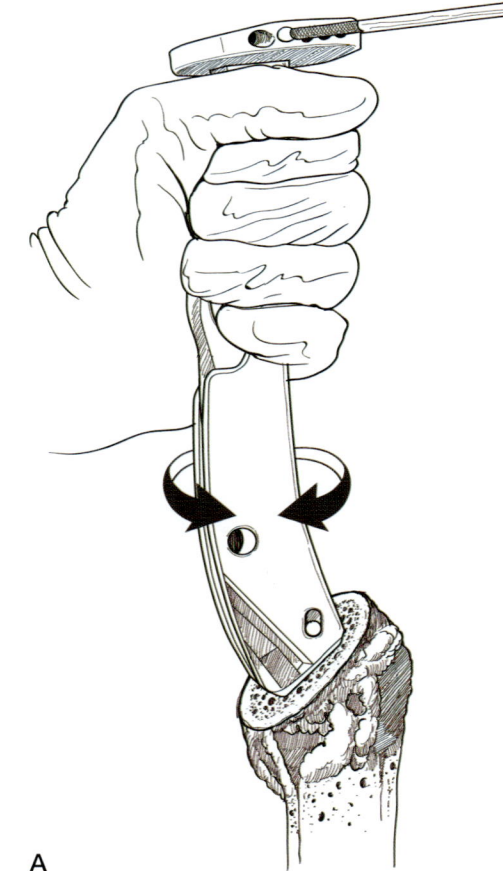
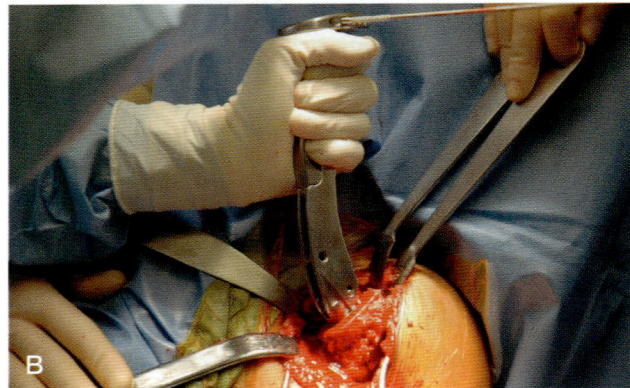

FIGURE 21.11 (A and B) The size and pressfit of the trial component can be tested with a "twist test," where the impactor handle is twisted to determine the press fit of the trial component.

Chapter 22. After the final glenoid components have been implanted, centered, low, or high offset humeral trial trays are tested to obtain optimal range of motion and stability. Additional humeral tray options include different humeral tray heights and polyethylene inserts (Fig. 21.13). We prefer to obtain lateral coverage with the humeral tray, but unlike the case involving an anatomic shoulder arthroplasty, the goal is not to cover the entire humeral cut surface with the humeral tray (Fig. 21.14). A slap hammer is used to remove the trial components after satisfactory trialing (see Chapter 23).

The final humeral implant is assembled on the back table (Fig. 21.15). The humeral stem and humeral tray can be combined and implanted without the final polyethylene

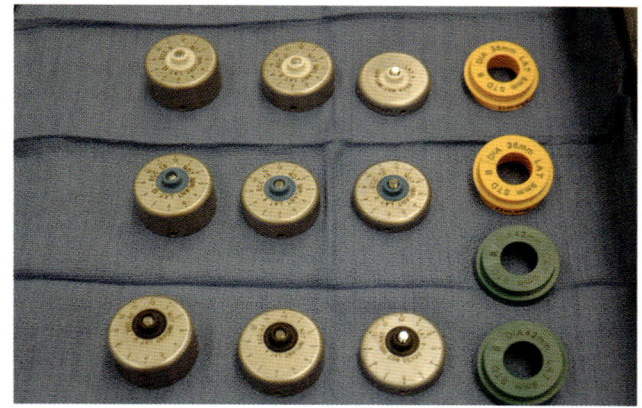

FIGURE 21.13 Different offsets and thicknesses of the humeral tray are available.

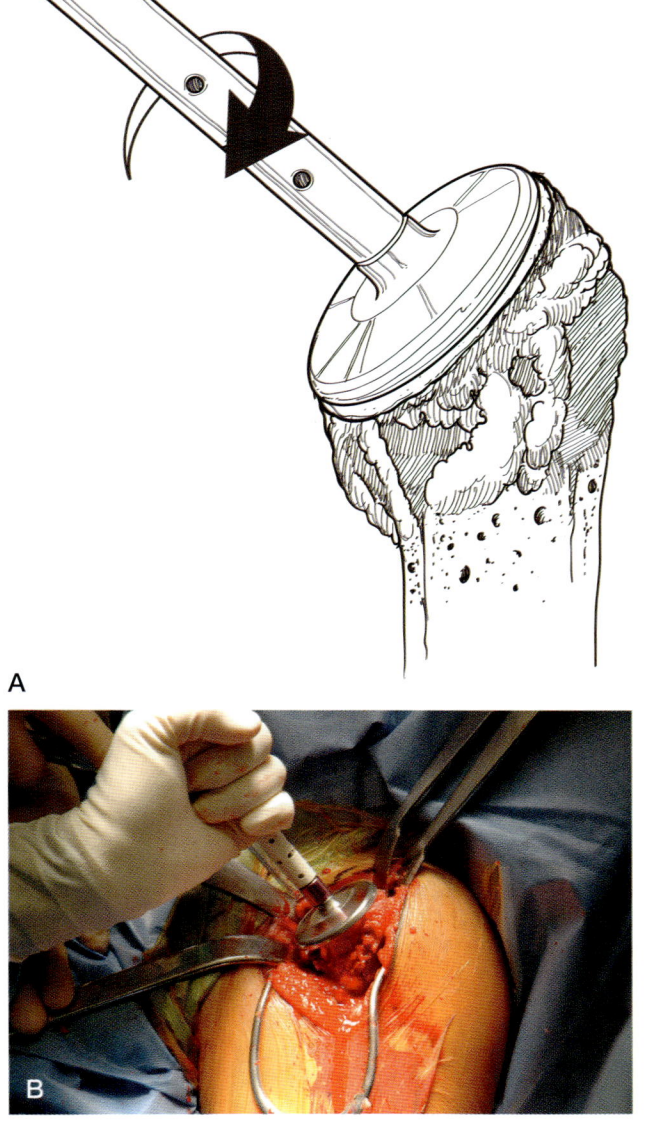

FIGURE 21.12 (A and B) A calcar planer or saw can be used to match the inclination and version of the cut surface of the humerus to the compactor surface if needed.

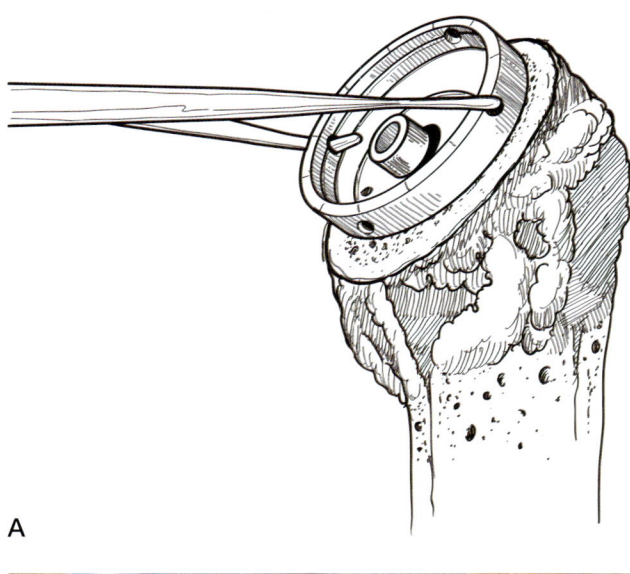

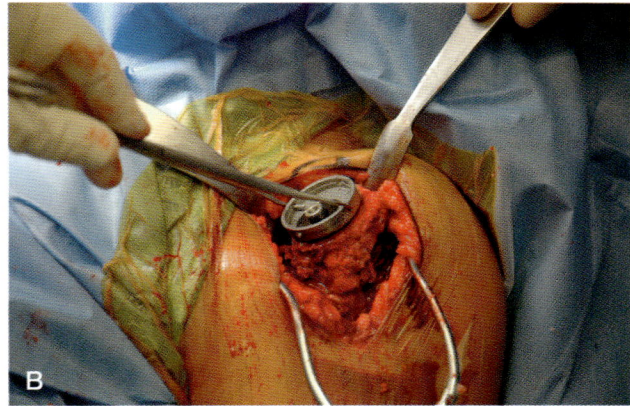

FIGURE 21.14 (A and B) The trial tray is rotated to a position flush with the lateral aspect of the cut surface, represented by the "6" index if using an offset tray.

component if additional trialing is desired. If the subscapularis is present, three transosseous no. 2 permanent braided sutures are placed through the stump of the subscapularis tendon and the lesser tuberosity for later use in reattaching the subscapularis. The final humeral prosthesis is impacted into place and care is taken to ensure that appropriate retroversion is maintained (Fig. 21.16).

There may be occasions when a press-fit long stem or a cemented humeral stem may be desired. We have found that the press-fit long stem is often not needed in primary reverse shoulder arthroplasty but is occasionally useful for revision cases. A cemented humeral stem for reverse shoulder arthroplasty is rarely utilized in our practice and is often reserved for very poor bone quality and sometimes in revision cases. The technique for a press-fit long stem is exactly the same as for the press-fit short stem. The technique for cementing a humeral stem involves first placing a cement restrictor at the appropriate level to create a 1-cm cement mantle distal to the tip of the stem (Fig. 21.17). The humeral canal is irrigated and dried. Fast-curing polymethylmethacrylate cement (DePuy CMW2 bone cement, DePuy, Inc., Warsaw, Indiana) is placed in the humeral canal with a catheter-tip 60-mL syringe that has been modified by cutting off the distal aspect of the plastic tip with heavy bandage scissors (Fig. 21.18). The final humeral component is placed at the appropriate height and version and the cement is allowed to cure prior to trialing.

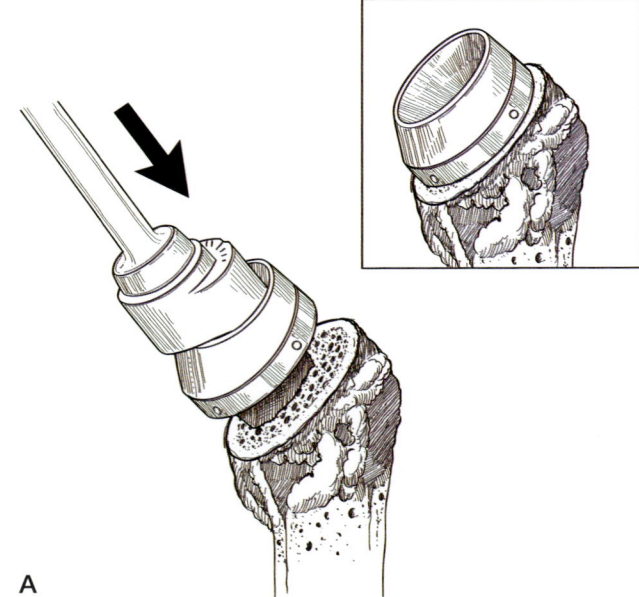

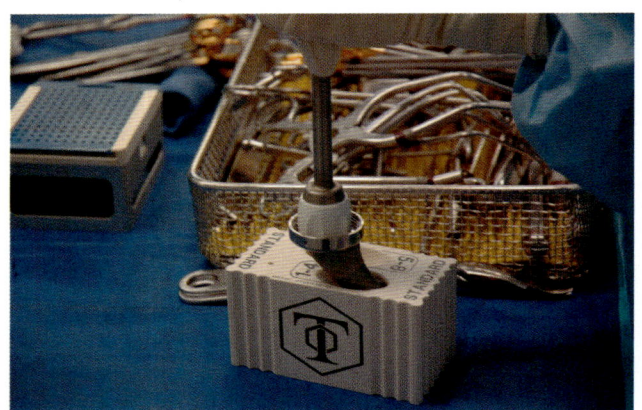

FIGURE 21.15 The final humeral implant is assembled on the backtable.

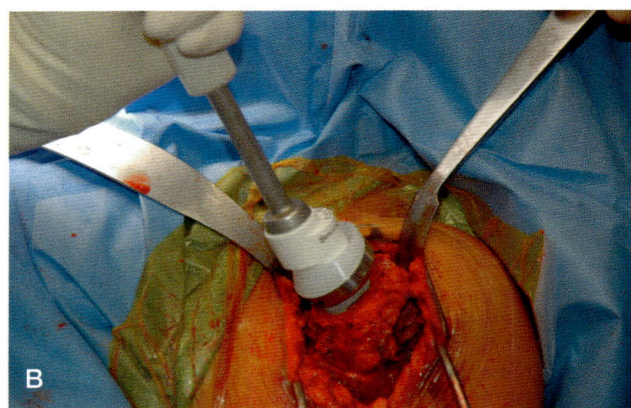

FIGURE 21.16 (A and B) Implantation of the final humeral prosthesis. The subscapularis tendon was absent in this case.

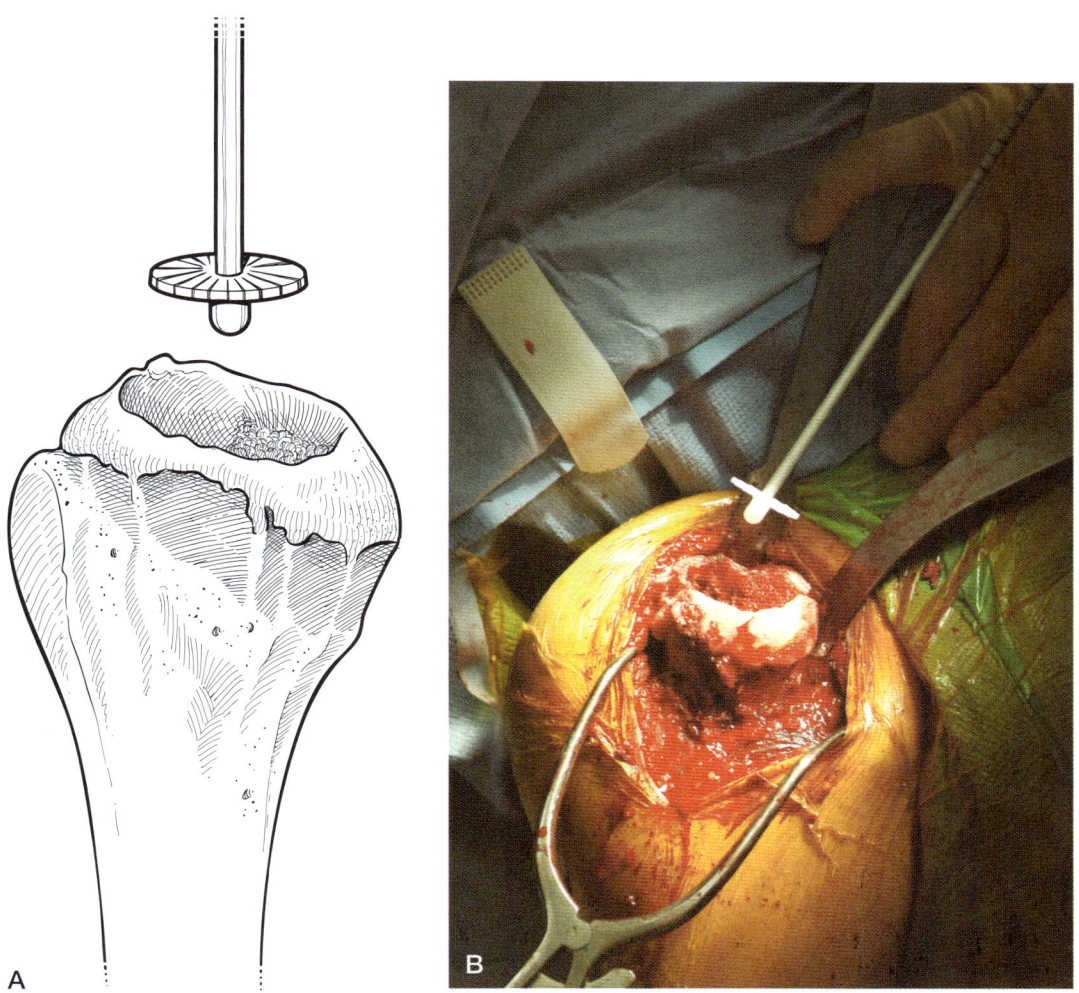

FIGURE 21.17 (A and B) Placement of a cement restrictor to a 1-cm distal cement mantle.

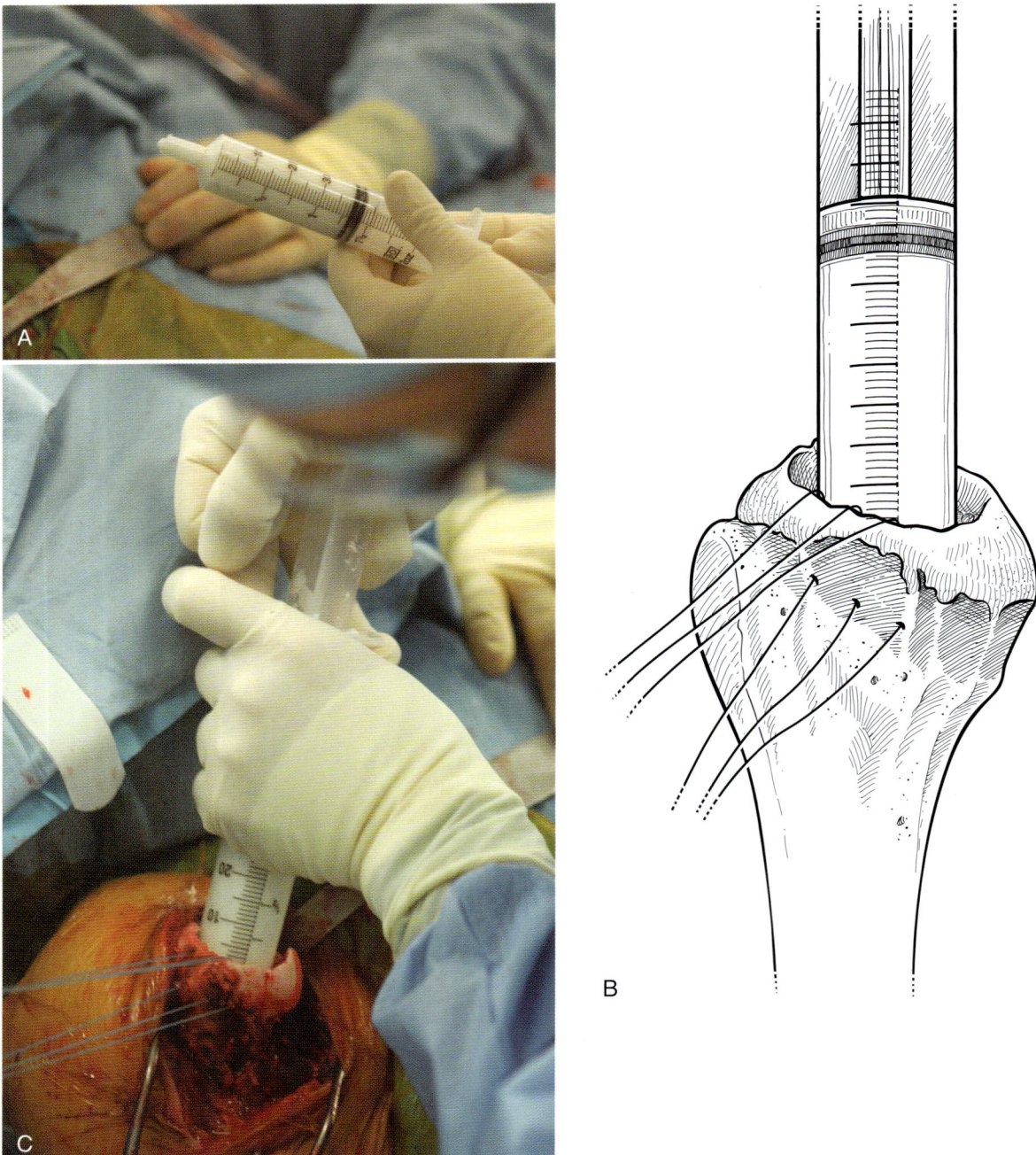

FIGURE 21.18 (A) Modified catheter-tip syringe used for application of the cement. (B and C) Insertion of cement into the humeral canal.

Glenoid component

CHAPTER 22

Unlike cases of unconstrained shoulder arthroplasty, in which placement of a glenoid component is optional, the glenoid component must be placed during reverse shoulder arthroplasty. As in unconstrained arthroplasty, adequate glenoid exposure is paramount in placement of the glenoid component; this is covered in Chapter 20. Many different implant companies are now manufacturing reverse-design shoulder prostheses. The glenoid components of the various brands generally consist of an uncemented metal base plate and a modular metallic glenosphere. The number and orientation of fixation screws used for the base plate and the design of the base plate (flat back vs. convex back) vary among manufacturers. The specific glenoid component implant with the longest and most successful follow-up is the Grammont-designed Delta (DePuy, France). Our preference is to use a glenoid component implant that does not differ appreciably from this clinically tested design. The Grammont-designed Delta base plate consists of a flat back with a central peg and is fixated with four peripheral cortical screws. The glenosphere is placed over the base plate to allow a medialized center of rotation. The technique described in this chapter is applicable to this type of reverse glenoid component.

GLENOID PREPARATION AND COMPONENT IMPLANTATION

After humeral preparation is complete (see Chapter 21), the proximal humerus is retracted posteriorly with a long Darrach retractor, a modified Trillat glenohumeral retractor, or a large glenoid rim retractor (see Chapter 3; Video 22.1). We avoid using a Fukuda glenohumeral retractor during implantation of a reverse prosthesis because the base-plate fixation screws may incarcerate the retractor (Fig. 22.1). After the glenoid is exposed by retracting the proximal humerus posteriorly, a drill hole is made with the inferior referencing guide provided; this is dependent upon selection of a 25-mm or 29-mm glenoid base plate. The guide is placed at the inferior border of the glenoid to align the inferior aspect of the glenosphere with the inferior aspect of the glenoid (Fig. 22.2). Placement of the glenosphere in this position will help to minimize the incidence of notching of the axillary border of the scapula as a result of the mechanical contact that occurs after implantation of the reverse prosthesis.

Reaming is performed at neutral tilt or while placing slight inferior pressure on the reamer to introduce approximately 10 degrees of inferior tilt to the surface of the glenoid.

This slight inferior tilt serves two purposes: it may increase the stability of the prosthesis by maximizing deltoid tension by distalization of the humerus (Fig. 22.3), and it helps avoid inadvertently placing the glenoid component in a superiorly oriented position, which can lead to early glenoid failure (Fig. 22.4). Although inferior tilt was also suspected to decrease scapular notching, we did not find a difference in scapular notching when comparing neutral versus 10 degrees of inferior tilt in a prospective randomized trial.[1]

Reaming is performed only to remove any remaining cartilage and flatten the glenoid surface. It is not necessary to ream to cancellous bone; such reaming should be avoided. Additionally, many patients undergoing implantation of a reverse prosthesis have osteopenic bone that is susceptible to fracture during glenoid preparation. To help avoid fracture, the reamer is always started before contacting the bone and then gradually and gently advanced to engage the bone and ream it to a flat surface (Fig. 22.5). Once reaming is complete, the cortical aperture of the glenoid hole is opened to a slightly larger diameter (7.6 mm) to accommodate the central peg of the glenoid base plate (Fig. 22.6). The glenoid base plate is oriented and introduced with the insertion handle (Fig. 22.7). A mallet is used to impact the base plate until it is flush with the glenoid bone circumferentially. The insertion handle is disengaged from the base plate, and the base plate is checked to ensure that it has been completely seated by inserting the tips of vascular forceps into each hole (Fig. 22.8). If any concern exists over incomplete seating of the base plate, a large smooth tamp may be used to further impact the base plate. Additionally, the peripheral inferior rim of the base plate should be confirmed to be in contact with the underlying glenoid. If the implant is not seated inferiorly, early glenoid loosening can occur. Occasionally the base plate will be larger in anteroposterior diameter than the native glenoid, as with bone loss or in a small patient (Fig. 22.9). This is not generally a problem as long as bone is visible in the anterior and posterior base-plate holes. If the bone loss is severe, bone graft reconstruction of the glenoid may be necessary (see the following section of this chapter).

The next step involves screw insertion to complete fixation of the base plate. Fixation of the glenoid base plate in our chosen prosthetic system involves the use of two different types of screws. The inferior and superior screws lock into a mobile variable-angle washer captured in the base plate to create a fixed-angle device once the screw is tightened. The anterior and posterior screws are placed through a

Text continued on p. 194

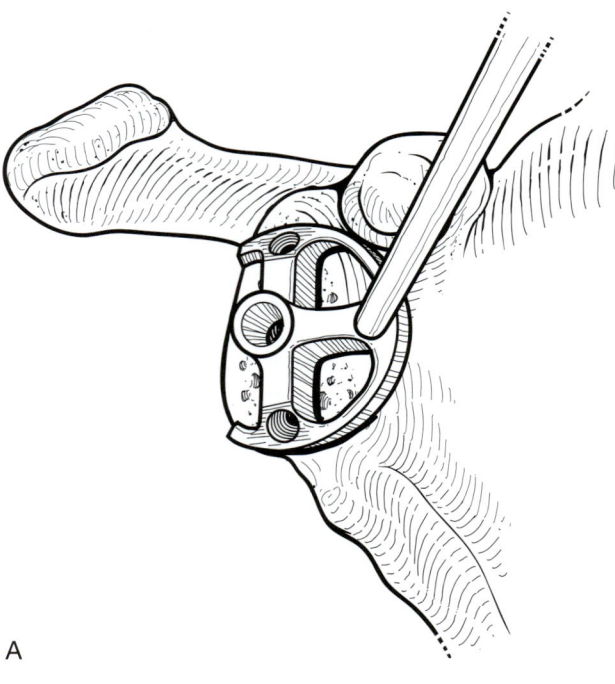

A

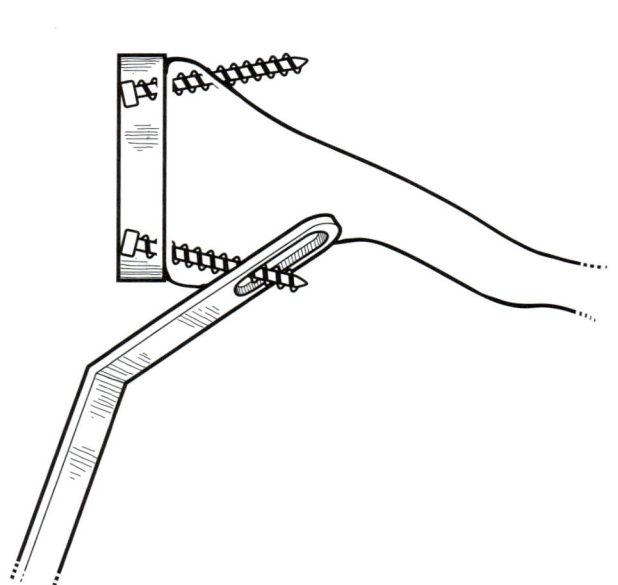

FIGURE 22.1 Mechanism by which a Fukuda-type humeral retractor may become incarcerated by a glenoid base-plate fixation screw.

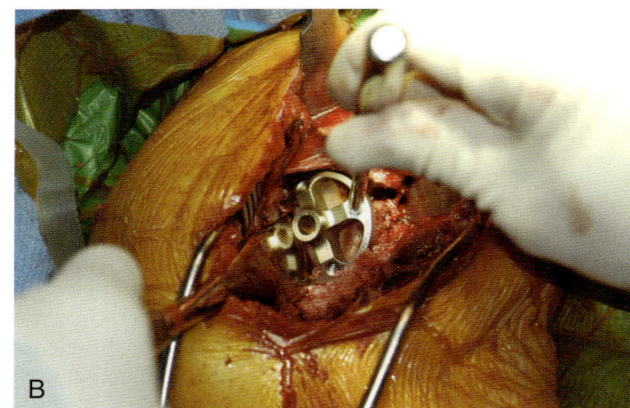

B

FIGURE 22.2 (A and B) Placement of the inferior referencing guide for drilling the initial hole in the glenoid face.

CHAPTER 22 ■ Glenoid Component

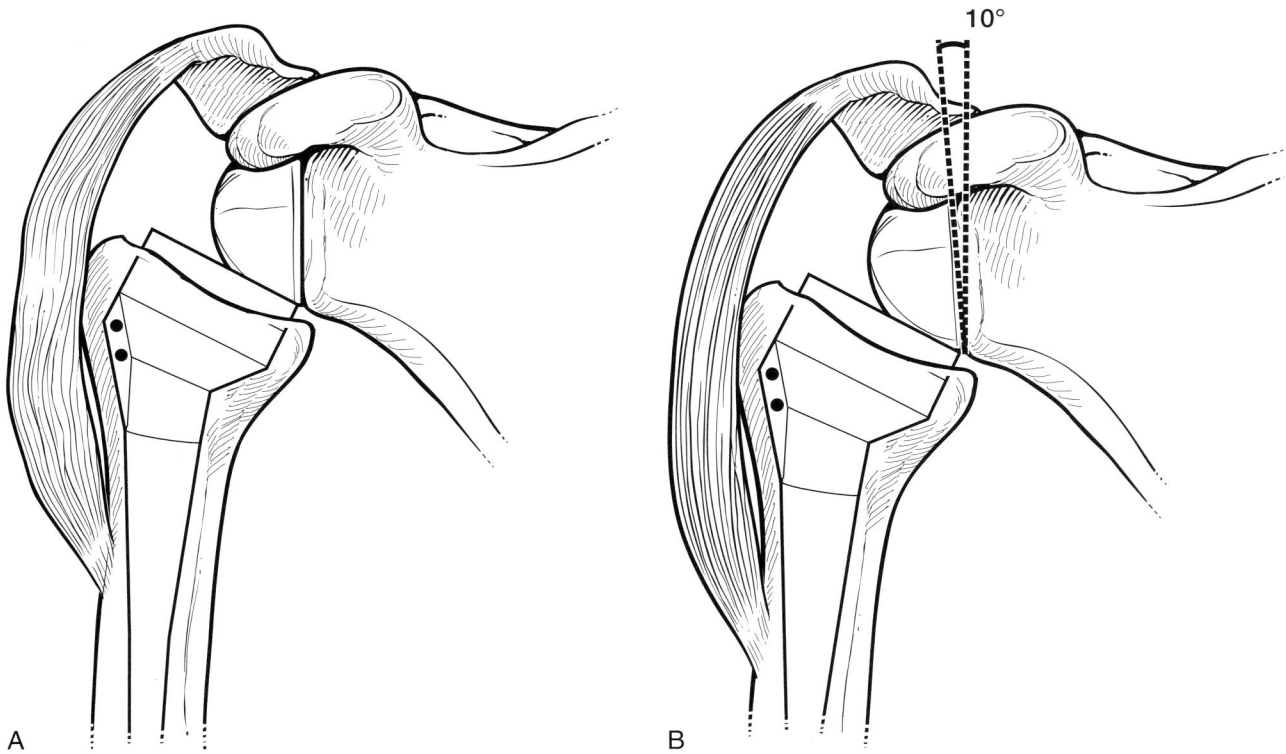

FIGURE 22.3 (A and B) Mechanism by which an inferiorly tilted glenoid component maximizes deltoid tension and thereby increases prosthetic stability.

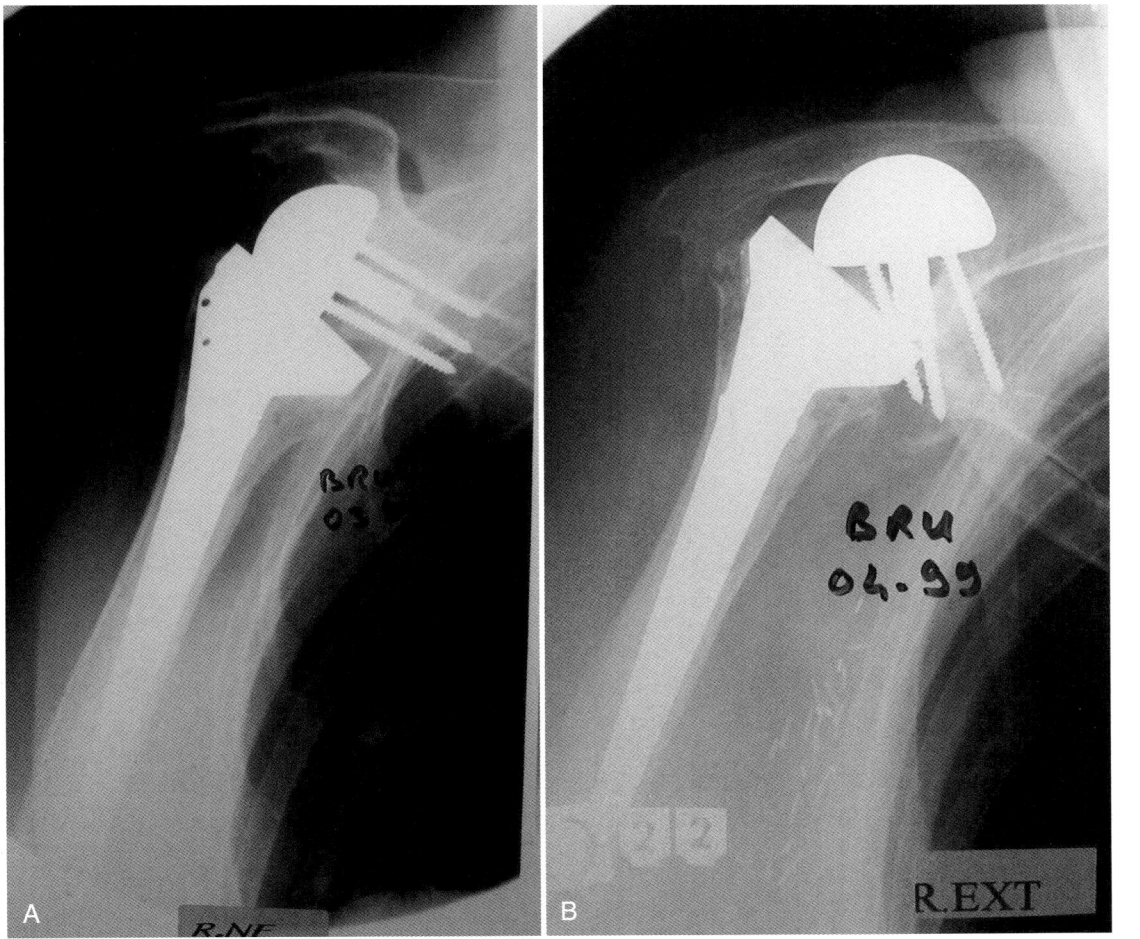

FIGURE 22.4 (A and B) Radiographs of a glenoid component inadvertently placed with superior tilt, resulting in early glenoid failure.

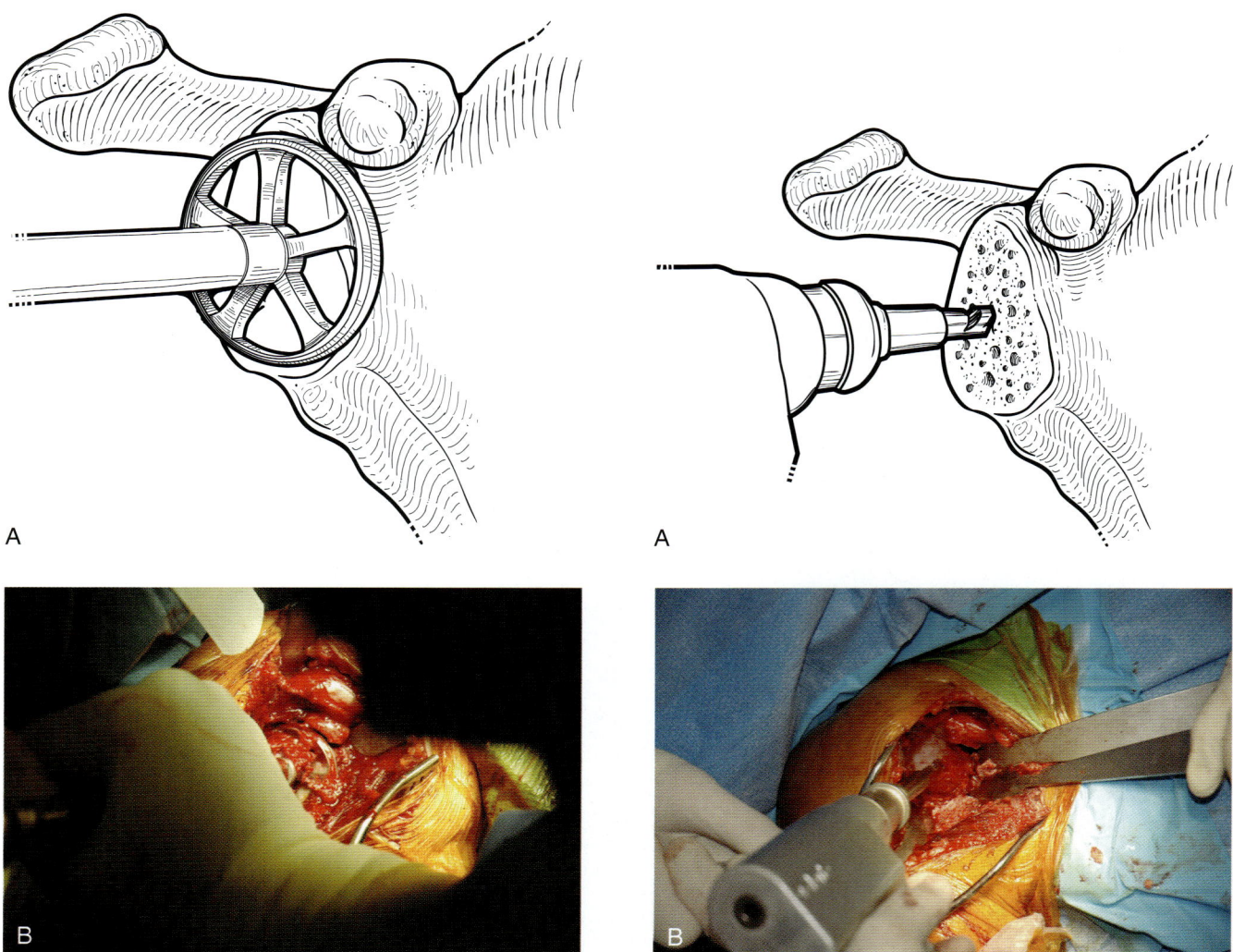

FIGURE 22.5 (A and B) Reaming of the glenoid to a flat surface.

FIGURE 22.6 (A and B) A 7.6-mm drill bit is used to enlarge the central peg hole for fixation of the base plate. This step can be omitted in patients with moderate to severe osteopenia.

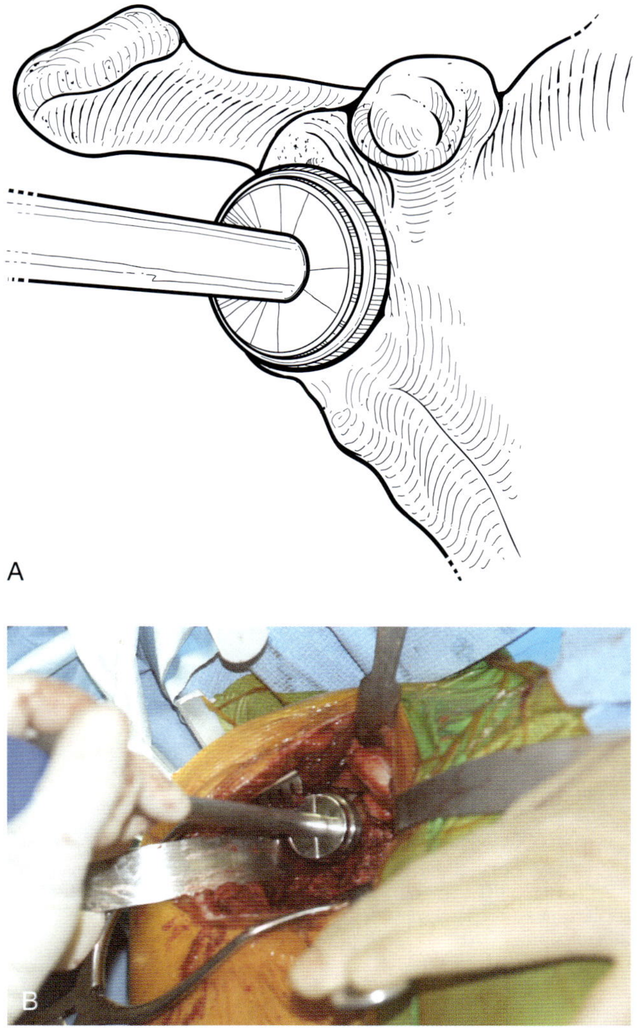

FIGURE 22.7 (A and B) The glenoid base plate is introduced with the insertion handle.

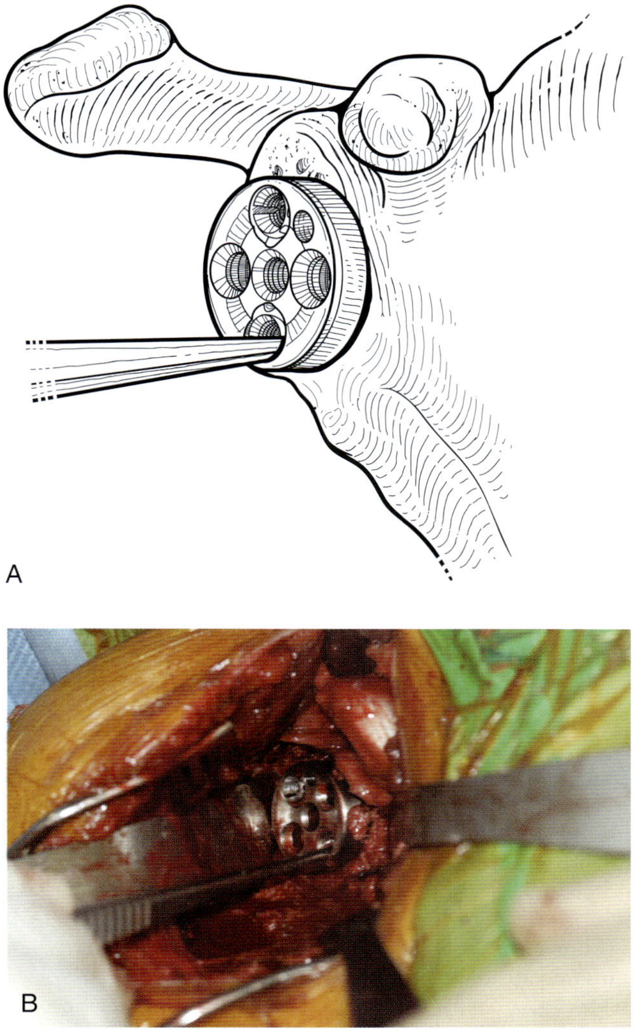

FIGURE 22.8 (A and B) Vascular forceps are used to ensure complete seating of the base plate.

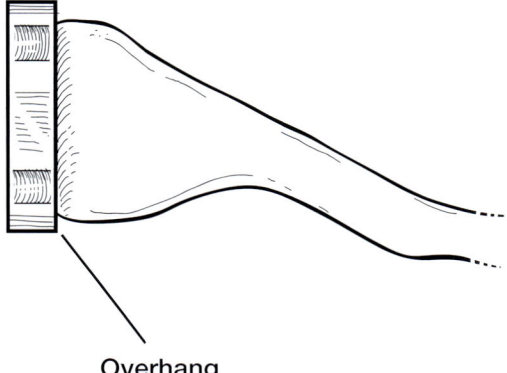

FIGURE 22.9 Base plate with anterior and posterior overhang caused by a small native glenoid.

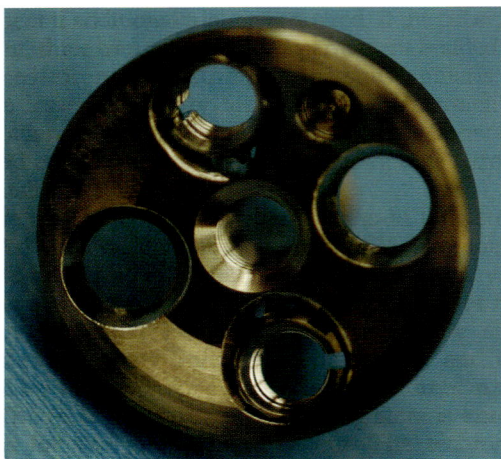

FIGURE 22.10 The screw holes for the base plate. The inferior and superior holes contain variable-angle locking washers that allow the screws to lock into the base plate as the screw heads are advanced into the washer, thereby fixing the angle of the screw within the base plate. The anterior and posterior screws do not lock into the base plate and serve to create compression between the base plate and the native glenoid.

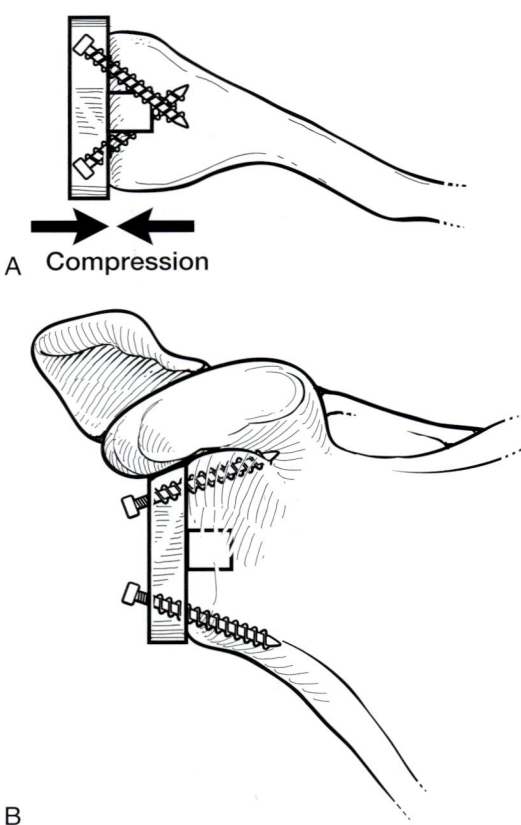

FIGURE 22.11 (A and B) Mechanism of base-plate screw fixation with anterior and posterior screws to initially compress the base plate to the native glenoid. The inferior and superior screws are then tightened to create a fixed-angle device.

standard hole within the base plate, which does not contain a locking mechanism (Fig. 22.10). The anterior and posterior screws can be placed at variable angles and allow compression of the base plate against the glenoid bone, whereas the inferior and superior screws "set" the distance between the implant and glenoid bone as soon as the threaded head engages the locking washer within the base plate (Fig. 22.11). Because of these special considerations, the screws are inserted and tightened in a specific order. The inferior screw is placed first to ensure maintenance of contact of the inferior aspect of the base plate with the underlying osseous glenoid. A drill guide is placed in the inferior hole of the base plate. A drill (3.0-mm bit) is used through the guide to create a bicortical hole (Fig. 22.12). The direction of the drill should be chosen to maximize screw length so that the strongest fixation possible is provided. Because of the inferior position of the base plate, if the drill is directed too inferiorly, it may exit the glenoid bone prematurely and result in poor fixation (Fig. 22.13). If the drill is passed perpendicular to the base plate, screw length may be shorter than desired (Fig. 22.14). We have found that directing the drill halfway between the perpendicular and the maximal inferior direction allowed by the mechanical constraints of the base plate permits consistent placement of a sufficiently long screw (Fig. 22.15).

After the second cortex has been penetrated by the drill bit, a depth gauge is used to determine screw length or the calibrated drill bit can be read to determine the length (Fig. 22.16). The obliquity of the scapula may cause too short a screw to be selected (Fig. 22.17). Therefore multiple measurements are obtained with the depth gauge and the longest measurement is taken. If the length measured is between two sizes, the longer size is always selected to ensure bicortical thread purchase. Muscle tissue overlies the point at which the screw tips exit the scapula; no neurovascular structures are at risk if the screw tip protrudes slightly beyond the scapular cortex. We have yet to witness symptoms caused by a screw that was radiographically too long. A 4.5-mm locking screw is introduced and tightened to just before the point at which the threaded screw head engages the washer of the base plate (Fig. 22.18). If the threaded head of the inferior screw engages the base-plate washer, no further compression between the base plate and glenoid bone can be obtained (Fig. 22.19). The advantage of partially inserting the inferior screw first is that it helps to maintain contact between the inferior aspect of the base plate and the native glenoid (Fig. 22.20). The drill for the superior locking screw is directed toward the base of the coracoid process (Fig. 22.21). The process of using the depth gauge is repeated for the superior locking screw. This screw is then inserted, once again making sure to not engage the base plate when the screw is advanced.

Placement of the anterior and posterior screws marks the final phase of insertion of the base plate. These nonlocking screws are placed at insertion angles judged to be optimal for cortical purchase. Whereas the inferior and superior screws are always divergent, the anterior and posterior screws are typically convergent. The drill is typically angled toward the central peg of the glenoid base plate and passes just superior or inferior to the central peg to perforate the opposite cortex (i.e., the anterior drill hole passes just superior to the central peg and perforates the posterior cortex deep within the glenoid vault, and the posterior drill hole passes

CHAPTER 22 ■ Glenoid Component

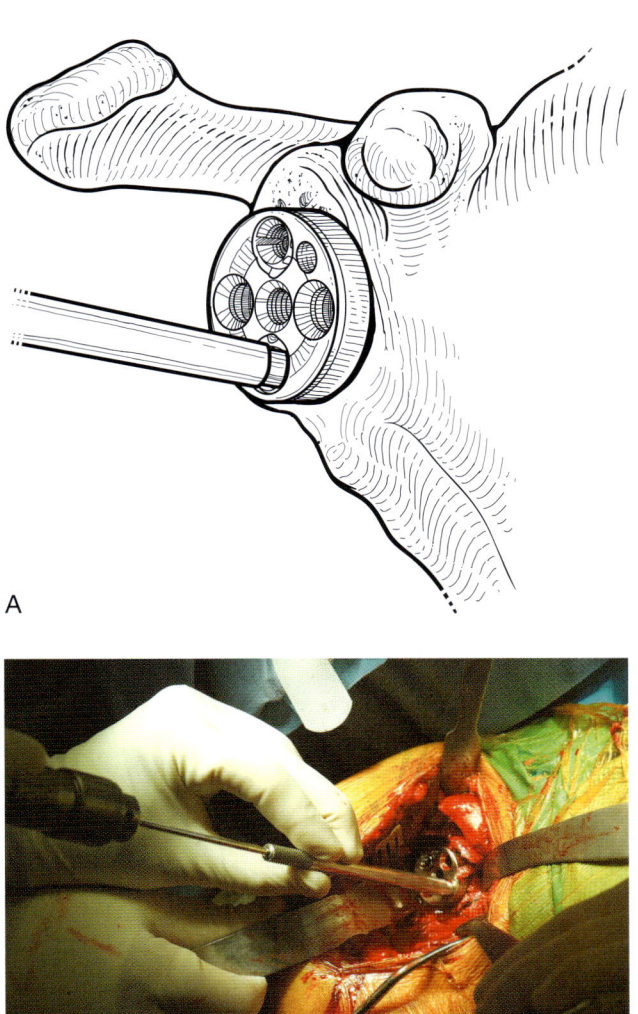

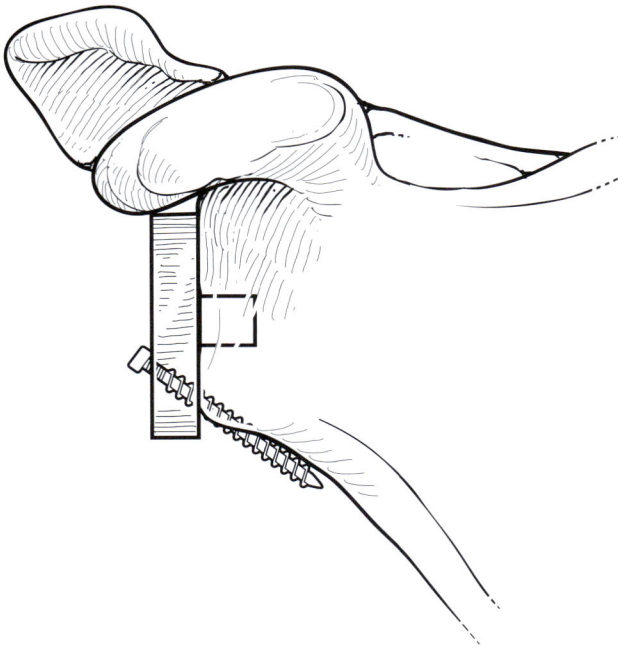

FIGURE 22.12 (A and B) A 3.0-mm drill bit is used to create the screw holes for base-plate fixation.

FIGURE 22.13 If the inferior base-plate screw is directed at too steep an angle, the screw may miss the glenoid bone.

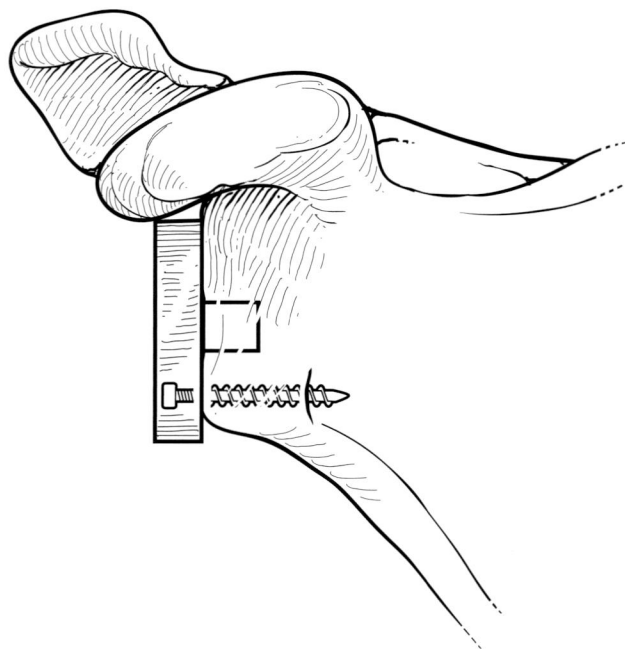

FIGURE 22.14 If the drill is directed perpendicular to the base plate, screw length may be shorter than desired.

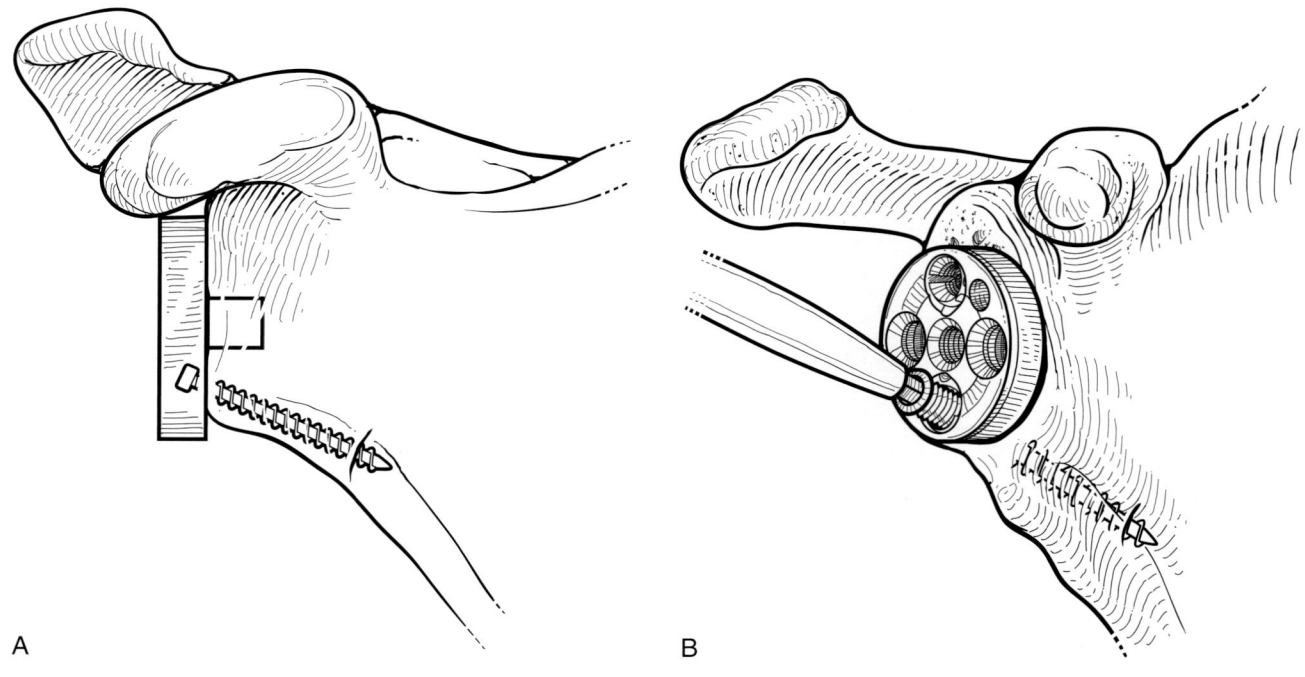

FIGURE 22.15 (A and B) Optimal inferior screw placement.

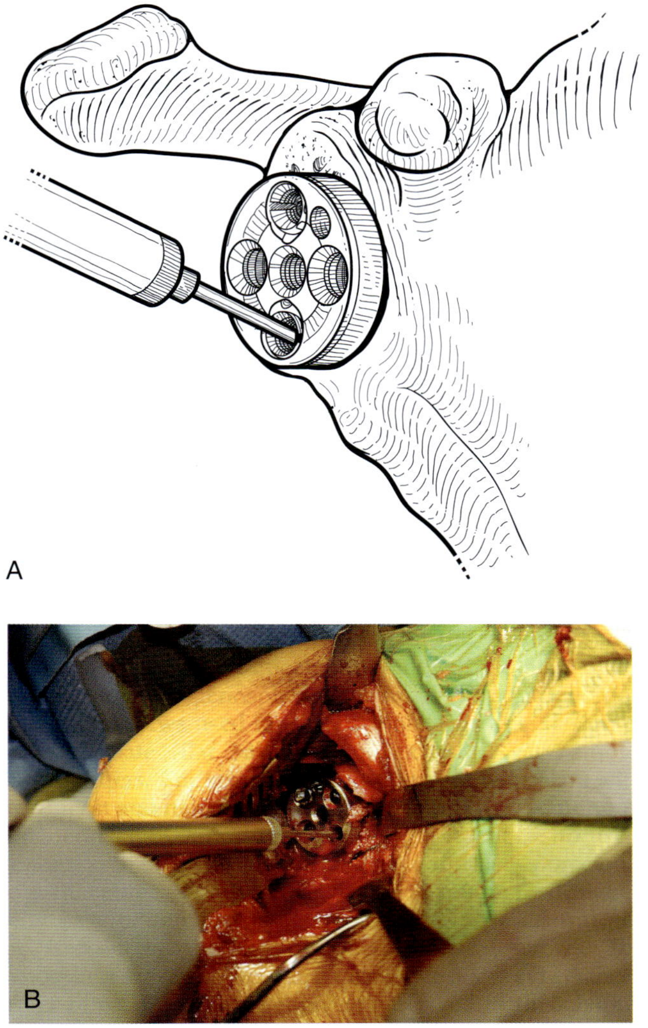

CHAPTER 22 ■ Glenoid Component

FIGURE 22.16 (A and B) A depth gauge is used to determine screw length.

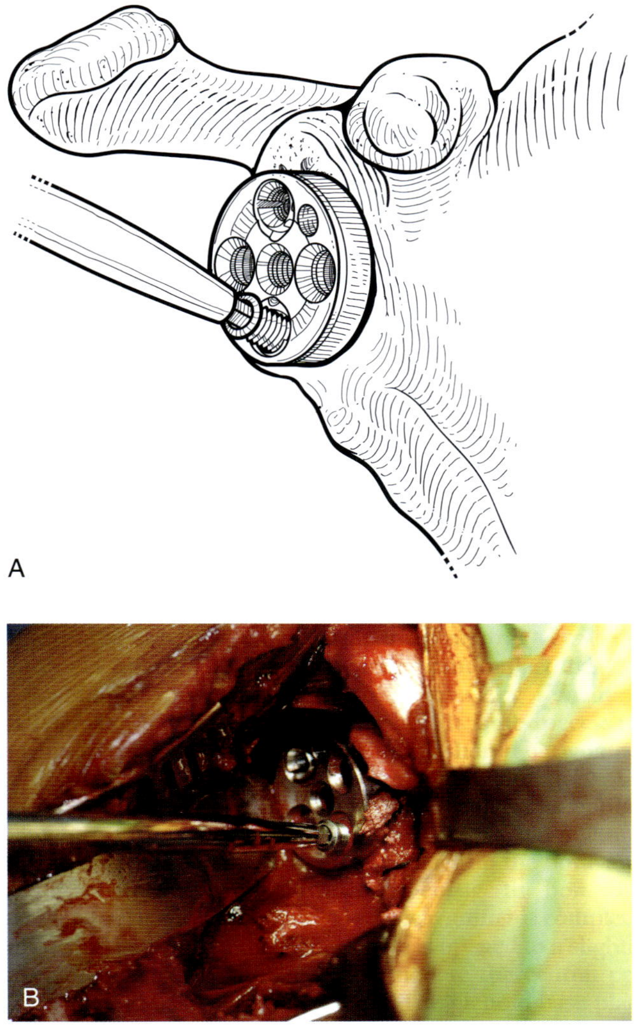

FIGURE 22.18 (A and B) Partial insertion of the inferior base-plate screw.

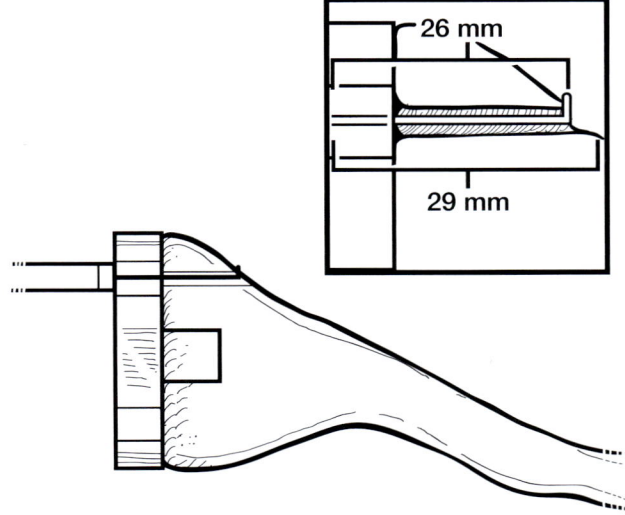

FIGURE 22.17 The obliquity of the scapula at the point where the screw tip exits the bone may cause too short a screw to be selected inadvertently.

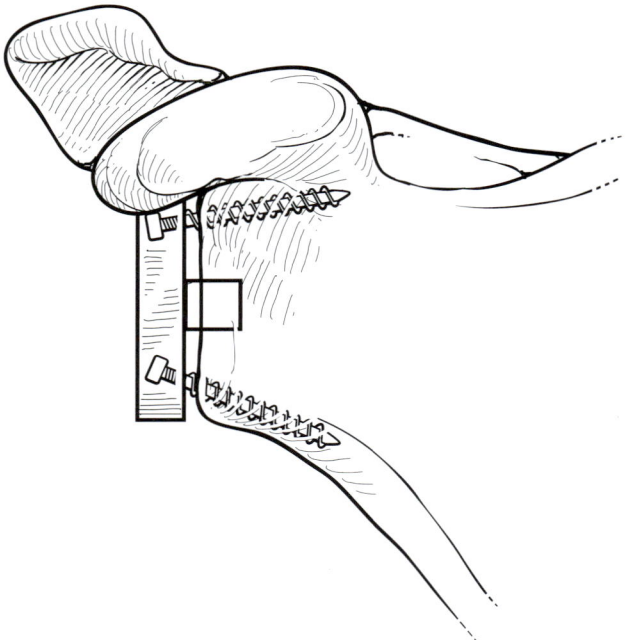

FIGURE 22.19 Mechanism by which compression of the base plate against the native glenoid is prohibited by completely seating the inferior or superior screw or both screws.

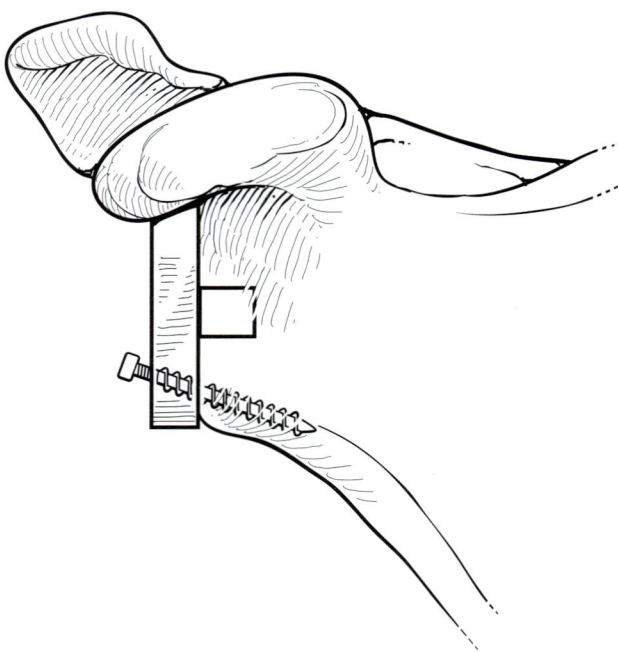

FIGURE 22.20 The base plate is prevented from tilting superiorly by the partially inserted inferior screw during fixation of the base plate.

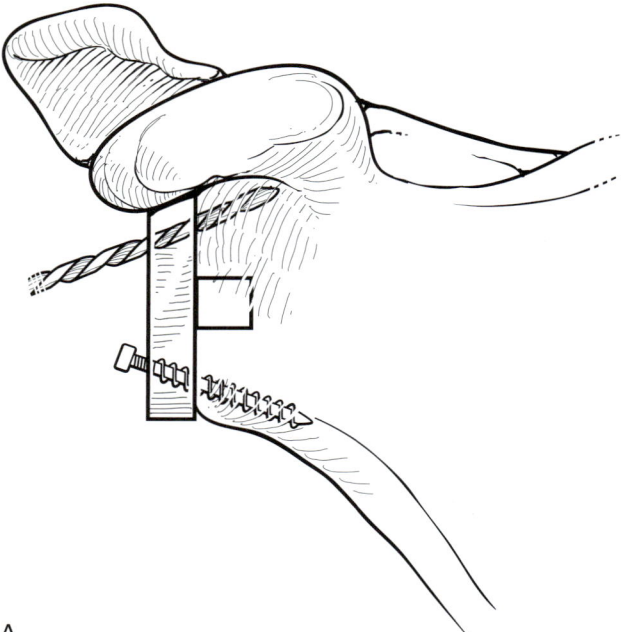
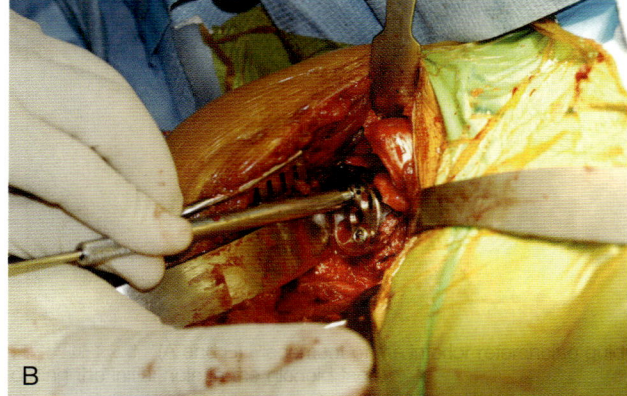

FIGURE 22.21 (A and B) Drill direction into the base of the coracoid for the superior locking screw.

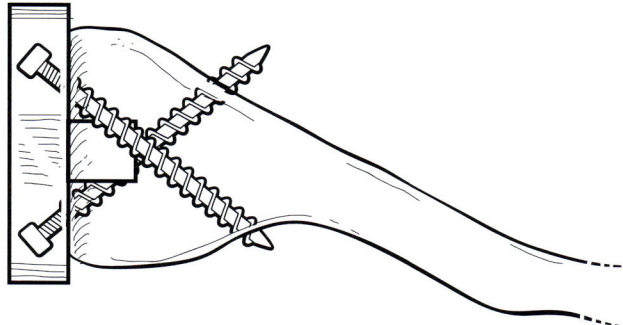

FIGURE 22.22 Optimal placement of the anterior and posterior compression screws.

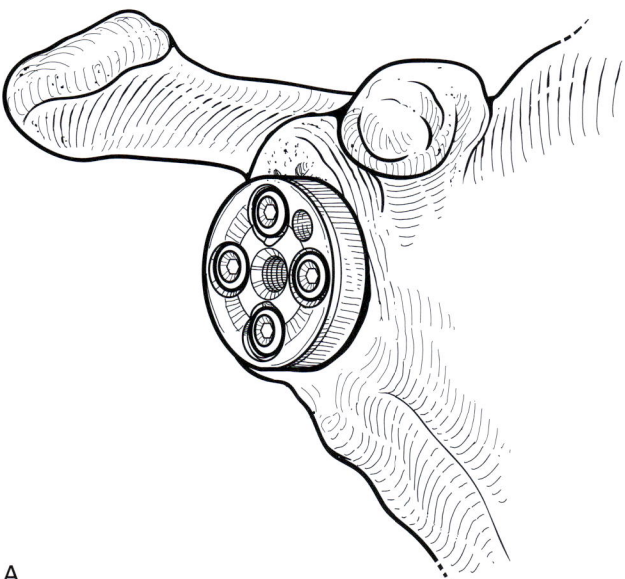

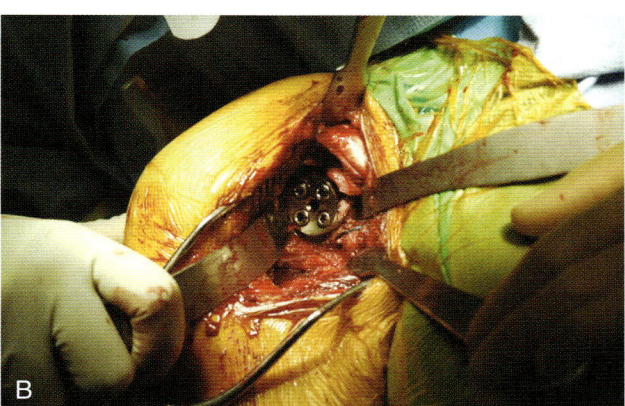

FIGURE 22.23 (A and B) Final tightening of the inferior and superior locking screws to complete fixation of the base plate.

just inferior to the central peg and perforates the anterior cortex deep within the glenoid vault; Fig. 22.22). The depth gauge is used to select screw length, and the anterior and posterior screws are inserted. In contrast to the inferior and superior screws, the anterior and posterior screws are fully tightened to provide compression between the base plate and the glenoid bone. After the anterior and posterior screws are fully seated, the inferior and then superior screws are fully tightened to engage and complete fixation of the base plate (Fig. 22.23). Occasionally the anterior or posterior screw will not obtain satisfactory osseous purchase because of underlying osteopenia. In this case the screw is left in place to provide interference-type resistance to loosening of the glenoid component.

The periphery and central hole of the base plate are cleared of soft tissue and blood, and the glenosphere component (36- or 42-mm glenosphere option) is positioned on the base plate with use of a screwdriver as an insertion device (Fig. 22.24). The glenosphere attaches to the base plate via a peripheral rim Morse taper and is further secured with a central safety screw (in the system that we use; Fig. 22.25). The glenosphere is impacted into place with the impaction device (Fig. 22.26), and the safety fixation screw is advanced to complete insertion of the glenoid component (Fig. 22.27).

GLENOID BASE-PLATE SELECTION—POST OR THREADED POST

The glenoid base-plate options include a press-fit post or a newer central threaded-post base plate. Our preference for the glenoid base plate is typically the 15-mm post, as described earlier. The threaded-post base plate is also available with a 25-mm post. This post is useful in the revision setting or for the bony increased offset reverse shoulder arthroplasty (BIO-RSA) technique, which is described later in this chapter and in Chapter 40.

The newer central threaded-post base-plate option is available for both primary and revision cases. The threaded post comes in various lengths to allow bicortical fixation; it can also accommodate a 10-mm bone graft when desired for BIO-RSA. Exposure for the threaded-post base plate is the same as described earlier. The threaded-post base plate may be used with or without a guide pin. The glenoid surface is prepared in the same manner for a threaded post as for a conventional post. A calibrated 6.5-mm drill bit is used to create the central glenoid hole and is drilled just past the far cortex (Fig. 22.28). The central glenoid hole is expanded using a cannulated 8.2-mm counterbore drill, which has a positive stop (Fig. 22.29). A tap can be used to prepare the central hole in case of hard bone. The tap is used manually; it has a depth stop that can be placed to the measured length. Tapping is considered an important step to prevent glenoid fracture during placement of the final implant. The base plate is manually threaded into the prepared central hole until it is flush to the glenoid surface (Fig. 22.30). The threaded-post base plate has four multidirectional locking screws, whereas the traditional central-peg baseplate has two nonlocking compression screws and two locking screws.

GLENOID BONE LOSS WITH A PRIMARY REVERSE PROSTHESIS

Glenoid bone loss is most commonly observed in two scenarios when a reverse prosthesis is being used in a primary

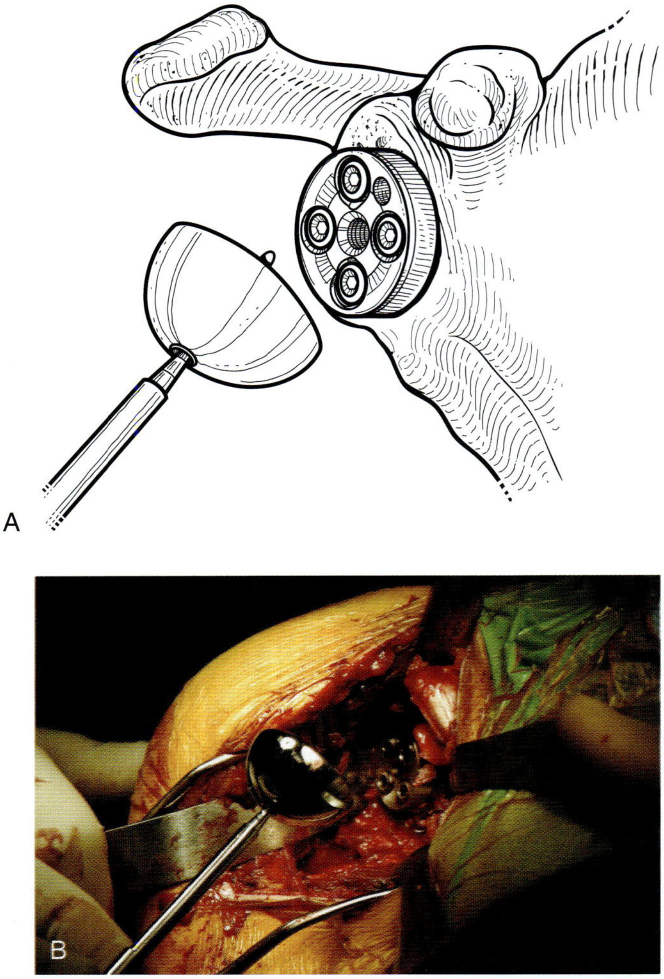

FIGURE 22.24 (A and B) Initial placement of the glenosphere.

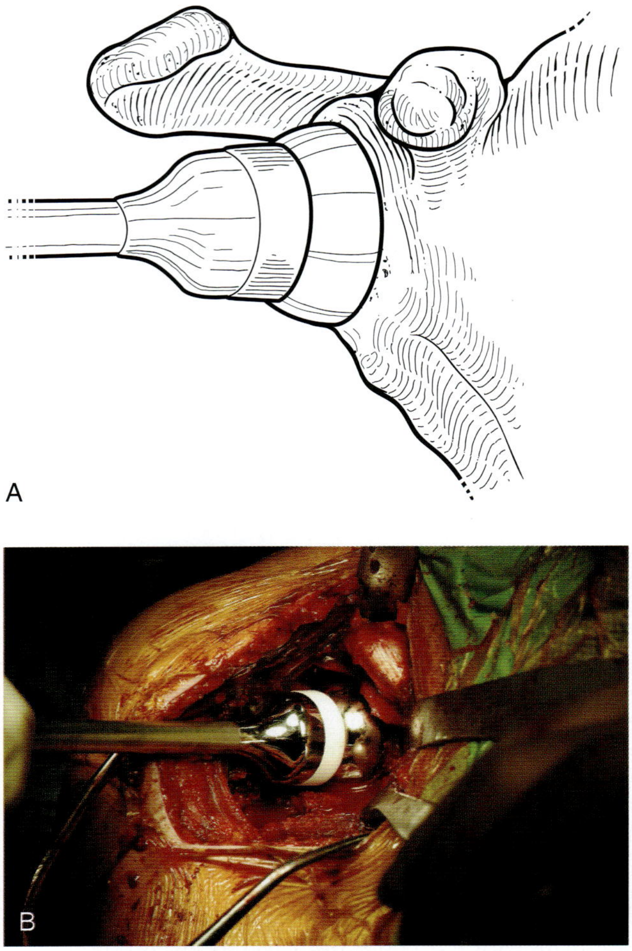

FIGURE 22.26 (A and B) The glenosphere is impacted into place by engaging the Morse taper.

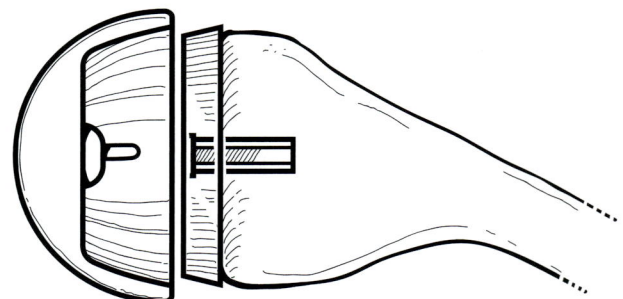

FIGURE 22.25 Mechanism of glenosphere fixation to the base plate.

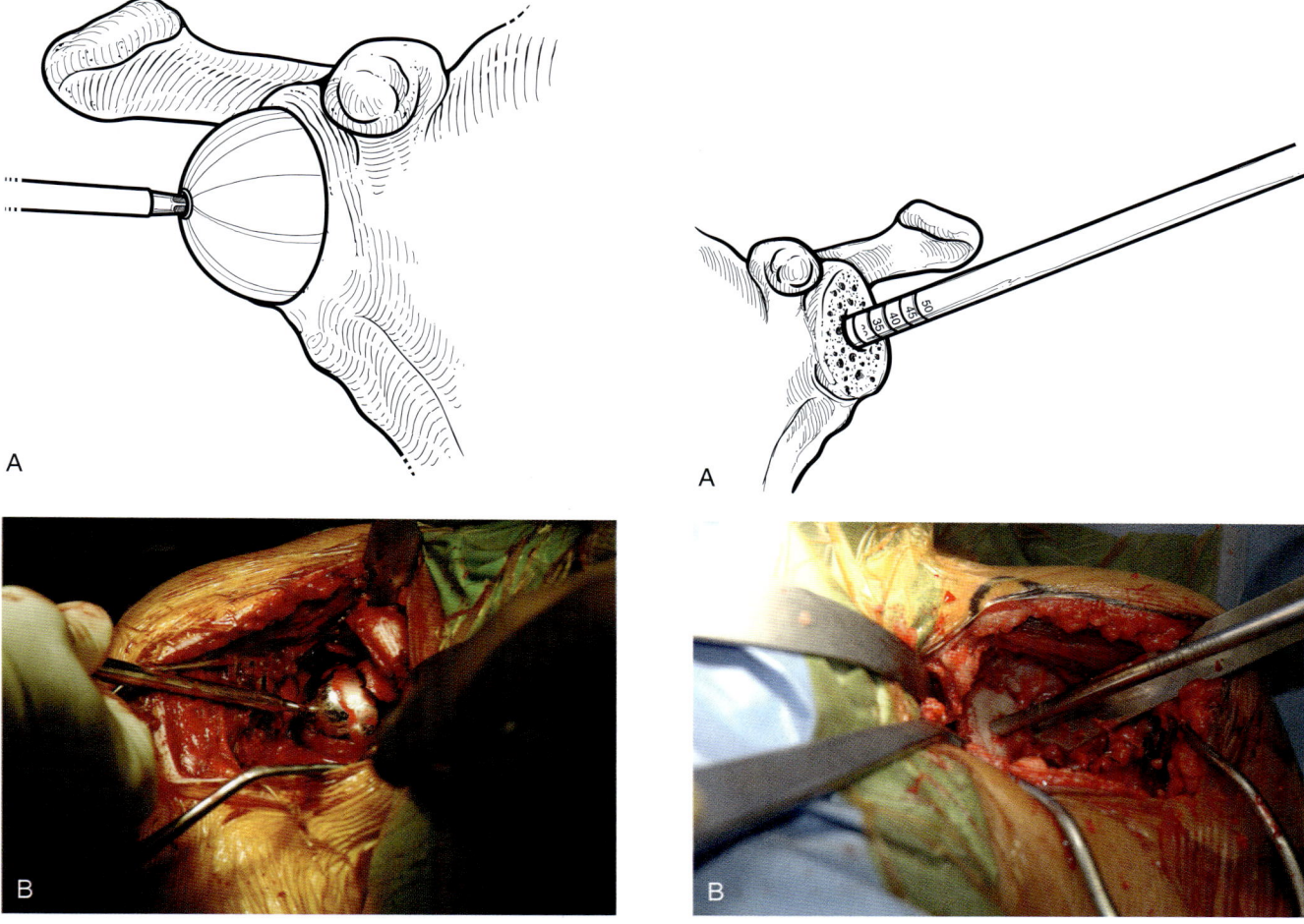

FIGURE 22.27 (A and B) The safety fixation screw is advanced to complete insertion of the reverse-prosthesis glenoid component.

FIGURE 22.28 (A and B) A calibrated 6.5-mm drill bit is used to create the central glenoid hole and is drilled just past the far cortex.

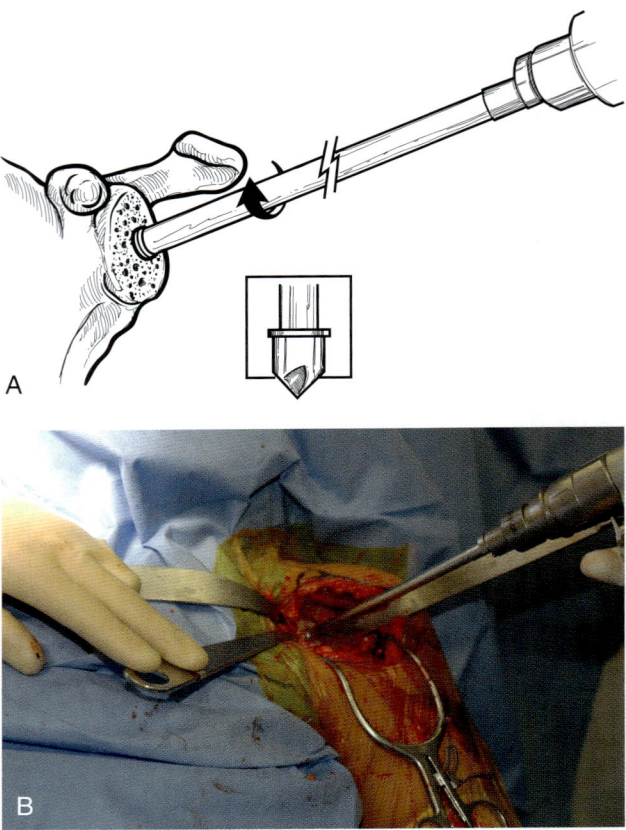

FIGURE 22.29 (A and B) The central glenoid hole is expanded using a cannulated 8.2-mm counterbore drill.

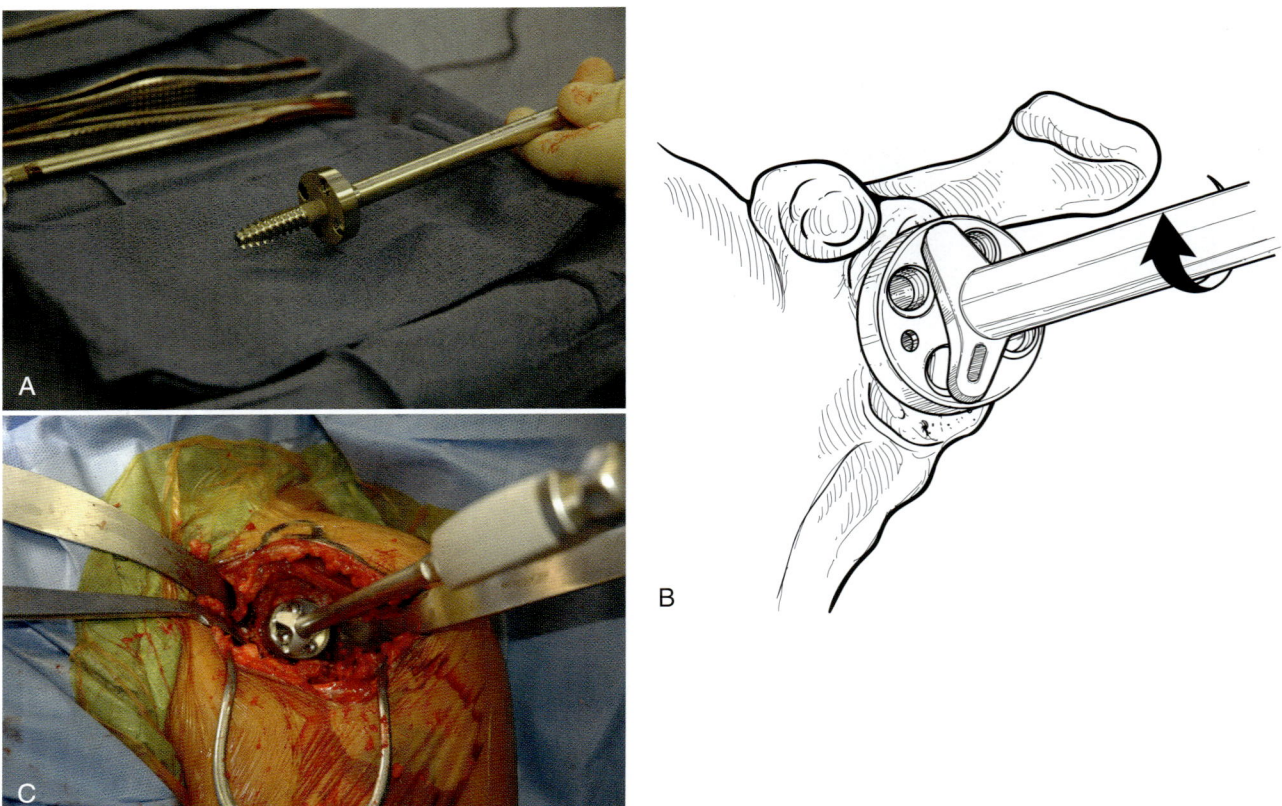

FIGURE 22.30 (A–C) The base plate is manually threaded into the prepared central hole until it is flush to the glenoid surface.

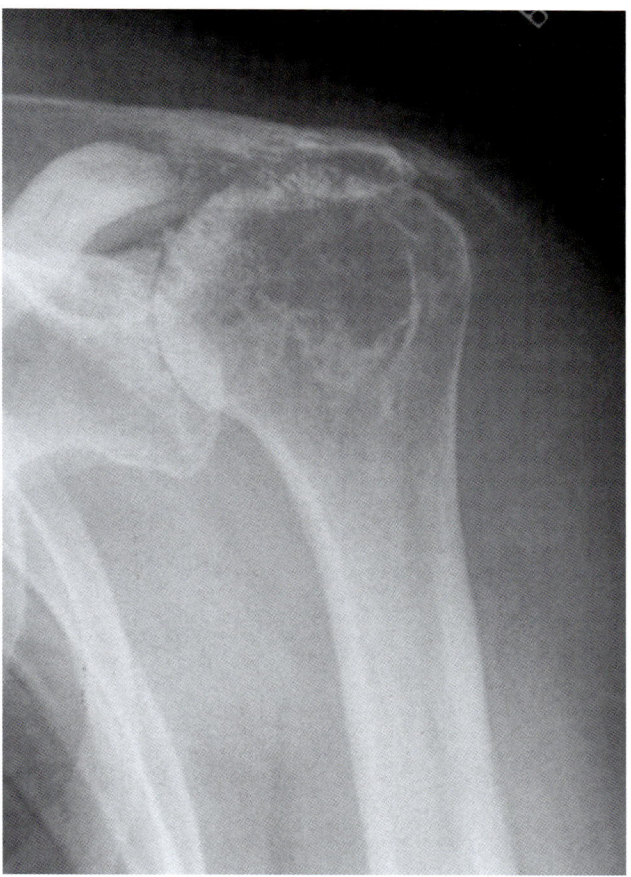

FIGURE 22.31 Radiograph showing superior erosion of the osseous glenoid.

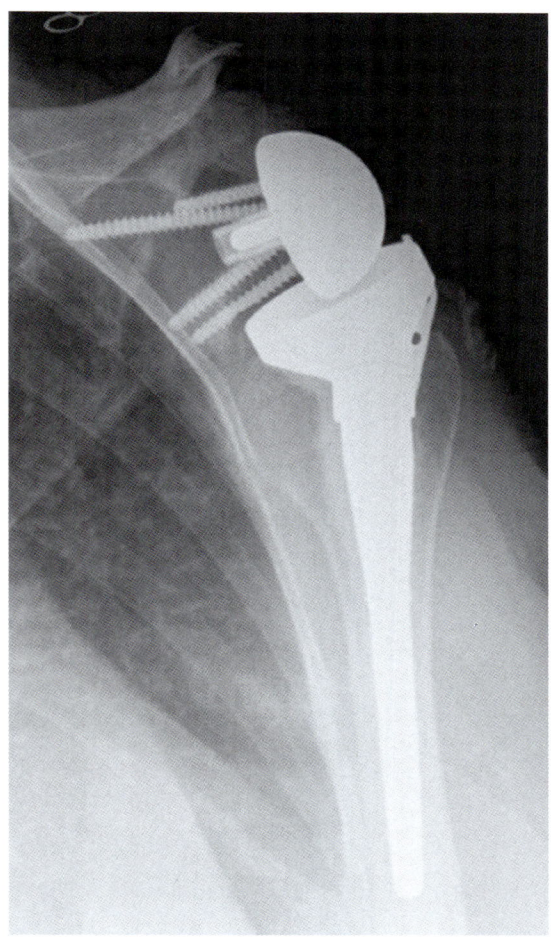

FIGURE 22.32 Inadvertent superior tilt of the glenoid component may be introduced by not appreciating superior glenoid erosion during glenoid preparation.

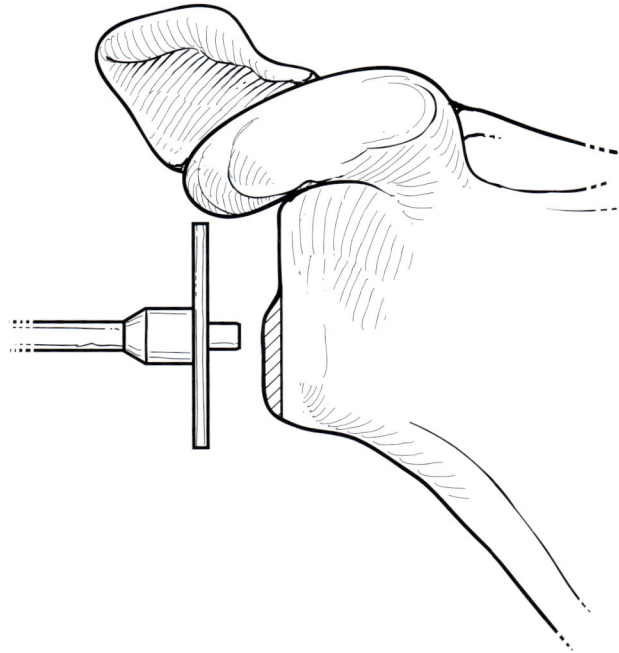

FIGURE 22.33 In mild cases of superior glenoid bone loss, preferential inferior reaming alone can correct the glenoid orientation.

shoulder arthroplasty. In patients with massive rotator cuff tears and glenohumeral arthritis, static superior migration of the humeral head may lead to nonconcentric glenoid wear and superior erosion of the osseous glenoid (Fig. 22.31). If this bone loss is not addressed, the glenoid component may inadvertently be implanted with superior tilt, thus risking glenoid failure (Fig. 22.32). In cases of mild superior bone loss, preferential inferior reaming alone can correct the glenoid orientation (Fig. 22.33).

In moderate cases of superior glenoid bone loss, the superior orientation of the glenoid is initially corrected by preferential inferior reaming. This leaves a superior biconcave glenoid deformity. In these cases, we utilize a bone graft harvested from the humeral head using specialized instrumentation, as described by Pascal Boileau and colleagues and labeled the BIO-RSA technique (Video 22.2).[2] Prior to resecting the humeral head, a guide pin is inserted into the proximal humerus using a specialized guide (Fig. 22.34). A bell saw is used over the guide pin (Fig. 22.35). A larger hole through the bone graft is drilled over the guidewire, which is then removed (Fig. 22.36). A cutting guide is impacted into the hole in the bone graft and an initial head resection is made with a saw, effectively harvesting the bone graft (Fig. 22.37). The bone graft is then placed on a longer central-peg base plate and contoured to fit the osseous defect in the glenoid (Fig. 22.38).

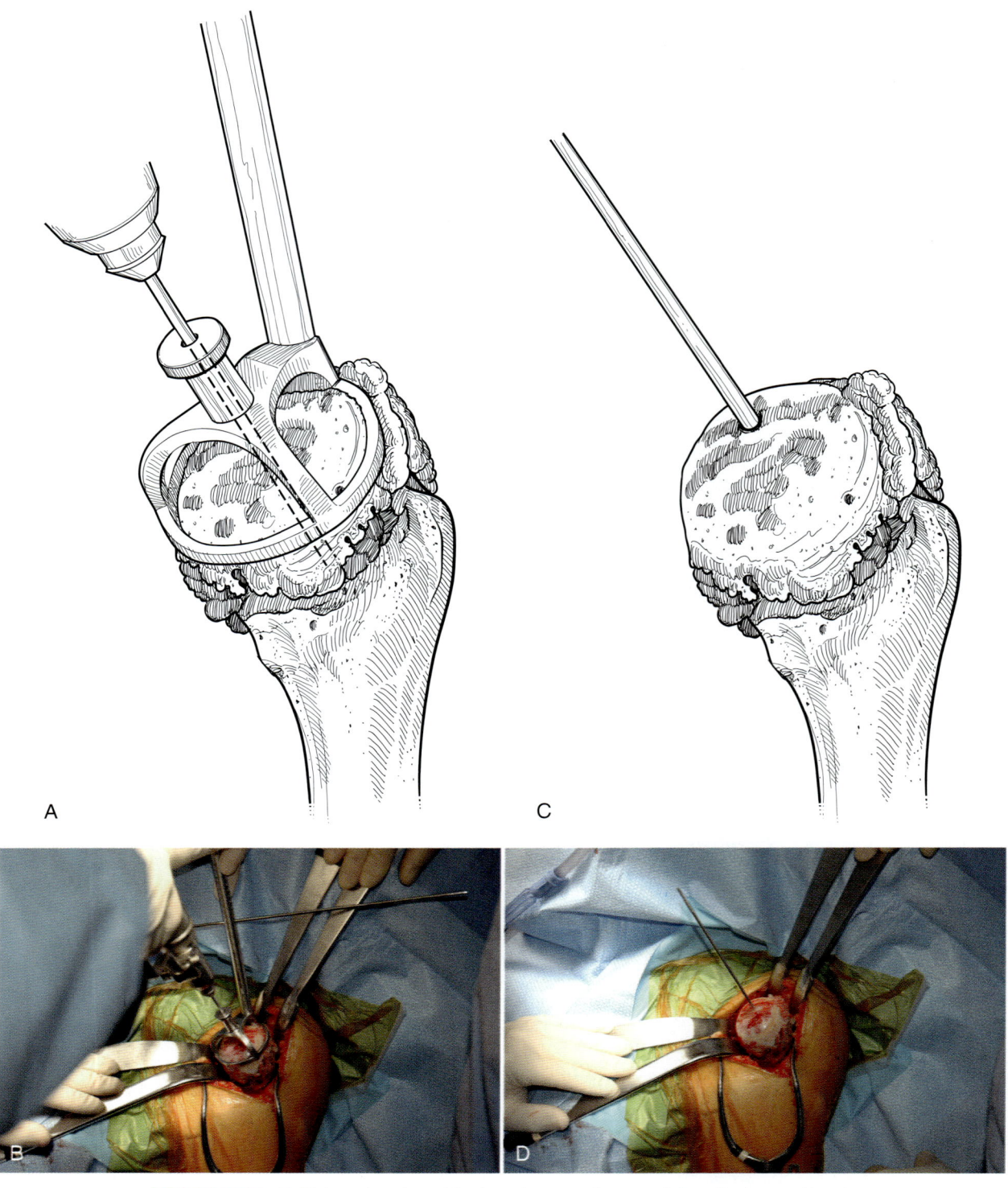

FIGURE 22.34 (A–D) Insertion of a guide pin to harvest a bone graft from the humeral head.

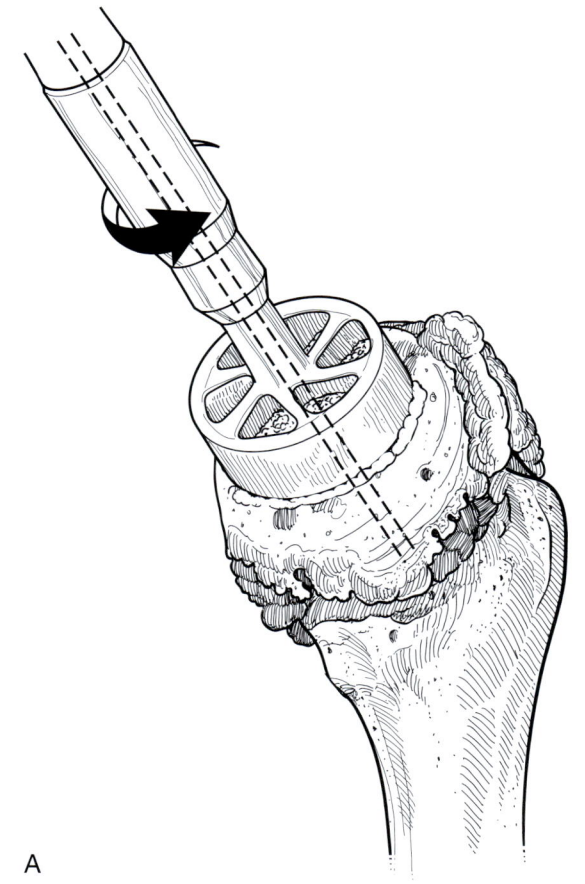
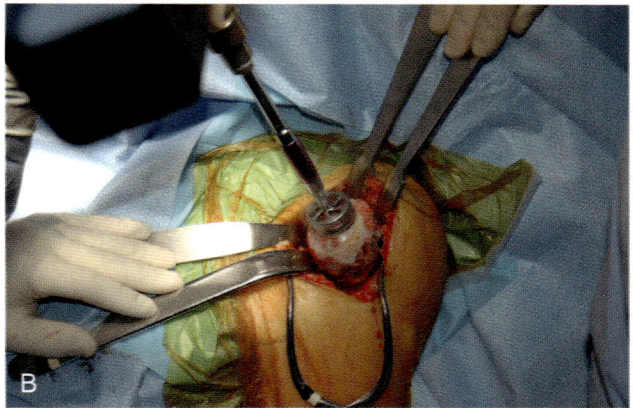

FIGURE 22.35 (A and B) A bell saw is used over the guide pin.

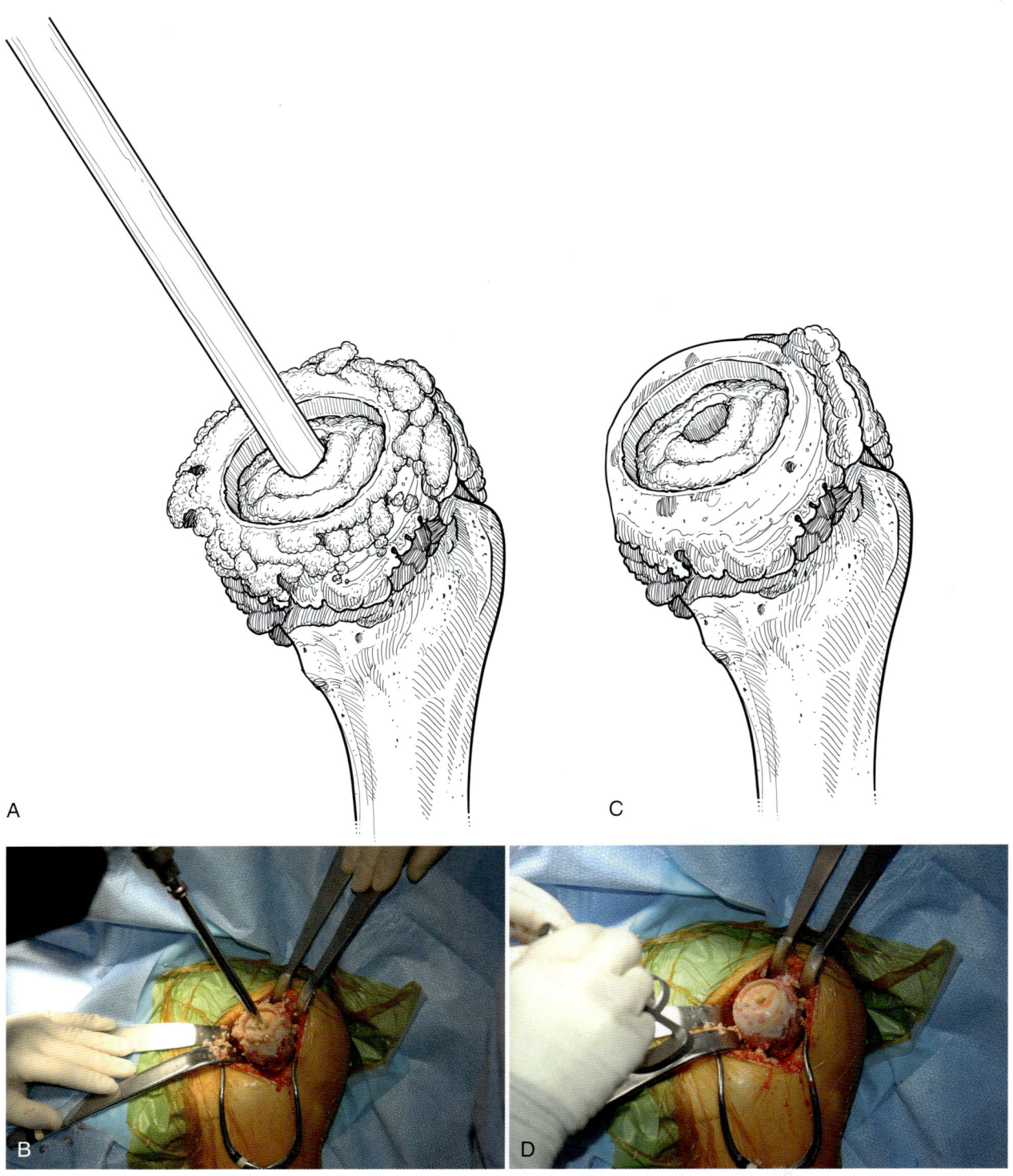

FIGURE 22.36 (A–D) A larger hole through the bone graft is drilled over the guidewire, and the guidewire is removed.

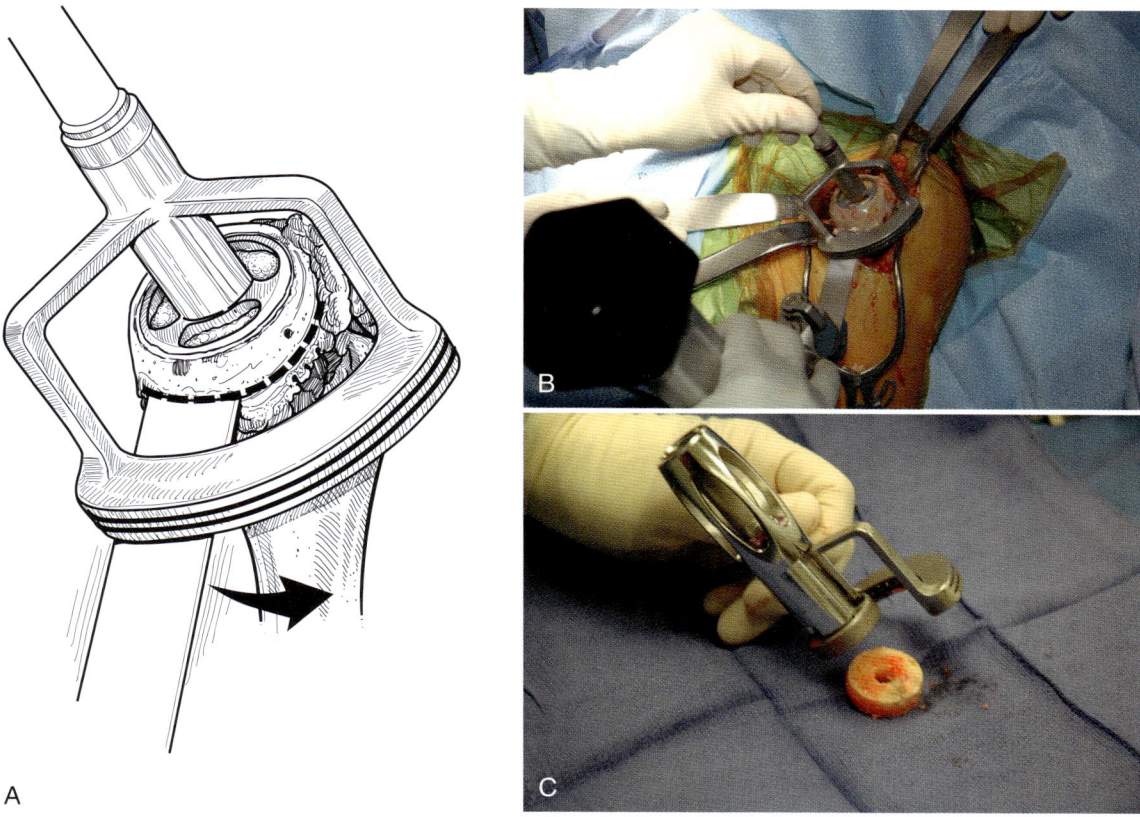

FIGURE 22.37 (A–C) A cutting guide is impacted into the hole in the bone graft and an initial head resection is made with a saw harvesting the bone graft.

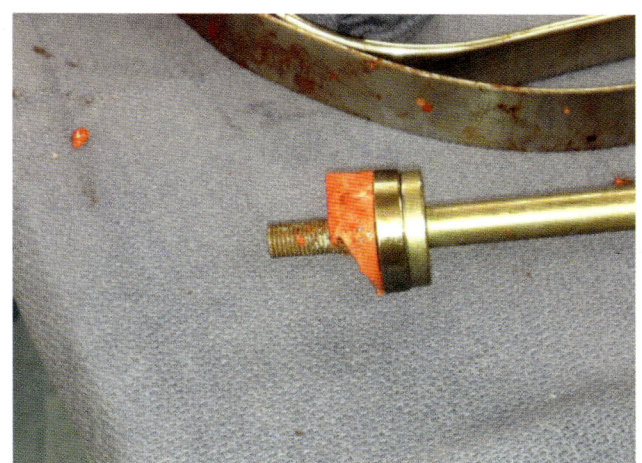

FIGURE 22.38 The bone graft is then placed on a longer central-peg base plate and contoured to fit the glenoid osseous defect.

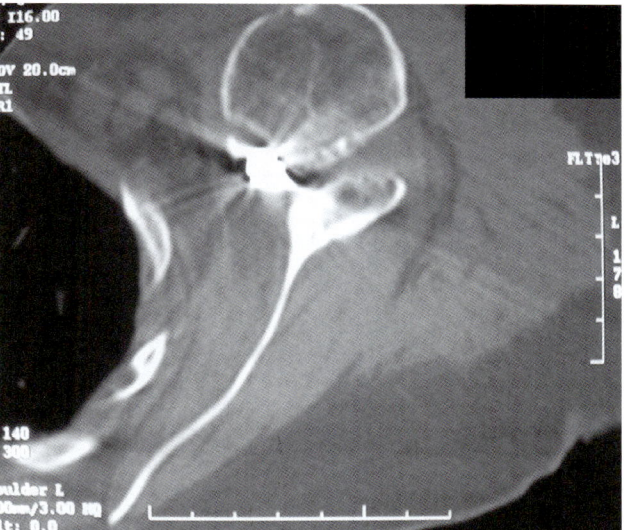

FIGURE 22.39 Preoperative computed tomography scan in a patient with a fixed anterior dislocation showing severe anterior glenoid bone loss requiring bone grafting at the time of insertion of the reverse prosthesis.

The less common scenario in which glenoid reconstruction may be necessary during implantation of a reverse prosthesis in a primary arthroplasty is for the treatment of fixed anterior glenohumeral dislocation. Chronic anterior shoulder dislocations in older patients often result in erosion of the anterior glenoid. When the severity of this erosion is such that no native glenoid is seen under the anterior base-plate screw hole, anterior glenoid reconstruction is required. The need for a bone graft is usually determined on the preoperative computed tomography scan (Fig. 22.39). In these cases the BIO-RSA bone graft/base-plate construct is shaped to fit the anterior defect.

REFERENCES

1. Edwards TB, Trappey GJ, Riley C, et al: Inferior tilt of the glenoid component does not decrease scapular notching in reverse shoulder arthroplasty: results of a prospective randomized study, *J Shoulder Elbow Surg* 21(5):641–646, 2012.
2. Boileau P, Moineau G, Roussanne Y, et al: Bony increased-offset reversed shoulder arthroplasty minimizing scapular impingement while maximizing glenoid fixation, *Clin Orthop Relat Res* 469:2558–2567, 2011.

Reduction and deltoid tensioning

CHAPTER 23

Perhaps the most important and yet most subjective portion of the surgical technique for implantation of a reverse prosthesis is proper tensioning of the deltoid. The most frequent complication of a reverse prosthesis that requires further treatment is dislocation of the glenohumeral prosthesis. Proper tensioning of the deltoid can help to minimize this complication.

HUMERAL COMPONENT TRIALING

After the humeral component has been inserted as described in Chapter 21, humeral component trialing begins. In patients with proximal humeral bone loss and in whom a cemented stem is used, component trialing should not begin before complete curing of the polymethylmethacrylate.

Trial reduction starts with insertion of the 6-mm polyethylene trial insert into the metaphyseal portion of the final implant (Fig. 23.1). The glenohumeral joint is reduced by applying longitudinal traction to the arm and placing a finger in the "cup" of the trial insert to guide the humeral component toward the glenosphere (Fig. 23.2). Gradually flexing the arm as traction is applied assists in reduction. Deltoid tension is evaluated by stabilizing the scapula and applying longitudinal traction to the arm in neutral position (Fig. 23.3). We have anesthesia personnel maintain neuromuscular paralysis during this portion of the procedure, the anterior glenoid rim retractor holding the conjoined tendon medially is relaxed, and any self-retaining retractors are also relaxed. A finger is placed at the interface of the humeral and glenoid components (Fig. 23.4). Minimal (<2 mm) "pistoning" should occur with this maneuver. If tension is inadequate with the 0-mm metallic tray and the 6-mm polyethylene trial insert, the 9-mm insert is placed and reduction and testing are repeated. Six millimeter and 12-mm metallic trays are also available to further increase tension if necessary (Fig. 23.5).

In addition to pistoning, we also put the shoulder through a full range of motion to assess stability and impingement, including forward flexion, abduction, external rotation at the side, external rotation, and internal rotation with the shoulder abducted to 90 degrees. Once appropriate tension is obtained and range of motion is satisfactory, it may be difficult to dislocate the implant with the trial polyethylene insert. We routinely use a bone hook on the edge of the trial insert to provide traction on the prosthesis (Fig. 23.6). After an insert of appropriate size is selected, the final polyethylene insert is impacted into the metaphyseal portion of the humeral component while taking care to align the laser mark on the insert appropriately (Fig. 23.7). When necessary, a thicker metallic metaphyseal tray is placed instead of the typical 0-mm tray (Fig. 23.8). The polyethylene insert is then impacted into the augment (Fig. 23.9). If present, the subscapularis is repaired with the previously placed transosseous sutures to further enhance prosthetic stability (Fig. 23.10).

SPECIAL CONSIDERATIONS—METAPHYSEAL BONE LOSS

Severe humeral metaphyseal bone loss merits special consideration during implantation of a reverse prosthesis. Most cases of prosthetic dislocation that we have observed have occurred in this situation. During primary arthroplasty with a reverse prosthesis, metaphyseal bone loss most commonly occurs when treating fracture sequelae (Fig. 23.11). With metaphyseal bone loss, no capsular or rotator cuff attachments exist between the scapula and humerus, thus leaving the large muscles of the shoulder girdle (deltoid, short head of the biceps, coracobrachialis) to provide nearly all the soft tissue tension and hence stability for the reverse prosthesis. Although the initial reduction of the reverse prosthesis may seem adequately tensioned, the biomechanical properties of these large muscles (compliance, stretch) allow them to lengthen over time and cause the initial tension to dissipate, thereby potentially leading to prosthetic instability (Fig. 23.12).

We address metaphyseal bone loss at the time of insertion of the reverse prosthesis by maximizing soft tissue tension during implantation and reduction of the prosthesis. In this situation, after insertion of the glenoid component, we reinsert the trial humeral stem with the 6-mm polyethylene insert and reduce the prosthetic glenohumeral joint. With longitudinal traction placed on the arm, the humeral component is manually telescoped maximally out of the humerus to the glenoid component (Fig. 23.13), and the level of the trial humeral implant with respect to the proximal humerus is marked (Fig. 23.14). The distance between the metaphyseal-diaphyseal prosthetic junction and the mark made with respect to the proximal humerus

Text continued on p. 218

SECTION III ■ Reverse Shoulder Arthroplasty

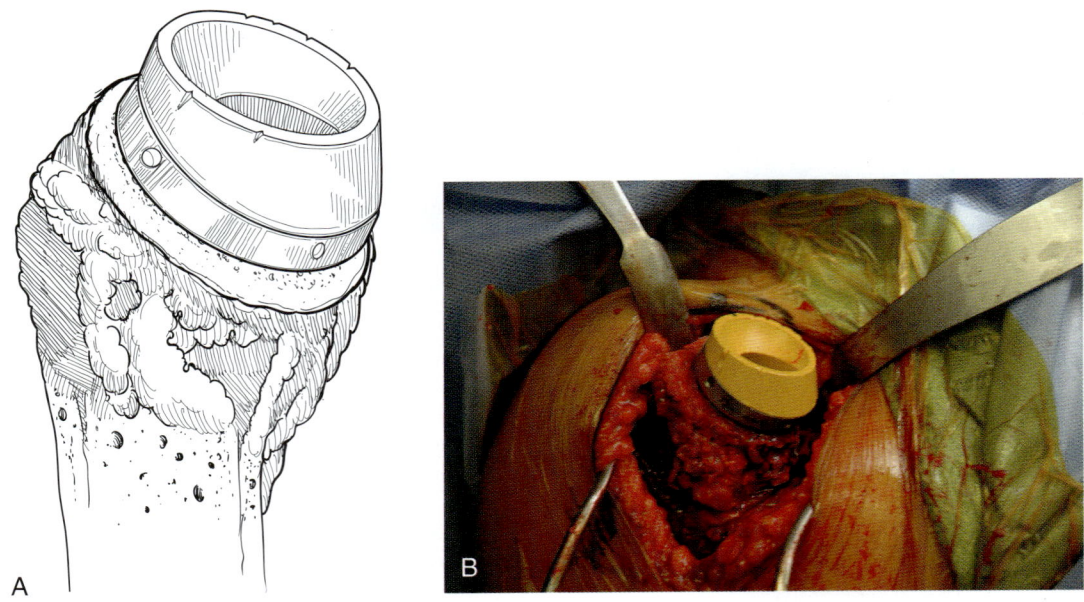

FIGURE 23.1 (A and B) Insertion of a trial insert into the humeral stem.

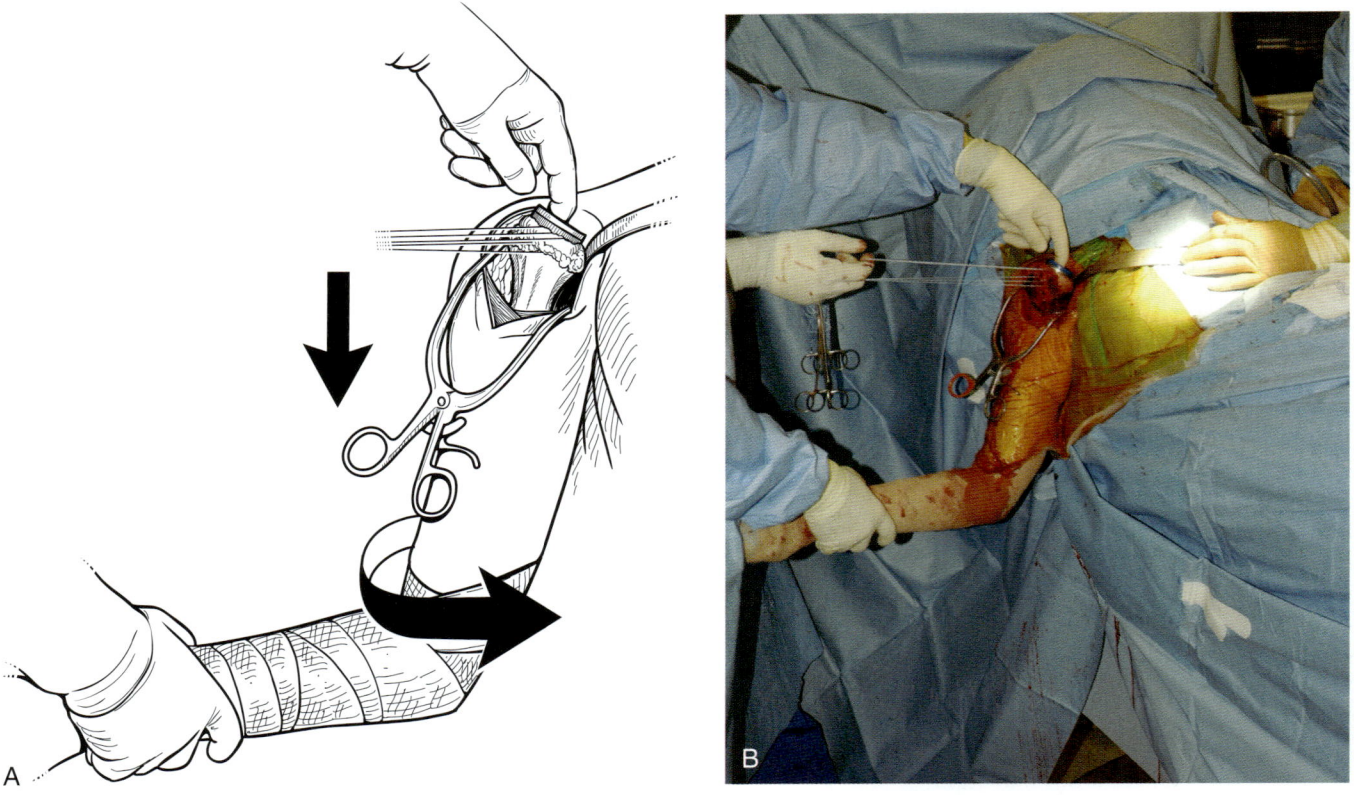

FIGURE 23.2 (A and B) Technique of trial reduction of a reverse prosthesis.

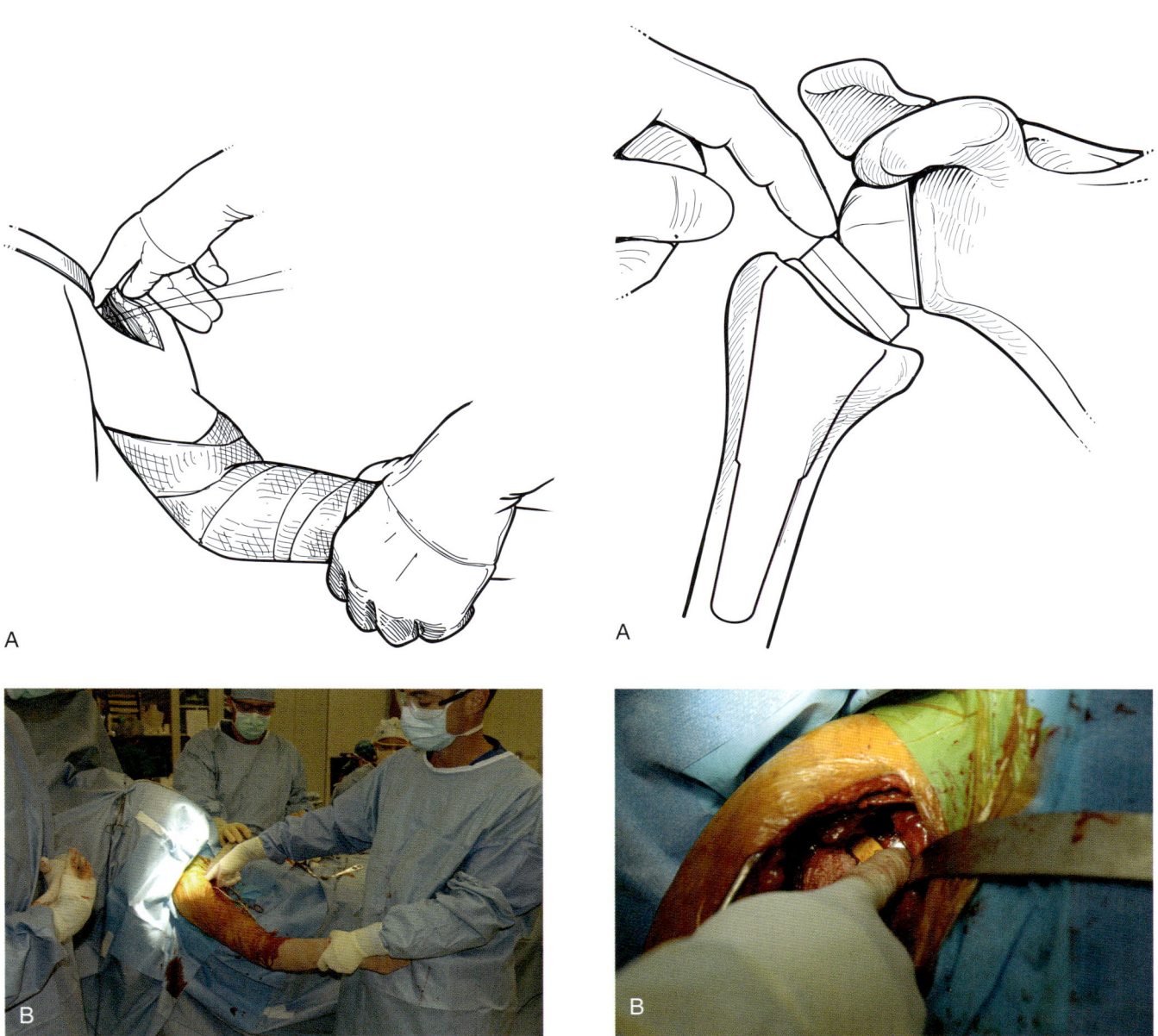

FIGURE 23.3 (A and B) Technique for evaluating deltoid tension.

FIGURE 23.4 (A and B) A finger is placed at the interface of the trial insert and the glenosphere to evaluate deltoid tension.

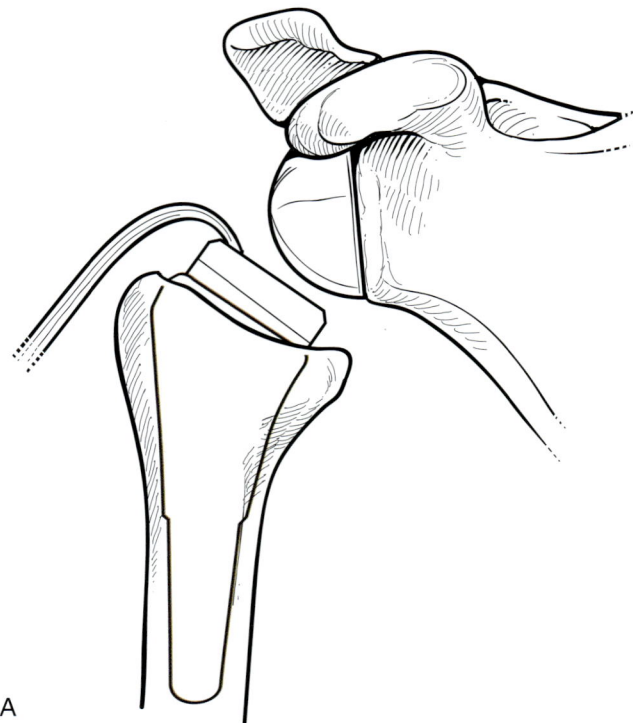

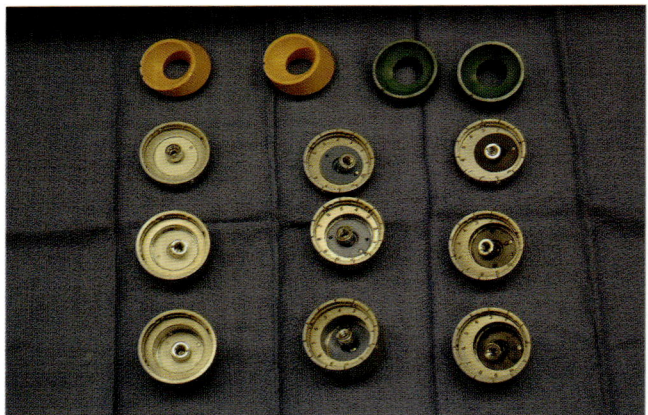

FIGURE 23.5 Different offsets and thicknesses of the humeral tray are available to increase deltoid tension.

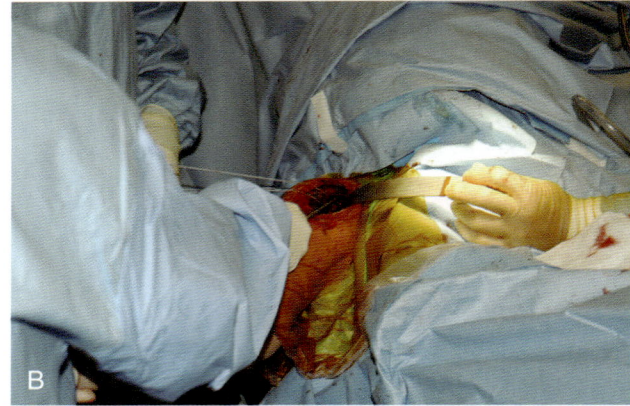

FIGURE 23.6 (A and B) Dislocation after trial reduction of an adequately tensioned reverse prosthesis with a bone hook.

CHAPTER 23 ■ Reduction and Deltoid Tensioning

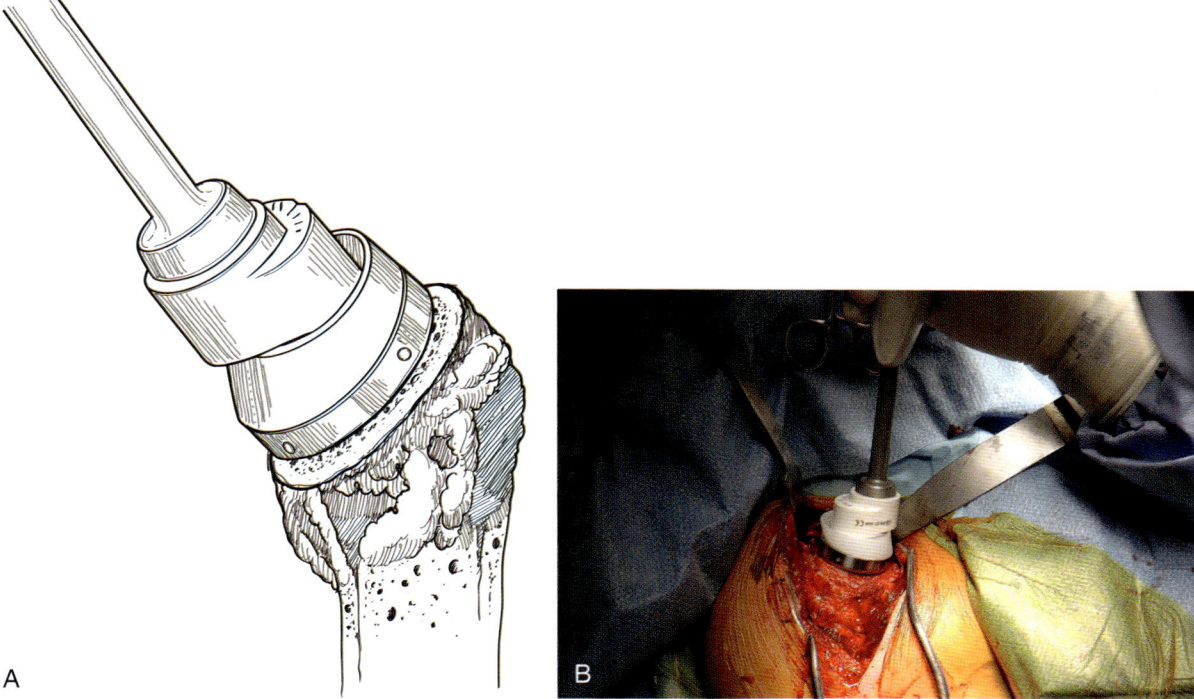

FIGURE 23.7 (A and B) Implantation of the final humeral polyethylene insert.

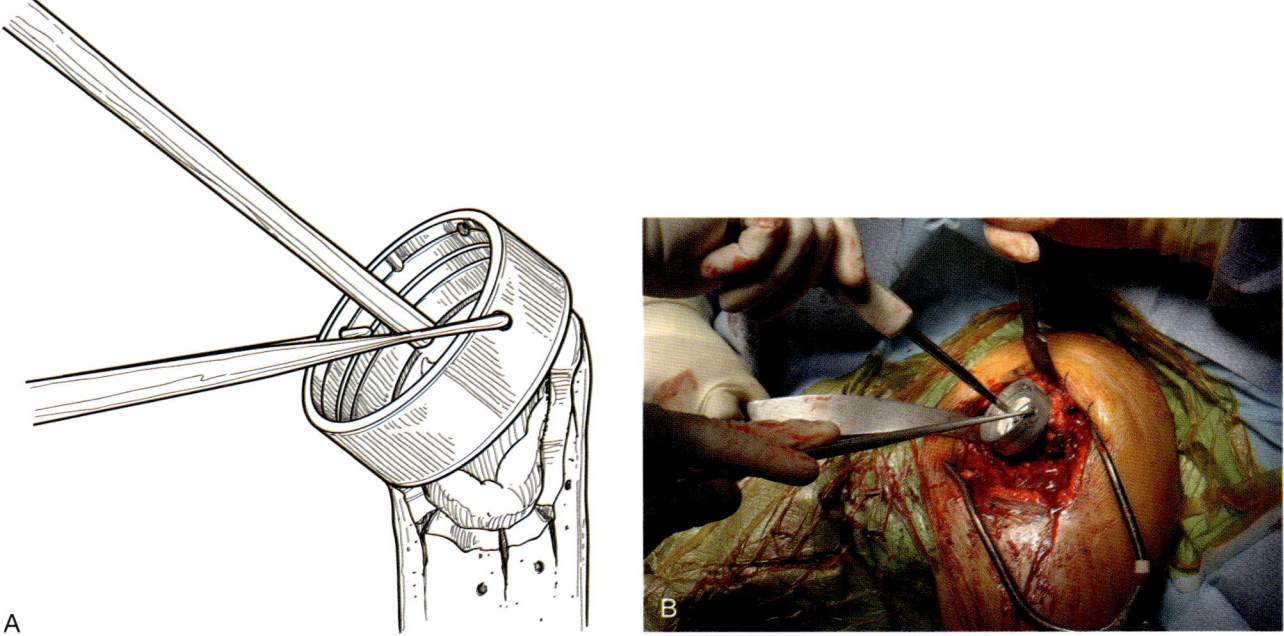

FIGURE 23.8 (A and B) Trialing with a thicker metallic tray to optimize soft tissue tension and stability.

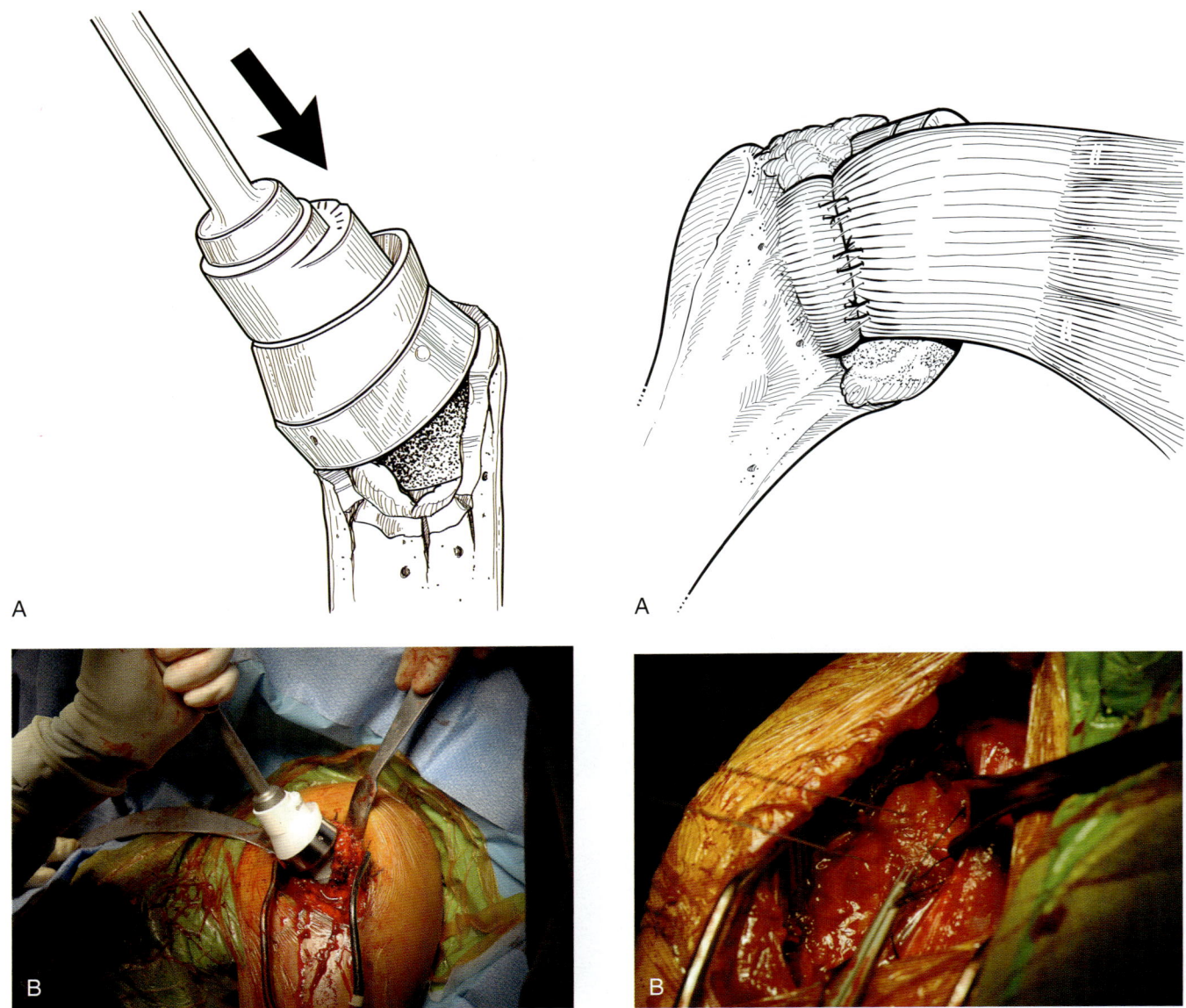

FIGURE 23.9 (A and B) The polyethylene insert and thicker metallic tray are impacted into the humerus.

FIGURE 23.10 (A and B) The subscapularis tendon, if present, is repaired.

CHAPTER 23 ■ Reduction and Deltoid Tensioning 215

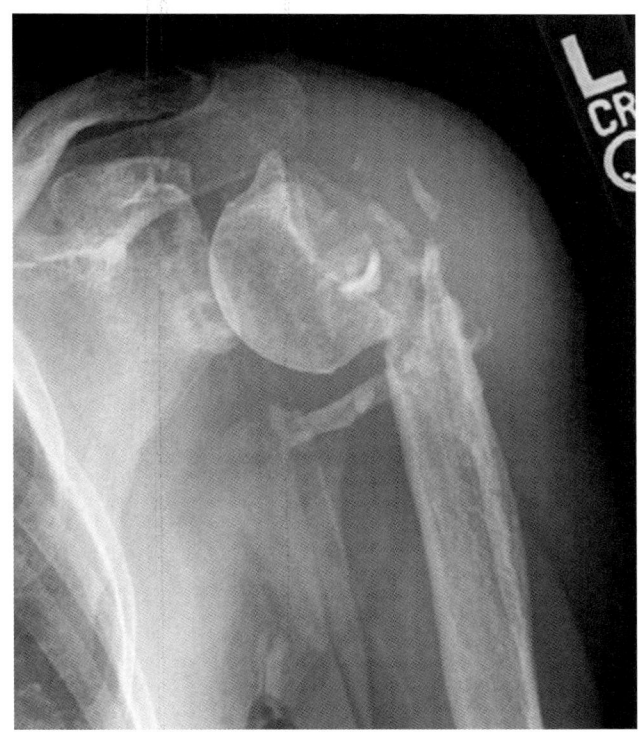

FIGURE 23.11 Case of fracture sequelae with proximal humeral bone loss.

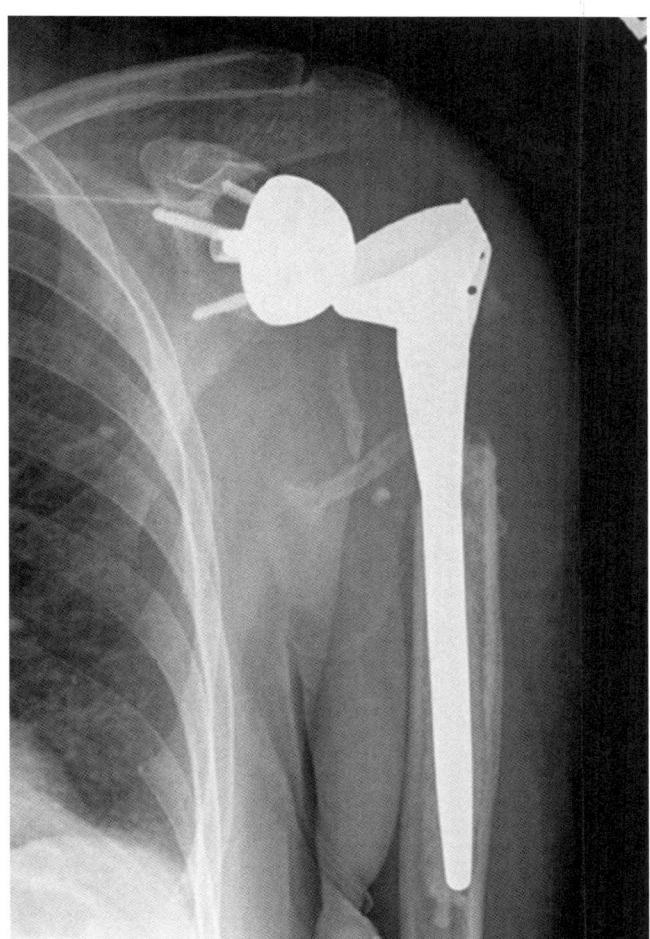

FIGURE 23.12 Case of prosthetic instability occurring in a patient with significant proximal humeral bone loss.

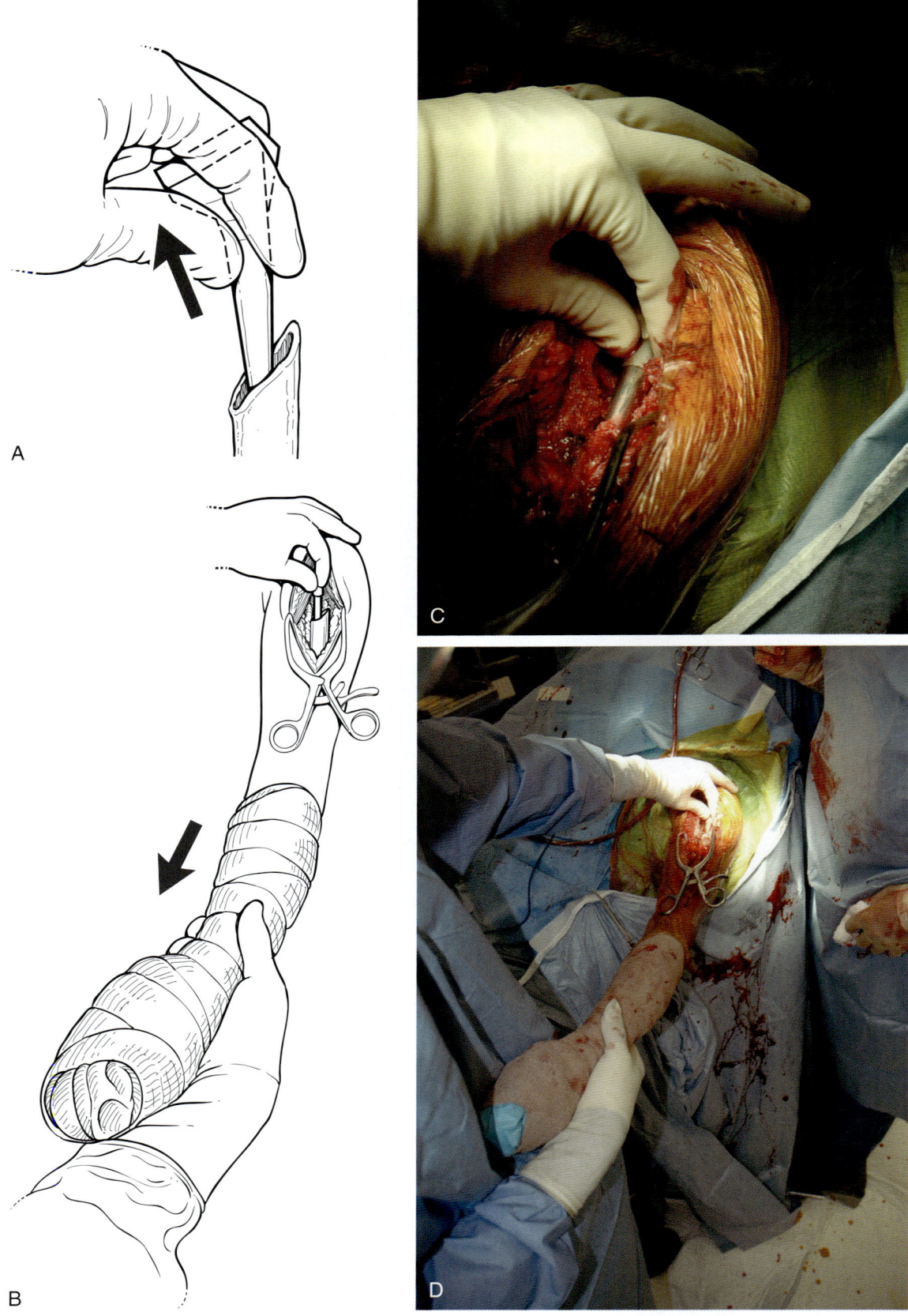

FIGURE 23.13 (A–D) Estimation of the appropriate height for implantation of the humeral component in a patient with significant proximal humeral bone loss.

CHAPTER 23 ■ Reduction and Deltoid Tensioning

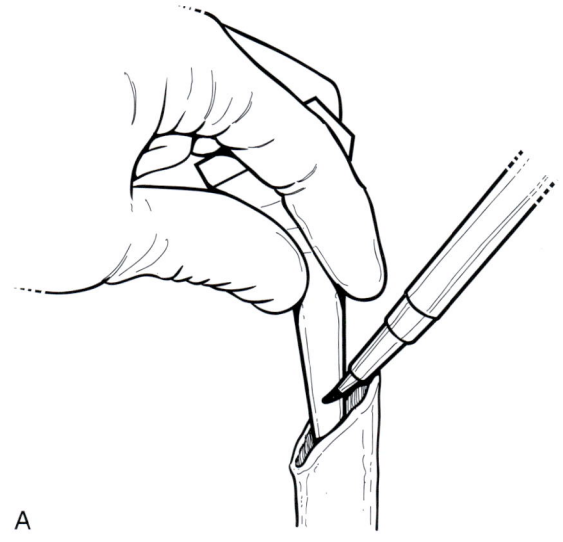

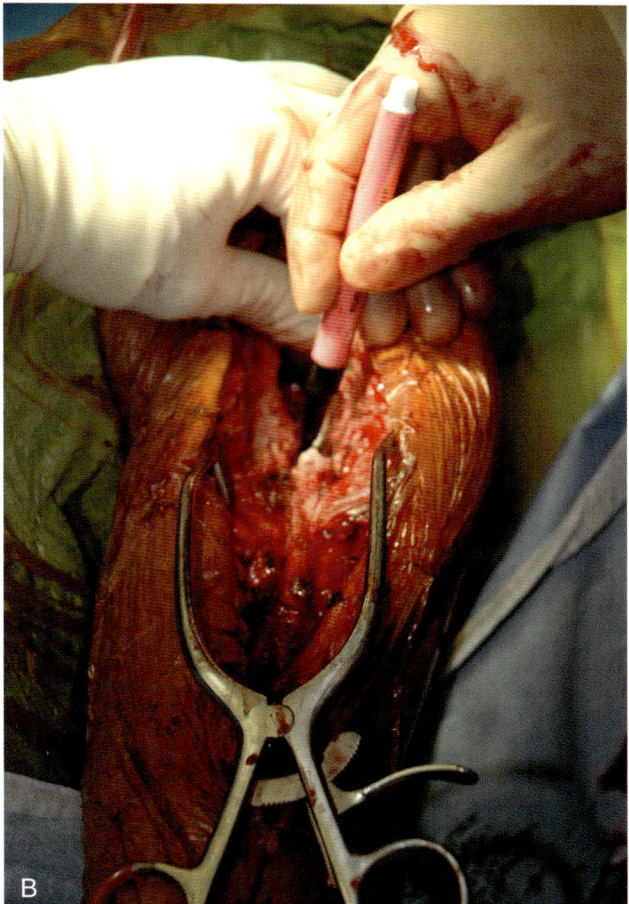

FIGURE 23.14 (A and B) The implant is marked to assist in placing the humeral component at the appropriate level.

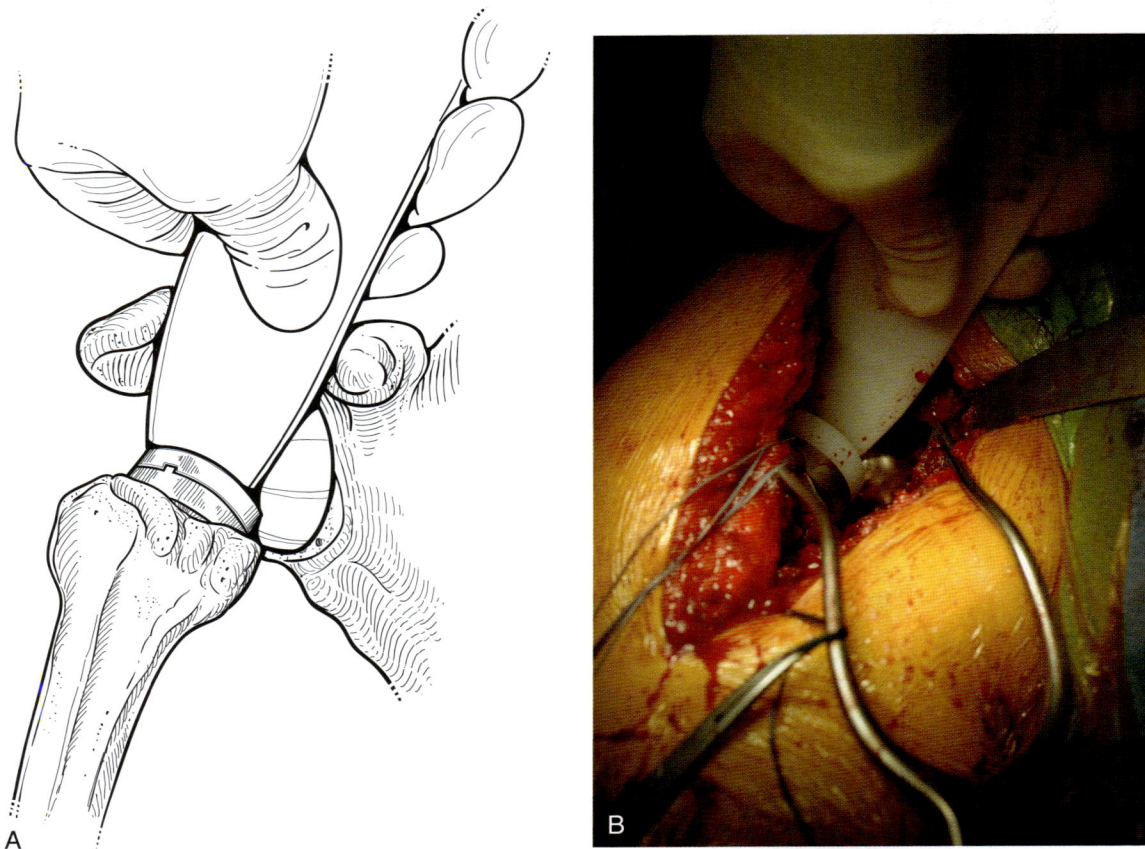

FIGURE 23.15 (A and B) Reduction of the reverse prosthesis with the "shoehorn" technique.

is compared with the distance templated preoperatively (see Chapter 18) to evaluate restoration of appropriate humeral length. This enables an estimation of the appropriate level at which to press fit or cement the humeral component. If the humeral component is implanted too distally within the humerus, adequate tension may not be obtainable. Conversely, if the humeral component is implanted too proximally within the humerus, the prosthetic joint may be irreducible.

After the humeral component has been implanted within the humerus, trialing of the various inserts commences as previously described. However, in the scenario of metaphyseal bone loss, no pistoning is accepted between the components. In addition, we often use a shoehorn instrument to aid in reduction by levering the humerus distally to engage the glenoid (Fig. 23.15). Once appropriate tension has been achieved, the final polyethylene insert is placed as described previously.

SPECIAL CONSIDERATIONS—NEW HUMERAL IMPLANTS FOR METAPHYSEAL BONE LOSS

Severe humeral metaphyseal bone loss clearly remains a challenge, and newer implants have been introduced to address the growing volume of revision reverse shoulder arthroplasty and reverse shoulder arthroplasty for malunion, nonunion, and tumor cases. Revision adjustable humeral implants are now available and are also available with press fit fixation (see Chapter 39). The press fit nature of these implants allows for use without cement fixation, thereby making any potential future revision surgery easier (Fig. 23.16). These adjustable humeral implants allow increased length options for severe humeral defects to improve deltoid tensioning. These implants sometimes need to be paired with proximal humeral allografts for severe bone loss cases.

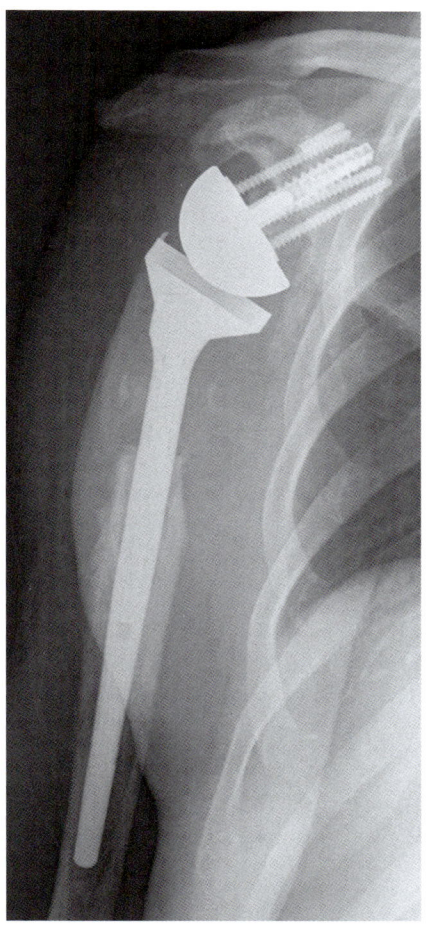

FIGURE 23.16 Diaphyseal press fit humeral implant used in a case of proximal humeral bone loss avoiding the introduction of cement.

CHAPTER 24

Wound closure and postoperative orthosis

The final steps in the operative procedure are wound closure and placement of the postoperative orthosis. Wound closure after implantation of a reverse prosthesis is performed as in cases of unconstrained shoulder arthroplasty. Because of the void created by lack of a rotator cuff, wound closure becomes more important after insertion of a reverse prosthesis than in cases of unconstrained arthroplasty because postoperative hematoma has been the most commonly reported complication after this procedure.[1]

WOUND CLOSURE TECHNIQUE

After reduction of the prosthesis and closure of the subscapularis, if present, the wound is irrigated with 800 mL of antibiotic-impregnated sterile saline (50,000 units bacitracin per liter sterile normal saline) via a bulb syringe. The wound is checked to ensure that adequate hemostasis has been obtained. The electrocautery is used as necessary to minimize any residual hemorrhage. A medium-sized closed suction drain is placed to help prevent postoperative hematoma formation. The trocar of the drain is used to puncture the soft tissue from inside the wound, and the skin is exited approximately 2 cm distal to the distal extent of the skin incision (Fig. 24.1). The drain is pulled through the skin until the transverse mark on the drain tube reaches the level of the skin (Fig. 24.2). The trocar is removed from the drain with scissors, and the other end of the drain is cut with scissors so that the tip of the drain rests in the void left by the absent rotator cuff (Fig. 24.3). When trimming the proximal end of the drain, care is taken to cut the drain between holes to minimize the risk of drainage tube breakage during removal (Fig. 24.4).

Wound closure is initiated by reapproximating the deep fascial layer with no. 0 braided absorbable suture in an interrupted figure-of-eight technique (Fig. 24.5). Just as in cases of unconstrained shoulder arthroplasty, we do not close the deltopectoral interval. The subcutaneous fascia is reapproximated with 2-0 braided absorbable suture in an interrupted figure-of-eight technique (Fig. 24.6). The skin is reapproximated with 3-0 undyed absorbable monofilament suture in a subcuticular running closure technique (Fig. 24.7).

After skin closure has been completed, the drain is checked to ensure that its position has been maintained. The occlusive draping is carefully removed from the site at which the drain tubing exits the skin. The skin in this area is cleaned and dried. Half-inch Steri-Strips are wrapped around the drain tubing to fix the drain to the skin and prevent inadvertent removal of the drain; we use two or three Steri-Strips (Fig. 24.8).

More of the occlusive draping is removed adjacent to the incision, and the skin is cleansed of blood with a saline-soaked sponge and then dried. Half-inch Steri-Strips are placed over the incision. Sterile gauze is then placed over the incision and a sterile absorbent pad is placed over the gauze. The dressing is secured with 3-inch foam tape. The remainder of the surgical drain is connected to the drainage tube, and the suction function of the drain is activated (Fig. 24.9). The remaining surgical drapes are then removed.

The surgical drain is removed the day after surgery regardless of the amount of drainage recorded. The dressing is maintained in place until postoperative day 3, at which time it is removed and not replaced. After removal of the dressing, the patient is allowed to shower, but submerging the incision in a bathtub is prohibited until 2 weeks postoperatively. The Steri-Strips are progressively removed by the patient as they lose their adhesion to the skin, typically after 10 to 14 days.

POSTOPERATIVE ORTHOSIS

The postoperative orthosis is placed in the operating room immediately after the dressing is applied. For a reverse prosthesis, we use a neutral-rotation sling (Ultrasling, Donjoy, Inc., Vista, California; Fig. 24.10). The patient is allowed to remove the sling for performance of hand, wrist, and elbow mobility exercises and for hygiene. The duration for which the orthosis is maintained is determined by the presence or absence of humeral metaphyseal bone loss. In uncomplicated cases with sufficient metaphyseal bone, the sling is discontinued and physical therapy initiated 3 weeks after surgery. In patients with humeral metaphyseal bone loss, the sling is maintained for an additional week, and physical therapy is initiated 4 weeks after surgery. Details of the postoperative rehabilitation regimen are provided in Chapter 43.

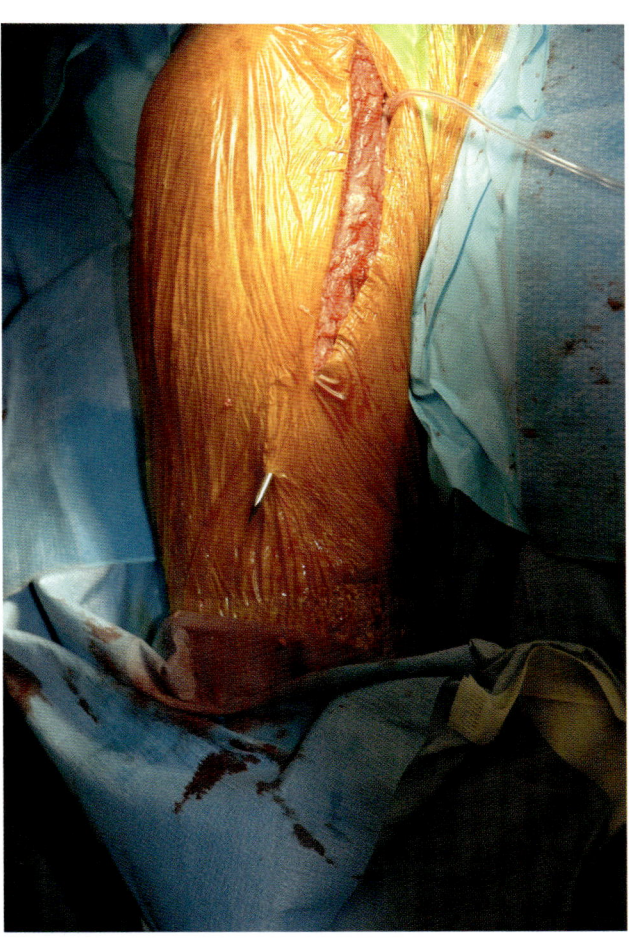

FIGURE 24.1 Placement of the drain tube with a sharp trocar.

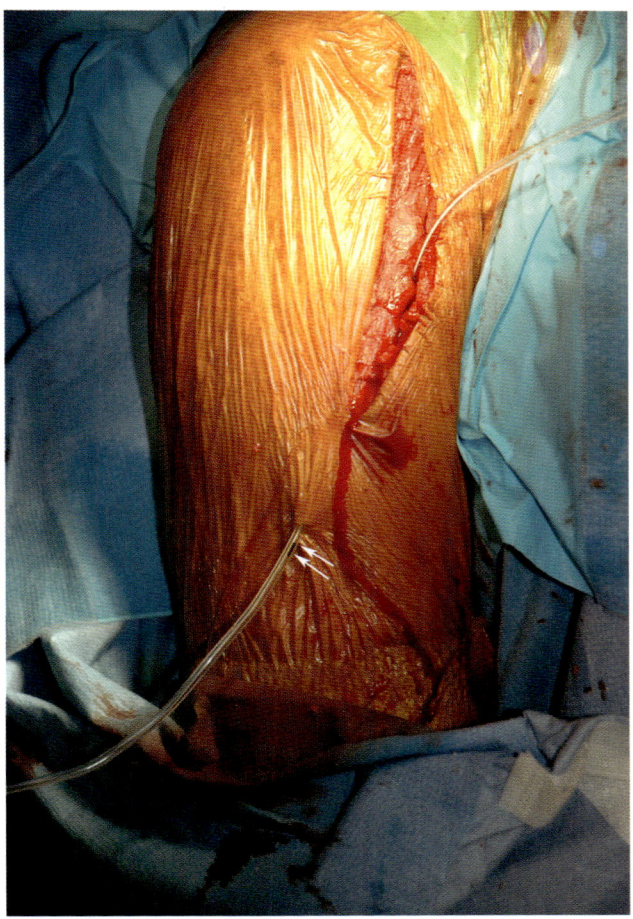

FIGURE 24.2 The drain is pulled through the skin until the transverse mark on the drain tube reaches the level of the skin *(arrows)*.

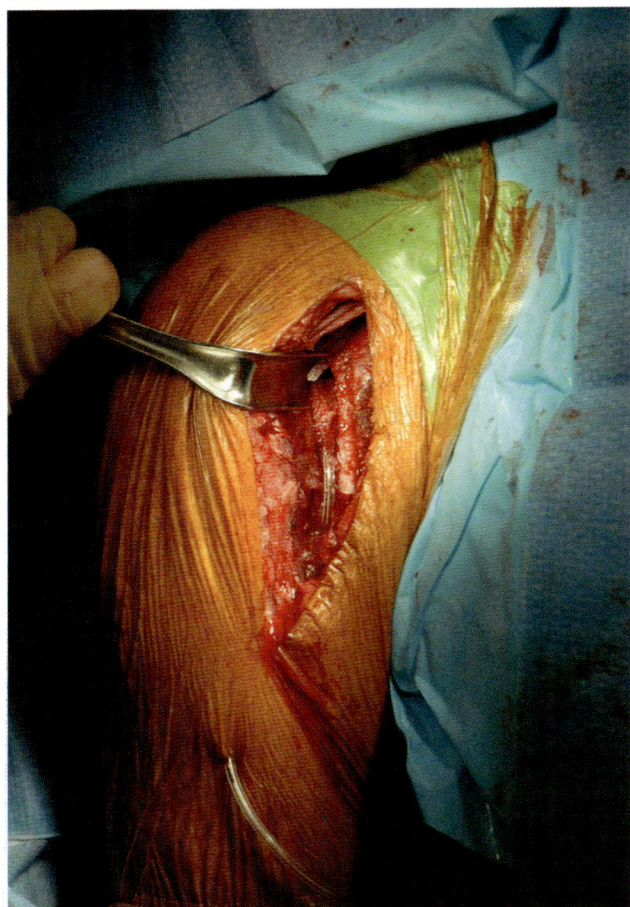

FIGURE 24.3 Placement of the drain in the surgical wound proximally.

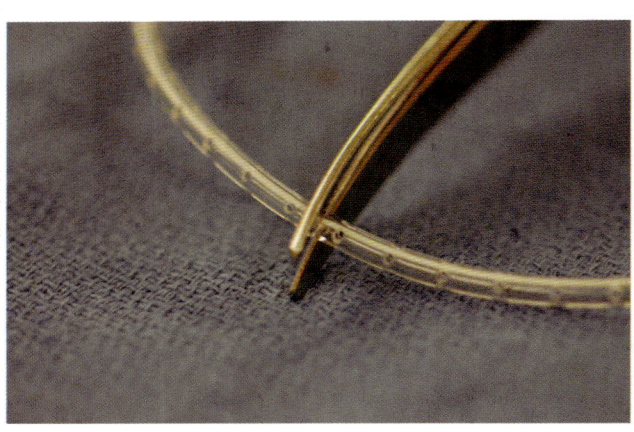

FIGURE 24.4 Proper trimming of the drain proximally to prevent breakage of the drain during removal.

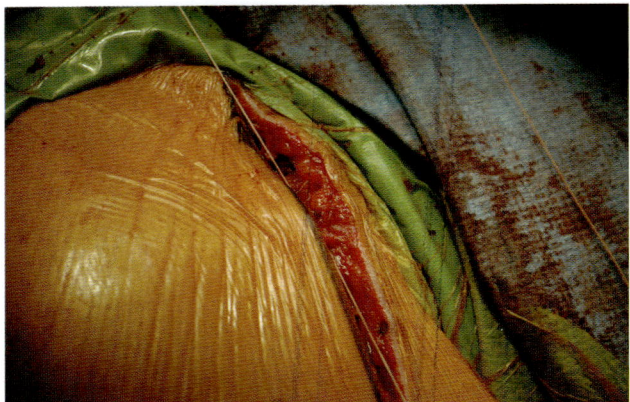

FIGURE 24.5 Closure of the deep fascial layer.

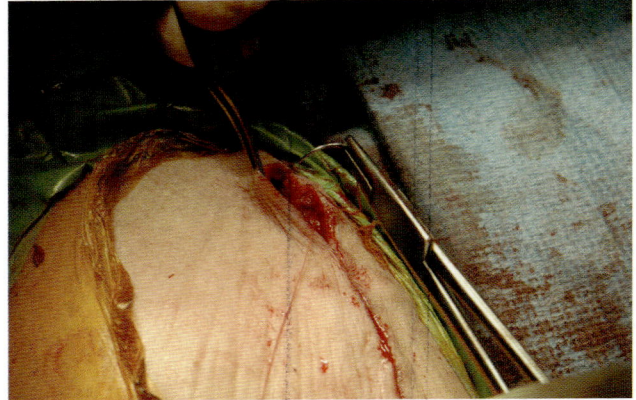

FIGURE 24.6 Closure of the subcutaneous fascia.

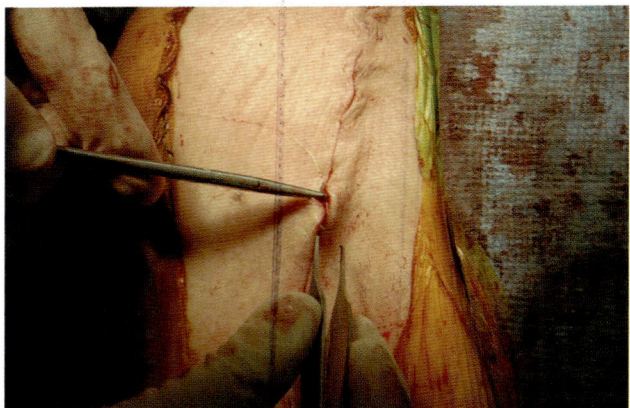

FIGURE 24.7 Subcuticular skin closure.

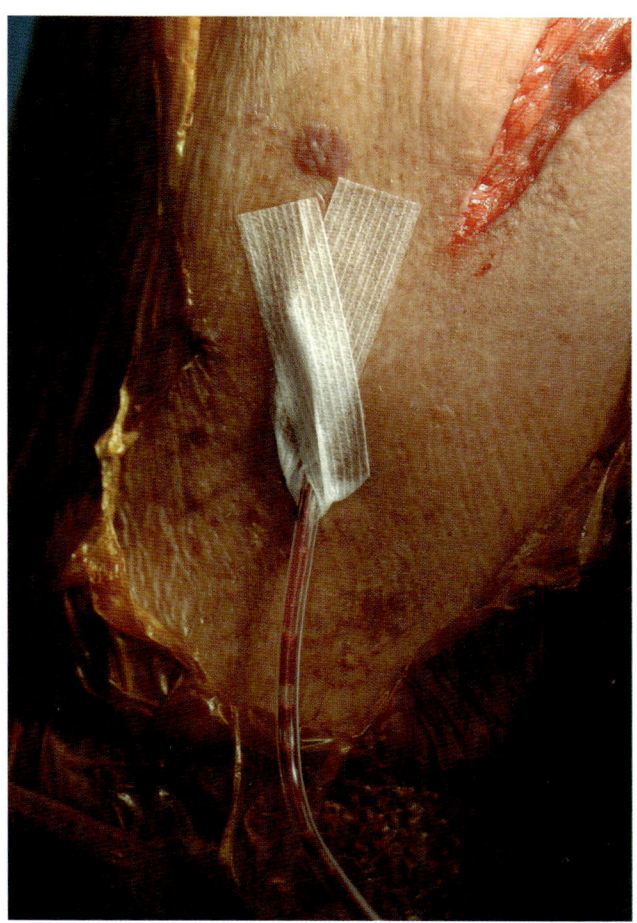

FIGURE 24.8 Fixation of the drainage tube with Steri-Strips.

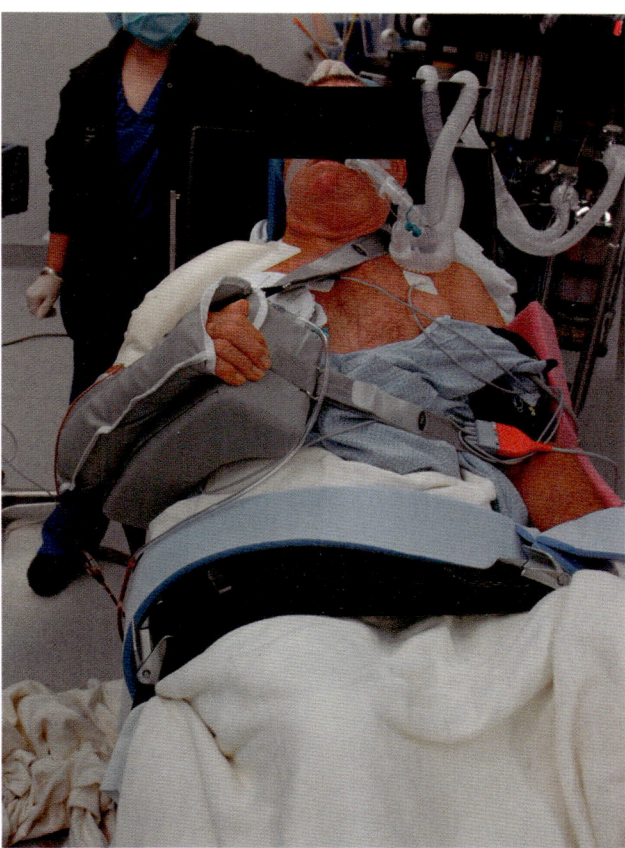

FIGURE 24.10 Neutral-rotation sling used after shoulder arthroplasty with a reverse prosthesis.

REFERENCE

1. Werner CM, Steinmann PA, Gilbart M, et al: Treatment of painful pseudoparesis due to irreparable rotator cuff dysfunction with the Delta III reverse-ball-and-socket total shoulder prosthesis, *J Bone Joint Surg Am* 87:1476–1486, 2005.

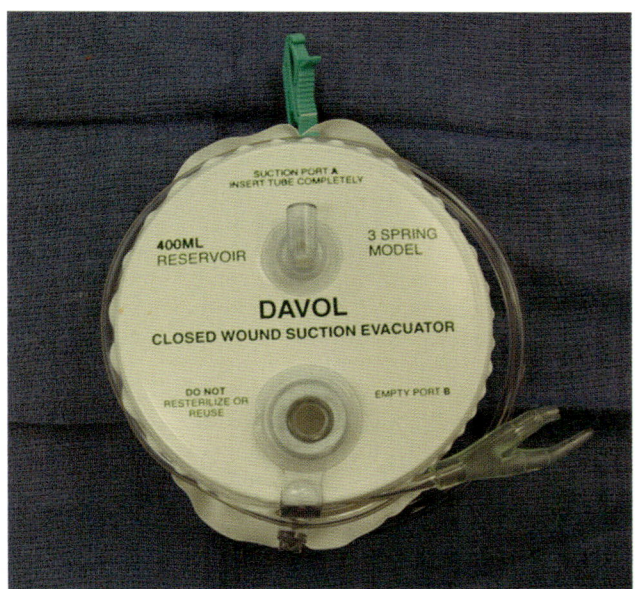

FIGURE 24.9 Surgical drain.

CHAPTER 25

Results and complications

Reports on the results of reverse shoulder arthroplasty are becoming more common as implantation of this type of shoulder arthroplasty increases. The results vary predominantly by the underlying indication for which the arthroplasty was performed. The results and complications presented in this chapter are drawn from our experience with this implant over the last 20 years, including the lead author's early experience in Europe.

RESULTS

The results of reverse shoulder arthroplasty vary mainly with the etiology for which the arthroplasty was performed. The best results are obtained in the treatment of osteoarthritis with a massive rotator cuff tear (rotator cuff tear arthropathy), whereas results are least satisfactory in patients with posttraumatic arthritis. Table 25.1 details the results of reverse shoulder arthroplasty for the most common surgical indications. Results are expressed in terms of active mobility; patient satisfaction; the Constant score, a shoulder-specific outcome measurement incorporating pain, mobility, activity, and strength; and the age- and gender-adjusted Constant score.[1,2]

INTRAOPERATIVE COMPLICATIONS

Intraoperative complications are more common during reverse shoulder arthroplasty than during unconstrained shoulder arthroplasty performed for chronic conditions; they may be divided into complications involving the humerus, glenoid, musculotendinous soft tissues (rotator cuff), and neurovascular structures.

Humerus

The most common humeral complication is iatrogenic fracture, which usually results from performing an overly aggressive dislocation maneuver without previous adequate soft tissue release. Many patients undergoing reverse shoulder arthroplasty have moderate to severe osteopenia, thus placing them at increased risk for this complication. Intraoperative tuberosity fractures during glenohumeral dislocation are less common during reverse shoulder arthroplasty than during unconstrained shoulder arthroplasty because of the lack of a rotator cuff attaching to the tuberosities, which could otherwise contribute to fracture during a dislocation maneuver. Fractures involving the humeral diaphysis should be reduced and a long-stem humeral implant placed. Allograft struts and cerclage cables may be added in patients with severe osteopenia (Fig. 25.1).

Intraoperative fractures involving the greater or lesser tuberosities (or both) are usually nondisplaced. Many of these fractures are stable or become stable once the humeral implant has been inserted. If a fragment of a greater tuberosity fracture that has maintained attachment of a substantial portion of the posterior rotator cuff is not satisfactorily stable, suture fixation of the tuberosity is performed and the postoperative rehabilitation adjusted accordingly to allow healing of the tuberosity. A fragment of a greater tuberosity fracture that is devoid of rotator cuff attachment and is unstable may simply be excised.

Intraoperative lesser tuberosity fractures can occur during retraction of the proximal humerus in the course of glenoid preparation and insertion. This fracture is without clinical consequence and can largely be ignored.

Glenoid

Intraoperative glenoid fractures are more detrimental than humeral injury. Frequently, surgeons who are beginning their experience in reverse shoulder arthroplasty do not have much proficiency in glenoid preparation because they have previously performed hemiarthroplasty for most cases where shoulder arthroplasty was indicated. Many surgeons initially attempt to ream the glenoid as though it were an acetabulum (i.e., overaggressively), which often leads to obliteration of the glenoid bone, glenoid fracture, or both. Patients undergoing reverse shoulder arthroplasty are at particular risk for intraoperative glenoid fracture because they tend to have more osteopenia than those undergoing unconstrained arthroplasty for nonfracture conditions. Fractures may involve only the peripheral glenoid rim or may extend significantly into the central portion of the glenoid. Adequate capsular release helps minimize the risk for glenoid fracture. Additionally, a motorized reamer (not a drill, because the speed and torque are different) should be used for preparation of the glenoid surface. The reamer should be started before the surgeon applies force to engage the reamer onto the glenoid face. This avoids having the reamer "catch" an edge of the glenoid, which may cause a fracture.

Fractures that involve only a small portion of the peripheral rim generally require no treatment, and the glenoid component can be inserted as planned. Glenoid fractures that extend

| TABLE 25.1 | Results of Primary Reverse Shoulder Arthroplasty According to Underlying Etiology in the Authors' Prospective Database From 2003 to 2014 |||||||||
| | Absolute Constant Score (Points) || Adjusted Constant Score (%) || Active Forward Flexion (Degrees) || Active External Rotation (Degrees) || Excellent/Good Subjective Results (%) |
Etiology	Preoperative	Postoperative	Preoperative	Postoperative	Preoperative	Postoperative	Preoperative	Postoperative	
Cuff tear arthropathy (n = 175)	17	63	24	87	46	130	9	29	82
Massive rotator cuff tear (n = 21)[a]	22	59	28	78	28	155	14	27	76
Rheumatoid arthritis (n = 12)	10	58	14	82	33	130	2	32	83
Posttraumatic arthritis (n = 28)	9	50	12	69	11	121	−1	13	86
Acute fracture (n = 37)	7	71	10	102	0	154	0	31	92
Other (n = 14)	10	52	13	68	14	128	4	25	86

[a]Includes patients with massive rotator cuff tears and chronic pseudoparalysis but without glenohumeral arthritis.

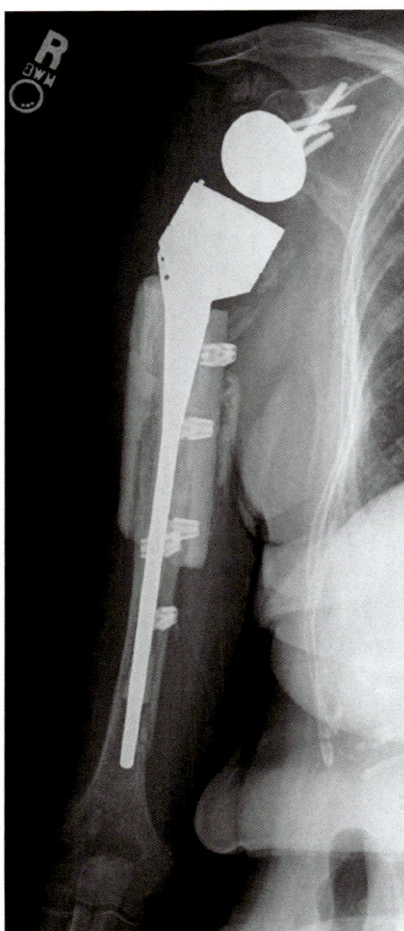

FIGURE 25.1 Patient with an intraoperative humeral diaphyseal fracture treated by placement of a long-stem humeral component and allograft struts fixed with cerclage cables.

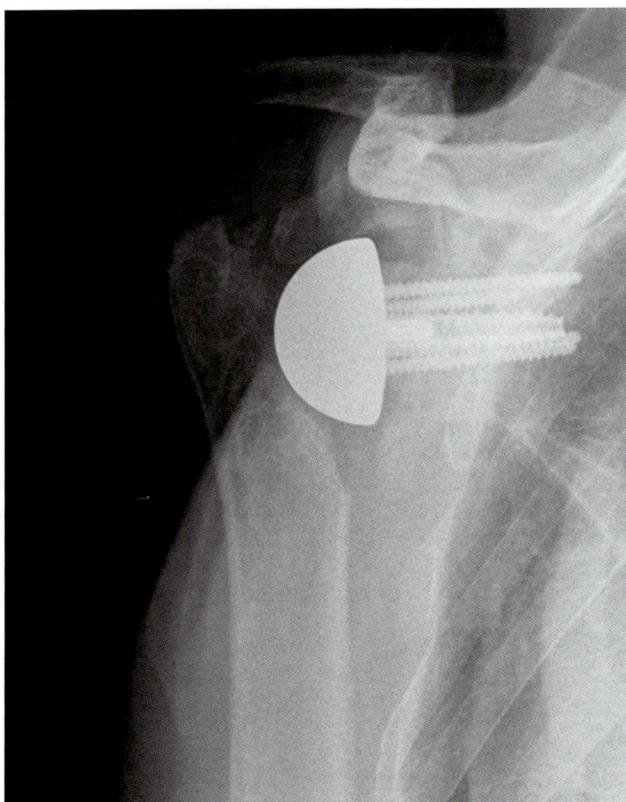

FIGURE 25.2 Case in which an intraoperative fracture of the glenoid was treated by bone grafting and placement of the glenoid component. Placement of the humeral component was delayed 6 months until the fracture had healed and remodeled.

into the central portion of the glenoid should be bone-grafted with the humeral head, and a long-posted revision-type base plate should be employed. The reverse glenoid component can be inserted to help secure the bone graft and fix the fracture internally. If the central post of the reverse component is firmly seated within native glenoid bone, consideration can be given to placing the humeral component in the same surgical setting. If the glenoid component does not seem secure or the central post of the glenoid base plate is not firmly seated in unfractured native glenoid bone, the humeral component should be initially omitted for 6 months to allow the fracture to heal. After 6 months, a humeral component can be placed as the second part of a two-stage procedure (Fig. 25.2).

Rotator Cuff

With proper exposure, intraoperative injury to the rotator cuff is rare. Although patients undergoing reverse shoulder arthroplasty have a compromised rotator cuff, every effort should be made to preserve any rotator cuff function that remains, both anteriorly and posteriorly. Repair of the subscapularis tendon after reverse shoulder arthroplasty has been shown to decrease postoperative dislocation for traditional Grammont-style implants. We always repair the subscapularis when a sufficient subscapularis tendon is present. Preservation of the posterior rotator cuff improves outcome by allowing active external rotation postoperatively. If the rotator cuff is adequately visualized, inadvertent damage to the rotator cuff during reverse shoulder arthroplasty can be avoided.

Neurovascular Structures

Catastrophic injury to the neurovascular structures around the shoulder is exceedingly rare during reverse shoulder arthroplasty. The neural structures most at risk during reverse shoulder arthroplasty are the axillary and musculocutaneous nerves. These nerves should not be at risk for transection during primary arthroplasty using accepted operative technique. Neuropraxic injury caused by stretch most commonly involves the axillary nerve, but any nerves within the brachial plexus can be affected. Care should be taken in positioning the patient so as to maintain the cervical spine in neutral alignment and avoid a stretch injury to the brachial plexus. We have yet to establish risk factors for neuropraxic injury to the axillary nerve. Intraoperative nerve monitoring studies have shown that nerve injury with anatomic shoulder arthroplasty may be increased with extremes of motion during the procedure and for patients with preoperative decreased passive external rotation, decreased forward flexion, and a history of prior open shoulder surgery.[3,4] These studies were based on intraoperative nerve monitoring and short-term electromyography and cannot definitively establish risk factors for long-term clinical implications. Logic would suggest that patients with the most stiffness creating difficulty in glenoid exposure would be at the highest risk for this type of complication. Our clinical experience has not borne this out, however, and we are currently unable to predict which patients are most likely to suffer this complication. Patient education preoperatively is of paramount importance in dealing with neuropraxia, inasmuch as patients are much more accepting if they have heard about the possibility of this complication before surgery. Axillary nerve (and other nerve) neuropraxia is treated by observation, with most patients recovering by 3 to 4 months postoperatively.

Although tearing of the cephalic vein is common and largely without consequence, significant arterial and venous injuries occurring during primary reverse shoulder arthroplasty performed for nonfracture indications are exceptionally rare. Injury to the major vessels of the upper extremity is usually caused by overzealous medial dissection, which is not needed during shoulder arthroplasty. Should such an injury occur, emergency intraoperative consultation with a vascular surgeon is required after cross-clamping of the injured vessel.

POSTOPERATIVE COMPLICATIONS

Postoperative complications are more common than intraoperative complications and historically have occurred in up to 50% of patients after reverse shoulder arthroplasty in some series.[5] Fortunately, complications after reverse shoulder arthroplasty generally appear to be decreasing over time, with more surgical experience with the implant and technique. The most common postoperative complications include wound problems (dehiscence, hematoma), glenoid problems, humeral problems, acromial problems, scapular notching, instability (dislocation), stiffness, and infection.

Wound Problems

Wound problems occur early after reverse shoulder arthroplasty. Hematoma is most easily avoided by extensive use of electrocautery during reverse shoulder arthroplasty and closed suction drainage for 24 hours postoperatively. The lack of a rotator cuff results in a large potential space in which a hematoma can form. Closed suction drainage minimizes hematoma formation and is highly recommended in reverse shoulder arthroplasty. Suture ligation, in addition to electrosurgical cauterization, of the anterior humeral circumflex vessels also minimizes the incidence of postoperative wound hematoma. When a hematoma occurs, it is managed by symptomatic nonoperative treatment (warm compresses, pain medication). Operative drainage is reserved for situations in which drainage persists beyond 1 week or infection is suspected (see later) and is rarely necessary.

Wound dehiscence occasionally occurs as a result of a reaction to dissolving subcutaneous sutures in susceptible patients. The presence of minimal serous drainage distinguishes this complication from the more serious deep infection. Superficial wound dehiscence is treated by local wound care, including removal of any residual dissolving suture material and chemical cauterization of any granulating tissue with silver nitrate applicators.

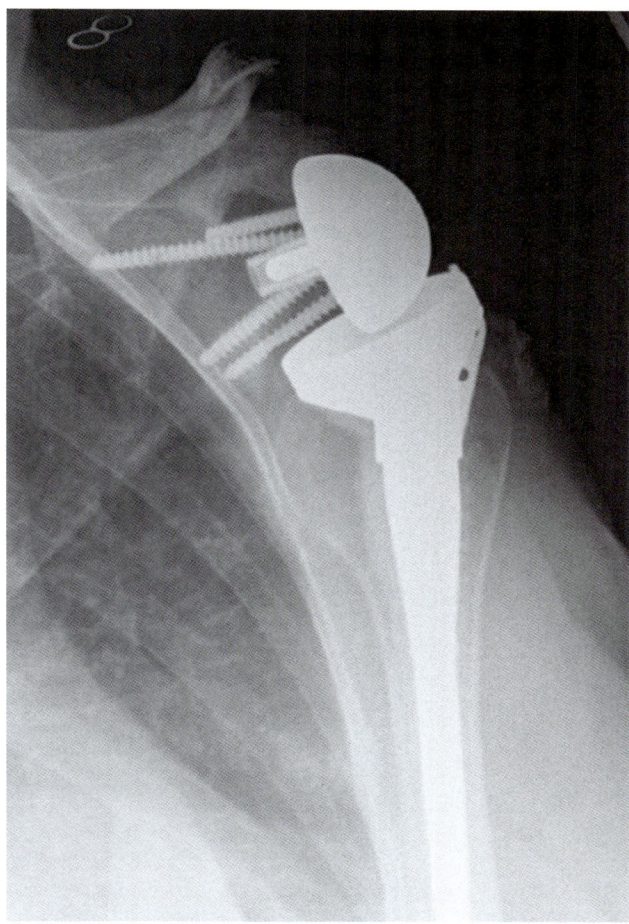

FIGURE 25.3 Placement of the glenoid component of a reverse prosthesis in a superiorly oriented position resulted in failure of the glenoid component.

Glenoid Problems

Glenoid problems after reverse shoulder arthroplasty are less common than after unconstrained total shoulder arthroplasty. In all cases of which we are aware, failure of the glenoid component after primary reverse shoulder arthroplasty has been associated with initial placement of the glenoid component in a superiorly oriented direction (Fig. 25.3), implantation of the prosthesis in the presence of an intraoperative glenoid fracture (Fig. 25.4), or lack of proper seating of the Morse taper between the glenosphere and the base plate. These complications are best avoided. We nearly always implant the reverse prosthesis through a deltopectoral approach to avoid inadvertent placement of the glenoid component in a superiorly oriented position, which can occur with use of the superolateral approach. If an intraoperative glenoid fracture occurs, we treat it as described previously in this chapter. In such an instance revision surgery—consisting of glenoid reconstruction and revision reverse shoulder arthroplasty, resection arthroplasty, or conversion to a hemiarthroplasty—is required (see Section VI).

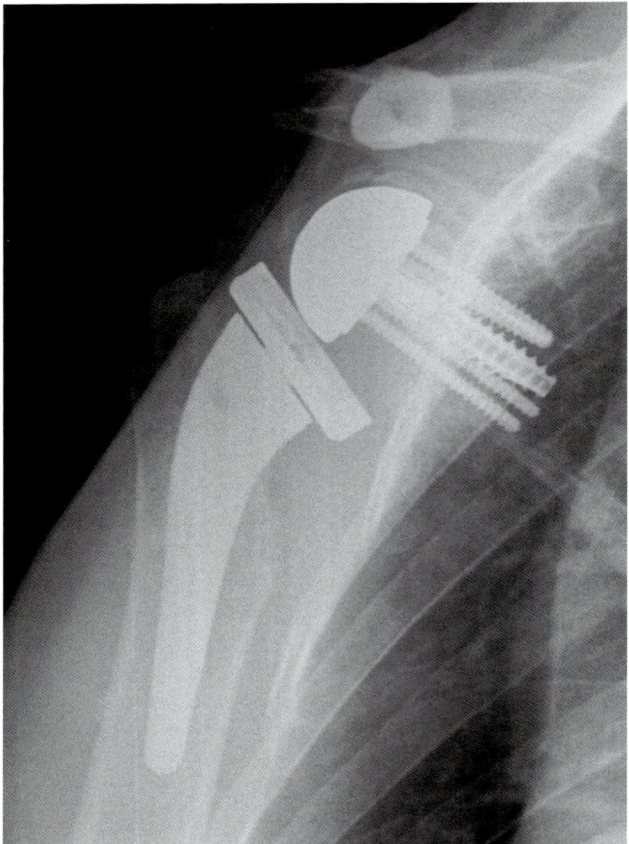

FIGURE 25.4 Placement of the glenoid component of a reverse prosthesis despite intraoperative glenoid fracture resulted in failure of the glenoid component.

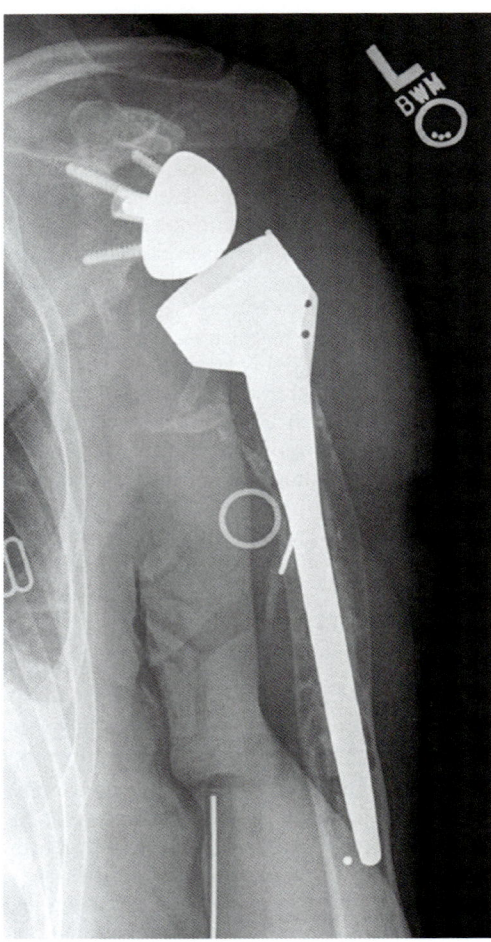

FIGURE 25.5 Aseptic loosening of a reverse humeral stem related to proximal humeral bone loss.

Humeral Problems

Humeral problems after reverse shoulder arthroplasty are rare and can be divided into loosening of the humeral component, mechanical problems of the humeral component (polyethylene dissociation and polyethylene wear), and periprosthetic humeral fracture. Aseptic loosening of the humeral stem of a reverse prosthesis occurs in less than 1% of cases. The predominant risk factor for aseptic loosening of the humeral stem is proximal humeral bone loss (Fig. 25.5). Whenever loosening of a humeral stem occurs, infection must be ruled out (see later). In the rare instance of symptomatic aseptic humeral component loosening, treatment consists of revision of the humeral stem, usually combined with allograft reconstruction of the proximal humerus to provide osseous support of the proximal portion of the revision stem (see Section VI).

Mechanical problems of the humeral component are exceedingly rare and are related to the polyethylene liner. We are aware of one case of dissociation of the polyethylene liner from the humeral stem that was most likely related to incomplete seating of the polyethylene component at the index arthroplasty. In this scenario, revision surgery with replacement of the polyethylene liner is indicated. Polyethylene wear occurs medially on the rim of the polyethylene liner in many patients, as noted at the time of revision surgery (Fig. 25.6). Such wear is related to scapular notching, as discussed later.

Periprosthetic humeral fractures are more common than loosening of the humeral component and are almost always the result of a fall or similar low-energy trauma (Fig. 25.7). The majority of these fractures occur just distal to the tip of the humeral stem, and most can be treated nonoperatively. Nonoperative treatment consists of fracture bracing, activity modification, pain medication, and frequent radiographic monitoring. If the fracture has not healed within 3 months, we will incorporate the use of an external bone stimulator (OL 1000 Bone Growth Stimulator, Donjoy Orthopedics, Vista, California). Despite these measures, periprosthetic humeral fractures treated nonoperatively may take longer than 9 months to heal.[6] Our criteria for recommending operative treatment of periprosthetic fractures (revision surgery; see Section VI) include complete displacement, angulation greater than 30 degrees, loosening or dislocation of the humeral component, or failure of nonoperative treatment (Fig. 25.8).

Acromial Problems

Occasionally, acromial stress fractures are seen after reverse shoulder arthroplasty; these fractures are likely more common

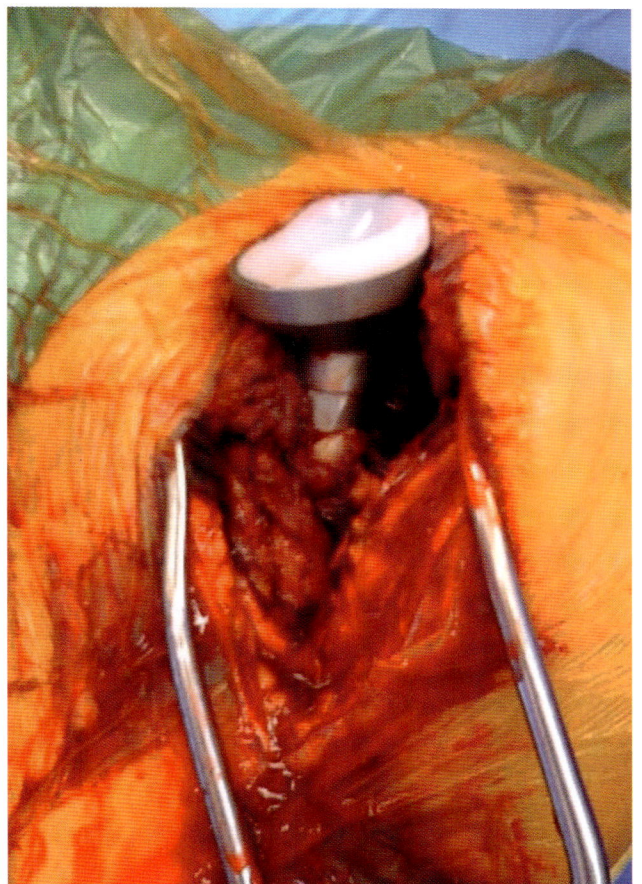

FIGURE 25.6 Polyethylene wear medially observed during revision surgery.

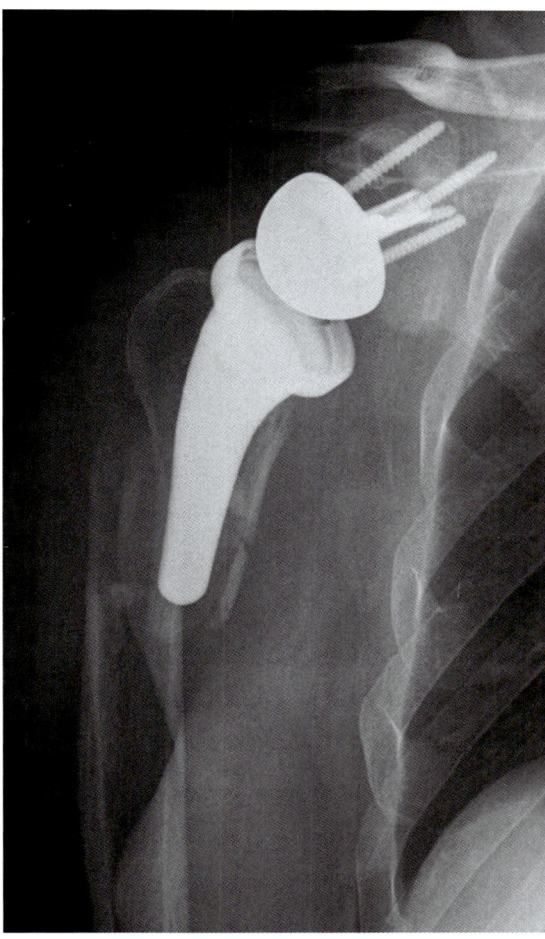

FIGURE 25.7 Periprosthetic humeral fracture, which occurred as a result of a fall, in a patient with a reverse prosthesis.

than initially suspected, with a reported incidence of up to 3% in one series (Fig. 25.9).[7] These fractures result from deltoid tension applied to osteopenic bone. Frequently these fractures are present preoperatively as a result of chronic superior migration of the humeral head with persistent acromiohumeral articulation. Postoperatively, deltoid tension may cause the fracture fragment to tilt inferiorly. We tend to see these fractures around 2 to 3 months postoperatively, with the reported series noting an average around 8 months postoperatively.[7] Acromial stress fractures are diagnosed with tenderness to palpation at the acromion and can sometimes be seen on radiographs. A computed tomography (CT) scan can be completed to confirm the fracture when desired but does not change our treatment approach. We treat postoperative acromial stress fractures nonoperatively with 6 weeks in a neutral rotation sling. We also obtain an endocrinology consultation to assess and treat osteoporosis, vitamin D deficiency, and other related causes. If the fracture has not healed within 3 months, we will incorporate the use of an external bone stimulator (OL 1000 Bone Growth Stimulator). Despite the occurrence of this complication, reported outcomes after acromial stress fracture note significant improvements in postoperative as compared with preoperative pain relief and function.[7]

Fractures of the Scapular Body and Scapular Spine

Fractures of the scapular body and scapular spine can occur after reverse shoulder arthroplasty and may vary in incidence with different prosthetic designs. One series reported an incidence of 1% of scapular spine fractures (classified as type III fractures) after reverse shoulder arthroplasty.[8] Similar to acromial stress fractures, scapular fractures are thought to be secondary to osteopenic bone and deltoid tension; they can potentially propagate through the superior screw of the base plate. The superior screw has been noted to be a potential stress riser for scapular fracture propagation, with some advocating avoiding placement of this screw when possible.[8] We also postulate that poor scapular motion may contribute to both acromial stress fractures as well as scapular spine fractures (see Chapter 44). Fractures of the scapular spine have become more frequent in our practice following the introduction of the "onlay" humeral prosthetic designs (Fig. 25.10). Although open reduction and internal fixation of these fractures has been advocated in this setting,[8] we treat them in the same way as we treat acromial fractures—nonoperatively with 6 weeks in a neutral rotation sling. We also obtain an endocrinology consultation to assess and treat

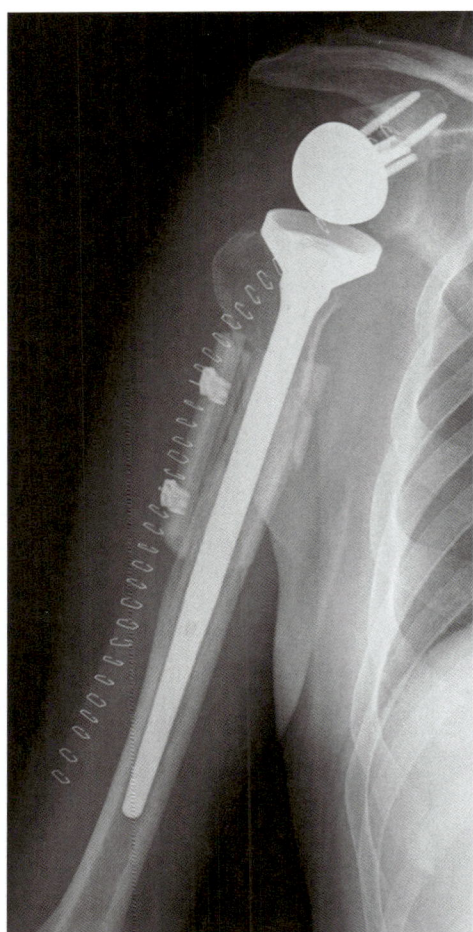

FIGURE 25.8 Operative treatment of a periprosthetic fracture in a patient with a reverse prosthesis.

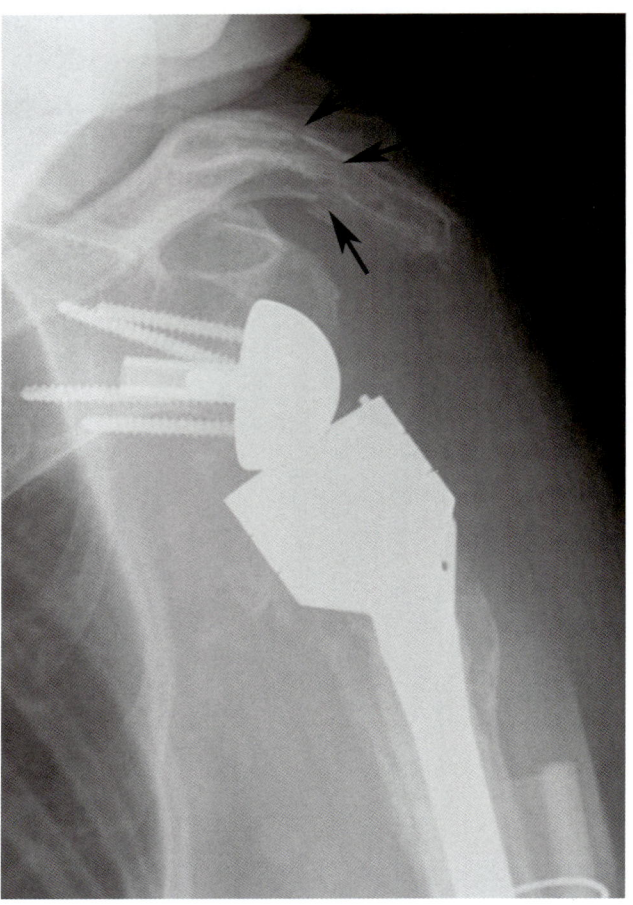

FIGURE 25.9 Acromial stress fracture *(arrows)* occurring after reverse shoulder arthroplasty.

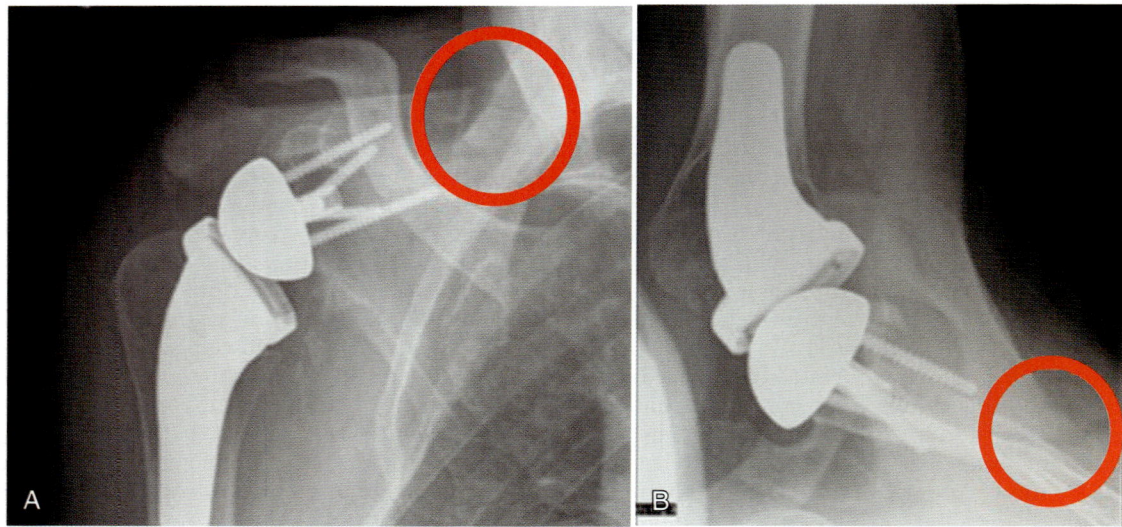

FIGURE 25.10 (A and B) Radiographs of a patient with a scapular spine stress fracture *(circles)*.

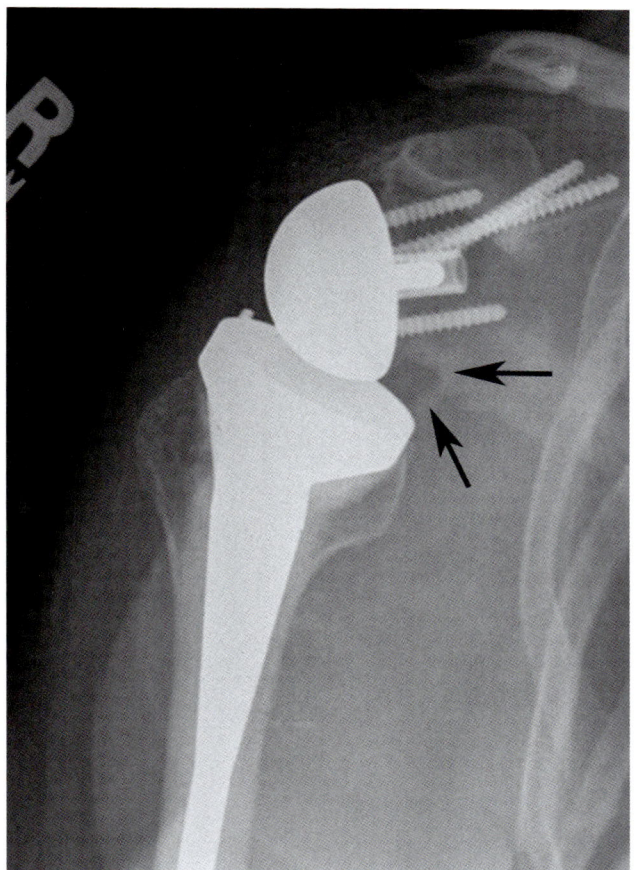

FIGURE 25.11 Inferior scapular notch (arrows), which commonly occurs in patients after reverse shoulder arthroplasty.

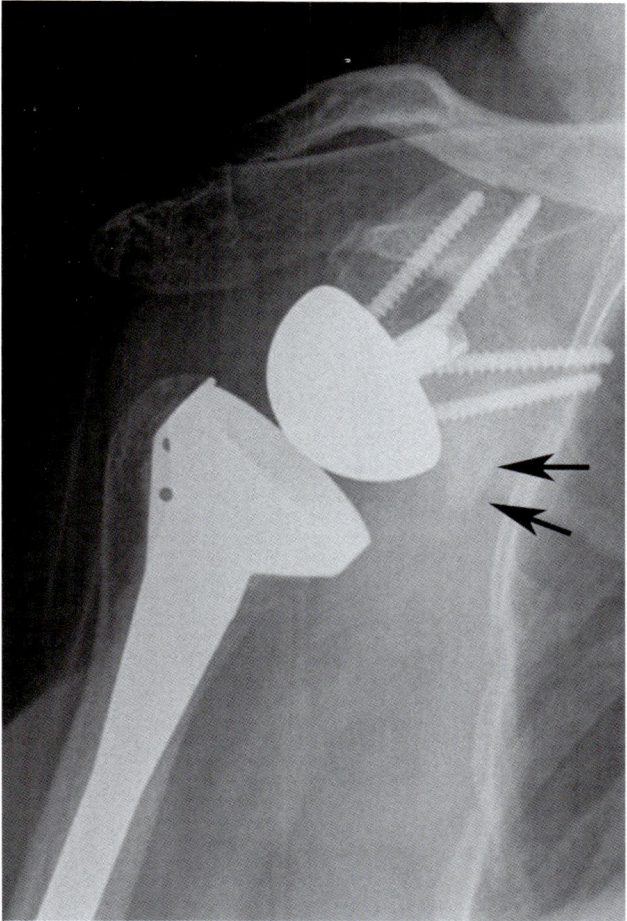

FIGURE 25.12 Scapular osteophyte (arrows) accompanying an inferior scapular notch after reverse shoulder arthroplasty.

osteoporosis, vitamin D deficiency, and other related causes. If the fracture has not healed within 3 months, we will incorporate the use of an external bone stimulator (OL 1000 Bone Growth Stimulator). As we feel this complication to be more common with onlay humeral designs, possibly because of increased deltoid tension, we try to avoid implanting onlay designs in excessive tension.

Scapular Notching

Though whether it should be considered a complication is debatable, notching of the scapula occurs within 2 years of surgery in about half of the patients who undergo reverse shoulder arthroplasty (Fig. 25.11). This radiographic finding most likely occurs as a result of mechanical impingement of the medial aspect of the humeral component and the lateral aspect of the scapula just inferior to the glenoid. The impingement is exacerbated when the patient rotates the shoulder internally. This theory of mechanical impingement is further supported by the observation that the internal rotation seems to improve as the scapular notch progresses, thus suggesting that the prosthesis must "carve out" a portion of the scapula to maximize postoperative internal rotation. Another view of the cause of scapular notching is polyethylene wear causing osteolysis, although this theory currently has less support than that involving mechanical impingement.

Scapular notching is commonly accompanied by a scapular osteophyte just medial to the notch, which may represent ossification within the triceps related to an incomplete inferior release (Fig. 25.12). The degree of scapular notching has also been graded by severity (Fig. 25.13).[9] The best way to avoid scapular notching was theorized to be by initially placing the glenoid component inferiorly on the glenoid face and introducing slight inferior tilt during glenoid reaming (Fig. 25.14); however, we did not find a difference in scapular notching after comparing neutral versus 10 degrees of inferior tilt in a prospective randomized trial.[10] More recently with the use of onlay humeral designs that introduce more lateralized offset, we noted a lower incidence of scapular notching following reverse shoulder arthroplasty. Despite the concerning appearance of scapular notching, its clinical implications are unclear, with most of the evidence suggesting no adverse consequence. As long as the glenoid component remains stable, no treatment of an asymptomatic scapular notch is indicated.

Instability

Instability after reverse shoulder arthroplasty is the most common complication we have observed in our practice,

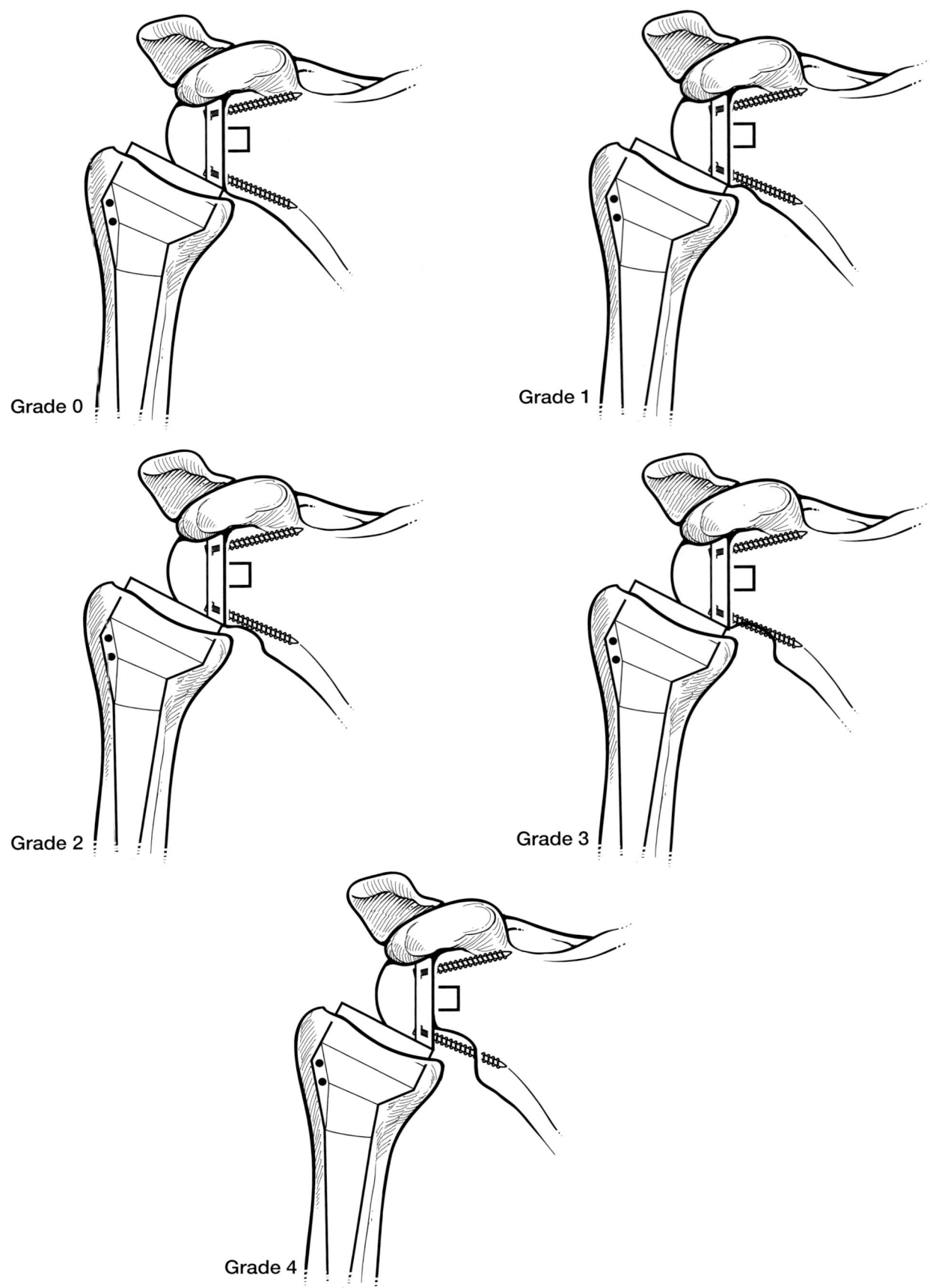

FIGURE 25.13 Classification of the inferior scapular notch occurring after reverse shoulder arthroplasty.

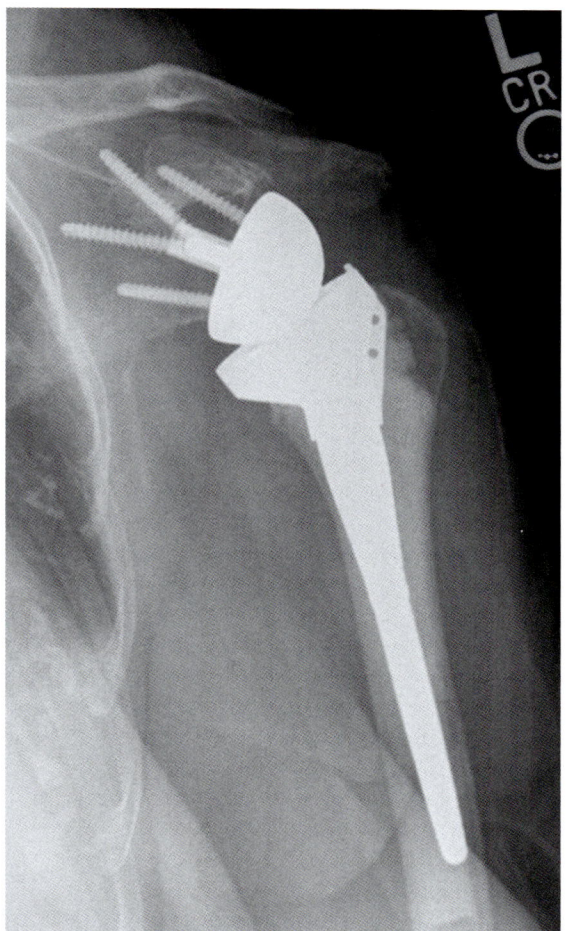

FIGURE 25.14 Avoidance of scapular notching by placing the glenoid component inferiorly on the glenoid face.

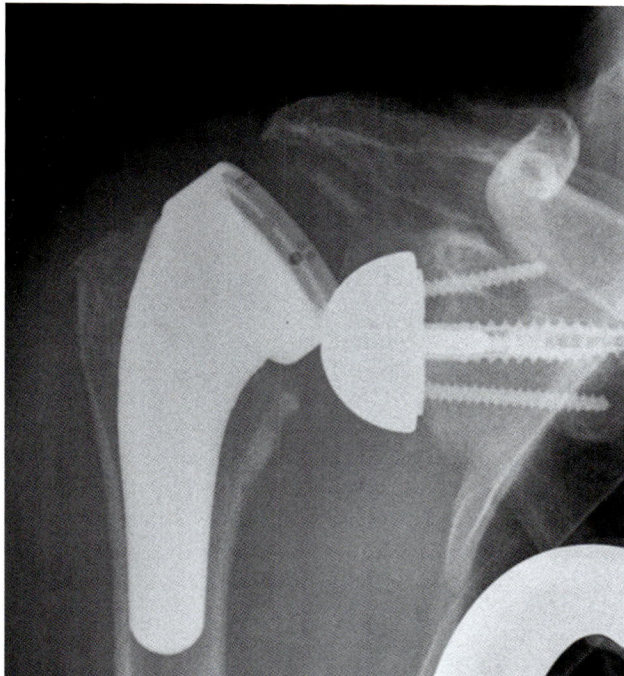

FIGURE 25.15 Dislocation of a reverse prosthesis.

occurring in approximately 5% of cases. Instability of a reverse prosthesis always occurs as a dislocation (Fig. 25.15). Most dislocations that we have observed have occurred within 6 weeks of reverse shoulder arthroplasty. The majority of patients do not realize that their shoulder is dislocated, with this being detected on radiography during routine follow-up. We have observed a few cases in which the patient could dislocate the prosthesis anteriorly with arm extension but could also perform a reduction maneuver to correct the dislocation (Fig. 25.16).

Instability of a reverse prosthesis can be related to various factors. In our experience, proximal humeral bone loss seems to be the greatest risk factor for dislocation of a reverse prosthesis. In this scenario, deltoid muscle tension is often solely responsible for stability of the implant because no rotator cuff or joint capsule exists to provide stability. Even if the deltoid is properly tensioned initially, it can gradually lose its tension and result in dislocation. A second major risk factor for dislocation of a reverse prosthesis is subscapularis insufficiency. All cases of dislocation that we have observed in our patients with the traditional Grammont-style implant have occurred in those without a reparable subscapularis. A less common factor contributing to dislocation of a reverse prosthesis is mechanical impingement causing the prosthetic socket to be levered away from the glenoid component. This impingement usually occurs inferiorly as the arm is adducted and is often related to positioning of the glenoid component too superior on the glenoid face (Fig. 25.17). Finally, we have observed two cases in which a patient had sustained a neuropraxic injury to the axillary nerve that resulted in prosthetic instability secondary to an inability to contract the deltoid. In most cases of dislocation, one or more of these factors are present.

In the majority of cases, initial treatment of a dislocated reverse prosthesis consists of closed reduction and a period of bracing. Closed reduction is performed in the operating room with the patient either heavily sedated or under general anesthesia. Under fluoroscopic guidance, an attempt is made to reduce the dislocation. If the prosthesis is successfully reduced, fluoroscopic examination is performed to ensure that mechanical impingement is not responsible for the instability. If the problem is not related to mechanical impingement and the prosthesis is reduced successfully, a brace is applied to maintain the arm with the humeral component centered on the glenoid component, generally in about 90 degrees of abduction with 30 degrees of forward flexion (Fig. 25.18). The patient maintains this brace at all times for 6 weeks, with radiographs performed in the brace every 7 to 10 days to confirm that the prosthesis has not dislocated (Fig. 25.19). After 6 weeks, the brace is discontinued and a normal rehabilitation regimen ensues.

If the prosthesis is not reducible by closed means, mechanical impingement is causing the dislocation, or closed reduction with bracing has failed, then open treatment and revision is indicated. Open reduction with insertion of a thicker and/or more constrained polyethylene spacer, insertion of an augmented metallic humeral tray, and upsizing the glenosphere component ensues (Fig. 25.20). Any mechanical

234 SECTION III ■ Reverse Shoulder Arthroplasty

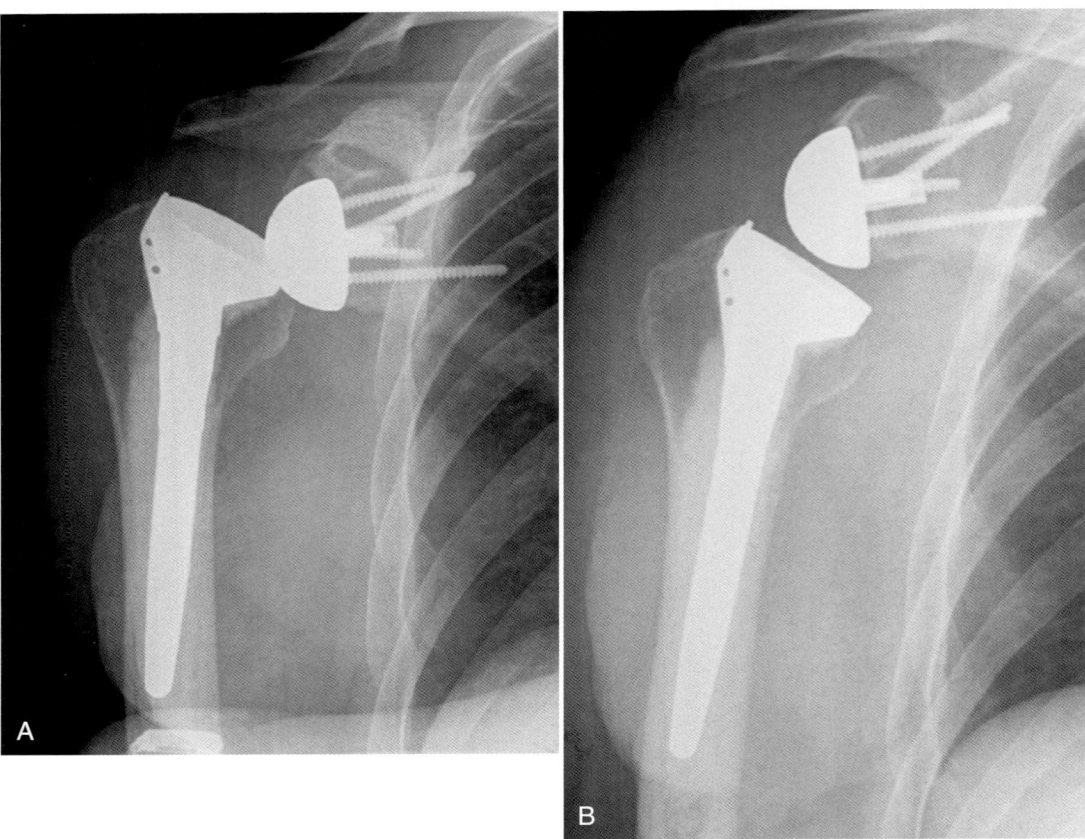

FIGURE 25.16 (A and B) Radiographs of a patient able to dislocate and relocate his reverse prosthesis because of inadequate deltoid tension.

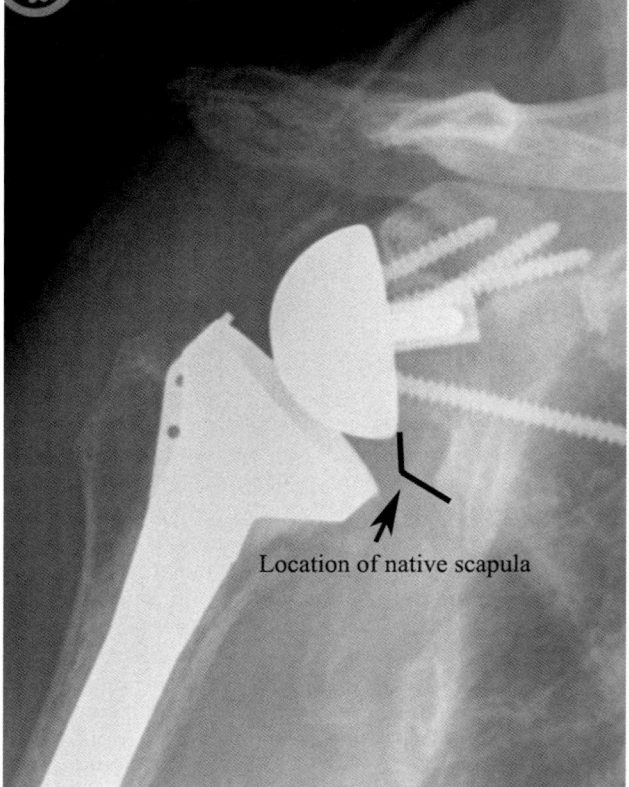

FIGURE 25.17 Positioning of the reverse glenoid component too superior on the glenoid face resulted in mechanical impingement.

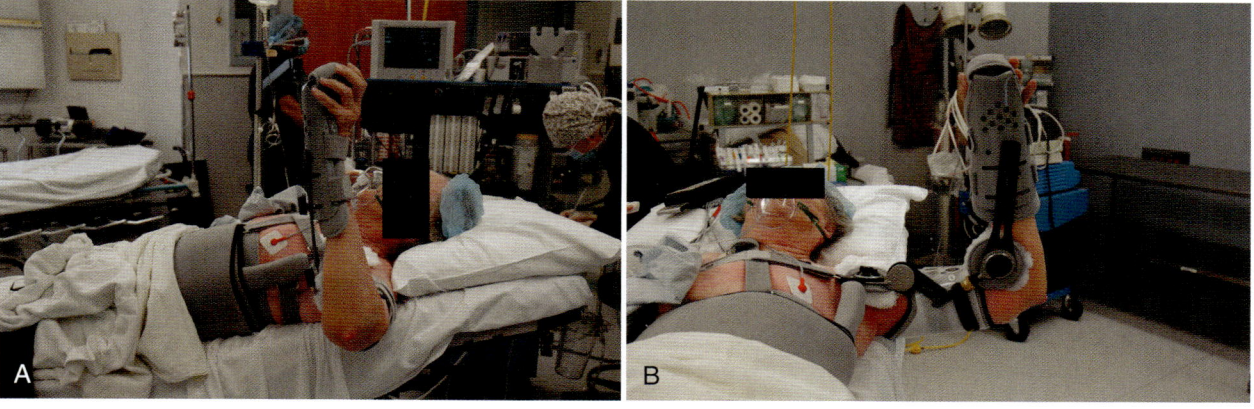

FIGURE 25.18 (A and B) Placement of a brace used for the treatment of a dislocated reverse prosthesis after closed reduction.

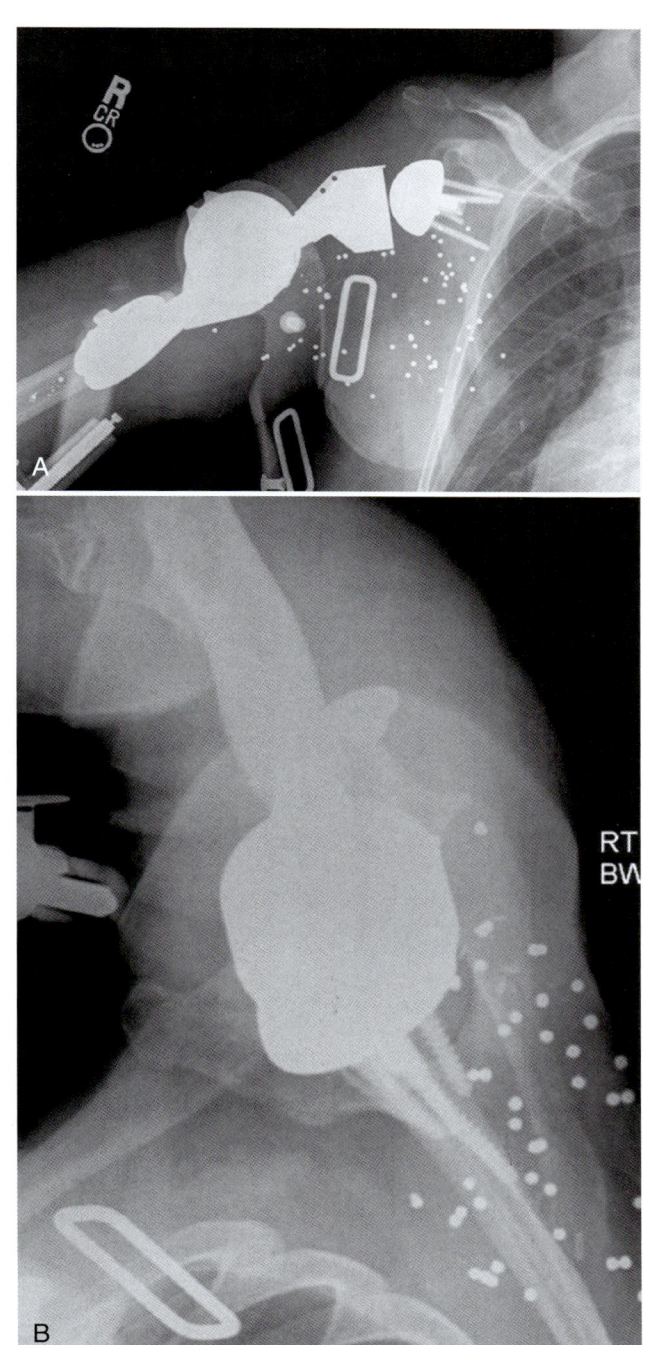

FIGURE 25.19 (A and B) Radiograph obtained in the brace, confirming maintenance of prosthetic reduction.

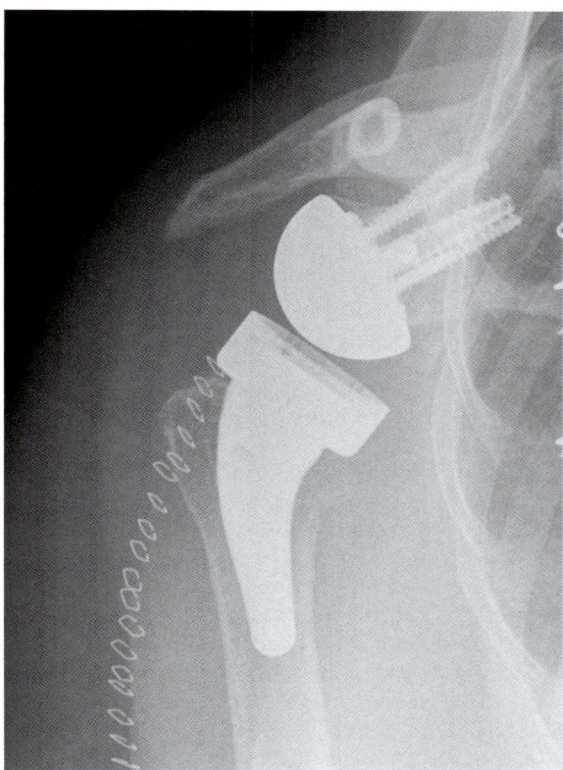

FIGURE 25.20 Treatment of a dislocated reverse prosthesis with insertion of a more constrained polyethylene spacer, insertion of an augmented metallic humeral tray, and upsizing of the glenosphere component.

impingement can simultaneously be addressed by careful removal of bone at the lateral aspect of the scapula just inferior to the glenoid component if necessary. Postoperatively, the patient is treated with the same bracing protocol used after closed reduction of a dislocated reverse prosthesis.

Stiffness

Glenohumeral stiffness after reverse shoulder arthroplasty is rare. Limitation of mobility after implantation of a reverse prosthesis is usually related to mechanical limitation of the prosthetic design and not capsular contracture. We personally have no experience in dealing with postoperative capsulitis after implantation of a reverse prosthesis.

Infection

Infection after primary reverse shoulder arthroplasty occurs at the same frequency as after unconstrained shoulder arthroplasty (<1% of cases). Patients most at risk for infection are those with systemic illness (diabetes mellitus), compromised soft tissues (radiation-induced osteonecrosis, posttraumatic arthritis), and inflammatory arthropathy (rheumatoid arthritis). These infections are most commonly caused by *Staphylococcus aureus* or *Propionibacterium acnes*. Infections after shoulder arthroplasty can be divided into perioperative (within 6 weeks of surgery) and late (hematogenous) infections.

Early perioperative infections are initially treated with two or three irrigation and débridement procedures and retention of the fixed components. With each irrigation and débridement procedure, the polyethylene liner of the humeral component is removed and the prosthesis is thoroughly cleaned. The original polyethylene liner is replaced after being cleaned during the initial one or two irrigation and débridement procedures. At the last planned irrigation and débridement procedure, absorbable antibiotic-impregnated beads (Osteoset, Wright Medical Technology, Inc., Memphis, Tennessee) are placed in the soft tissues around the shoulder and the polyethylene liner is replaced. Consultation with an infectious disease specialist is obtained, and a minimum of 6 weeks of intravenous antibiotics tailored to the specific organism causing the infection (or covering the most likely offending organisms if cultures remain negative despite obvious infection) is usually recommended. If this regimen fails, prosthetic removal ensues, as detailed in Section VI.

Late-appearing infections are treated by removal of the prosthesis, placement of antibiotic spacer, and intravenous administration of antibiotics as detailed in Section VI. The decision as to whether to place a revision shoulder arthroplasty or continue with a resection arthroplasty is patient-specific.

REFERENCES

1. Constant CR, Murley AH: A clinical method of functional assessment of the shoulder, *Clin Orthop Relat Res* 214:160–164, 1987.
2. Constant CR: Assessment of shoulder function. In Gazielly D, Gleyze P, Thomas T, editors: *The cuff*, New York, 1997, Elsevier, pp 39–44.
3. Nagda SH, Rogers KJ, Sestokas AK, et al: Neer Award 2005: peripheral nerve function during shoulder arthroplasty using intraoperative nerve monitoring, *J Shoulder Elbow Surg* 16(3 Suppl):S2–S8, 2007.
4. Parisien RL, Yi PH, Hou L, et al: The risk of nerve injury during anatomical and reverse total shoulder arthroplasty: an intraoperative neuromonitoring study, *J Shoulder Elbow Surg* 25(7):1122–1127, 2016.
5. Werner CML, Steinmann PA, Gilbart M, et al: Treatment of painful pseudoparesis due to irreparable rotator cuff dysfunction with the Delta III reverse-ball-and-socket total shoulder prosthesis, *J Bone Joint Surg Am* 87:1476–1486, 2005.
6. Kumar S, Sperling JW, Haidukewych GH, et al: Periprosthetic humeral fractures after shoulder arthroplasty, *J Bone Joint Surg Am* 86:680–689, 2004.
7. Teusink MJ, Otto RJ, Cottrell BJ, et al: What is the effect of postoperative scapular fracture on outcomes of reverse shoulder arthroplasty? *J Shoulder Elbow Surg* 23:782–790, 2014.
8. Crosby LA, Hamilton A, Twiss T: Scapula fractures after reverse total shoulder arthroplasty: classification and treatment, *Clin Orthop Relat Res* 469:2544–2549, 2011.
9. Valenti P, Boutens D, Nerot C: Delta 3 reversed prosthesis for osteoarthritis with massive rotator cuff tear: long term results (>5 years). In Walch G, Boileau P, Molé D, editors: *2000 Prosthèses d'Epaule ... Recul de 2 à 10 Ans*, Paris, 2001, Sauramps Medical, pp 253–259.
10. Edwards TB, Trappey GJ, Riley C, et al: Inferior tilt of the glenoid component does not decrease scapular notching in reverse shoulder arthroplasty: results of a prospective randomized study, *J Shoulder Elbow Surg* 21(5):641–646, 2012.

SECTION IV
SHOULDER ARTHROPLASTY FOR FRACTURE

CHAPTER 26
Indications and contraindications

The use of unconstrained humeral head replacement or reverse shoulder arthroplasty in cases involving acute fracture represents perhaps the most difficult indication for shoulder arthroplasty. Patients who are candidates for arthroplasty after proximal humeral fracture tend to be older, with age-related osteopenia. Complications, both systemic and shoulder-specific, are more common in this patient population than in patients undergoing unconstrained and reverse shoulder arthroplasty for chronic conditions. These factors contribute to the difficulty of treating proximal humeral fractures with unconstrained and reverse shoulder arthroplasty.

Neer popularized the use of humeral head replacement for the treatment of complex proximal humeral fractures.[1] Neer's classification of these fractures is the most commonly used scheme. Unfortunately, this classification system has been shown to have poor interobserver and intraobserver reliability.[2] Other classification schemes have been introduced, but their complexity has limited their usefulness. For us, the most important, readily observable factor that indicates the need for shoulder arthroplasty after proximal humeral fracture is the condition of the humeral head articular fragment (soft tissue attachments, bone quality, dislocation, head splitting). In all cases in which we are anticipating possible shoulder arthroplasty for the treatment of proximal humeral fracture, we obtain a computed tomography scan. Because of the widespread use of Neer's classification scheme, this chapter discusses our indications for unconstrained or reverse shoulder arthroplasty based on the condition of the humeral head fragment within the context of the Neer classification as determined by computed tomography.

FOUR-PART PROXIMAL HUMERAL FRACTURES

The most common indication for unconstrained or reverse shoulder arthroplasty for proximal humeral fracture is a four-part fracture. This refers to a fracture involving four distinct fragments, including a humeral head fragment, a greater tuberosity fragment, a lesser tuberosity fragment, and a humeral shaft fragment (Fig. 26.1). Neer did not consider a fragment to constitute a "part" unless it was displaced greater than 1 cm or angulated more than 45 degrees.[1] We have found strict application of these criteria to be difficult because determination of fragment angulation and even displacement can be complex despite the use of computed tomography. In any fracture that contains fracture lines separating the proximal humerus into four parts for which we plan operative treatment consisting of open reduction and internal fixation, we will be prepared to perform a hemiarthroplasty or reverse shoulder arthroplasty for fracture should the need arise intraoperatively. The two principal circumstances that make us opt for hemiarthroplasty or reverse shoulder arthroplasty, even in cases in which the tuberosities are displaced less than 1 cm, are when the humeral head fragment is discovered to be completely devoid of soft tissue attachment (Fig. 26.2) and when the bone in the humeral head is too severely osteopenic to permit any sort of fixation. In cases where each fragment is clearly displaced more than 1 cm, we plan to perform hemiarthroplasty or reverse shoulder arthroplasty for fracture from the outset (Fig. 26.3).

THREE-PART PROXIMAL HUMERAL FRACTURES

A less common indication for unconstrained shoulder arthroplasty for the treatment of proximal humeral fracture is a three-part fracture. This refers to a fracture involving three distinct fragments, including a humeral head fragment, a greater (more common) or lesser (less common) tuberosity fragment, and a humeral shaft fragment (Fig. 26.4). The majority of these fractures can be treated successfully with open reduction and internal fixation. In any fracture that contains fracture

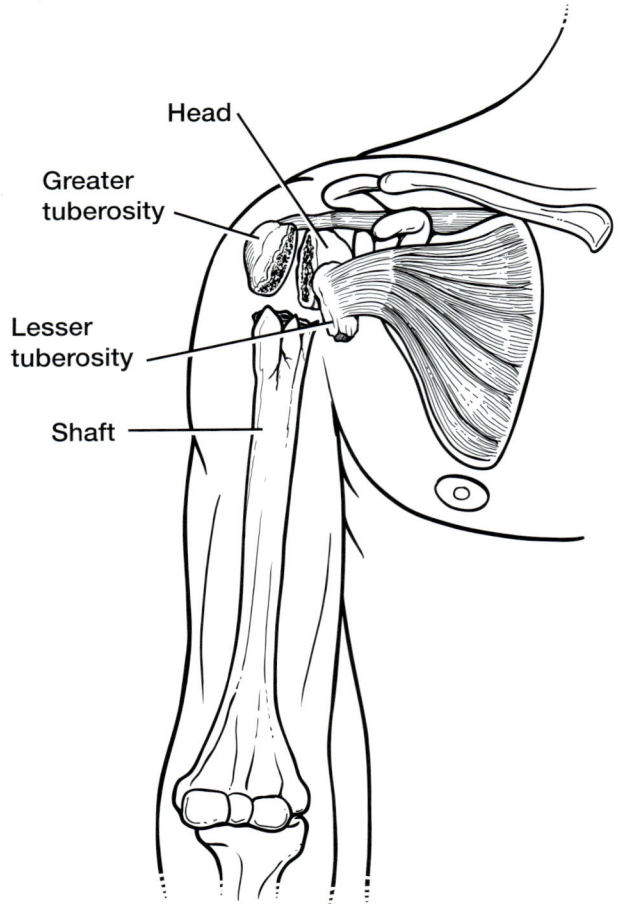

FIGURE 26.1 Schematic of the typical four-part proximal humeral fracture.

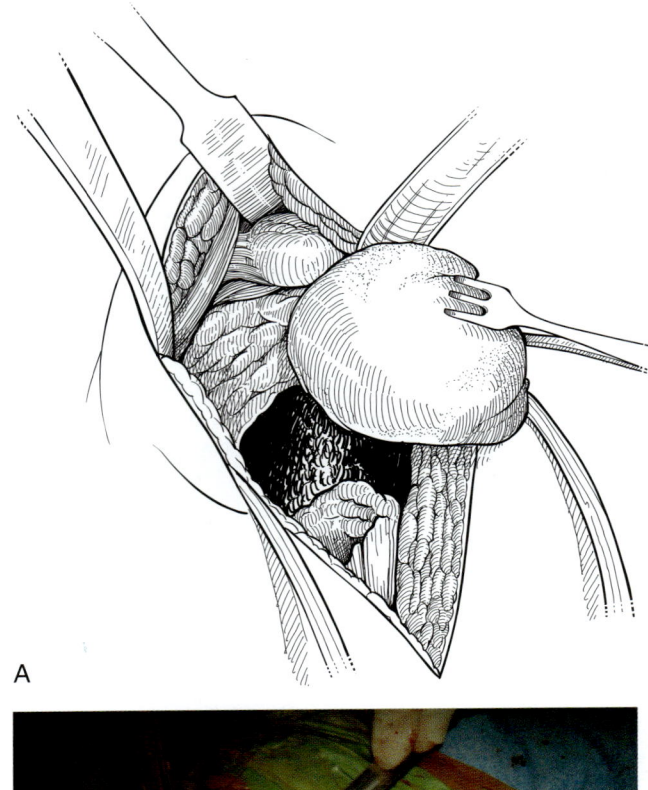

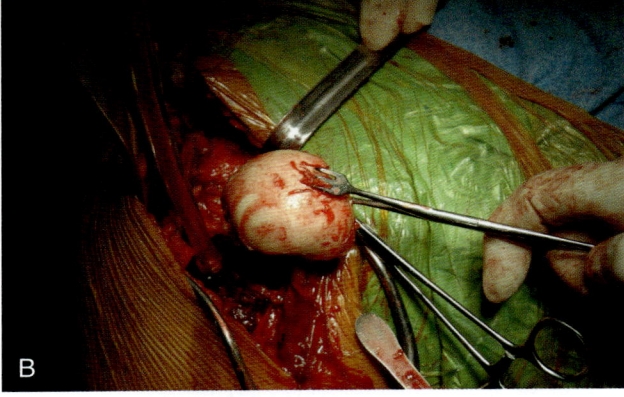

FIGURE 26.2 (A and B) Drawing and intraoperative photograph of a humeral head devoid of soft tissue attachment.

lines separating the proximal humerus into three parts for which we plan operative treatment consisting of open reduction and internal fixation, we will be prepared to perform a hemiarthroplasty or reverse shoulder arthroplasty should the need arise intraoperatively. The principal circumstance that makes us opt for hemiarthroplasty or reverse shoulder arthroplasty in three-part fractures, even in cases in which the tuberosities are displaced less than 1 cm, is when the bone in the humeral head is too severely osteopenic to permit any sort of fixation (Fig. 26.5). These cases require osteotomy of the lesser tuberosity at the time of arthroplasty.

FRACTURE-DISLOCATION

Occasionally a four- or three-part fracture will be accompanied by dislocation of the humeral head (Fig. 26.6). In these cases, we nearly always opt for arthroplasty over open reduction and internal fixation because the humeral head fragment is nearly always devoid of significant soft tissue attachment.

HEAD-SPLITTING FRACTURE

In fractures where the proximal humeral articular surface has been split, we opt for humeral hemiarthroplasty or reverse shoulder arthroplasty (Fig. 26.7). These cases nearly always occur with a greater or lesser tuberosity fracture (or both). Occasionally, dislocation of all or part of the proximal humeral articular surface will be present.

SPECIAL SITUATIONS

Severe Osteopenia

Severe osteopenia in an elderly patient is occasionally a contraindication to open reduction and internal fixation of a comminuted proximal humeral fracture (Fig. 26.8). Additionally, severe proximal humeral osteopenia may prevent healing of the tuberosities. In our practice, severe proximal humeral osteopenia and a proximal humeral fracture with indications for replacement is a relative indication for use of a reverse shoulder arthroplasty for fracture combined with fixation of the tuberosities. In this circumstance, in the event

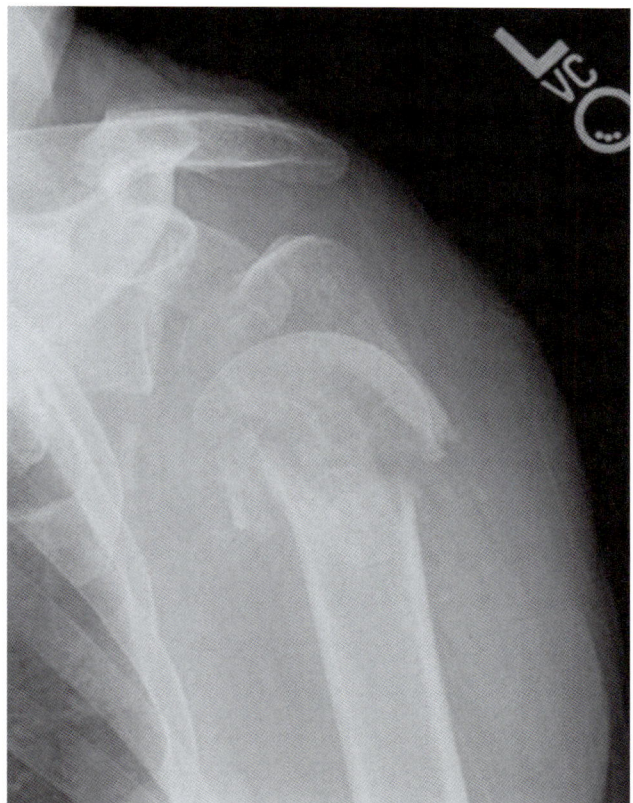

FIGURE 26.3 Displaced four-part proximal humeral fracture.

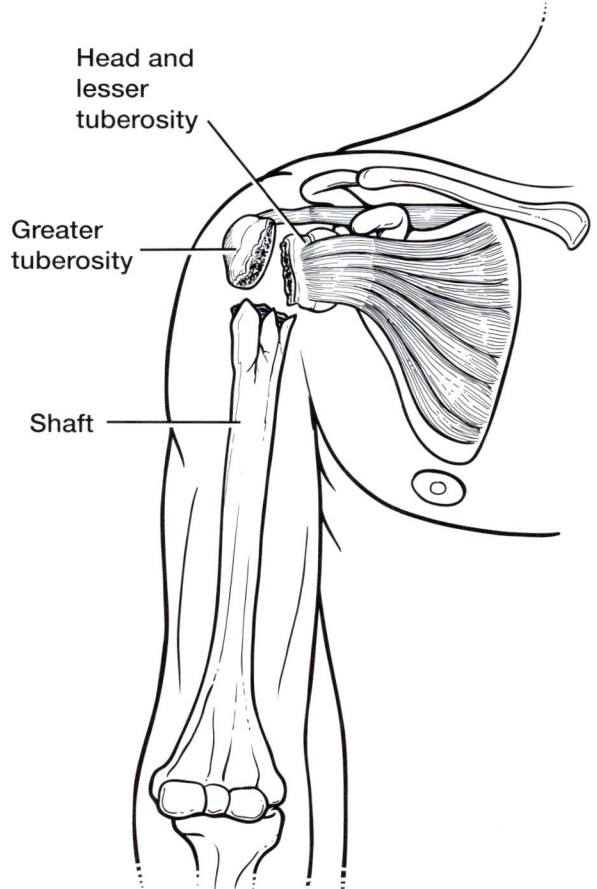

FIGURE 26.4 Schematic of the typical three-part proximal humeral fracture.

that the tuberosities do not heal, elevation may still be possible and prevent the need for further surgery.

Neural Injury

Many patients with proximal humeral fractures have signs of neural injury, most commonly deficits of the motor branch of the axillary nerve. These injuries are nearly always neuropraxias that spontaneously recover and do not represent a contraindication to arthroplasty for fracture. The patients need to be educated about this finding, however.

Glenoid Issues

In contrast to unconstrained shoulder arthroplasty performed for chronic conditions, in which we usually resurface the glenoid, we nearly always perform hemiarthroplasty without resurfacing the glenoid in cases of acute fracture. The only circumstance in the past that we would consider concomitant insertion of a glenoid component is a fracture occurring in the presence of end-stage glenohumeral arthritis. In our experience, this situation is exceedingly rare. Currently in this situation we would opt to treat with a reverse shoulder arthroplasty rather than a hemiarthroplasty with glenoid resurfacing.

Although it is true that glenoid erosion will develop in some patients after unconstrained hemiarthroplasty, the number of patients facing this problem is small relative to those who will experience nonunion or malunion of the tuberosity fragments. If tuberosity fixation failure occurs, the humerus will inevitably subluxate statically. Such subluxation causes nonconcentric loading of a glenoid component if it has been implanted and ultimately leads to failure of the glenoid component via the "rocking horse" phenomenon.[3] Additionally, revision to a reverse prosthesis in a patient with tuberosity fixation failure (our usual treatment in this scenario) is more easily performed if the native glenoid has not been previously violated. For these reasons, we prefer isolated humeral hemiarthroplasty in cases in which we use unconstrained shoulder arthroplasty for the treatment of proximal humeral fractures.

Rotator Cuff Pathology

Rarely, a patient with a massive rotator cuff tear that has been relatively asymptomatic will sustain a proximal humeral fracture requiring operative treatment. In this scenario, we opt for use of a reverse prosthesis with fixation of the tuberosities if some rotator cuff is still attached.

CONTRAINDICATIONS TO SHOULDER ARTHROPLASTY FOR FRACTURE

Contraindications to shoulder arthroplasty for acute proximal humeral fracture are listed in Table 26.1. Some of these contraindications are absolute, whereas others are relative.

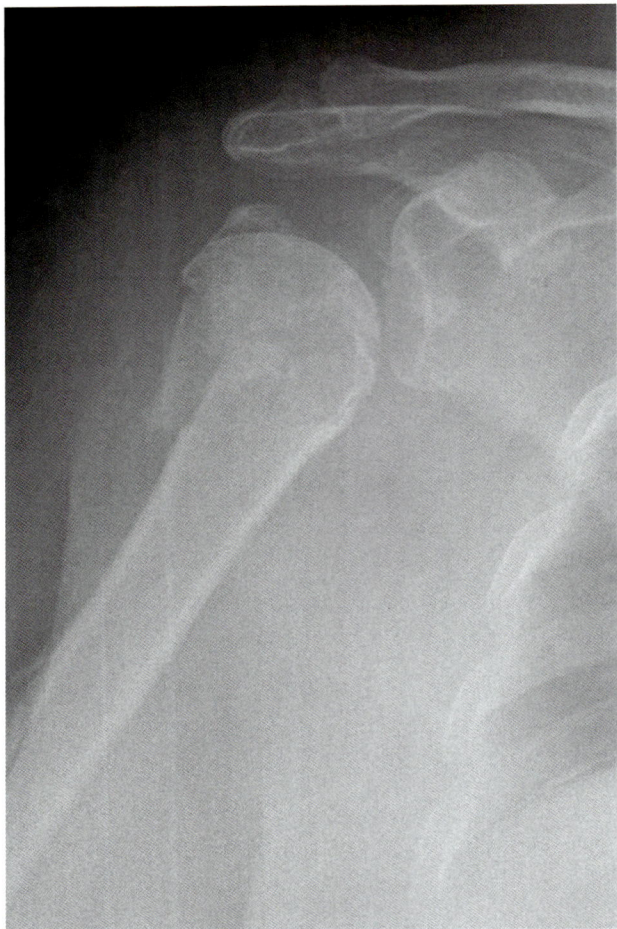

FIGURE 26.5 Severe osteopenia of the humeral head fragment in a three-part proximal humeral fracture, precluding open reduction and internal fixation.

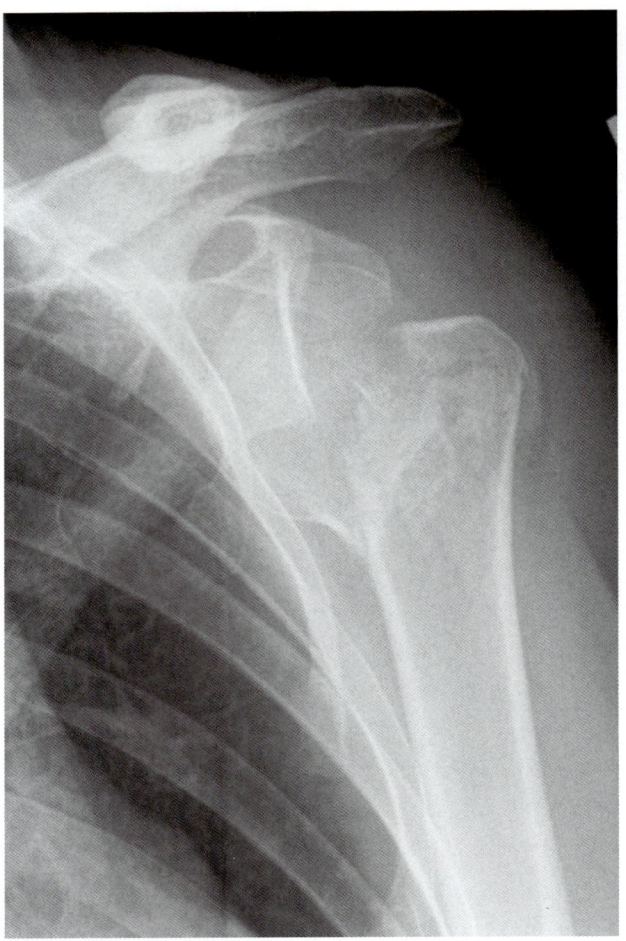

FIGURE 26.6 Proximal humeral fracture-dislocation.

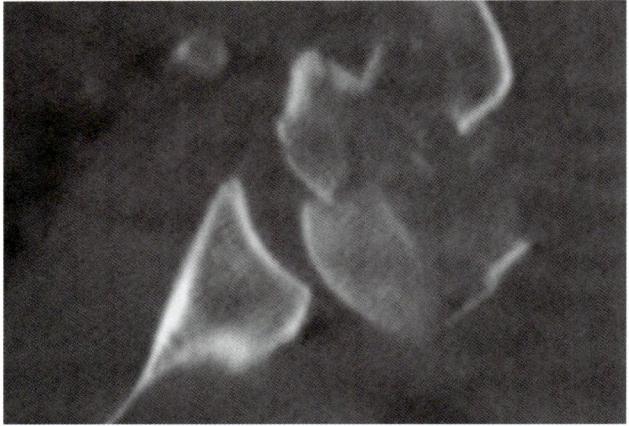

FIGURE 26.7 Head-splitting fracture of the proximal humerus.

CHOOSING UNCONSTRAINED HUMERAL HEAD REPLACEMENT OR REVERSE SHOULDER ARTHROPLASTY FOR PROXIMAL HUMERAL FRACTURE

As noted in the preceding discussion, there are some clear indications for shoulder arthroplasty for proximal humeral fracture. However, there continues to be debate about the best treatment choice between unconstrained humeral head replacement or reverse shoulder arthroplasty. Tuberosity healing is critical for the function of unconstrained humeral head replacement, while it is less critical for good functional results after reverse shoulder arthroplasty. Furthermore, reverse shoulder arthroplasty has typically shown better tuberosity healing rates and lower tuberosity resorption compared to unconstrained humeral head replacement. A consecutive series of 53 elderly patients (average age 74.4 years) with complex three- or four-part proximal humeral fractures underwent either unconstrained humeral head replacement (26 patients) or reverse shoulder arthroplasty (27 patients).[4] The study showed better forward flexion, patient outcomes, and satisfaction for reverse shoulder arthroplasty with a similar complication rate. A blinded prospective randomized study with 62 patients comparing unconstrained humeral head replacement to reverse shoulder

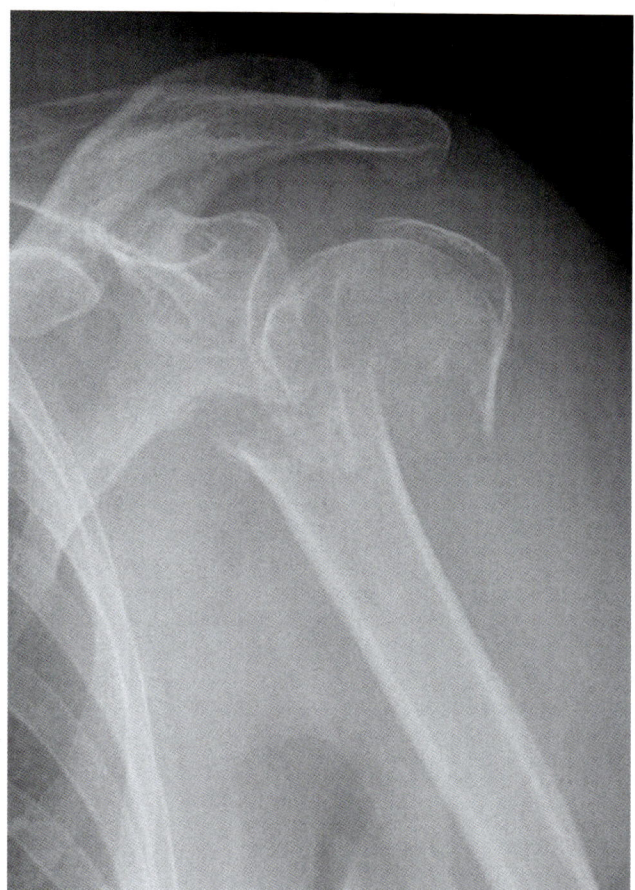

FIGURE 26.8 Severe proximal humeral osteopenia in an elderly patient with a proximal humeral fracture. In such a patient, we would consider use of a reverse prosthesis for treatment of the fracture acutely.

TABLE 26.1	Contraindications to Shoulder Arthroplasty for Acute Proximal Humeral Fractures	
Contraindication	Absolute or Relative	Comments
Nondisplaced fracture	Absolute	Nonoperative treatment
Fracture amenable to ORIF	Absolute	Should be treated by ORIF
Poor generalized health	Relative	Appropriate perioperative medical treatment required
Active infection	Absolute	
Massive rotator cuff tear	Relative	Relative contraindication for unconstrained arthroplasty and better suited for reverse prosthesis
Upper motor neuron lesion	Relative	Absolute contraindication if the patient has uncontrolled shoulder spasticity
Poor patient motivation	Relative	May best be treated nonoperatively; consider resection arthroplasty if the shoulder remains symptomatic

ORIF, Open reduction with internal fixation.

arthroplasty showed similar results in favor of reverse shoulder arthroplasty, with better pain and functional scores and a lower revision rate.[5]

We prefer reverse shoulder arthroplasty for fracture instead of unconstrained humeral head replacement for older patients with proximal humeral fractures following low-energy trauma. We have examined our own data comparing unconstrained humeral head replacement and reverse shoulder arthroplasty and have found better tuberosity healing and better results following reverse shoulder arthroplasty in this population (see Chapter 32). Unconstrained humeral head replacement would typically be reserved in our practice for younger patients with a high-energy injury in the setting of a fracture type described earlier that is not amenable to open reduction and internal fixation.

REFERENCES

1. Neer CS, II: Displaced proximal humeral fractures: Part 1: classification and evaluation, *J Bone Joint Surg Am* 52:1077–1089, 1970.
2. Siebenrock KA, Gerber C: The reproducibility of classification of fractures of the proximal end of the humerus, *J Bone Joint Surg Am* 75:1751–1755, 1993.
3. Franklin JL, Barrett WP, Jackins SE, et al: Glenoid loosening in total shoulder arthroplasty: association with rotator cuff deficiency, *J Arthroplasty* 3:39–46, 1988.
4. Cuff DJ, Pupello DR: Comparison of hemiarthroplasty and reverse shoulder arthroplasty for the treatment of proximal humeral fractures in elderly patients, *J Bone Joint Surg Am* 95(22):2050–2055, 2013.
5. Sebastiá-Forcada E, Cebrián-Gómez R, Lizaur-Utrilla A, et al: Reverse shoulder arthroplasty versus hemiarthroplasty for acute proximal humeral fractures. A blinded, randomized, controlled, prospective study, *J Shoulder Elbow Surg* 23(10):1419–1426, 2014.

CHAPTER 27
Preoperative planning and imaging

Preoperative planning is important for all shoulder arthroplasty indications, but it is most crucial for fracture cases. Although proximal humeral anatomy may be somewhat distorted by prolonged wear and osteophyte formation in cases of chronic disease for which shoulder arthroplasty is performed, most reliable anatomic landmarks remain consistent despite the disease process. In fracture cases, however, these normally reliable landmarks are often displaced, thus making them useless as points of reference. Because of the lack of recognizable landmarks, preoperative planning is critical to establish the proper position for humeral stem implantation. Thorough preoperative planning minimizes the risk of placing the humeral stem at the incorrect height or version.[1] Preoperative planning is of paramount importance and is detailed in this chapter. Additionally, important aspects of the clinical history and physical examination, the radiographic examination, and secondary imaging studies are highlighted.

CLINICAL HISTORY AND EXAMINATION

A thorough history is taken of the antecedent trauma responsible for the fracture. Most often, these proximal humeral fractures are caused by a fall from a standing position. Elucidation of the reason for the fall should be sought to assist in evaluating any underlying contributing medical conditions (i.e., syncope as a symptom of cardiac arrhythmia). The presence of any shoulder problems before the fracture should be noted in the history. A previous history of shoulder pathology, such as a massive rotator cuff tear or glenohumeral arthritis, influences surgical decision making (i.e., the type of prosthesis to be implanted, such as an unconstrained fracture prosthesis or reverse shoulder prosthesis).

Physical examination in a patient with an acute proximal humeral fracture is limited so that the patient will not be subjected to pain unnecessarily. A detailed neurovascular examination is performed with specific attention to the sensory and motor function of the axillary nerve. The sensory function of the axillary nerve can always be evaluated by testing sensibility to touch of the posterior aspect of the upper part of the arm (superior lateral brachial cutaneous branch of the axillary nerve). Motor function of the axillary nerve may be more difficult to evaluate because pain induced by the fracture may inhibit deltoid contraction. The condition of the soft tissues, particularly anterior at the planned surgical site, is meticulously evaluated.

RADIOGRAPHY

Three radiographic views are obtained in all patients with a proximal humeral fracture. We prefer the same radiographic views that we obtain for patients being considered for unconstrained shoulder arthroplasty for chronic conditions: an anteroposterior view of the glenohumeral joint with the arm in neutral rotation (Fig. 27.1), an axillary view (Fig. 27.2), and a scapular outlet view (Fig. 27.3). These radiographs are used to evaluate the fracture pattern (two-, three-, and four-part fractures), the amount of displacement of the fracture fragments, the presence of humeral head dislocation and of a split in the humeral head fragment. Frequently the patient has radiographs obtained in an emergency department that are of poor quality. We always repeat these radiographs to obtain better-quality films and to assess for progressive displacement. Once it is determined that the patient is a potential candidate for shoulder arthroplasty, anteroposterior full-length radiographs of both humeri taken with the arm in neutral rotation are obtained for use in preoperative determination of appropriate humeral head height. These radiographs must include the entire length of the humerus and must be controlled for magnification (Fig. 27.4).

SECONDARY IMAGING

Computed tomography is performed in all patients with substantially displaced proximal humeral fractures (Fig. 27.5). This study allows further elucidation of the fracture pattern and assessment of the amount of displacement of the fracture fragments. Additionally, the position of the tuberosities and humeral head is visualized, thereby allowing easier identification at the time of surgery. Any comminution of the tuberosities can also be identified with computed tomography.

PROSTHETIC POSITIONING FOR UNCONSTRAINED HUMERAL HEAD REPLACEMENT FOR FRACTURE—THE GOTHIC ARCH TECHNIQUE

Placement of the prosthesis at the correct height and version remains one of the most difficult challenges in performing shoulder arthroplasty for fracture, especially with unconstrained humeral head replacement. Sumant "Butch" Krishnan has developed a technique for prosthetic positioning that

CHAPTER 27 ■ Preoperative Planning and Imaging 243

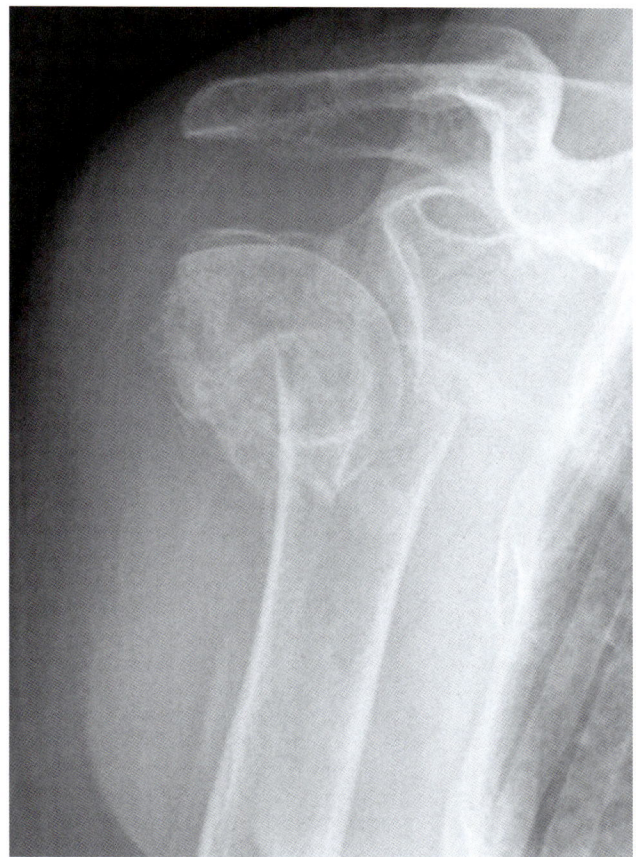

FIGURE 27.1 Anteroposterior radiograph in a patient with a comminuted proximal humeral fracture.

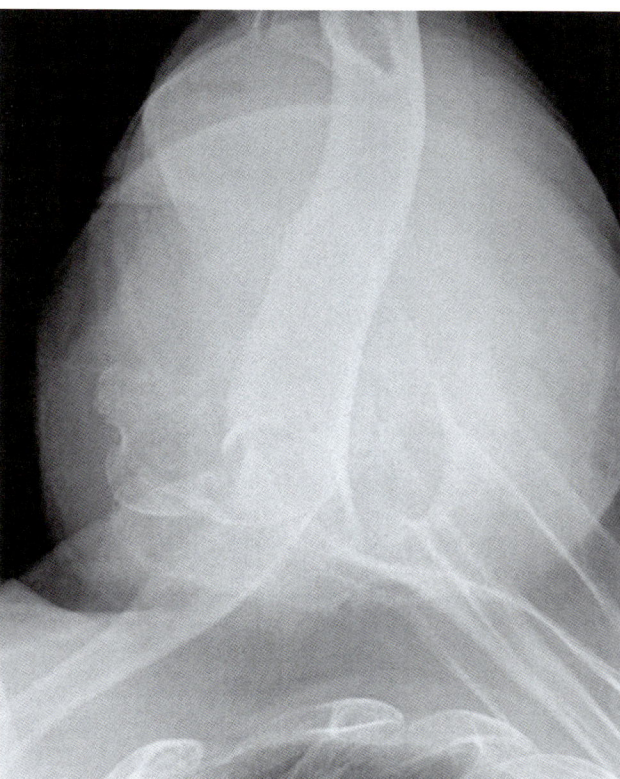

FIGURE 27.2 Axillary radiograph in a patient with a comminuted proximal humeral fracture.

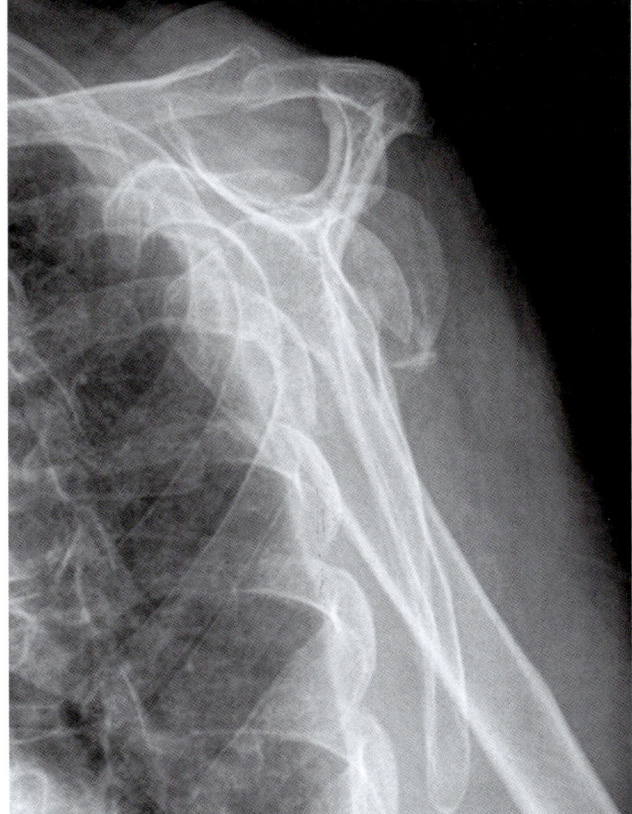

FIGURE 27.3 Scapular outlet radiograph in a patient with a comminuted proximal humeral fracture.

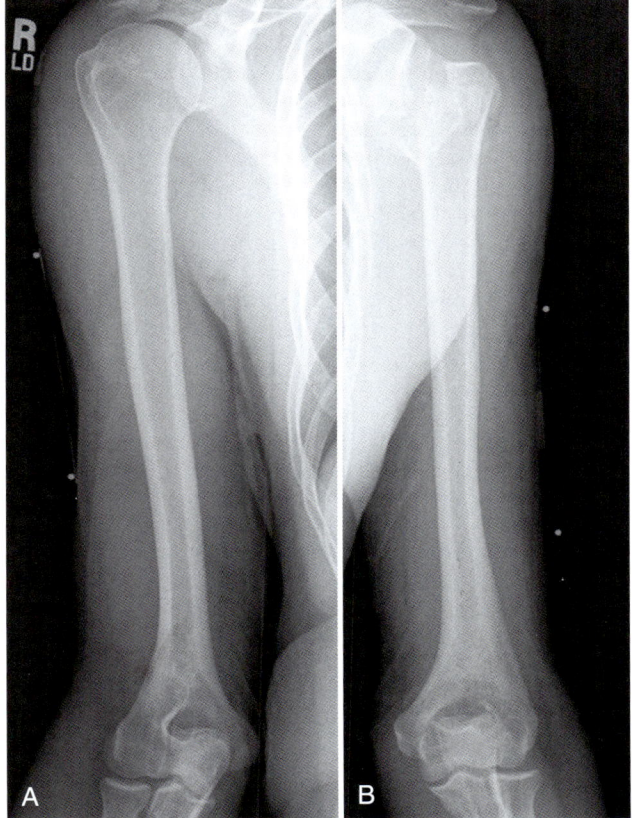

FIGURE 27.4 (A and B) Bilateral anteroposterior humeral radiographs that have been controlled for magnification.

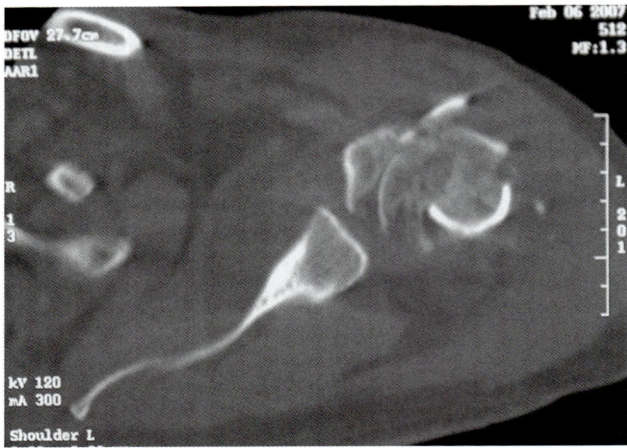

FIGURE 27.5 Computed tomography scan of a comminuted proximal humeral fracture being evaluated for hemiarthroplasty.

we have found useful and reproducible; he terms the technique "restoration of the Gothic arch."[2]

When using this technique it is necessary to perform preoperative planning with anteroposterior radiographs of the affected and unaffected humeri. From this radiograph, the length of the humerus from the superior aspect of the humeral head to the transepicondylar axis is measured and normalized for magnification. This measurement is obtained by first establishing the prosthetic axis proximally within the humeral canal. This is done by measuring the center point of the proximal diaphysis at two locations and connecting these points with a line running the length of the humerus. Next, a line perpendicular to the prosthetic axis is drawn at the superior aspect of the humeral head (Fig. 27.6). A third line intersecting the prosthetic axis is drawn at the transepicondylar axis of the distal humerus. The distance between the superior aspect of the humeral head and the transepicondylar axis is measured in centimeters along the prosthetic axis (Fig. 27.7). This value is corrected for magnification if necessary (a digital radiography system does this step automatically at our institution) by using the mathematical formula shown in the example in Fig. 27.8.

By using the anteroposterior humeral radiograph of the affected extremity, the prosthetic axis and transepicondylar axis are established (Fig. 27.9). A line perpendicular to the prosthetic axis is drawn at the level of the fracture medially (Fig. 27.10). The distance between the medial fracture line and the transepicondylar axis (residual humeral length) is measured and corrected for magnification if necessary (Fig. 27.11). In cases where the greater tuberosity is visible as a single fragment, the length of the greater tuberosity is measured and corrected for magnification (Fig. 27.12). The difference between humeral length measured on the unaffected radiograph and residual humeral length measured on the affected radiograph is calculated (Fig. 27.13). This difference is marked on the humeral implant to establish the height at which the humeral stem should be positioned with respect to the medial fracture line (Fig. 27.14). The length of the

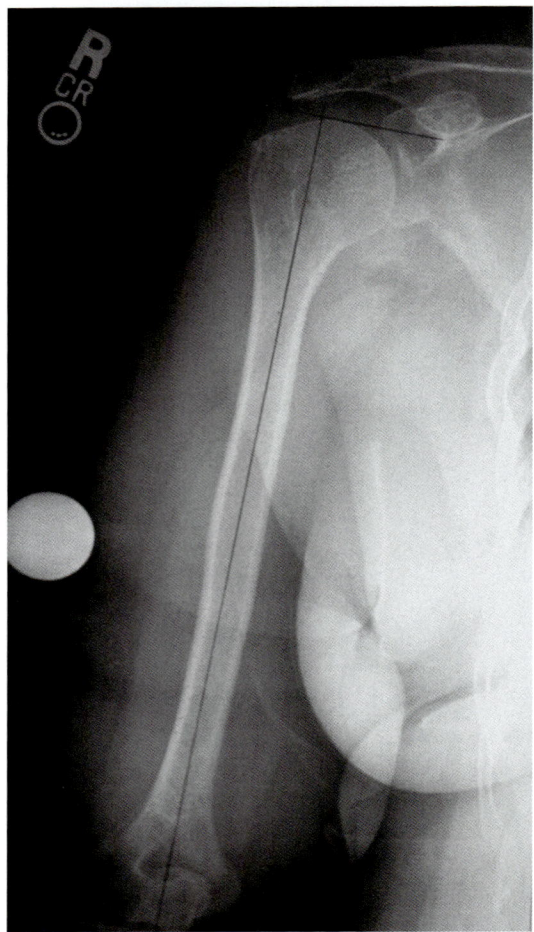

FIGURE 27.6 When using the Gothic arch technique, a perpendicular line to the prosthetic axis is drawn at the superior aspect of the humeral head.

greater tuberosity, when available, is used as a check rein. When the length of the greater tuberosity is added to length of the residual humerus, the sum should be approximately 3 to 5 mm less than the humeral length measured on the radiograph of the unaffected humerus (Fig. 27.15).

PROSTHETIC POSITIONING FOR REVERSE SHOULDER ARTHROPLASTY FOR FRACTURE WITH ANCILLARY INSTRUMENTATION

Placement of the prosthesis at the correct height and version is critical for reverse shoulder arthroplasty for fracture. Use of specialized instrumentation enhances the surgeon's ability to place the prosthesis at the correct height and version to help ensure stability of the reverse prosthesis. A height gauge that attaches to the humeral trial implant and the final humeral implant is used to reproduce humeral height and humeral version (see Chapter 29).

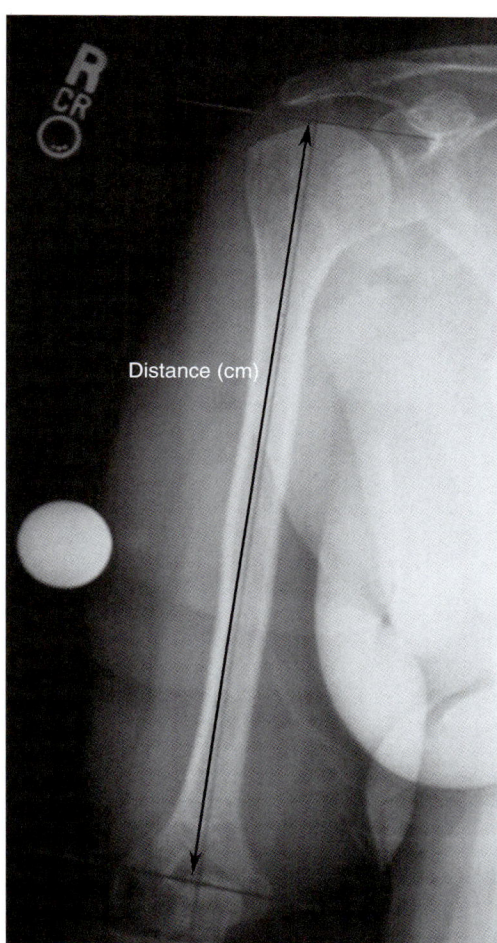

FIGURE 27.7 In the Gothic arch technique, the distance between the superior aspect of the humeral head and the transepicondylar axis is measured in centimeters along the prosthetic axis.

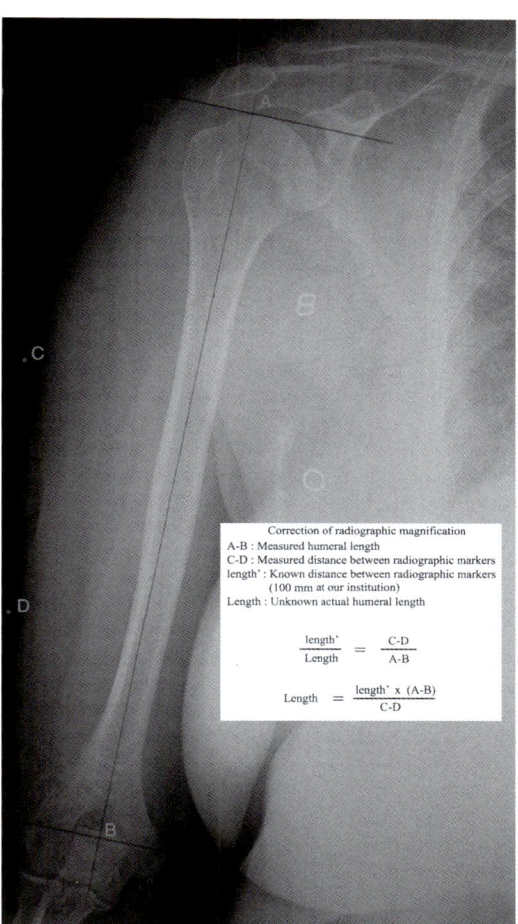

FIGURE 27.8 Example of correction for radiographic magnification.

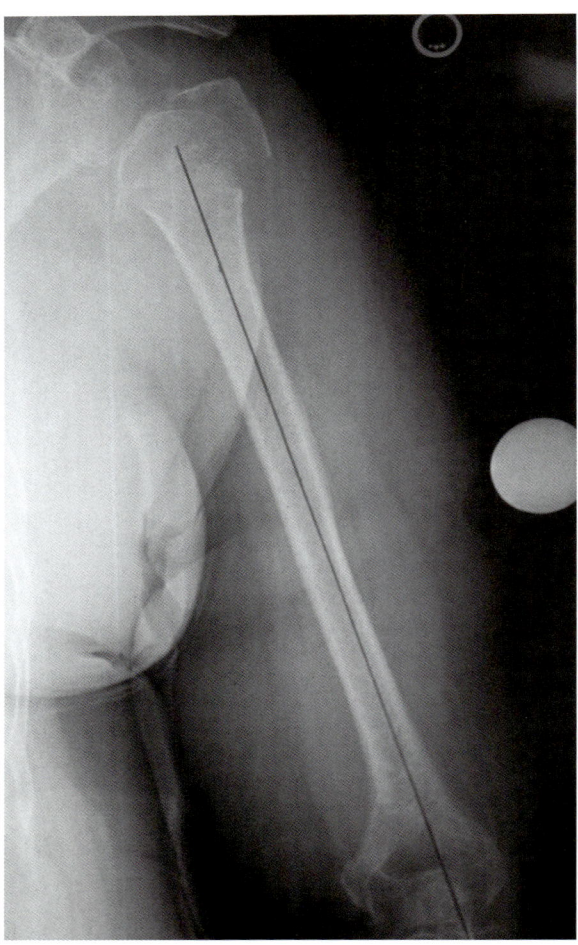

FIGURE 27.9 By using an anteroposterior humeral radiograph of the affected extremity, the prosthetic axis and transepicondylar axis are established for the Gothic arch technique.

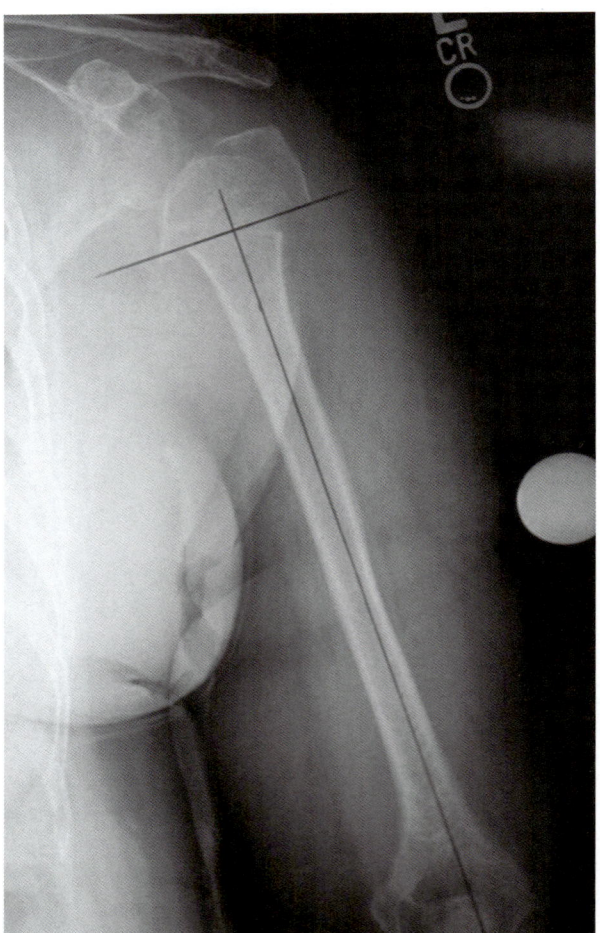

FIGURE 27.10 A perpendicular line to the prosthetic axis is constructed at the level of the fracture medially for the Gothic arch technique.

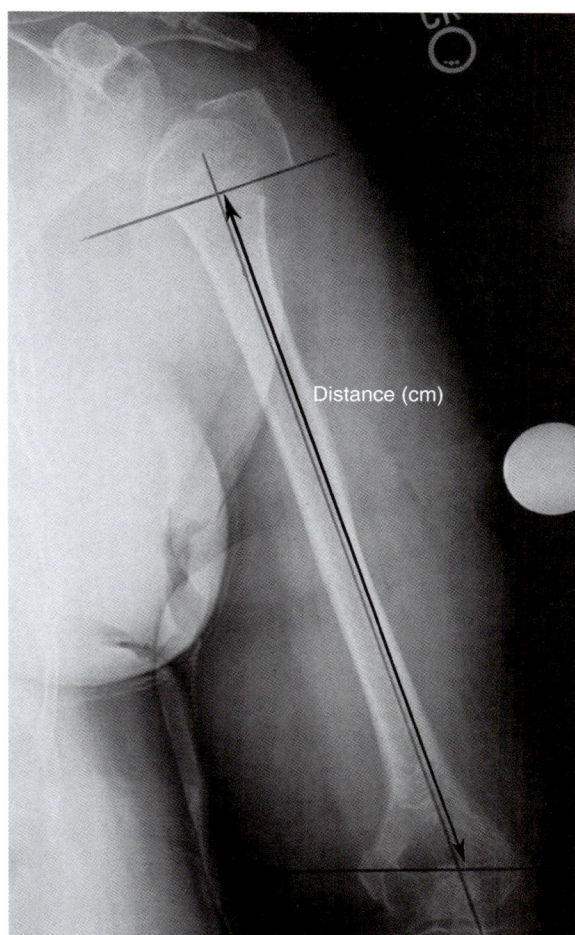

FIGURE 27.11 The distance between the medial fracture line and the transepicondylar axis (residual humeral length) is measured and corrected for magnification if necessary.

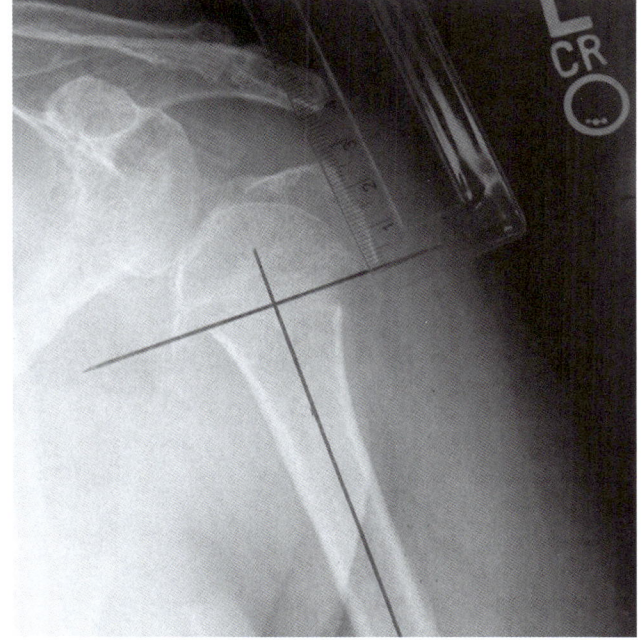

FIGURE 27.12 The length of the greater tuberosity is measured and corrected for magnification.

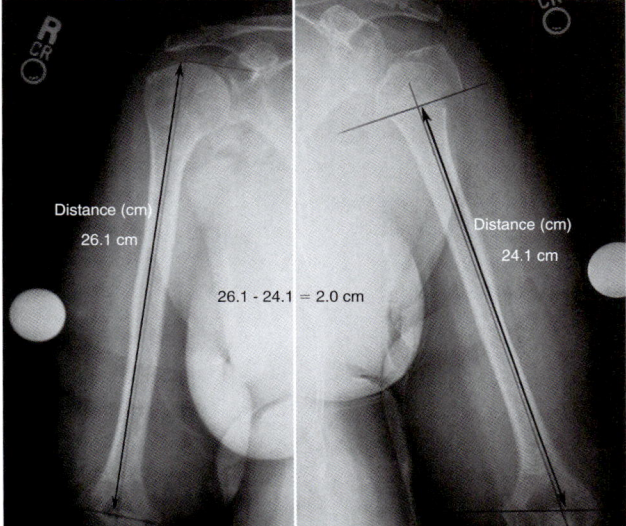

FIGURE 27.13 The difference between the humeral length measured from the unaffected radiograph and the residual humeral length measured from the affected radiograph is calculated.

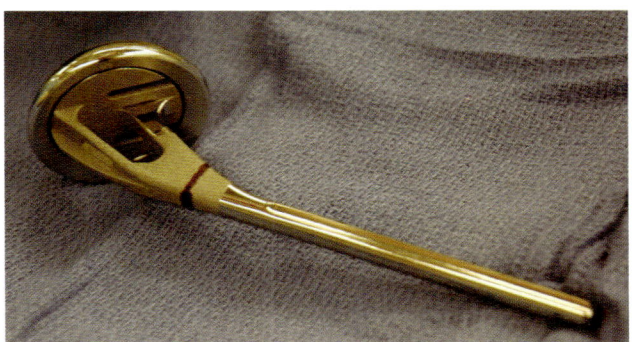

FIGURE 27.14 The difference between the humeral length measured on the unaffected humeral radiograph and the residual humeral length measured on the affected humeral radiograph is marked on the humeral implant to establish the height at which the humeral stem should be positioned with respect to the medial fracture line.

REFERENCES

1. Boileau P, Coste JS, Ahrens PM, et al: Prosthetic shoulder replacement for fracture: results of the multicentre study. In Walch G, Boileau P, Molé D, editors: *2000 Prosthèses d'Epaule ... Recul de 2 à 10 Ans*, Paris, 2001, Sauramps Medical, pp 561–578.
2. Krishnan SG, Pennington SD, Burkhead WZ, et al: Shoulder arthroplasty for fracture: restoration of the "gothic arch," *Tech Shoulder Elbow Surg* 6:57–66, 2005.

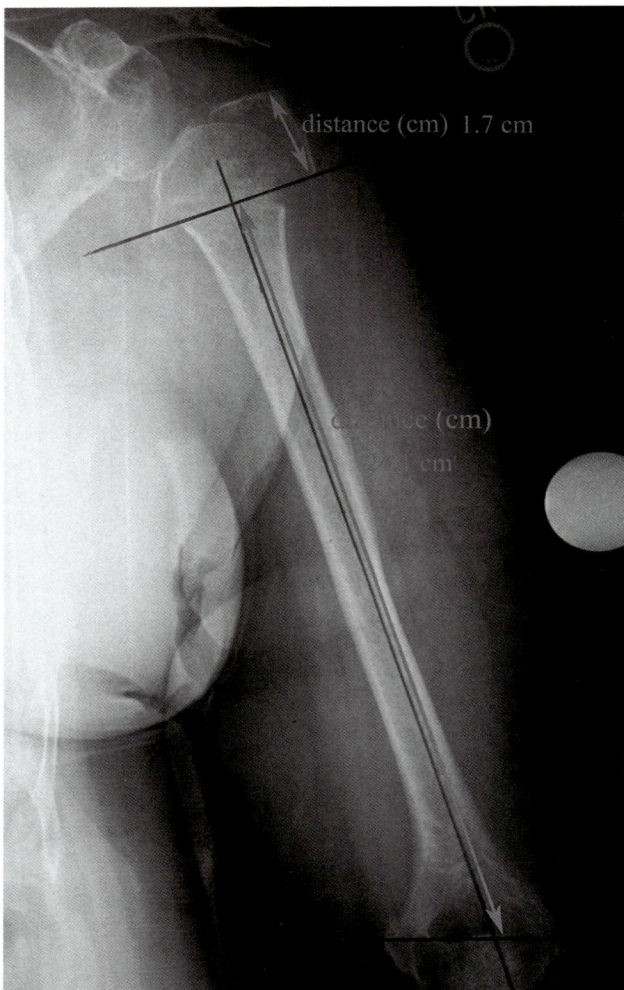

Residual humeral length: 24.1 cm
Greater tuberosity length: 1.7 cm
24.1 cm + 1.7 cm = 25.8 cm

Length of unaffected humerus: 26.1 cm
26.1 − 25.8 = 0.3 cm

FIGURE 27.15 The length of the greater tuberosity is used as a check rein. When the length of the greater tuberosity is added to the residual length of the humerus measured on the affected humeral radiograph, this calculation should be approximately 3 to 5 mm less than the humeral length measured on the unaffected humeral radiograph.

Surgical approach and handling of the tuberosities

CHAPTER 28

SURGICAL APPROACH

In shoulder arthroplasty for fracture (Video 28.1), operating room setup, anesthesia, patient positioning, surgical site preparation, and sterile draping (Chapters 3 and 4) are essentially the same as for nonfracture cases.

A standard deltopectoral approach is used for exposure, as in arthroplasty surgery performed for chronic conditions. The skin incision starts at the tip of the coracoid process and extends distally and laterally approximately 10 to 15 cm, depending on the size of the patient. A needle-tip electrocautery is used for deep dissection throughout the procedure in order to minimize hemorrhage. The interval between the deltoid and pectoralis major is identified by locating the cephalic vein. Once the cephalic vein has been identified, it is retracted laterally with the deltoid muscle. The superior centimeter of the pectoralis major tendon is divided with the electrocautery to further enhance exposure. A self-retaining deltopectoral retractor is placed to maintain exposure during the procedure. The conjoined tendon is identified and traced to its insertion on the coracoid process. The tip of a Hohmann-type retractor is placed behind the base of the coracoid process to provide proximal retraction. With the arm abducted and externally rotated, the apex formed by the insertion of the coracoacromial ligament and the conjoined tendon onto the coracoid process is identified. The conjoined tendon is retracted medially to expose the proximal humeral fracture (Fig. 28.1).

IDENTIFICATION AND HANDLING OF THE TUBEROSITY

A Cobb elevator is used to perform blunt dissection and begin the process of identification of the tuberosities (Fig. 28.2). In the prototypical four-part fracture pattern, the lesser tuberosity with the attached subscapularis represents one fragment, the greater tuberosity with the attached posterior superior rotator cuff represents a second fragment, the humeral head represents a third fragment, and the humeral shaft represents the final fragment. Various combinations exist; however, the most common fracture pattern for which arthroplasty is indicated involves these major fracture fragments. Control of the lesser tuberosity is achieved by identifying the tuberosity and subscapularis tendon anteriorly in the shoulder just posterior to the conjoined tendon. Stay sutures of no. 1 polyester are placed through the subscapularis tendon just medial to its osseous insertion on the lesser tuberosity. One suture is placed superiorly and a second suture is placed inferiorly if necessary (Fig. 28.3). Sutures are not placed through the lesser tuberosity because it is usually osteopenic and does not support transosseous sutures sufficiently. These sutures will also aid in retracting the lesser tuberosity to gain access to the humeral head fragment. The humeral head fragment is identified and may be dislocated or split into two or more fragments. The humeral head is removed with locking forceps (Lahey type) and kept on the sterile field for later use as bone graft material (Fig. 28.4).

Removal of the humeral head facilitates identification of the greater tuberosity, which is located posteriorly in the shoulder. Frequently, especially in elderly patients in whom these fractures are most common, the greater tuberosity is a mere shell of thin cortical bone and must be handled with care to avoid further fracture (Fig. 28.5). Control of the greater tuberosity and attached posterior superior rotator cuff is obtained by passing no. 2 braided looped permanent sutures through the rotator cuff tendons just medial to their insertion on the greater tuberosity. One looped suture is passed through the rotator cuff at the junction of the supraspinatus and infraspinatus. A second looped suture is passed through the rotator cuff at the junction of the infraspinatus and teres minor (Fig. 28.6). These sutures provide immediate control of the greater tuberosity and are used later as passing sutures for fixation of both the greater and lesser tuberosities. As with the lesser tuberosity, sutures are not placed through the greater tuberosity because it is usually osteopenic and does not support transosseous sutures sufficiently. Occasionally it is necessary to temporarily grasp the greater tuberosity with Lahey forceps to provide traction and enable suture placement. This should always be done gently and with great care to avoid further fracture of the tuberosity.

Rarely, arthroplasty is indicated in patients in whom the greater or lesser tuberosity remains attached to the humeral head (fracture-dislocation, head-splitting fracture). In these cases the tuberosity must be detached from the humeral head fragment. A 1-inch osteotome is used while leaving as much bone with the tuberosity fragment as possible (Fig. 28.7). The tuberosity is then handled as with a four-part fracture, as described earlier.

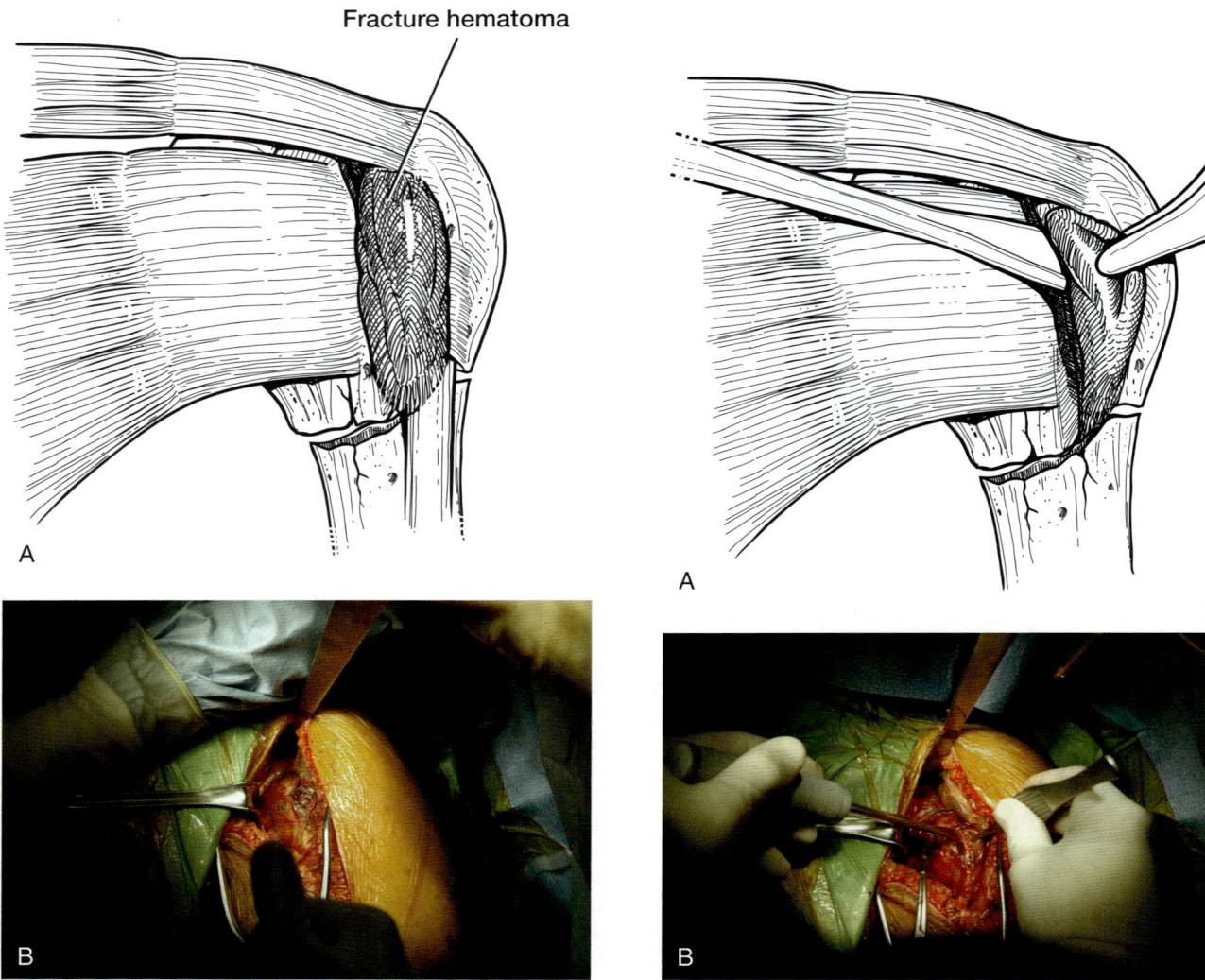

FIGURE 28.1 (A and B) Identification of the proximal humeral fracture.

FIGURE 28.2 (A and B) Development of fracture planes with a Cobb elevator.

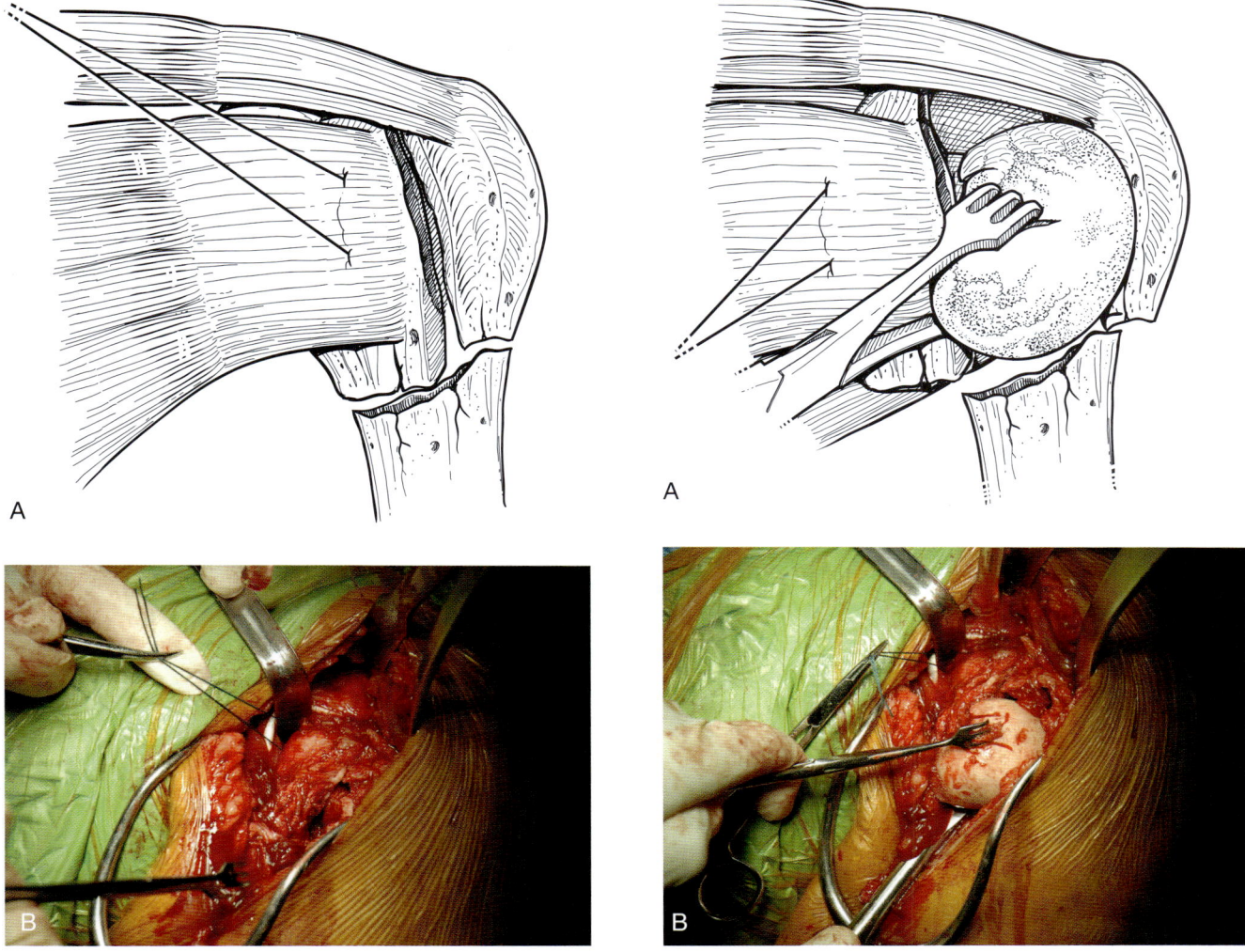

FIGURE 28.3 (A and B) Control of the lesser tuberosity with stay sutures placed through the subscapularis tendon.

FIGURE 28.4 (A and B) Removal of the humeral head fragment.

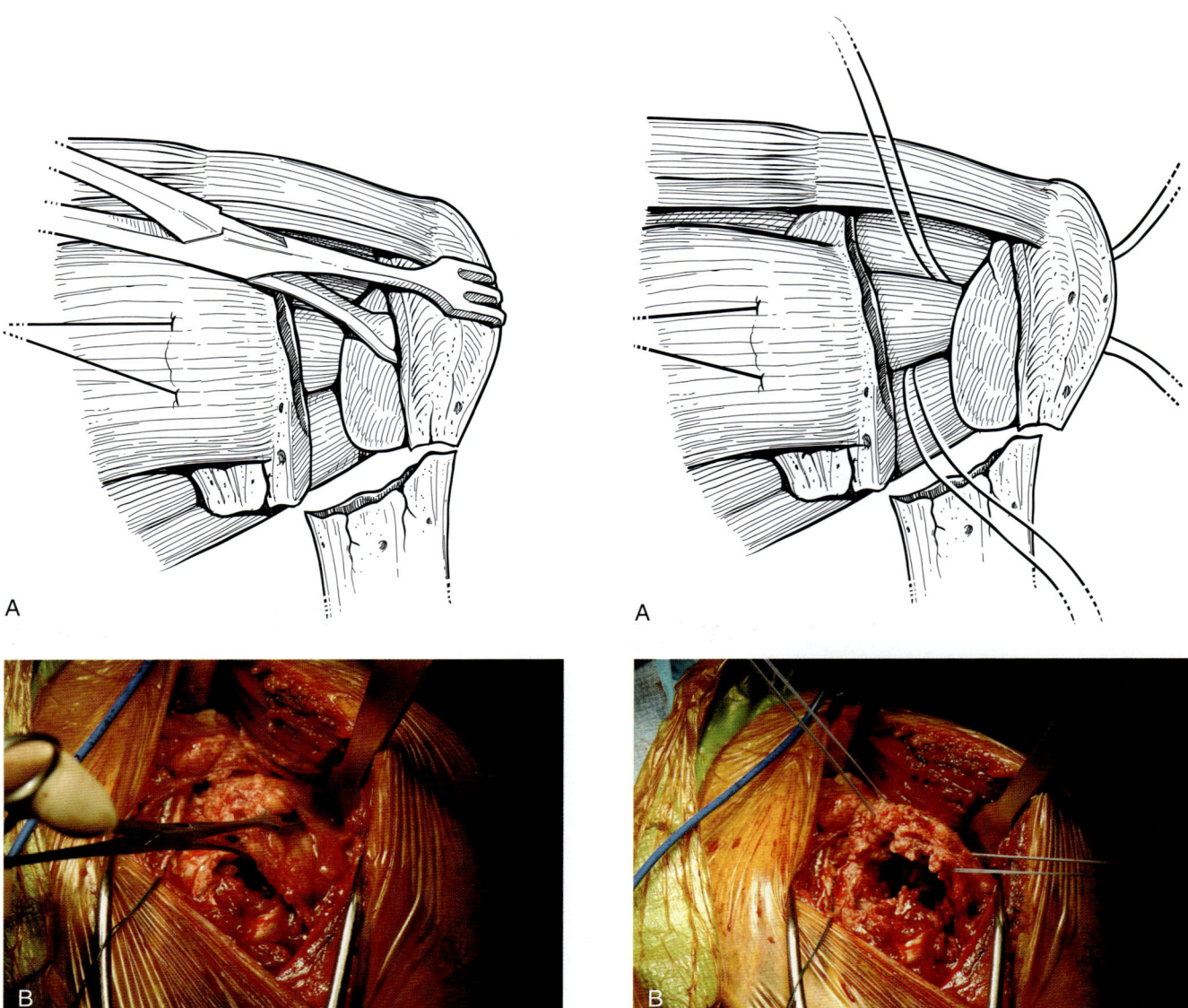

FIGURE 28.5 (A and B) Thin shell of cortical bone representing what remains of the greater tuberosity after a proximal humeral fracture.

FIGURE 28.6 (A and B) Control of the greater tuberosity by passing no. 2 braided permanent suture through the rotator cuff tendons just medial to their insertion on the greater tuberosity.

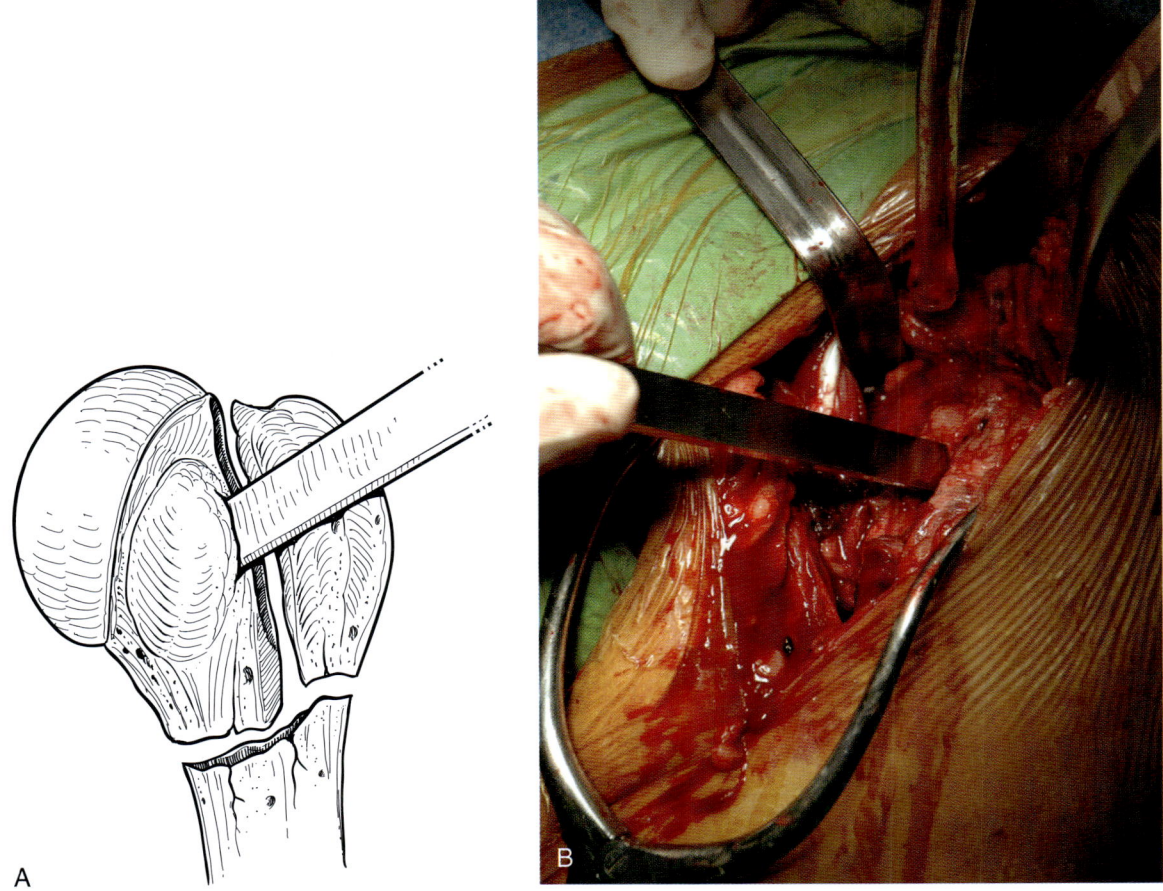

FIGURE 28.7 (A and B) Technique for separating the greater or lesser tuberosity from the head fragment with an osteotome.

CHAPTER 29

Humeral prosthetic positioning

Humeral prosthetic positioning remains the most difficult step in performing unconstrained humeral head arthroplasty or reverse shoulder arthroplasty for fracture. Placing the humeral component excessively proud or in excessive retroversion may result in loss of fixation and subsequent migration of the greater tuberosity (Figs. 29.1 and 29.2). The complication of tuberosity migration has been found to be a key factor in poor results after unconstrained shoulder arthroplasty performed for the treatment of proximal humeral fractures.[1] Tuberosity healing appears to be less critical for reverse shoulder arthroplasty for fracture but is important nonetheless. Tuberosity healing in reverse shoulder arthroplasty can improve functional results and improve stability. This chapter details humeral prosthetic positioning for both unconstrained and reverse shoulder arthroplasty.

UNCONSTRAINED HUMERAL HEAD REPLACEMENT FOR FRACTURE

Identification and Preparation of the Humeral Diaphysis for Unconstrained Humeral Head Replacement for Fracture

After control of both tuberosities has been achieved, the humeral shaft is identified. The humeral shaft is progressively reamed until the reamer that is used corresponds to the diameter of the prosthesis to be implanted (Fig. 29.3). Using the largest diaphyseal reamer that is possible to advance down the humeral canal without difficulty avoids selecting too small a diameter of the humeral implant, which can inadvertently be positioned in valgus or varus (Fig. 29.4). However, because most of these patients are severely osteopenic, no effort is made to force too large a reamer down the humeral canal for fear of iatrogenic fracture. The bicipital groove is located and two 2-mm holes are drilled in the humeral shaft approximately 1 cm distal to the fracture site, one on each side of the bicipital groove, for use later in tuberosity fixation (Fig. 29.5). The intraarticular portion of the long head of the biceps, which is frequently at least partially torn, is excised, and suture tenodesis of the remaining stump to the pectoralis major tendon is carried out with no. 1 nonabsorbable braided suture in a figure-of-eight stitch as described in Chapter 5.[2]

Selection of the Humeral Implant for Unconstrained Humeral Head Replacement for Fracture

The trial humeral implant is then assembled by selecting a stem with a diameter corresponding to the largest diaphyseal reamer used and a head size corresponding to the size of the removed head fracture fragment. The humeral head fragment is usually slightly ovoid and has a lesser and greater diameter. A head size corresponding to the lesser diameter is selected to avoid insertion of too large a component, which can lead to nonunion of the tuberosities (Fig. 29.6). The prosthetic system that we use allows variation of the posterior and medial offset of the humeral head seen in normal anatomy. We have found it most useful to place the offset laterally at the "1" position because this has consistently given us the most nearly anatomic reconstruction radiographically (Fig. 29.7). The trial implant is attached to the prosthetic holder (Fig. 29.8).

Prosthetic Positioning for Unconstrained Humeral Head Replacement for Fracture—the Gothic Arch Technique

Placement of the prosthesis at the correct height and version remains one of the most difficult challenges when performing shoulder arthroplasty for fracture. The Gothic arch technique is a method of determining appropriate height and version.[3] In this technique, prosthetic height is based on preoperative planning, as described in Chapter 27. With these calculations, the position on the humeral trial implant that should correspond to the position of the medial aspect of the fracture is marked (Fig. 29.9). The trial humeral implant is placed in the humeral canal at the desired height with the prosthetic holder. Humeral retroversion is set between 20 and 30 degrees by judging the angle formed by the prosthetic holder and the forearm (Fig. 29.10). The glenohumeral joint is reduced while the trial implant is held at the desired height and version with the prosthetic holder. The humeral head should be directed into the center of the glenoid fossa with the arm held in neutral rotation. After proper version is determined, an electrocautery is used to mark the position of the prosthetic fin on the humeral diaphysis (Fig. 29.11). An assistant can reduce the tuberosities around the trial

Text continued on p. 260

CHAPTER 29 ■ Humeral Prosthetic Positioning

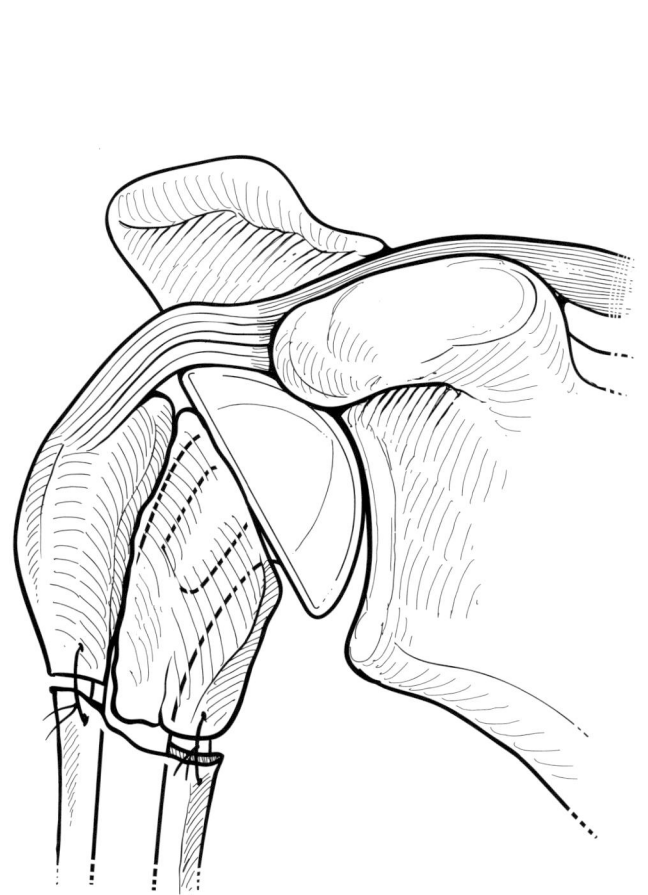

FIGURE 29.1 Placement of the humeral prosthesis excessively proud can result in loss of greater tuberosity fixation.

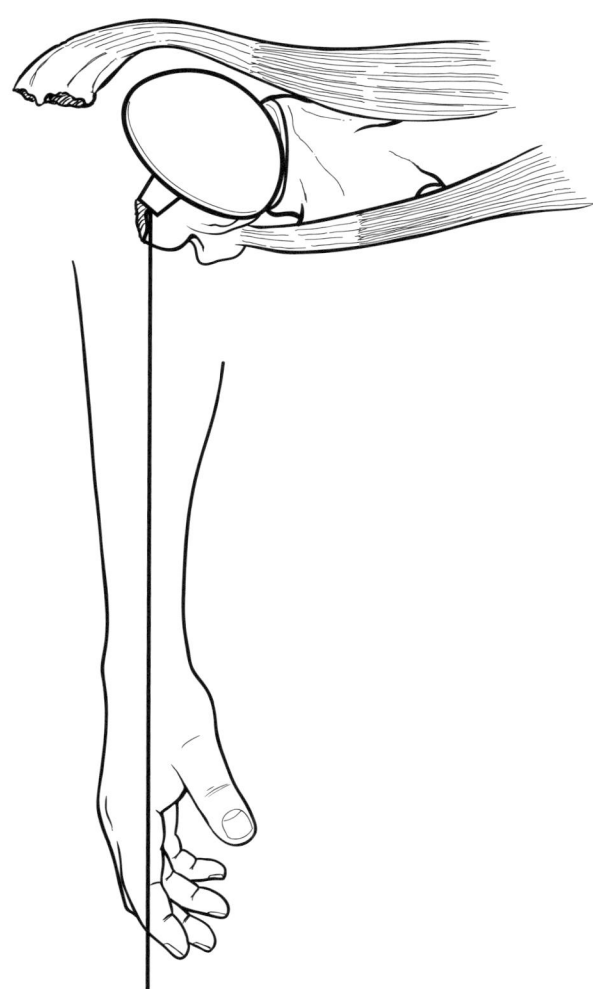

FIGURE 29.2 Placement of the humeral prosthesis in excessive retroversion can result in loss of greater tuberosity fixation.

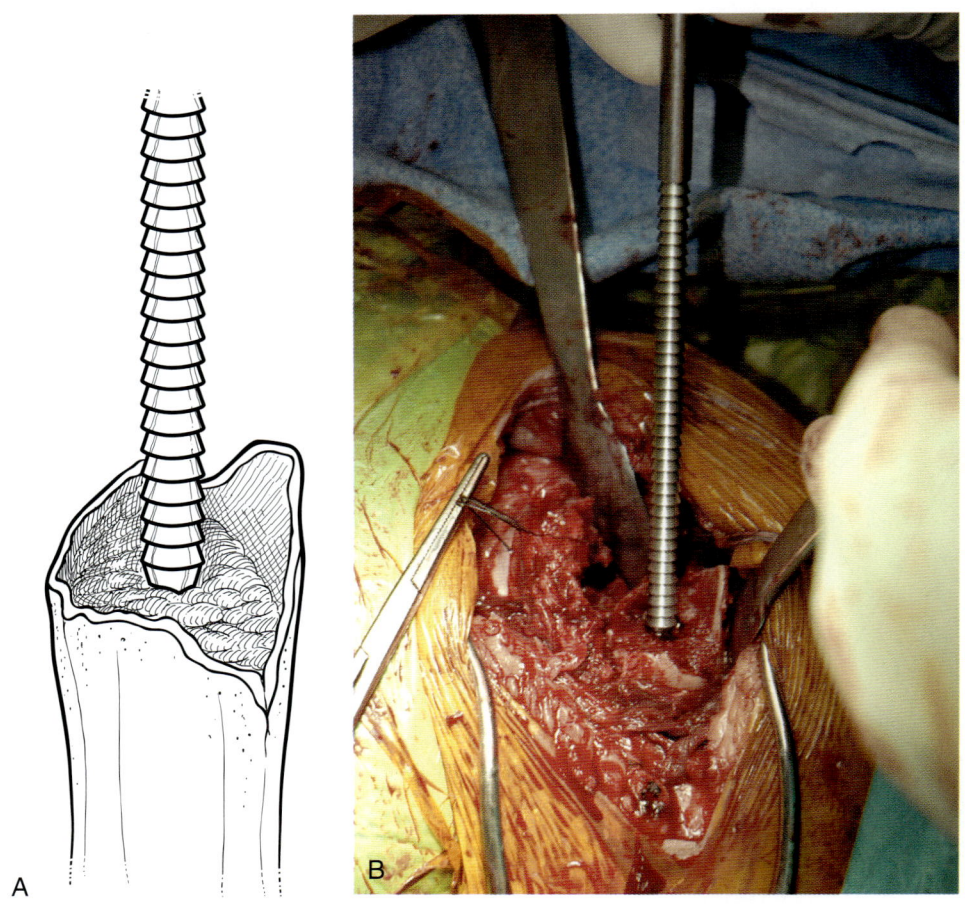

FIGURE 29.3 (A and B) Reaming of the humeral shaft.

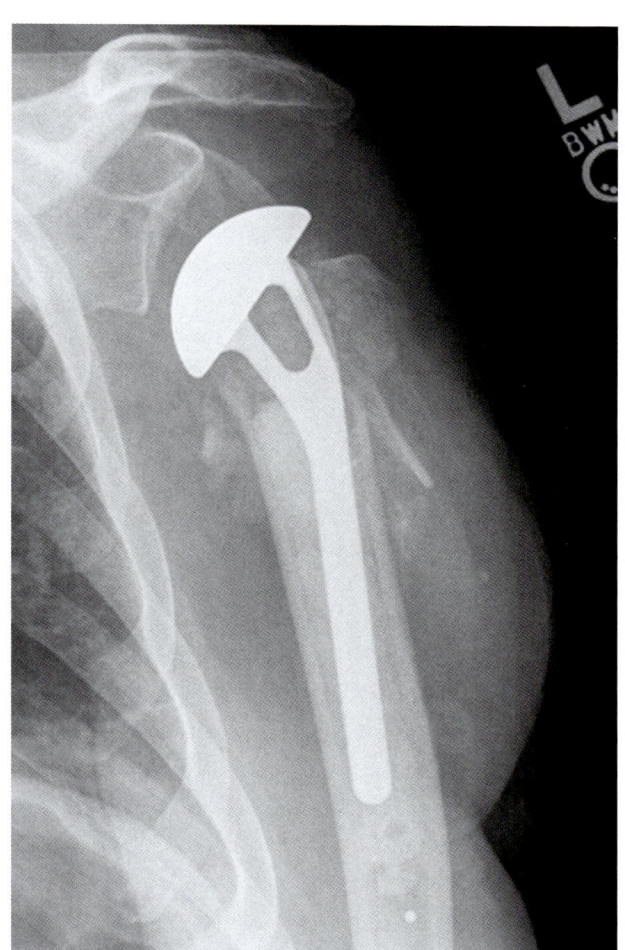

FIGURE 29.4 Radiograph of a humeral implant placed in valgus. Use of a larger-diameter implant would potentially have avoided this problem.

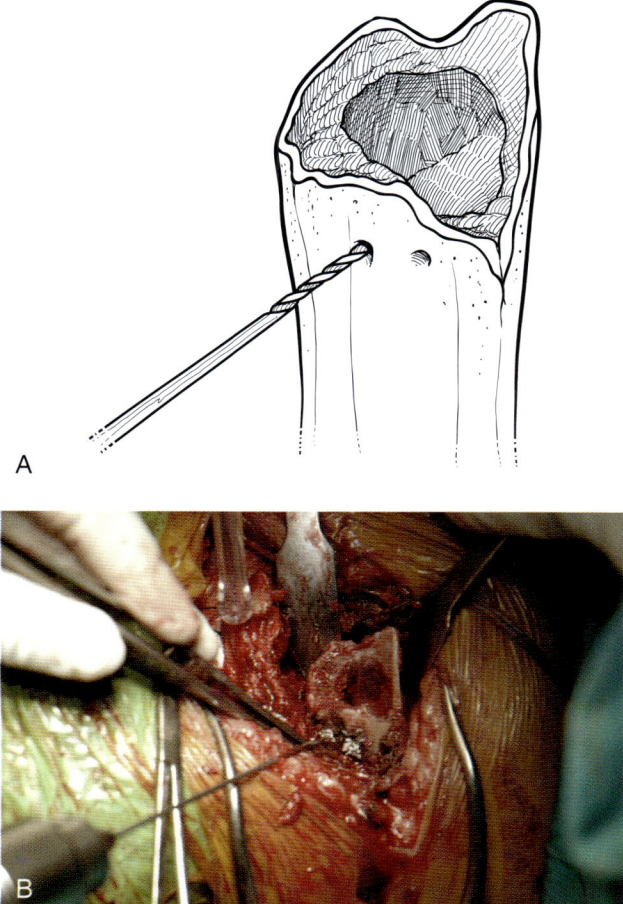

FIGURE 29.5 (A and B) Holes are drilled on each side of the bicipital groove in the humeral shaft for later fixation of the tuberosities.

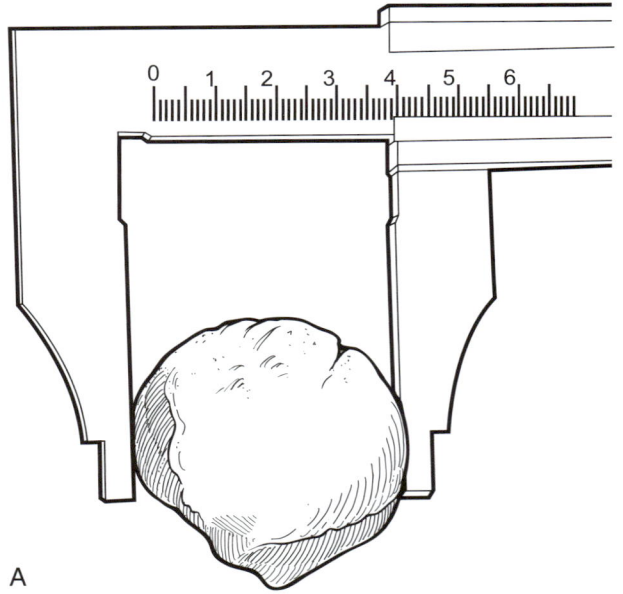

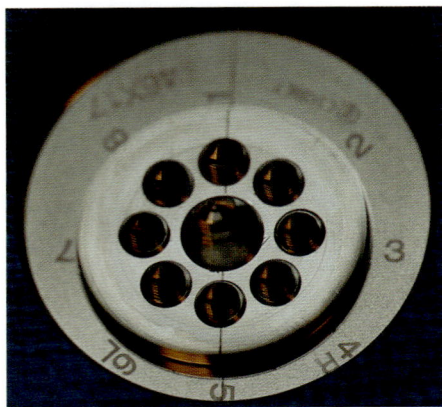

FIGURE 29.7 The "1" position corresponding to lateral offset of the humeral head is selected in fracture cases.

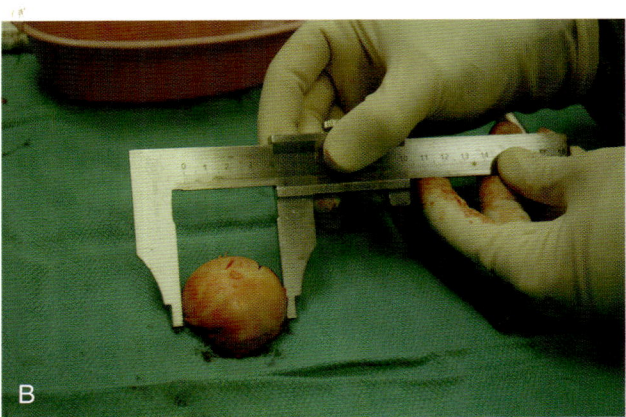

FIGURE 29.6 (A and B) Selection of the appropriate humeral head prosthetic diameter. The lesser diameter from the native humeral head is selected.

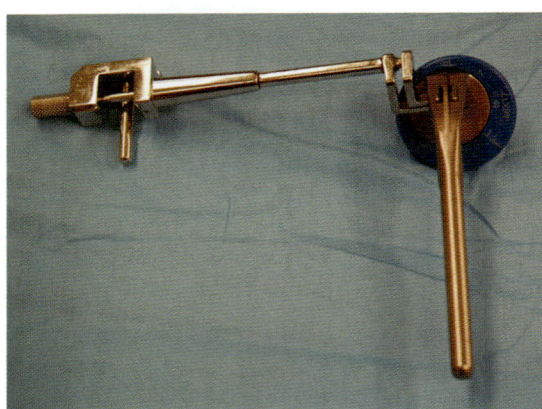

FIGURE 29.8 Trial implant attached to the prosthetic holder.

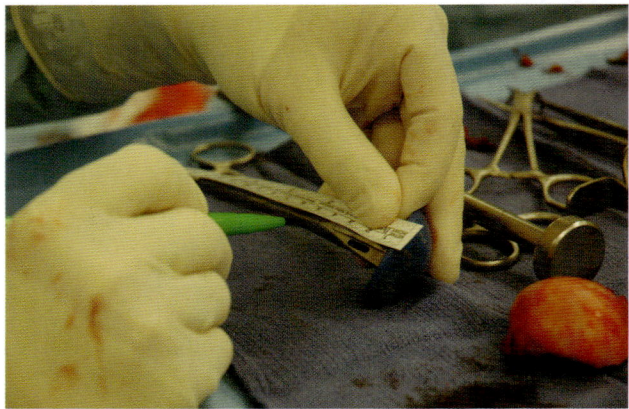

FIGURE 29.9 When using the Gothic arch technique, the position on the humeral trial implant that should correspond to the position of the medial aspect of the fracture is marked.

CHAPTER 29 ■ Humeral Prosthetic Positioning

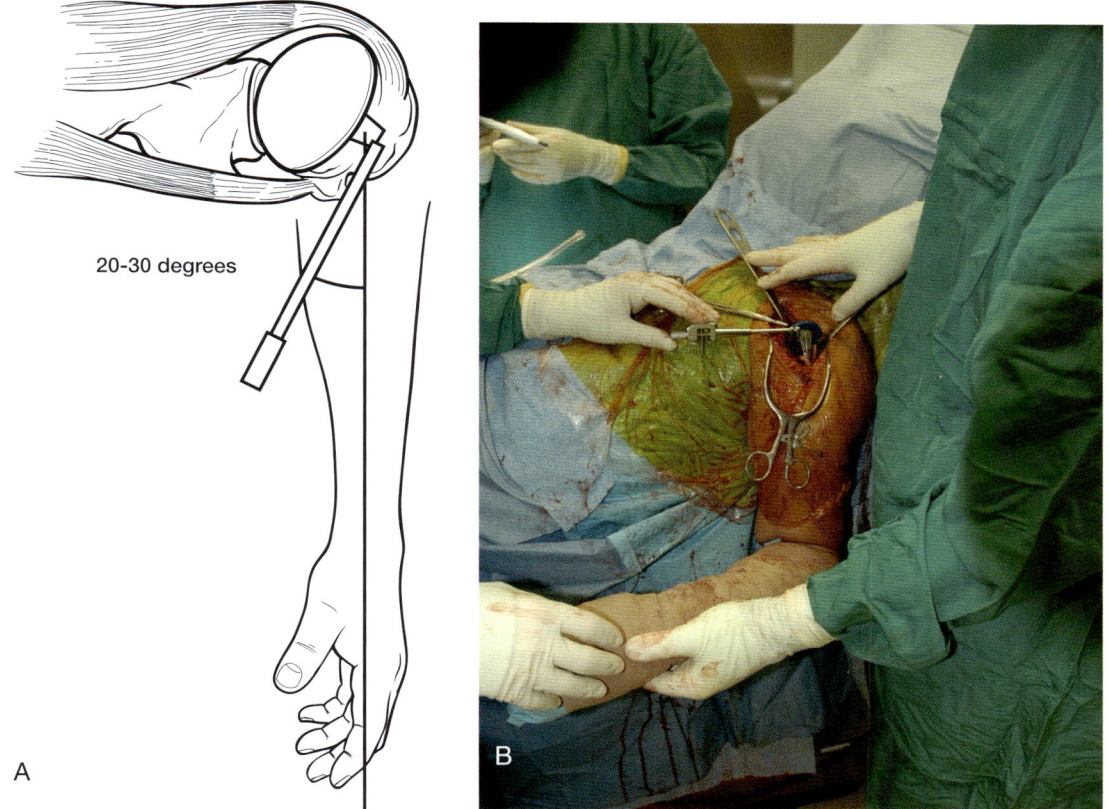

FIGURE 29.10 (A and B) Humeral retroversion is set between 20 and 30 degrees by judging the angle formed by the prosthetic holder and the forearm.

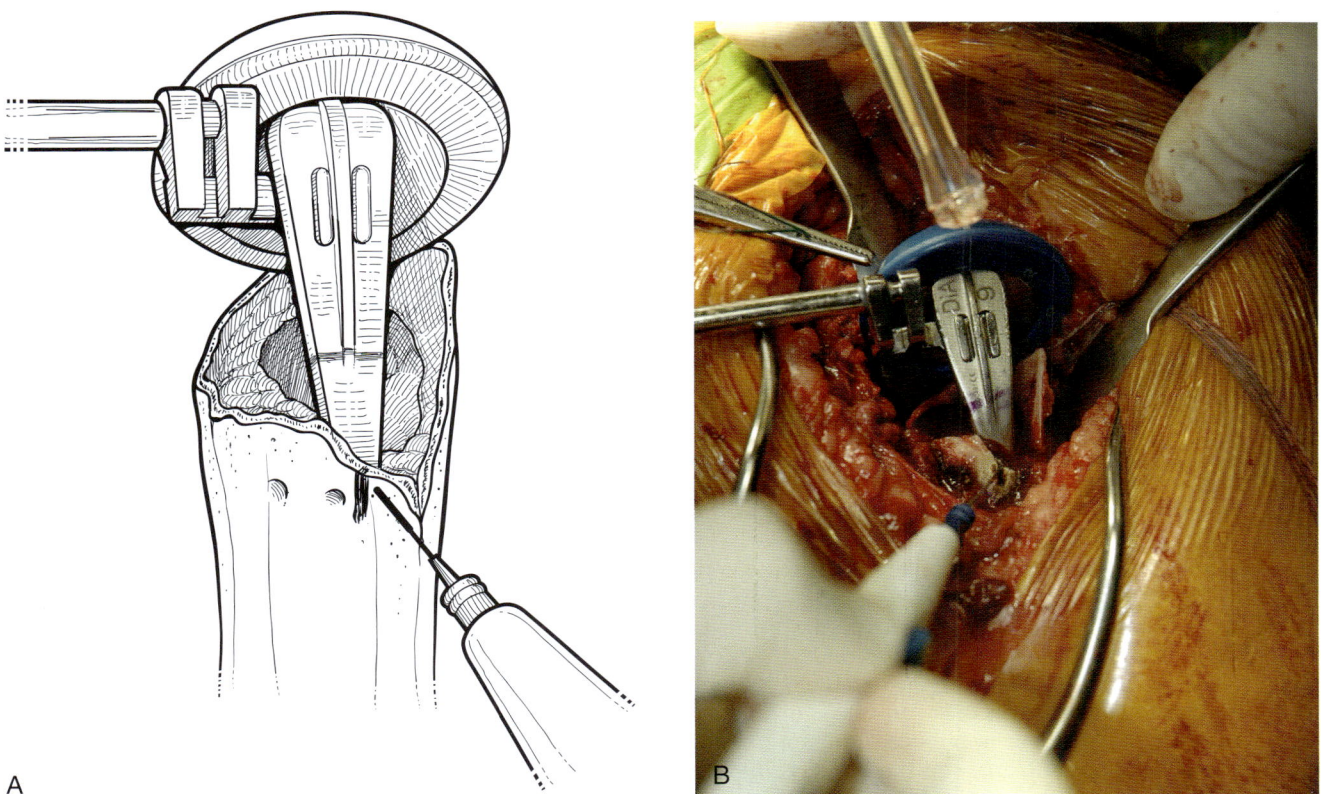

FIGURE 29.11 (A and B) After proper version is determined, the diaphysis is marked with an electrocautery.

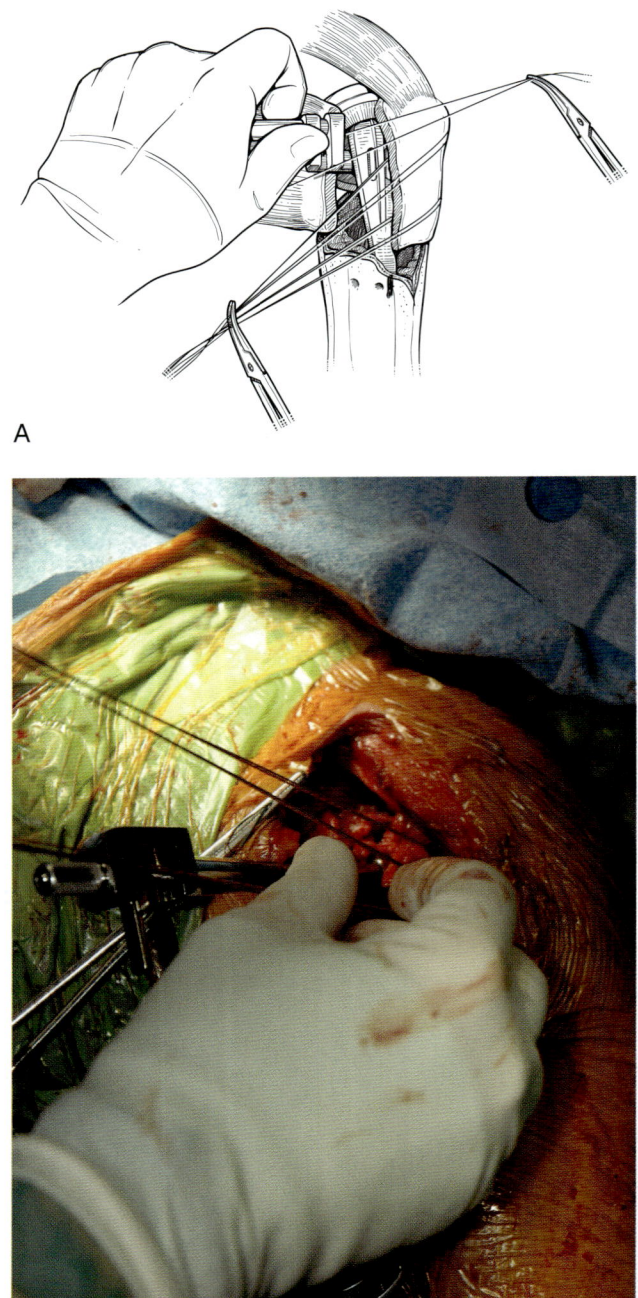

FIGURE 29.12 (A and B) Trial reduction of the tuberosities by an assistant while the trial prosthesis is held with the prosthesis holder by the surgeon.

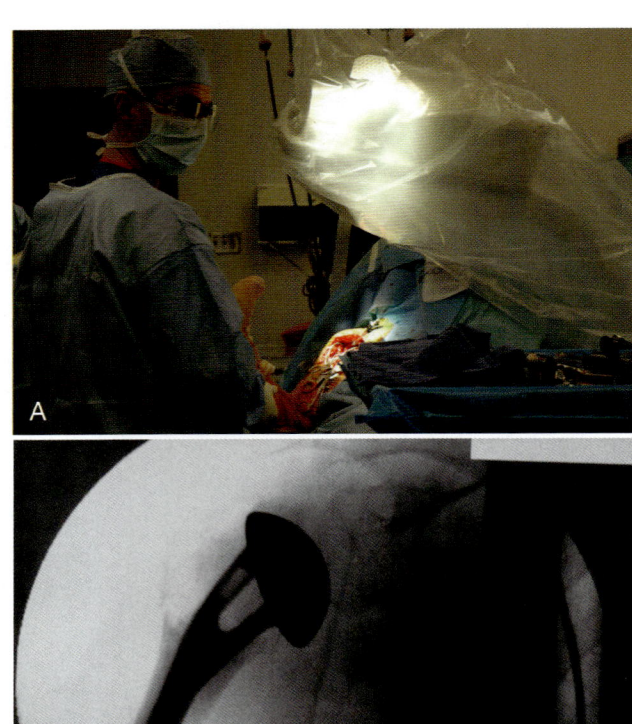

FIGURE 29.13 (A and B) Evaluation of humeral trial position via intraoperative fluoroscopy.

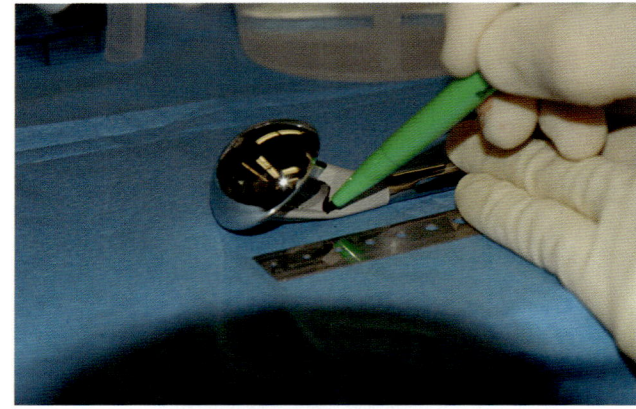

FIGURE 29.14 The final humeral implant is marked at the level that should correspond to the medial fracture line.

implant, thereby further confirming appropriate prosthetic position (Fig. 29.12). Finally, intraoperative fluoroscopy can be used to help confirm appropriate prosthetic position. Because the plastic trial humeral head is radiolucent, we use the actual humeral implant when judging prosthetic position with fluoroscopy (Fig. 29.13). Once prosthetic position is found acceptable, the implant is removed, the appropriate height is marked on the implant, and the humeral implant is attached to the prosthetic holder (Fig. 29.14).

Preparation of Bone Graft for Unconstrained Humeral Head Replacement for Fracture

Autogenous bone graft is taken from the humeral head fragment and serves two purposes. First, the bone graft enhances healing between the greater and lesser tuberosities and between the tuberosities and the humeral diaphysis. Second, because the greater tuberosity fragment is often no more than a thin shell of bone, the bone graft acts to position the greater tuberosity laterally in a more anatomic position.

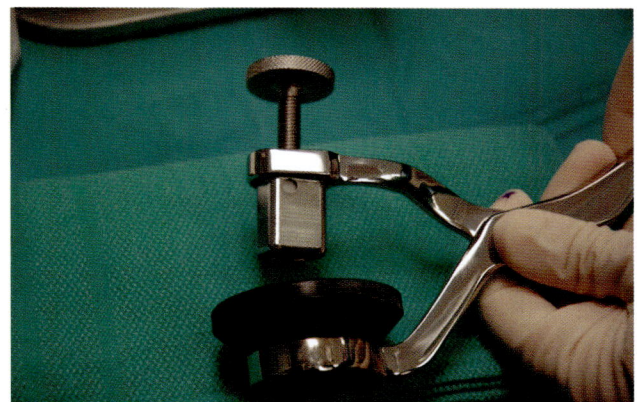

FIGURE 29.15 Bone graft cutter with the thumbscrew completely recessed.

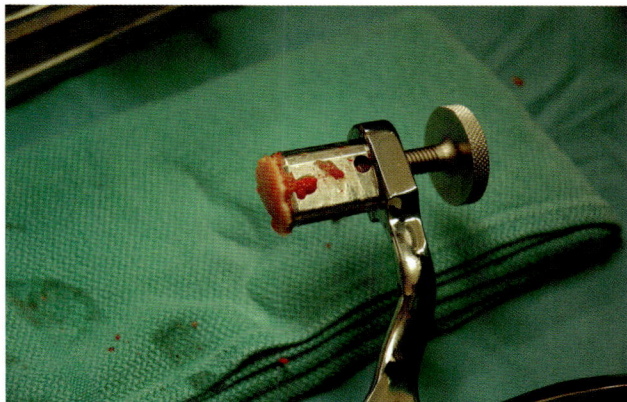

FIGURE 29.17 The thumbscrew of the bone graft cutter is advanced slightly to extrude just the portion of the bone graft plug covered with articular cartilage.

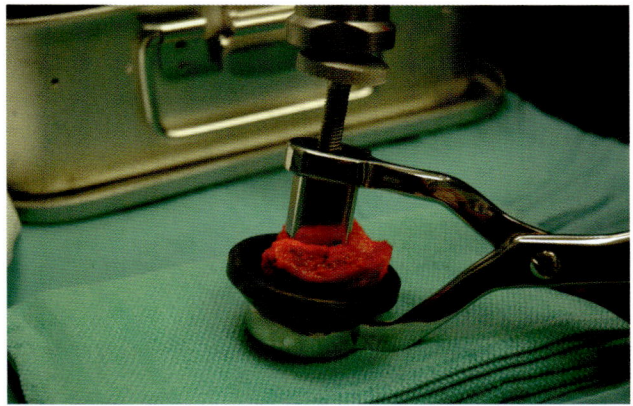

FIGURE 29.16 Advancing the bone graft cutter through the humeral head.

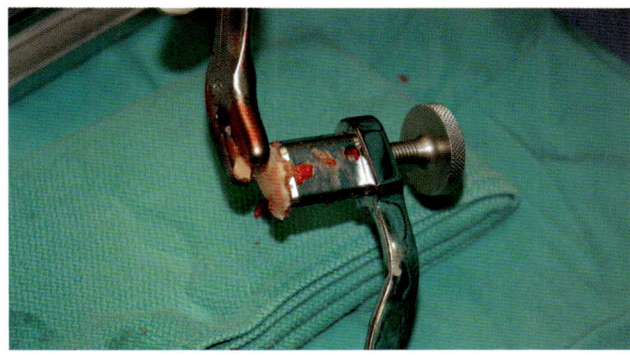

FIGURE 29.18 The articular cartilage is removed from the bone graft plug with a large biting rongeur.

We prefer to insert the bone graft into the fracture specific implant prior implantation.

A specially designed bone graft cutter is used to harvest bone graft plugs from the humeral head fragment. The thumbscrew of the bone graft cutter is completely recessed, and the cutting edge is advanced through the humeral head from cancellous surface to articular surface with a mallet (Figs. 29.15 and 29.16). After the cutting edge of the bone graft cutter has been advanced completely through the humeral head, the remaining humeral head is removed from the cutter and preserved. The thumbscrew of the bone graft cutter is advanced slightly to extrude just the portion of the bone graft plug covered with articular cartilage (Fig. 29.17). The articular cartilage is removed from the bone graft plug with a large biting rongeur (Fig. 29.18). The bone graft plug is then fully extruded from the bone graft cutter (Fig. 29.19). This process is repeated for a second bone graft plug for unconstrained humeral head replacement for fracture.

The remaining cancellous bone in the humeral head fragment is removed with a large biting rongeur and morselized (Fig. 29.20). Care is taken to not include articular cartilage in the morselized bone graft. One of the bone graft plugs is gently impacted into the fenestration of the humeral prosthesis, and the second bone graft plug is reserved for placement between the prosthesis and the greater tuberosity laterally.

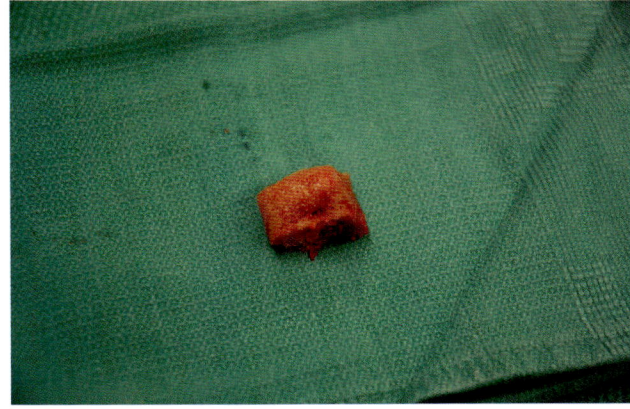

FIGURE 29.19 Bone graft plug harvested with the bone graft cutter.

Implantation of the Humeral Component for Unconstrained Humeral Head Replacement for Fracture

A cement restrictor is placed in the humeral canal to create a 1-cm distal cement mantle (Fig. 29.21). Two looped strands of no. 2 nonabsorbable braided suture are passed in an outside-to-inside direction through one of the holes previously drilled in the humeral shaft adjacent to the bicipital groove.

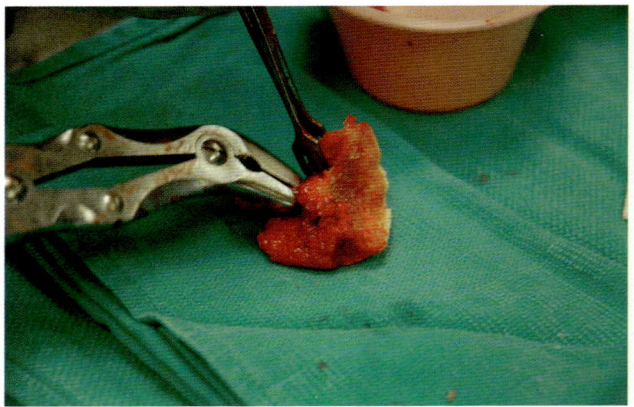

FIGURE 29.20 Removal of any remaining cancellous bone from the humeral head fragment.

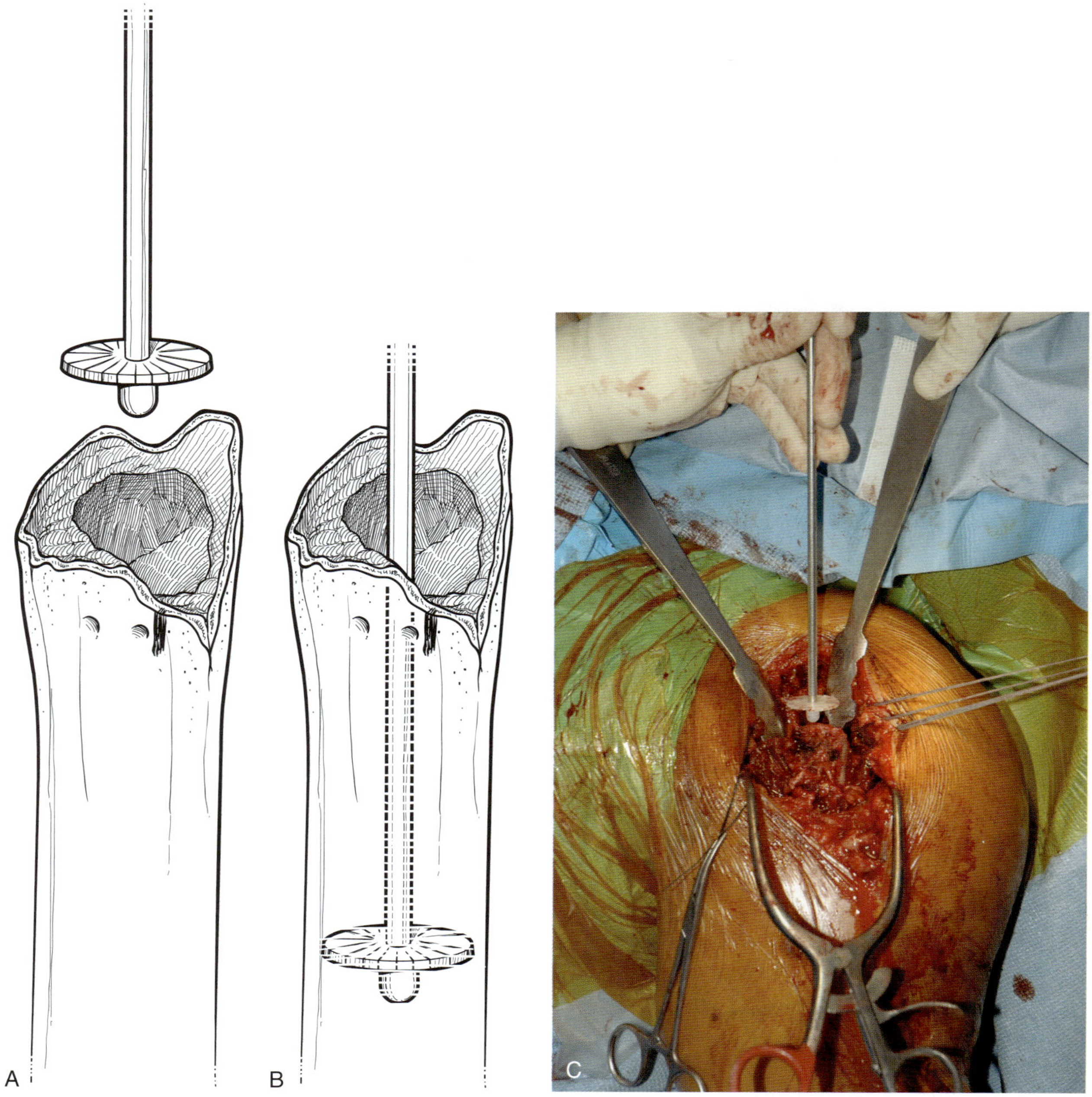

FIGURE 29.21 (A–C) Placement of a diaphyseal cement restrictor to create a 1-cm distal cement mantle.

Humeral Prosthetic Positioning

The humeral implant attached to the prosthetic holder is introduced into the humeral shaft to the appropriate level marked on the implant and at the version marked on the humeral diaphysis (Fig. 29.23). The position of the prosthesis is continually checked to ensure that no movement occurs as the cement cures.

All excess cement is removed, with special attention to removing cement in the fenestration of the prosthesis and at the diaphyseal fracture site. After the appropriate prosthetic position is confirmed and excess cement has been removed, the cement is allowed to fully cure, thus completing insertion of the humeral component.

REVERSE SHOULDER ARTHROPLASTY FOR FRACTURE

Identification and Preparation of the Humeral Diaphysis for Reverse Shoulder Arthroplasty for Fracture

Identification and preparation of the humeral diaphysis for reverse shoulder arthroplasty for fracture is the nearly the same as described previously for unconstrained humeral head replacement for fracture. After control of both tuberosities has been achieved, the humeral shaft is identified. The humeral shaft is progressively reamed until the reamer that is used corresponds to the diameter of the prosthesis to be implanted (Fig. 29.24). However, because most of these patients are severely osteopenic, no effort is made to force too large a reamer down the humeral canal for fear of iatrogenic fracture. The bicipital groove is located, and two 2-mm holes are drilled in the humeral shaft approximately 1 cm distal to the fracture site, one on each side of the bicipital groove, for use later in tuberosity fixation (see Fig. 29.5). The intraarticular portion of the long head of the biceps, which is frequently at least partially torn, is excised, and suture tenodesis of the remaining stump to the pectoralis major tendon is carried out with no. 1 nonabsorbable braided suture in a figure-of-eight stitch as described in Chapter 5.[2]

Selection of the Humeral Implant and Prosthetic Positioning for Reverse Shoulder Arthroplasty for Fracture

The trial humeral implant is selected using a stem with a diameter corresponding to the largest diaphyseal reamer used. Placement of the prosthesis at the correct height and version remains one of the most difficult challenges when performing reverse shoulder arthroplasty for fracture. The humeral trial is systematically placed in 25 degrees of retroversion using a version rod placed on the humeral prosthetic insertion device (Fig. 29.25). The version rod should align with the patient's forearm. After proper version is determined, an electrocautery is used to mark the position of the prosthetic fin on the humeral diaphysis. The ideal humeral height and tensioning is determined during trialing, which can also include the use of variable thickness polyethylene trials. An assistant can reduce the tuberosities around the trial implant, thereby further confirming appropriate prosthetic position. A height gauge that attaches to humeral prosthetic

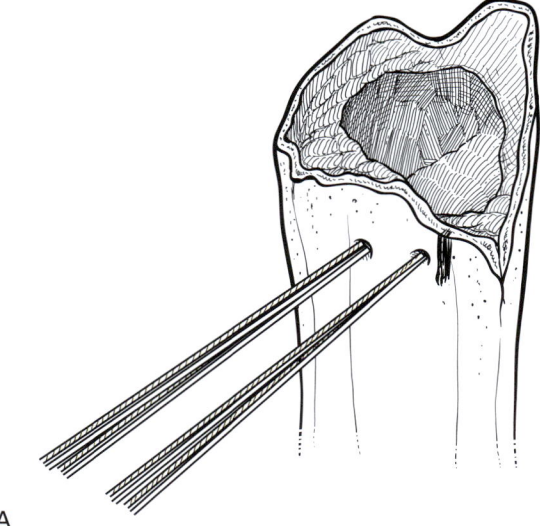

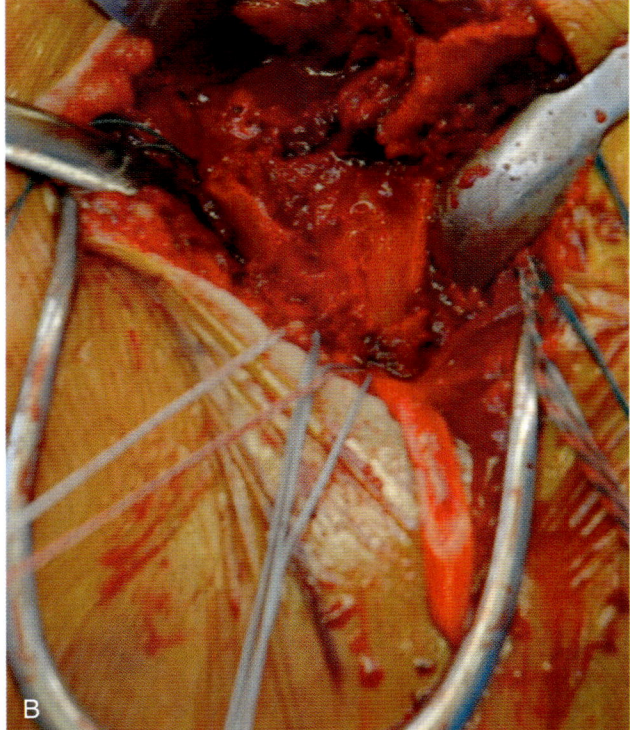

FIGURE 29.22 (A and B) Two looped strands of no. 2 nonabsorbable braided suture are passed in an outside-to-inside direction through one of the holes previously drilled in the humeral shaft adjacent to the bicipital groove. These sutures are then passed from inside to outside through the other hole previously drilled in the humeral shaft adjacent to the bicipital groove.

These sutures are then passed from inside to outside though the other hole previously drilled in the humeral shaft adjacent to the bicipital groove (Fig. 29.22). The humeral canal is irrigated and dried thoroughly. Bone cement (we prefer to use DePuy CMW 2 bone cement [DePuy, Inc., Warsaw, Indiana] because of its accelerated curing time of less than 8 minutes) is mixed and introduced into the humeral shaft with a catheter tip syringe.

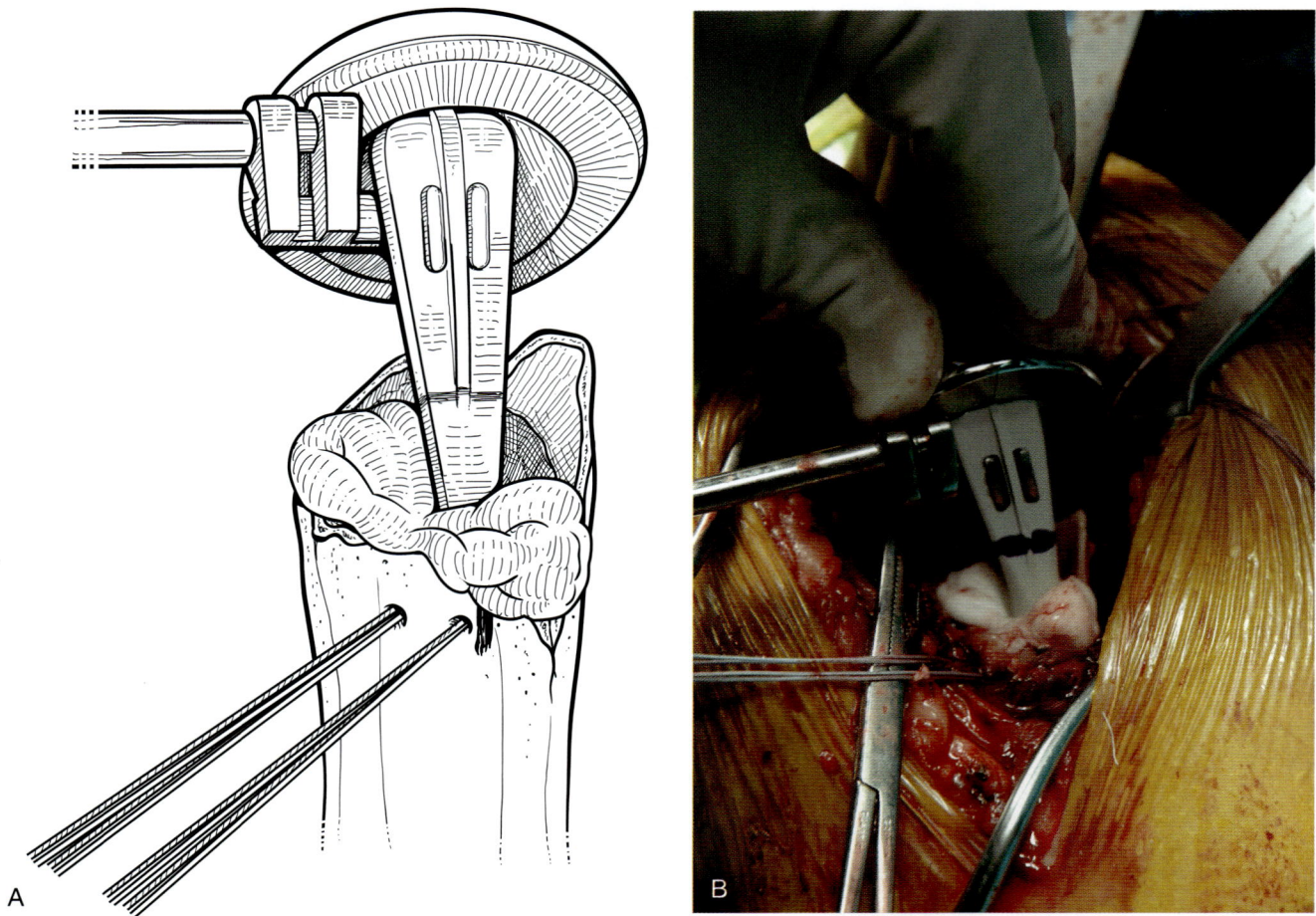

FIGURE 29.23 (A and B) Implantation of the humeral prosthesis at the appropriate height via the Gothic arch technique.

insertion device is used to reproduce the appropriate height upon insertion of the final humeral component (Fig. 29.26).

Preparation of Bone Graft for Reverse Shoulder Arthroplasty for Fracture

Preparation for bone graft for reverse shoulder arthroplasty for fracture is the same as described previously for unconstrained humeral head replacement for fracture, with the exception that only one bone graft plug is used for reverse shoulder arthroplasty for fracture instead of two bone plugs used for unconstrained humeral head replacement for fracture. Figs. 29.15–29.20 demonstrate the harvesting and preparation of this bone graft.

Implantation of the Humeral Component for Reverse Shoulder Arthroplasty for Fracture

The cement technique for reverse shoulder arthroplasty for fracture is the same as described previously for unconstrained humeral head replacement for fracture. A cement restrictor is placed in the humeral canal to create a 1-cm distal cement mantle. Two looped strands of no. 2 nonabsorbable braided suture are passed in an outside-to-inside direction through one of the holes previously drilled in the humeral shaft adjacent to the bicipital groove. These sutures are then passed from inside to outside though the other hole previously drilled in the humeral shaft adjacent to the bicipital groove. The humeral canal is irrigated and dried thoroughly. Bone cement is mixed and introduced into the humeral shaft with a catheter tip syringe.

The humeral implant is attached to the prosthetic holder with the predetermined height gauge set and the version rod set at 25 degrees. The implant is introduced into the humeral shaft to the appropriate height as set by the height gauge and at the retroversion determined with the version rod (Fig. 29.27). The position of the prosthesis is continually checked to ensure that no movement occurs as the cement cures.

All excess cement is removed, with special attention to removing cement in the fenestration of the prosthesis and at the diaphyseal fracture site. After the appropriate prosthetic position is confirmed and excess cement has been removed, the cement is allowed to fully cure. At this point, trial polyethylene inserts can be used to confirm the appropriate soft tissue tension (Fig. 29.28). After the final polyethylene insert size is selected, the insert is impacted into place (Fig. 29.29), completing insertion of the reverse humeral component.

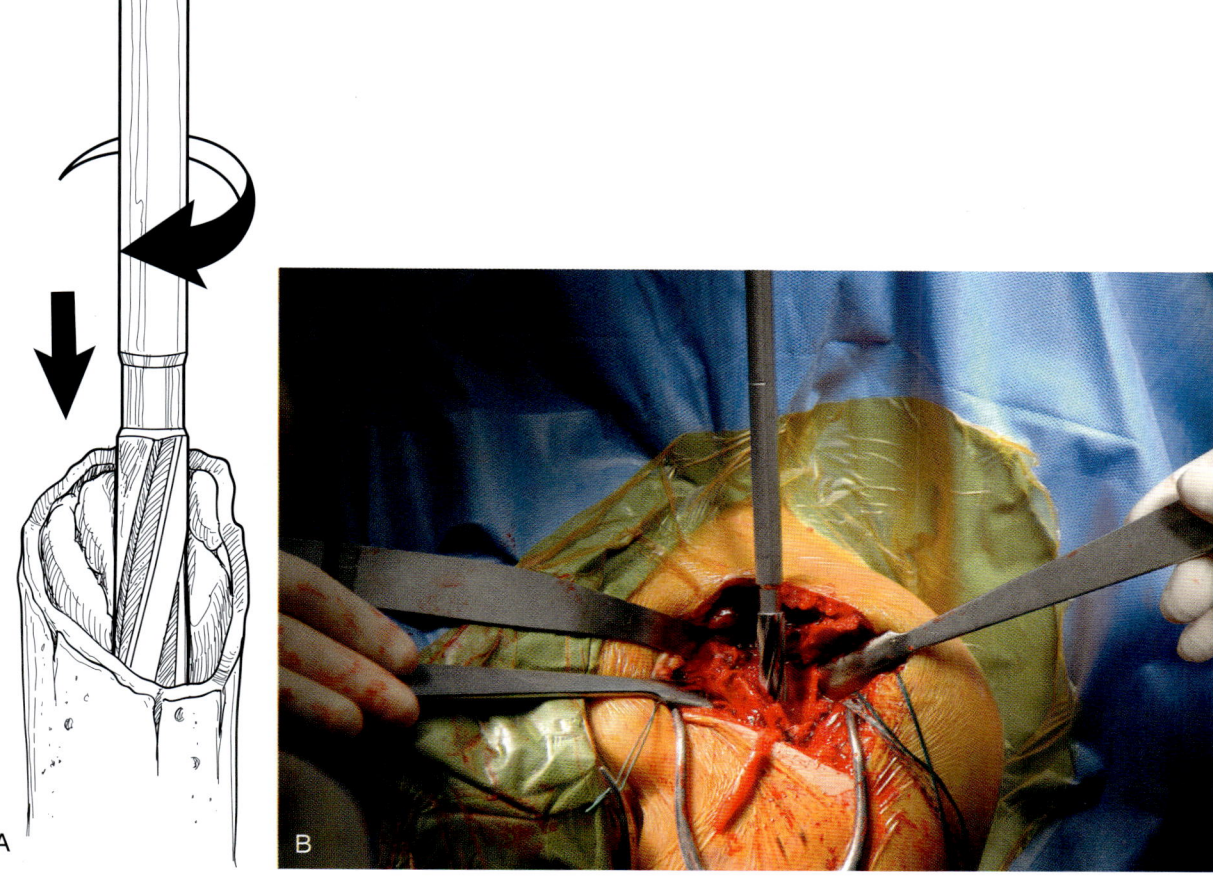

FIGURE 29.24 (A and B) The humeral shaft is progressively reamed until the reamer that is used corresponds to the diameter of the prosthesis to be implanted.

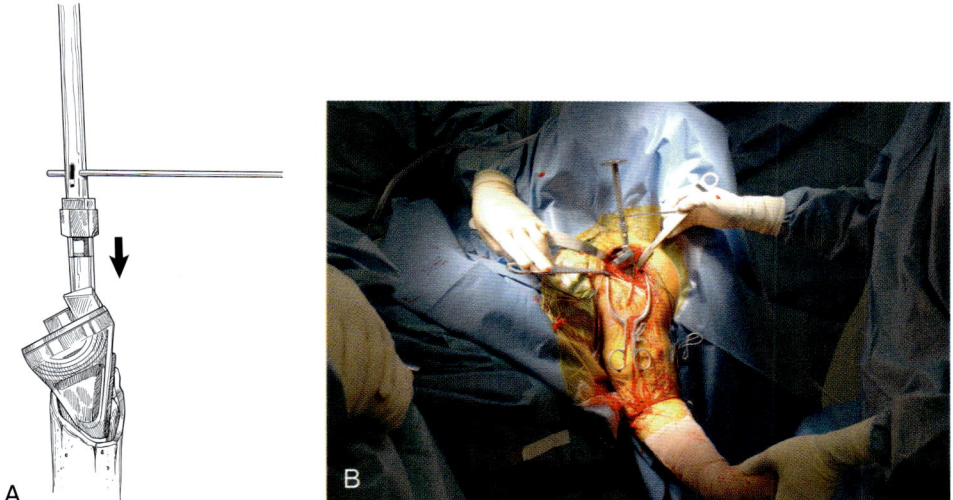

FIGURE 29.25 (A and B) The humeral trial is systematically placed in 25 degrees of retroversion using a version rod placed on the humeral prosthetic insertion device. The version rod should align with the patient's forearm.

266 SECTION IV ■ Shoulder Arthroplasty for Fracture

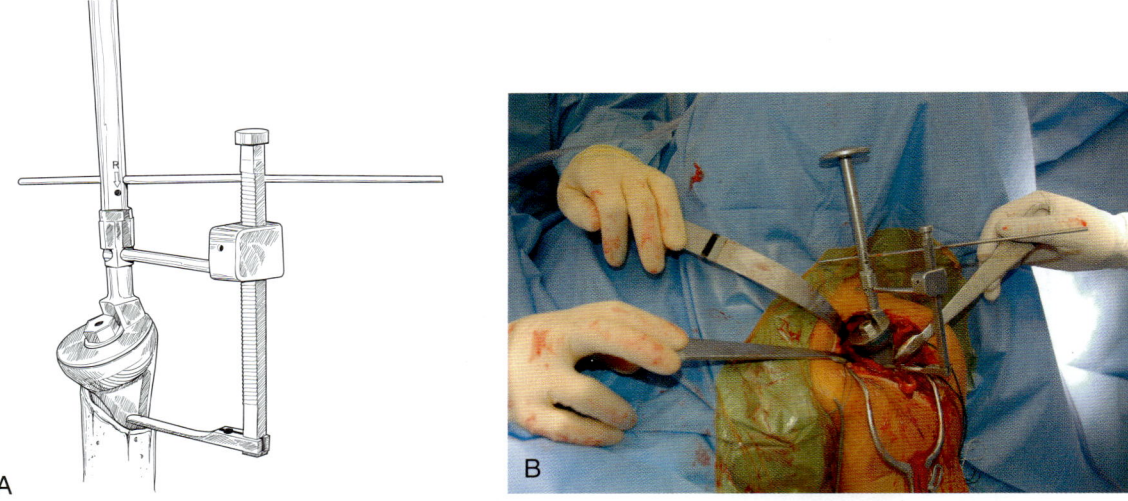

FIGURE 29.26 (A and B) A height gauge that attaches to humeral prosthetic insertion device is used to reproduce the appropriate height upon insertion of the final humeral component.

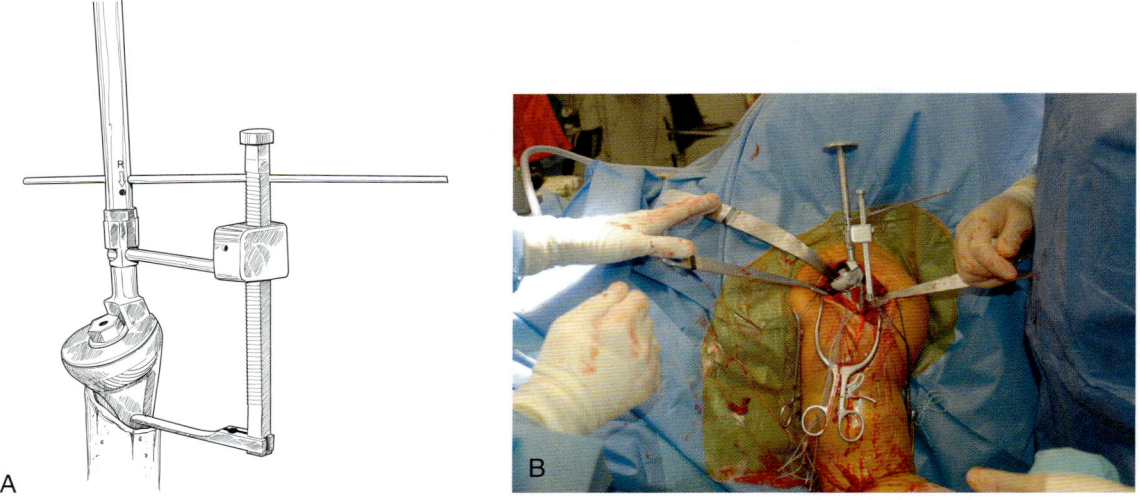

FIGURE 29.27 (A and B) The final humeral stem is cemented into place using the insertion guide.

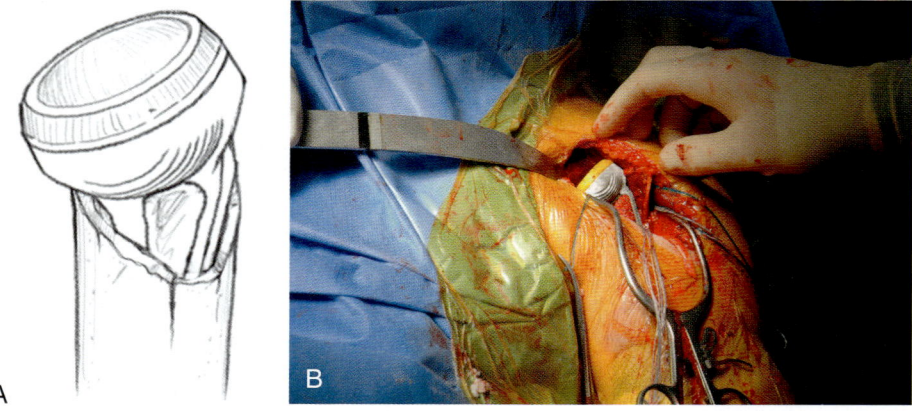

FIGURE 29.28 (A and B) Trial polyethylene inserts can be used to confirm the appropriate soft tissue tension.

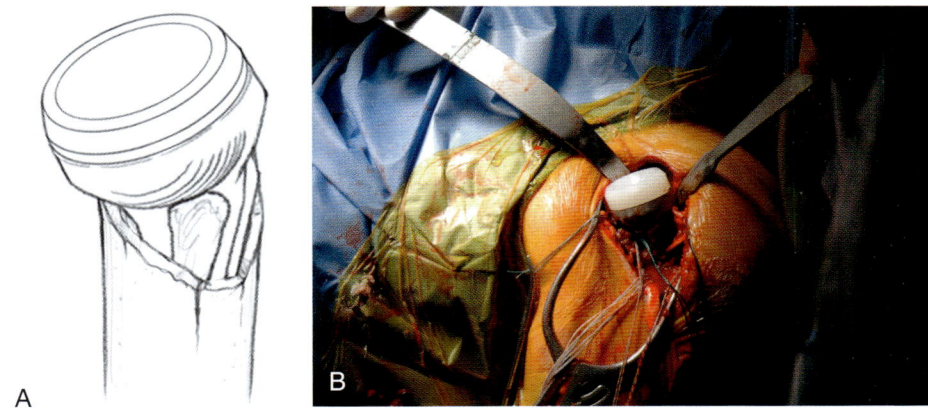

FIGURE 29.29 (A and B) Completed insertion of the reverse humeral component.

REFERENCES

1. Boileau P, Coste JS, Ahrens PM, et al: Prosthetic shoulder replacement for fracture: Results of the multicentre study. In Walch G, Boileau P, Molé D, editors: *2000 Prosthèses d'Epaule…Recul de 2 à 10 Ans*, Paris, 2001, Sauramps Medical, pp 561–578.
2. Dines D, Hersch J: Long head of the biceps lesions after shoulder arthroplasty. *Paper presented at the 8th International Congress on Surgery of the Shoulder*, April 2001, Cape Town, South Africa.
3. Krishnan SG, Pennington SD, Burkhead WZ, et al: Shoulder arthroplasty for fracture: Restoration of the "gothic arch," *Tech Shoulder Elbow Surg* 6:57–66, 2005.

CHAPTER 30

Tuberosity reduction and fixation

Greater and lesser tuberosity complications are primary obstacles to achieving a satisfactory result after shoulder arthroplasty for the treatment of proximal humeral fractures.[1] Tuberosity malunion and nonunion are situations to be avoided. The first step in avoiding these complications is placement of the tuberosities at their correct anatomic location through proper preoperative planning and accurate humeral prosthetic positioning (Chapters 27 and 29). The second step in avoiding these complications is through tuberosity fixation. Tuberosity fixation consists of two major components: use of a reliable and reproducible suture fixation technique to provide initial fracture stability, and use of bone graft to assist in tuberosity healing and provide long-term fracture stability (Chapter 29). This chapter details our preferred tuberosity fixation technique and the use of bone graft to enhance tuberosity position and healing. Our tuberosity reduction and fixation technique is the same for unconstrained humeral head replacement for fracture and reverse shoulder arthroplasty for fracture.

TECHNIQUE FOR REDUCTION AND FIXATION OF THE TUBEROSITIES

Fixation of the tuberosities is achieved with a reproducible suture fixation technique consisting of four looped horizontal cerclage sutures (two looped sutures around the greater tuberosity and two looped around the greater and lesser tuberosities) and two vertical looped cerclage sutures (Fig. 30.1). The passing sutures to be used for horizontal cerclage were previously placed when control of the greater tuberosity was initially achieved (Chapter 28) and consisted of a looped no. 2 braided permanent suture placed through the rotator cuff at the junction of the supraspinatus and infraspinatus and a looped strand of no. 2 braided permanent suture placed through the rotator cuff at the junction of the infraspinatus and teres minor. The vertical cerclage sutures consist of the two looped strands of no. 2 nonabsorbable braided suture placed in the humeral diaphysis before humeral implant cementation, as described in Chapter 29.

The sutures controlling the greater tuberosity are passed around the smooth polished medial aspect of the prosthetic neck (Fig. 30.2). In unconstrained arthroplasty, a bone graft plug is placed lateral to the neck of the prosthesis to accommodate for bone loss in the greater tuberosity and to place the greater tuberosity in a more anatomic lateral position (Fig. 30.3). The morselized bone graft is placed along the diaphyseal fracture line to promote healing of the greater and lesser tuberosities to the humeral shaft (Fig. 30.4). The looped sutures are then used as passing sutures to shuttle two looped sutures, each leaving two looped sutures passing around the superior aspect of the greater tuberosity and two looped sutures passing around the inferior aspect of the greater tuberosity (Fig. 30.5). All passed sutures are depicted in Fig. 30.6. The four looped sutures that are passed have needles attached. Two of the needles are removed. The greater tuberosity is gently grasped with Lahey forceps and reduced into position (Fig. 30.7). Two of the looped sutures controlling the greater tuberosity, one superior and one inferior, are tied in a "racking hitch" fashion to fixate the greater tuberosity (Fig. 30.8).[2,3] The sequential steps of the "racking hitch" technique are described and shown in Figs. 30.9 to 30.12.[2,3] A loop is created (see Fig. 30.9) and the free ends of the suture are passed through the loop, which creates the racking hitch (see Fig. 30.10). The free ends of the suture are pulled simultaneously and then each suture end individually if needed to tighten the racking hitch (see Fig. 30.11). The racking hitch is then backed up with four half hitches. Four half hitches have shown increased knot security and are superior to 1, 2, or 3 half hitches for the racking hitch knot (see Fig. 30.12).[3]

The remaining two looped sutures, with needles attached and controlling the greater tuberosity, one superior and one inferior, are passed through the subscapularis tendon with a free needle just medial to its osseous insertion on the lesser tuberosity. The lesser tuberosity is reduced with the previously placed stay sutures, and the circumferential sutures are tied using a racking hitch knot to secure the tuberosity (Fig. 30.13). Vertical tuberosity fixation is completed with the two looped sutures previously placed through drill holes in the humeral diaphysis. One looped suture is passed with a free needle through the infraspinatus and supraspinatus tendons just medial to their osseous insertion and then secured using a racking hitch knot (Fig. 30.14). The second looped suture is passed with a free needle through the subscapularis and supraspinatus tendons just medial to their osseous insertion and then secured using a racking hitch knot (Fig. 30.15). Security of the tuberosities must be evaluated by checking the mobility of the shoulder after tuberosity repair. The tuberosities and humeral prosthesis should move as one unit.

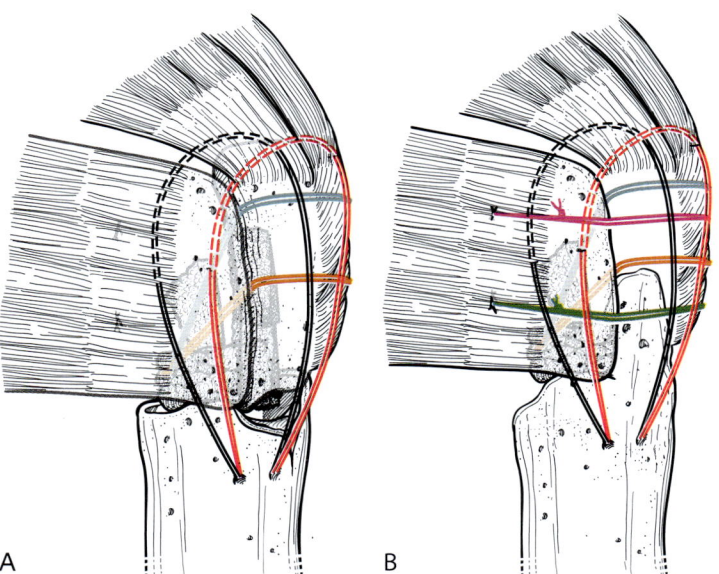

FIGURE 30.1 Overview of the suture fixation technique used for the greater and lesser tuberosities around an unconstrained humeral head replacement (A) and a reverse arthroplasty (B).

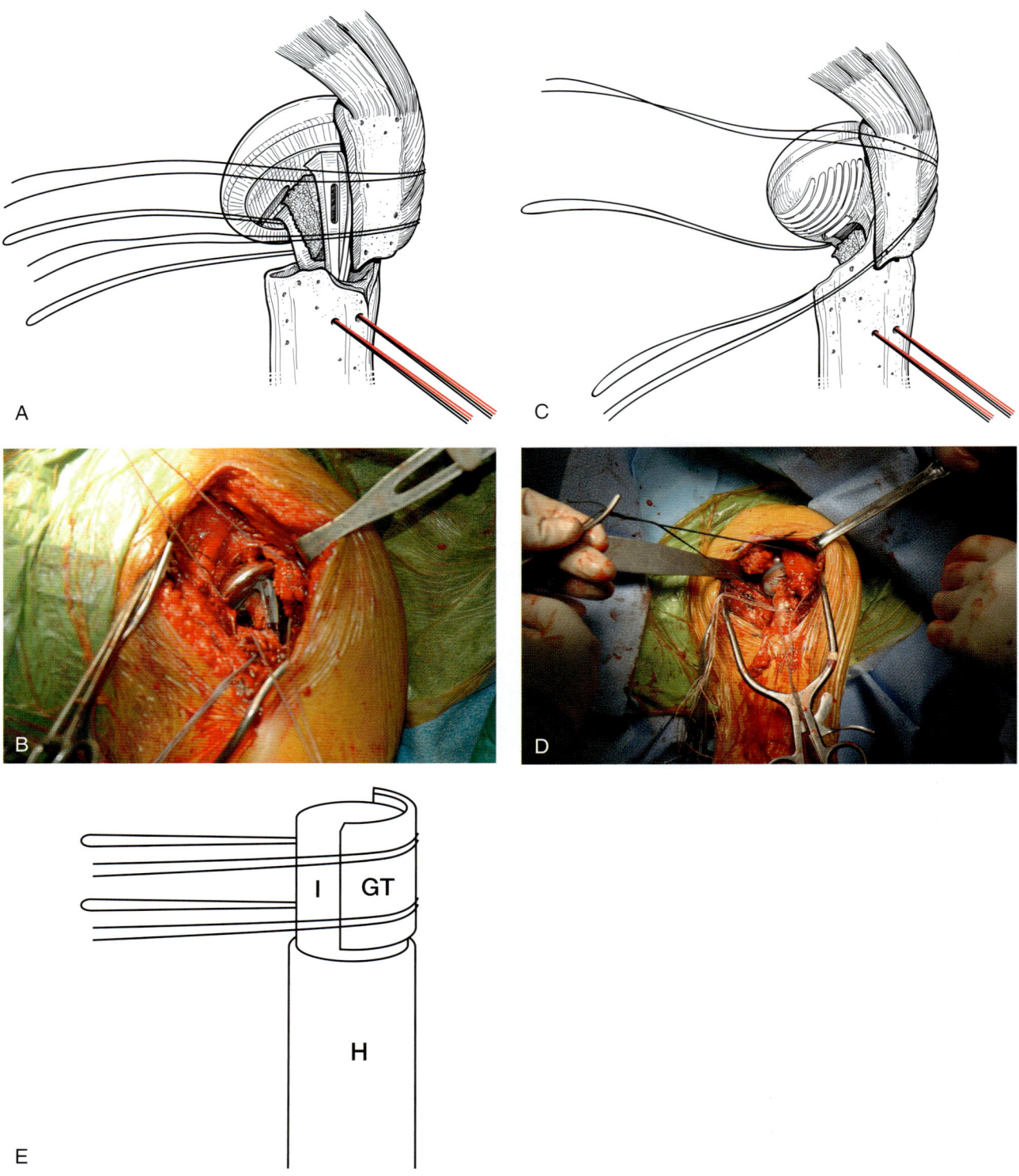

FIGURE 30.2 The sutures controlling the greater tuberosity are passed around the smooth polished medial aspect of the humeral prosthetic neck of either an unconstrained arthroplasty (A and B) or a reverse arthroplasty (C and D). (E) depicts a schematic of suture position. *GT*, Greater tuberosity; *H*, humeral shaft; *I*, implant.

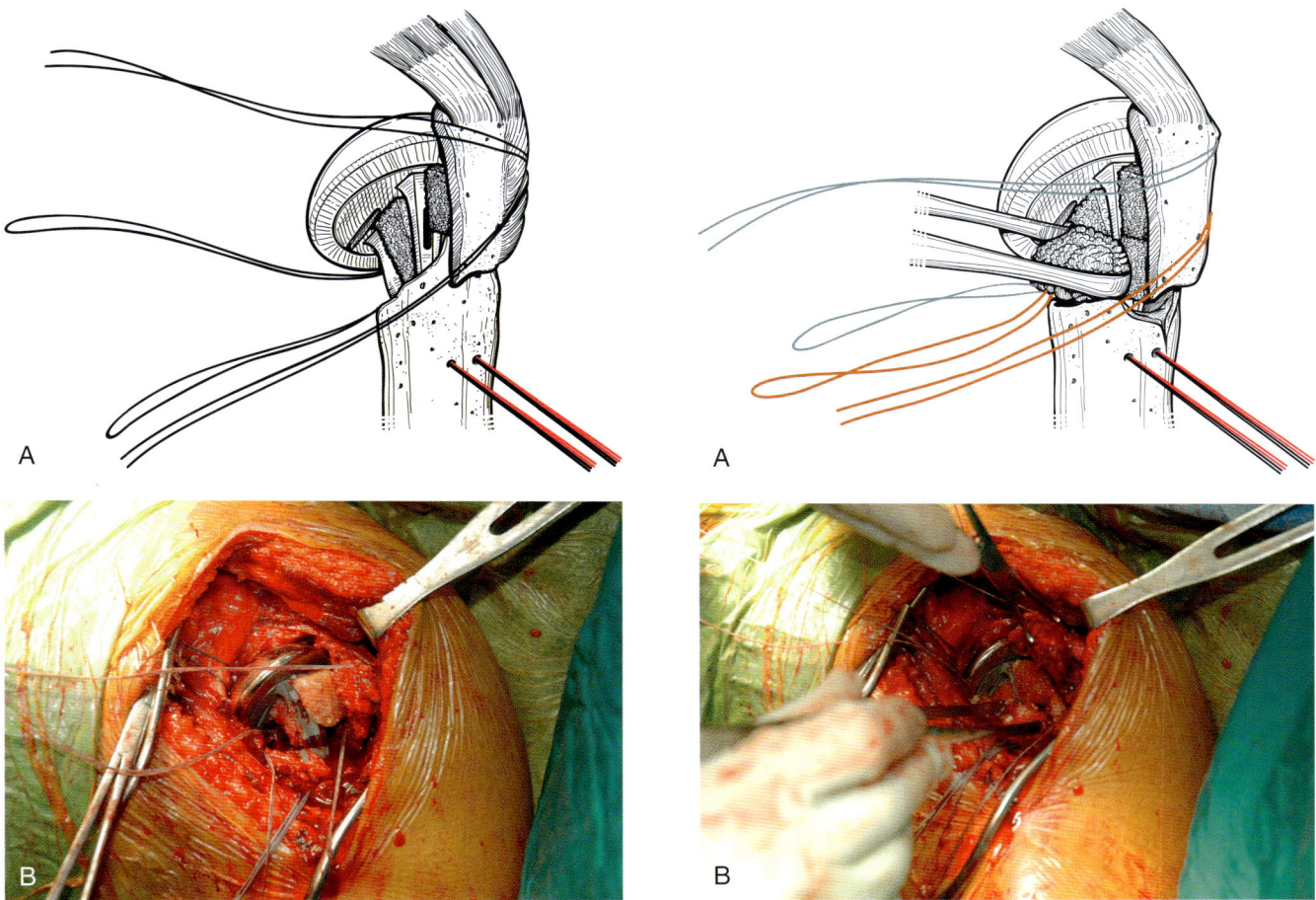

FIGURE 30.3 (A and B) A bone graft plug is placed lateral to the neck of the prosthesis to accommodate for bone loss in the greater tuberosity and place the greater tuberosity in a more anatomic lateral position when using an unconstrained arthroplasty.

FIGURE 30.4 (A and B) Morselized bone graft is placed along the diaphyseal fracture line to promote healing of the greater and lesser tuberosities to the humeral shaft.

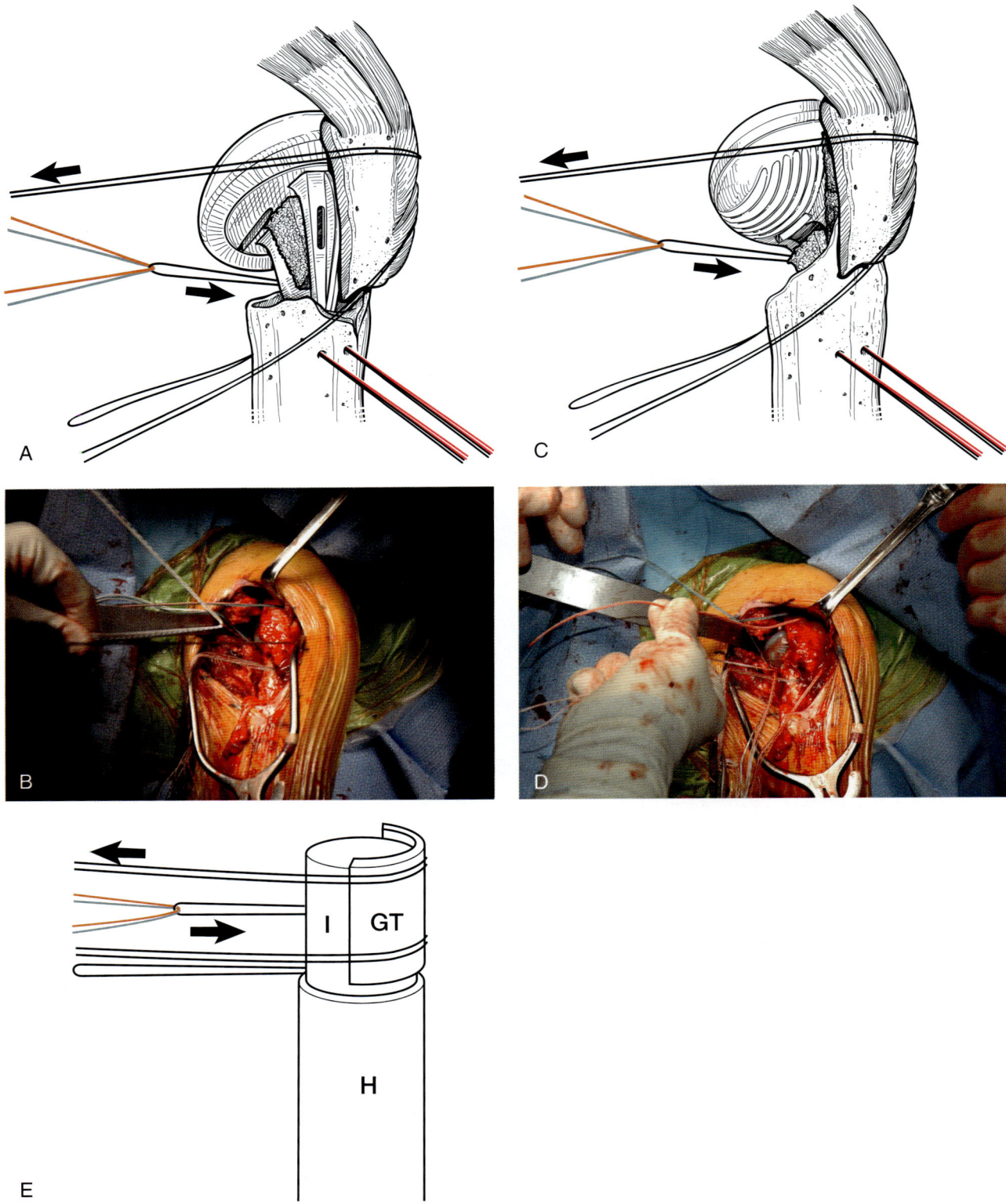

FIGURE 30.5 The looped sutures are then used as passing sutures to shuttle two looped sutures, each leaving two looped sutures passing around the superior aspect of the greater tuberosity and two looped sutures passing around the inferior aspect of the greater tuberosity and the humeral prosthetic neck of either an unconstrained arthroplasty (A and B) or a reverse arthroplasty (C and D). (E) Depicts a schematic of suture position. *GT*, Greater tuberosity; *H*, humeral shaft; *I*, implant.

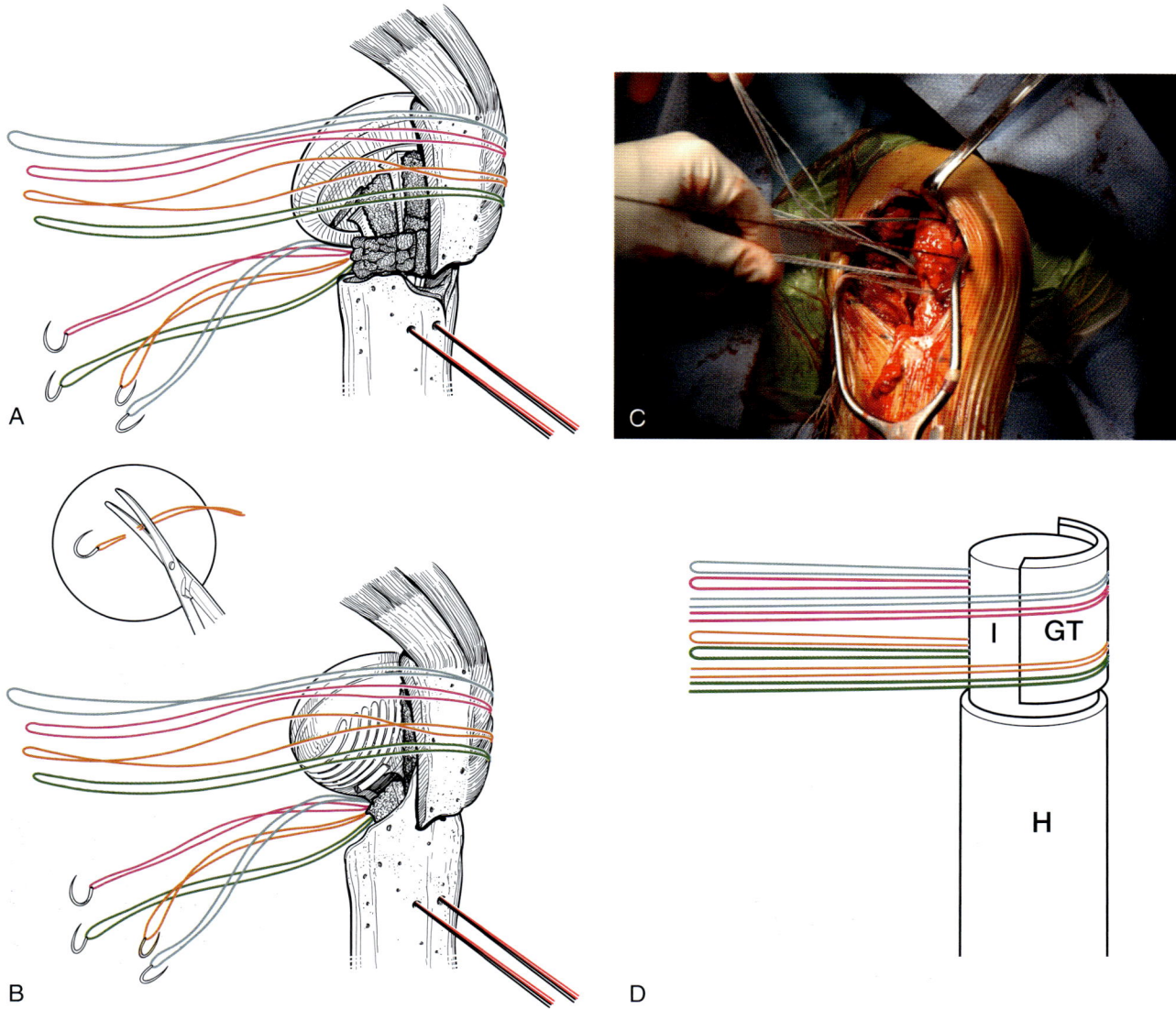

FIGURE 30.6 All passed sutures with either an unconstrained arthroplasty (A) or a reverse arthroplasty (B and C). (Inset) The four looped sutures have needles attached. The needle is cut off one of the superior looped sutures and off one of the inferior looped sutures. (D) Depicts a schematic of suture position. *GT*, Greater tuberosity; *H*, humeral shaft; *I*, implant.

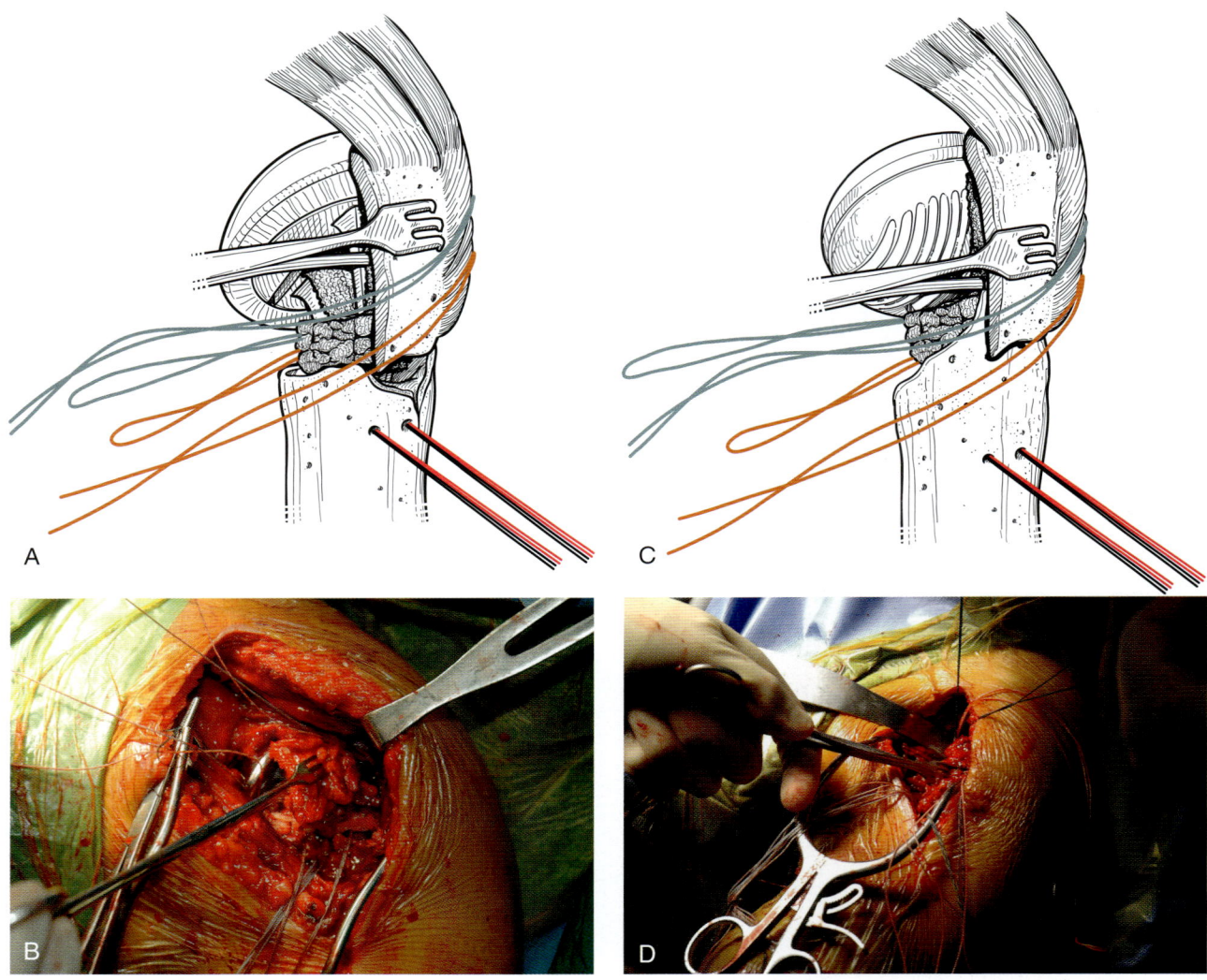

FIGURE 30.7 The greater tuberosity is gently grasped with Lahey forceps and reduced into position for an unconstrained arthroplasty (A and B) or a reverse arthroplasty (C and D).

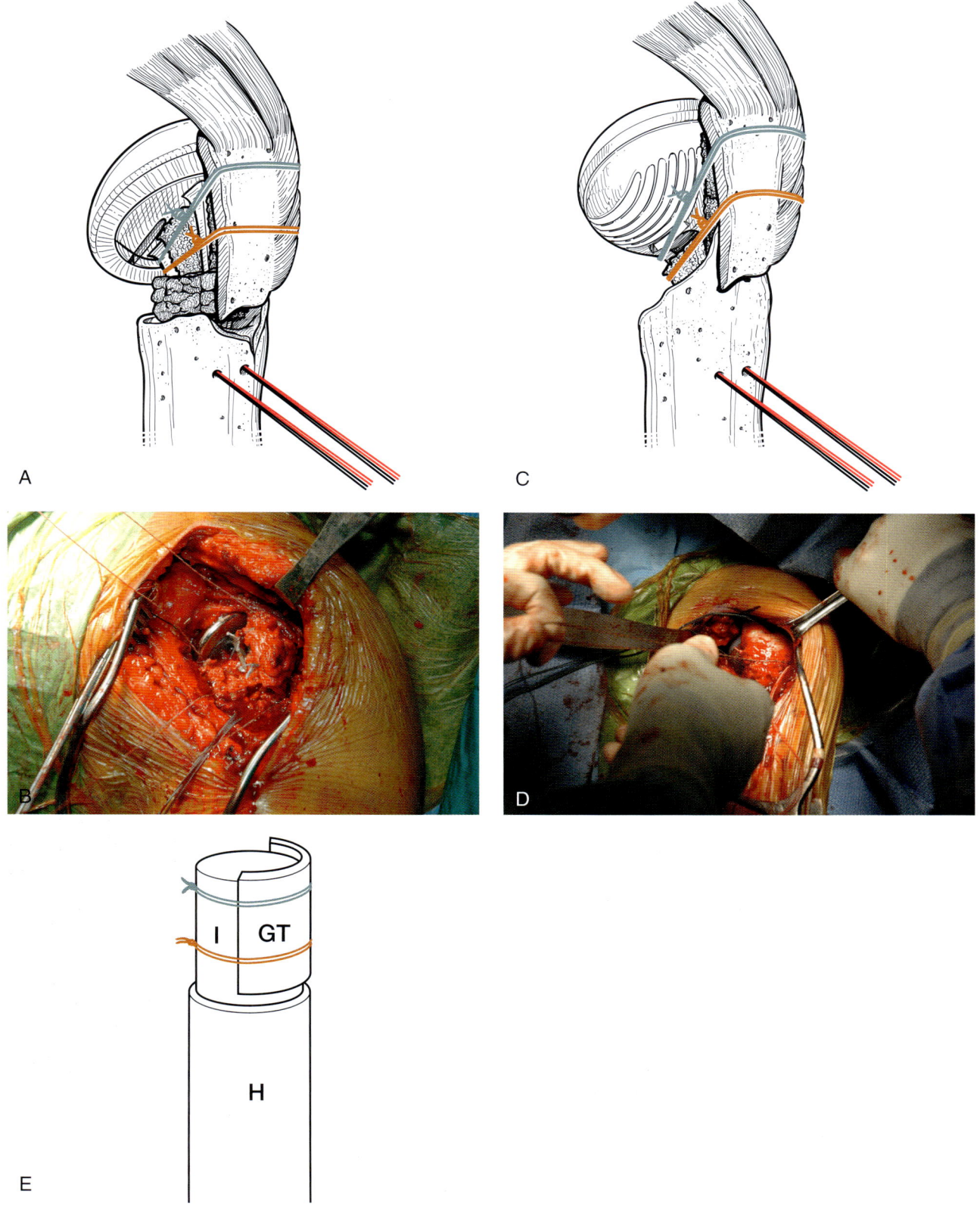

FIGURE 30.8 The sutures controlling the greater tuberosity, one superior and one inferior, are tied to fixate the greater tuberosity around either an unconstrained arthroplasty (A and B) or a reverse arthroplasty (C and D). (E) Depicts a schematic of suture position. *GT*, Greater tuberosity; *H*, humeral shaft; *I*, implant.

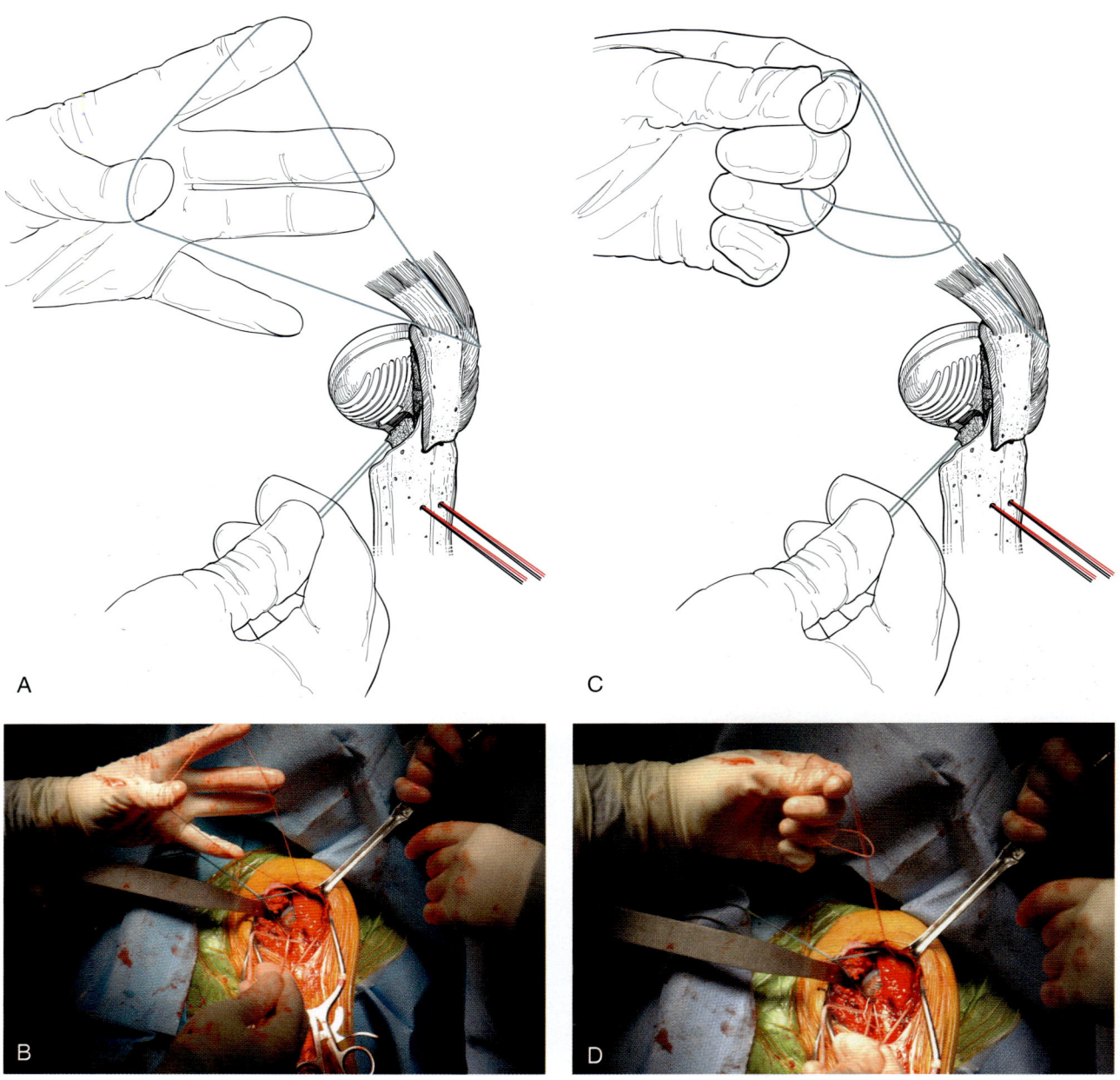

FIGURE 30.9 (A to D) The first step of the racking hitch: creation of a loop.

CHAPTER 30 ■ Tuberosity Reduction and Fixation 277

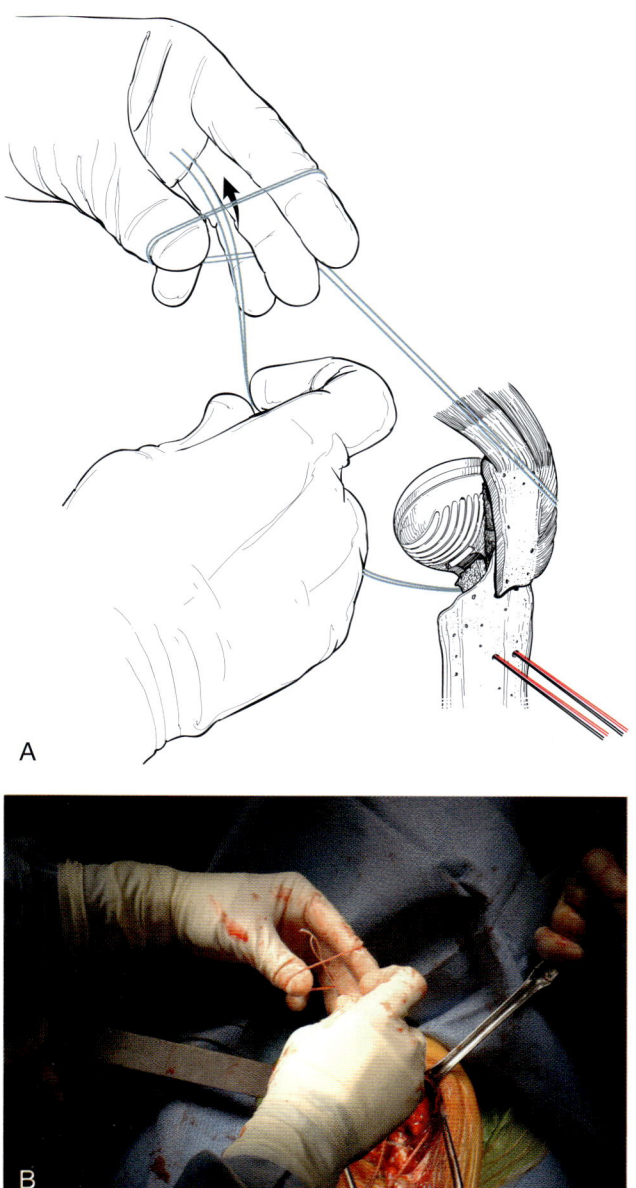

FIGURE 30.10 (A and B) The second step of the racking hitch: passing the free ends through the loop.

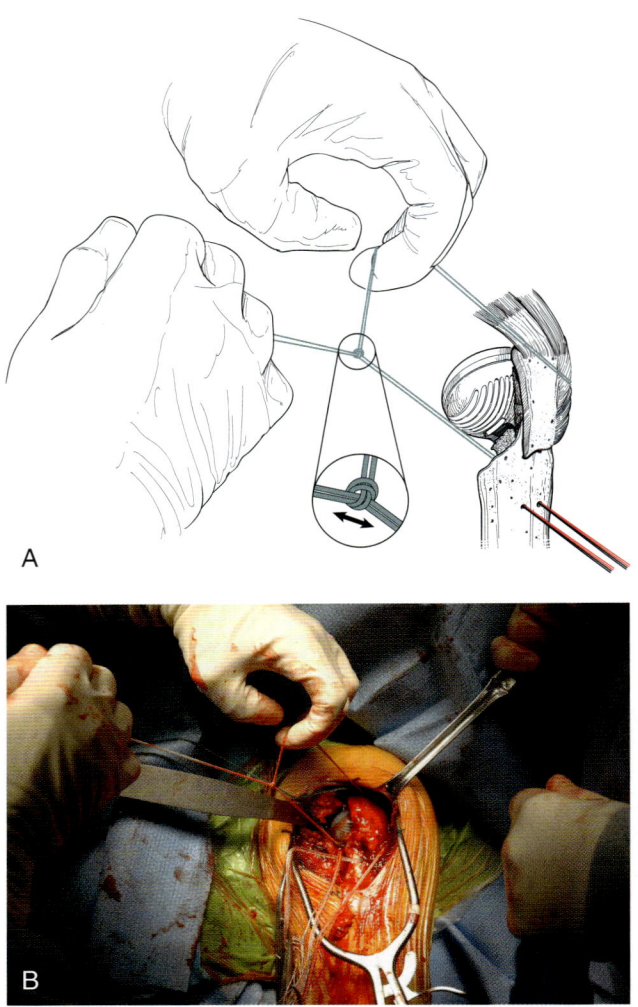

FIGURE 30.11 (A and B) The third step of the racking hitch: the free ends are pulled to tighten the racking hitch.

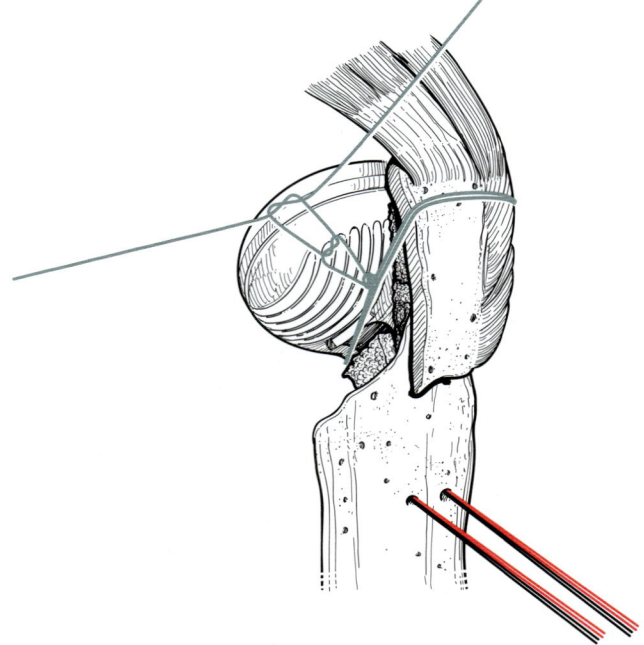

FIGURE 30.12 The racking hitch is then backed up with 4 half hitches.

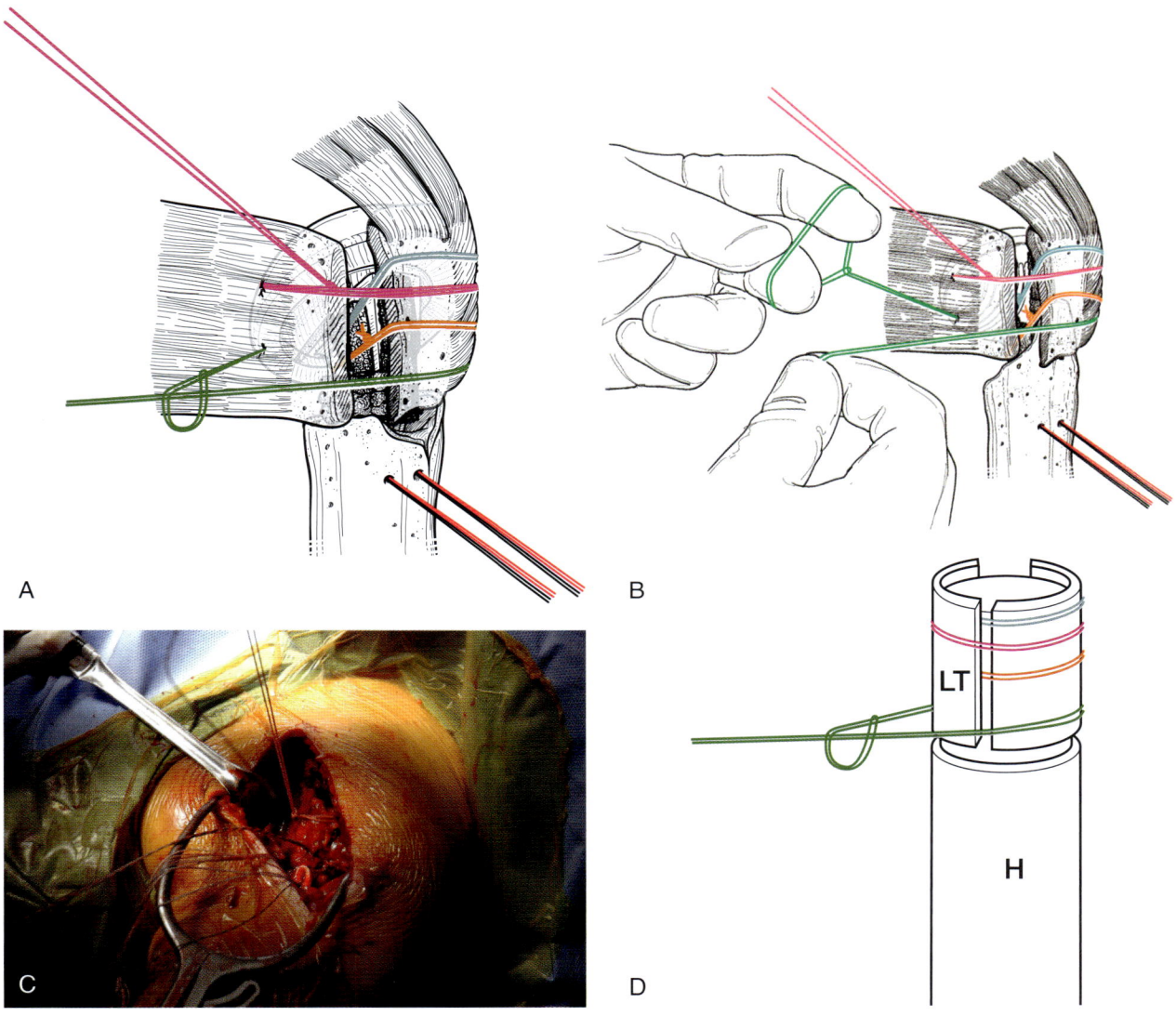

FIGURE 30.13 The remaining two looped sutures controlling the greater tuberosity, one superior and one inferior, are passed through the subscapularis tendon with a free needle just medial to its osseous insertion on the lesser tuberosity in unconstrained arthroplasty (A) or reverse arthroplasty (B and C). The lesser tuberosity is reduced with the previously placed stay sutures, and the circumferential sutures are tied using a racking hitch knot to secure the tuberosity. (D to G) depict illustrations, photos, and a schematic of the fixation of the lesser tuberosity. *GT,* Greater tuberosity; *H,* humeral shaft; *I,* implant.

Continued

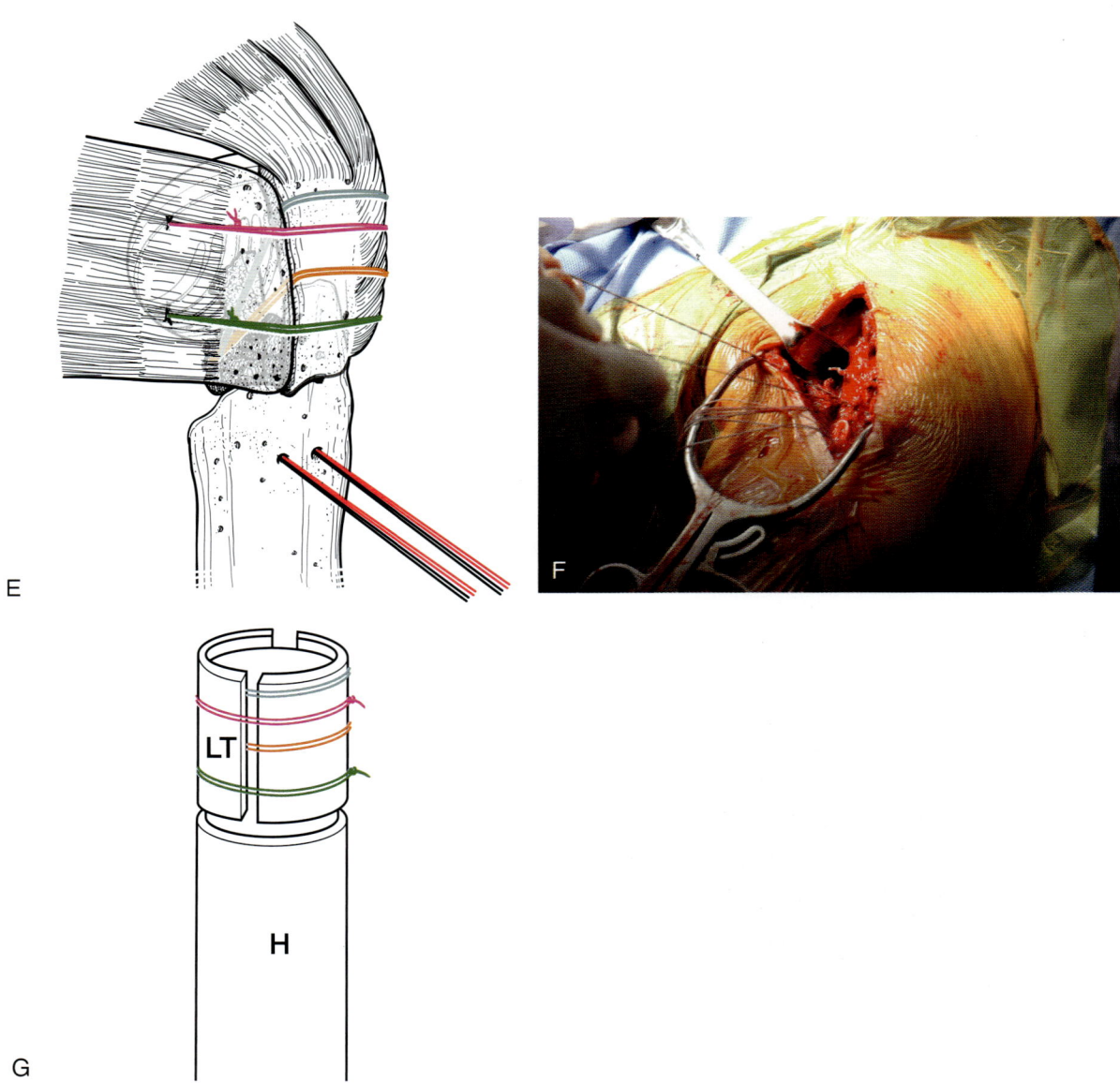

FIGURE 30.13, cont'd

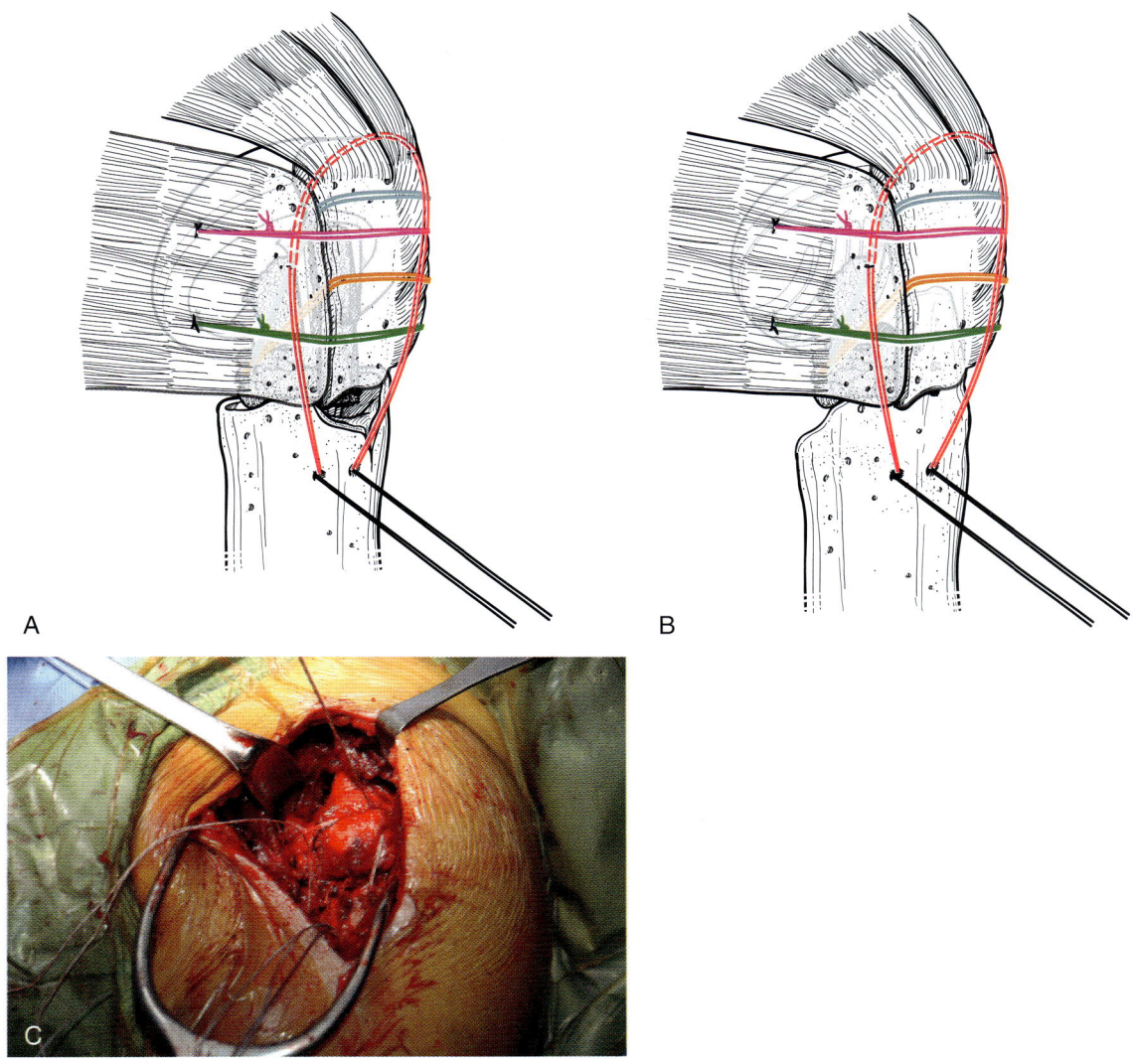

FIGURE 30.14 Vertical tuberosity fixation. One looped suture is passed with a free needle through the infraspinatus and supraspinatus tendons just medial to their osseous insertion and then secured using a racking hitch knot with either an unconstrained arthroplasty (A) or a reverse arthroplasty (B and C).

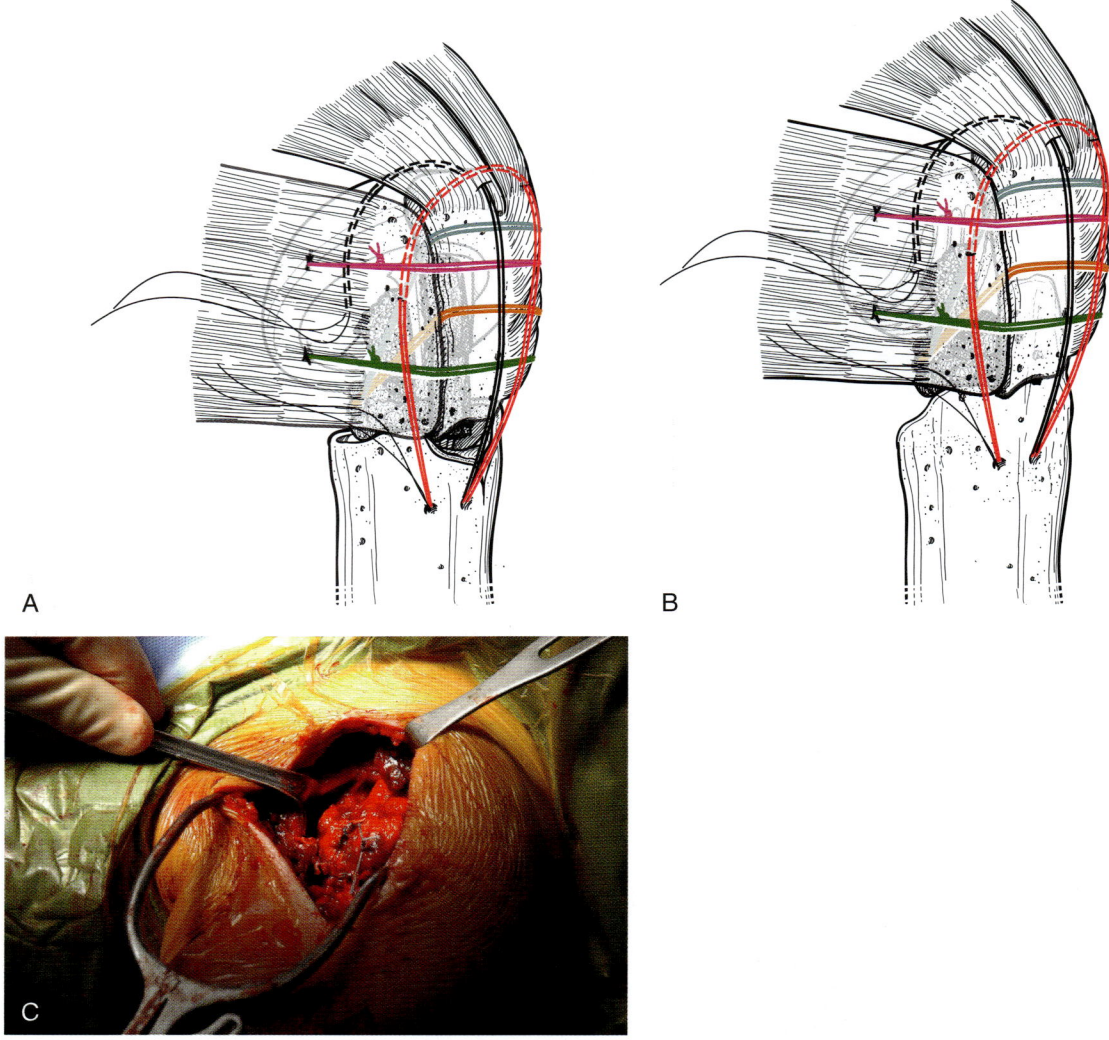

FIGURE 30.15 Vertical tuberosity fixation. A second looped suture is passed with a free needle through the subscapularis and supraspinatus tendons just medial to their osseous insertion and then secured using a racking hitch knot with either an unconstrained arthroplasty (A) or a reverse arthroplasty (B and C).

REFERENCES

1. Boileau P, Coste JS, Ahrens PM, et al: Prosthetic shoulder replacement for fracture: Results of the multicentre study. In Walch G, Boileau P, Molé D, editors: *2000 Prosthèses d'Epaule … Recul de 2 à 10 Ans*, Paris, 2001, Sauramps Medical, pp 561–578.
2. Chokshi BV, Ishak C, Iesaka K, et al: The modified racking hitch (MRH) knot—a new sliding knot for arthroscopic surgery, *Bull NYU Hosp Jt Dis* 65(4):306–307, 2007.
3. Kelly JD, Vaishnav S, Saunders BM, et al: Optimization of the racking hitch knot: How many half hitches and which suture material provide the preatest security?, *Clin Orthop Relat Res* 472:1930–1935, 2014.

The final steps of the operative procedure are wound closure and placement of the postoperative orthosis. The major difference from patients undergoing shoulder arthroplasty performed for chronic disease is the type of postoperative orthosis used.

TECHNIQUE FOR WOUND CLOSURE

After fixation of the tuberosities, the wound is irrigated with 800 mL of antibiotic-impregnated sterile saline (50,000 units of bacitracin per liter sterile normal saline) via a bulb syringe. The wound is checked to ensure that adequate hemostasis has been achieved. An electrocautery is used as necessary to minimize any residual hemorrhage. A drain is routinely used for arthroplasty for fracture cases. We use a medium closed wound suction drain (Bard, Inc., Covington, Georgia) for 24 hours after surgery (Fig. 31.1). The drain is placed deep to the deltopectoral interval with the trocar provided and exits the skin approximately 3 cm distal to the terminal extent of the skin incision (Fig. 31.2). The proximal extent of the drain tubing is trimmed with heavy scissors to allow the proximal tip of the drain to reach the superior aspect of the humerus (Fig. 31.3). Care is taken to not cut the drain tubing through a side portal because this risks fracture of the drain during removal (Fig. 31.4). Uncut half-inch Steri-Strips are applied immediately to secure the drain distally to skin (Fig. 31.5).

Wound closure is performed in the same manner as described for unconstrained arthroplasty (Chapter 15). We do not close the deltopectoral interval but initiate our closure with the overlying fascial layer. This layer is reapproximated with no. 0 braided absorbable suture in an interrupted figure-of-eight technique. Care is taken to avoid passing a suture through or around the drain. After sutures have been placed in the fascia, the drain should always be checked to make sure that it slides freely. The subcutaneous fascia is reapproximated with 2-0 braided absorbable suture via an interrupted figure-of-eight technique. The skin is reapproximated with 3-0 undyed absorbable monofilament suture in a subcuticular running closure.

The occlusive draping is removed adjacent to the incision and the skin is cleansed of blood with a saline-soaked sponge and then dried. Half-inch Steri-Strips are placed over the incision. Sterile gauze is placed over the incision and a sterile absorbent pad is placed over the gauze. The dressing is secured with 3-inch foam tape. The remaining surgical drapes are then removed.

The dressing is maintained in place until postoperative day 3, at which time it is removed. The distal extent of the dressing is loosened to allow drain removal the morning after surgery. After removal of the dressing on postoperative day 3, the patient is allowed to shower, but submerging the incision in a bathtub is prohibited until 2 weeks postoperatively. The Steri-Strips are progressively removed by the patient as they lose their adhesion to the skin, typically 10 to 14 days after surgery.

POSTOPERATIVE ORTHOSIS

The postoperative orthosis is placed in the operating room immediately after the dressing; it consists of a neutral-rotation sling (Fig. 31.6). This sling avoids internal rotation, a situation that places increased tension on the greater tuberosity fixation (Fig. 31.7). The sling is maintained for 4 to 6 weeks to protect the tuberosity repair. In patients with good bone quality and secure tuberosity fixation, the sling is discontinued at 4 weeks. In patients with poor bone quality or less secure tuberosity fixation (or both), the sling is maintained until 6 weeks postoperatively. Patients are allowed to remove the sling only for hygiene and rehabilitation exercises. Patients are discouraged from internally rotating or adducting the arm before the postoperative orthosis has been discontinued because of the potential for tuberosity migration.

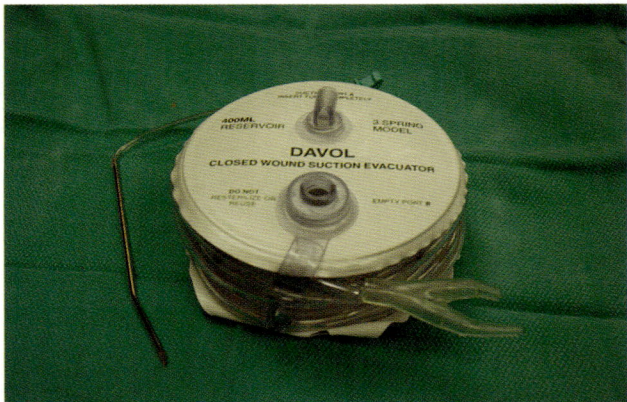

FIGURE 31.1 The type of medium suction drain used in arthroplasty for fracture cases.

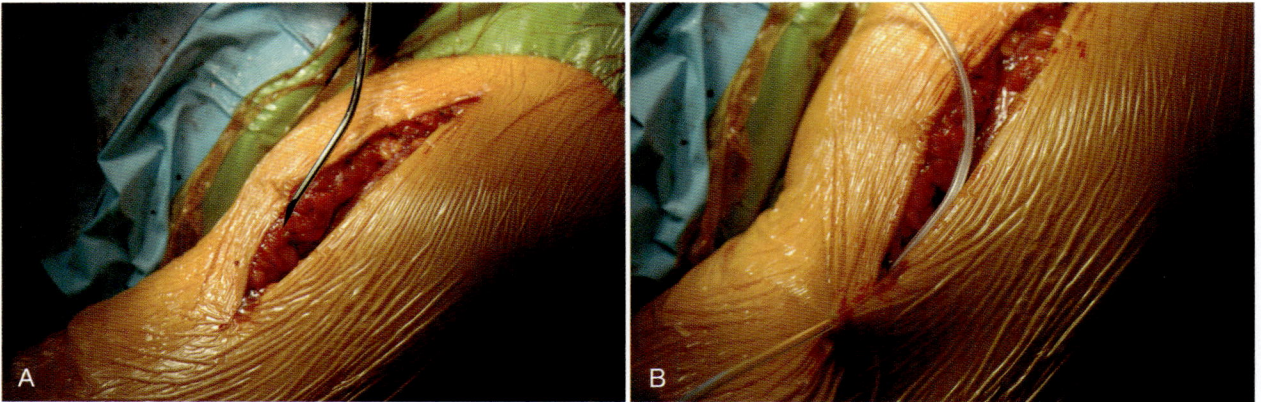

FIGURE 31.2 (A and B) Placement of the drain with the trocar provided.

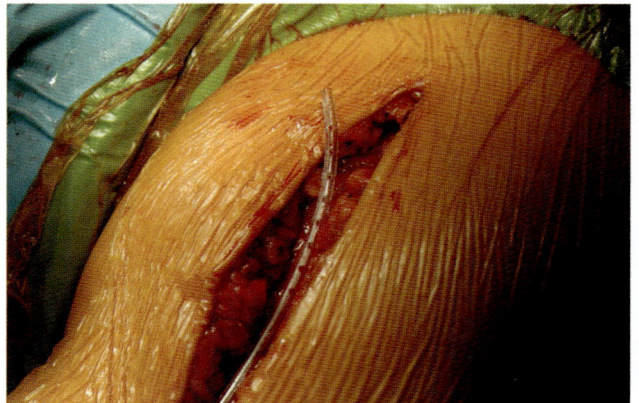

FIGURE 31.3 Proximal extent of the drain.

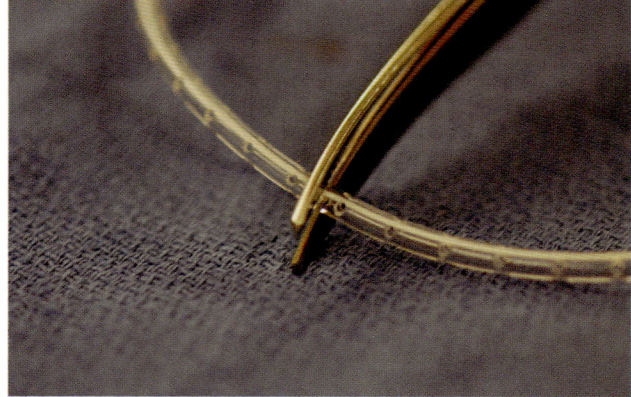

FIGURE 31.4 Care is taken to not cut the drain tubing through a side portal because this risks fracture of the drain during removal.

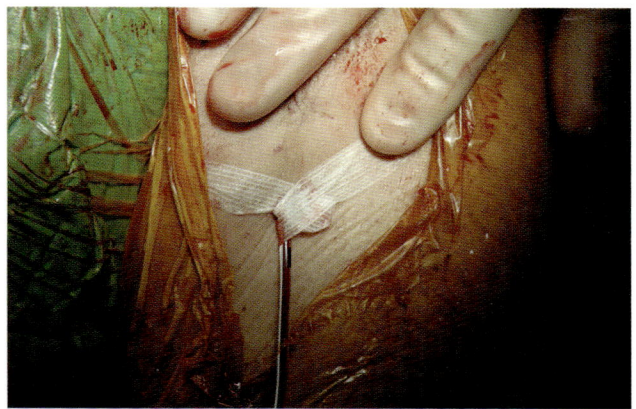

FIGURE 31.5 Uncut half-inch Steri-Strips are used immediately to secure the drain distally to the skin.

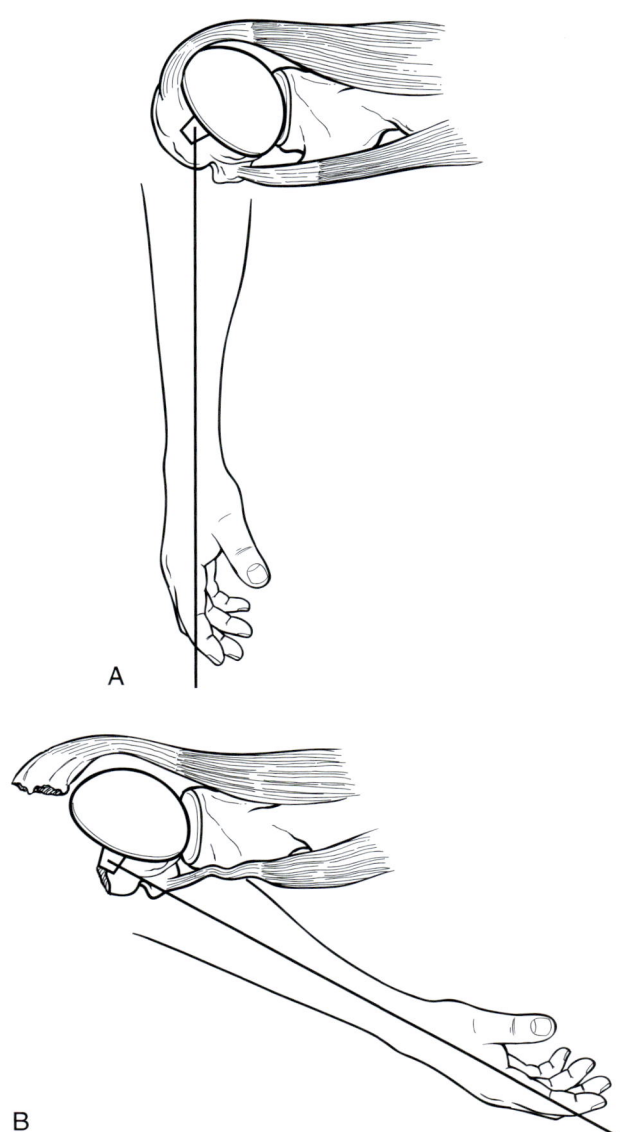

FIGURE 31.7 (A and B) Tension placed on the greater tuberosity repair when positioning the arm in internal rotation.

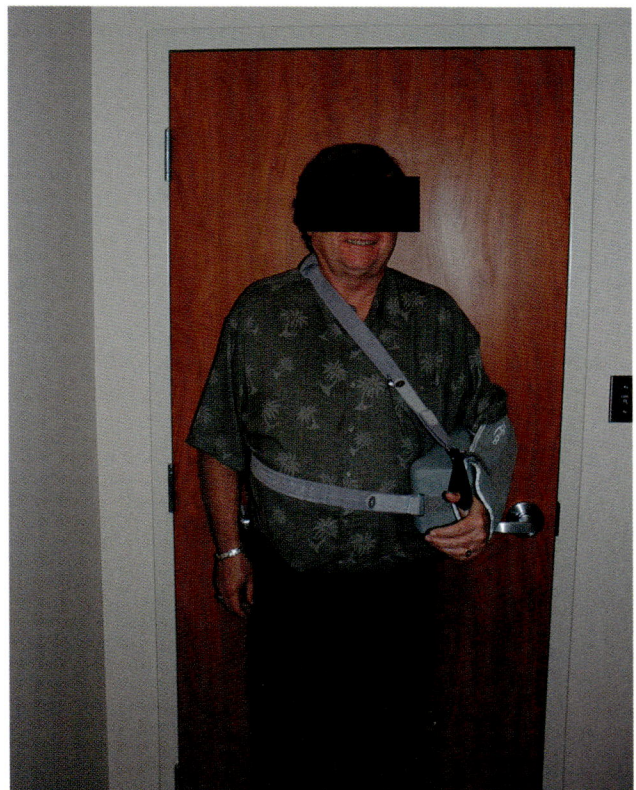

FIGURE 31.6 Neutral rotation sling used after shoulder arthroplasty for fracture.

CHAPTER 32
Results and complications

The results of unconstrained shoulder arthroplasty for fracture have been reported by multiple investigators. The overall results have been very disappointing and are not comparable with those obtained for chronic conditions such as primary osteoarthritis. The advances in unconstrained arthroplasty implants and techniques for fracture described in this section have greatly improved the results. Fortunately, results from reverse shoulder arthroplasty for fracture are promising, with improved early outcomes compared with unconstrained shoulder arthroplasty for fracture. To our knowledge, the largest reported database of results of unconstrained shoulder arthroplasty for fracture was presented in Nice, France, in 2001.[1] Because of the large number of patients enrolled, this multicenter study has allowed meaningful conclusions to be made about the outcomes and complications of unconstrained shoulder arthroplasty for the treatment of fracture. Our results have largely mirrored those reported in the Nice study. This chapter reports the results of unconstrained shoulder arthroplasty and reverse shoulder arthroplasty for the treatment of proximal humerus fractures by drawing from information in the Nice database and our arthroplasty database that was prospectively established in 2003. In addition, the most frequent complications and their treatment are outlined.

RESULTS

The results of unconstrained shoulder arthroplasty for fracture are largely related to two prognostic factors: age and the presence of tuberosity complications (nonunion, malunion). These two factors are related in that older patients are more likely to have osteopenia of the tuberosities and hence complications with tuberosity healing. Although age-related osteopenia is beyond the surgeon's control, advances in prosthetic design and tuberosity fixation techniques continue to decrease the rate of tuberosity-related complications. Table 32.1 details the results of unconstrained and reverse shoulder arthroplasty in the treatment of proximal humeral fracture.[2] This table expresses the results in terms of active mobility; patient satisfaction; the Constant score, a shoulder-specific outcomes device incorporating pain, mobility, activity, and strength; and the age- and gender-adjusted Constant score.[3,4]

INTRAOPERATIVE COMPLICATIONS

Intraoperative complications are uncommon during shoulder arthroplasty for proximal humeral fractures and are usually related to neurovascular injury or iatrogenic humeral shaft fracture.

Neurovascular Structures

Catastrophic injury to neurovascular structures around the shoulder, although rare, is more common during performance of shoulder arthroplasty for fracture than for performance of shoulder arthroplasty for nonfracture indications. Many patients with proximal humeral fractures suffer neuropraxic injury to the axillary nerve, and this should be documented on clinical examination before surgery. In addition, the implications of axillary nerve injury secondary to fracture should be discussed with the patient extensively before surgery. Treatment of axillary nerve injury is observation, with less than 2% of patients sustaining a permanent axillary nerve deficit.[5]

Vascular injuries during shoulder arthroplasty performed for fracture most often involve injury to the axillary artery. Such injury is usually a consequence of overzealous medial dissection or retraction (or both), combined with vasculature that has been compromised by aging (plaques, calcification). Should one of these injuries occur, after cross-clamping of the injured structure, emergency intraoperative consultation with a vascular surgeon is required.

Humeral Shaft Fracture

Intraoperative humeral shaft fractures are very rare when performing shoulder arthroplasty for the treatment of proximal humeral fractures. Intraoperative stiffness is rarely a problem in these cases, thus minimizing the torsional stress placed on the humeral shaft during manipulation of the arm. More commonly, humeral injury occurs during reaming of the humeral shaft. The diaphyseal cortex in many elderly patients is very thin and hence has an increased risk of diaphyseal penetration. When this complication occurs, it is often unrecognized (Fig. 32.1).

Glenoid Fracture

In proximal humeral fracture cases, intraoperative fractures occur only with reverse shoulder arthroplasty; however, they can be more detrimental than humeral injury. Intraoperative glenoid fractures occurring in this setting should be handled similar to intraoperative glenoid fractures occurring in reverse shoulder arthroplasty cases for nonfracture conditions (see Chapter 25).

CHAPTER 32 ■ Results and Complications

TABLE 32.1	Results of Unconstrained and Reverse Shoulder Arthroplasty in the Treatment of Proximal Humeral Fractures				
	Absolute Constant Score (Points) (Postoperative)	Adjusted Constant Score (%) (Postoperative)	Active Forward Flexion (Degrees) (Postoperative)	Active External Rotation (Degrees) (Postoperative)	Excellent/Good Subjective Results (%)
Nice series (n = 300)[2]					
Hemiarthroplasty for fracture (n = 300)	54	74	103	21	39
Author's prospective database (n = 76)					
Hemiarthroplasty for fracture (n = 39)	49	62	106	25	68
Reverse shoulder arthroplasty for fracture (n = 37)	71	102	154	31	92

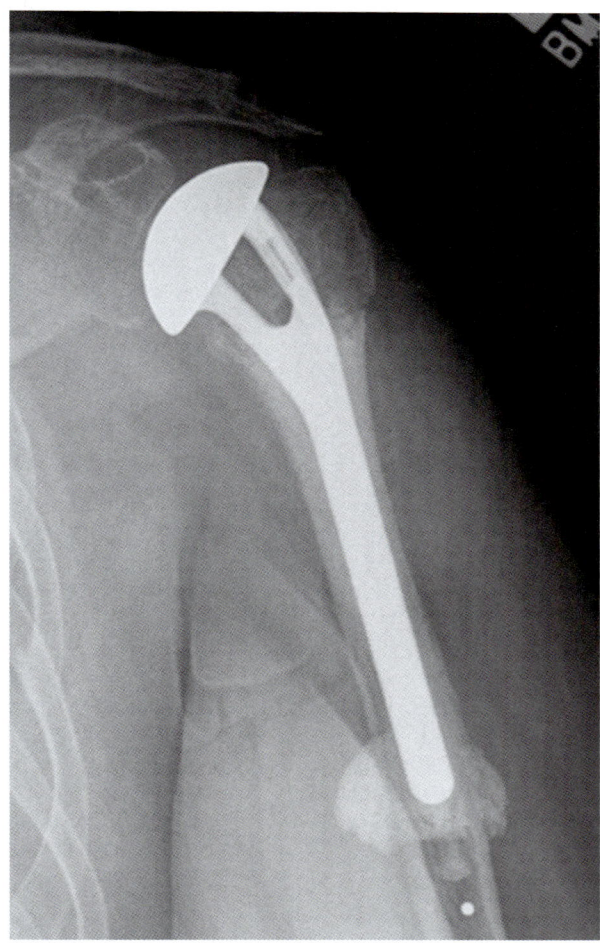

FIGURE 32.1 Radiograph of cement extravasation after unrecognized diaphyseal perforation during insertion of a humeral stem for a proximal humeral fracture.

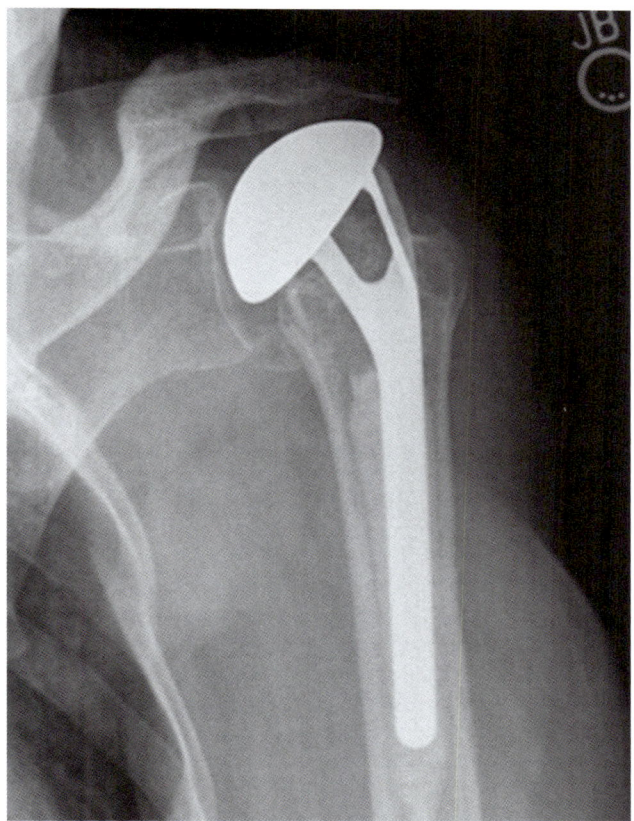

FIGURE 32.2 Migration of the greater tuberosity after unconstrained shoulder arthroplasty performed for a proximal humeral fracture.

POSTOPERATIVE COMPLICATIONS

Postoperative complications are much more common than intraoperative complications and occur in up to 50% of cases of unconstrained shoulder arthroplasty performed for fracture and in a high percentage (up to 20%) of reverse shoulder arthroplasty for fracture cases.[5,6] Most complications involve the greater or lesser tuberosities (or both) but also may include wound problems (dehiscence, hematoma), glenoid problems, humeral problems, instability, stiffness, and infection.

Tuberosity Complications

Nonunion and malunion of the greater and lesser tuberosities are the most common complications after shoulder arthroplasty for fracture cases, especially for unconstrained shoulder arthroplasty for fracture (Fig. 32.2). The occurrence of a tuberosity complication compromises the outcome

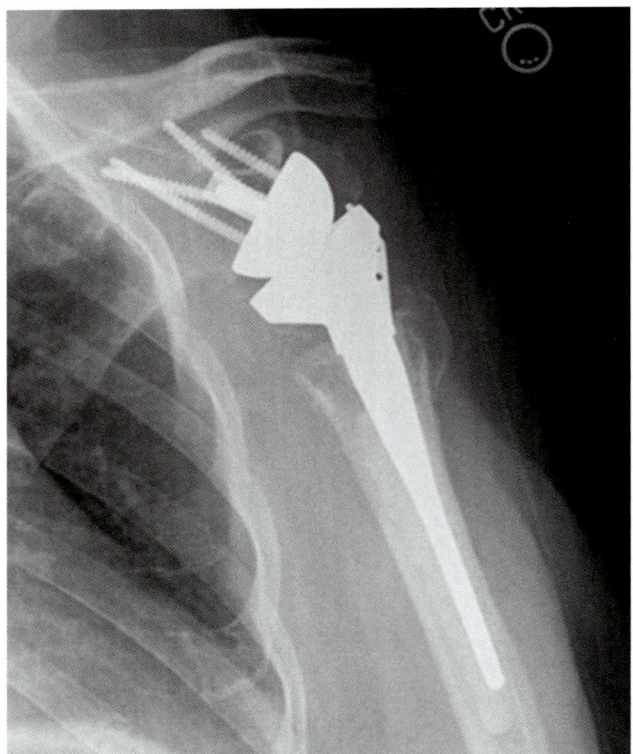

FIGURE 32.3 Revision of a hemiarthroplasty to a reverse prosthesis for the treatment of greater tuberosity migration.

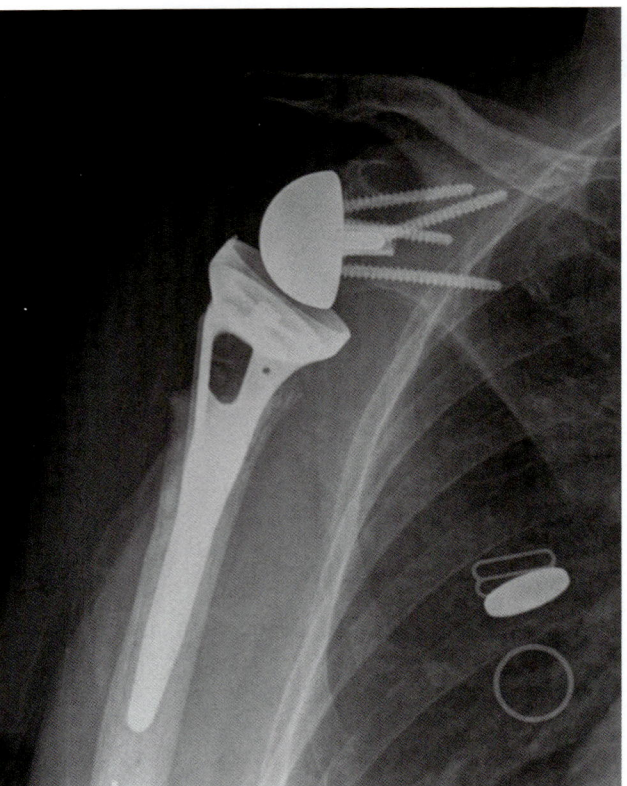

FIGURE 32.4 Migration of the greater tuberosity after reverse shoulder arthroplasty performed for a proximal humeral fracture. Treatment of this patient is with observation.

significantly in unconstrained shoulder arthroplasty and to less degree in reverse shoulder arthroplasty for fracture cases. The best way to handle tuberosity complications is to avoid them by using the techniques described in this section. When tuberosity complications do occur, there is no simple solution that provides a reliable result. Even early recognition and reattachment of a migrated tuberosity yields unsatisfactory results in nearly all cases. Similarly, tuberosity osteotomy produces poor results in cases of malunion. The most predictable results for tuberosity complications after unconstrained shoulder arthroplasty for fracture are obtained with revision arthroplasty to a reverse prosthesis (Fig. 32.3; see Section VI).

Tuberosity complications following reverse shoulder arthroplasty for fracture are uncommon. For reasons not completely understood, the tuberosities seem to heal more readily following reverse shoulder arthroplasty for fracture compared with unconstrained shoulder arthroplasty for fracture. In the uncommon event that the greater tuberosity does not heal following reverse shoulder arthroplasty for fracture, treatment is simply observation. It is important to educate these patients that, although their active elevation will be acceptable, active external rotation will likely be compromised (Fig. 32.4).

Wound Problems

Wound problems occur early after shoulder arthroplasty for fracture. Hematoma is most easily avoided by extensive use of electrocautery during the procedure and closed suction drainage for 24 hours postoperatively. When a hematoma occurs, it is managed by symptomatic nonoperative treatment (warm compresses, pain medication). Operative drainage is reserved for situations in which drainage persists beyond 1 week or infection is suspected (see later) and is rarely necessary.

Wound dehiscence occurs occasionally when susceptible patients have a reaction to dissolving subcutaneous sutures. The presence of minimal serous drainage distinguishes this complication from the more serious deep infection. Superficial wound dehiscence is treated with local wound care, including removal of any residual dissolving suture material and chemical cauterization of any granulating tissue with silver nitrate applicators.

Glenoid Problems

Glenoid problems after unconstrained shoulder arthroplasty for fracture are exceedingly rare. After hemiarthroplasty for fracture, erosion of the glenoid articular cartilage and osseous glenoid can occur. Successful treatment of glenoid erosion usually requires revision surgery with resurfacing of the glenoid or conversion to reverse shoulder arthroplasty.

Glenoid problems after reverse shoulder arthroplasty for fracture are uncommon and no different than expected in a standard reverse shoulder arthroplasty. Glenoid complications following reverse shoulder arthroplasty for fracture should be handled similar to glenoid complications occurring in reverse shoulder arthroplasty cases for nonfracture conditions (see Chapter 25).

Humeral Diaphysis Problems

Humeral diaphysis problems after shoulder arthroplasty for fracture are rare and consist of loosening of the humeral component or periprosthetic humeral fracture.

Aseptic loosening of the humeral stem occurs more frequently in fracture cases than in nonfracture cases, mainly because of the lack of metaphyseal support of the implant. Use of cement is recommended in fracture cases to help prevent this potential complication. Whenever a humeral stem loosens, infection must be ruled out (see later). In the rare instance of symptomatic aseptic loosening of the humeral component in an unconstrained shoulder arthroplasty for fracture, treatment is revision of the humeral stem, often with a reverse prosthesis, because this complication is generally accompanied by tuberosity nonunion (see Section VI).

Periprosthetic humeral fractures are almost always the result of a fall or similar low-energy trauma. The majority of these fractures occur just distal to the tip of the humeral stem, and most can be treated nonoperatively. Nonoperative treatment consists of fracture bracing, activity modification, pain medication, and frequent radiographic monitoring. If the fracture has not healed within 3 months, we incorporate the use of an external bone stimulator (OL 1000 Bone Growth Stimulator, Donjoy Orthopedics, Vista, California). Despite these measures, periprosthetic humeral fractures treated nonoperatively may take longer than 9 months to heal.[7] Our criteria for recommending operative treatment of periprosthetic fractures (revision surgery; see Section VI) include complete displacement, angulation of greater than 30 degrees, loosening of the humeral component, or failure of nonoperative treatment.

Instability

Instability after unconstrained shoulder arthroplasty for fracture is usually related to tuberosity nonunion or, less commonly, prosthetic malalignment. Tuberosity nonunion may result in static migration of the humerus superiorly or anterosuperiorly, similar to the situation in a patient with rotator cuff tear arthropathy that has undergone hemiarthroplasty. In most cases, reattachment of the tuberosities does not resolve the instability, so we treat these patients by revision to a reverse shoulder arthroplasty (Fig. 32.5; see Section VI).

Less commonly, prosthetic malposition will lead to instability despite healing of the tuberosities. The instability is caused by version malalignment (excessive retroversion causing posterior instability or excessive anteversion causing anterior instability) or by the humeral stem's being implanted at an improper level with the humeral shaft (Fig. 32.6). In this scenario, revision of the humeral stem to change prosthetic position is necessary (see Section VI). If the prosthetic malalignment has resulted in wear of the glenoid cartilage, resurfacing of the glenoid should be considered as well.

Although common when treating nonfracture conditions, instability after reverse shoulder arthroplasty for fracture is exceedingly rare in our practice. We feel that appropriate tuberosity management with the described surgical technique and appropriate tensioning will minimize the occurrence of instability in reverse arthroplasty for fracture cases. The biggest suspected cause of instability in reverse arthroplasty for fracture cases would be inappropriate humeral prosthesis height and lack of tuberosity fixation. See Chapter 25 for more information on causes and treatment of instability after reverse shoulder arthroplasty.

Stiffness

Glenohumeral stiffness is a common complication after unconstrained shoulder arthroplasty for fracture and is related to capsular contracture or the prosthesis (or both). Prosthetic problems resulting in stiffness are almost always the result of implantation of too large a humeral component or placement of the humeral component in the wrong position, as described earlier. Rehabilitation with capsular stretching can be attempted in an effort to improve mobility. If rehabilitation fails (no improvement over a 6-month period), revision surgery is indicated, consisting of realignment of the humeral component or downsizing of the humeral head with open release of any capsular contractures that are present.

Stiffness related to capsular contracture almost always responds to nonoperative management with aquatic-based rehabilitation (see Chapter 43). If the patient shows no improvement in mobility over a 6-month course of rehabilitation and has no obvious prosthetic problem, we consider the patient a candidate for arthroscopic capsular contracture release.

Glenohumeral stiffness after reverse shoulder arthroplasty for fracture is rare. Limitation of mobility after implantation of a reverse prosthesis is usually related to mechanical limitation of the prosthetic design and not capsular contracture. We personally have no experience in dealing with postoperative capsulitis after implantation of a reverse prosthesis.

Scapular Notching

Although whether it should be considered a complication is debatable, notching of the scapula occurs within 2 years of surgery in up to half the patients who undergo reverse shoulder arthroplasty. Scapular notching can occur after reverse for fracture no differently than after other indications for reverse shoulder arthroplasty (see Chapter 25).

Infection

Infection after shoulder arthroplasty for fracture is rare, although more common than with other indications for primary arthroplasty. Patients most at risk for infection are those with systemic illness (diabetes mellitus) and those with compromised soft tissues (open fractures). These infections are most commonly caused by *Staphylococcus aureus* or *Propionibacterium acnes*. Infections after shoulder arthroplasty can be divided into perioperative (within 6 weeks of surgery) and late (hematogenous) infections.

Early perioperative infections are initially treated with multiple (two or three) irrigation and débridement procedures and retention of the humeral component if the tuberosity repair remains intact. At the last planned irrigation and

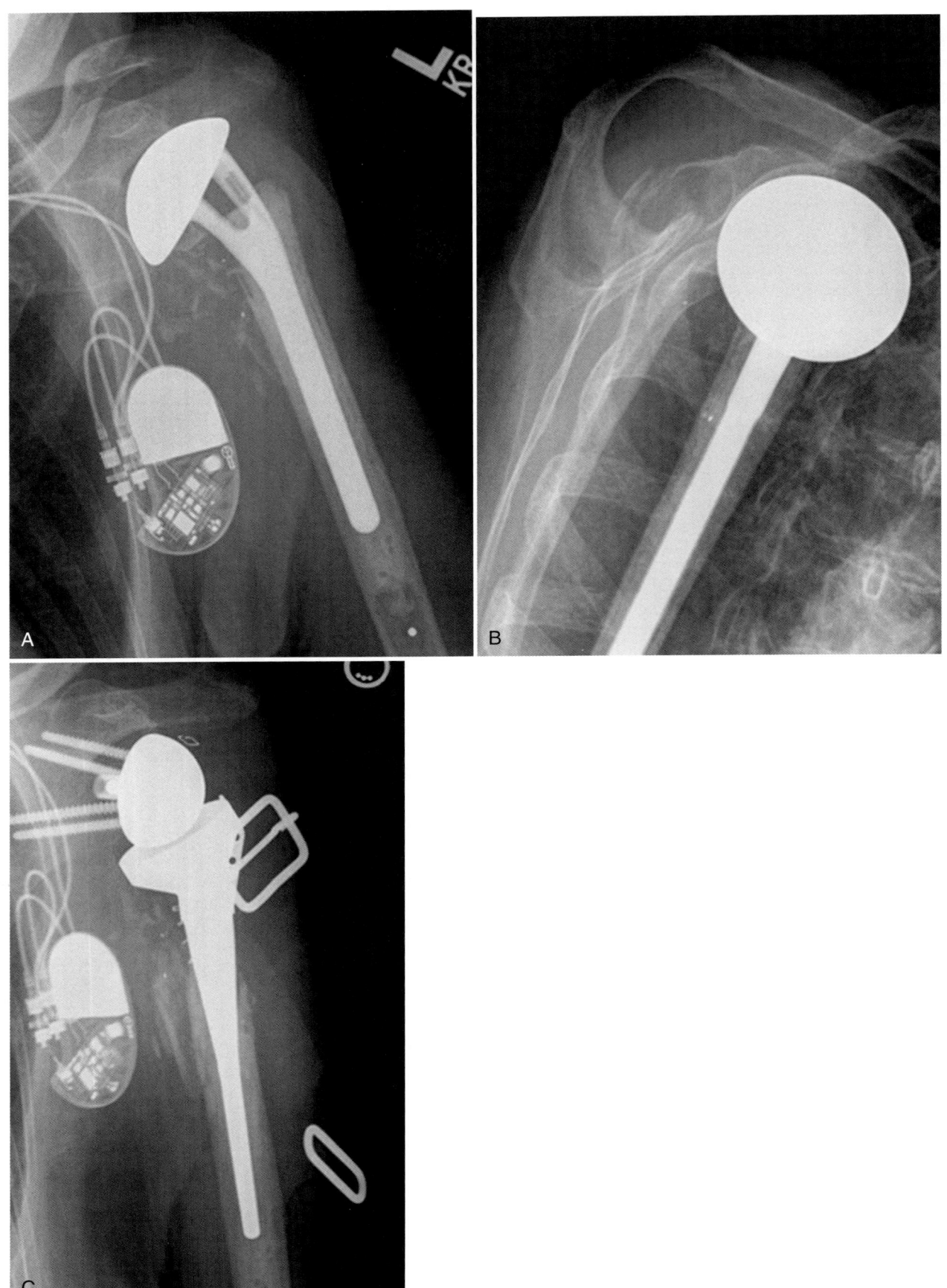

FIGURE 32.5 (A–C) Anterosuperior instability of a hemiarthroplasty used in the treatment of a proximal humeral fracture necessitated revision with a reverse prosthesis.

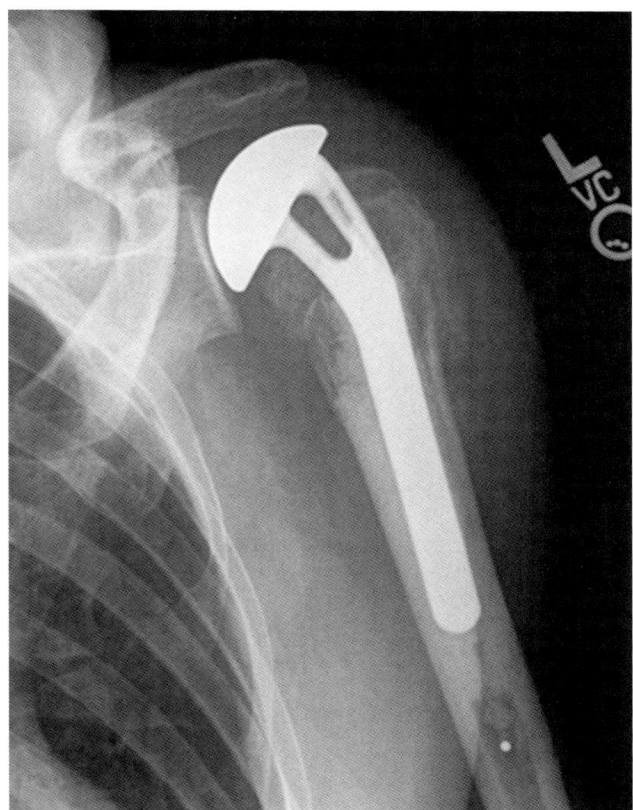

FIGURE 32.6 A humeral stem implanted too proximally within the humeral shaft resulted in instability.

débridement procedure, absorbable antibiotic-impregnated beads (Osteoset, Wright Medical Technology, Inc., Memphis, TN) are placed in the soft tissues around the shoulder. Consultation with an infectious disease specialist is obtained, and a minimum of 6 weeks of intravenous antibiotics tailored to the specific organism causing the infection (or covering the most likely offending organisms, if cultures remain negative despite obvious infection) is usually recommended. If this regimen fails or if the tuberosity repair fails because of the infection, the humeral component is removed and the patient is treated in the same manner as for a late-appearing infection.

Late-appearing infections are treated by removal of the prosthesis and intravenous antibiotics, as detailed in Section VI. The decision whether to perform a revision shoulder arthroplasty or continue with a resection arthroplasty is patient specific. See Chapter 36 for additional information of the diagnosis and treatment of periprosthetic infection.

REFERENCES

1. Walch G, Boileau P: Presentation of the multicentric study. In Walch G, Boileau P, Molé D, editors: *2000 Prosthèses d'Epaule…Recul de 2 à 10 Ans*, Paris, 2001, Sauramps Medical, pp 11–20.
2. Hubert L, Dayez J: Results of the standard Aequalis prosthesis for proximal humeral fractures: The entire series. In Walch G, Boileau P, Molé D, editors: *2000 Prosthèses d'Epaule…Recul de 2 à 10 Ans*, Paris, 2001, Sauramps Medical, pp 527–529.
3. Constant CR, Murley AH: A clinical method of functional assessment of the shoulder, *Clin Orthop Relat Res* 214:160–164, 1987.
4. Constant CR: Assessment of shoulder function. In Gazielly D, Gleyze P, Thomas T, editors: *The cuff*, New York, 1997, Elsevier, pp 39–44.
5. Schild F, Burger B, Willems J: Complications of prostheses for fractures. In Walch G, Boileau P, Molé D, editors: *2000 Prosthèses d'Epaule…Recul de 2 à 10 Ans*, Paris, 2001, Sauramps Medical, pp 539–544.
6. Namdari S, Horneff JG, Baldwin K: Comparison of hemiarthroplasty and reverse arthroplasty for treatment of proximal humeral fractures: a systematic review, *J Bone Joint Surg Am* 95(18):1701–1708, 2013.
7. Kumar S, Sperling JW, Haidukewych GH, et al: Periprosthetic humeral fractures after shoulder arthroplasty, *J Bone Joint Surg Am* 86:680–689, 2004.

SECTION V
ALTERNATIVES TO CONVENTIONAL SHOULDER ARTHROPLASTY

CHAPTER 33
Stemless shoulder arthroplasty

The modern-day shoulder arthroplasty design has evolved from Dr. Charles Neer's design dating back to the 1950s.[1–3] The humeral side has classically been a stemmed implant. The size of the stemmed implant has evolved over time from long stems to shorter stems that are now more commonly used. Most consider the current humeral stems to be the fourth generation.[2]

Dr. Stephen Copeland pioneered humeral head resurfacing in the 1980s.[4] Humeral head resurfacing involves retaining the humeral head but using a reamer over the existing native humeral head and impacting a metallic humeral resurfacing cap. The advantage of complete surface replacement of the humeral head lies mainly in preservation of subchondral bone.[4]

It is important to distinguish humeral head resurfacing with a metallic cap from a stemless or canal-sparing humeral implant. Humeral head resurfacing involves retaining the humeral head, whereas utilization of a stemless humeral implant involves making a standard humeral head cut along the anatomic neck, as described in Chapter 11. Making the humeral head cut along the anatomic neck for a stemless humeral implant enables the same exposure for prosthetic glenoid implantation as one would achieve for total shoulder arthroplasty with a stemmed humeral implant. Situations in our practice in which humeral head resurfacing is more advantageous than conventional humeral head replacement with a stemmed or stemless humeral implant are increasingly rare.

Stemless or canal-sparing humeral components first became commercially available in Europe in 2004.[3] Stemless humeral components achieve metaphyseal fixation and do not violate the humeral canal. Stemless implants have been offered as an alternative to help decrease complications with stemmed implants. Although the humeral side is a rare mode of failure in shoulder arthroplasty, there are some theoretical advantages of a stemless implant, including decreased intraoperative and postoperative humeral fractures, facilitation of revision arthroplasty, and bone preservation.[3] Stemless humeral components also permit anatomic placement and sizing of the humeral head that is not dependent on the stem or the metaphyseal-diaphyseal relationship.[3] Stemmed humeral components rarely exhibit aseptic loosening; however, longer-term follow-up of stemmed humeral implants shows medial calcar bone loss, and it is unclear if this is secondary to stress shielding or osteolysis from glenoid component polyethylene wear.[3,5] It remains to be seen whether the canal-sparing humeral implants will reduce the incidence of medial calcar bone loss noted with stemmed humeral implants. The only published results in the United States on stemless humeral implants for unconstrained total shoulder arthroplasty showed good clinical results in a prospective 2-year multicenter study with no evidence of humeral component migration, subsidence, osteolysis, or loosening.[3]

Mid-term follow-up (5-year minimum follow-up) is available from a single stemless humeral component used for unconstrained total shoulder arthroplasty in Europe.[6,7] Functional outcomes were good, and there were no revisions due to humeral prosthetic loosening; however, 34.9% demonstrated "decreased density of cancellous bone in the greater tuberosity."[6] Similar findings were noted with a stemless humeral implant in unconstrained total shoulder arthroplasty, with 17 of 47 patients (36.2%) demonstrating radiolucent lines superior and lateral to the implant that appeared to be static.[8] There were no revisions for humeral loosening.[8] The radiographic findings in stemless humeral components were subsequently studied in a cadaveric model with computed tomography.[9] The study concluded that the radiolucencies appear to be "imaging artifact" and the radiographic "halo" disappears with adjustments in the imaging sequence voltage.

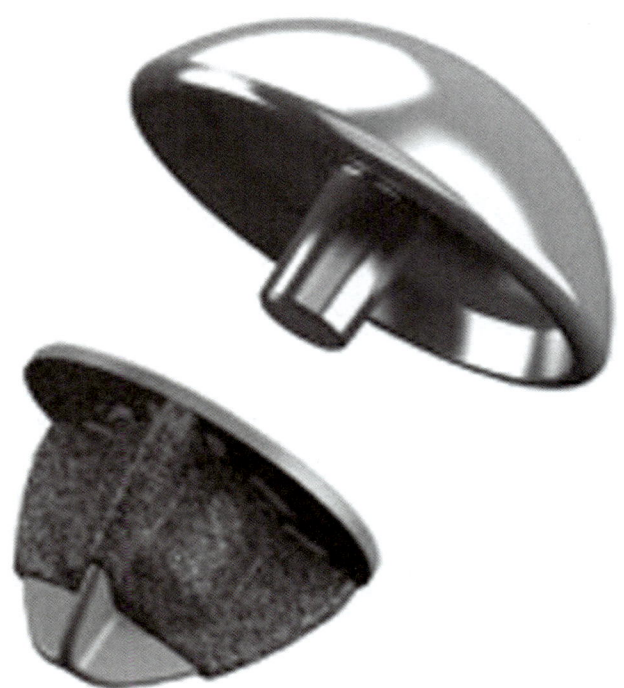

FIGURE 33.1 Simpliciti stemless shoulder arthroplasty. (Wright Medical N.V.)

The "halo effect" was more pronounced in specimens with decreased bone density.[9] Early clinical results from stemless appear to be promising, but longer-term follow-up is needed to confirm the early radiographic and clinical findings.

The number of stemless implant options is growing, with at least eight available in Europe.[7] There is currently one stemless implant commercially available in the United States. Two additional stemless implants are part of US Food and Drug Administration (FDA) Investigational Device Exemption study protocols.[7] There are currently no available stemless humeral implants in the United States for reverse shoulder arthroplasty.

In addition, reverse shoulder arthroplasty with a stemless humeral component has been reported in Europe dating back to at least 2006.[7] Results appear promising; however, little is known about mid-term or long-term radiographic findings and implant survival.

We present our experience and technique for unconstrained total shoulder arthroplasty with the only commercially available stemless component in the United States (Fig. 33.1).

INDICATIONS AND CONTRAINDICATIONS FOR STEMLESS UNCONSTRAINED TOTAL SHOULDER ARTHROPLASTY

Published indications for unconstrained shoulder arthroplasty with a stemless humeral component have been limited thus far with the experience in the United States, but widening indications are expected over time as more results are published. Currently, the only published study in the United States included patients with primary osteoarthritis or posttraumatic arthritis.[3] Part of the published European experience also included instability arthropathy and postinfectious arthritis with rheumatoid arthritis, osteoporosis, and large humeral subchondral cysts considered contraindications.[6] In addition to the standard contraindications to unconstrained shoulder arthroplasty (see Chapter 6), we consider any condition jeopardizing implant humeral fixation to be a contraindication to stemless humeral component use (i.e., humeral bone loss, extensive proximal humeral osteonecrosis). The published operative technique for the United States experience noted that the metaphyseal bone was inspected after the anatomic neck cut and cystic formation or bone voids were considered contraindications to stemless humeral implantation.[3] Furthermore, a "thumb test" was suggested, in which the surgeon attempted to compress the metaphyseal cut surface.[3] Bone that was easily compressible was not considered acceptable for stemless component implantation.

TECHNIQUE FOR STEMLESS UNCONSTRAINED TOTAL SHOULDER ARTHROPLASTY

The operating room setup, anesthesia, patient positioning, skin preparation, surgical draping, and surgical approach are identical to that for unconstrained shoulder arthroplasty with a stemmed implant (see Chapters 3, 4, and 8).

After the inferior capsule is released from the neck of the glenoid as described in Chapter 10, humeral preparation begins. The humeral head retractor is removed, and the humeral head is dislocated by externally rotating and extending the arm. A Hohmann retractor positioned superior to the coracoid process is moved to the margin of the bare area of the humeral head articular surface (junction of the supraspinatus and infraspinatus), and a modified Hohmann retractor is placed inferiorly and medially at the surgical neck of the humerus. This completes the proximal humeral exposure (Fig. 33.2). The presence and extent of humeral head osteophytes vary with the underlying diagnosis. Although conditions such as primary osteoarthritis typically have large osteophytes, other conditions such as rheumatoid arthritis have a paucity of osteophytes. The anteroposterior radiograph is helpful in determining the presence and extent of humeral osteophytes. To identify the true anatomic neck of the humerus, the osteophytes are removed with a ½-inch straight osteotome (Fig. 33.3). Typically, a layer of adipose tissue is present between the osteophytes and the native humerus and aids in identification of the normal margin of the humeral head articular surface (Fig. 33.4). The insertion of the infraspinatus tendon should be readily visible on the posterior aspect of the humerus. It is critical to visualize the infraspinatus to prevent damage to the posterior rotator cuff during humeral head resection. In addition, when using a prosthesis with an anatomic design including a stemless humeral component, the location of the posterior rotator cuff (infraspinatus) defines humeral version (which varies from 7 degrees of anteversion to 48 degrees of retroversion) and, consequently, version of the humeral head cut.[10] After identification of the insertion of the infraspinatus, the humeral head is removed at the anatomic neck of the humerus with an oscillating saw (Fig. 33.5).

CHAPTER 33 ■ Stemless Shoulder Arthroplasty

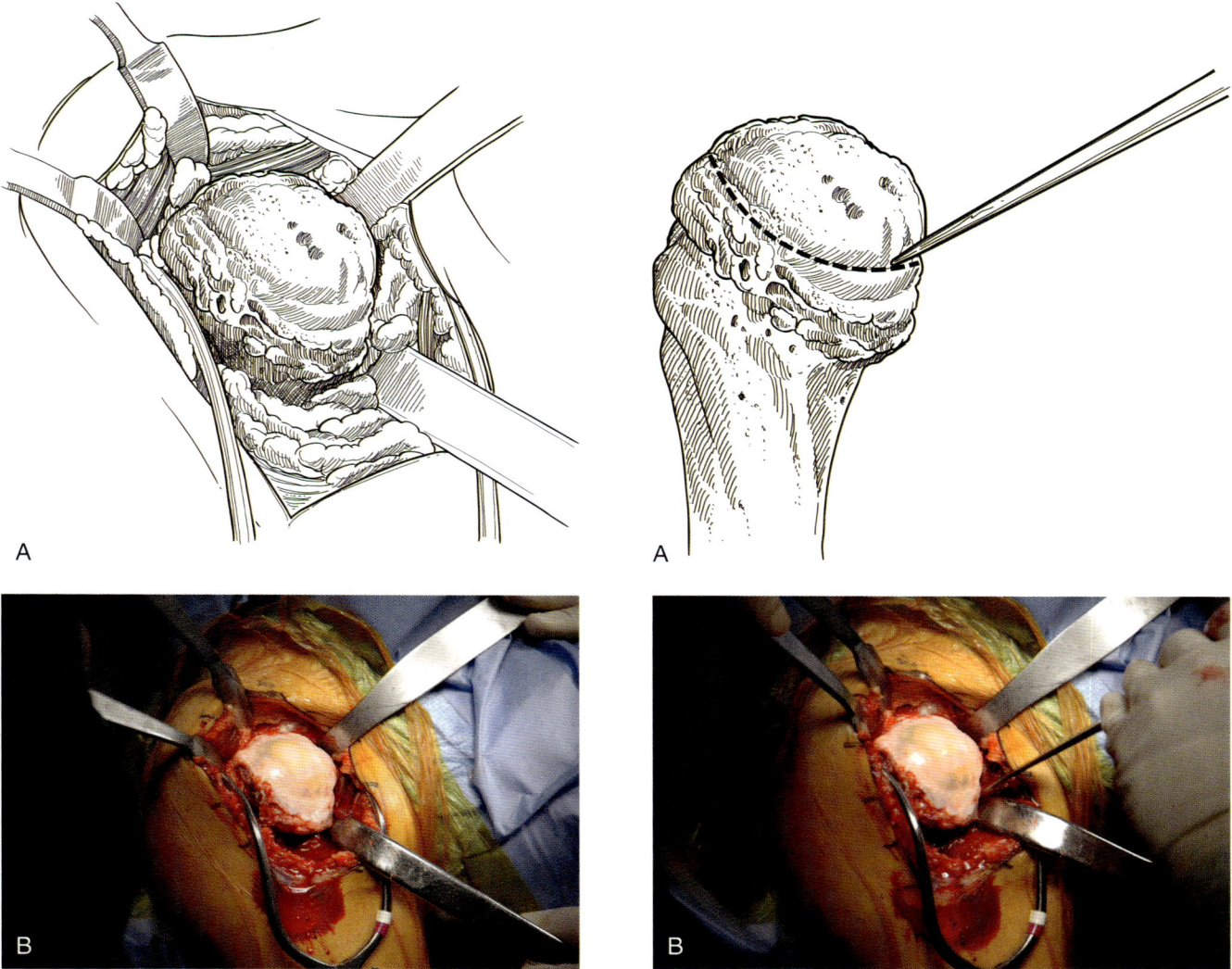

FIGURE 33.2 (A and B) The dislocated proximal humerus reveals peripheral osteophytes.

FIGURE 33.3 (A and B) Peripheral humeral osteophytes are removed with an osteotome to expose the anatomic neck of the humerus.

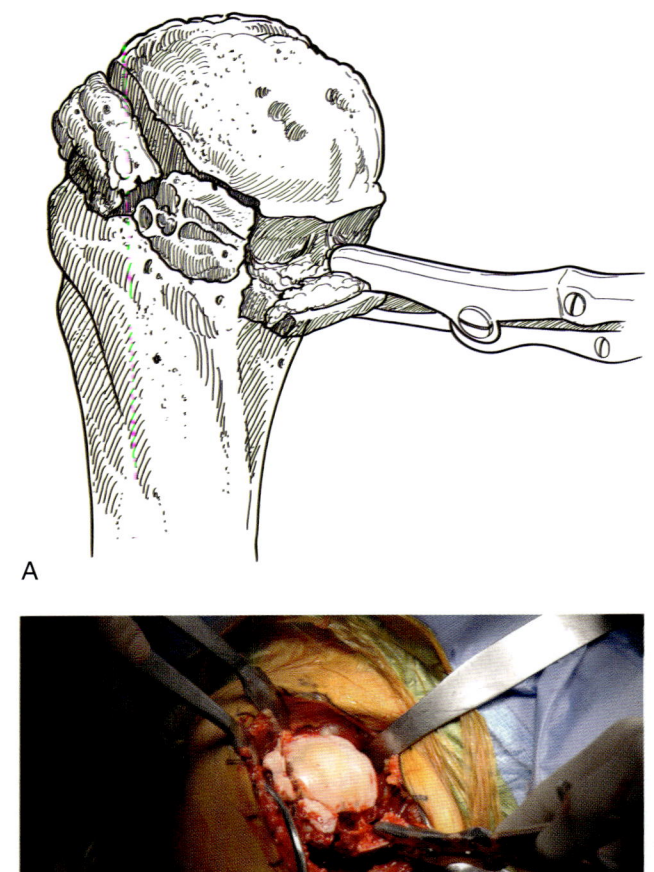

A

B

FIGURE 33.4 (A and B) Layer of adipose tissue interposed between the osteophytes and the native humerus.

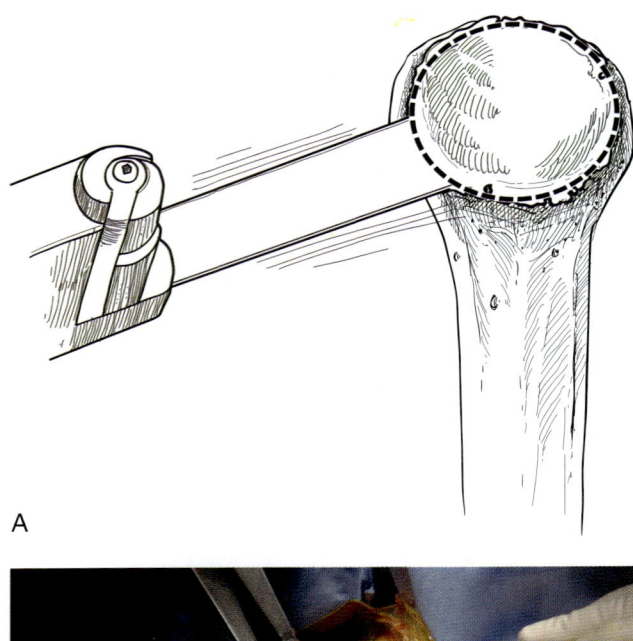

A

B

FIGURE 33.5 (A and B) Resection of the humeral head with an oscillating saw.

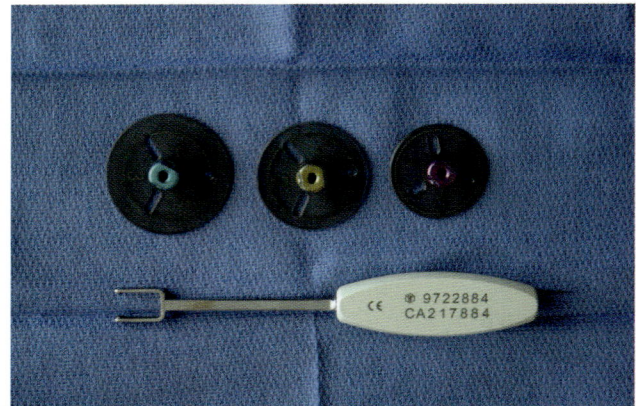

FIGURE 33.6 Three different sizer disks are available to determine the appropriate sized component.

We currently use the only commercially available stemless humeral implant in the United States (Tornier Simpliciti, Wright Medical Group N.V.). Stemless humeral prosthesis preparation begins following anatomic resection of the humeral head, as long as the cut surface is examined and deemed appropriate for a stemless implant. As noted previously, the metaphyseal bone is inspected at this point after the anatomic neck cut and cystic formation or bone voids are considered contraindications to stemless humeral implantation.[3] Furthermore, a "thumb test" is suggested at this point, in which the surgeon attempts to compress the metaphyseal cut surface.[3] Bone that is easily compressible is not considered acceptable for stemless component implantation.

Three different sizer disks are available to determine the appropriate sized component (1, 2, or 3; Fig. 33.6). The largest sized disk that does not overhang beyond the humeral cortex at any point should be selected (Fig. 33.7). The appropriately sized disk should be centered on the cut humeral surface, and a guide pin is place through the central hole of the disk until it engages the lateral cortex (Fig. 33.8). The disk sizer shoulder be removed and the guide pin

CHAPTER 33 ■ Stemless Shoulder Arthroplasty

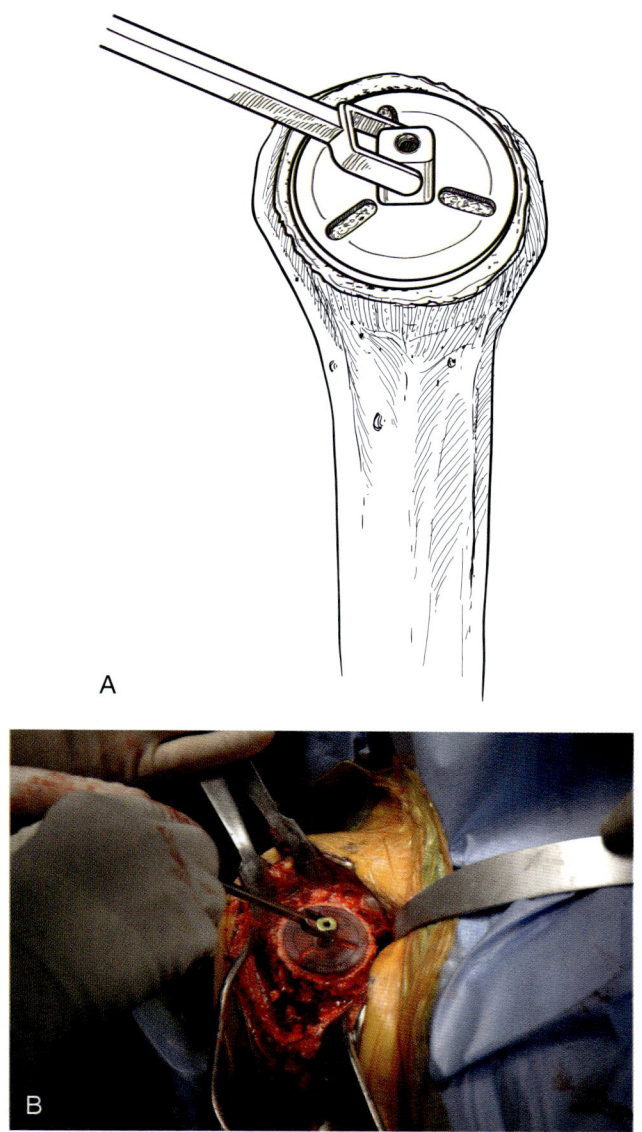

FIGURE 33.7 (A and B) The largest sized disk that does not overhang beyond the humeral cortex is selected.

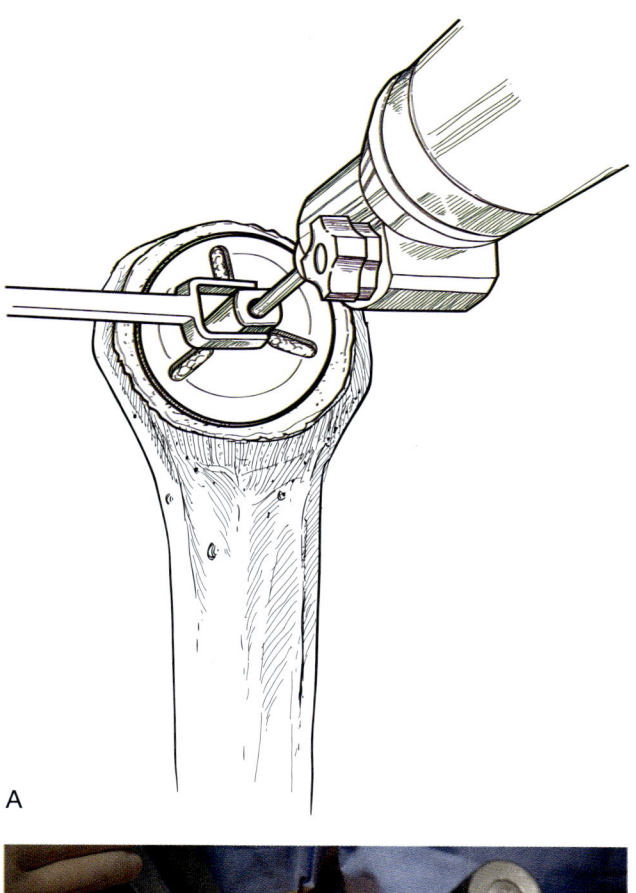

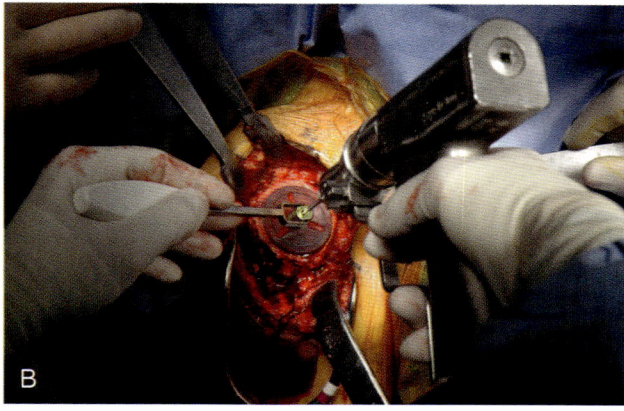

FIGURE 33.8 (A and B) The appropriate sized disk should be centered on the cut humeral surface and a guide pin is place through the central hole of the disk until it engages the lateral cortex.

inspected to ensure that it is centered on the cut humeral surface and that the guide pin trajectory is perpendicular to the cut surface (Fig. 33.9).

A surface planar is used to prepare the metaphyseal surface. The cannulated surface planar size corresponding to the proper disk size (1, 2, or 3) is used (Fig. 33.10). The planer is initiated over the guide pin on "ream" and is started off of the bone. The planer has windows to allow visualization of the reamed surface and to view for concentric witness marks on the metaphyseal surface to ensure appropriate reaming. The reamed surface is visualized to ensure proper reaming technique and depth with a flat surface. A cannulated core drill is advanced over the guide pin on power until the collar is flush with the cut humeral surface (Fig. 33.11).

The metaphyseal fin tracts for the implant are created with a three-finned blazer that is impacted into the metaphyseal bone oriented with one fin pointing superolaterally (Fig. 33.12). The fin blazer must correspond to the matching disk size (1, 2, or 3). The fin blazer is advanced until the collar reaches the cut humeral surface (Fig. 33.13). Do not overimpact the collar of the fin blazer into the metaphyseal bone. The quality of the metaphyseal bone is checked again at this point. If the blazer is deemed unstable, the bone is considered unacceptable for a stemless humeral implant and preparations are made for a stemmed humeral component. If the blazer is stable, the bone is considered acceptable for a stemless implant and the humeral preparation continues.

If a glenoid component is to be inserted, the cut humeral surface is covered with a humeral cut protector to prevent

Text continued on p. 301

298   SECTION V ■ Alternatives to Conventional Shoulder Arthroplasty

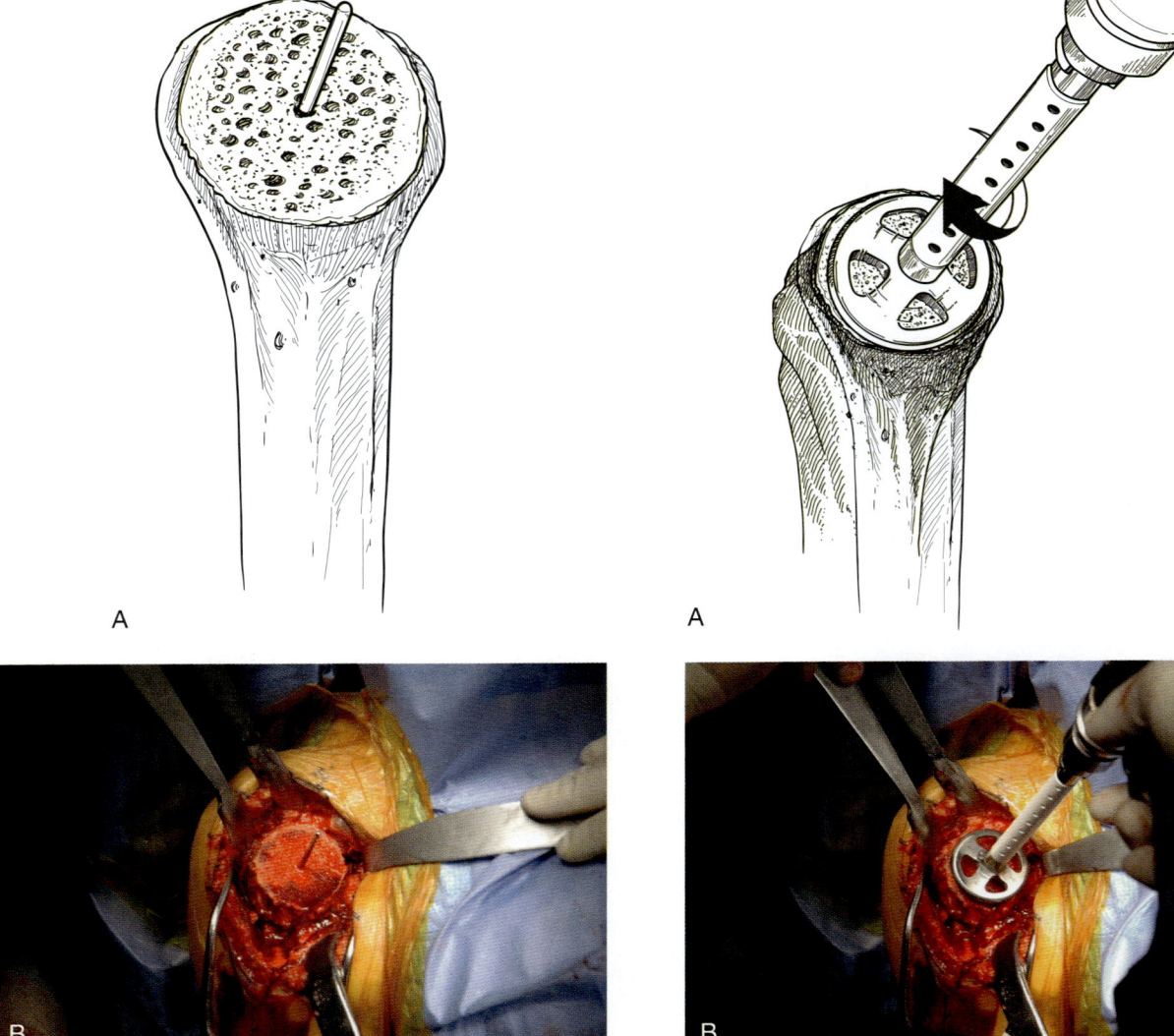

FIGURE 33.9 (A and B) Final location of the guide pin.

FIGURE 33.10 (A and B) A surface planar is used to prepare the metaphyseal surface.

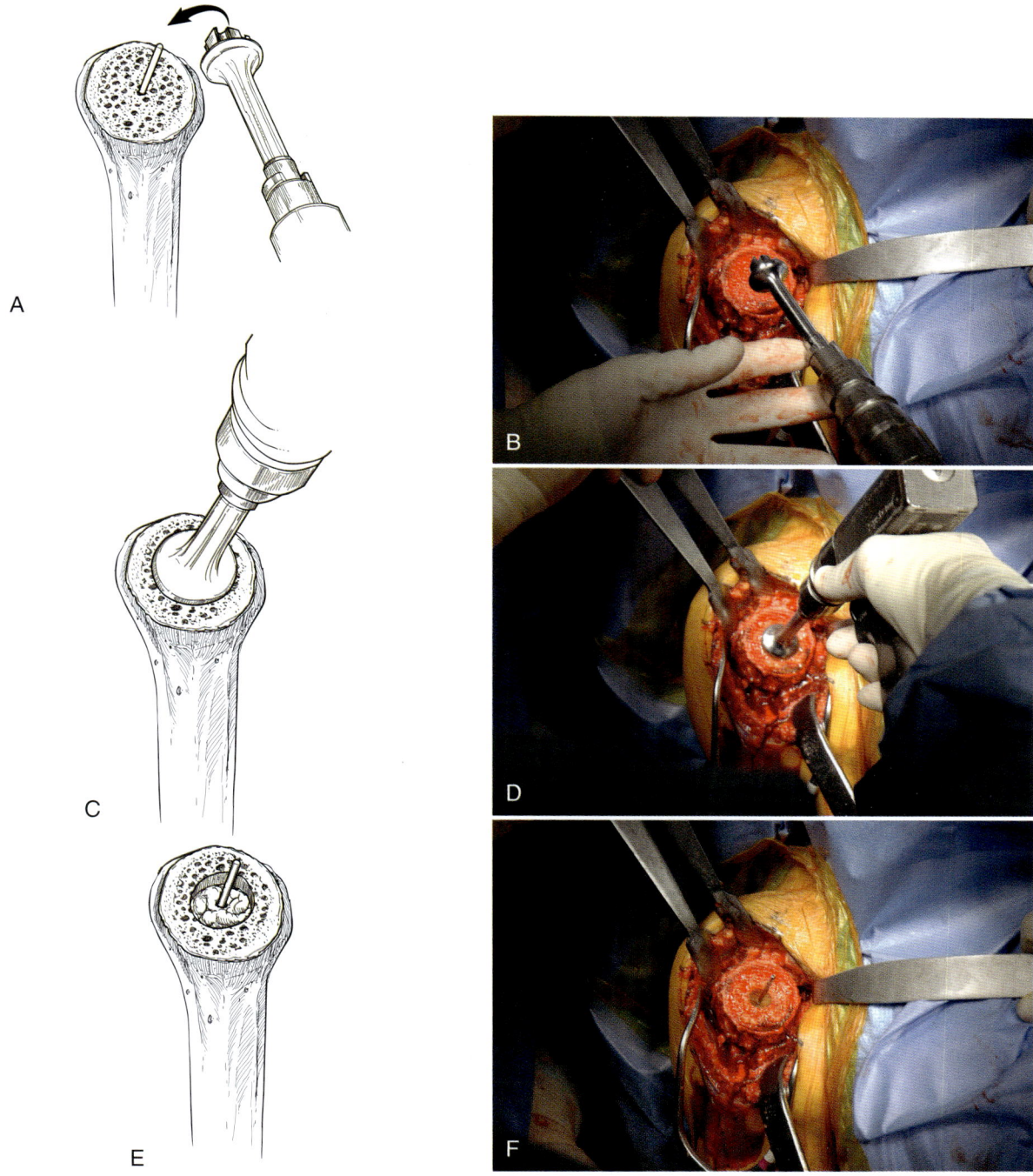

FIGURE 33.11 (A–F) A cannulated core drill is advanced over the guide pin on power until the collar is flush with the cut humeral surface.

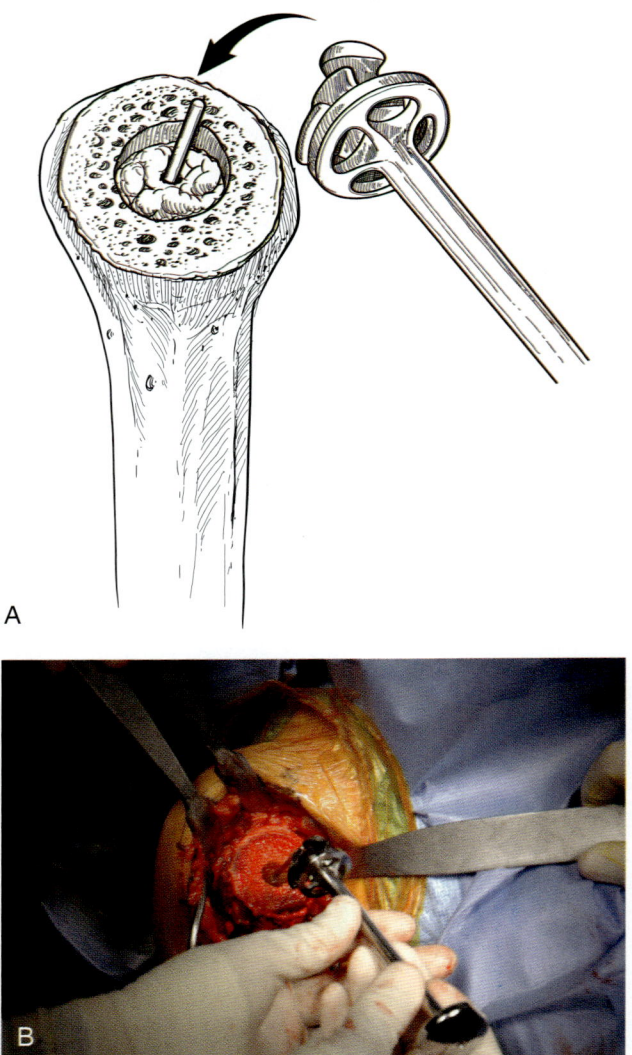

FIGURE 33.12 (A and B) A three-finned blazer is impacted into the metaphyseal bone.

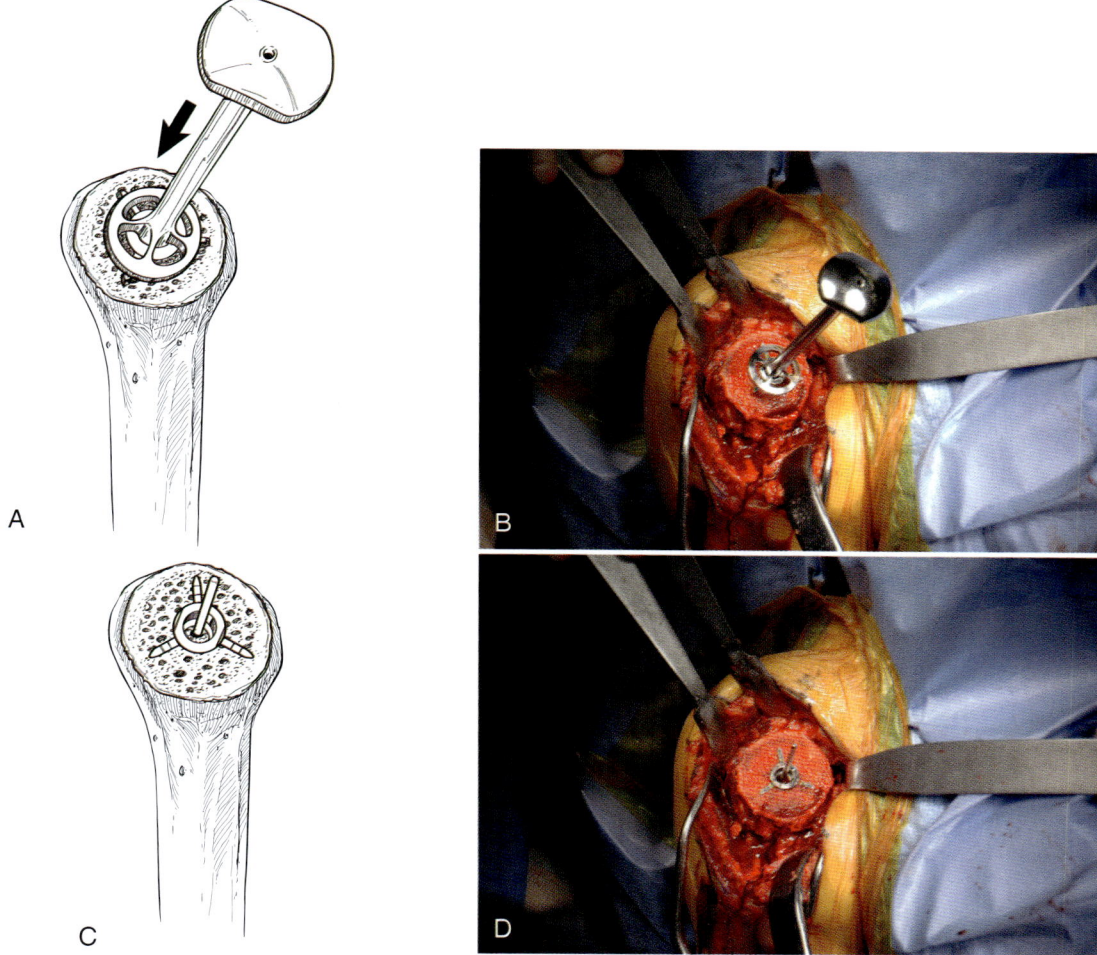

FIGURE 33.13 (A–D) The fin blazer is advanced until the collar reaches the cut humeral surface.

deformation of the humeral cut surface during glenoid preparation and implantation (Fig. 33.14) to allow transition to the glenoid instrumentation.

A trial prosthetic humeral head is selected to match the size of the resected humeral head (Fig. 33.15). Most humeral heads are slightly elliptical; if this is the case, the smaller diameter is selected. In addition, if the resected humeral head is between the sizes available in the prosthetic system, the smaller size is initially selected to avoid "overstuffing" the glenohumeral joint. The appropriate sized trial prosthesis is placed to determine proper fit (Fig. 33.16). Care is taken to avoid overhang of the prosthetic head anteriorly, superiorly, and posteriorly to prevent impingement of the rotator cuff. Inferior overhang, although not ideal, is acceptable. If a large amount of overhang is observed, the selected head is probably too large. In areas in which the prosthetic head does not quite cover the cut humeral surface, a rongeur can be used to trim the cut surface and create a better fit.

Tenotomy or tenodesis of the biceps tendon is performed (as described in Chapter 5), the glenoid is addressed (as described in Chapter 12), and soft tissue balancing is completed (as described in Chapter 13) in cases of total shoulder arthroplasty. The humeral implant is then impacted into place while making sure to avoid inadvertent rotation or inadvertent tilt of the component during insertion (Fig. 33.17). Three no. 2 nonabsorbable braided sutures are placed first through the humeral stump of the subscapularis tendon, into the lesser tuberosity, and out through the cut surface of the humerus to be used in later reattachment of the subscapularis (Fig. 33.18). These sutures are tagged with three different types of hemostats to identify the sutures as superior, middle, and inferior (we use a curved Kelly hemostat superiorly, a mosquito hemostat on the middle suture, and a regular hemostat inferiorly). The final humeral head prosthesis in manually placed (Fig. 33.19). The humeral head impactor is used to seat the Morse taper and complete seating of the implant onto the humeral cut surface.

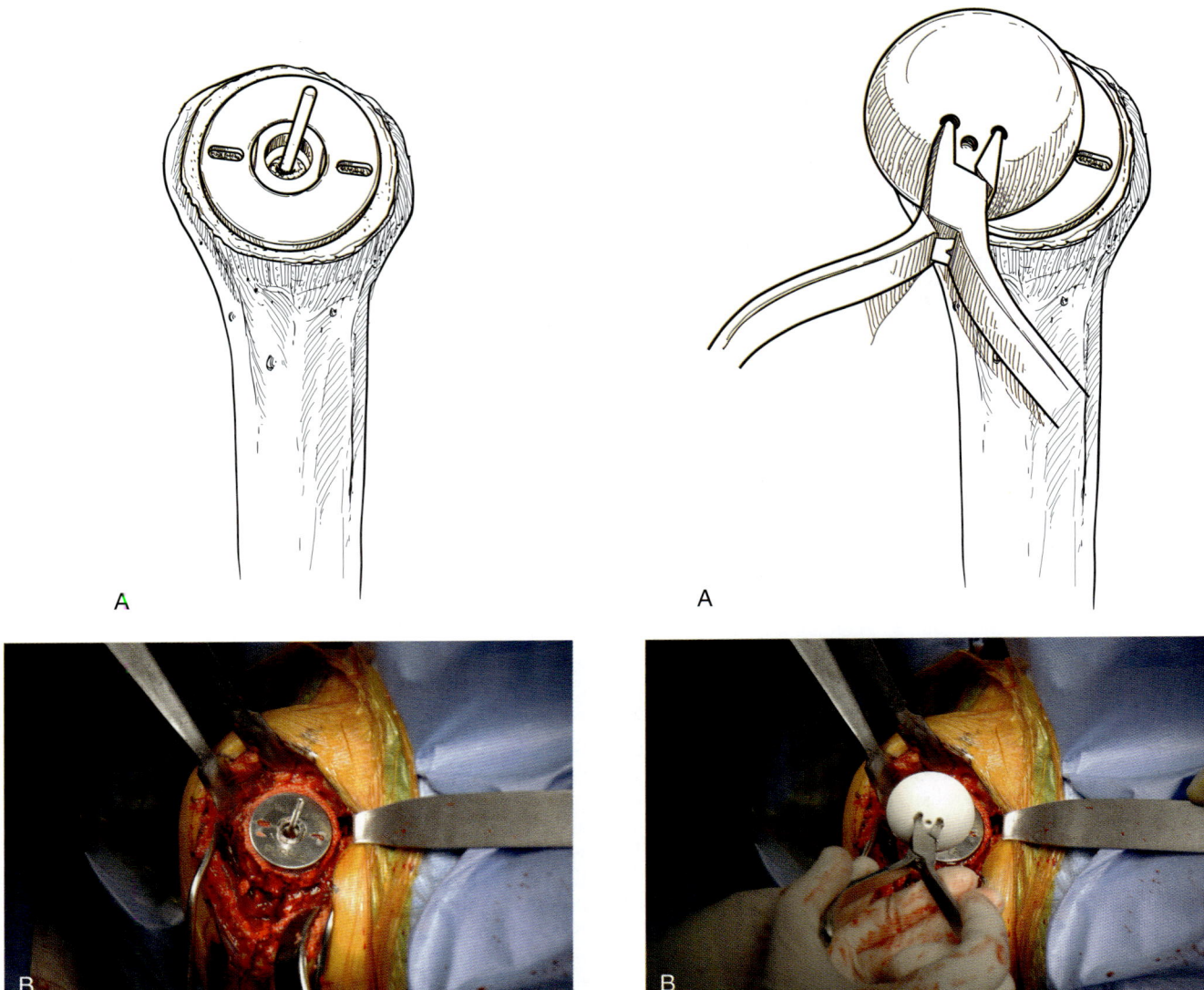

FIGURE 33.14 (A and B) The cut humeral surface is covered with a humeral cut protector.

FIGURE 33.15 (A and B) A trial prosthetic humeral head is selected to match the size of the resected humeral head.

CHAPTER 33 ■ Stemless Shoulder Arthroplasty

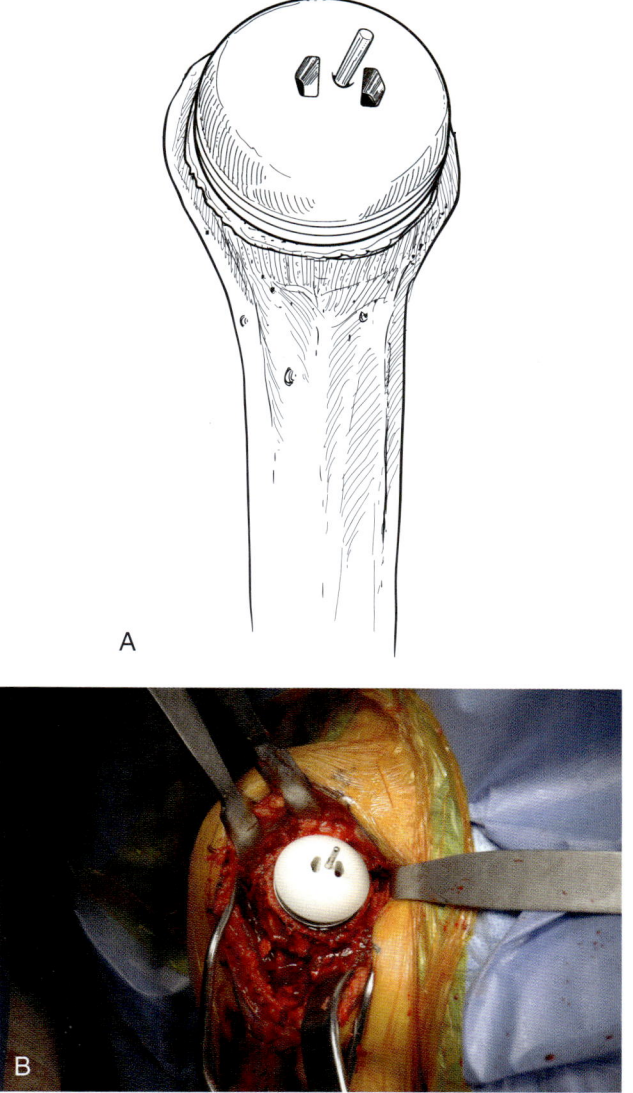

FIGURE 33.16 (A and B) Placement of the trial prosthetic humeral head.

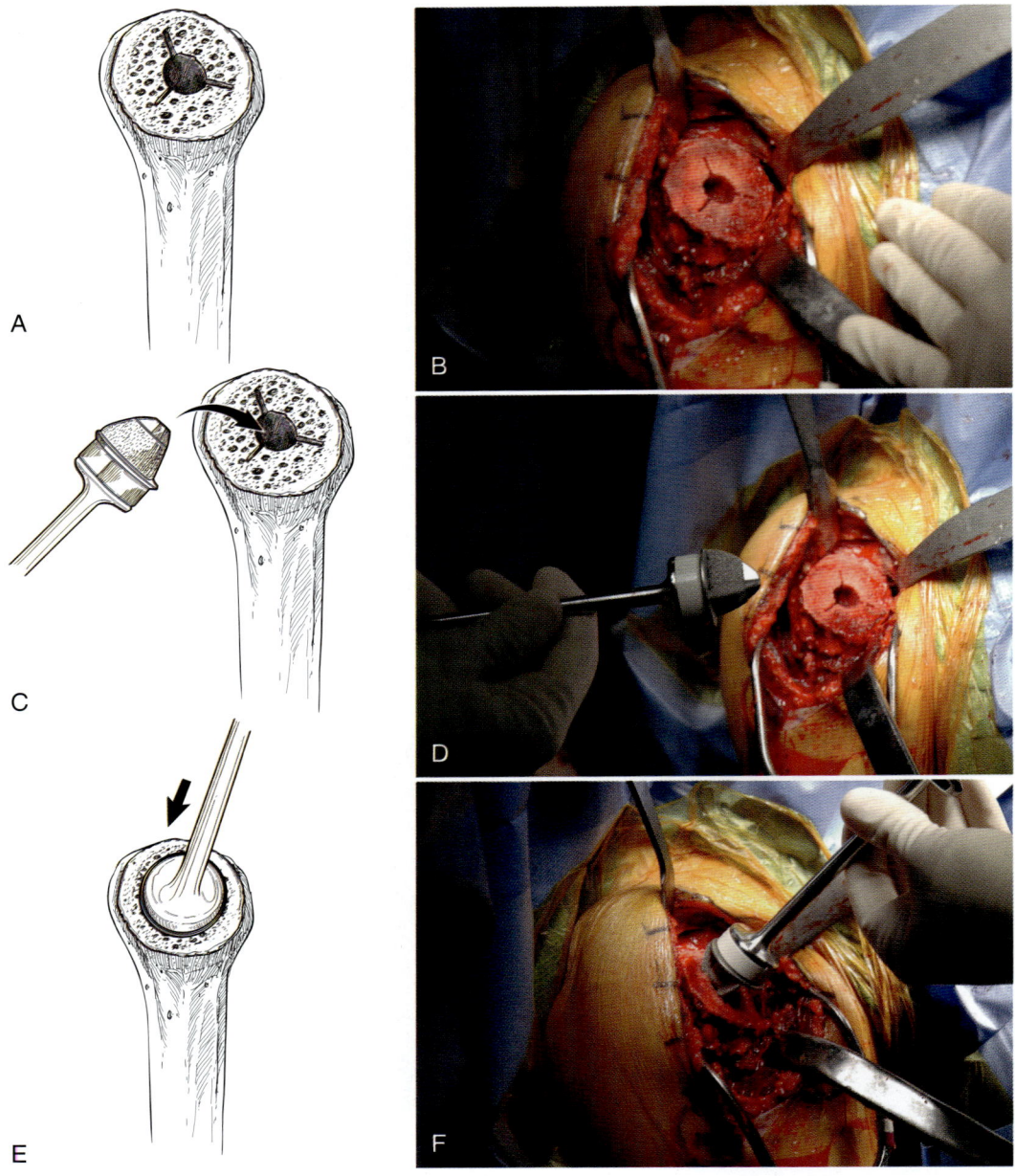

FIGURE 33.17 (A to F) The humeral implant is then impacted into place.

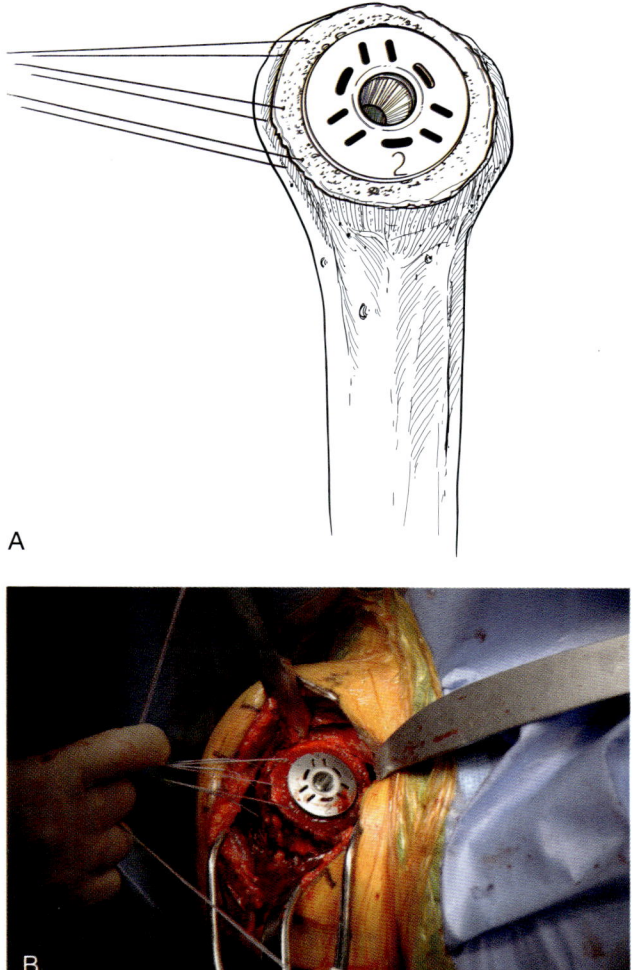

FIGURE 33.18 (A and B) Three no. 2 nonabsorbable braided sutures are placed first through the humeral stump of the subscapularis tendon, into the lesser tuberosity, and out through the cut surface of the humerus.

306 SECTION V ■ Alternatives to Conventional Shoulder Arthroplasty

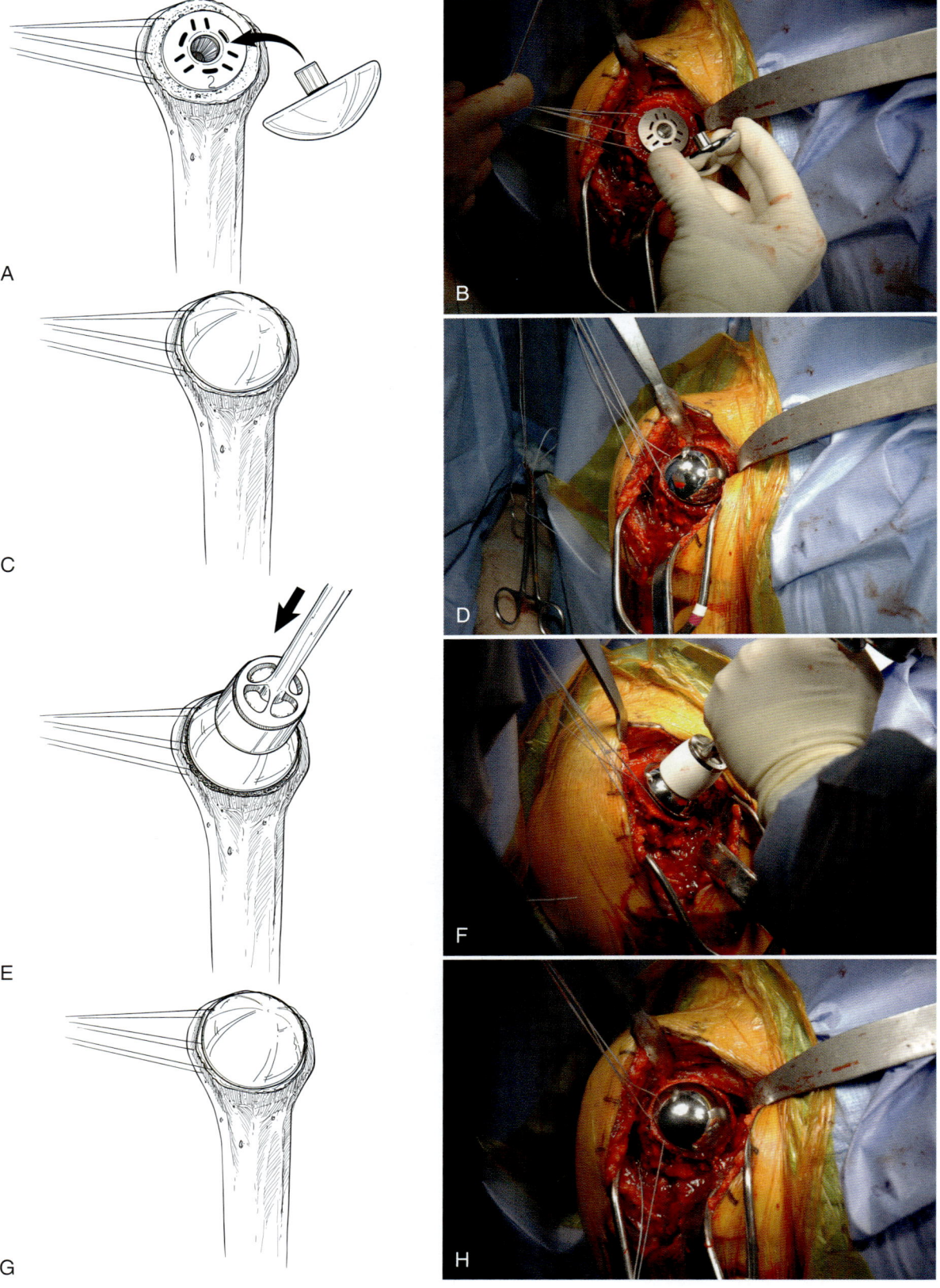

FIGURE 33.19 (A–H) The final humeral head prosthesis is placed.

REFERENCES

1. Neer CS, II: Articular replacement for the humeral head, *J Bone Joint Surg Am* 37:215–228, 1955.
2. Churchill RS: Stemless shoulder arthroplasty: current status, *J Shoulder Elbow Surg* 23:1409–1414, 2014.
3. Churchill RS, Chuinard C, Wiater JM, et al: Clinical and radiographic outcomes of the Simpliciti canal-sparing shoulder arthroplasty system a prospective two-year multicenter study, *J Bone Joint Surg Am* 98:552–560, 2016.
4. Levy O, Copeland SA: Cementless surface replacement arthroplasty of the shoulder. 5- to 10-year results with the Copeland Mark-2 prosthesis, *J Bone Joint Surg Br* 83:213–221, 2001.
5. Raiss P, Edwards TB, Deutsch A, et al: Radiographic changes around humeral components in shoulder arthroplasty, *J Bone Joint Surg Am* 96:e54(1-9), 2014.
6. Habermeyer P, Lichtenberg S, Tauber M, et al: Midterm results of stemless shoulder arthroplasty: a prospective study, *J Shoulder Elbow Surg* 24:1463–1472, 2015.
7. Churchill RS, Athwal GS: Stemless shoulder arthroplasty—current results and designs, *Curr Rev Musculoskelet Med* 9:10–16, 2016.
8. Collin P, Matsukawa1 T, Boileau P, et al: Is the humeral stem useful in anatomic total shoulder arthroplasty?, *Int Orthop* 41(5):1035–1039, 2017.
9. Hudek R, Werner B, Abdelkawi AF, et al: Radiolucency in stemless shoulder arthroplasty is associated with an imaging phenomenon, *J Orthop Res* 35(9):2040–2050, 2017.
10. Boileau P, Walch G: Anatomical study of the proximal humerus: surgical technique consideration and prosthetic design rationale. In Walch G, Boileau P, editors: *Shoulder arthroplasty*, Berlin, 1999, Springer, pp 69–82.

CHAPTER 34

Biologic alternatives to shoulder arthroplasty

In our practice, few situations exist in which biologic surface replacement of the humeral head is more advantageous than conventional humeral head replacement with a stemmed or new stemless implant. In addition, use of biologic replacement hinders glenoid exposure and thus prevents implantation of a prosthetic glenoid implant in many cases. However, there are some indications for biologic humeral resurfacing for focal loss of humeral head articular cartilage. Similarly, in our practice, few situations exist in which biologic glenoid resurfacing is more advantageous than conventional glenoid resurfacing with a polyethylene glenoid component.

This chapter outlines our preferred use of biologic humeral resurfacing and biologic glenoid resurfacing and the situations in which these techniques would be used.

BIOLOGIC HUMERAL RESURFACING

Biologic subtotal resurfacing of the humeral head is an option for focal loss of humeral head articular cartilage. Situations in which subtotal resurfacing of the humeral head are indicated are rare, but biologic implants can prove useful in certain scenarios.

Biologic surface replacement is indicated in young patients (<30 years) with localized full-thickness defects of the articular cartilage of the humeral head who have failed other treatments. When young patients with full-thickness articular cartilage lesions of the humeral head are seen in our practice, we initially treat them nonoperatively with nonsteroidal antiinflammatory medications, selective rest, and activity modification for a period of 6 to 12 weeks. If such treatment proves unsuccessful, we offer arthroscopic treatment of the lesion with débridement and drilling of subchondral bone to stimulate the formation of fibrocartilage. If patients remain symptomatic 6 months after arthroscopic treatment, we will offer them biologic surface replacement with a matched osteochondral allograft. In our experience, it is rare for a patient to fail arthroscopic treatment of these localized articular cartilage lesions, thus minimizing the indications for partial surface replacement.

Contraindications specific to biologic surface replacement include cartilaginous lesions larger than 35 mm in diameter, the presence of nonlocalized disease, and the absence of sufficient bone quality to support the osteochondral allograft.

TECHNIQUE FOR BIOLOGIC RESURFACING

The operating room setup, anesthesia, patient positioning, skin preparation, surgical draping, and surgical approach are identical to that for humeral surface replacement and other shoulder arthroplasties (see Chapters 3, 4, and 8). Handling of the subscapularis is the same as for stemless shoulder replacement, as described previously in Chapter 33. Biologic resurfacing necessitates greater preoperative planning in that it is necessary for the company supplying the proximal humeral allograft to locate an appropriately sized specimen (we use the Musculoskeletal Transplant Foundation). Magnification-controlled radiographs and computed tomography scans of the proximal humerus are provided to the allograft supplier to allow appropriate specimen selection. Our supplier has usually been able to provide specimens within 6 weeks of receiving the preoperative imaging studies. After the specimen has been obtained, surgery is scheduled.

The humeral head is dislocated to expose the articular cartilage lesion (Fig. 34.1). The size of the lesion is measured with a templating device from the instrumentation set (Arthrex, Inc., Naples, Florida; Fig. 34.2), and a guide pin is placed in the humeral head at the center of the articular cartilage lesion with the templating device used as a guide (Fig. 34.3). A specialized cannulated drill is used to score the periphery of the lesion (Fig. 34.4), and a cannulated triflange reamer is used to create an osseous defect in which to place the osteochondral allograft (Fig. 34.5). If associated osteonecrosis is present in addition to the articular cartilage lesion, the reamer is advanced to a depth sufficient to eliminate the necrotic bone as determined on preoperative imaging studies. If no or minimal osteonecrosis is present, the reamer is advanced a minimum of 10 mm deep to provide an adequate interference fit for the osteochondral allograft. Fig. 34.6 shows the humerus after reaming has been completed.

The proximal humeral allograft is positioned in the cutting jig, and the selected donor site is marked with a surgical marker (Fig. 34.7). A cutting guide of appropriate diameter is assembled onto the cutting jig, and a coring drill is used to harvest the osteochondral allograft plug (Fig. 34.8). The allograft plug is placed in a specialized clamp, and a saw is used to trim the deep surface of the allograft to match the depth penetrated by the triflange reamer (Fig. 34.9). The

CHAPTER 34 ■ Biologic Alternatives to Shoulder Arthroplasty

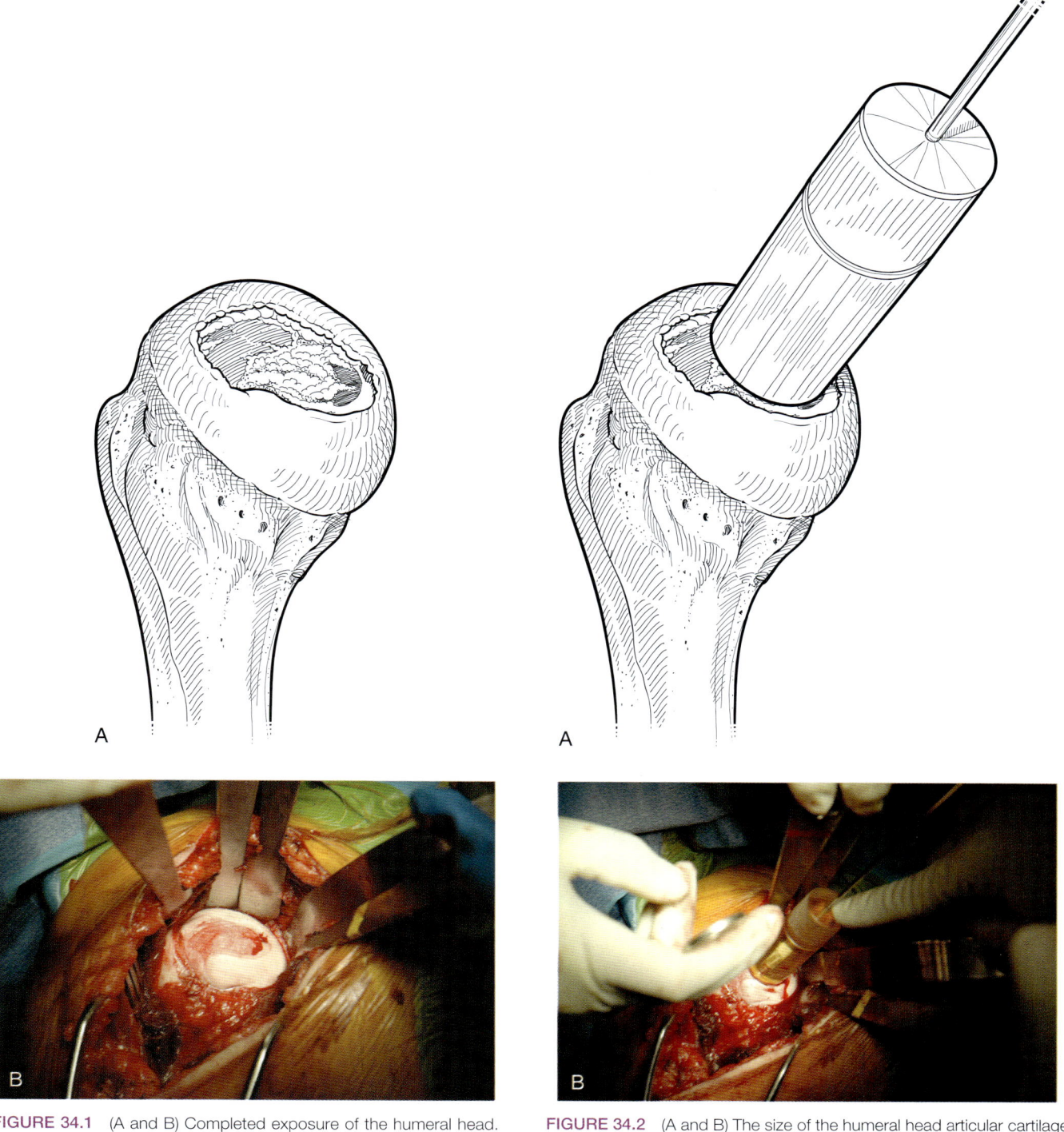

FIGURE 34.1 (A and B) Completed exposure of the humeral head.

FIGURE 34.2 (A and B) The size of the humeral head articular cartilage lesion is measured.

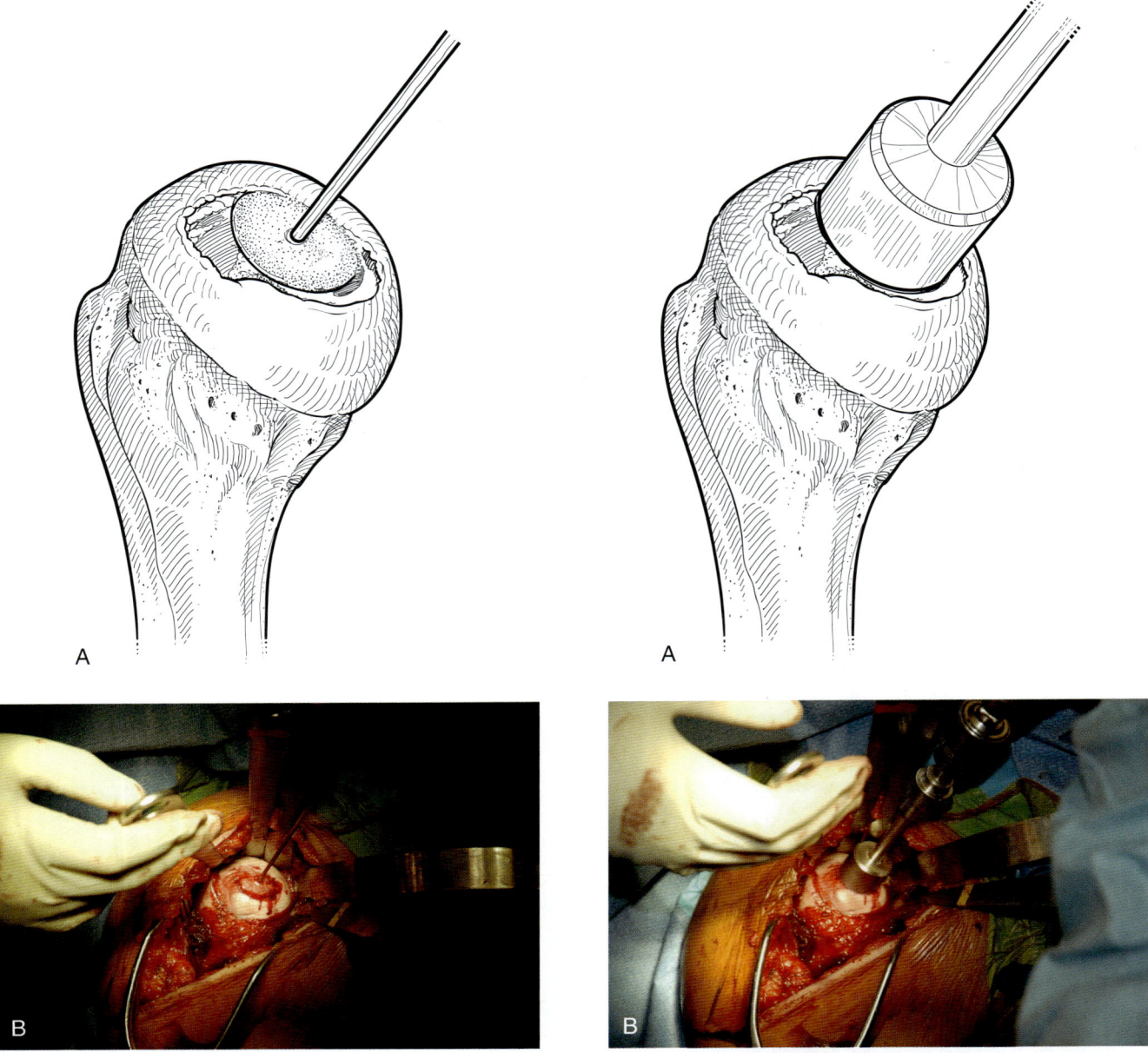

FIGURE 34.3 (A and B) Placement of the guide pin in the center of the lesion.

FIGURE 34.4 (A and B) The periphery of the lesion is scored with a special instrument.

CHAPTER 34 ■ Biologic Alternatives to Shoulder Arthroplasty

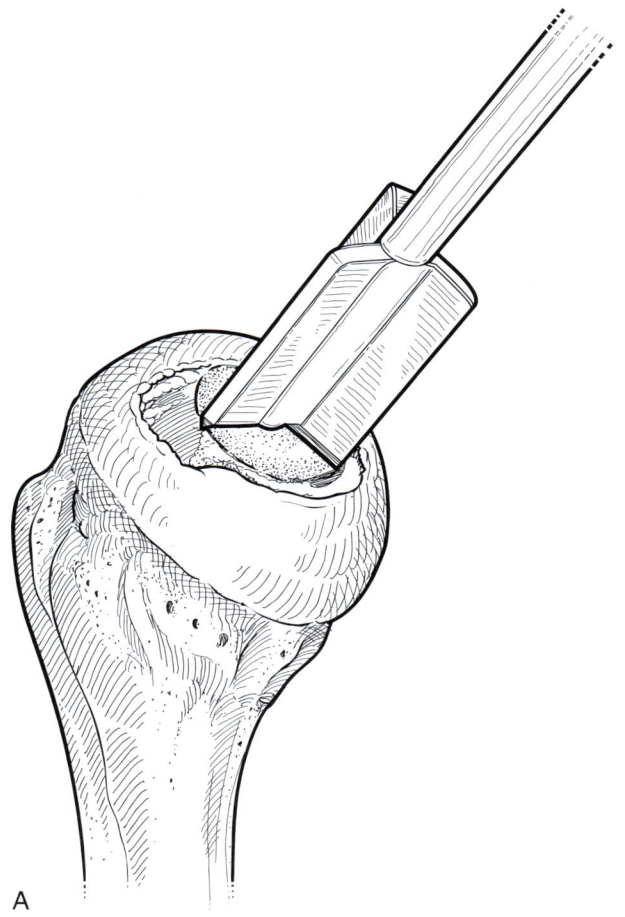
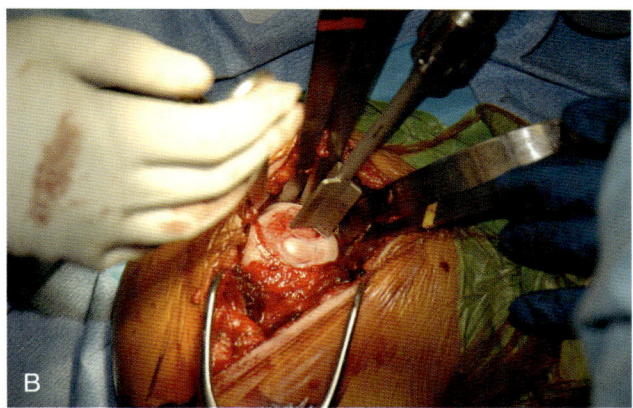

FIGURE 34.5 (A and B) Reaming of the humeral head with a triflange reamer.

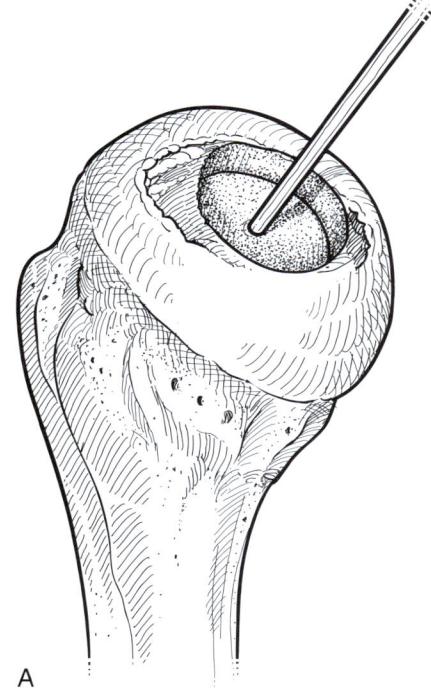
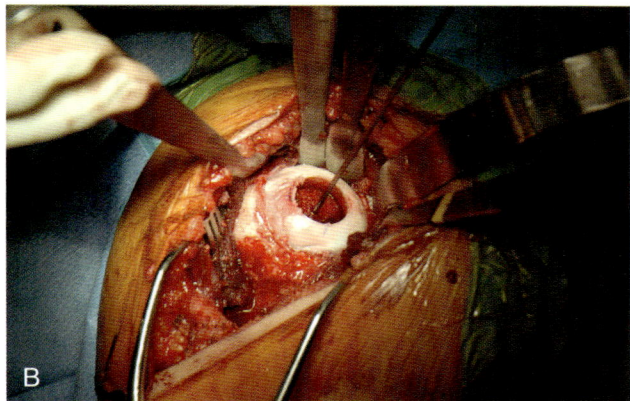

FIGURE 34.6 (A and B) Completed humeral preparation.

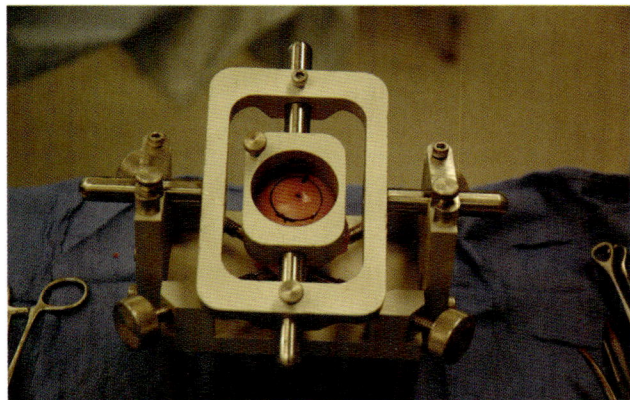

FIGURE 34.7 Placement of the proximal humeral allograft in the cutting jig.

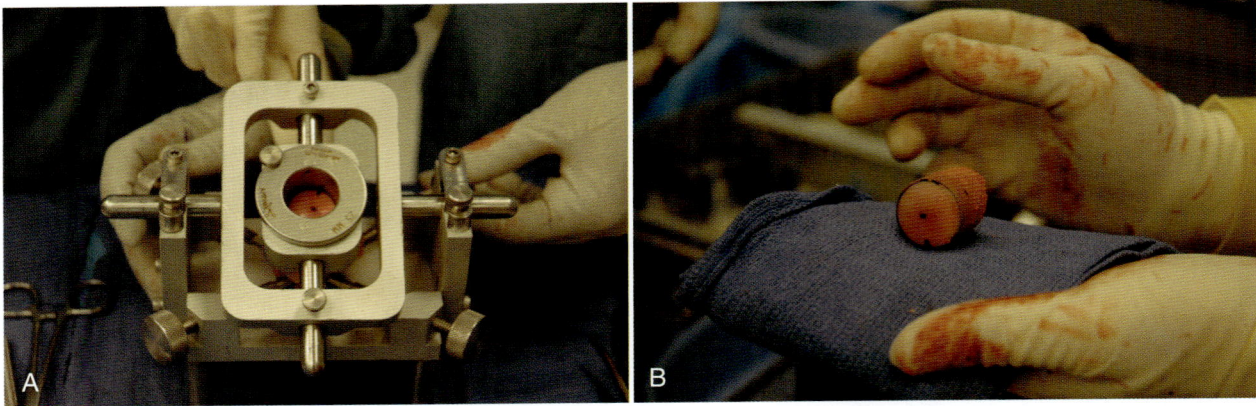

FIGURE 34.8 (A and B) A coring drill is used to harvest the osteocartilaginous allograft plug.

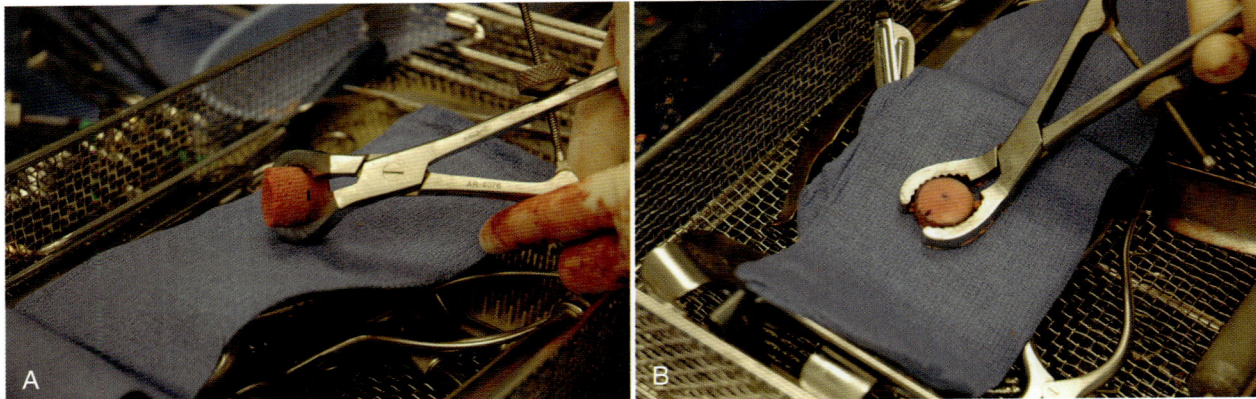

FIGURE 34.9 (A and B) The deep surface of the allograft plug is trimmed with a saw.

bone plug is progressively impacted into the prepared humeral defect until it is fully seated (Fig. 34.10).

The subscapularis is closed with interrupted no. 2 braided permanent tendon-to-tendon suture. The closure is reinforced with running no. 1 braided absorbable suture. The wound is then closed as for other cases of shoulder arthroplasty.

BIOLOGIC GLENOID RESURFACING

Biologic resurfacing of the glenoid has been performed with various materials, including fascia lata autograft, fascia lata allograft, meniscal allograft, and Achilles tendon allograft.[1] The main advantage of biologic glenoid resurfacing lies in providing a new articulating surface for the glenoid while avoiding potential late-term complications associated with polyethylene wear and failure. Consequently, consideration of biologic glenoid resurfacing is most reasonable in younger patients. Biologic glenoid resurfacing also allows resurfacing of localized glenoid articular cartilage lesions that may result from trauma in young patients. In our practice, we almost always combine biologic glenoid resurfacing with humeral head arthroplasty (hemiarthroplasty or biologic surface replacement) because our patients with glenoid articular cartilage disease almost always have associated humeral head articular cartilage disease.

Of the available tissues for use in biologic glenoid resurfacing, we prefer autogenous fascia lata. Use of the patient's own tissue minimizes the risk of graft rejection, a phenomenon that we have observed with allografts. In addition, the morbidity associated with harvest of a fascia lata autograft is minimal.

INDICATIONS AND CONTRAINDICATIONS

Indications in our practice for biologic glenoid resurfacing are limited to a young patient (<40 years old) with glenoid disease; in an older patient, the use of a prosthetic glenoid component would be indicated. We have performed biologic resurfacing most commonly in patients with a generalized arthritic condition (i.e., glenohumeral chondrolysis; Fig. 34.11) but have also used it for localized traumatic glenoid articular cartilage lesions. One situation in which we opt for a prosthetic glenoid component in a young patient is a diagnosis of juvenile rheumatoid arthritis.

A rare situation in which we use biologic glenoid resurfacing is a revision case with a competent rotator cuff in which hemiarthroplasty has resulted in symptomatic glenoid erosion and insufficient bone exists to permit prosthetic resurfacing (Fig. 34.12). In these scenarios, biologic resurfacing represents an alternative to resection arthroplasty (see Chapter 35 for more on indications for revision shoulder arthroplasty). In most primary cases in older patients in whom unconstrained arthroplasty is indicated yet insufficient glenoid bone exists

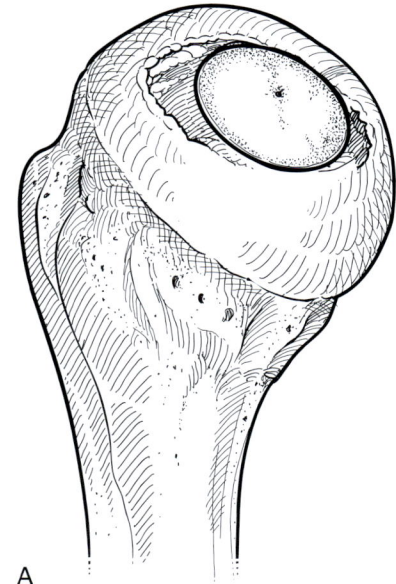

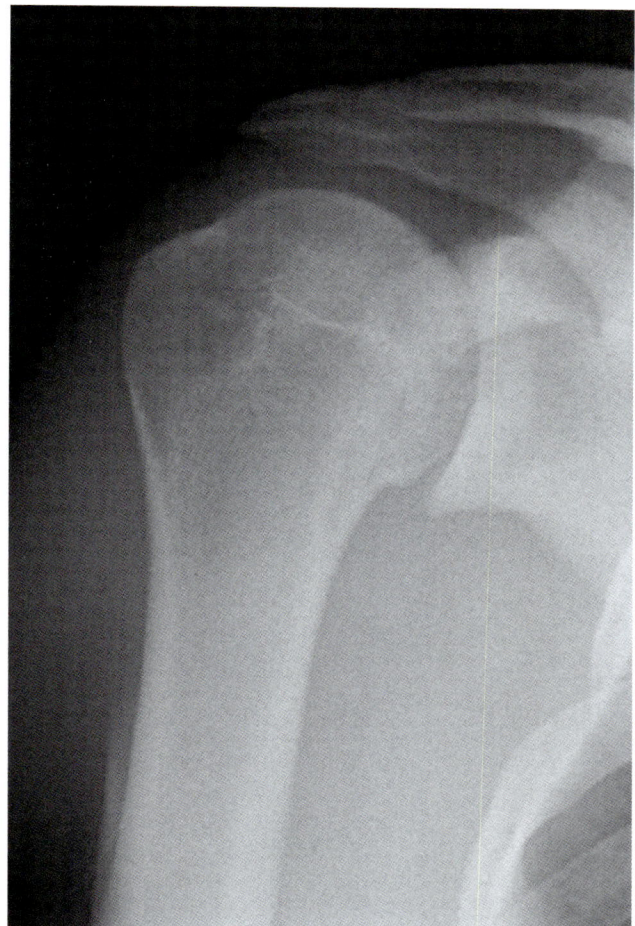

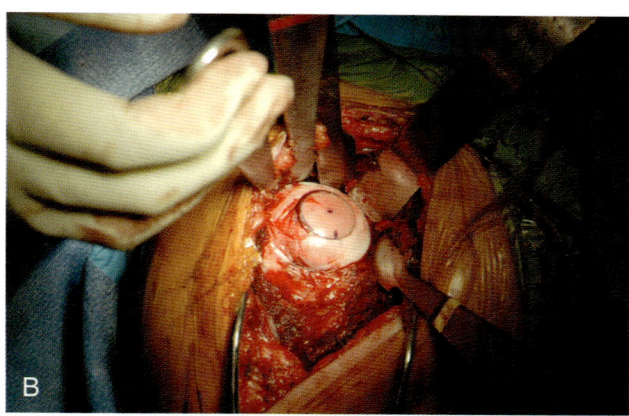

FIGURE 34.10 (A and B) The allograft plug is seated into the prepared humerus.

FIGURE 34.11 Radiograph of a young patient with glenohumeral joint chondrolysis after shoulder arthroscopy.

for prosthetic resurfacing, we generally perform isolated hemiarthroplasty because most of these patients obtain satisfactory pain relief and function (although these results are inferior to those obtained with total shoulder arthroplasty) without prosthetic or biologic glenoid resurfacing.

Contraindications to biologic glenoid resurfacing include the standard contraindications to unconstrained shoulder arthroplasty. In addition, any situation in which the native glenoid is insufficient to allow anchorage of the biologic tissue is a contraindication to biologic resurfacing (Fig. 34.13).

TECHNIQUE FOR BIOLOGIC GLENOID RESURFACING

Autogenous Fascia Lata Harvest

The operating room setup, anesthesia, patient positioning, skin preparation, surgical draping, and surgical approach are identical to that for other shoulder arthroplasties. In addition, the contralateral lower extremity and hip region are prepared and draped (Fig. 34.14). Using the contralateral lower extremity permits an assistant to close the fascia lata harvest wound while the approach is made to the shoulder. An 8-cm incision is started 3 cm distal to the greater trochanter of the femur and extended distally along the longitudinal axis of the femur (Fig. 34.15). A needle tip electrocautery is used to obtain hemostasis and aids in dissection through the subcutaneous layer down to the fascia lata. The fascia lata is cleared of the overlying subcutaneous fat to complete the exposure (Fig. 34.16). A scalpel is used to harvest a segment of fascia lata 8 cm long by 3 cm wide (Fig. 34.17). The wound is irrigated; it is not necessary to close the residual defect in the fascia lata (Fig. 34.18). The subcutaneous tissue is closed with 2-0 absorbable braided suture in an interrupted technique. The skin is closed with 3-0 absorbable monofilament suture in a continuous running subcuticular technique. Steri-Strips and sterile dressings are applied. The fascia lata is folded to double its thickness. Braided 2-0 absorbable suture is used to suture the perimeter of the autograft (Fig. 34.19).

Implantation of the Fascia Lata Autograft

A standard deltopectoral approach is performed as described in Chapter 8. The subscapularis is treated as described in

314 SECTION V ■ Alternatives to Conventional Shoulder Arthroplasty

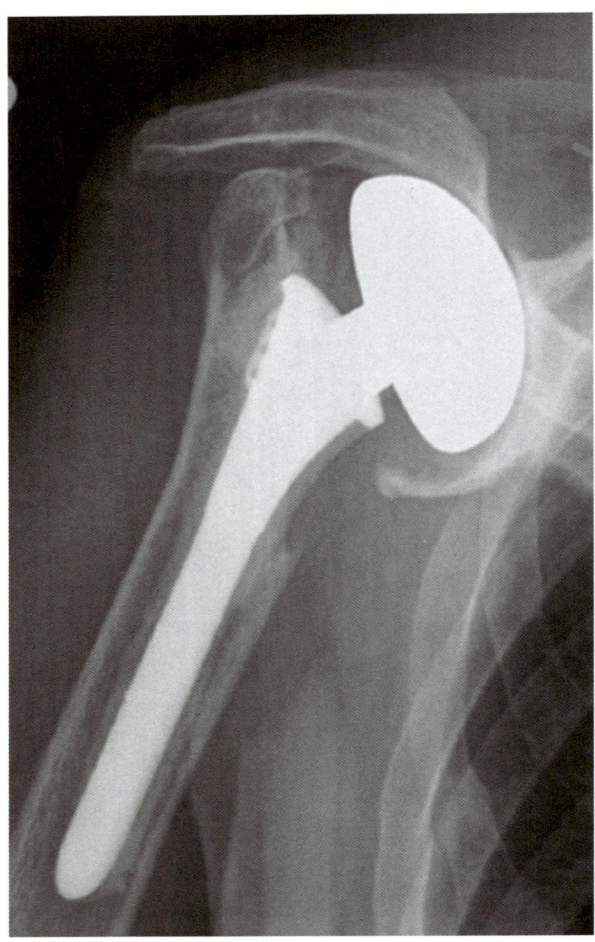

FIGURE 34.12 Glenoid erosion after hemiarthroplasty. The residual glenoid bone is insufficient to permit insertion of a prosthetic glenoid component.

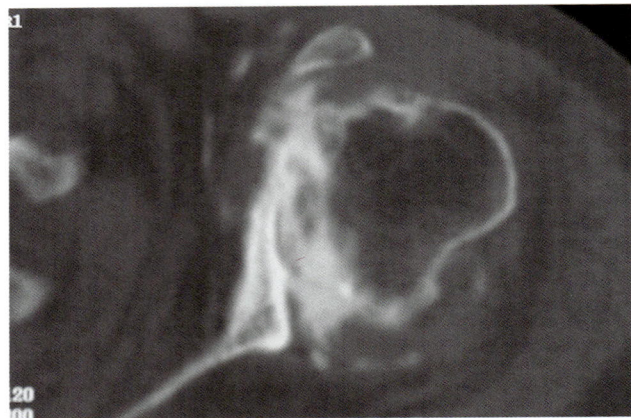

FIGURE 34.13 Glenoid insufficiency preventing anchorage of a biologic resurfacing graft.

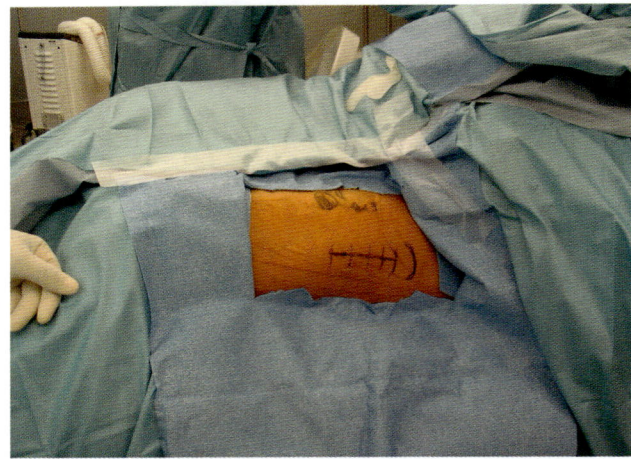

FIGURE 34.14 Preparation and draping for harvest of an autogenous fascia lata graft.

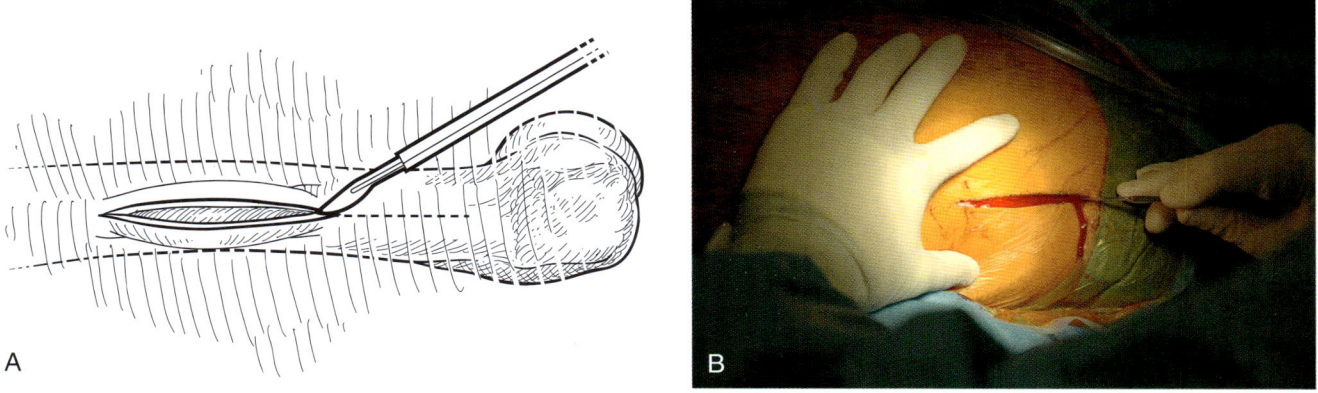

FIGURE 34.15 (A and B) Incision for harvest of an autogenous fascia lata graft.

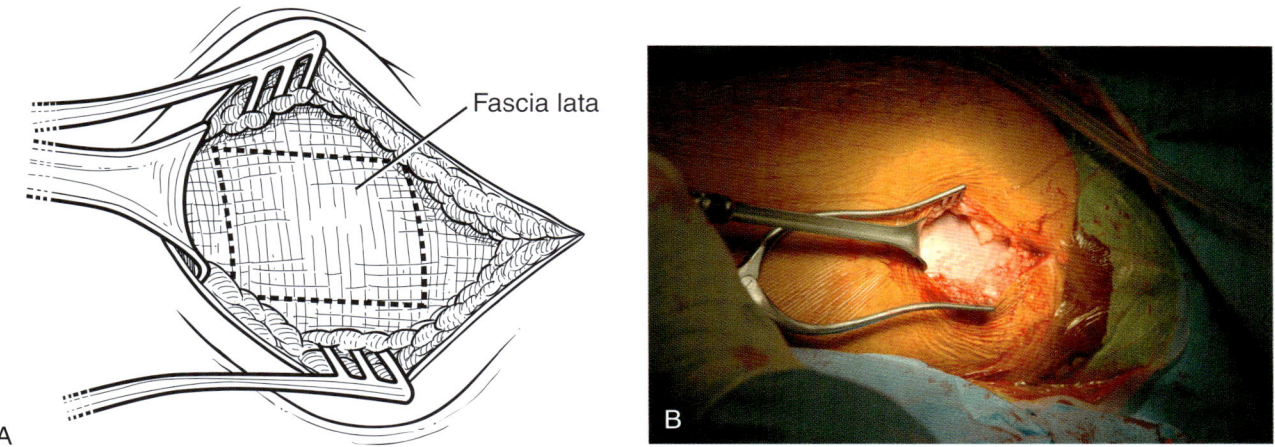

FIGURE 34.16 (A and B) Completed exposure of the fascia lata graft.

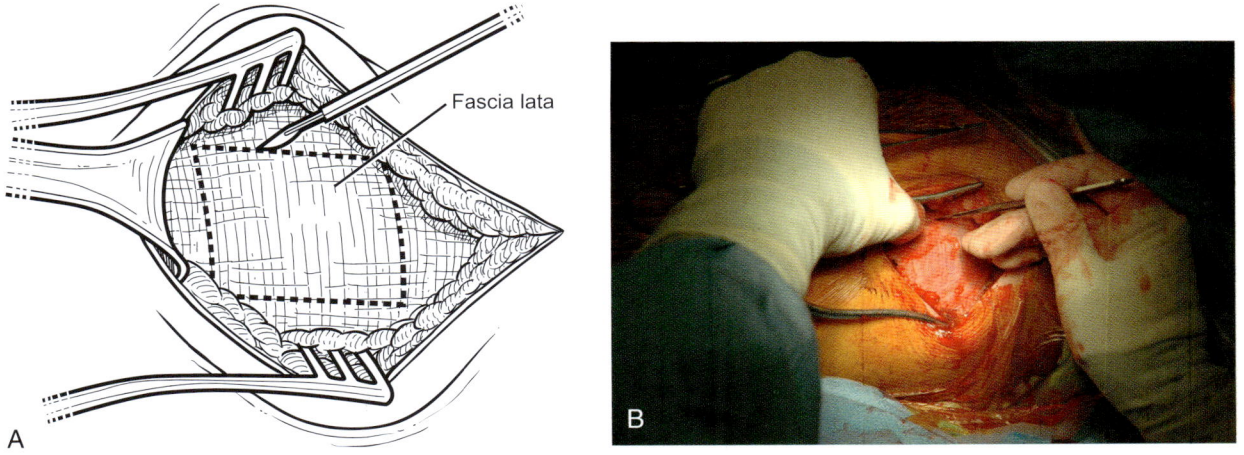

FIGURE 34.17 (A and B) Harvesting of the fascia lata graft with a scalpel.

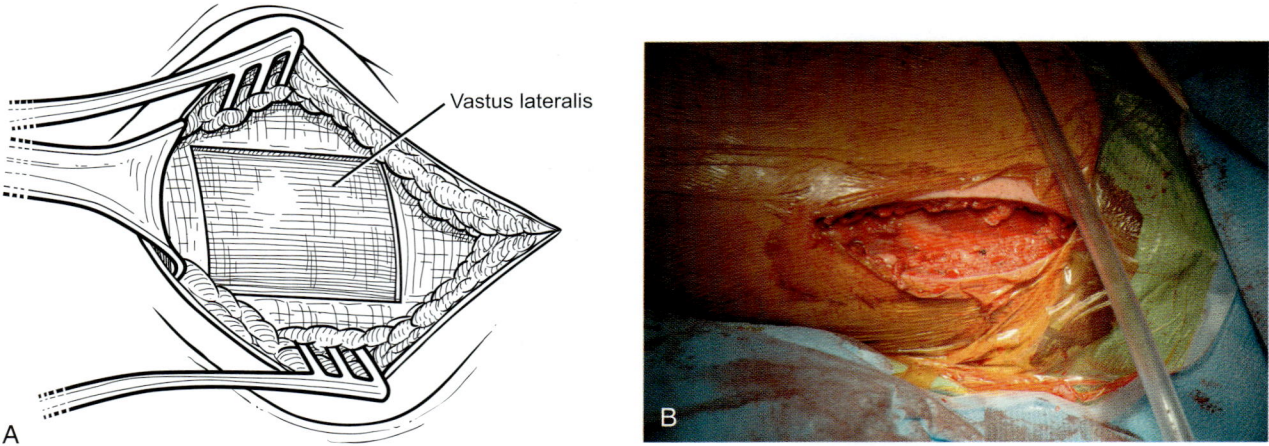

FIGURE 34.18 (A and B) The residual defect in the fascia lata is left open.

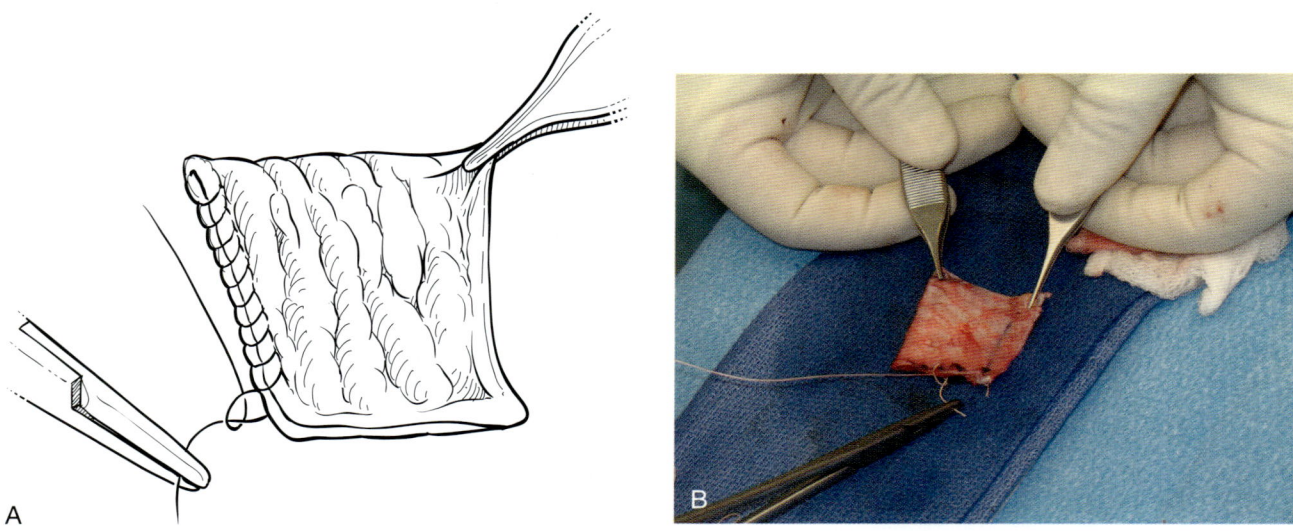

FIGURE 34.19 (A and B) Preparation of the fascia lata graft by doubling it and suturing the three "free" sides.

Chapter 9 if hemiarthroplasty is planned. If biologic humeral head resurfacing is planned, the anterior humeral circumflex vessels are preserved. The glenoid is exposed by releasing the inferior glenohumeral joint capsule from the glenoid neck (Fig. 34.20). The glenoid joint surface is prepared by removing any residual articular cartilage with a Cobb elevator or motorized burr, if necessary. Any nonconcentric wear is corrected with the burr or a reamer (see Chapter 12), if needed. Two options exist for graft fixation. If the glenoid labrum is intact circumferentially, the autograft can be sutured directly to the intact glenoid labrum. If the glenoid labrum is absent or diseased to the extent that graft fixation would be compromised, bioabsorbable suture anchor fixation is used to secure the graft (we use a 2.9-mm Bioraptor anchor, Smith Nephew, Inc., Andover, Massachusetts).

In patients with an intact glenoid labrum, no. 2 braided permanent sutures are placed through the labrum at the 12, 2, 4, 6, 8, and 10 o'clock positions (Fig. 34.21). These sutures are kept separate by tagging them with hemostats. The autograft is oriented so that the nonsutured side of the graft is superior. The glenoid side suture at each location is passed through the perimeter of the graft at each position (12, 2, 4, 6, 8, and 10 o'clock; Fig. 34.22). The graft is then passed down the sutures until it rests on the glenoid surface (Fig. 34.23). The sutures are tied sequentially to complete the resurfacing (Fig. 34.24). Alternatively, in patients with an insufficient labrum, a doubly loaded bioabsorbable suture anchor can be placed on the glenoid margin in each quadrant of the glenoid (a total of four anchors), and the same suturing process used (Fig. 34.25). When using anchor fixation, a 2.9-mm hole is predrilled at each location and the anchors placed via standard insertion technique.

We have also performed biologic glenoid resurfacing for incomplete defects of glenoid articular cartilage. In this circumstance, only the area of full-thickness cartilage loss is prepared with the Cobb elevator or motorized burr. The fascia lata autograft is prepared as previously described, except that it is trimmed to fit the glenoid articular cartilage defect (Fig. 34.26). In this circumstance it is often helpful to use suture anchors to fix the graft at the location immediately adjacent to the remaining intact glenoid articular cartilage (Fig. 34.27). Fig. 34.28 shows the final construct after resurfacing of the superior half of the glenoid.

Text continued on p. 321

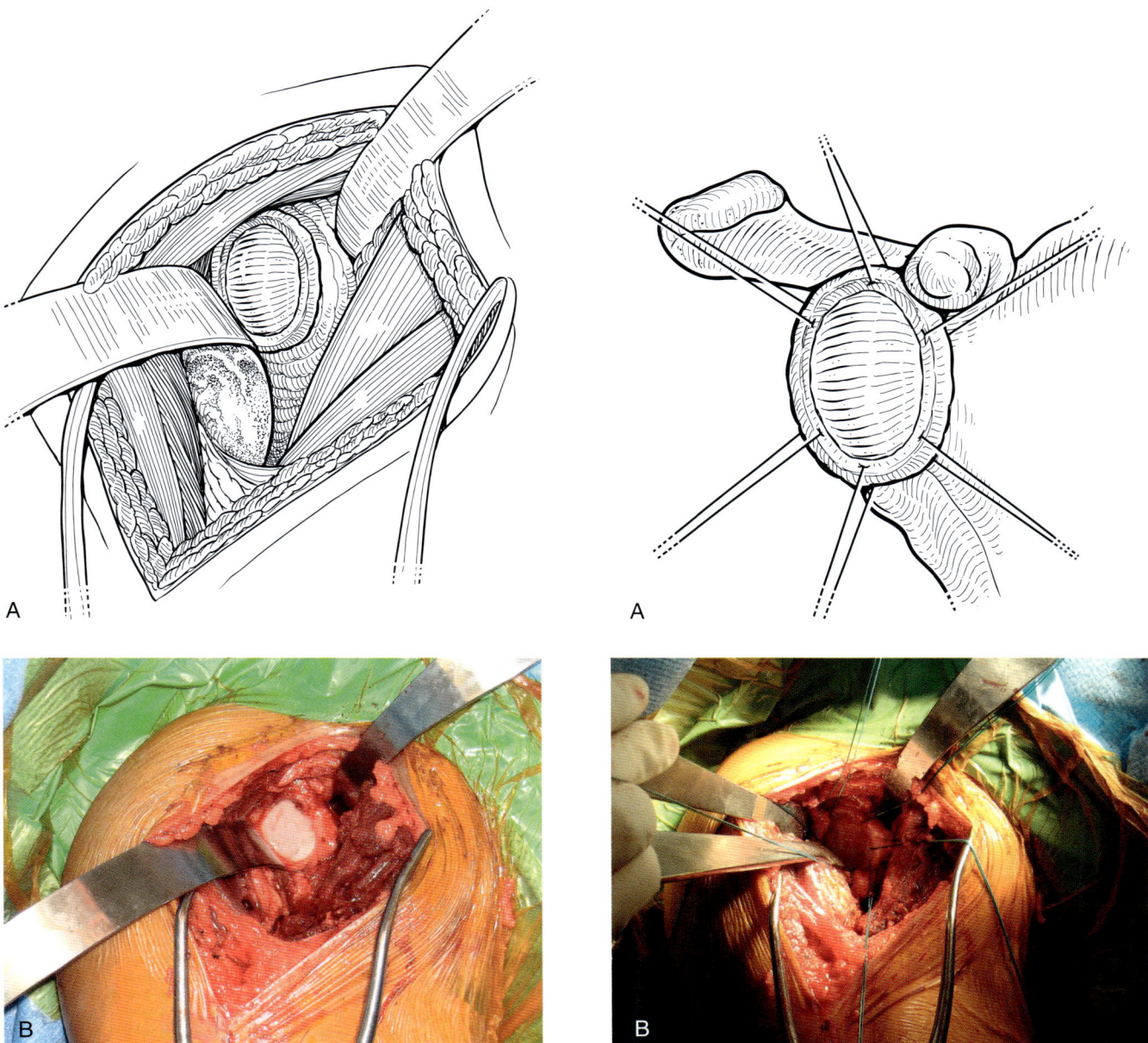

FIGURE 34.20 (A and B) Exposure of the glenoid before biologic resurfacing.

FIGURE 34.21 (A and B) Sutures placed circumferentially around the labrum for use in fixation of the autogenous fascia lata.

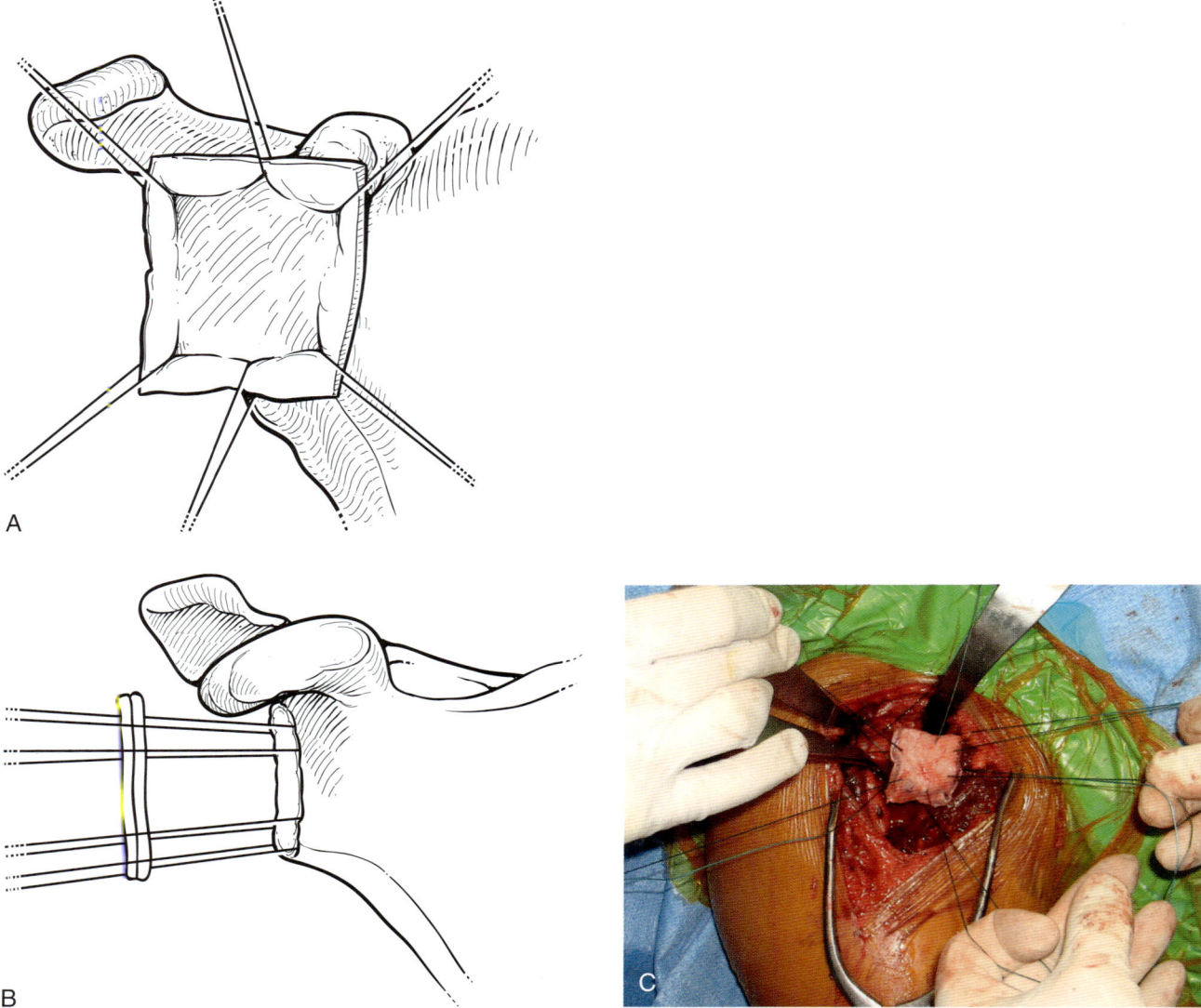

FIGURE 34.22 (A–C) Sutures are passed through the autograft outside the wound to facilitate graft placement and fixation.

CHAPTER 34 ■ Biologic Alternatives to Shoulder Arthroplasty 319

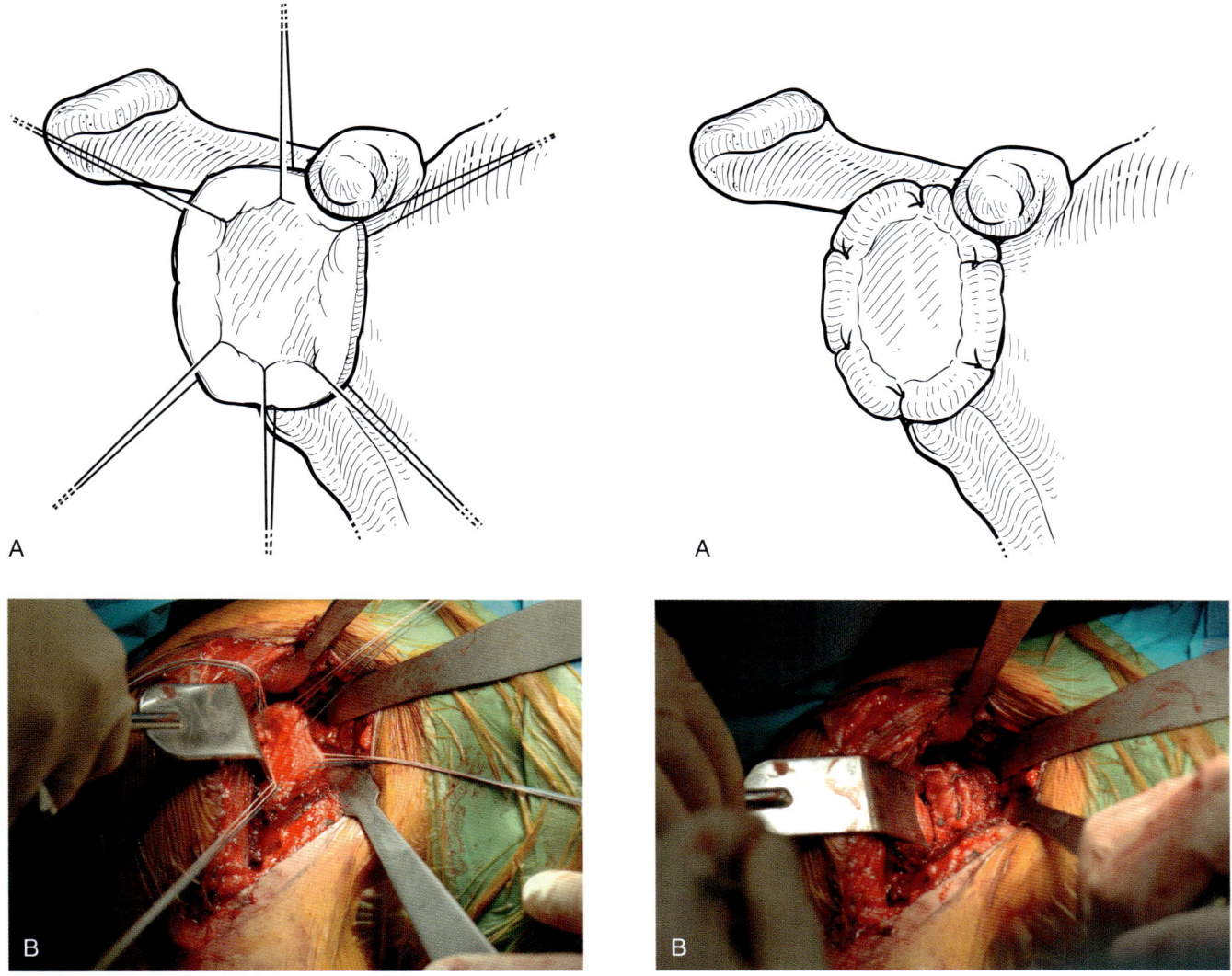

FIGURE 34.23 (A and B) The graft is shuttled down the sutures to the glenoid face.

FIGURE 34.24 (A and B) Final glenoid resurfacing after all sutures are tied.

320 SECTION V ■ Alternatives to Conventional Shoulder Arthroplasty

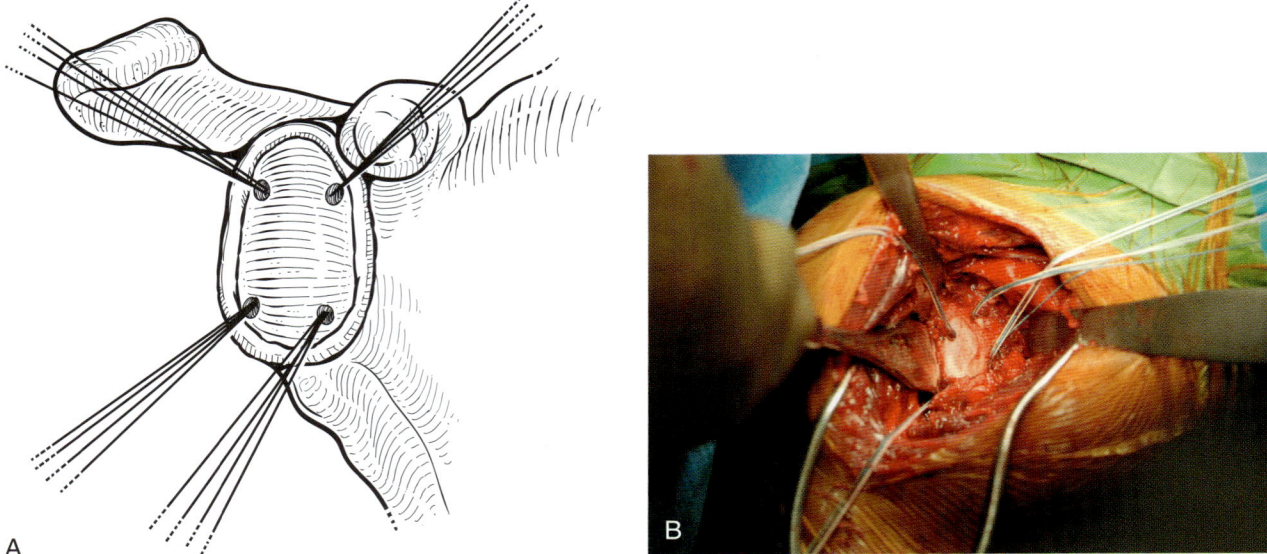

FIGURE 34.25 (A and B) Suture anchor placement for biologic glenoid resurfacing in a patient with a deficient labrum.

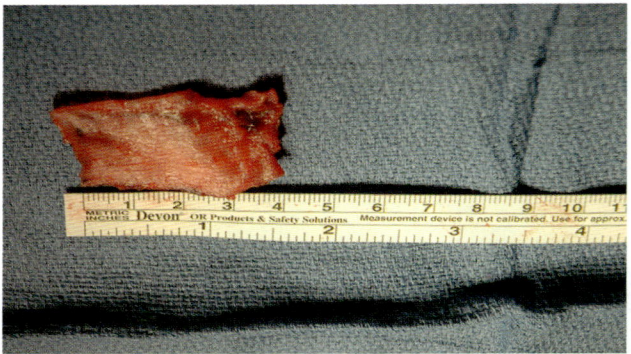

FIGURE 34.26 Fascia lata autograft used for resurfacing the superior half of the glenoid in a young patient in whom the inferior half of the glenoid articular cartilage is intact.

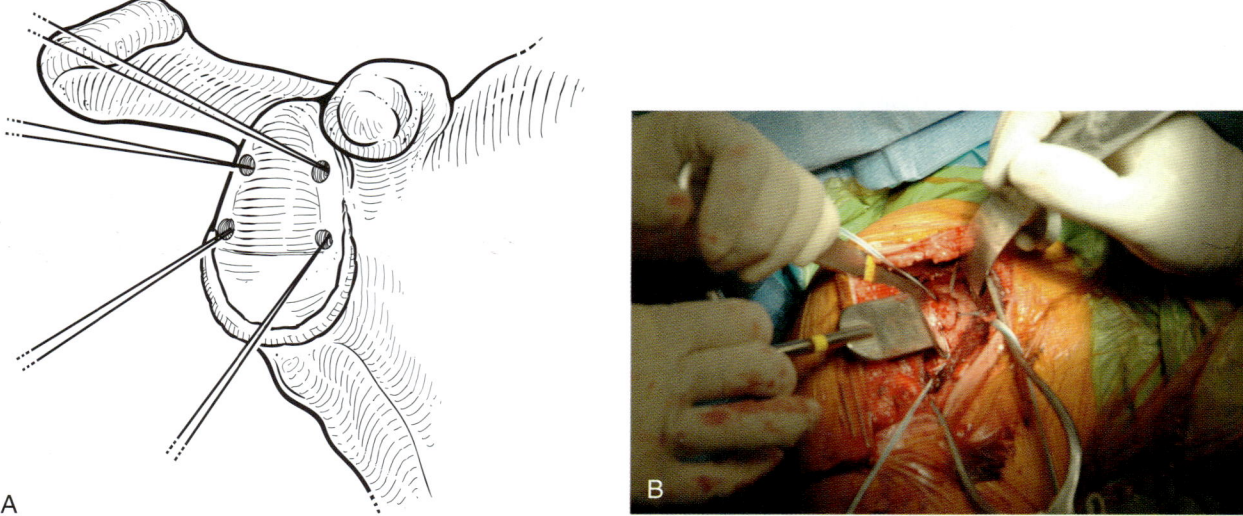

FIGURE 34.27 (A and B) Suture anchor placement for fixation of a fascia lata autograft used for resurfacing the superior half of the glenoid.

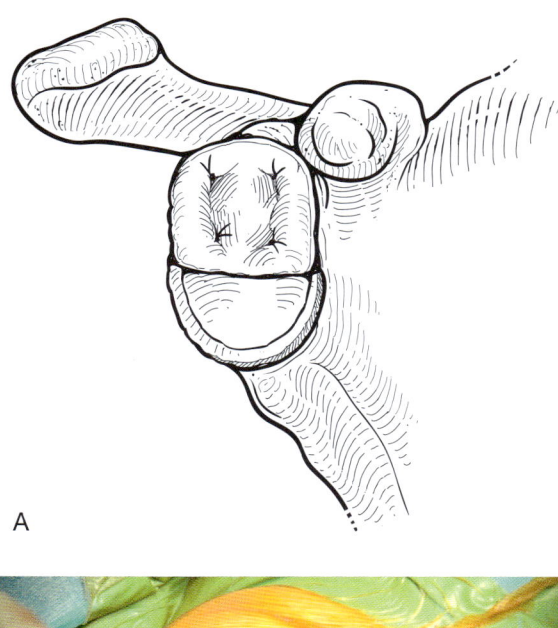

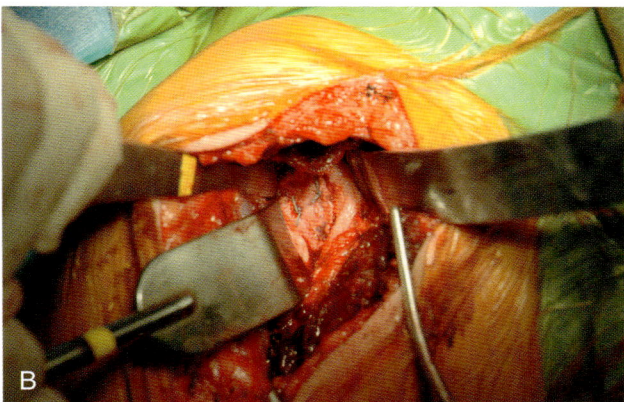

FIGURE 34.28 (A and B) Final construct after resurfacing of the superior half of the glenoid.

After biologic glenoid resurfacing is complete, the humeral portion of the surgery is performed and the subscapularis and wound are closed as for unconstrained shoulder arthroplasty.

REFERENCE

1. Burkhead WZ, Jr, Hutton KS: Biologic resurfacing of the glenoid with hemiarthroplasty of the shoulder, *J Shoulder Elbow Surg* 4:263–270, 1995.

SECTION VI

REVISION SHOULDER ARTHROPLASTY

CHAPTER 35

Indications and contraindications

Just as with hip and knee arthroplasty, as the volume of shoulder arthroplasties performed each year increases, so will the number of patients requiring revision shoulder arthroplasty. Indications for performing revision shoulder arthroplasty are variable and numerous and can include problems related to the glenoid, problems related to the humerus, and problems related to the soft tissues (rotator cuff, instability). Rarely, infection, either early postoperative or late-appearing hematogenous, is an indication for revision arthroplasty. Complications related to healing of the greater and lesser tuberosities can be observed after unconstrained shoulder arthroplasty performed for proximal humeral fractures. Finally, certain periprosthetic humeral fractures are an indication for revision shoulder arthroplasty. This chapter details our specific indications and contraindications for revision shoulder arthroplasty.

PROBLEMS RELATED TO THE GLENOID

Problems related to the glenoid are the most common indications for revision shoulder arthroplasty in our practice. One category consists of patients with problems of their native glenoid (glenoid erosion following hemiarthroplasty), and a second category includes patients who have problems with a previously placed glenoid component following total shoulder arthroplasty.

Glenoid Erosion

Glenoid erosion after hemiarthroplasty is a multifactorial problem.[1] It may occur early or late and does not seem to be related to any readily identifiable risk factor. This problem occurs when the metallic prosthetic humeral head erodes into the softer glenoid bone (Fig. 35.1). Initially, pain may be the sole manifestation of this problem. As the erosion progresses medially, the normal length-tension relationships of the rotator cuff may become compromised and result in substantial weakness (Fig. 35.2).

Glenoid erosion may be central or peripheral. If the rotator cuff is intact, as in primary osteoarthritis, the erosion is usually central or, less commonly, posterior (Fig. 35.3). If the rotator cuff is deficient, the erosion is generally superior (Fig. 35.4) or, less commonly, anterior (if the subscapularis is deficient; Fig. 35.5).

Glenoid erosion is best treated by resurfacing of the glenoid if sufficient native glenoid bone is available for implantation of a glenoid component (see Chapter 36). Frequently, the humeral component will require revision for glenoid exposure, and two options are available to the surgeon. We may exchange the component for a smaller head size in an unconstrained arthroplasty (Fig. 35.6) or change to a reverse-design arthroplasty. In general, with a functioning rotator cuff, an unconstrained arthroplasty is performed for revision arthroplasty. If rotator cuff function is significantly compromised, revision to a reverse prosthesis is performed.

Glenoid Component Failure

Glenoid component failure can vary from subtle loosening to migration of the component with severe glenoid bone loss (Fig. 35.7). Additionally, mechanical failure of the implant can necessitate revision surgery (Fig. 35.8). When considering revision surgery for failure of a glenoid component, the surgeon must first decide whether to simply remove the failed glenoid component or to remove the failed glenoid component and reconstruct the osseous glenoid. In debilitated patients seeking mainly pain relief without significant concern for function, isolated removal of the glenoid component is usually the best treatment option. Isolated removal of the glenoid component can be completed arthroscopically or with an open procedure. In other patients, glenoid reconstruction with iliac crest bone graft is indicated. For patients undergoing revision with an unconstrained prosthesis, we reconstruct the glenoid with an iliac crest bone graft as the first stage. Four to six months later, after complete incorporation of the bone graft, if the shoulder is still painful, we perform the second stage, which consists of placement of a

Text continued on p. 326

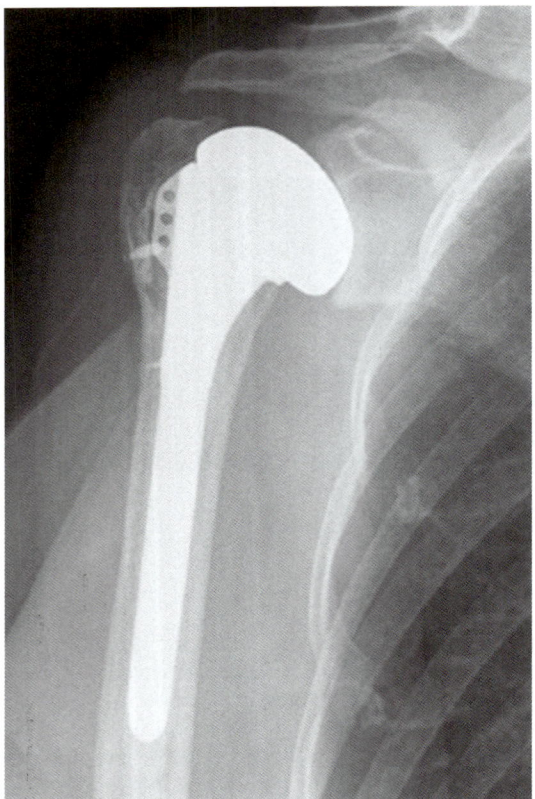

FIGURE 35.1 Radiograph demonstrating osseous glenoid erosion after hemiarthroplasty.

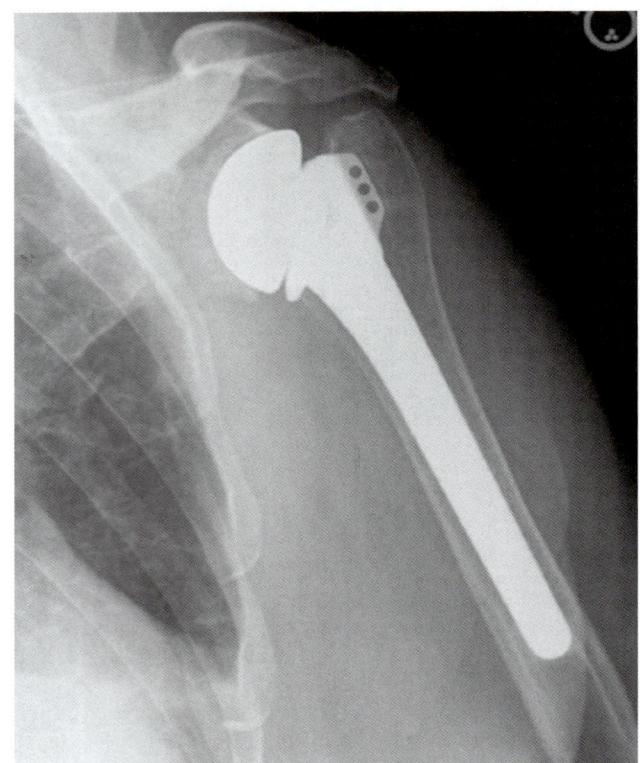

FIGURE 35.2 Severe medialization of the humeral head caused by progressive glenoid erosion.

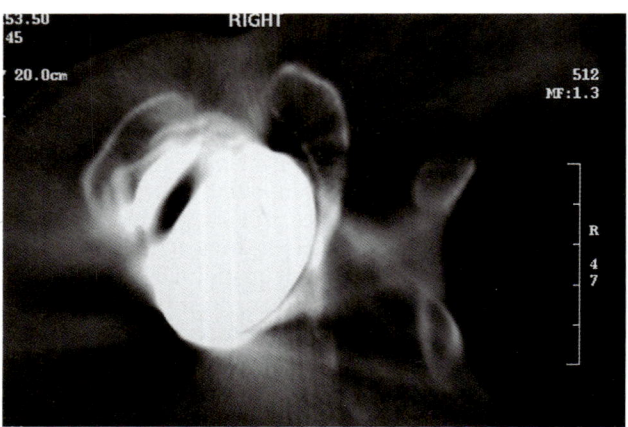

FIGURE 35.3 Computed tomography scan demonstrating central glenoid erosion after hemiarthroplasty for primary osteoarthritis.

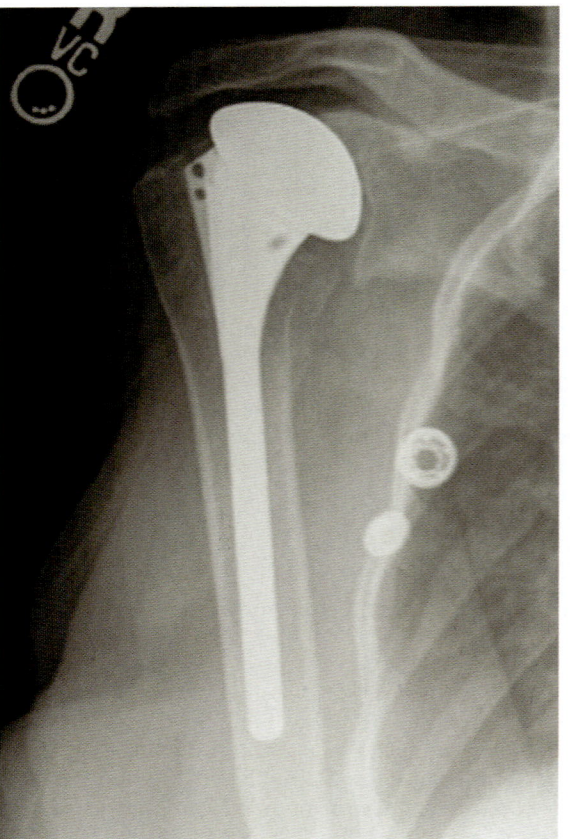

FIGURE 35.4 Superior glenoid erosion in a patient who has undergone hemiarthroplasty for rotator cuff tear arthropathy.

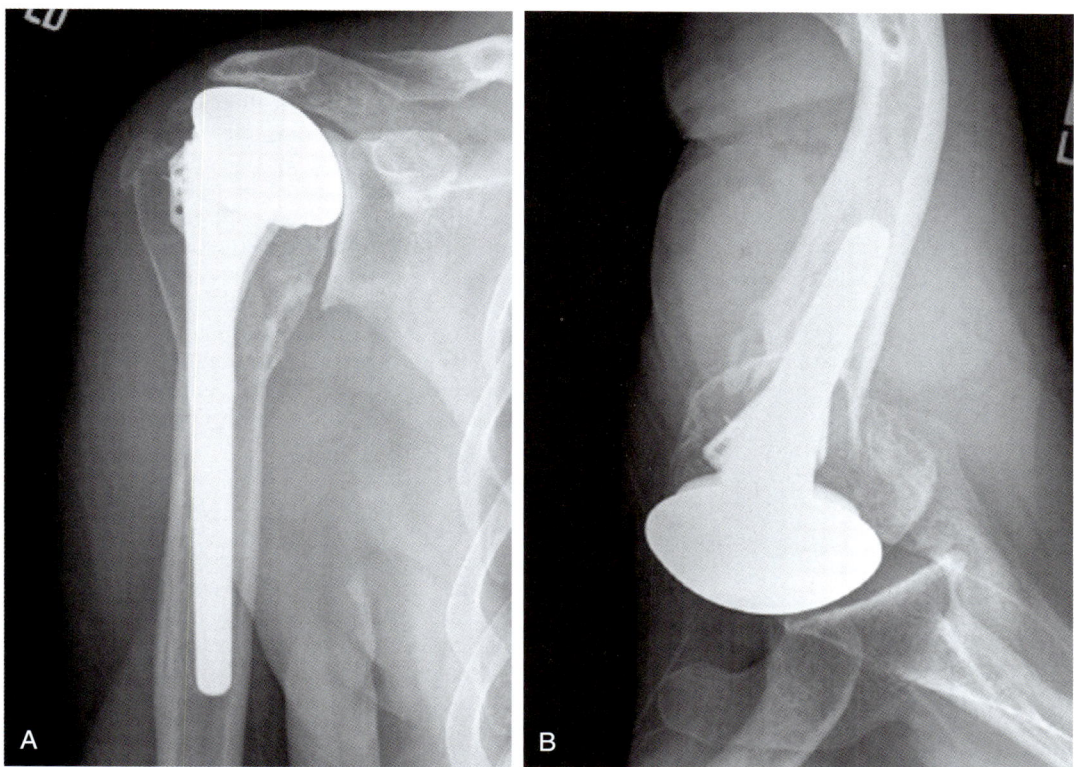

FIGURE 35.5 (A and B) Anterior superior glenoid erosion in a patient who has undergone hemiarthroplasty for anterior superior rotator cuff insufficiency.

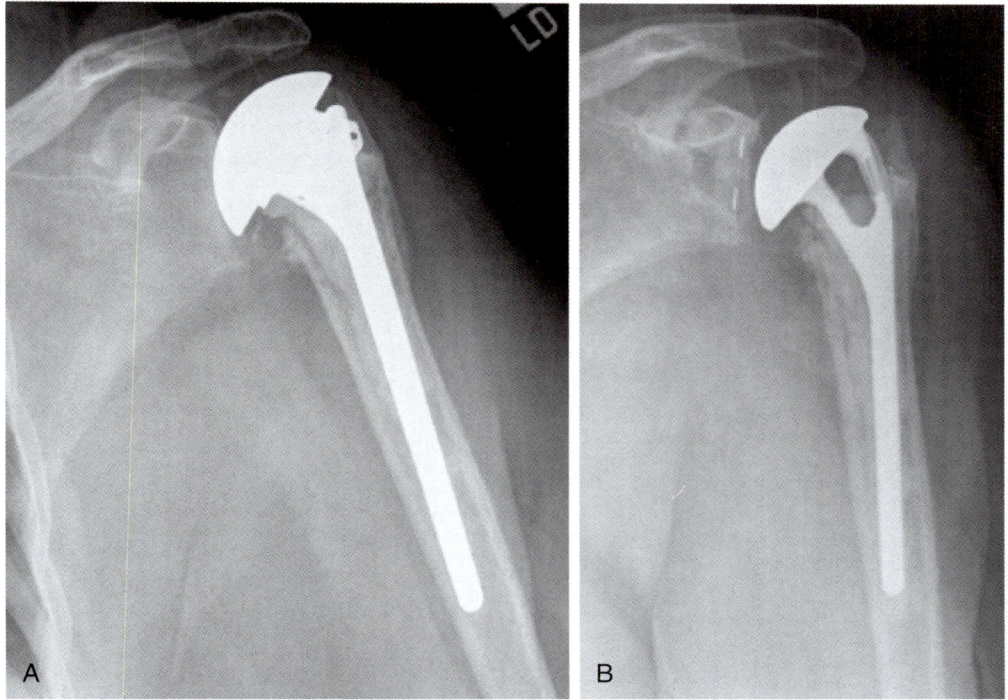

FIGURE 35.6 (A) Pre-revision radiograph. (B) Humeral revision in which the humeral stem has been exchanged and the humeral head exchanged for a smaller size.

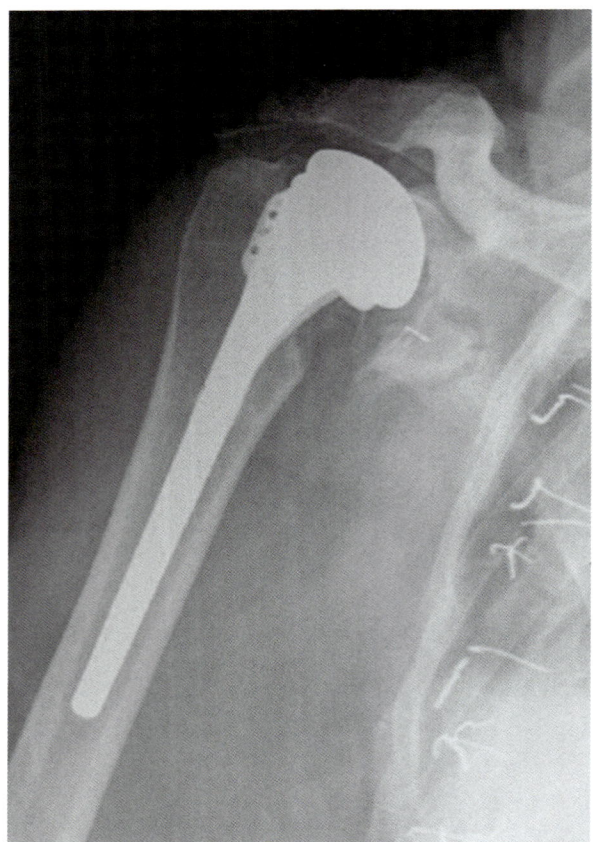

FIGURE 35.7 Radiograph showing loosening of a glenoid component.

new glenoid component (Fig. 35.9). When performing revision surgery with a reverse-design prosthesis, glenoid reconstruction and revision can often be performed as a single stage, provided that the central post or screw of the revision glenoid component can be firmly fixed in native glenoid bone (Fig. 35.10).

Just as in cases of glenoid erosion, patients requiring revision surgery for a problem with the glenoid component often require revision of the humeral component for glenoid exposure, and the surgeon can exchange the component for a smaller head size in an unconstrained arthroplasty or change to a reverse-design arthroplasty. As previously mentioned, in a patient with a functioning rotator cuff, an unconstrained arthroplasty is used for revision arthroplasty. If rotator cuff function is significantly compromised, revision to a reverse prosthesis is performed.

Reverse Glenoid Component

In our experience, failure of the glenoid component of a reverse prosthesis is far less common than failure of the glenoid component of an unconstrained shoulder arthroplasty. The most common problem that we observe is inadvertent placement of the glenoid component in a superiorly oriented position (Fig. 35.11). This usually occurs when a superior surgical approach has been used to place the reverse prosthesis. Although this radiographic finding does not merit revision surgery in and of itself, revision is indicated if this problem evolves into early glenoid loosening (Fig. 35.12).

Another radiographic finding related to a reverse glenoid component is inferior scapular notching. This finding can be related to excessive superior placement of the reverse glenoid component (Fig. 35.13). Notching, even when it is severe, has not been shown to cause loosening of the glenoid component, and revision surgery is unnecessary in the absence of glenoid loosening.

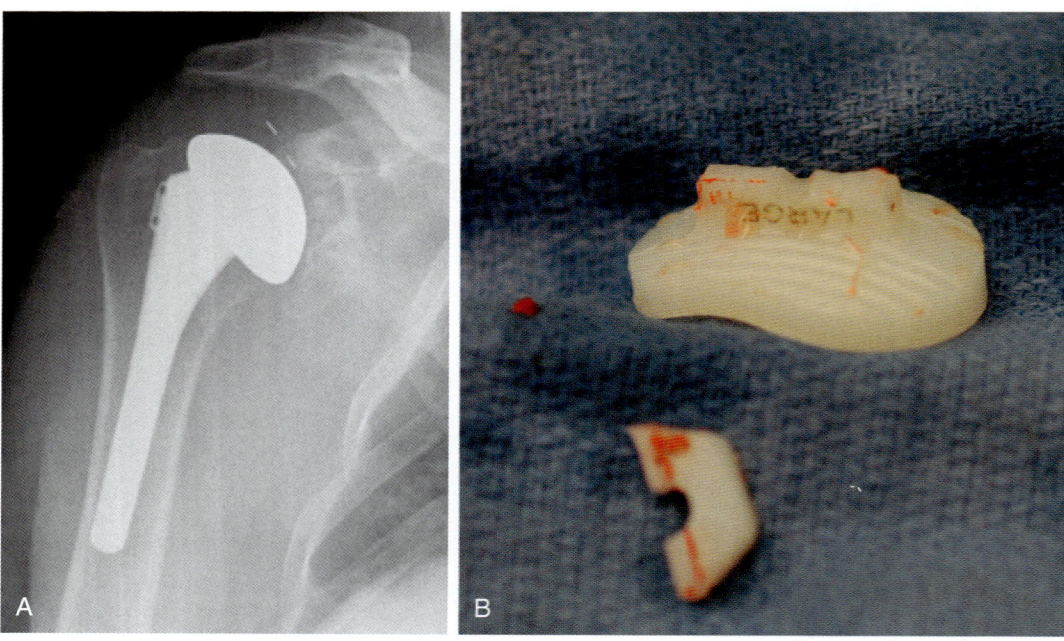

FIGURE 35.8 (A and B) Mechanical failure of a glenoid implant.

CHAPTER 35 ■ Indications and Contraindications 327

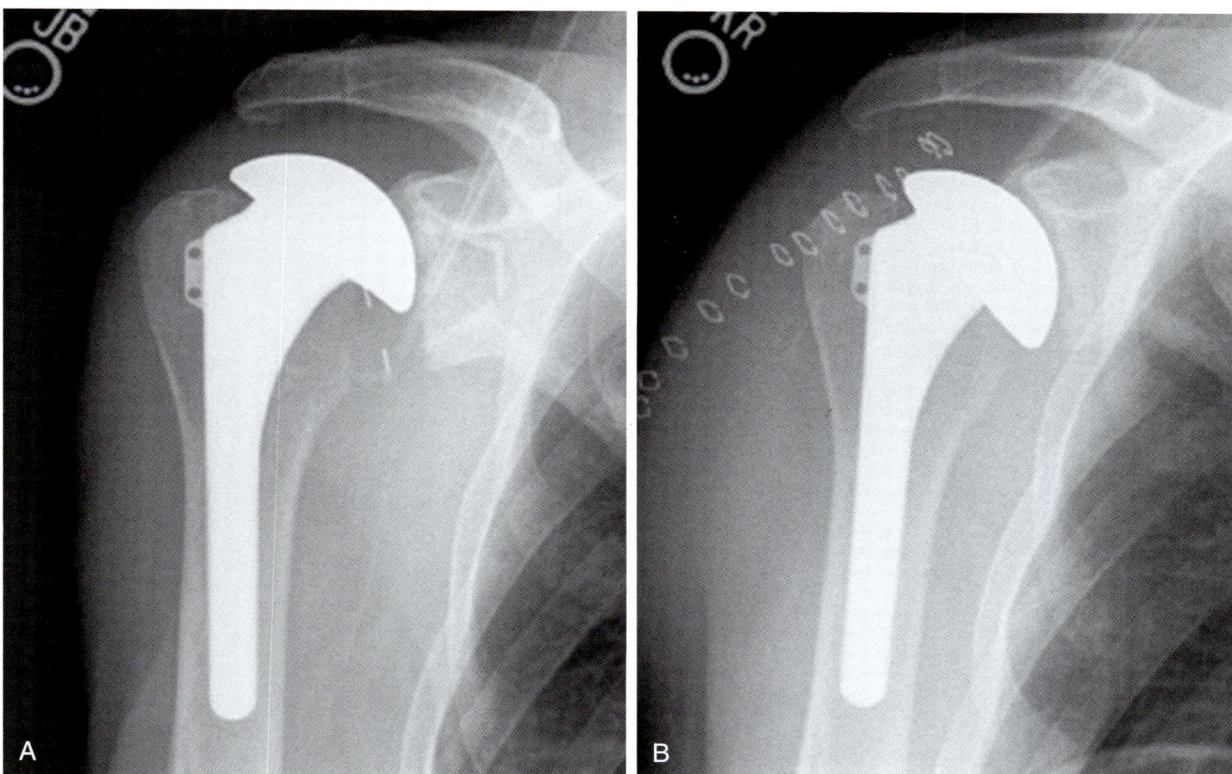

FIGURE 35.9 Preoperative radiograph (A) and postoperative radiograph (B) after removal of a loose glenoid component and bone grafting of the residual osseous defect in the glenoid.

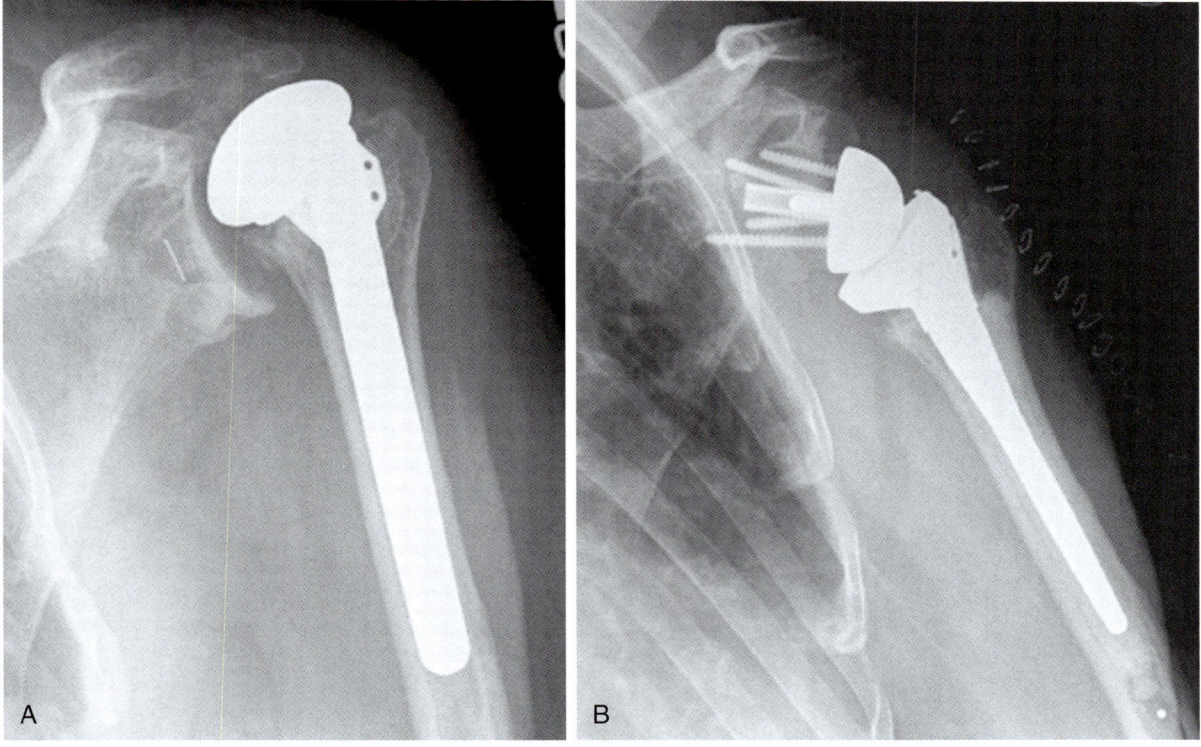

FIGURE 35.10 (A) Preoperative radiograph. (B) Postoperative radiograph after revision of a failed unconstrained shoulder arthroplasty to a reverse shoulder arthroplasty with bone grafting of the glenoid.

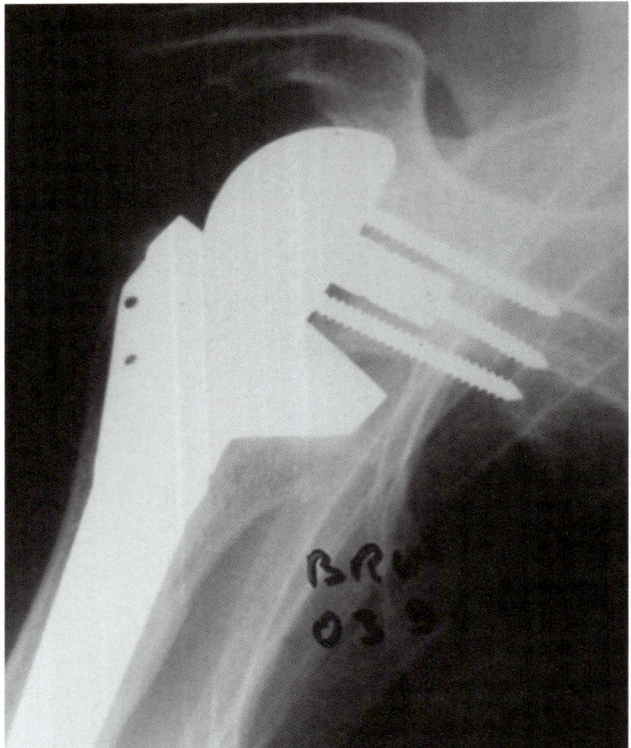

FIGURE 35.11 Superiorly oriented glenoid component after reverse shoulder arthroplasty performed through a superior approach.

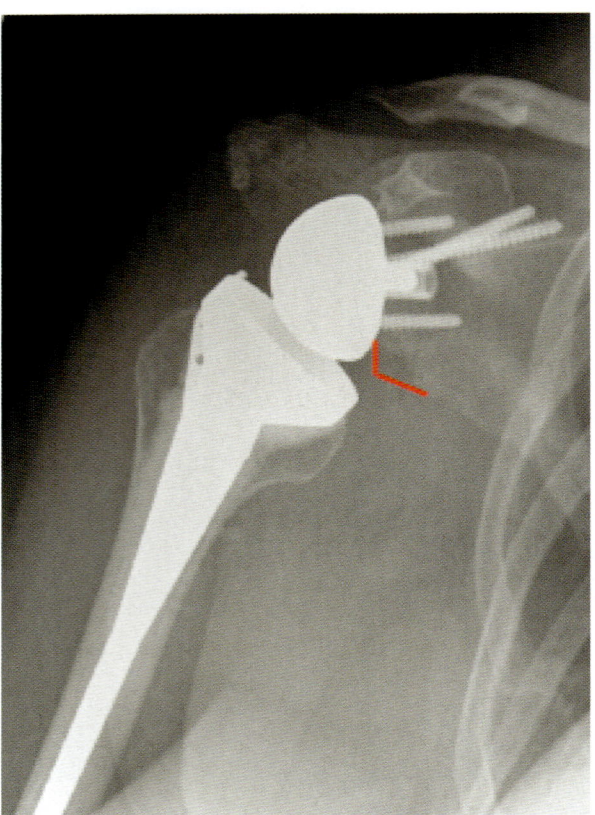

FIGURE 35.13 Scapular notching after reverse shoulder arthroplasty in which the glenoid component was placed superiorly on the glenoid face. The red line indicates the original border of the glenoid.

Rarely, a traumatic injury can result in mechanical failure of the glenoid component of the reverse prosthesis (Fig. 35.14). In these cases, revision is indicated to resolve the problem.

PROBLEMS RELATED TO THE HUMERUS

Humeral component problems requiring revision surgery are much less common than glenoid problems. Specifically, aseptic loosening of both unconstrained and reverse humeral components is rare. More commonly, revision surgery for a humeral component problem results from positioning or size of the humeral component.

Unconstrained Humeral Components

The main problem that leads us to revise an unconstrained humeral component is placement of a humeral head prosthesis that is too large (Fig. 35.15). This can lead to stiffness, glenoid problems, and rotator cuff problems. If the stem of the humeral implant is acceptably positioned, the humeral head is simply exchanged for a smaller size.

Less frequently, a humeral implant will be improperly positioned, generally with respect to humeral version. Problems with humeral component version can lead to instability of the component; nonconcentric glenoid loading, wear, and loosening; and failure of subscapularis repair. These scenarios are indications for revision of the humeral component.

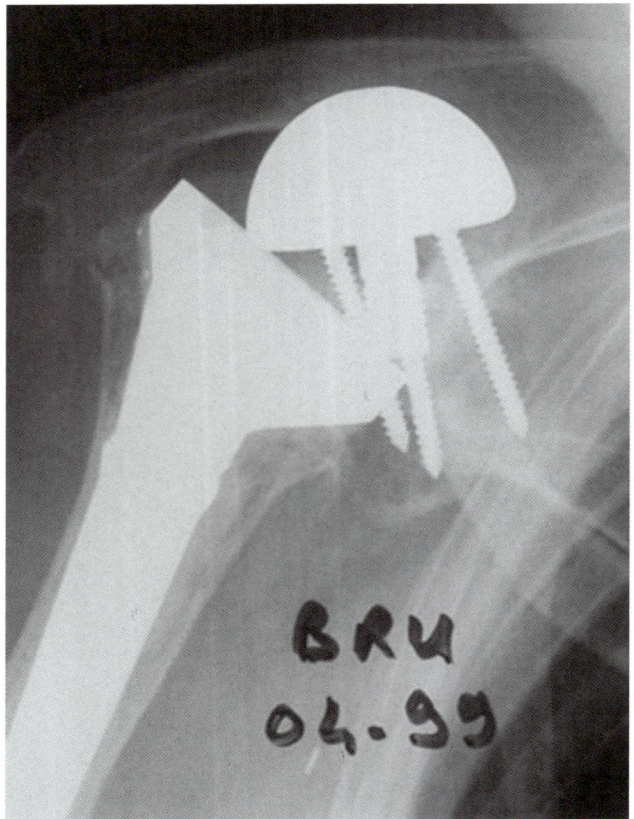

FIGURE 35.12 Failure of the glenoid component in reverse shoulder arthroplasty. The glenoid component was initially placed in a superiorly directed orientation.

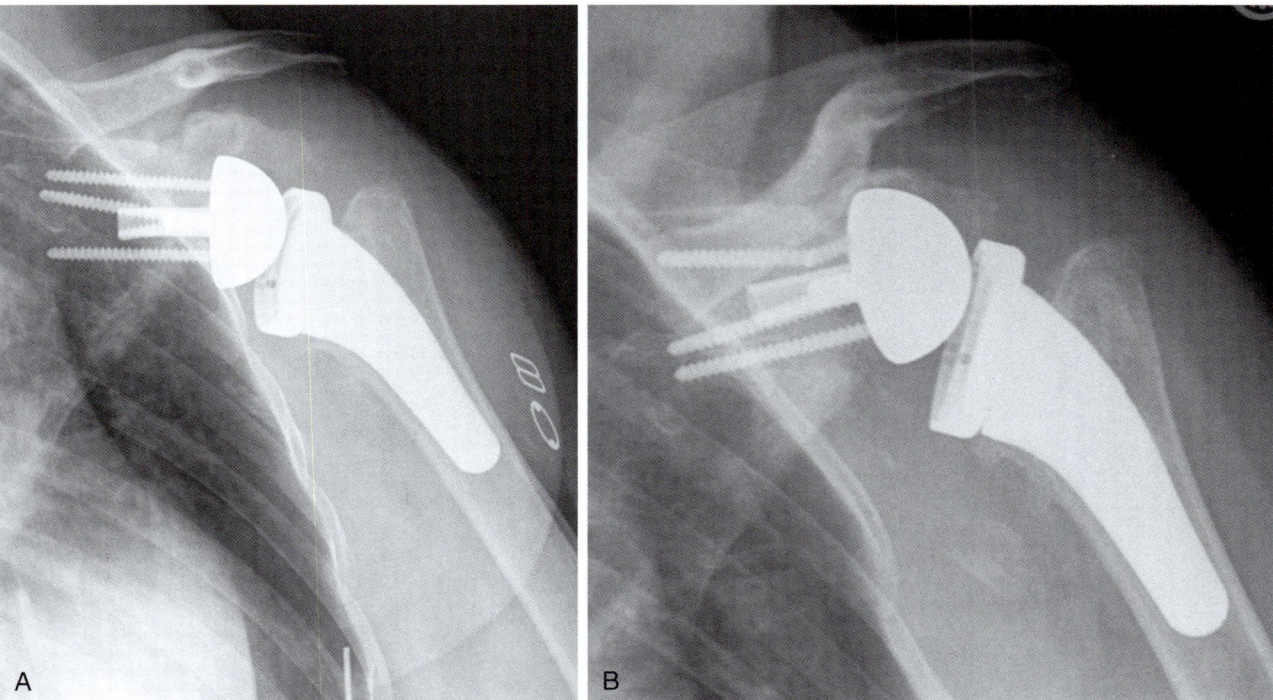

FIGURE 35.14 (A and B) Traumatic failure of a reverse glenoid component occurring from a motor vehicle crash.

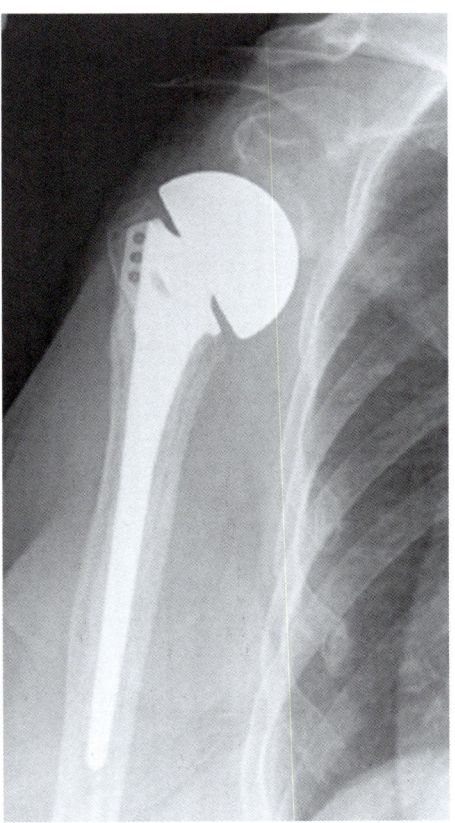

FIGURE 35.15 Unconstrained shoulder arthroplasty with an excessively large humeral head component.

Reverse Humeral Components

Even in cases in which a reverse humeral component is properly positioned, the deltoid muscle can "stretch out" and result in loss of prosthetic stability and, ultimately, dislocation. Patients most at risk for this complication are those with proximal humeral bone loss (Fig. 35.16). In such cases, it is sometimes necessary to add more length to the humeral component to restore prosthetic stability via restoration of deltoid tension. This can usually be accomplished by exchanging the primarily placed polyethylene liner for a thicker, more constrained liner or adding a thicker metallic tray, or both (Fig. 35.17). Tensioning the deltoid by adding length to the prosthesis almost never requires removal of the humeral stem. In cases in which use of a metallic augment and the thickest polyethylene liner fails to stabilize the prosthesis, the glenosphere size may be increased to further increase stability (Fig. 35.18).

Rarely, proximal humeral bone loss during revision surgery is sufficiently severe to necessitate use of a custom implant or proximal humeral composite bone graft (allograft-prosthesis composite reconstruction) (Fig. 35.19).

PROBLEMS RELATED TO SOFT TISSUE

Soft tissue problems necessitating revision shoulder arthroplasty can be divided into those related to instability and those related to the rotator cuff. These problems often occur concomitantly because rotator cuff insufficiency can lead to glenohumeral prosthetic instability.

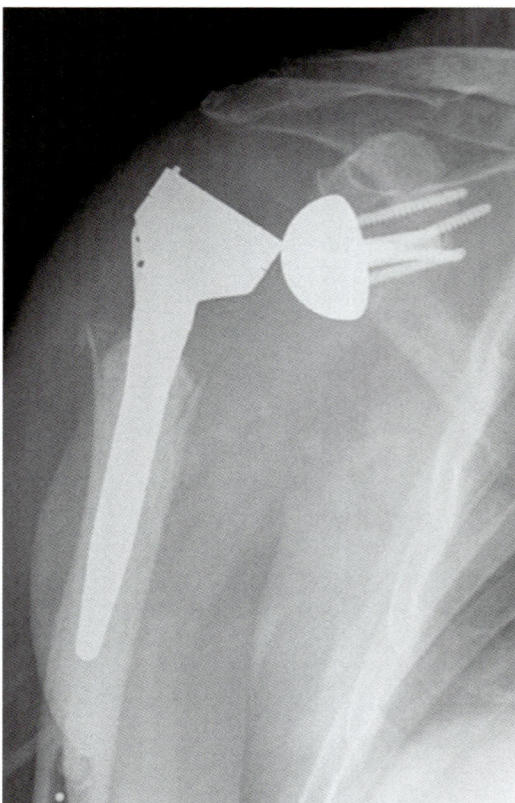

FIGURE 35.16 Patient with severe proximal humeral bone loss resulting in dislocation of the reverse prosthesis.

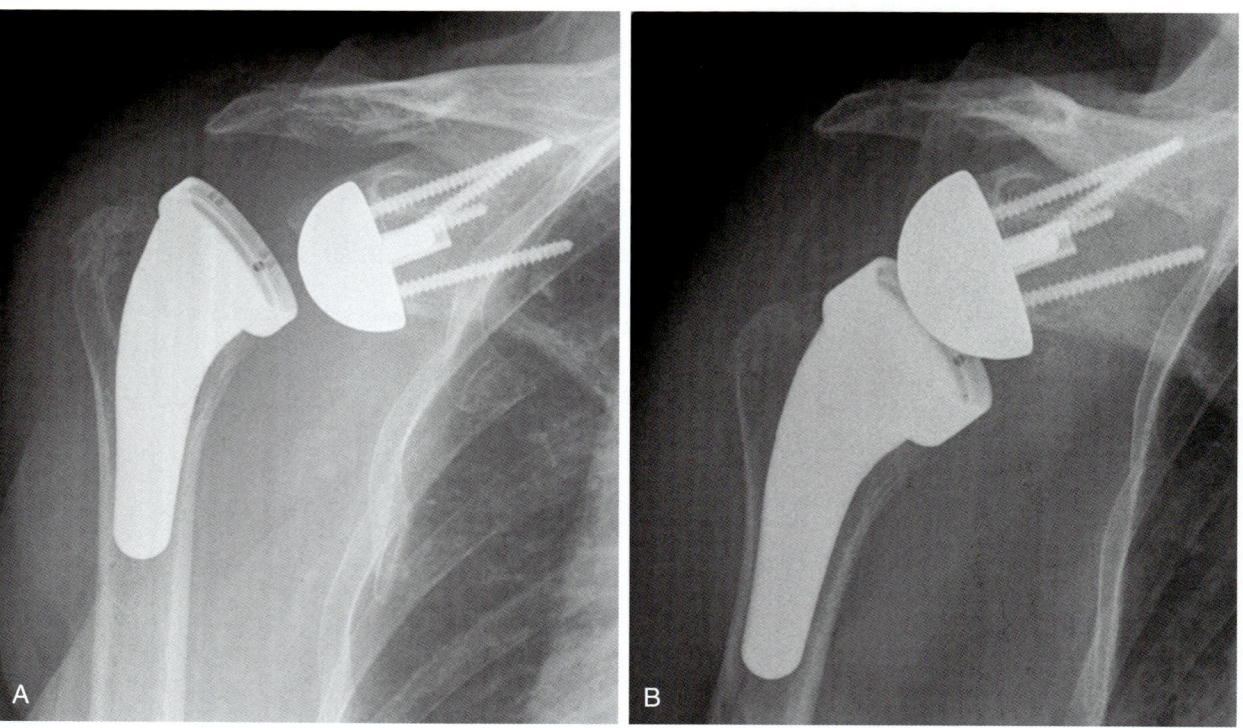

FIGURE 35.17 (A) Pre-revision radiograph. (B) Radiograph after revision of a dislocated reverse prosthesis by adding a thicker metallic tray with a thicker, more constrained polyethylene spacer to increase deltoid tension and prosthetic stability.

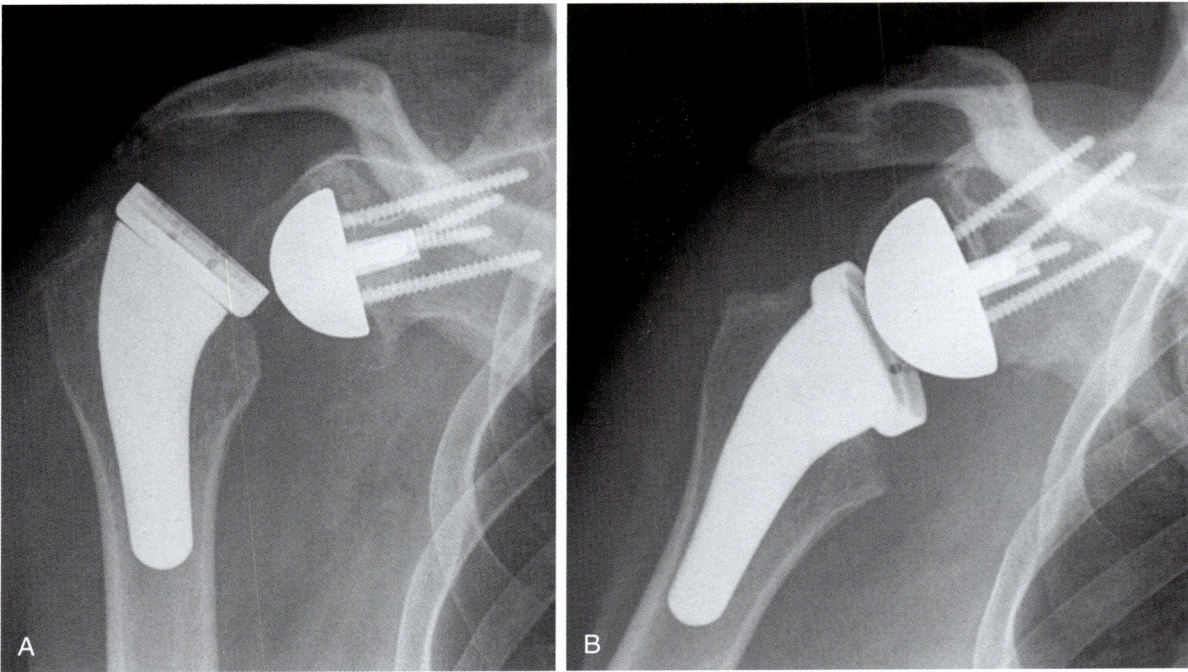

FIGURE 35.18 (A) Pre-revision radiograph. (B) Radiograph after revision of a dislocated reverse prosthesis by changing to a larger diameter glenosphere and adding a thicker, more constrained polyethylene spacer to increase prosthetic stability.

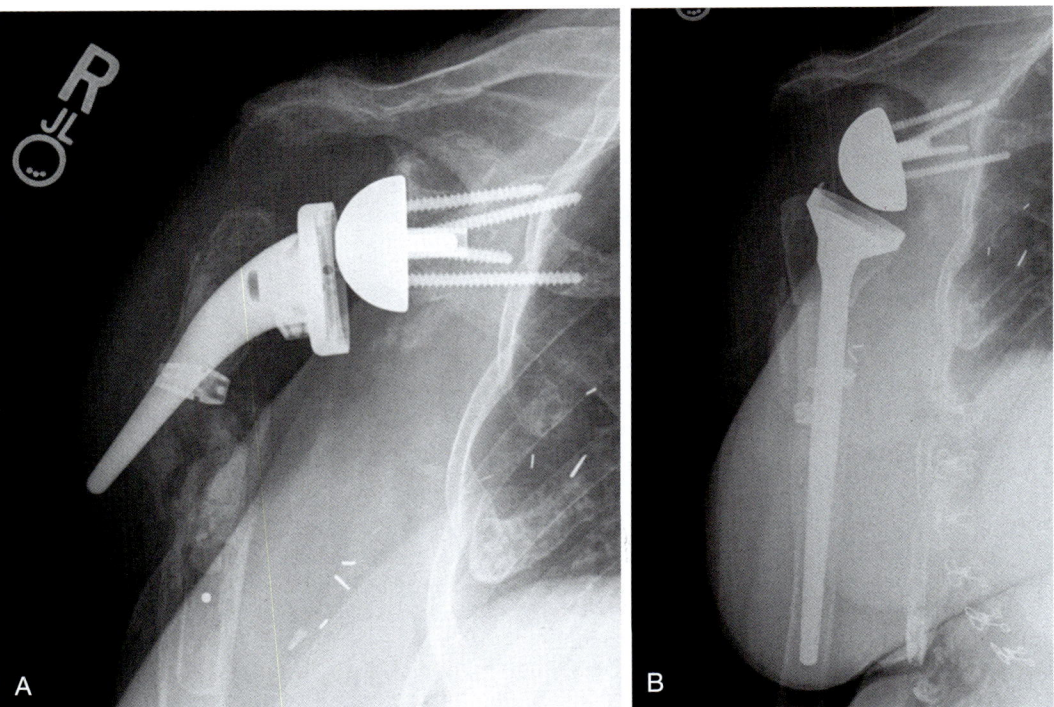

FIGURE 35.19 (A and B) Proximal humeral bone loss sufficiently severe to necessitate use of a proximal humeral composite bone graft (allograft-prosthesis composite reconstruction).

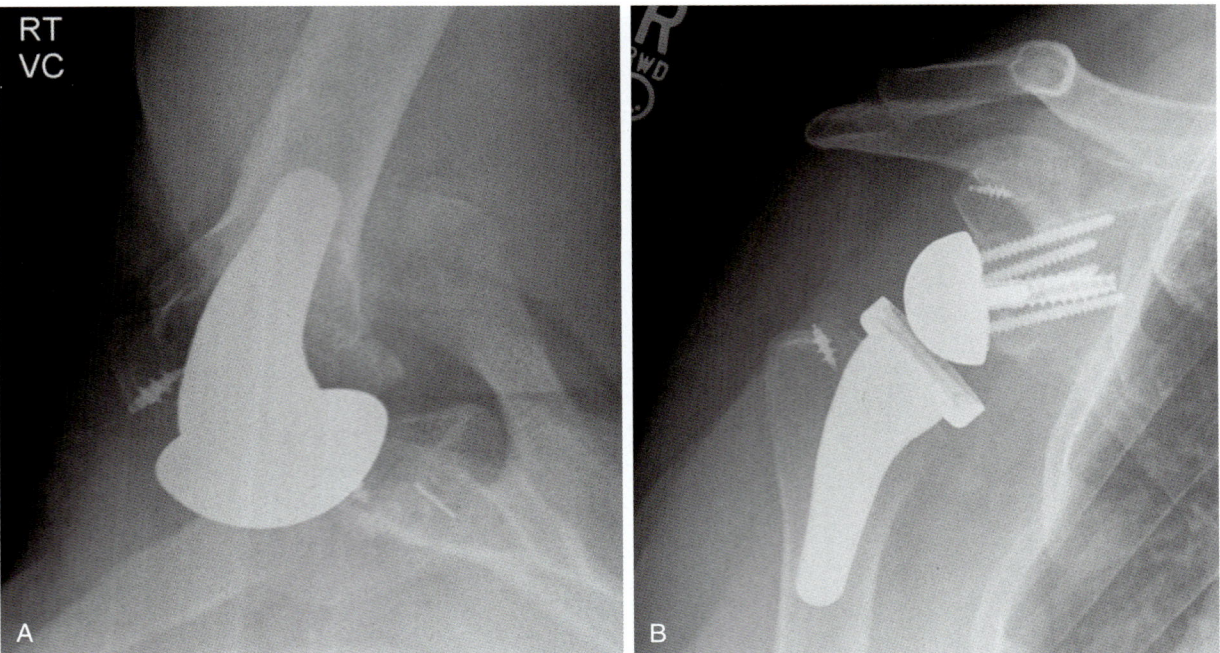

FIGURE 35.20 Case in which a patient with subscapularis insufficiency and dynamic glenohumeral prosthetic instability (A) underwent revision to a reverse prosthesis with a convertible stem (B).

Subscapularis Problems

Occasionally, subscapularis dehiscence will develop after unconstrained shoulder arthroplasty. In many circumstances, postoperative failure of a subscapularis repair will be asymptomatic or minimally symptomatic and is a contraindication to revision surgery. If the patient has early (<6 weeks postoperatively) subscapularis failure without instability, subscapularis repair with retention of all components can be considered, provided that they are appropriately sized and positioned. If the patient complains only of weakness and pain without instability and has chronic subscapularis insufficiency, a subcoracoid pectoralis major transfer with retention of all components can be considered, provided that they are appropriately sized and positioned.

If subscapularis insufficiency is coupled with either dynamic or static anterior instability after unconstrained shoulder arthroplasty, our experience has been that revision to a reverse-design prosthesis is the only reliable way of restoring glenohumeral stability (Fig. 35.20).

Other Rotator Cuff Problems

The development of rotator cuff insufficiency after unconstrained shoulder arthroplasty is very rare. In cases in which a patient has sustained a massive (two or more tendons) rotator cuff tear after unconstrained shoulder arthroplasty that has resulted in severe dysfunction and static or dynamic glenohumeral prosthetic instability, revision to a reverse-design prosthesis can be considered (Fig. 35.21).

Instability

Glenohumeral instability after unconstrained shoulder arthroplasty usually occurs in one of two scenarios. First, instability can occur with rotator cuff insufficiency, as previously mentioned. Second, instability can occur in patients who have undergone unconstrained shoulder arthroplasty for primary osteoarthritis with posterior glenoid wear and posterior capsular distention (Fig. 35.22). In these cases, we have found soft tissue procedures unpredictable in restoration of glenohumeral stability. We opt for revision to a reverse-design prosthesis (Fig. 35.23).

A less common problem causing instability is an unconstrained humeral implant positioned in incorrect version (Fig. 35.24). This is an indication for revision of the humeral component and placement of the revision component in correct humeral version.

INFECTION

Infections after shoulder arthroplasty can be divided into perioperative (within 6 weeks of surgery) and late (hematogenous) infections. Early perioperative infections are initially treated with two or three irrigation and débridement procedures, retention of the fixed components, and exchange of any nonfixed modular components (i.e., polyethylene liner, humeral head). At the last planned irrigation and débridement procedure, absorbable antibiotic-impregnated beads (Stimulan, Biocomposites, Inc., Staffordshire, England) are placed in the soft tissues around the shoulder, and the final nonfixed components are replaced. Consultation with an infectious disease specialist is obtained, and a minimum of 6 weeks of intravenous antibiotics tailored to the specific organism causing the infection (or covering the most likely offending organisms, if cultures remain negative despite obvious infection) is usually recommended. If this regimen fails, prosthetic removal ensues, followed by staged revision or resection arthroplasty, depending on the specific circumstances of the patient.

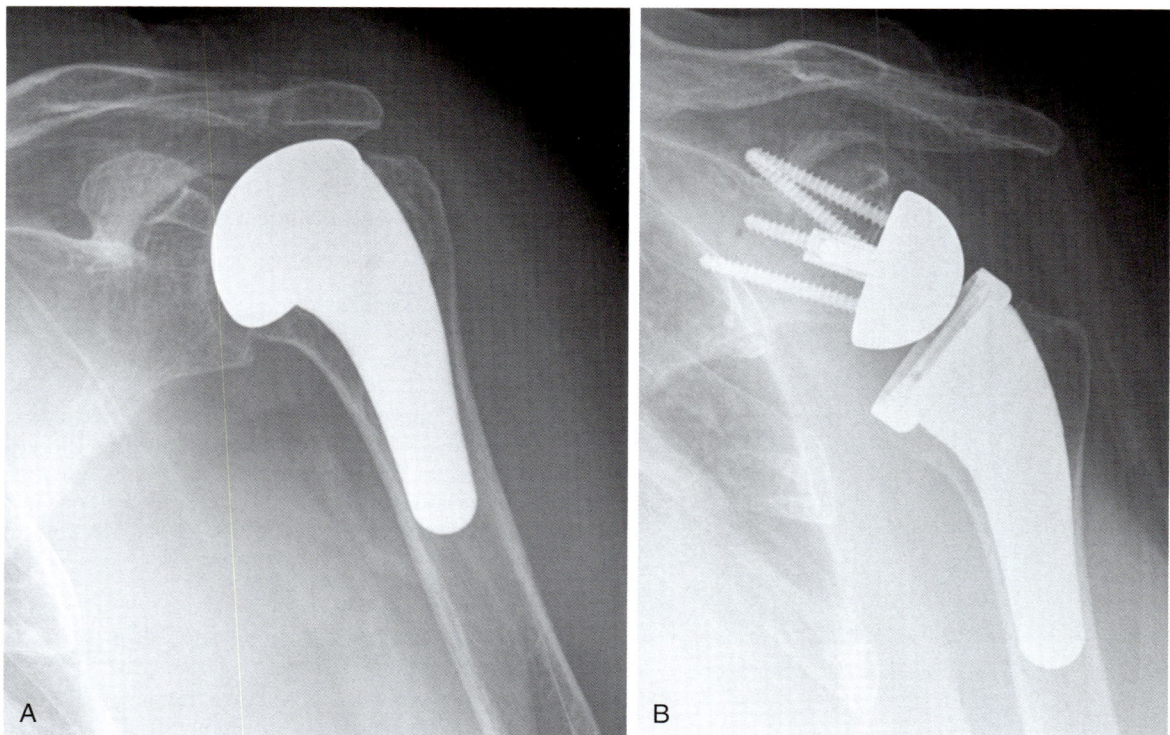

FIGURE 35.21 (A) Patient with a massive irreparable rotator cuff tear after an unconstrained shoulder arthroplasty. (B) Static superior migration of the humerus required revision to a reverse prosthesis.

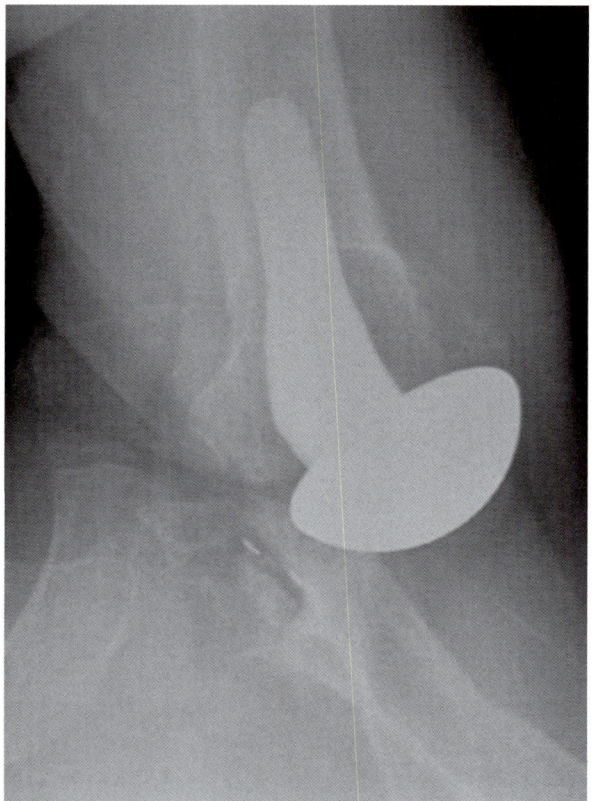

FIGURE 35.22 Posterior dislocation of a total shoulder arthroplasty performed for primary osteoarthritis in a patient with severe posterior glenoid wear.

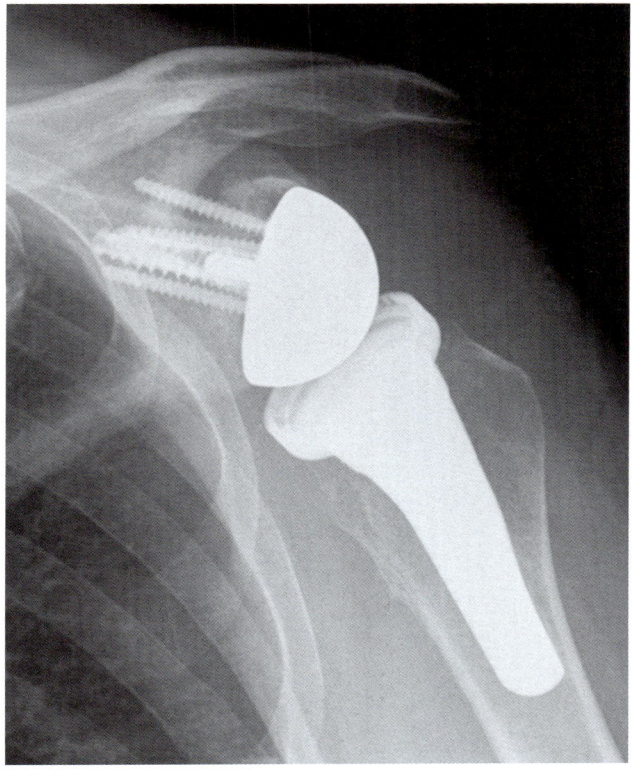

FIGURE 35.23 Revision of a posteriorly dislocated unconstrained total shoulder arthroplasty to a reverse prosthesis.

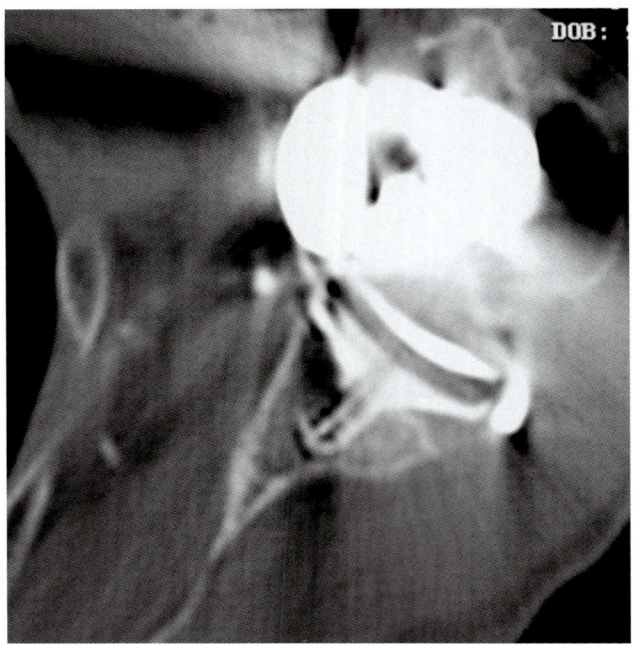

FIGURE 35.24 Computed tomography scan of a patient with a humeral component placed in excessive anteversion that resulted in anterior instability.

Late-appearing infections are treated by removal of the prosthesis, placement of antibiotic spacer, and intravenous administration of antibiotics. The decision whether to place a revision shoulder arthroplasty or continue with a resection arthroplasty is patient specific. Revision arthroplasty can be considered as a second stage after appropriate treatment of the infection (Fig. 35.25). See Chapter 7 for additional information of the diagnosis and treatment of periprosthetic infection.

SPECIAL SITUATION—TUBEROSITY PROBLEMS AFTER UNCONSTRAINED ARTHROPLASTY FOR FRACTURE

Tuberosity malunion and nonunion after unconstrained shoulder arthroplasty for proximal humeral fracture are an indication for revision shoulder arthroplasty with a reverse-design prosthesis (Fig. 35.26). Our experience in achieving reliable tuberosity union once tuberosity migration has occurred has not been favorable.

PERIPROSTHETIC FRACTURE

Displaced periprosthetic fractures not amenable to nonoperative treatment or treatment by open reduction and internal fixation because of inability to achieve adequate fixation proximally are an indication for revision shoulder arthroplasty (Fig. 35.27). In this scenario, we believe it best to remove

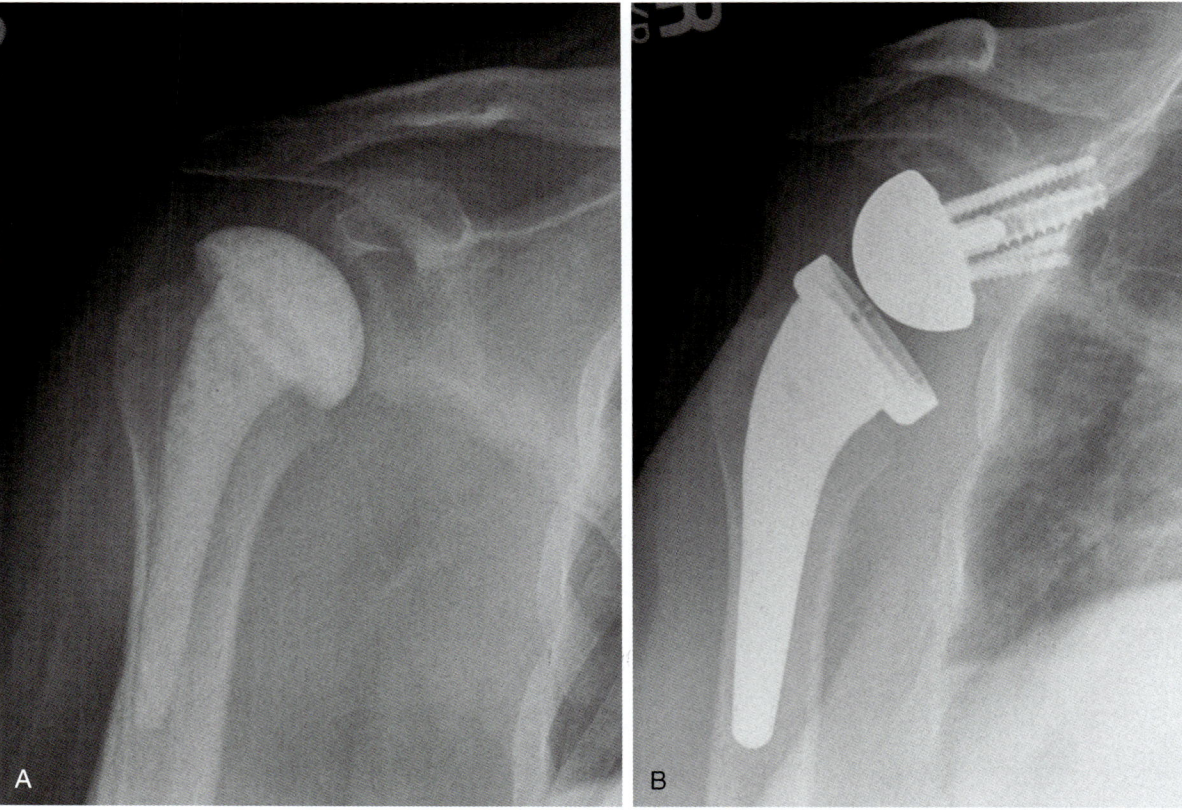

FIGURE 35.25 Infection of the primary arthroplasty with placement of an antibiotic spacer (A) required revision shoulder arthroplasty (B).

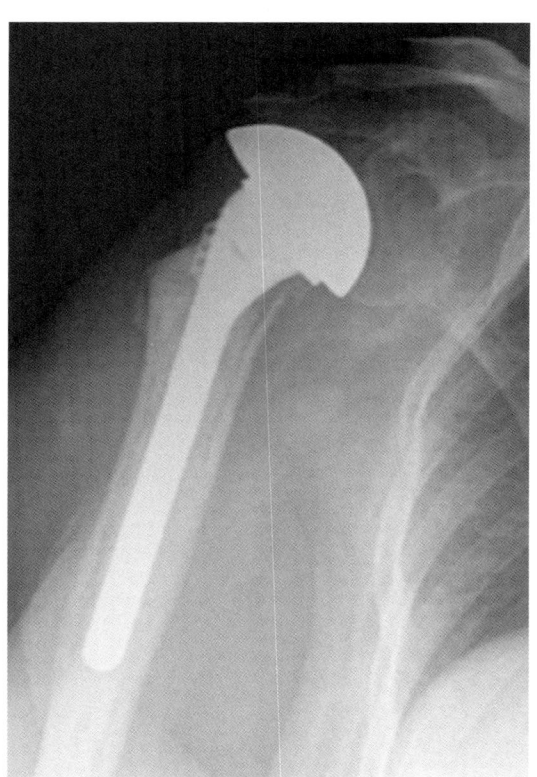

FIGURE 35.26 Tuberosity nonunion after hemiarthroplasty for the treatment of a proximal humeral fracture.

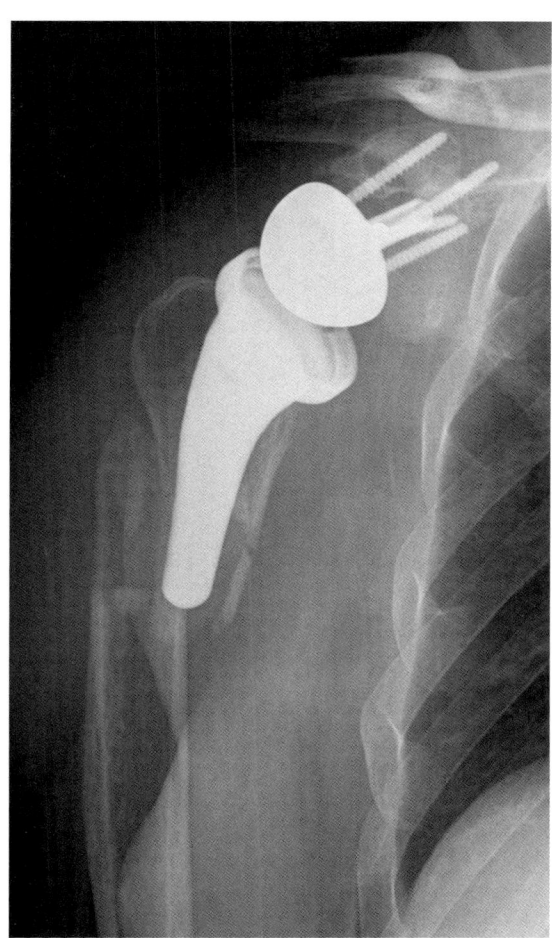

FIGURE 35.27 Displaced periprosthetic humeral fracture.

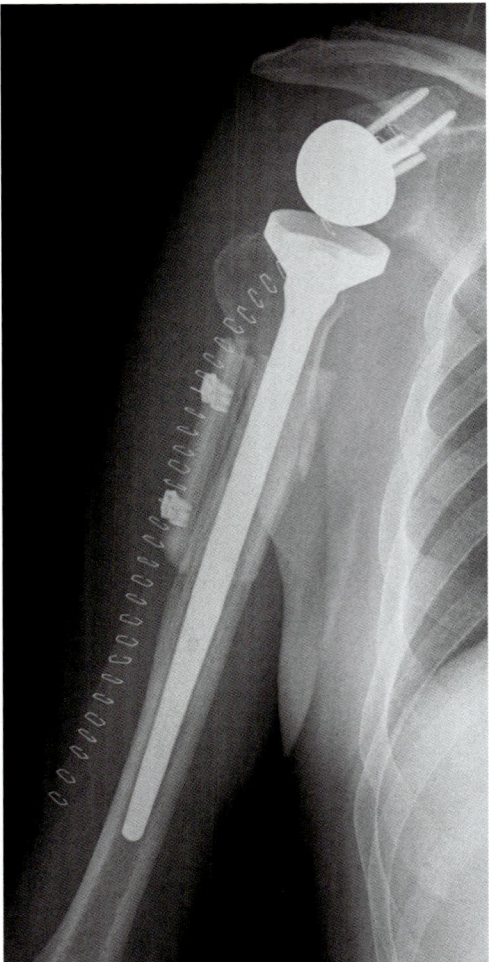

FIGURE 35.28 Revision arthroplasty for the treatment of a periprosthetic fracture.

TABLE 35.1	Contraindications to Revision Shoulder Arthroplasty	
Contraindication	Absolute or Relative	Comments
Poor generalized health	Relative	Appropriate perioperative medical treatment required
Active infection	Absolute	Must clear infection first. May be candidate for revision as a second stage
Axillary nerve palsy	Absolute	Better suited for resection arthroplasty
Deltoid insufficiency	Absolute	Better suited for resection arthroplasty
Insufficient humeral bone stock	Relative	May be able to restore bone stock with a proximal humeral reconstruction
Insufficient glenoid bone stock	Relative	May be able to restore bone stock with a staged procedure
Poor patient motivation	Absolute	

CONTRAINDICATIONS TO REVISION SHOULDER ARTHROPLASTY

Contraindications to revision shoulder arthroplasty are listed in Table 35.1. Some of these contraindications are absolute, whereas others are relative.

REFERENCE

1. Hertel R, Lehmann O: Glenoid erosion after hemiarthroplasty of the shoulder. In Walch G, Boileau P, Molé D, editors: *2000 Prosthèses d'Epaule ... Recul de 2 à 10 Ans*, Paris, 2001, Sauramps Medical, pp 417–423.

the existing humeral stem and revise to a long-stem humeral component to act as an intramedullary fixation device. This is combined with allograft struts placed peripherally at the fracture site and fixated with cerclage cables (Fig. 35.28). In addition to this scenario, any periprosthetic fracture in which the humeral stem is loose is an indication for revision of the humeral component via the same technique.

Preoperative planning, imaging, and special tests

CHAPTER 36

Revision shoulder arthroplasty is more challenging overall than primary shoulder arthroplasty. Preoperative planning for a revision arthroplasty case is critically important and is initiated as soon as revision arthroplasty is being considered; it should never be an afterthought the morning of surgery. Preoperative planning for revision shoulder arthroplasty is similar to, albeit more complex than, planning for primary shoulder arthroplasty and consists of reviewing the patient's clinical history and physical examination, radiographs, and secondary imaging studies, as well as any special tests obtained. This chapter reviews our approach to preoperative planning for revision shoulder arthroplasty.

CLINICAL HISTORY AND EXAMINATION

Although description of a detailed shoulder history and examination are beyond the scope of this textbook, certain aspects of the history and physical examination are important in preoperative planning for revision shoulder arthroplasty. The patient's complaints are reviewed, such as the type of symptoms (pain, stiffness, weakness), duration of symptoms (weeks, months, years), indication for the primary arthroplasty, initial results of the primary arthroplasty (relief of all symptoms, relief of some symptoms, no improvement from surgery), and the presence of any symptoms of infection (previous history of infection, fevers, wound redness, wound drainage). These shoulder-specific complaints help the surgeon decide which patients are candidates for revision shoulder arthroplasty. A patient with complaints of only mild pain, mild weakness, or mild stiffness may initially best be treated with nonoperative modalities even if radiographs demonstrate positive findings such as glenoid erosion after hemiarthroplasty. Similarly, a patient with a sudden onset of symptoms of a short duration to date may be experiencing a transient acute rotator cuff tendinitis not directly related to the shoulder replacement. In this situation, a period of nonoperative treatment would certainly be indicated. Special attention is given to factors that could make the operative procedure more difficult. The number and type of all previous shoulder surgeries, arthroplasty and nonarthroplasty, should be recorded in the patient's history. Chronic use of nonsteroidal antiinflammatory medications can result in excessive operative blood loss, so these medications should be discontinued the week before surgery.

Any medical history of systemic illness (diabetes mellitus, cardiac problems) should be considered in preoperative planning. Although these factors may not affect the actual surgical procedure, they may necessitate special considerations in the patient's postoperative care. Appropriate medical consultations should be obtained well in advance of the surgery date. The availability of appropriate care of these systemic illnesses, including the availability of consultants, should be confirmed before surgery.

All of our patients undergo a thorough shoulder examination, much of which is detailed in Chapter 7. The visual appearance of the shoulder yields useful information in candidates for revision shoulder arthroplasty. The presence and location of surgical scars are noted. The preoperative plan should include whether all or part of a previous skin incision site is to be used or whether a completely new incision is to be created (Fig. 36.1). In thin patients, anterior superior escape of a prosthetic humeral head caused by anterior superior rotator cuff deficiency may be obvious (Fig. 36.2). Special attention should be paid to the condition of the deltoid, especially if it has previously been surgically violated (Fig. 36.3). Atrophy of the supraspinatus and infraspinatus should be noted as well (Fig. 36.4).

Both active and passive mobility is recorded, as detailed in Chapter 7. Special attention should be paid to evaluation of the deltoid muscle. If deltoid contractility appears to be compromised, further evaluation with electromyography and nerve conduction studies should be performed before revision shoulder arthroplasty.

The integrity of the rotator cuff is tested (see Chapter 7). Details of this examination are of paramount importance in preoperative planning for revision surgery. Although a minor rotator cuff deficiency such as an isolated supraspinatus tendon tear may have little influence on preoperative planning, larger rotator cuff tears (two-, three-, and four-tendon tears), especially when coupled with static or dynamic glenohumeral instability, may change the type of revision prosthesis to be inserted (reverse instead of unconstrained).

The results of the clinical history and examination are documented in the patient's chart and reviewed well in advance of surgery as part of preoperative planning.

RADIOGRAPHY

Recent (within 3 months) magnification- and fluoroscopy-controlled radiographs are obtained in all patients who are candidates for revision shoulder arthroplasty. The same views obtained for primary arthroplasty, including an anteroposterior view of the glenohumeral joint with the arm in neutral rotation, an axillary view, and a scapular outlet view, are

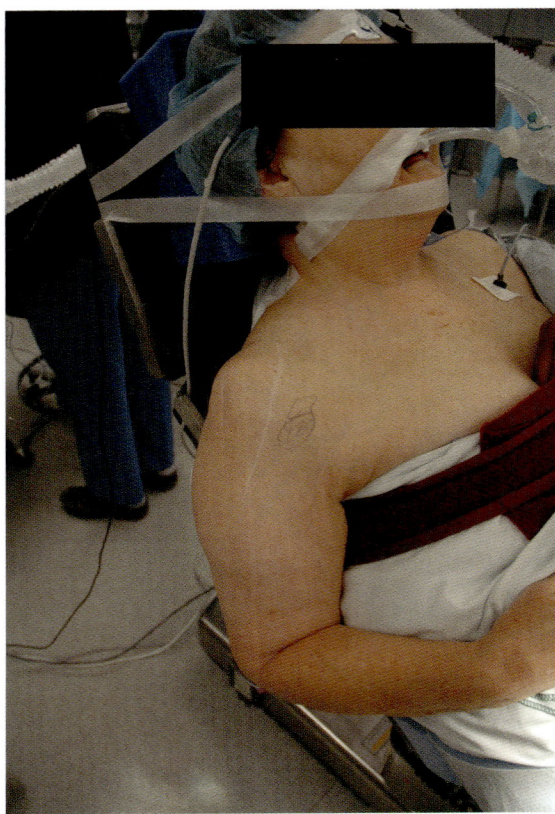

FIGURE 36.1 Previous skin incision used in primary shoulder arthroplasty.

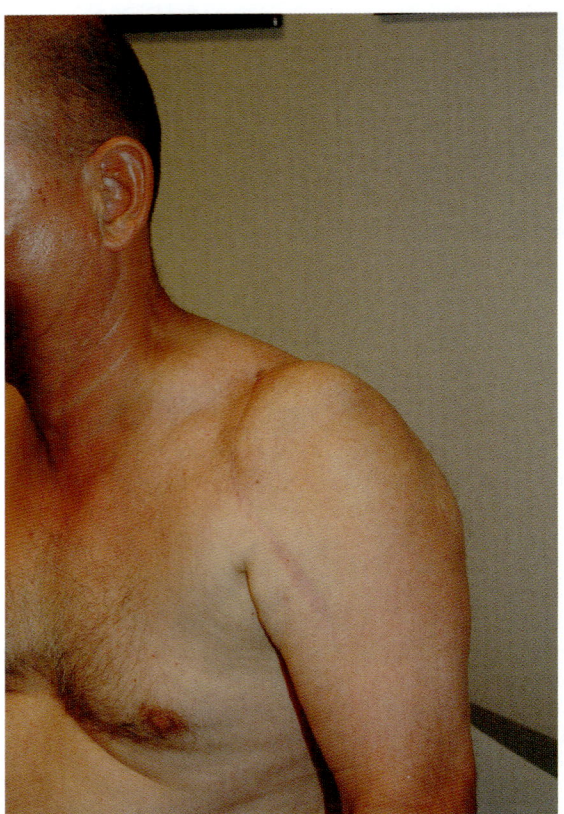

FIGURE 36.2 Hemiarthroplasty located subcutaneously secondary to anterior superior escape.

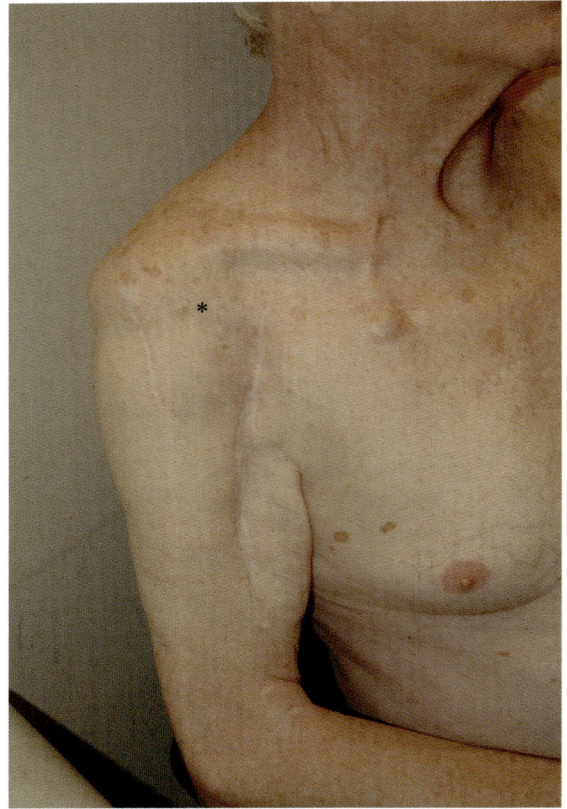

FIGURE 36.3 Atrophy (asterisk) of the anterior deltoid.

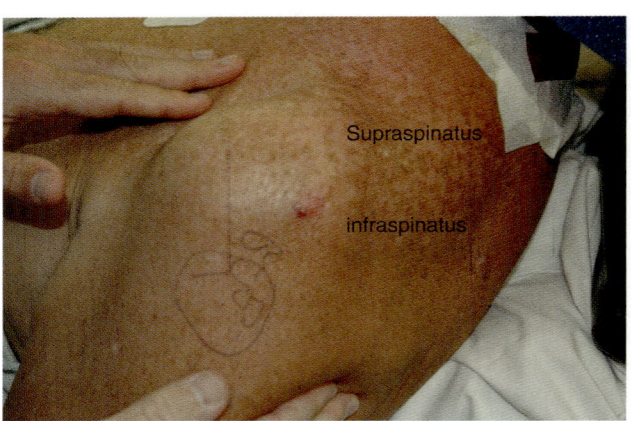

FIGURE 36.4 Atrophy of the supraspinatus and infraspinatus.

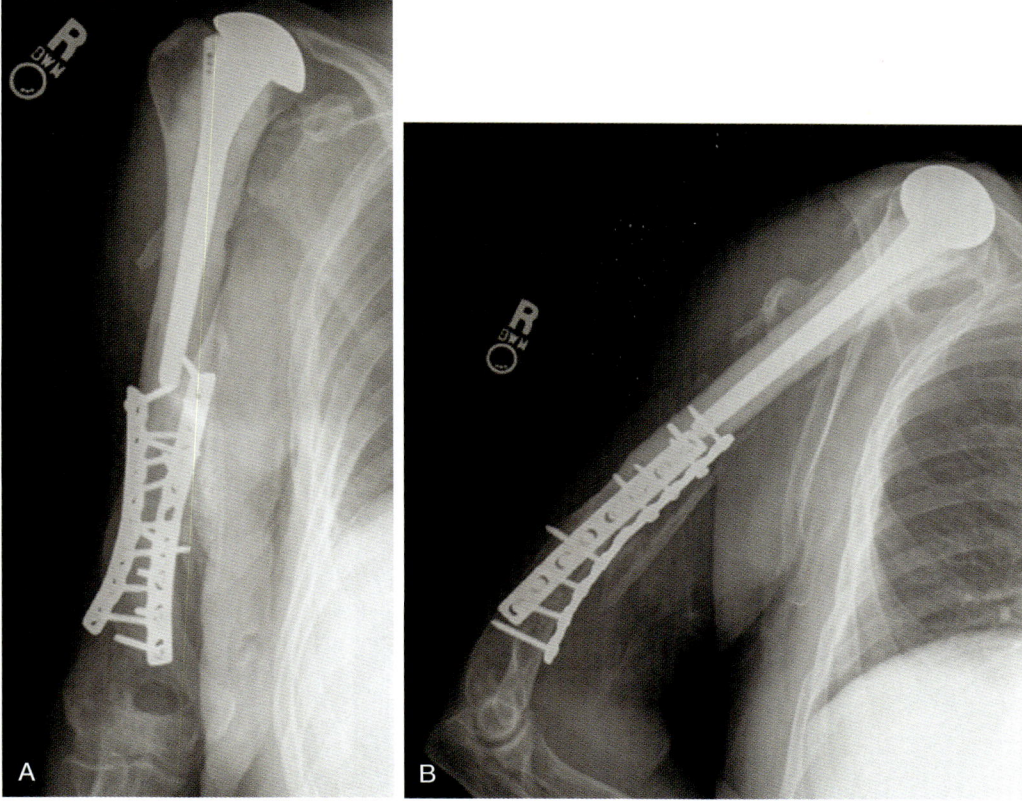

FIGURE 36.5 (A and B) Full-length orthogonal radiographic views of the humerus taken before revision shoulder arthroplasty.

obtained in the revision scenario. Additionally, full-length orthogonal views of the humerus (anteroposterior and lateral) are obtained to evaluate diaphyseal cortical bone quality (Fig. 36.5). The previous arthroplasty is inspected on these radiographs for signs of loosening of the glenoid and humeral components, signs of mechanical failure of components (Fig. 36.6), appropriateness of component size and position, signs of static or dynamic instability (Fig. 36.7), and signs of infection (Fig. 36.8).

Preoperative radiographic templating can be useful in planning revision shoulder arthroplasty, especially in cases of proximal humeral deficiency. In most of these cases, the proximal humeral deficiency with resultant rotator cuff compromise constitutes an indication for revision with a reverse-design prosthesis. In patients demonstrating proximal humeral bone loss, bilateral full-length magnification-controlled anteroposterior humeral radiographs are obtained. These radiographs are used to help select the height at which to implant the humeral stem and the length of proximal humeral allograft to employ if indicated. Using the full-length humeral radiographs, the desired position of the reverse prosthesis is templated on the radiograph of the unaffected humerus, and the level of the metaphyseal-diaphyseal junction of the humeral component is marked (Fig. 36.9). The distance from the transepicondylar axis at the elbow to this point is measured (Fig. 36.10). A mark is made at the same distance from the transepicondylar axis on the affected radiograph. A second mark is made at the most proximal extent of the humeral shaft (Fig. 36.11). The distance between the desired prosthetic level at the metaphyseal-diaphyseal junction and the proximal extent of the humeral shaft is measured (Fig. 36.12). A ruler is used during surgery to measure the distance and mark the level on the humeral stem or humeral allograft to obtain the desired prosthetic position (Fig. 36.13). This technique of preoperative planning provides only a guideline and may be superseded by intraoperative observations.

SECONDARY IMAGING

A computed tomography arthrography is obtained in all patients for evaluation of the rotator cuff tendons and musculature before revision shoulder arthroplasty (Fig. 36.14). This study further assists in evaluation of possible component loosening. Many patients exhibit radiolucent lines around the glenoid component after unconstrained total shoulder arthroplasty. Use of computed tomography arthrography assists in determining whether these components are indeed loose by demonstrating radiographic contrast material around the base of the component (Fig. 36.15). Computed tomography also provides the greatest osseous detail of the glenoid and can show the presence and extent of bony glenoid deficiency. Bony deficiencies can occur after erosion from hemiarthroplasty (Fig. 36.16). In these cases the computed tomography scan helps determine whether

Text continued on p. 344

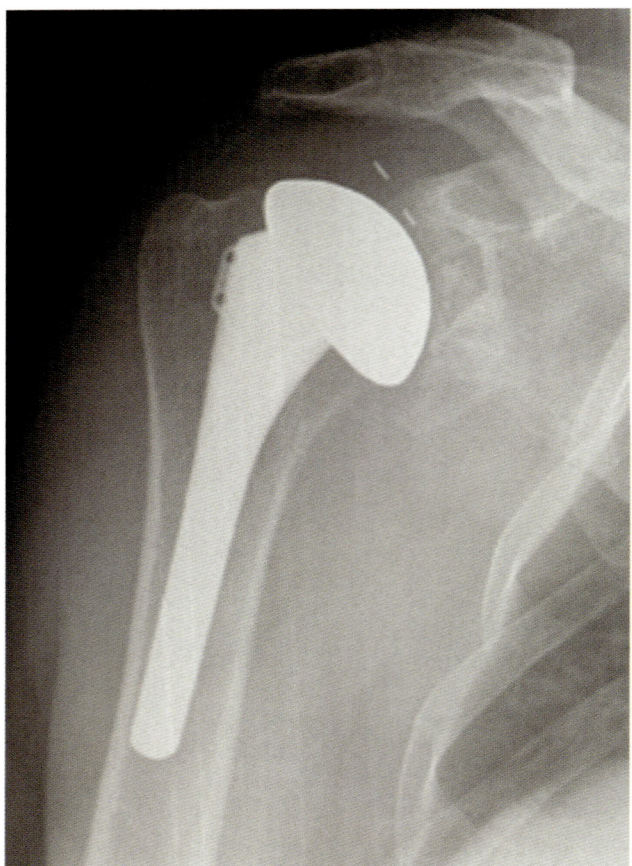

FIGURE 36.6 Mechanical failure of a keeled glenoid component detected on anteroposterior radiography.

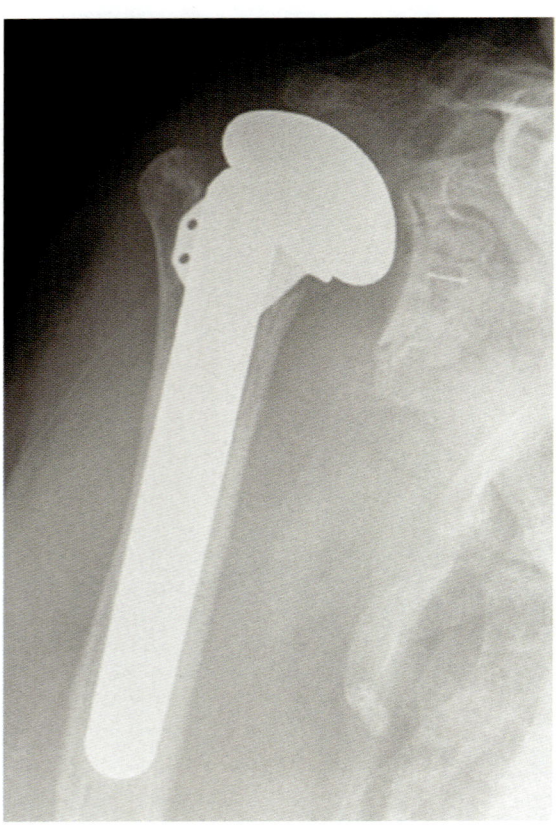

FIGURE 36.7 Static superior migration after total shoulder arthroplasty.

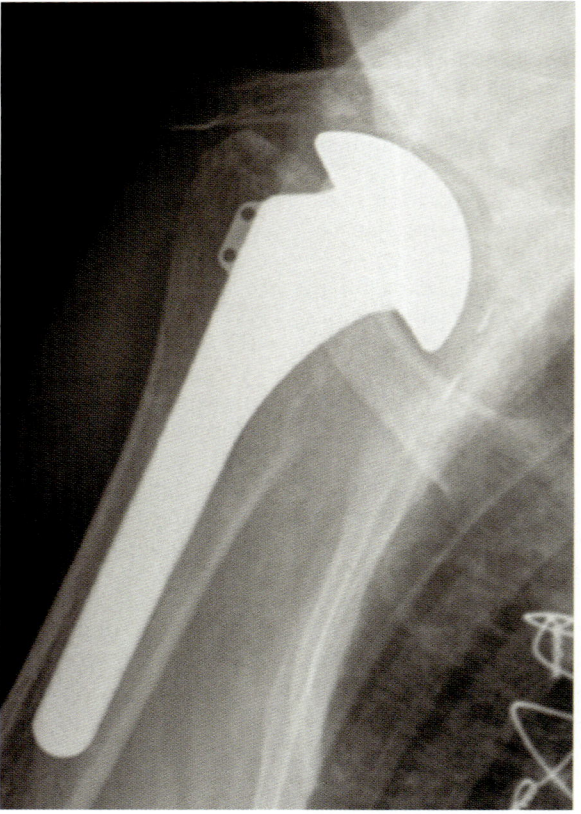

FIGURE 36.8 Osteolysis around both the glenoid and humeral components is strongly suggestive of infection.

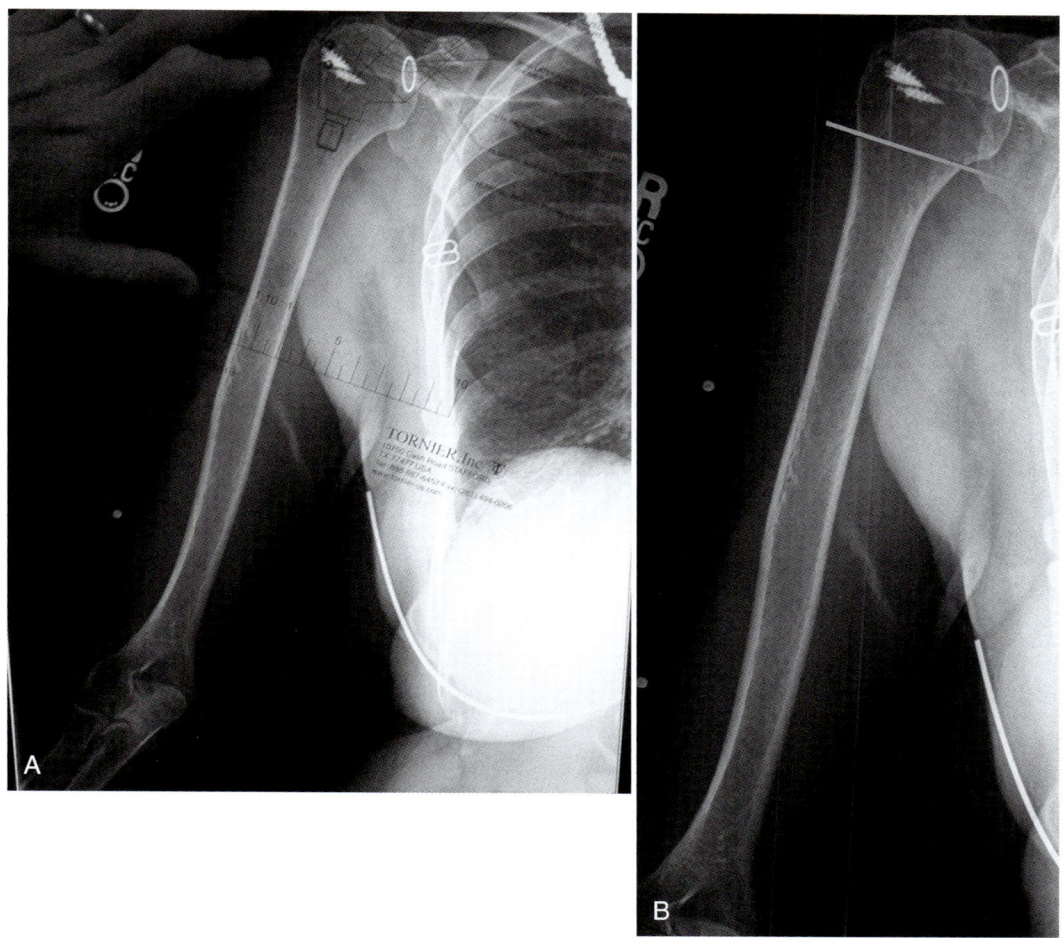

FIGURE 36.9 The desired position of the reverse prosthesis is templated on the unaffected humeral radiograph (A), and the level of the metaphyseal-diaphyseal junction of the humeral component is marked (B).

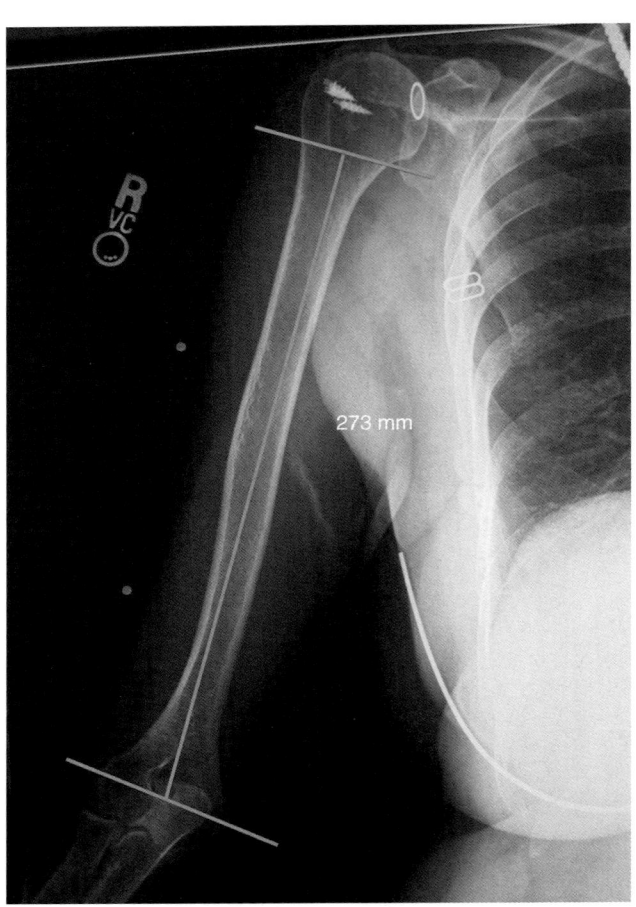

FIGURE 36.10 The distance from the transepicondylar axis at the elbow to the desired level of the metaphyseal-diaphyseal junction of the humeral component is measured.

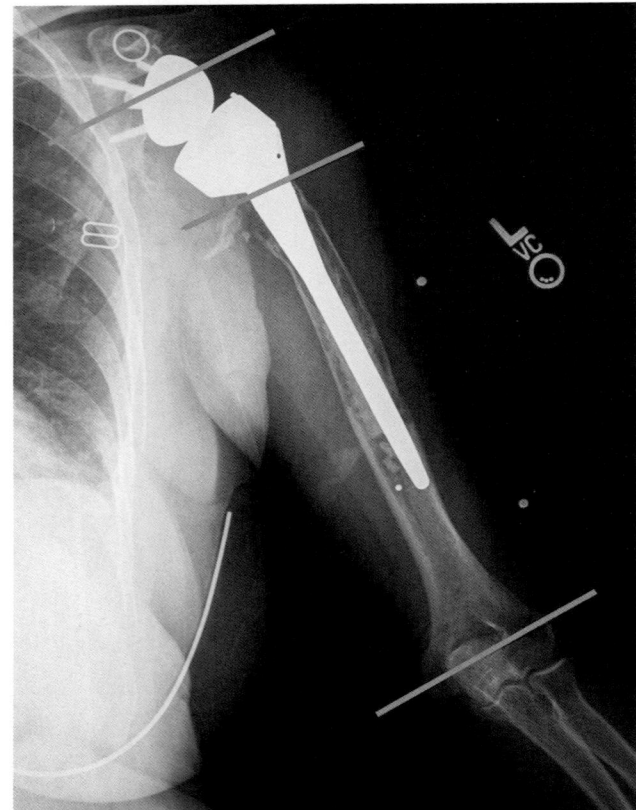

FIGURE 36.11 A mark is made at the same distance from the transepicondylar axis on the affected radiograph. A second mark is made at the most proximal extent of the humeral shaft.

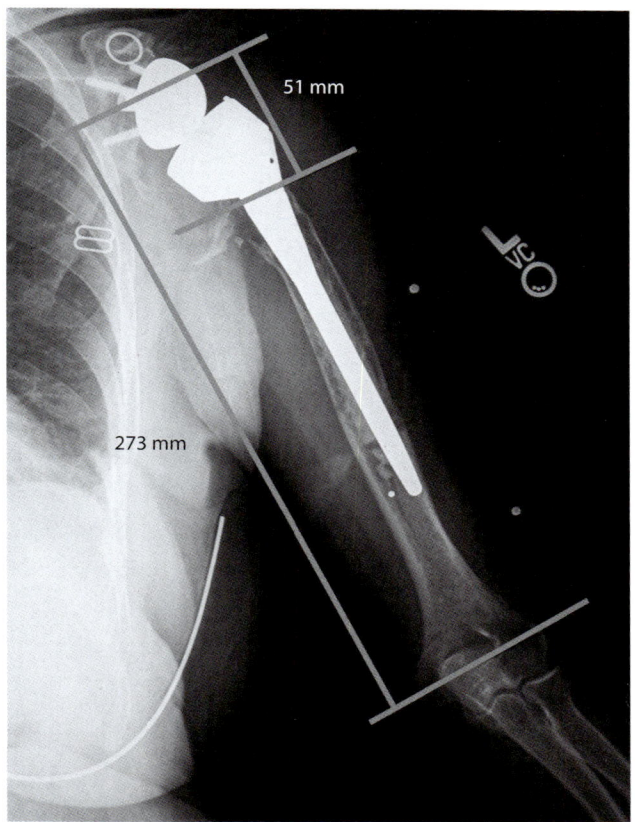

FIGURE 36.12 The distance between the desired prosthetic level at the metaphyseal-diaphyseal junction and the proximal extent of the humeral shaft is measured.

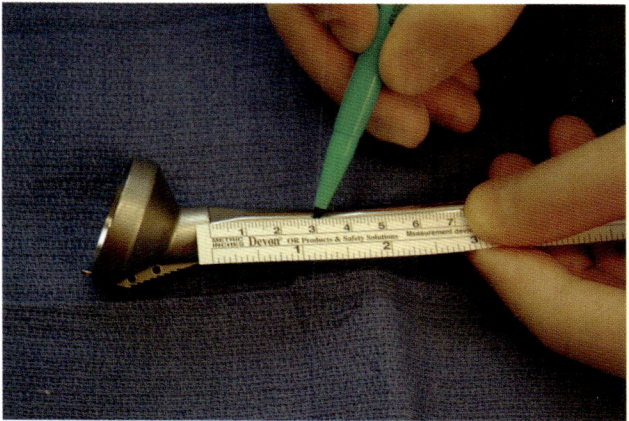

FIGURE 36.13 A ruler is used during surgery to measure the distance and mark the level on the proximal humeral allograft to achieve the desired prosthetic position.

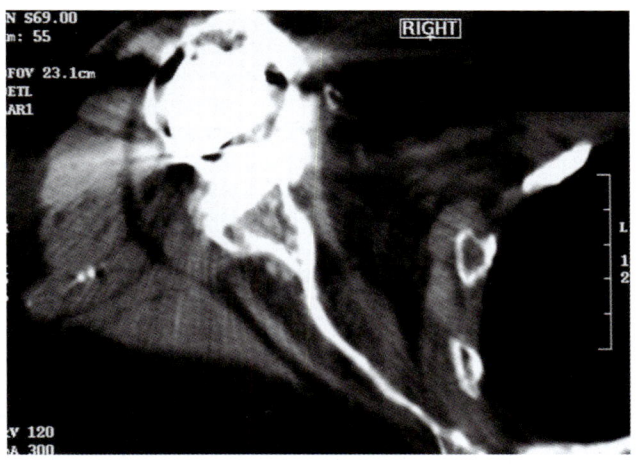

FIGURE 36.14 Evaluation of the rotator cuff tendons and musculature with computed tomography arthrography.

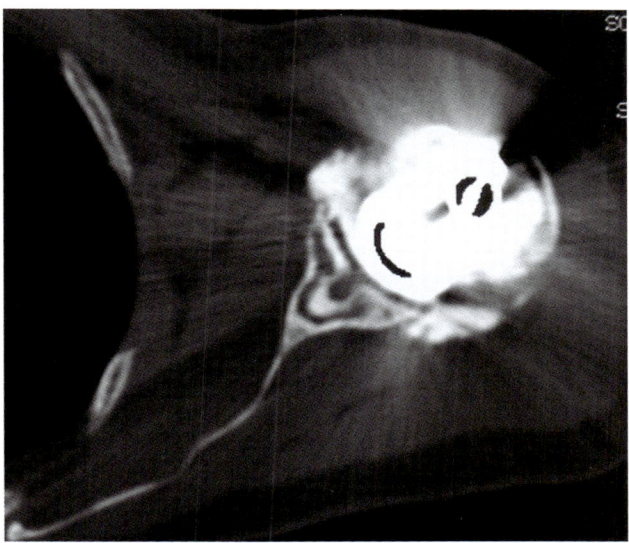

FIGURE 36.15 Glenoid component loosening identified on computed tomography arthrography. Note the contrast material located around the keel of the glenoid component.

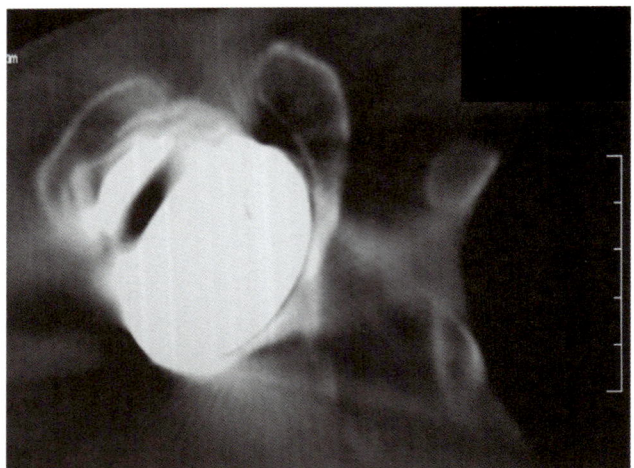

FIGURE 36.16 Central glenoid bony deficiency caused by glenoid erosion after hemiarthroplasty.

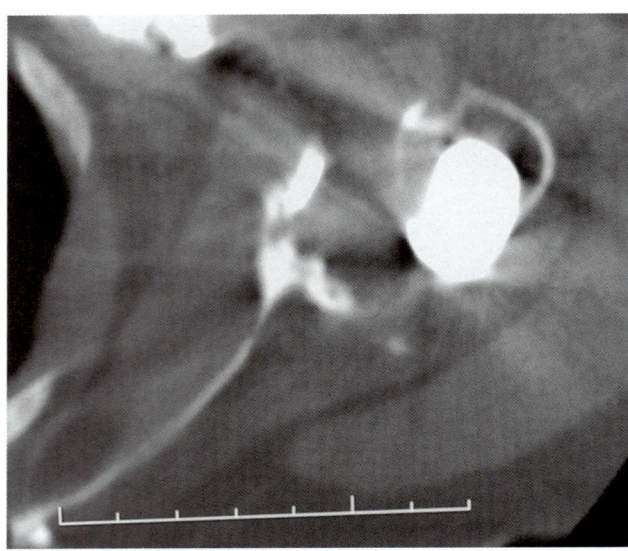

FIGURE 36.17 Bony glenoid deficiency caused by loosening of the glenoid component.

the existing glenoid bone is sufficient to allow implantation of a glenoid component. Bony deficiencies more commonly occur concomitantly with loosening of the glenoid component (Fig. 36.17). In these cases the computed tomography scan allows the bony deficiency to be classified as contained or uncontained (Fig. 36.18).[1]

The rotator cuff is evaluated, including assessment of tendinous integrity and muscle quality (fatty infiltration). The condition of the long head of the biceps tendon is noted, particularly its position (centered, subluxated, dislocated, ruptured), to assist in identifying it at the time of surgery.

SPECIAL TESTS

In all candidates for revision shoulder arthroplasty, regardless of whether signs of infection are present, a preoperative infection workup is indicated, including hematologic evaluation consisting of a complete blood cell count with differential, a sedimentation rate, and C-reactive protein. Additionally, a fluoroscopically guided shoulder aspiration is performed at the time of computed tomography arthrography and the specimen is submitted for aerobic, anaerobic, fungal, and mycobacterial culture and the cultures are held for 21 days to allow for detection of *Propionibacterium acnes* and *Staphylococcus epidermidis*. The aspirate is also sent for alpha defensin (Synovasure Alpha Defensin Test [Zimmer, Inc., Warsaw, IN]), which is used to detect infection. If the findings are suggestive of infection (increased sedimentation rate, increased C-reactive protein, leukocytosis, moderate to many leukocytes observed in aspirated joint fluid), intraoperative frozen histologic sections are planned at the time of revision shoulder arthroplasty. The patient is educated that the revision surgery may be staged if infection is further suspected by the results of intraoperative histologic tissue analysis. If the preoperative infection workup yields a positive culture from the aspirate or is positive for alpha defensin, infection is considered present and the treatment plan proceeds accordingly. In all patients with an infected shoulder arthroplasty, consultation with an infectious disease specialist is obtained preoperatively.

Electromyography and nerve conduction studies are performed in any patient with a suggestion of neurologic deficiencies on physical examination. Specifically, all patients unable to reliably contract the deltoid should undergo neurologic testing before revision shoulder arthroplasty. If the deltoid is compromised, neurologic consultation is obtained. Revision shoulder arthroplasty is reserved until the time of deltoid/axillary nerve recovery. In patients with permanent deltoid insufficiency, revision arthroplasty is contraindicated and resection arthroplasty is considered.

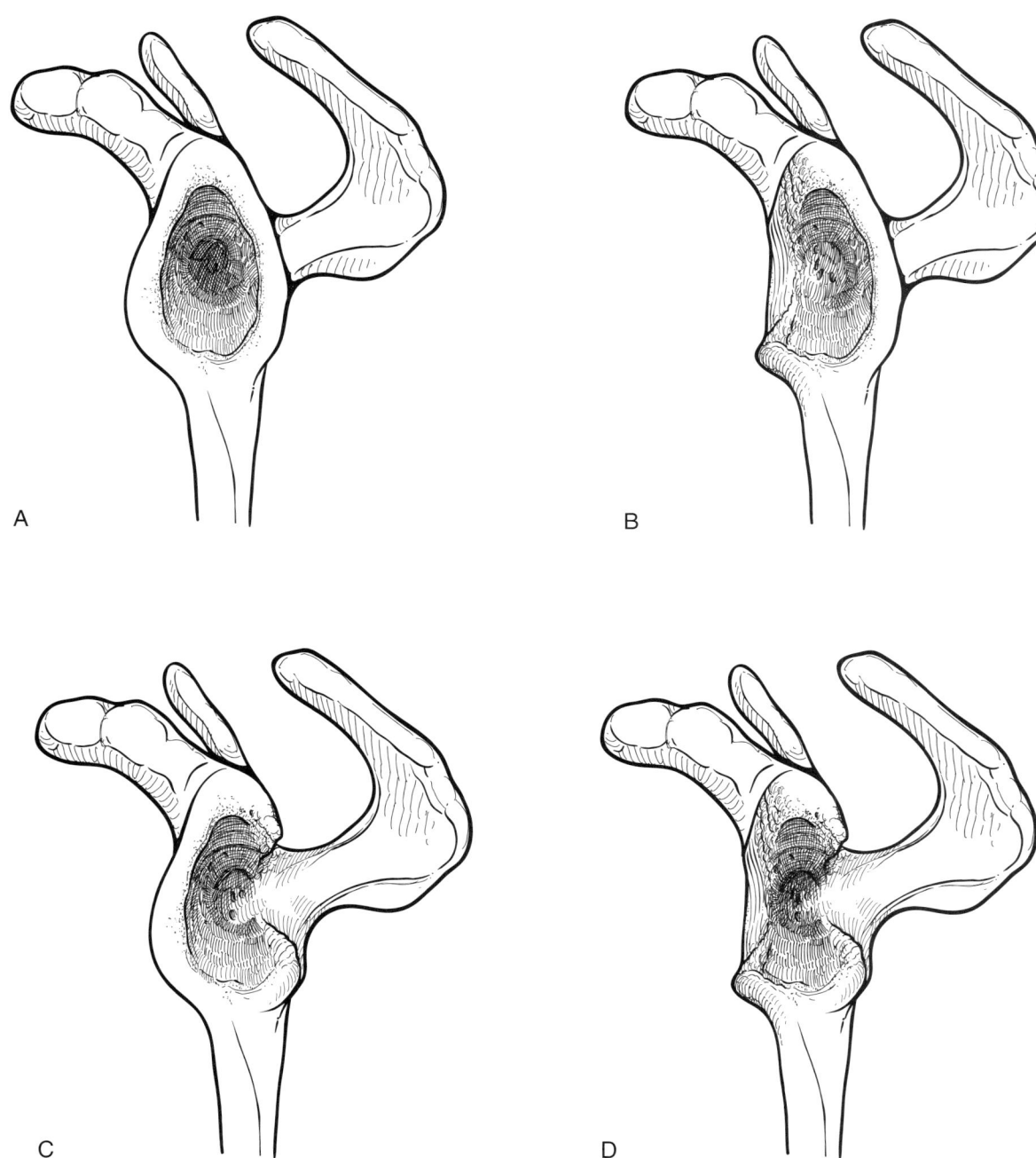

FIGURE 36.18 Classification of bony glenoid deficiency. (A) Contained. (B) Uncontained—anterior. (C) Uncontained—posterior. (D) Uncontained—combined.

REFERENCE

1. Antuna SA, Sperling JW, Cofield RH, et al: Glenoid revision surgery after total shoulder arthroplasty, *J Shoulder Elbow Surg* 10:217–224, 2001.

CHAPTER 37

Surgical approach

All revision shoulder arthroplasty in our practice is performed through a deltopectoral approach. The utilitarian nature of this approach makes it ideal for use in revision shoulder arthroplasty. The deltopectoral approach is easily extended into an anterolateral approach to the humeral diaphysis should it be necessary for extraction of a humeral component or for fixation of a periprosthetic fracture.

The most difficult portion of the deltopectoral approach performed in the revision scenario is dealing with scar tissue from previous surgery because it obscures the normal tissue planes easily identified during primary arthroplasty. The extent of scarring present and the amount of difficulty encountered in identifying soft tissue planes vary greatly among patients, and we have yet to identify any reliable preoperative factors to assist in determining which dissections will be especially difficult. Scarring may be present throughout the surgical approach and commonly obscures the deltopectoral interval, the plane between the pectoralis major and conjoined tendon of the short head of the biceps and coracobrachialis, and the plane between the conjoined tendon and the subscapularis. In addition, subdeltoid adhesions are commonly present at the time of revision surgery.

When performing revision shoulder arthroplasty, the surgeon must be able to approach the humeral shaft, which is done by extending the deltopectoral approach into an anterolateral approach to the humeral diaphysis. Use of the extensile portion of this approach is necessary when performing a humeral osteotomy for removal of the humeral stem or in the operative treatment of a periprosthetic fracture. In these scenarios, it is often necessary to perform some type of cerclage fixation of the humeral diaphysis. Before performing cerclage fixation of the humeral diaphysis, it is mandatory that the radial nerve be identified so that it can be protected throughout this portion of the procedure. The surgeon must be able to perform radial nerve dissection to safely perform revision shoulder arthroplasty.

TECHNIQUE FOR THE DELTOPECTORAL APPROACH

The deltopectoral approach used for revision shoulder arthroplasty follows the same technical principles described for primary shoulder arthroplasty (see Chapter 8). Patient positioning is the same as for primary shoulder arthroplasty. Draping differs in revision arthroplasty in that the stockinet is placed only up to the elbow to allow distal extension of the surgical approach if necessary (Fig. 37.1). Any previous skin incisions are delineated with a sterile surgical marking pen (Fig. 37.2). This makes these incisional scars more visible after skin preparation and placement of the occlusive drape. The previous skin incision is used if possible. If the previous incision is topographically positioned within 5 cm of our standard deltopectoral skin incision, as described in Chapter 8, we will use the previous incision site (Fig. 37.3). If the previous incision deviates substantially from our standard deltopectoral incision, we will make a new incision altogether. If the previous incision has resulted in a hypertrophic scar, the scar is elliptically excised with a no. 10 scalpel blade (Fig. 37.4). The incision extends for 10 to 15 cm, depending on the size of the patient. Occasionally, the original incision is longer than what we consider necessary. In that situation we use only a portion of the original incision. To minimize hemorrhage, we use a needle tip electrocautery for subcutaneous dissection and for most of the deep dissection throughout the procedure. Medium-size skin rakes are used for retraction during this portion of the approach.

The cephalic vein, when present, is located to identify the interval between the deltoid and pectoralis major. In many cases the cephalic vein is not identified during revision shoulder arthroplasty. If such is the case, the deltopectoral interval can be readily located proximally by identifying a small triangular area devoid of muscle tissue between the proximal portions of the deltoid and pectoralis major muscles (Fig. 37.5). If located, the cephalic vein is dissected free of the pectoralis major muscle with Metzenbaum scissors. We prefer to retract the cephalic vein laterally with the deltoid because most of the branches of the cephalic vein are deltoid-based. Medial retraction of the cephalic vein with the pectoralis major disrupts these deltoid branches and introduces unwanted hemorrhage.

The deltopectoral interval is developed through somewhat tedious dissection, depending on the severity of scarring, with a combination of Metzenbaum scissors and needle tip electrocautery. After the deltopectoral interval has been developed, Army-Navy retractors are used to maintain the interval. The humeral insertion of the pectoralis major tendon is identified. Dividing the superior centimeter of the pectoralis major tendon enhances exposure of the inferior aspect of the subscapularis and axillary nerve (Fig. 37.6). The deltoid is frequently adherent to the subdeltoid bursa and lateral aspect of the proximal humerus. If so, the deltoid is progressively released from the subdeltoid bursa with electrocautery

Text continued on p. 350

CHAPTER 37 ■ Surgical Approach 347

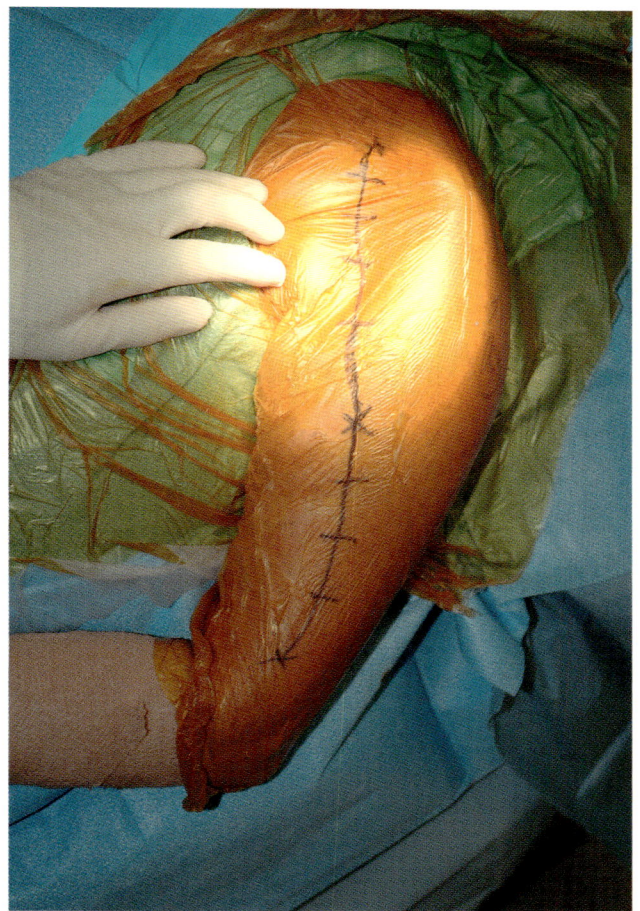

FIGURE 37.1 Draping for revision shoulder arthroplasty while leaving the distal part of the arm accessible to allow an extensile exposure.

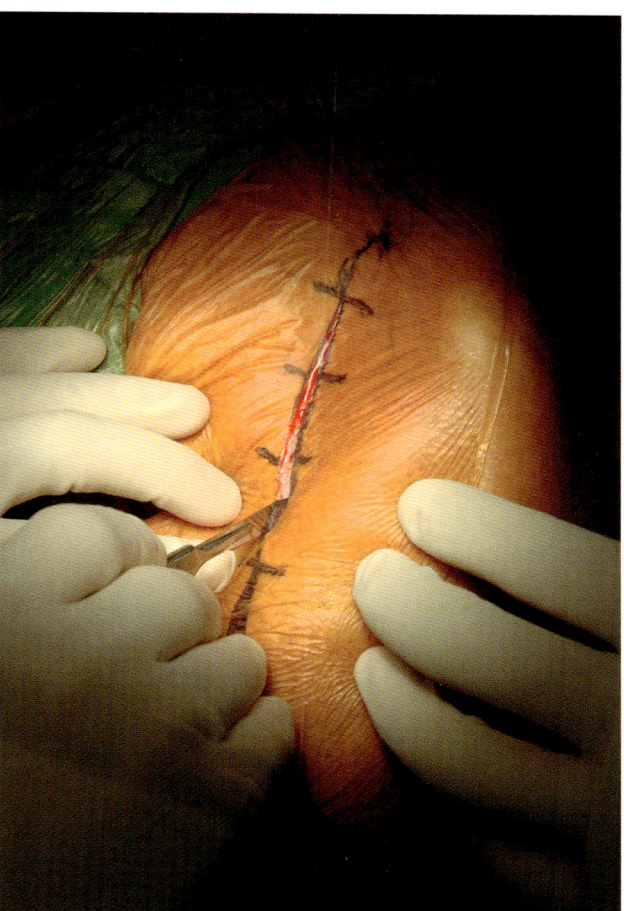

FIGURE 37.3 Use of the previous incision for the deltopectoral approach during revision shoulder arthroplasty.

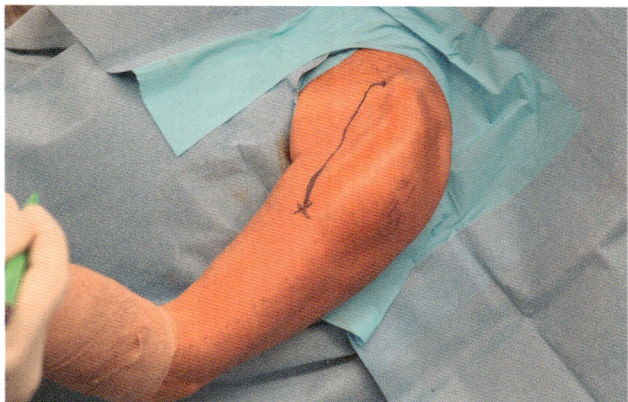

FIGURE 37.2 Previous incisions are marked before placing the occlusive drape.

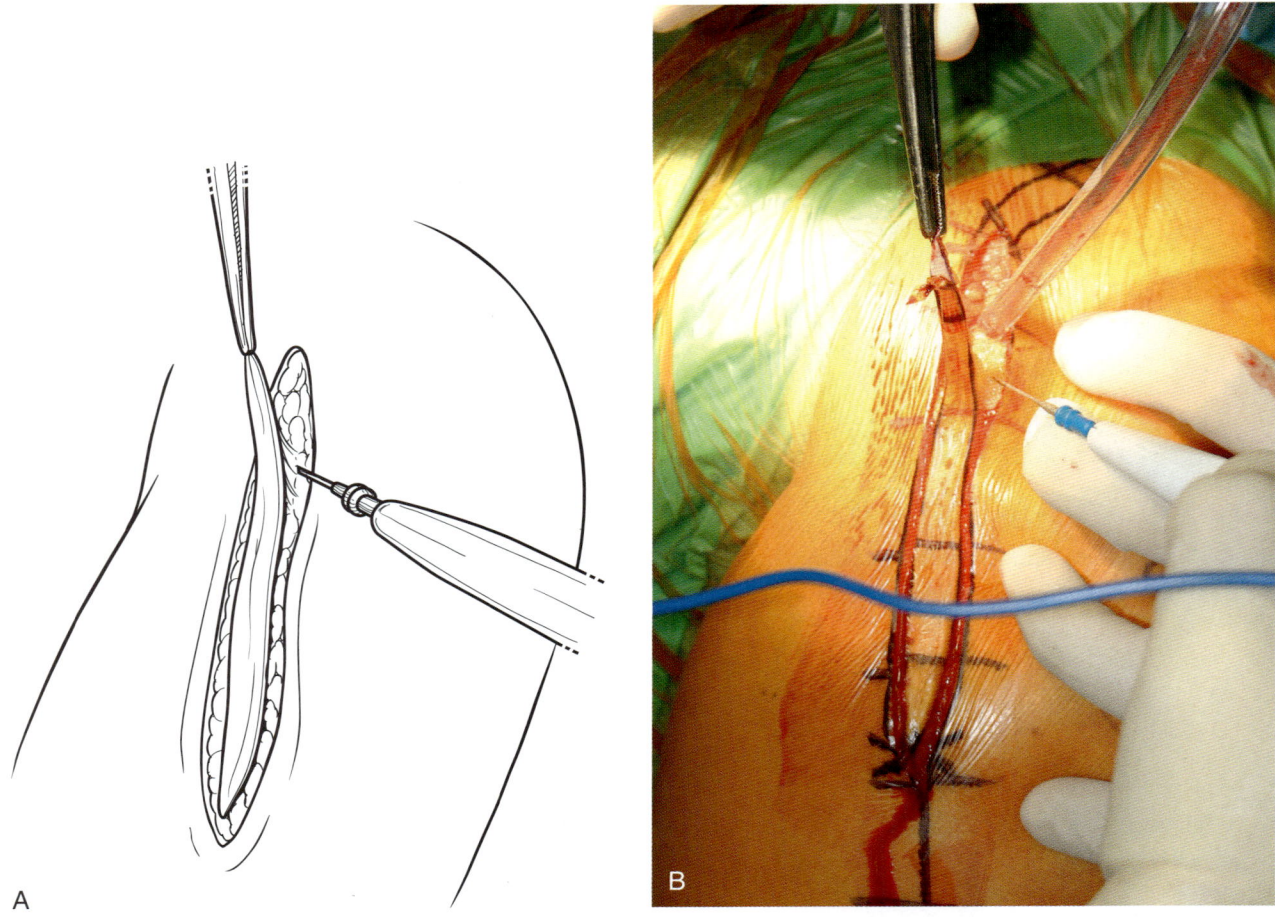

FIGURE 37.4 (A and B) Excision of a previous hypertrophic skin scar.

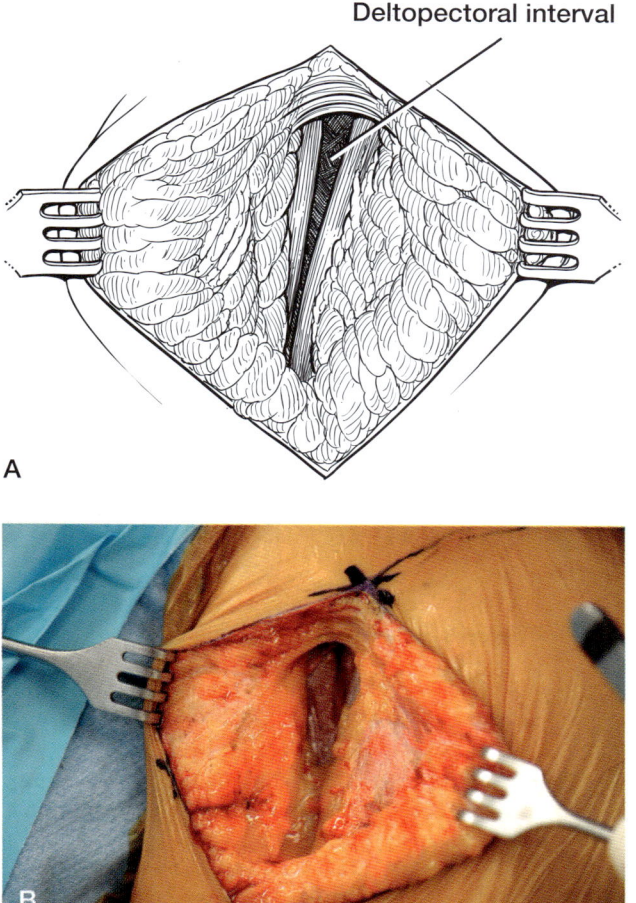

FIGURE 37.5 (A and B) Identification of the deltopectoral interval proximally in a patient without an identifiable cephalic vein by locating the area proximally devoid of muscle.

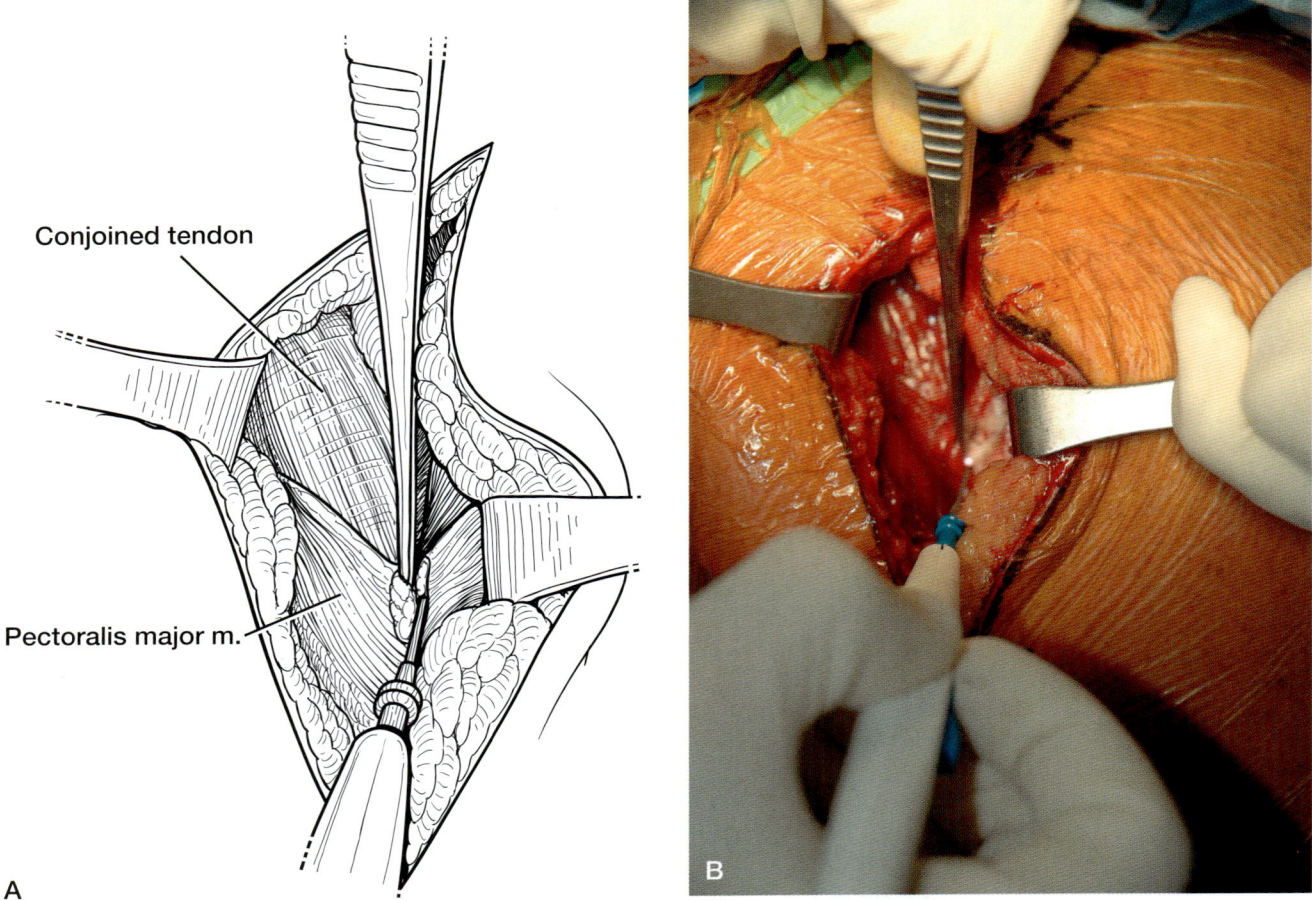

FIGURE 37.6 (A and B) Release of the superior aspect of the pectoralis major tendon to enhance exposure of the inferior subscapularis.

as the arm is progressively internally rotated (Fig. 37.7). A self-retaining cerebellar-type deltopectoral retractor is inserted to maintain the deltopectoral interval. Next, the conjoined tendon is identified and traced proximally to its insertion on the coracoid process. Large curved Mayo scissors are used to create a space superior to the coracoid process by placing the scissors just over the top of the coracoid and spreading the blades open. The tip of a Hohmann retractor is placed in the space behind the base of the coracoid process to allow proximal retraction (Fig. 37.8). The pectoralis major muscle is frequently adherent to the conjoined tendon during revision shoulder arthroplasty. If this is the case, the pectoralis major muscle is released from the conjoined tendon with Metzenbaum scissors or a Cobb elevator (Fig. 37.9).

The arm is placed in an abducted and externally rotated position, and the apex that is formed by the insertions of the coracoacromial ligament and the conjoined tendon on the coracoid process is identified. This apex is developed with the needle tip electrocautery. If an unconstrained implant is planned, the coracoacromial ligament is retained. If a reverse prosthesis is the implant to be used in the revision, the coracoacromial ligament is released with the electrocautery to further enhance visualization, particularly if superior migration of the humerus is noted. The lateral aspect of the conjoined tendon is released with the electrocautery to expose the subscapularis tendon, if present. Scar tissue is nearly always present between the deep surface of the conjoined tendon and the anterior surface of the subscapularis tendon, and surgical release of the scar tissue is necessary. The release is performed carefully with Metzenbaum scissors or a Cobb elevator along the surface of the subscapularis tendon (Fig. 37.10). Extreme caution is exercised to avoid injury to the musculocutaneous nerve, which may enter the coracobrachialis within 4 cm distal to the tip of the coracoid process. After this release, the conjoined tendon is retracted medially with a narrow Richardson retractor to expose the subscapularis tendon, when present. The anterior humeral circumflex vessels (the "three sisters") are usually absent at the time of revision shoulder arthroplasty. With the arm externally rotated, the anterior humeral circumflex vessels, when present, are suture-ligated together at the inferior border of the subscapularis with no. 0 dyed absorbable braided suture, as in cases of primary shoulder arthroplasty.

The axillary nerve can be identified at this point, if desired, through direct visualization. The narrow Richardson retractor is moved slightly inferiorly along the conjoined tendon to a point just below the inferior aspect of the subscapularis. The arm is flexed forward in neutral rotation, and blunt dissection

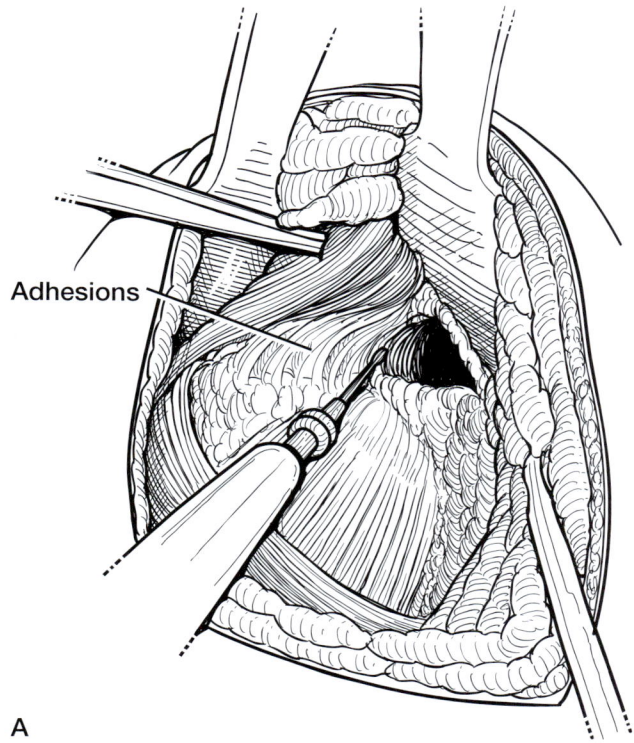
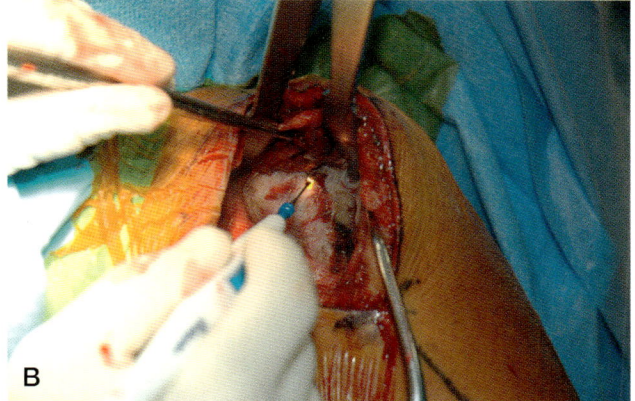

FIGURE 37.7 (A and B) Release of subdeltoid adhesions.

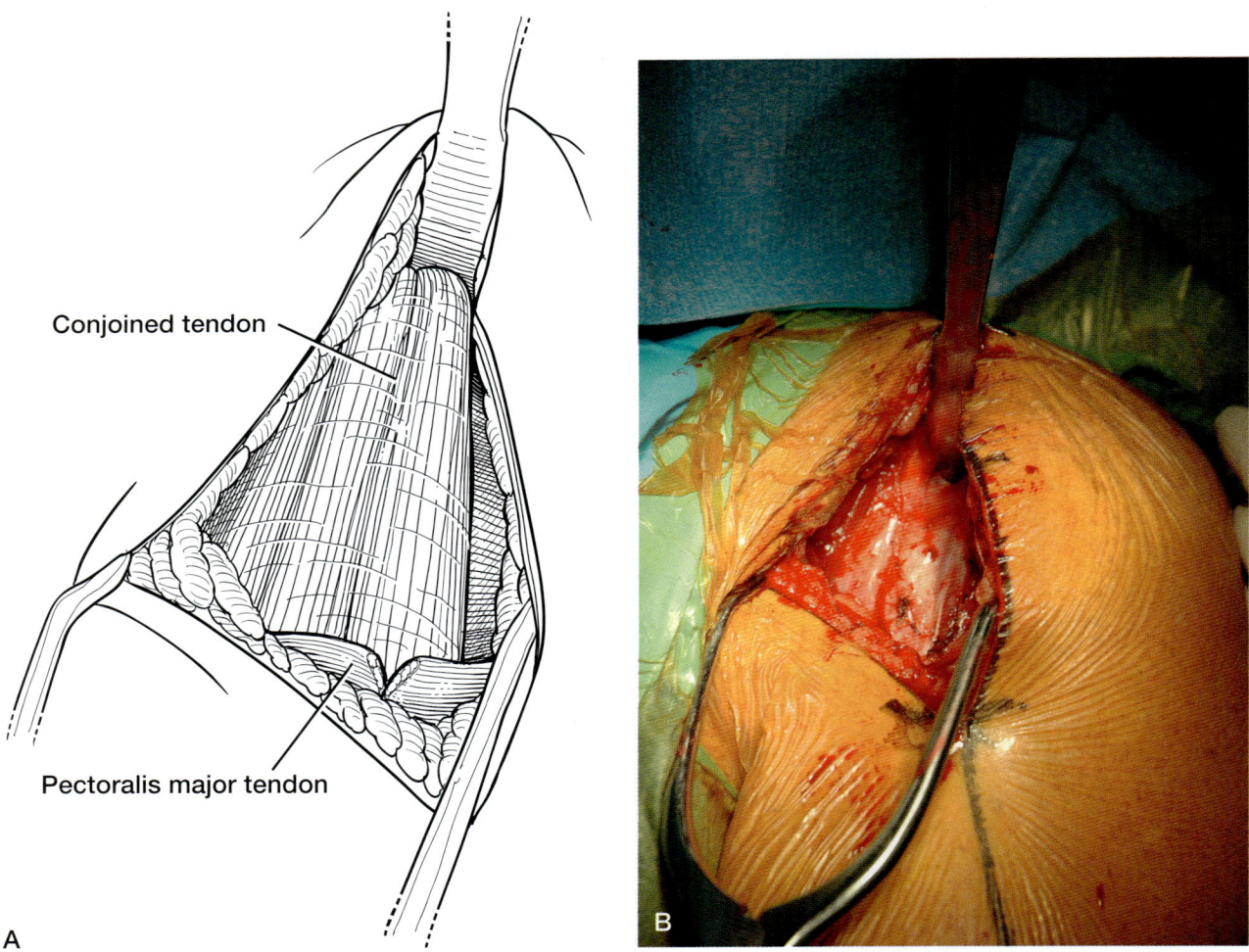

FIGURE 37.8 (A and B) Proximal retraction with a Hohmann retractor behind the coracoid process.

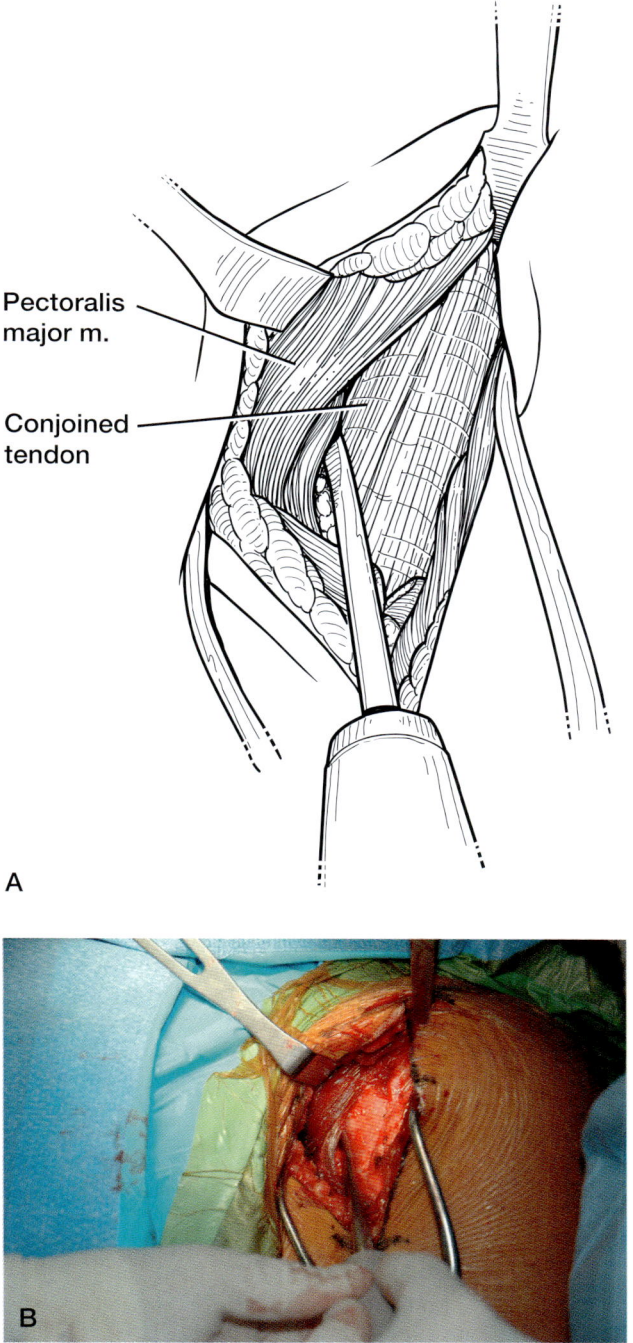

FIGURE 37.9 (A and B) Release of the undersurface of the pectoralis major muscle from the underlying conjoined tendon.

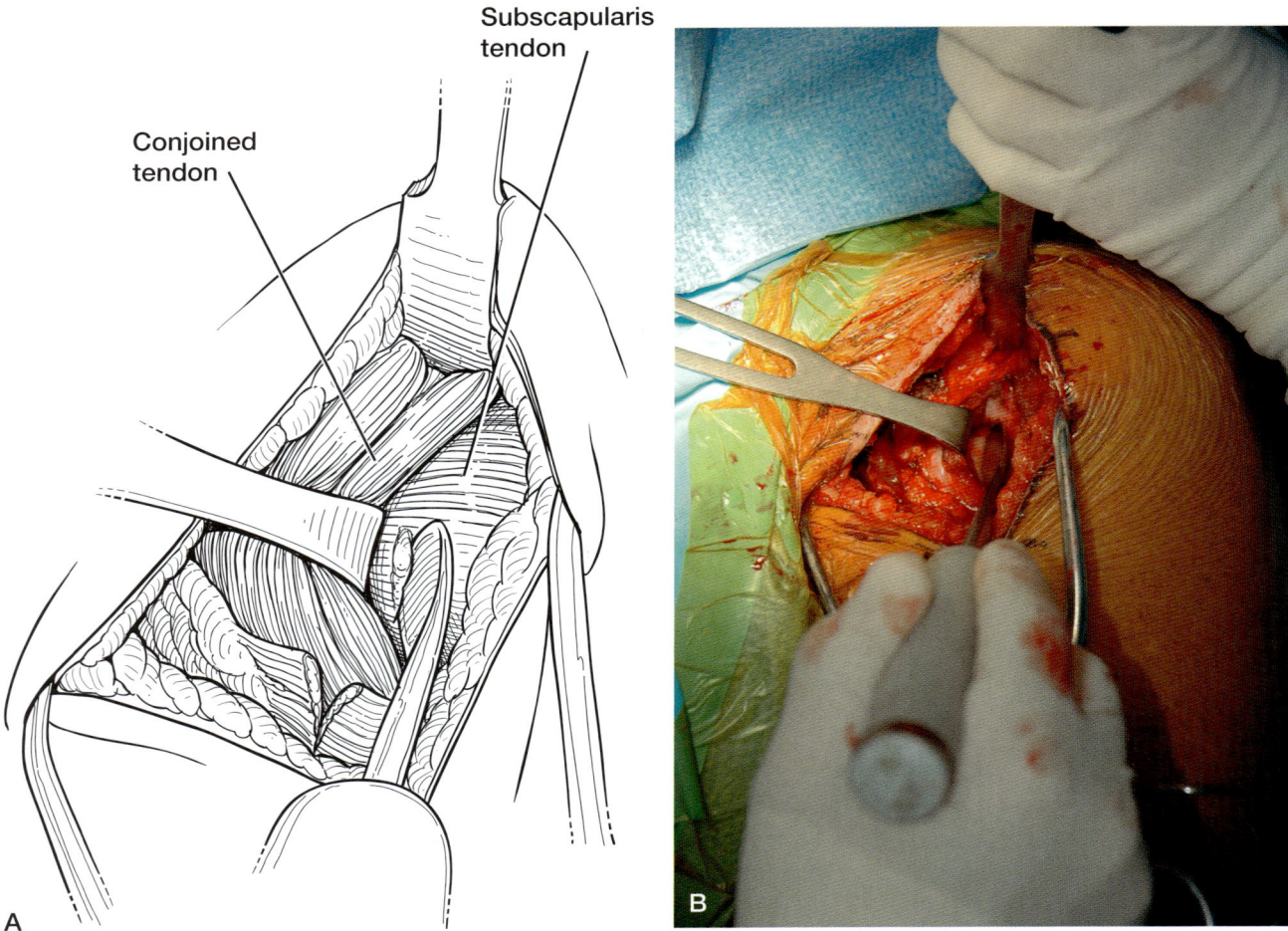

FIGURE 37.10 (A and B) Release of the conjoined tendon from the underlying subscapularis tendon.

is undertaken by spreading the tips of Metzenbaum scissors in the axillary fat inferior and deep to the subscapularis. Identification of the axillary nerve can be helpful in some cases to identify and protect it throughout the procedure.

In cases in which the subscapularis is intact, it is handled identically to cases of primary shoulder arthroplasty. Two stay sutures of no. 2 polyester are placed in the subscapularis tendon near the musculotendinous junction. The neck of the humeral prosthesis is identified, and a scalpel is used to transect the subscapularis tendon and joint capsule along the prosthetic humeral neck. If permanent sutures from earlier subscapularis repair at the time of the previous arthroplasty are present and appear to be in the appropriate location along the prosthetic neck, they are used as a guide for subscapularis tenotomy (Fig. 37.11). The electrocautery replaces the scalpel at the inferior portion of the subscapularis to cauterize the previously ligated anterior humeral circumflex vessels, when present. A humeral head retractor is placed in the glenohumeral joint and used to retract the prosthetic humeral head posteriorly. Circumferential release of the subscapularis tendon is performed, along with release of the superior, middle, and inferior glenohumeral ligaments, as in unconstrained shoulder arthroplasty. The subscapularis is then tucked into the subscapularis fossa with forceps and held with a glenoid rim retractor. If a reverse prosthesis is to be used as the revision implant, no sponge is placed in the subscapularis fossa because insertion of the screws for fixation of the glenoid base plate risks entrapment of the sponge with screws as they penetrate the anterior scapular cortex. If the subscapularis tendon is not present, the remaining subscapularis bursa is excised to expose the glenohumeral joint, and the humeral head retractor and glenoid rim retractor are inserted. If present, the intraarticular portion of the long head of the biceps tendon is handled as described in Chapter 5 (tenotomy or tenodesis).

TECHNIQUE FOR EXTENSION OF THE DELTOPECTORAL APPROACH INTO AN ANTEROLATERAL APPROACH TO THE HUMERAL DIAPHYSIS

During revision shoulder arthroplasty, it is frequently necessary to extend the deltopectoral approach distally to obtain access to the mid-humeral diaphysis. The main indications for using an extensile approach in revision shoulder arthroplasty are extraction of a well-fixated humeral stem and management of periprosthetic fractures. The surgeon should

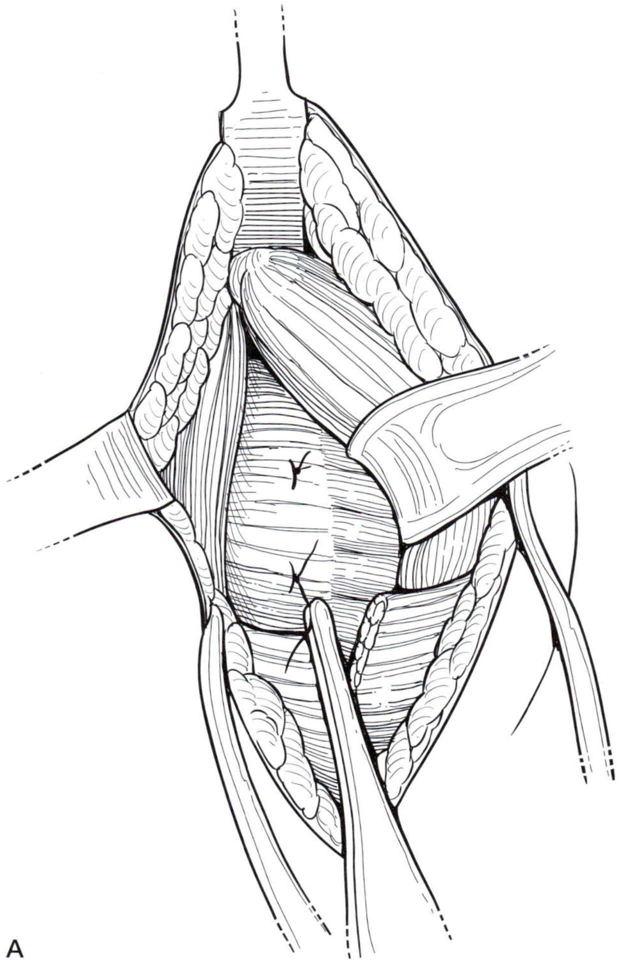

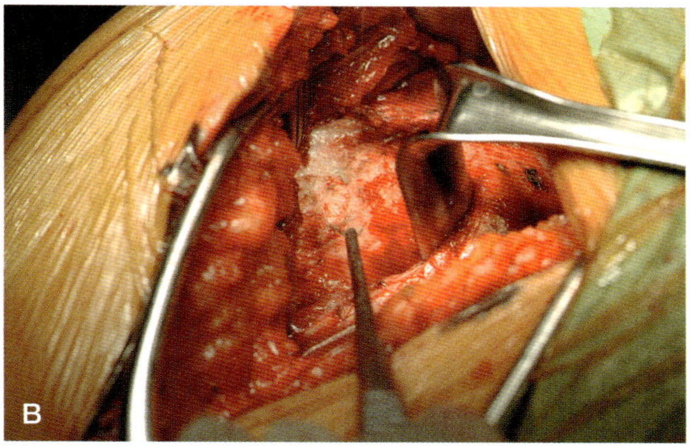

FIGURE 37.11 (A and B) Line of permanent sutures placed during repair of the subscapularis at the time of primary arthroplasty.

be prepared to perform this extended approach for any revision shoulder arthroplasty.

After marking the primary incision site and the planned deltopectoral portion of the revision incision (these are often the same), the marking pen is used to delineate the proposed skin incision for extending the skin incision distally along the lateral border of the biceps brachii for an anterolateral approach to the humeral diaphysis (Fig. 37.12). After it is determined that an extensile approach is necessary, the skin incision is extended with a no. 10 scalpel blade (Fig. 37.13). The needle tip electrocautery is used to dissect through subcutaneous tissue and around the lateral border of the biceps brachii (Fig. 37.14). The brachialis muscle is next encountered along the anterolateral humeral shaft. The brachialis is split longitudinally to expose the humeral shaft (Fig. 37.15). Subperiosteal dissection can be carried out around the humeral shaft if necessary to complete the exposure (Fig. 37.16). More proximally, the humeral insertion of the deltoid should be identified and protected (Fig. 37.17).

In some cases, particularly those involving a periprosthetic fracture, it may be necessary to place cerclage cables around the humeral shaft in the middle diaphysis. In such cases the radial nerve should be visualized and protected to avoid transection or incarceration by a cable. In these cases, it is

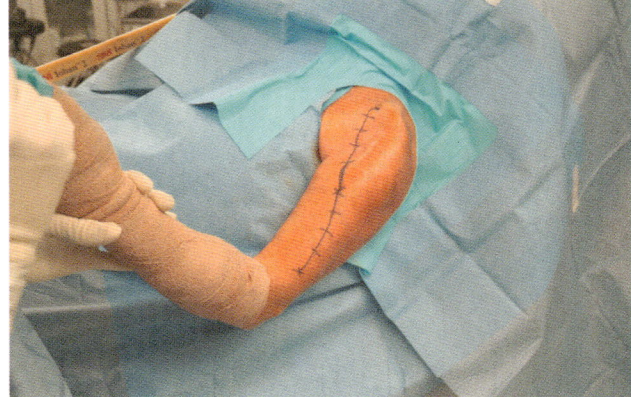

FIGURE 37.12 Planned skin incision for extending the deltopectoral approach into an anterolateral approach to the humeral shaft.

easiest to identify the radial nerve distally and trace its course proximally and posteriorly. The nerve is identified just proximal to the elbow as it courses between the brachialis and brachioradialis muscles (Fig. 37.18). From this point, it is traced proximally and protected from any cerclage devices placed around the humeral diaphysis (Fig. 37.19).

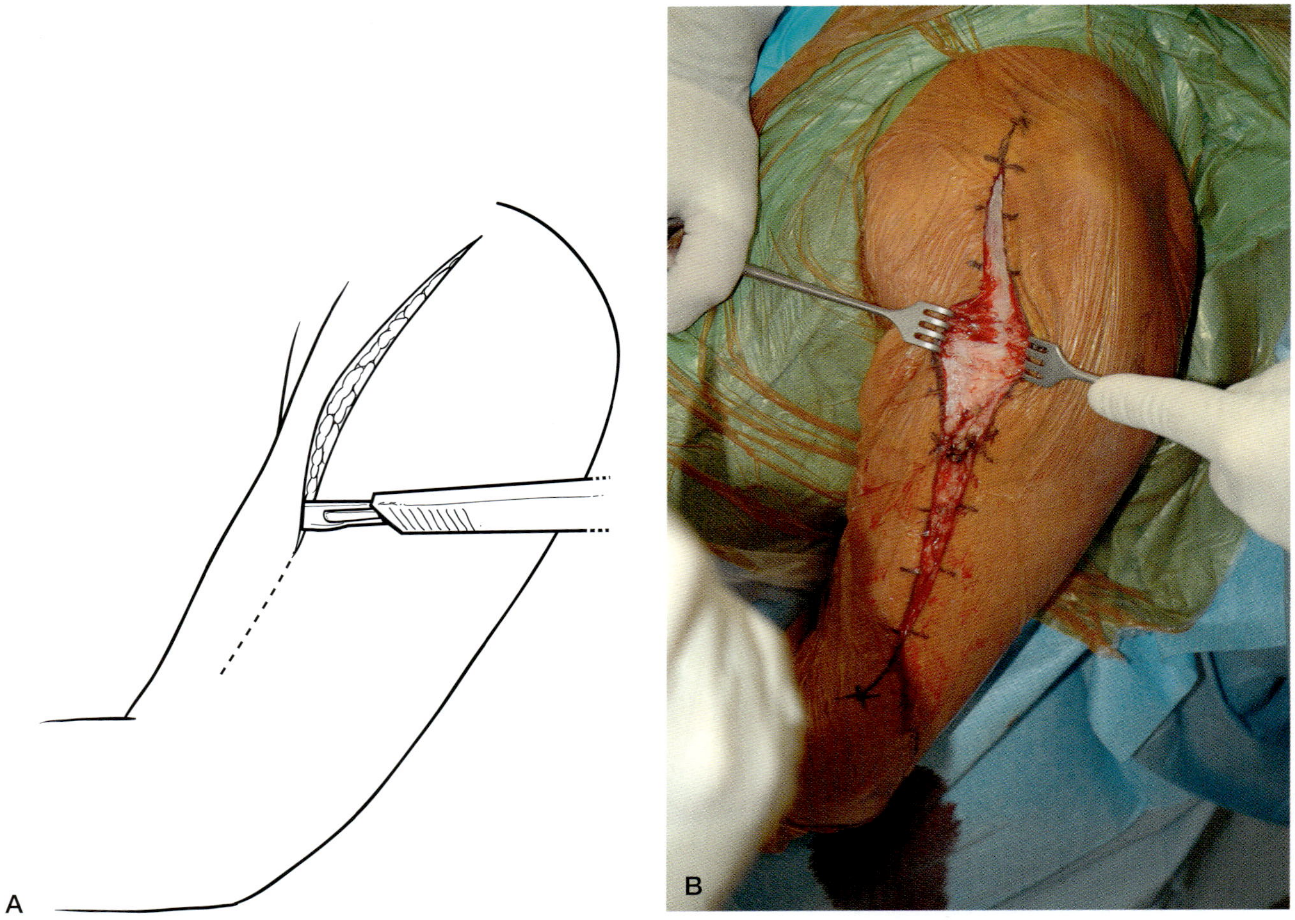

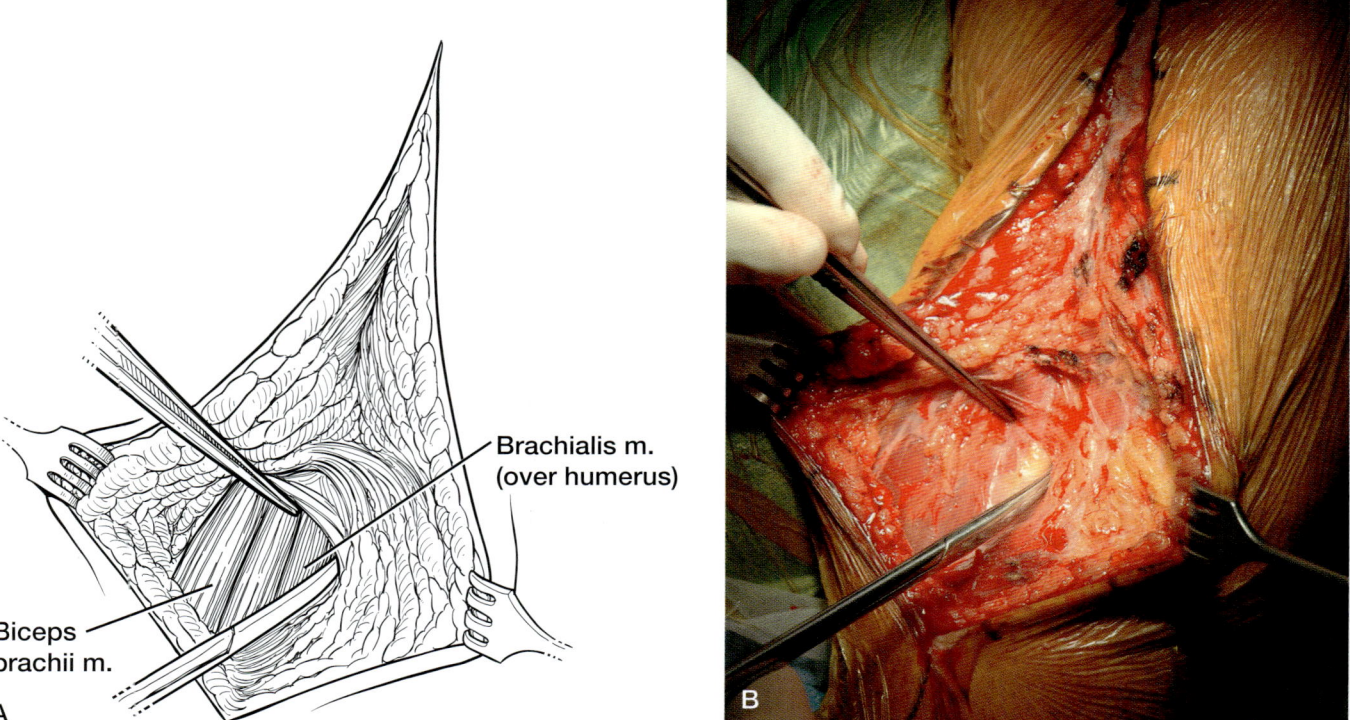

FIGURE 37.13 (A and B) Extension of the skin incision for the anterolateral approach to the humeral shaft.

FIGURE 37.14 (A and B) Dissection lateral to the biceps brachii.

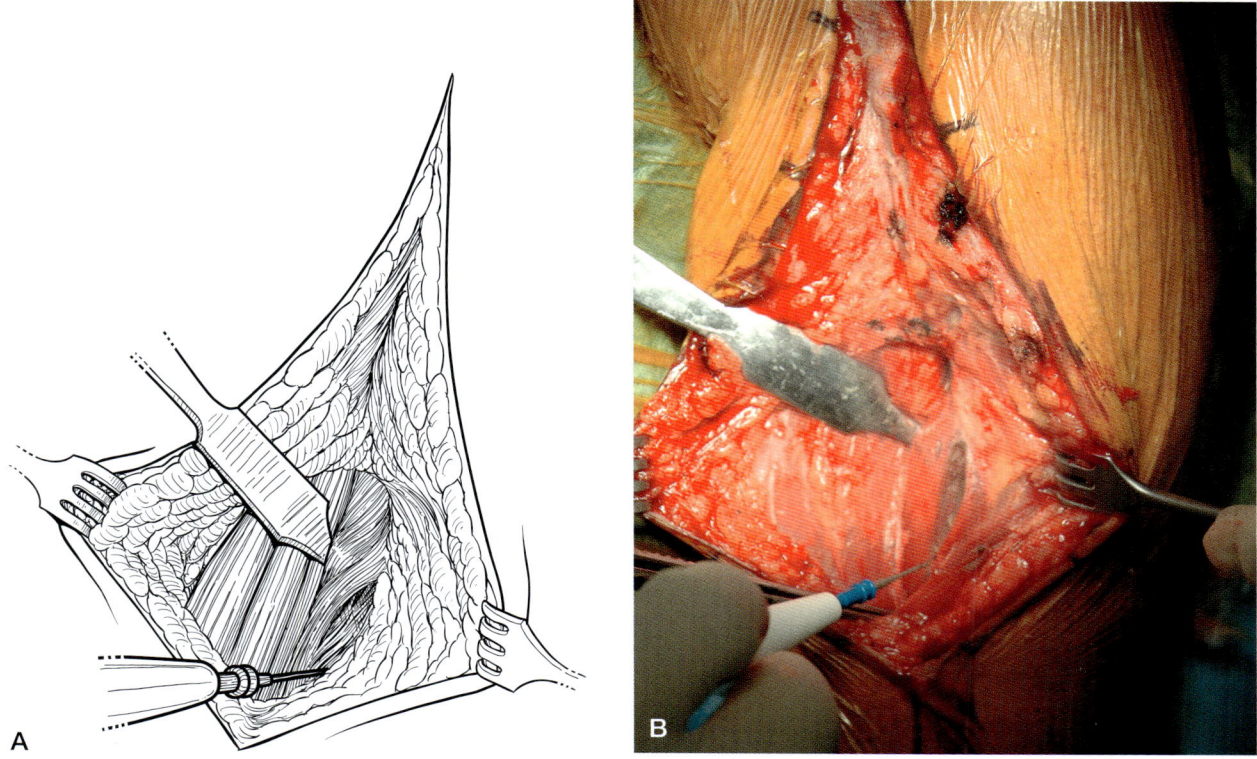

FIGURE 37.15 (A and B) Splitting of the brachialis to expose the humeral shaft.

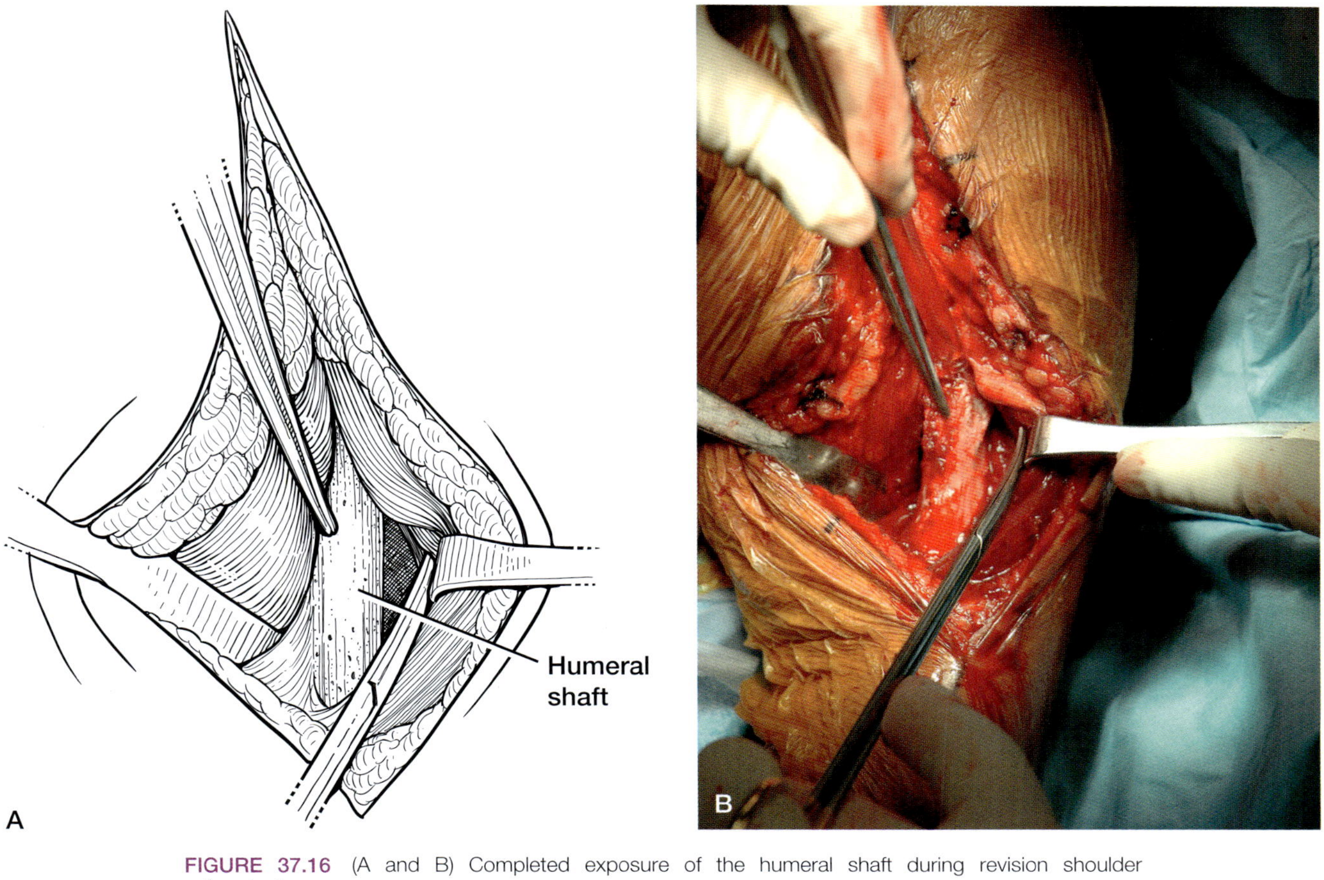

FIGURE 37.16 (A and B) Completed exposure of the humeral shaft during revision shoulder arthroplasty.

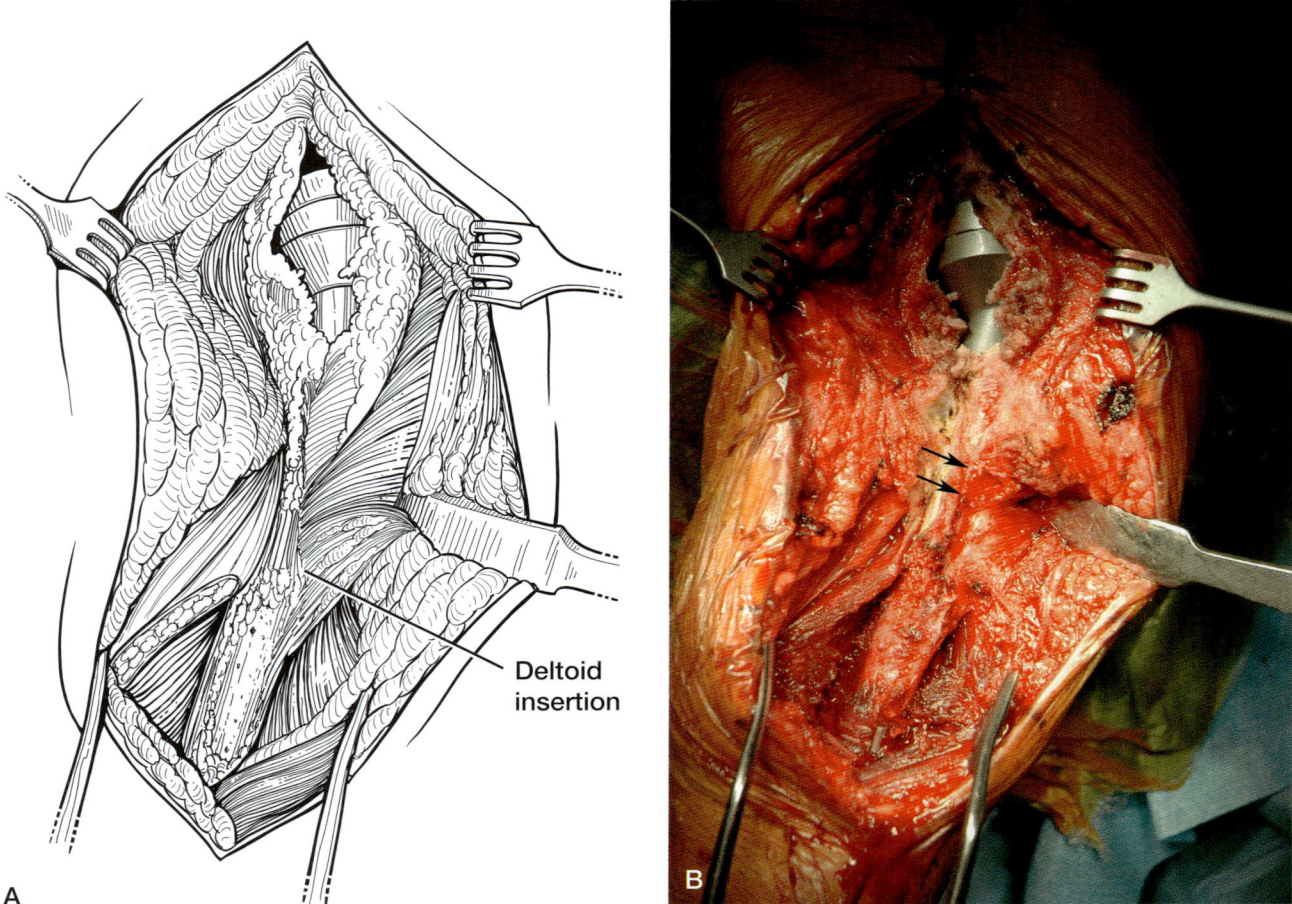

FIGURE 37.17 (A and B) The humeral insertion of the deltoid *(arrows)* is protected during the extensile approach used for revision shoulder arthroplasty.

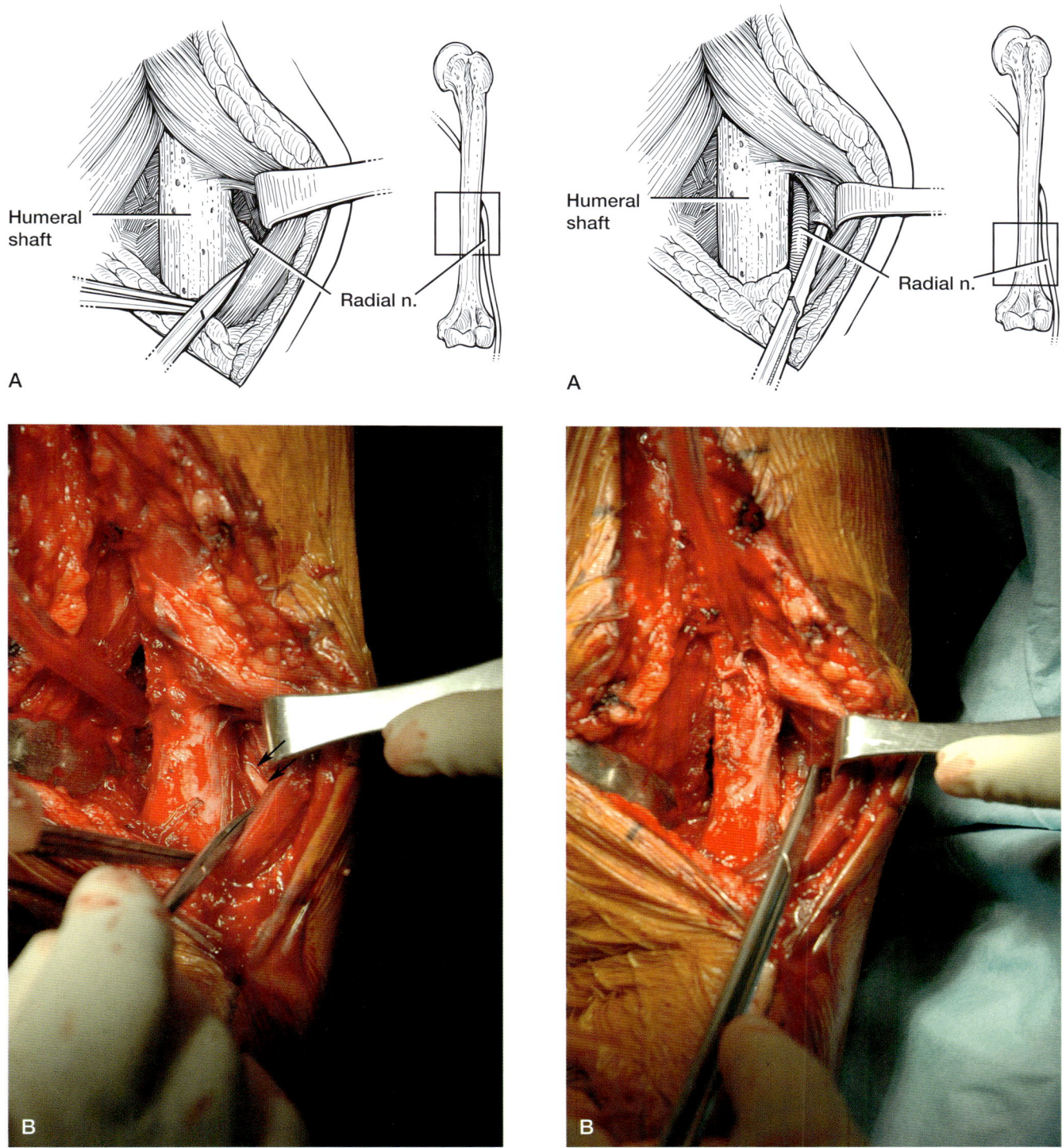

FIGURE 37.18 (A and B) The radial nerve *(arrows)* is identified between the brachialis and brachioradialis distally in the incision.

FIGURE 37.19 (A and B) The radial nerve is traced proximally and protected throughout the procedure.

CHAPTER 38

Humeral stem removal and glenoid exposure

Humeral stem removal can be simple or one of the most difficult and time-consuming aspects of revision shoulder arthroplasty. Preoperative planning becomes very important in facilitating removal of the humeral stem during revision shoulder arthroplasty. Although relatively smooth press fit humeral stems may be easy to remove, extensively porous-coated stems can be especially difficult to extract, particularly when they have been inserted with bone cement. Identification of the brand and type of implant used in the primary shoulder arthroplasty by radiographs or the primary arthroplasty operative report (or both) allows the surgeon to have an instrument set available to assist in extraction of the humeral implant (Fig. 38.1). Controlled extraction of the humeral implant, even if a humeral osteotomy is required, is certainly preferable to an intraoperative fracture of the proximal humerus caused by ill-fated attempts at extracting a well-fixated humeral stem without performing an osteotomy.

After the humeral stem is removed, glenoid exposure proceeds in much the same manner as for primary shoulder arthroplasty (see Chapter 10). This chapter details our techniques for humeral stem removal and glenoid exposure during revision shoulder arthroplasty.

TECHNIQUE FOR HUMERAL STEM REMOVAL

Tenotomy of the subscapularis with subsequent release of the superior, middle, and inferior glenohumeral ligaments (see Chapters 9 and 37) is performed if the subscapularis is intact. If the subscapularis is absent, any subscapularis bursa is excised to expose the anterior aspect of the humeral component (Fig. 38.2). A humeral head retractor is placed for retraction of the proximal humerus posteriorly (Fig. 38.3). If this provides sufficient visualization of the anterior glenoid and inferior capsule, inferior capsular release is performed, as described in the following section on glenoid exposure. However, because of its size, the humeral implant frequently sufficiently hinders glenoid visualization to prevent inferior capsular release. In these cases, it is necessary to remove the humeral stem before proceeding with glenoid exposure.

The proximal humerus must be dislocated before attempts at removal of the humeral stem. The dislocation must be done with great care to avoid humeral injury. Frequently, capsular stiffness prevents dislocation by simple external rotation and extension of the arm. If this maneuver is not initially successful, a humeral-based inferior capsular release is performed (Fig. 38.4). Progressive release of the inferior medial capsule from the humerus with the needle tip electrocautery allows dislocation of the proximal humerus. Care must be taken to keep the electrocautery in contact with the humerus to avoid injury to the axillary nerve. Dislocation maneuvers must be done slowly and with great care in revision cases to prevent humeral fracture because the humerus is often osteopenic and compromised (Fig. 38.5).

After the humerus has been dislocated, the humeral head portion of the arthroplasty is circumferentially exposed by removing any fibrous tissue at its margins with the needle tip electrocautery (Fig. 38.6). Nearly all implants currently encountered during revision surgery have a modular head fixed onto a stem via a Morse taper mechanism. However, it is important for a surgeon unfamiliar with the type of implant being removed to obtain any information available about the implant from the manufacturer. The surgeon must discover whether the implant is modular or monoblock and whether any accessory mechanisms have been used to fix the humeral head to the stem portion of the component. If the humeral component is modular with only Morse taper fixation of the humeral head portion to the stem portion of the component, the humeral head is usually easily removed by disimpacting the humeral head from the stem with a Cobb elevator at the inferior aspect of the humeral head component (Fig. 38.7). Often, fibrous tissue covers the proximal aspect of the stem portion of the component (Fig. 38.8). This fibrous tissue is completely removed with the needle tip electrocautery to delineate the peripheral proximal portion of the stem circumferentially (Fig. 38.9). The condition of the superior and posterior rotator cuff tendons can be evaluated at this point (Fig. 38.10).

After all soft tissue has been released peripherally from the proximal aspect of the stem portion of the implant, the extraction device specific for the implant, if available, is attached (Fig. 38.11). Attempts are made with the extraction device (generally with an attached slap hammer). If attempts to extract the implant are initially unsuccessful, the extraction device is removed and small, thin osteotomes are used to delicately separate the proximal humerus from the proximal aspect of the humeral implant (Fig. 38.12). The extraction device is reattached, and additional attempts are made to remove the humeral component. If these attempts are unsuccessful, a humeral osteotomy is performed for removal of the humeral implant (see later).

Text continued on p. 367

CHAPTER 38 ■ Humeral Stem Removal and Glenoid Exposure 361

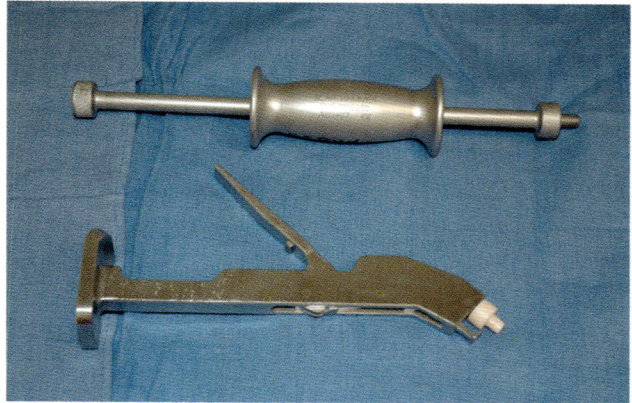

FIGURE 38.1 Specialized instruments for humeral stem extraction specific for a single brand and model of humeral implant.

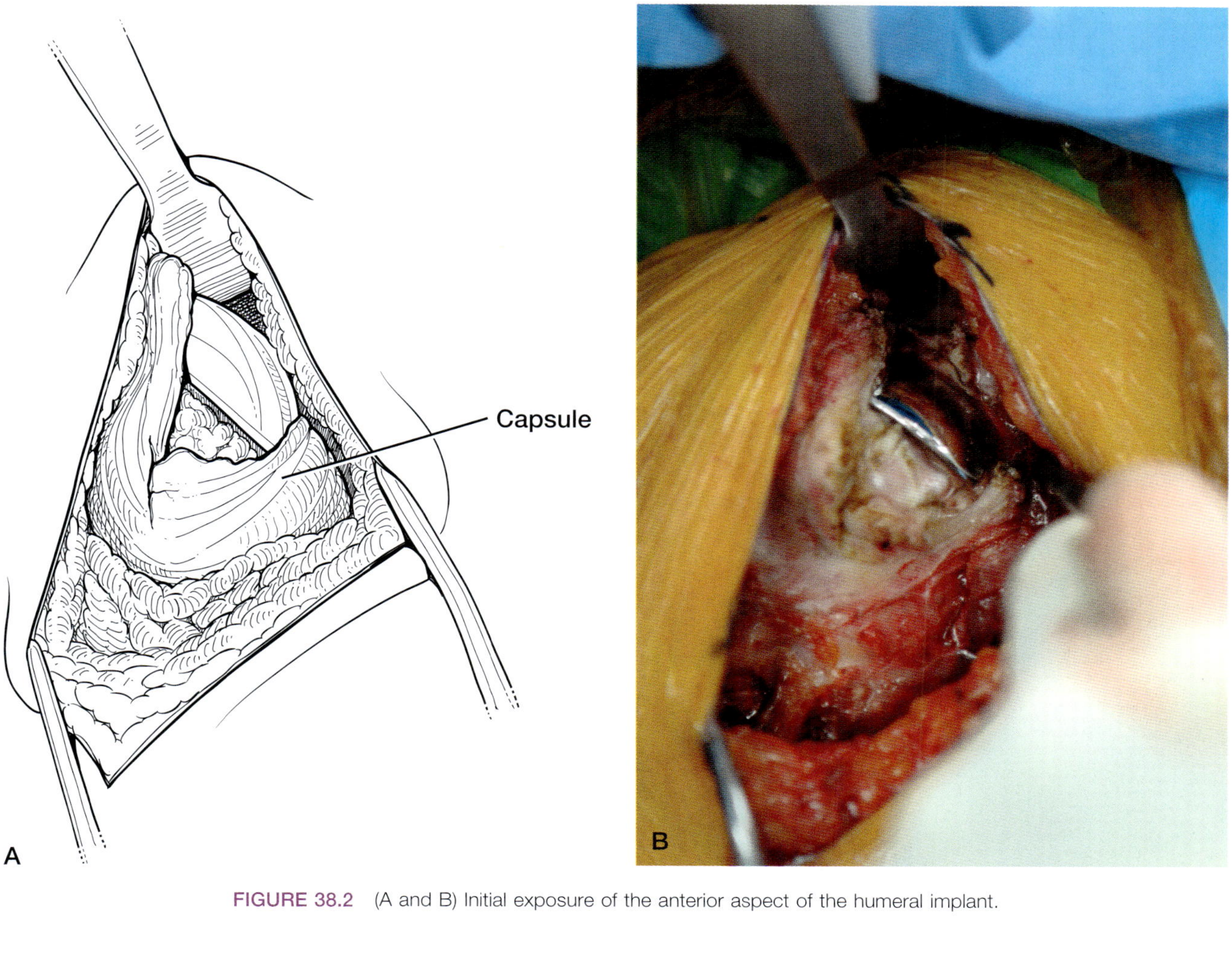

FIGURE 38.2 (A and B) Initial exposure of the anterior aspect of the humeral implant.

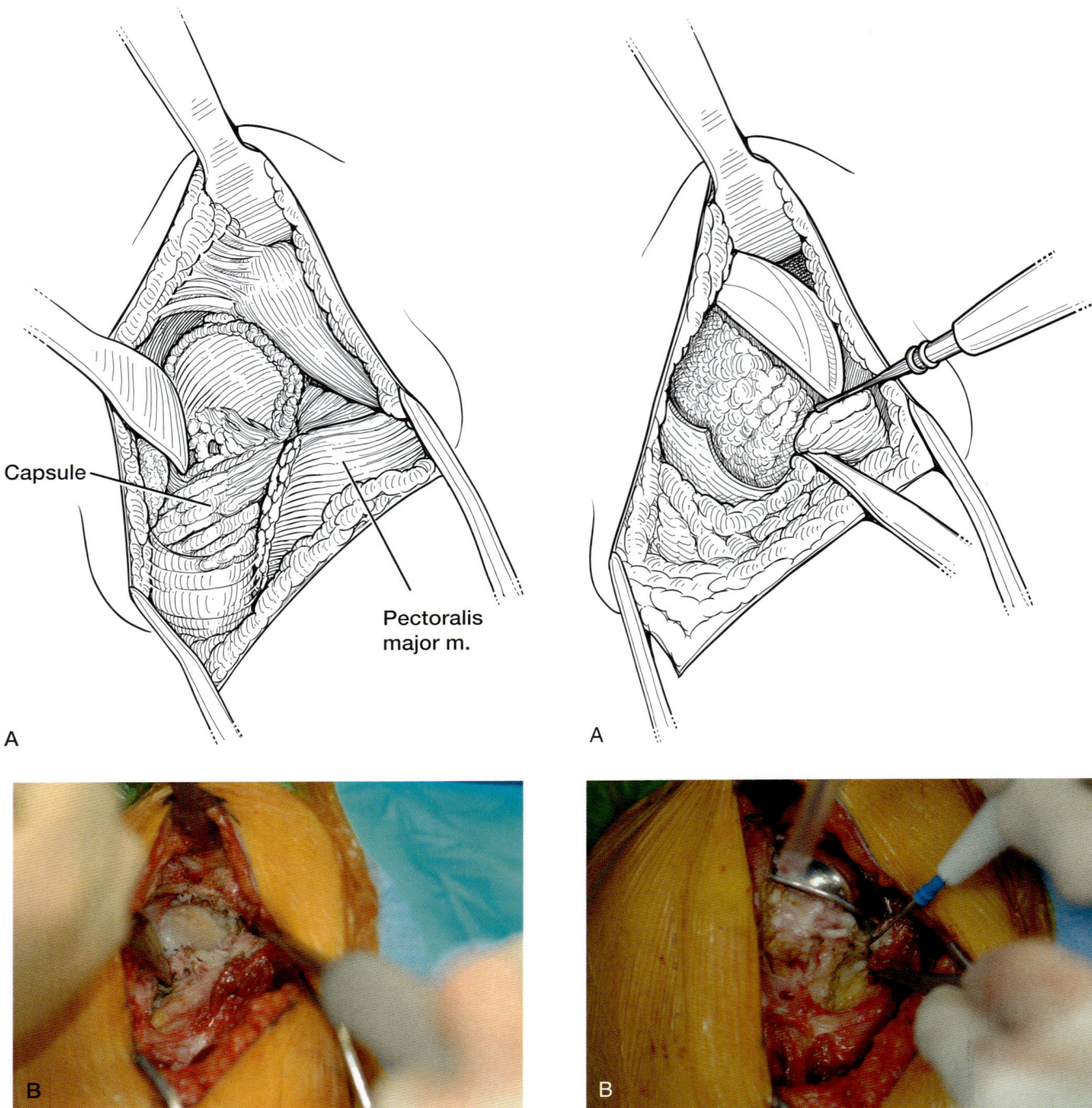

FIGURE 38.3 (A and B) Retraction of the proximal humerus posteriorly with a humeral head retractor before extraction of the primary humeral prosthesis.

FIGURE 38.4 (A and B) Performance of a humeral-based inferior capsular release with the needle tip electrocautery to allow dislocation of the proximal humerus.

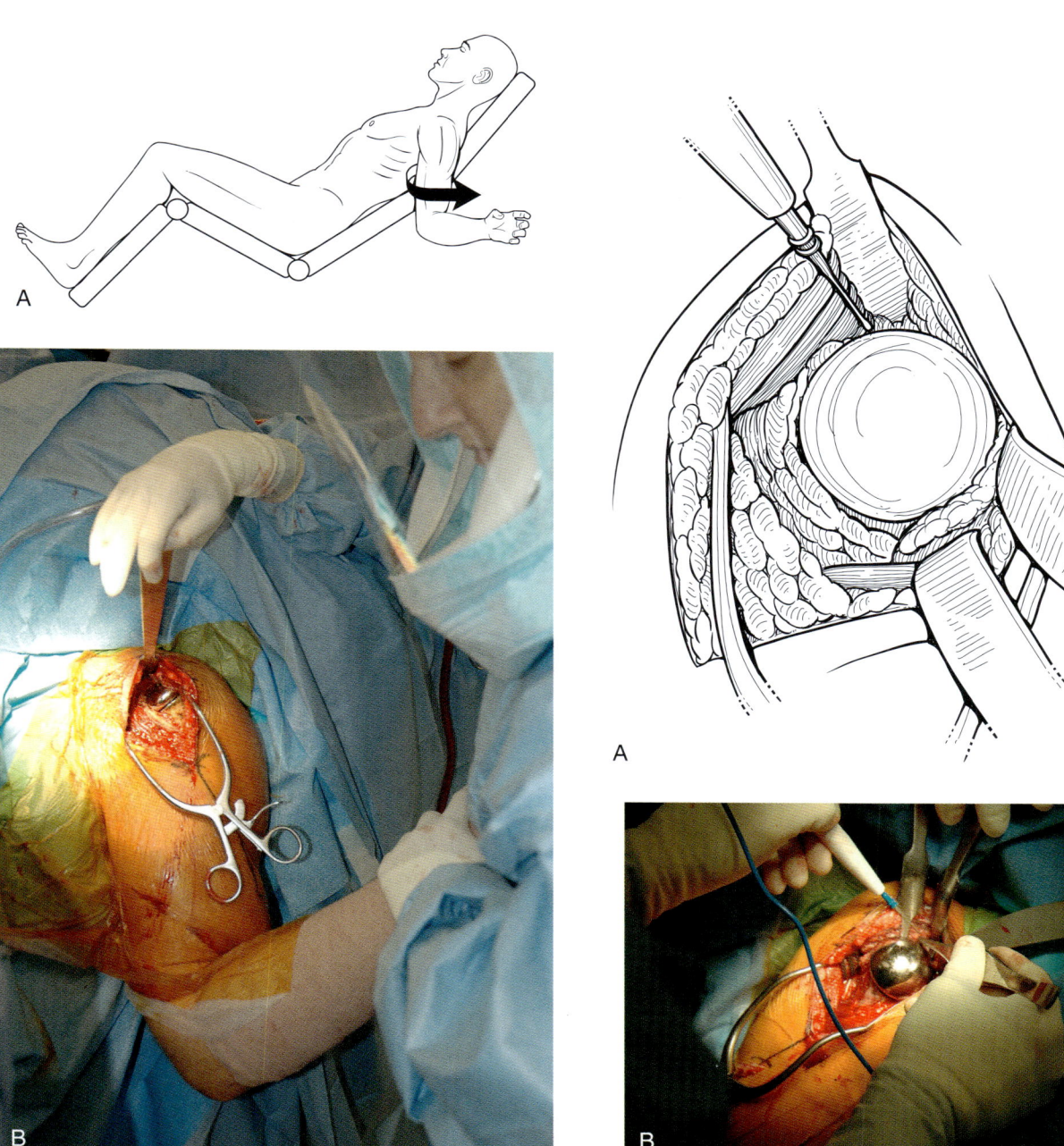

FIGURE 38.5 (A and B) Gentle dislocation maneuver consisting of external rotation and extension of the arm.

FIGURE 38.6 (A and B) After the glenohumeral joint is dislocated, any fibrous tissue at the margins of the humeral implant proximally is removed with the electrocautery.

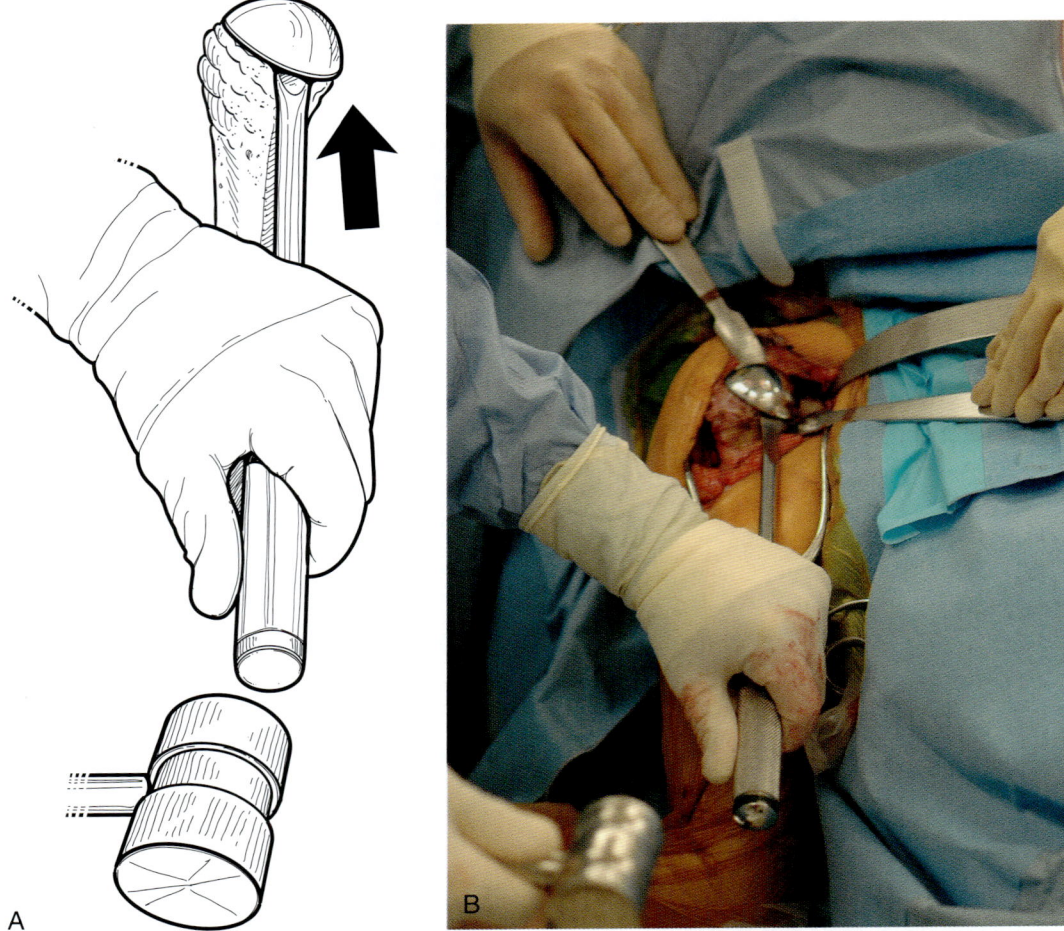

FIGURE 38.7 (A and B) A Morse taper–secured humeral head of a modular humeral implant is usually easily removed with a Cobb elevator as an impactor.

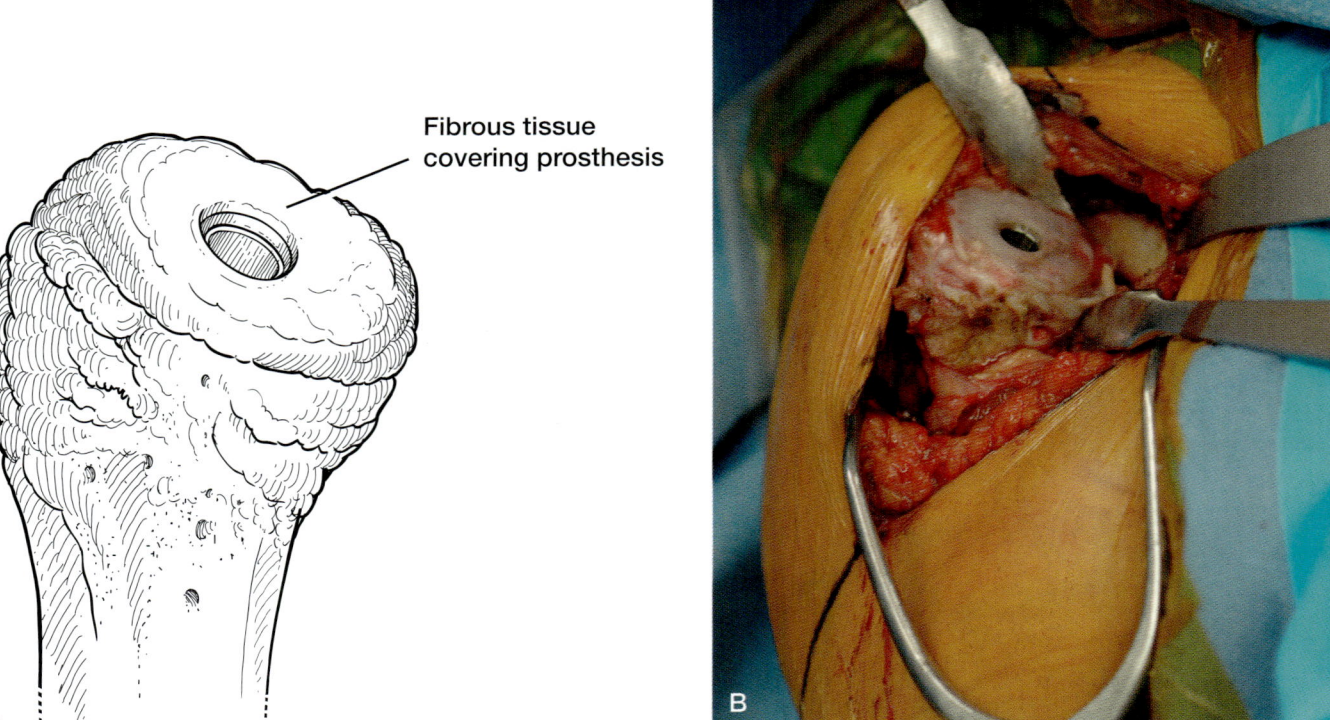

FIGURE 38.8 (A and B) Fibrous tissue covering the proximal aspect of the stem portion of the humeral prosthesis after removal of a modular humeral head.

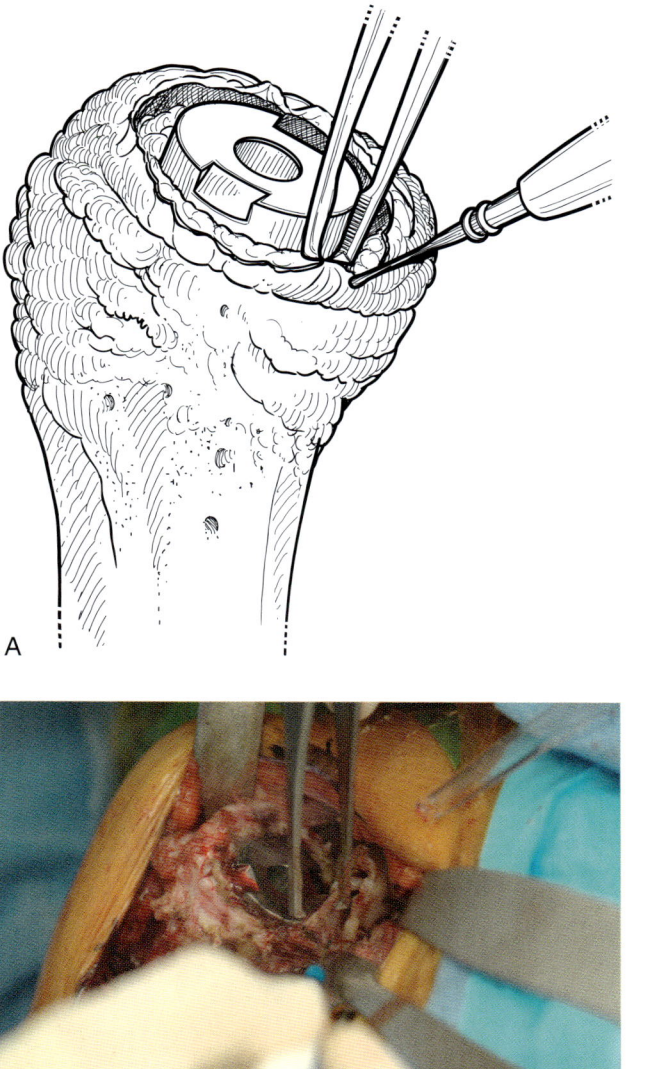

FIGURE 38.9 (A and B) Removal of the fibrous tissue covering the proximal aspect of the stem portion of the humeral prosthesis with a needle tip electrocautery.

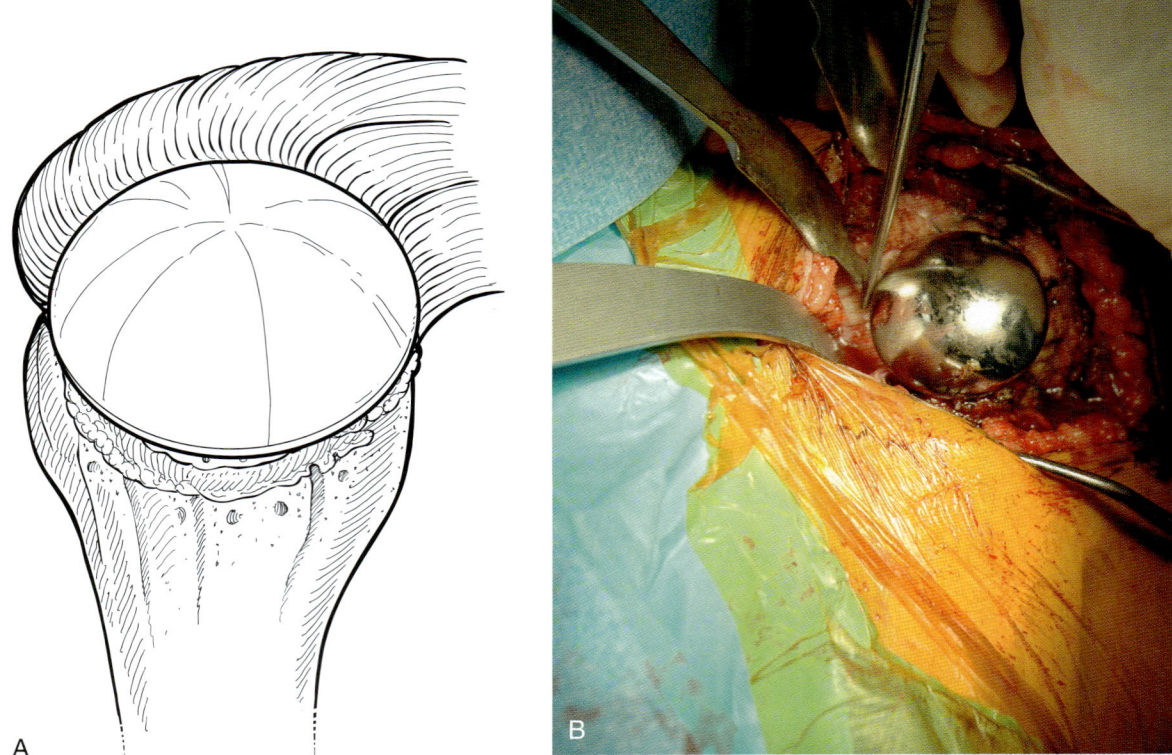

FIGURE 38.10 (A and B) Inspection of the rotator cuff before extraction of the humeral stem.

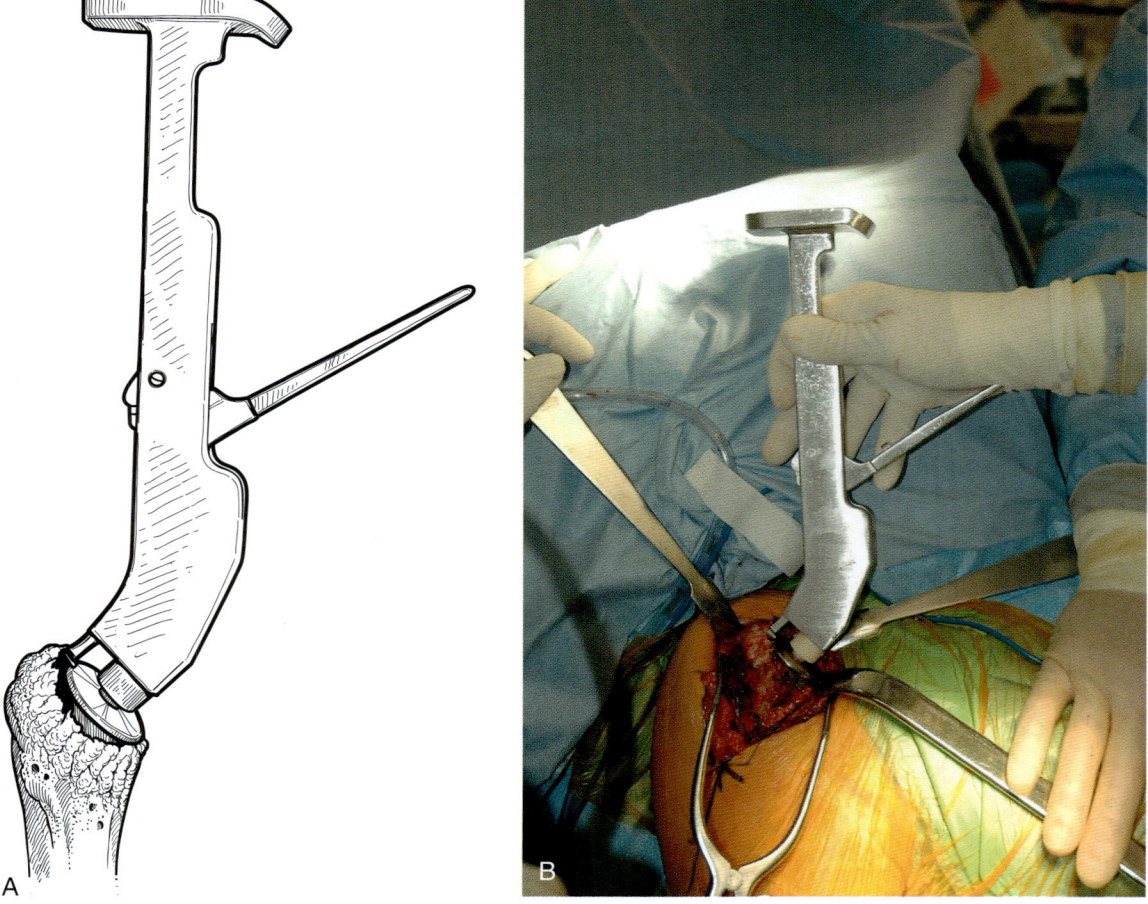

FIGURE 38.11 (A and B) Attachment of an extraction device to the stem portion of the primary humeral stem.

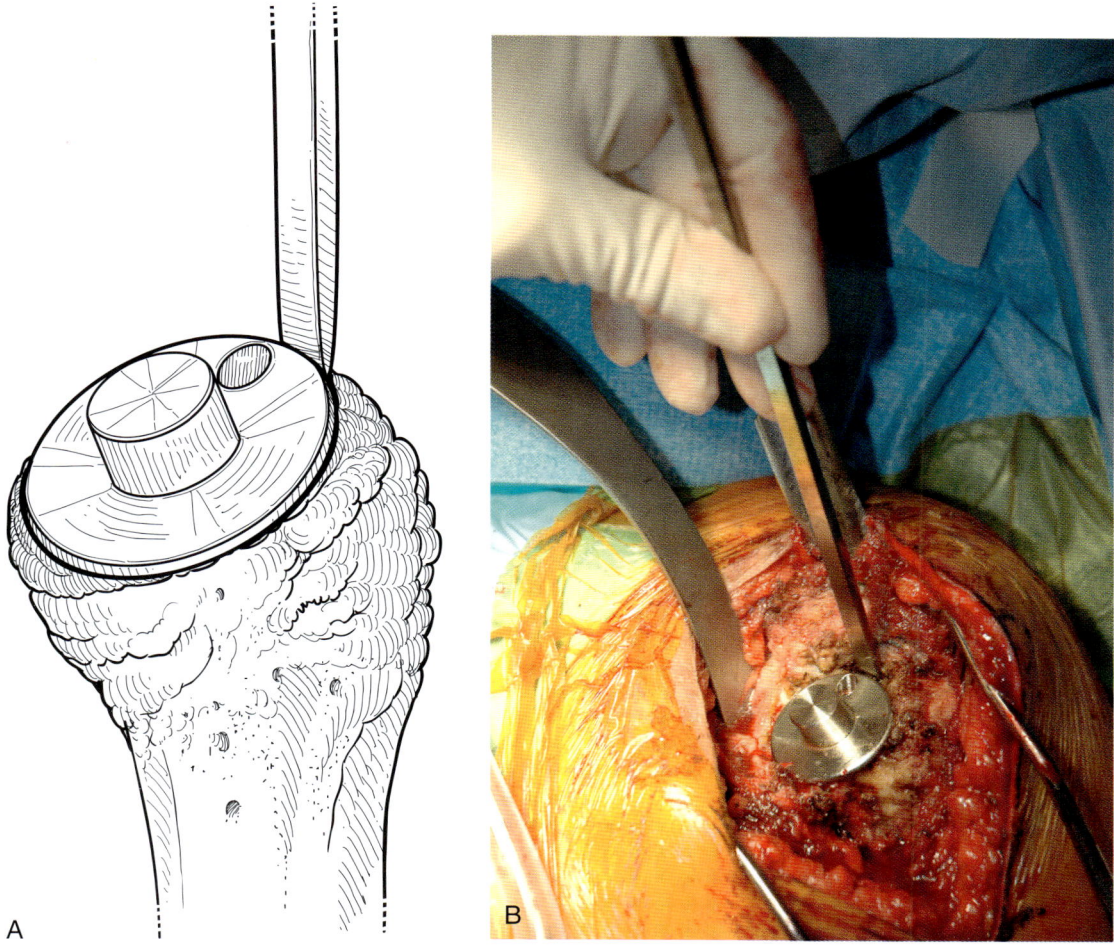

FIGURE 38.12 (A and B) Small, thin osteotomes are used to delicately separate the proximal humerus from the proximal aspect of the humeral implant.

If no extraction device for the type of implant being removed exists, small, thin osteotomes are used to delicately separate the proximal humerus from the proximal aspect of the humeral implant after all soft tissue has been released peripherally from the proximal portion of the stem portion of the implant. A large Cobb elevator is used to disimpact the humeral implant from the proximal humerus by striking it at its medial portion (Fig. 38.13). The Cobb elevator is directed as parallel as possible to the humeral implant stem. If attempts at implant extraction are unsuccessful with this technique, humeral osteotomy should be performed.

Humeral Osteotomy

After the necessity for humeral osteotomy is established, the surgical approach is extended distally, as detailed in Chapter 37. The humerus is exposed from its proximal aspect to the area distal to the pectoralis major insertion (Fig. 38.14). The planned osteotomy site is demarcated with the needle tip electrocautery and extended along the anterior humerus by starting just medial to the bicipital groove and continuing distally between the pectoralis major insertion and the deltoid insertion (Fig. 38.15). The distal extent of the osteotomy is determined by the length of the humeral stem to be removed.

Before performing the osteotomy, cerclage cables are placed for subsequent osteotomy fixation. Depending on the length of the osteotomy, we place two or three cables composed of a nylon monofilament core wrapped in braided ultrahigh-molecular-weight polyethylene (Kinamed Inc., Camarillo, California). The cables are placed subperiosteally with the cable-passing instrumentation provided (Fig. 38.16). In cases in which the osteotomy extends beyond the junction of the proximal third and middle third of the humeral shaft, the radial nerve must be identified and protected before passing cables posterior to the humerus (see Chapter 37). After the cables are passed, the free ends of each cable are clamped together with Kocher clamps (Fig. 38.17).

A unicortical humeral osteotomy is performed by penetration of the anterior cortex with a sagittal saw along the humerus at the demarcated osteotomy site down to the humeral implant (Fig. 38.18). A 1½-inch straight osteotome is impacted into the osteotomy site proximally (Fig. 38.19). The osteotome is turned to open the osteotomy by plastically deforming the proximal humerus (Fig. 38.20). The humeral stem can then be removed with the extraction instrumentation provided or by disimpaction with a Cobb elevator, as described earlier (Fig. 38.21).

Text continued on p. 373

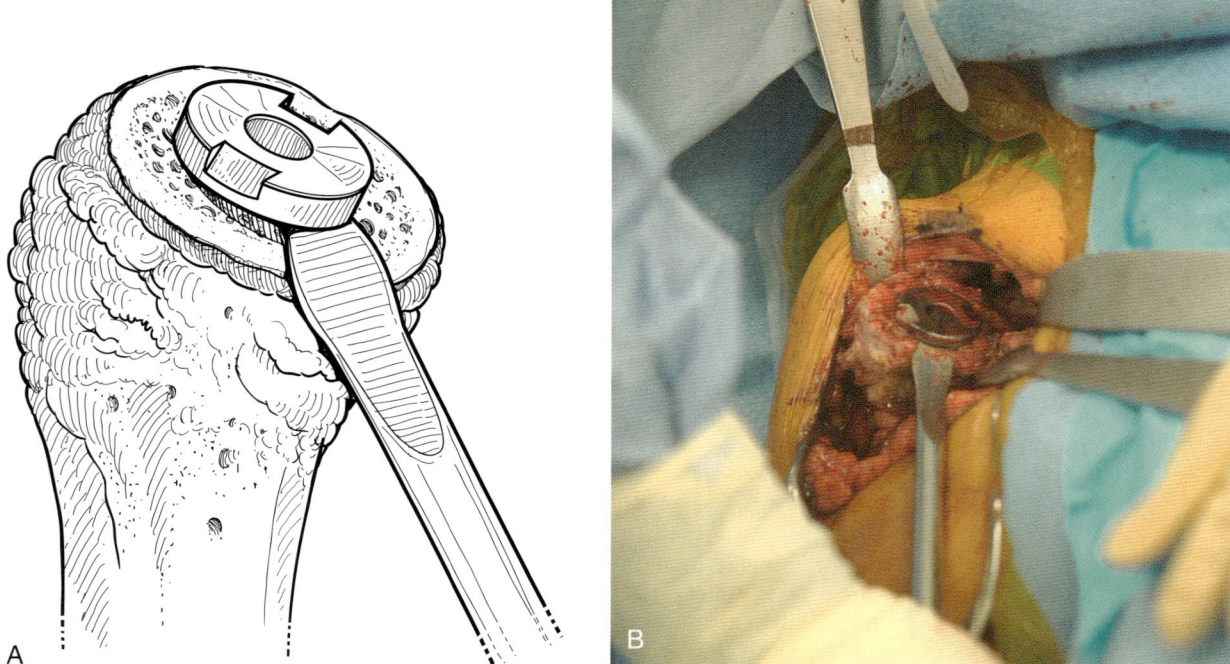

FIGURE 38.13 (A and B) A large Cobb elevator is used to disimpact the humeral implant from the proximal humerus by striking it at its medial portion.

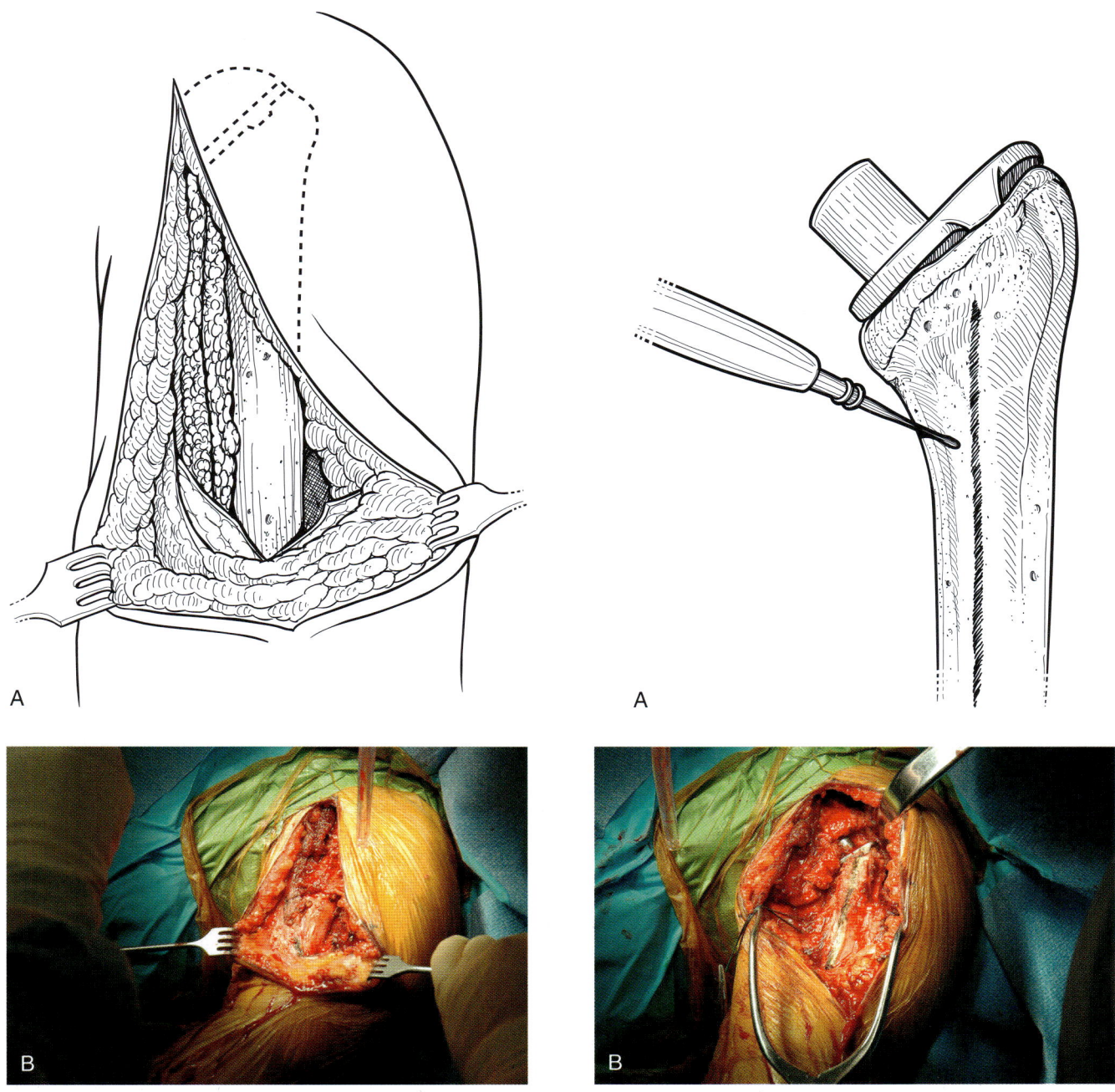

FIGURE 38.14 (A and B) Exposure of the humerus in preparation for humeral osteotomy.

FIGURE 38.15 (A and B) The planned osteotomy site is demarcated with a needle tip electrocautery.

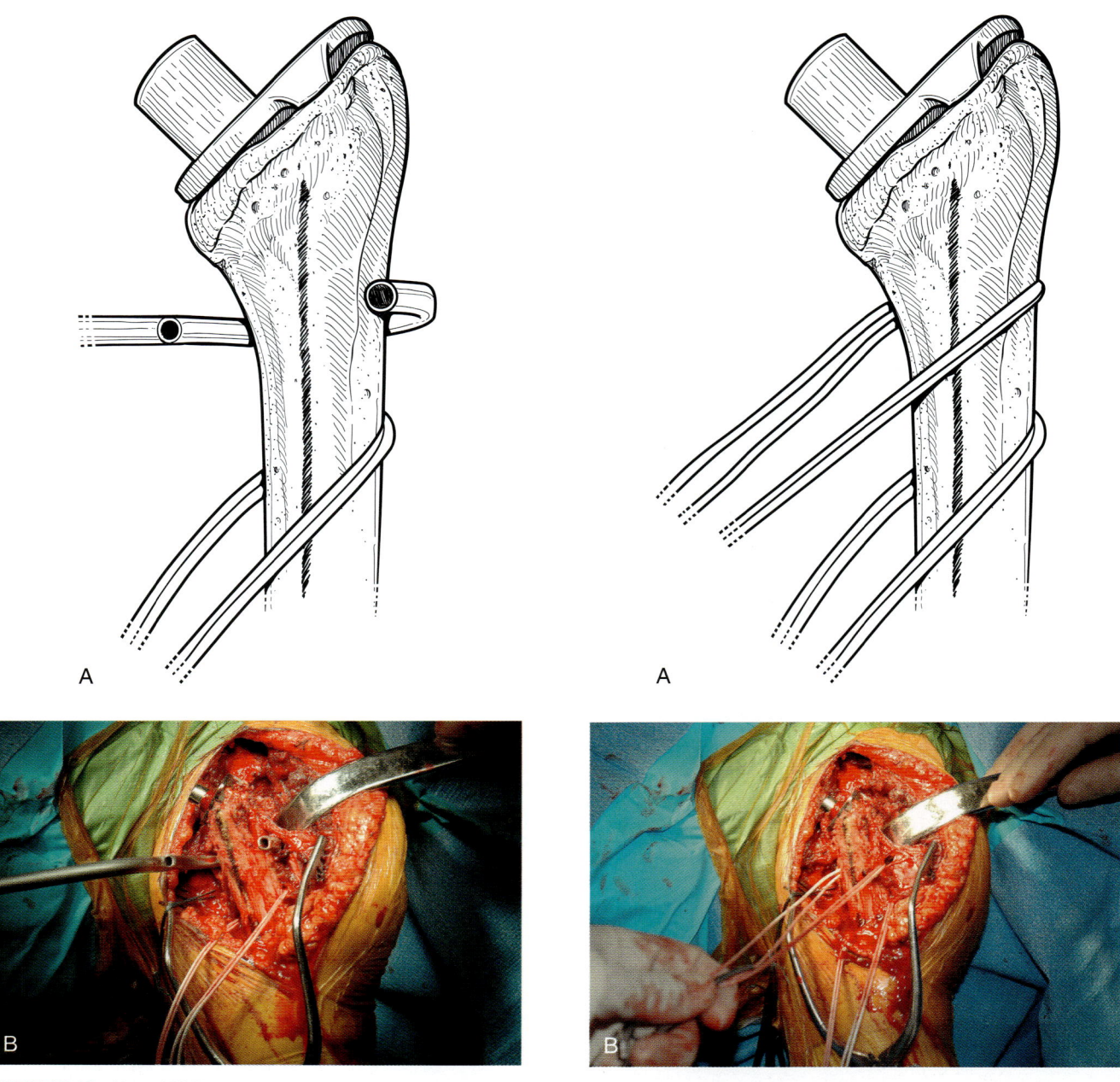

FIGURE 38.16 (A and B) Placement of cables for later fixation of the humeral osteotomy.

FIGURE 38.17 (A and B) Final placement of the cables, which are held temporarily with Kocher clamps.

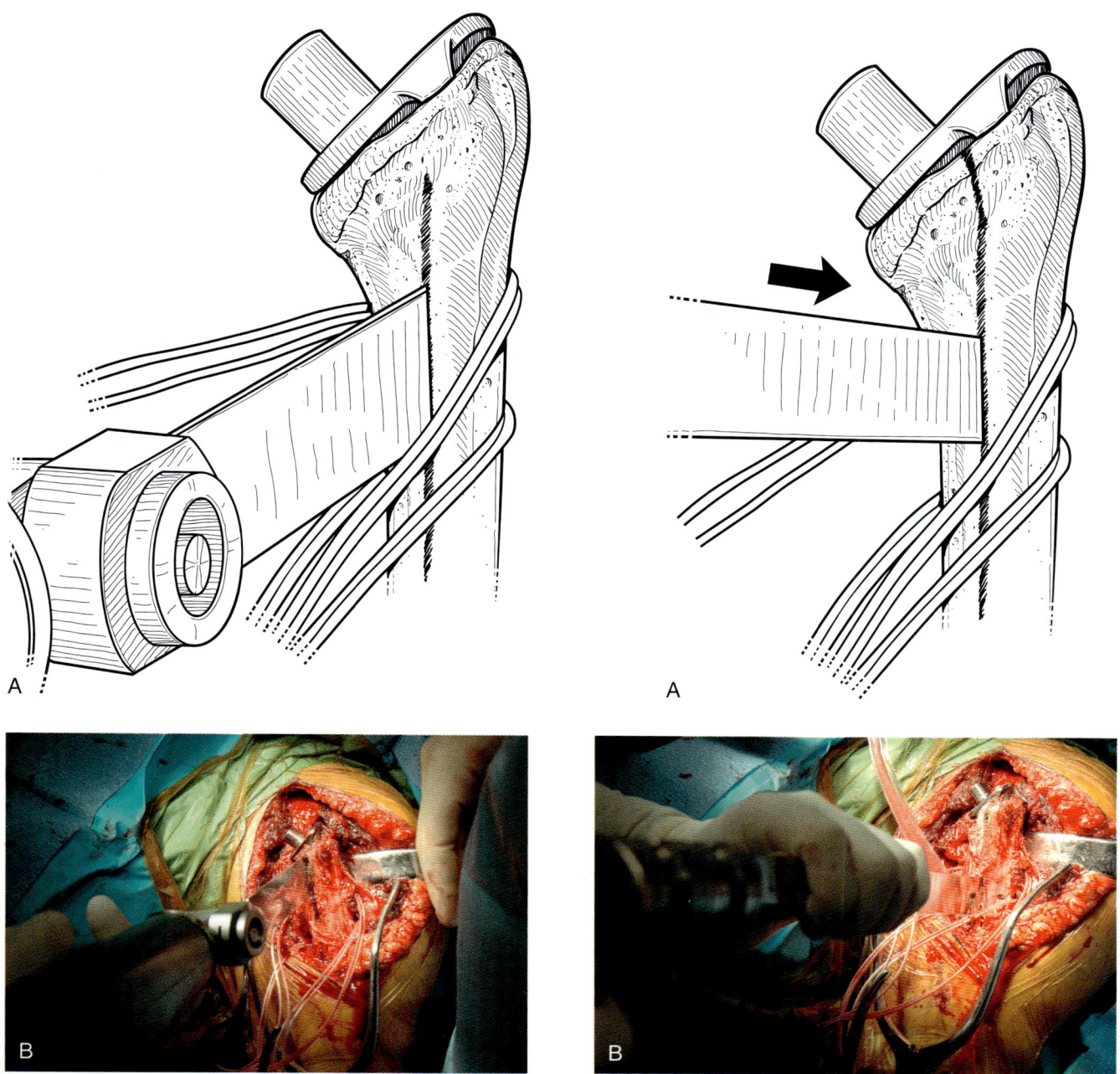

FIGURE 38.18 (A and B) The osteotomy is performed with a saw along the anterior humerus.

FIGURE 38.19 (A and B) An osteotome is impacted into the osteotomy site proximally.

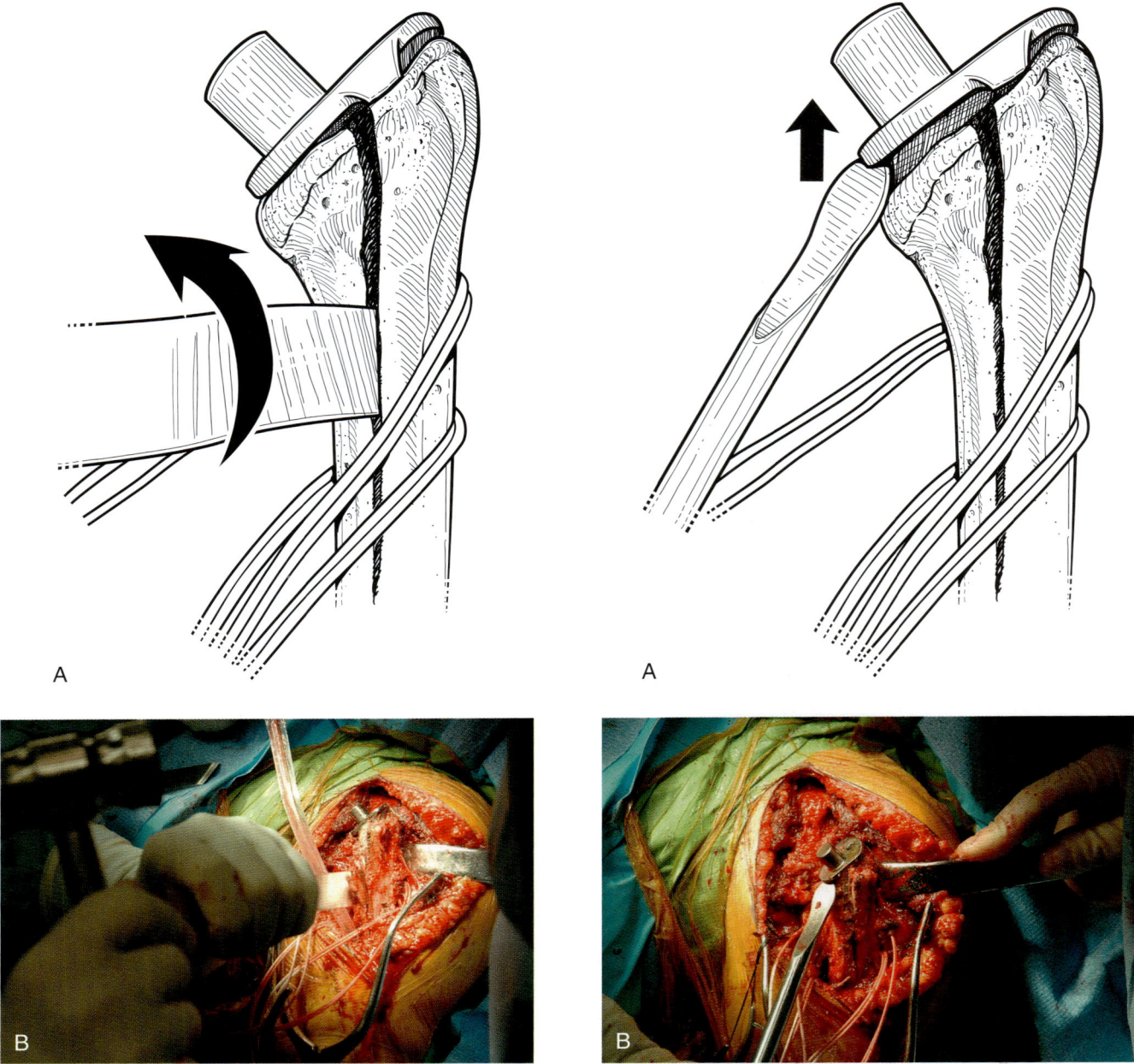

FIGURE 38.20 (A and B) The osteotome is turned to open the osteotomy site by plastic deformation.

FIGURE 38.21 (A and B) The humeral stem is removed.

Cement Removal

When removing a cemented humeral stem, residual cement is removed for two reasons—if it is loose within the humerus and if it prevents insertion of the revision humeral stem. Any residual cement that is well fixed within the humeral canal and does not interfere with insertion of the revision humeral stem is left in place. The revision humeral stem can be successfully fixated into a stable residual cement mantle.[1]

Loose cement within the humeral canal is easily removed with pituitary-type forceps (Fig. 38.24). Removing cement that is well fixed within the humeral canal to make room for the revision humeral component is more challenging. We use a set of specialized cement-removing osteotomes (Moreland osteotomes) that come in a variety of shapes and sizes (Fig. 38.25). A combination of curved and straight Moreland osteotomes is used to remove the proximal cement mantle (Fig. 38.26). Any cement fragments that fall into the humeral canal are removed with pituitary forceps. Only enough cement is removed to permit insertion of the revision humeral stem. The trial stem is inserted intermittently during the cement removal process to evaluate the sufficiency of cement removal.

Occasionally, it is necessary to remove a distal cement plug to permit insertion of the revision humeral stem. If this is the case, it will often be necessary to perform a humeral osteotomy to permit removal of the cement plug without perforating and damaging the humeral diaphysis. After the humeral osteotomy is performed and extended distal to the cement plug, the osteotomy is plastically opened distally with an osteotome and the cement plug is removed from the humeral canal with pituitary forceps. If a cement restrictor is present, it is removed with the pituitary forceps.

TECHNIQUE FOR GLENOID EXPOSURE

After the humeral component is removed, attention is turned to glenoid exposure. In cases in which no glenoid component has previously been implanted, any remaining labrum is excised from the base of the coracoid process extending inferiorly to the 5 o'clock position in a right shoulder (7 o'clock in a left shoulder) with the needle tip electrocautery. This allows identification of the osseous anterior margin of the glenoid. In nearly all cases, proper exposure of the glenoid requires release of the inferior capsule. The tip of the electrocautery is used to release the inferior capsule directly off the rim of the glenoid bone, just as in primary total shoulder arthroplasty. To help prevent injury to the axillary nerve, the tip of the electrocautery should be kept in contact with glenoid bone. This release is extended sufficiently medially to completely transect the capsule and expose the muscular fibers of the long head of the triceps inserting on the inferior osseous glenoid. The amount of posterior subluxation present on preoperative secondary imaging studies (computed tomography, magnetic resonance imaging) determines the posterior extent of release. In shoulders without posterior subluxation, the release continues posteriorly to the 8 o'clock position for right shoulders (4 o'clock position for left shoulders). In shoulders that have preexisting posterior subluxation, either with or without posterior glenoid erosion,

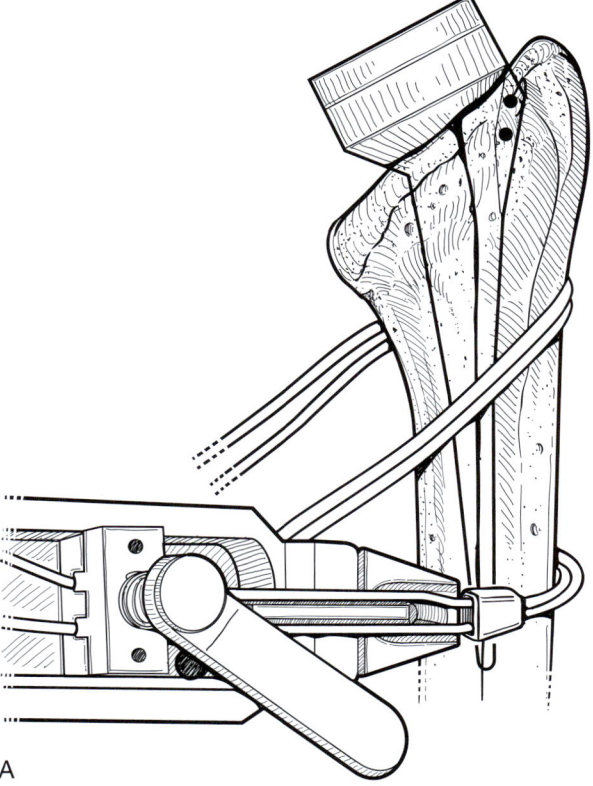
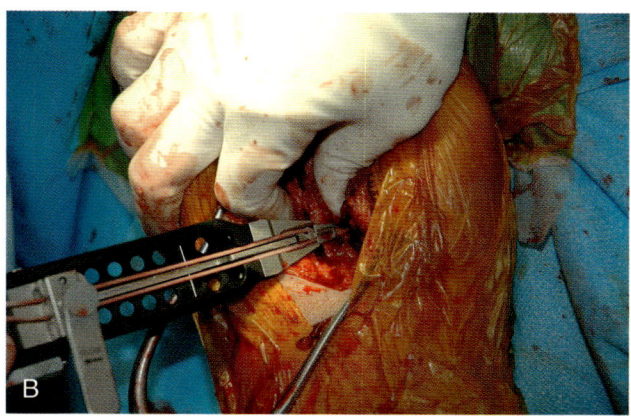

FIGURE 38.22 (A and B) The cables are tightened over the trial stem.

After the humeral stem and any necessary cement (see later) are removed, the osteotomy must be fixated. This is performed by first preparing the proximal humerus for insertion of the revision humeral component with the instrumentation provided. The trial humeral stem is inserted, and the cables are tightened with the tensioning device provided (Fig. 38.22). The cables are tightened in a distal-to-proximal direction. In cases in which the native humeral cortex is excessively thin, fresh frozen allograft cortical struts are placed around the native humerus beneath the cables before tightening to provide additional support to the proximal humerus (Fig. 38.23).

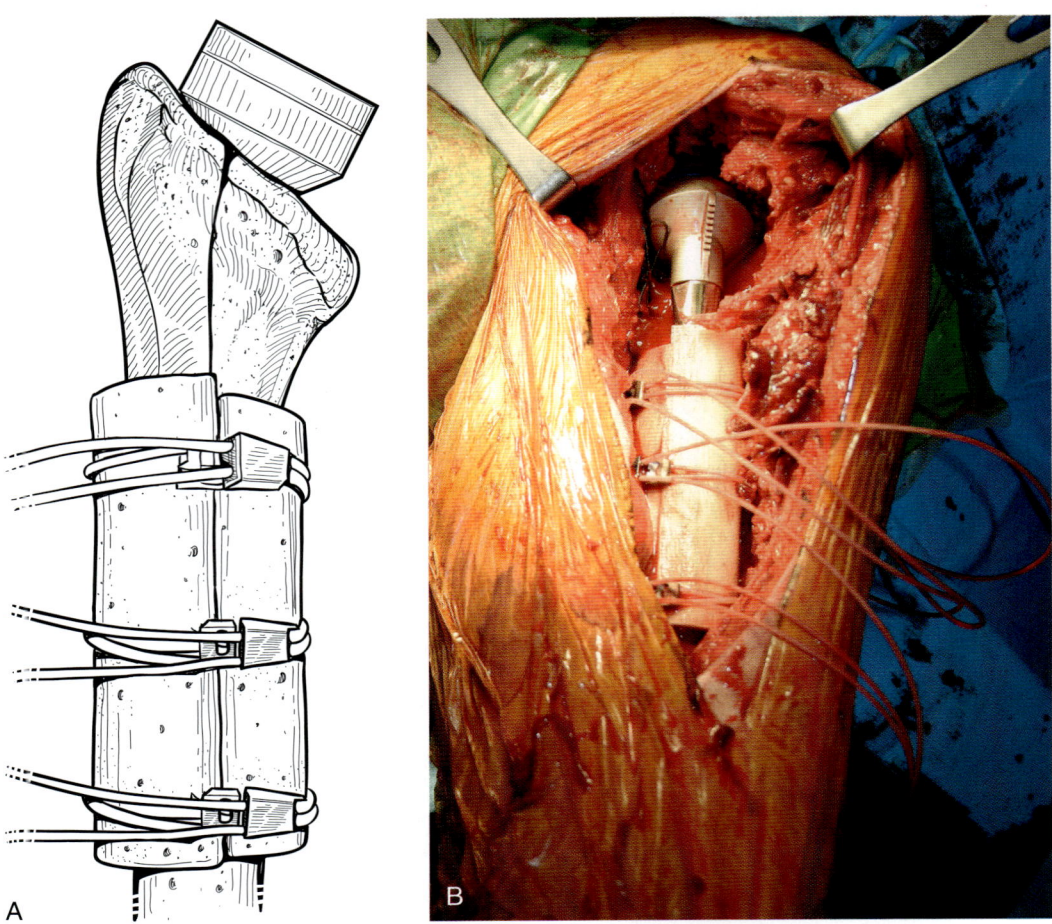

FIGURE 38.23 (A and B) Cortical allograft struts can be used to reinforce the proximal humerus in patients with severe osteopenia.

the release continues initially to only the 6 o'clock position. These patients often have a distended posterior capsule, so no more release is performed than is absolutely necessary to avoid compromising these posterior structures further. If release to only the 6 o'clock position proves inadequate later in the procedure during glenoid reaming, the release can be extended at that time. A Cobb elevator can be used to check the release for completeness.

If a glenoid component has previously been placed, removal is usually simple because most of these components are loose in the revision scenario. After the humeral component has been removed, the proximal humerus is retracted posteriorly with a humeral head retractor. Soft tissue is removed circumferentially from around the glenoid component with the needle tip electrocautery (Fig. 38.27). The inferior capsule is released just as in cases in which no glenoid component has previously been placed. After the periphery of the glenoid component has been cleared of soft tissue, a half-inch curved osteotome is used to lever the glenoid component gently out of the native glenoid (Fig. 38.28). Loose cement fragments and fibrous tissue are removed with forceps and a rongeur. Any residual cement fixed to the native glenoid is removed with a quarter-inch straight osteotome. Only when all residual cement and fibrous tissue have been removed can the osseous defect in the remaining native glenoid be properly evaluated and classified as contained or uncontained (Fig. 38.29).

SPECIAL SITUATIONS

Periprosthetic Fracture

If a periprosthetic fracture is encountered either preoperatively or intraoperatively, the fracture site may be used for removal of the humeral stem. The radial nerve must be identified and protected. Working through the fracture site, the humeral stem may be removed by striking the distal tip of the humeral component with a mallet and bone tamp (Fig. 38.30). This should be performed only after proper exposure plus release of the proximal humerus has been achieved. This technique may eliminate the need for a humeral osteotomy.

Infection

In cases of confirmed or suspected infection (based on the preoperative infection work-up; see Chapter 36), no preoperative antibiotics are administered. After the glenohumeral joint is opened, samples are taken for multiple cultures, including aerobic, anaerobic, fungal, and mycobacterial, and

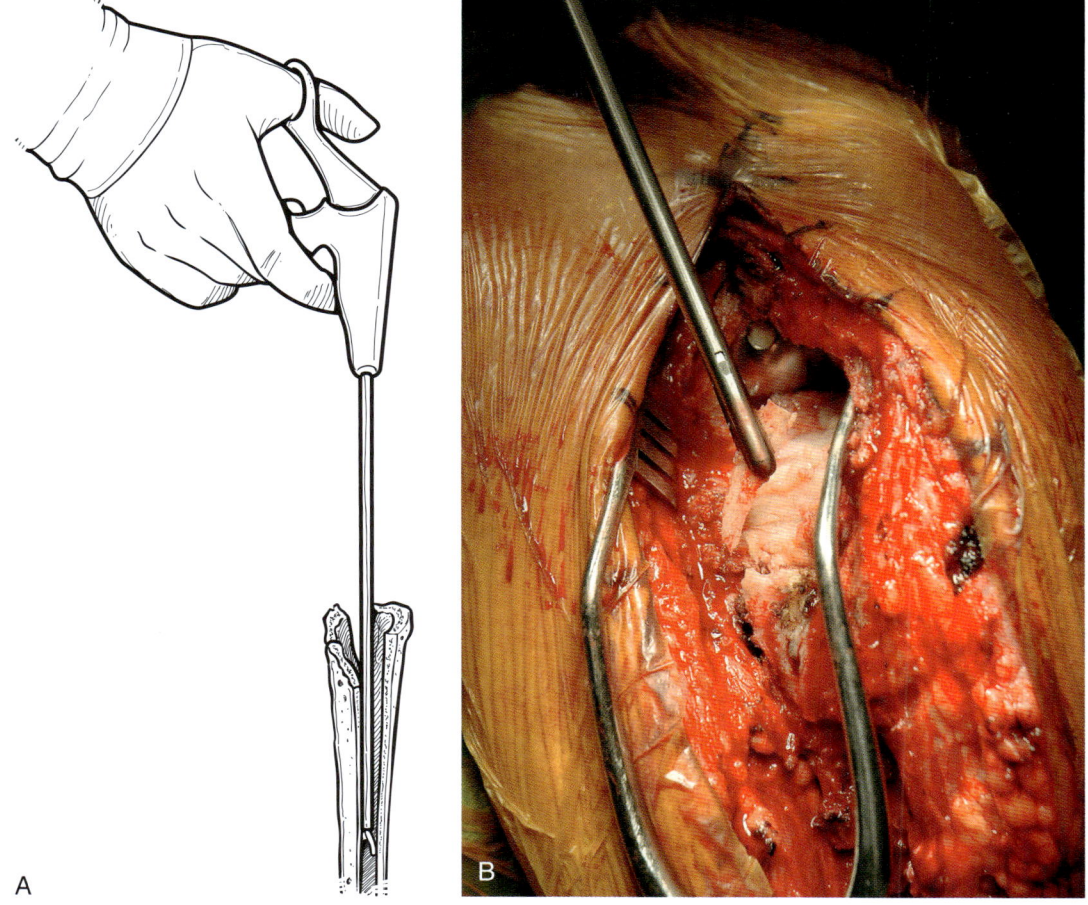

FIGURE 38.24 (A and B) Loose cement within the humeral canal is removed with pituitary-type forceps.

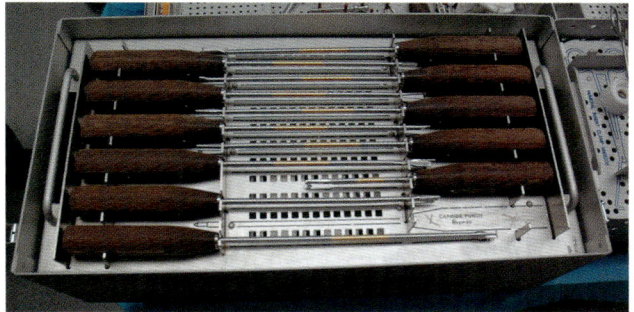

FIGURE 38.25 Cement removal osteotomes.

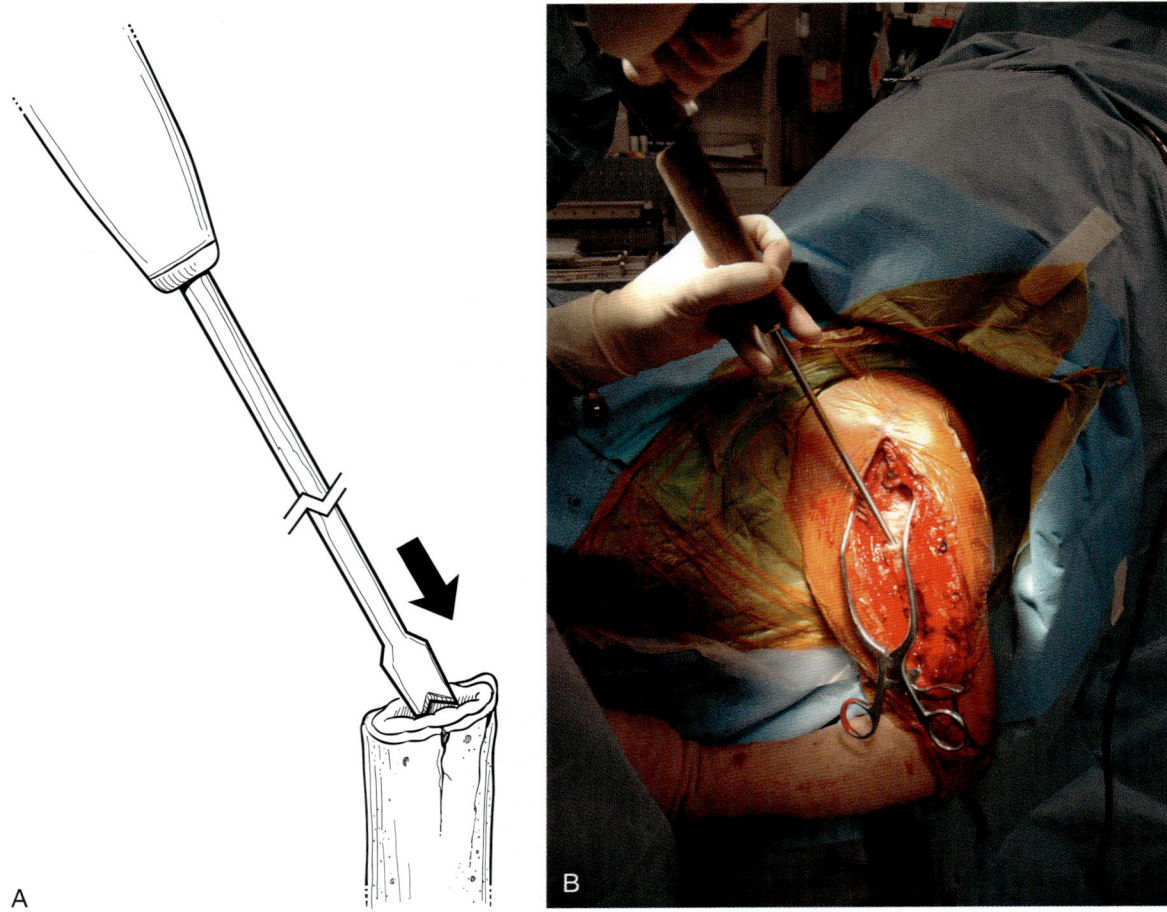

FIGURE 38.26 (A and B) Removal of the proximal cement mantle with specialized osteotomes.

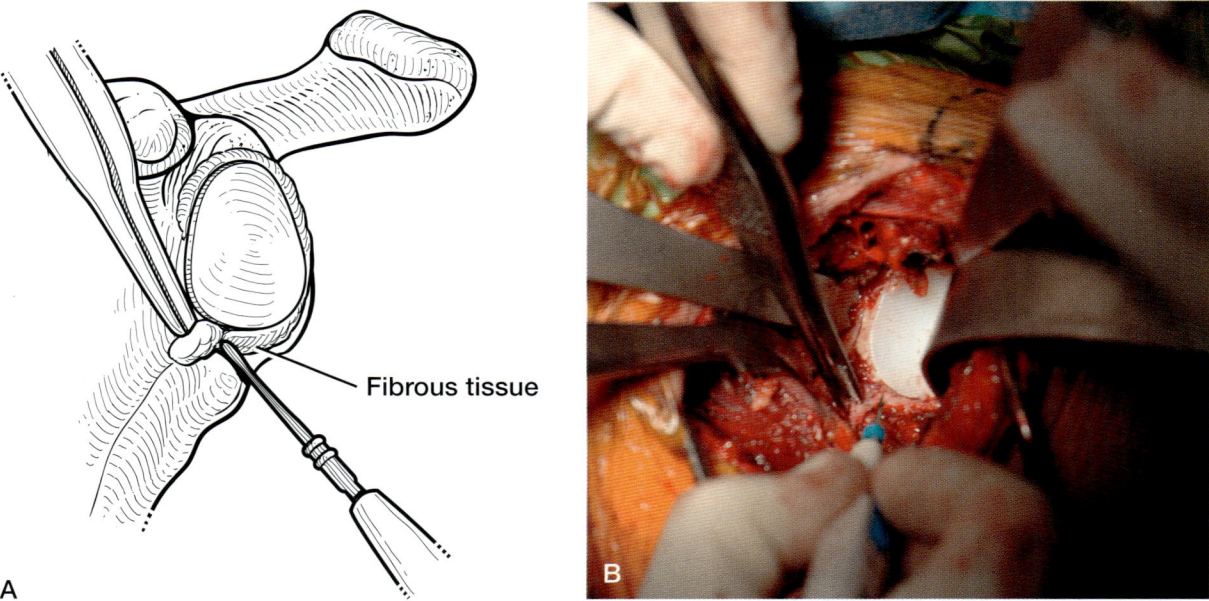

FIGURE 38.27 (A and B) Soft tissue is removed circumferentially from around the glenoid component.

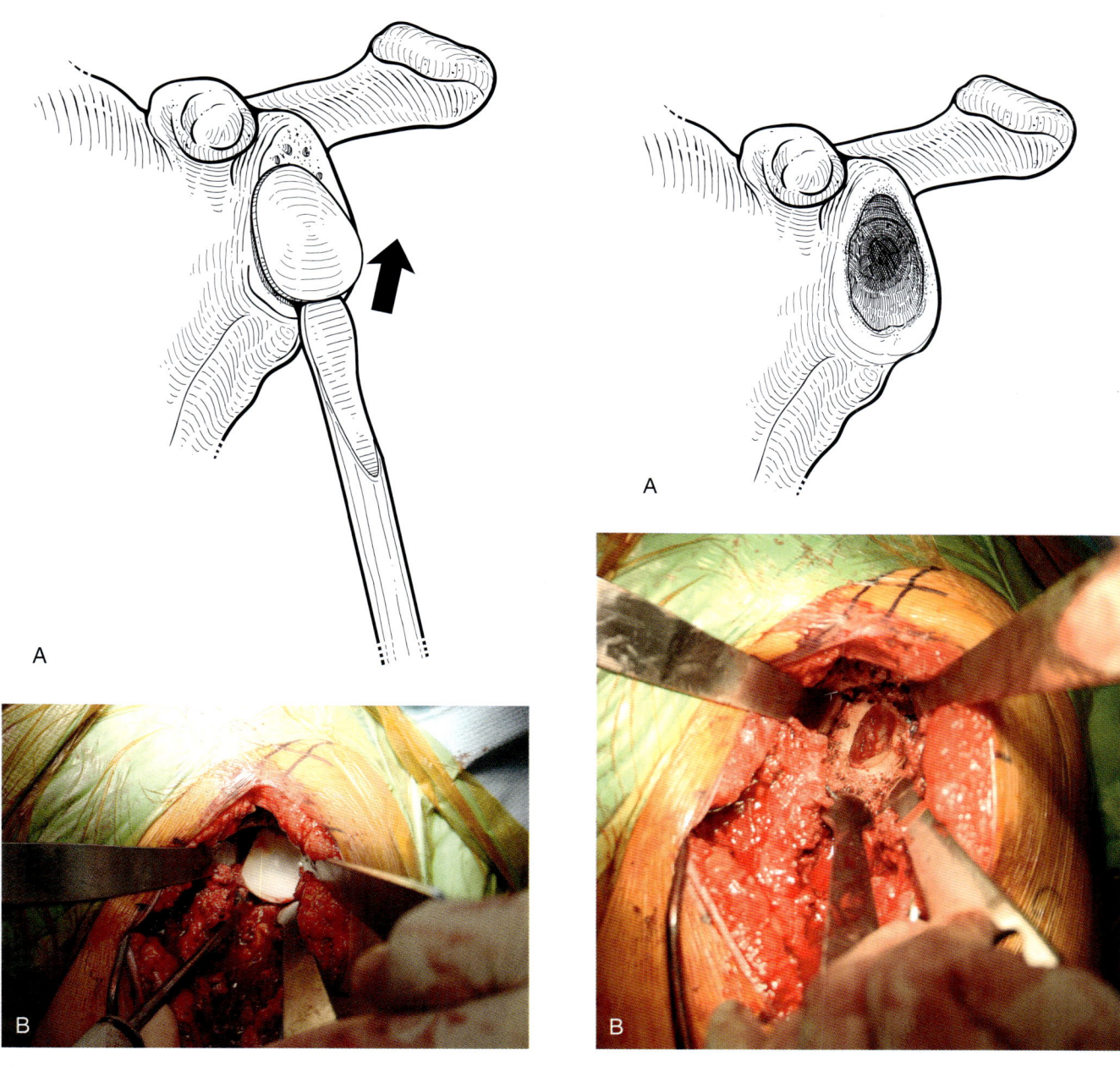

FIGURE 38.28 (A and B) A curved osteotome is used to gently lever the glenoid implant from the native glenoid bone.

FIGURE 38.29 (A and B) Osseous defect remaining in the glenoid after removal of the glenoid component and cement.

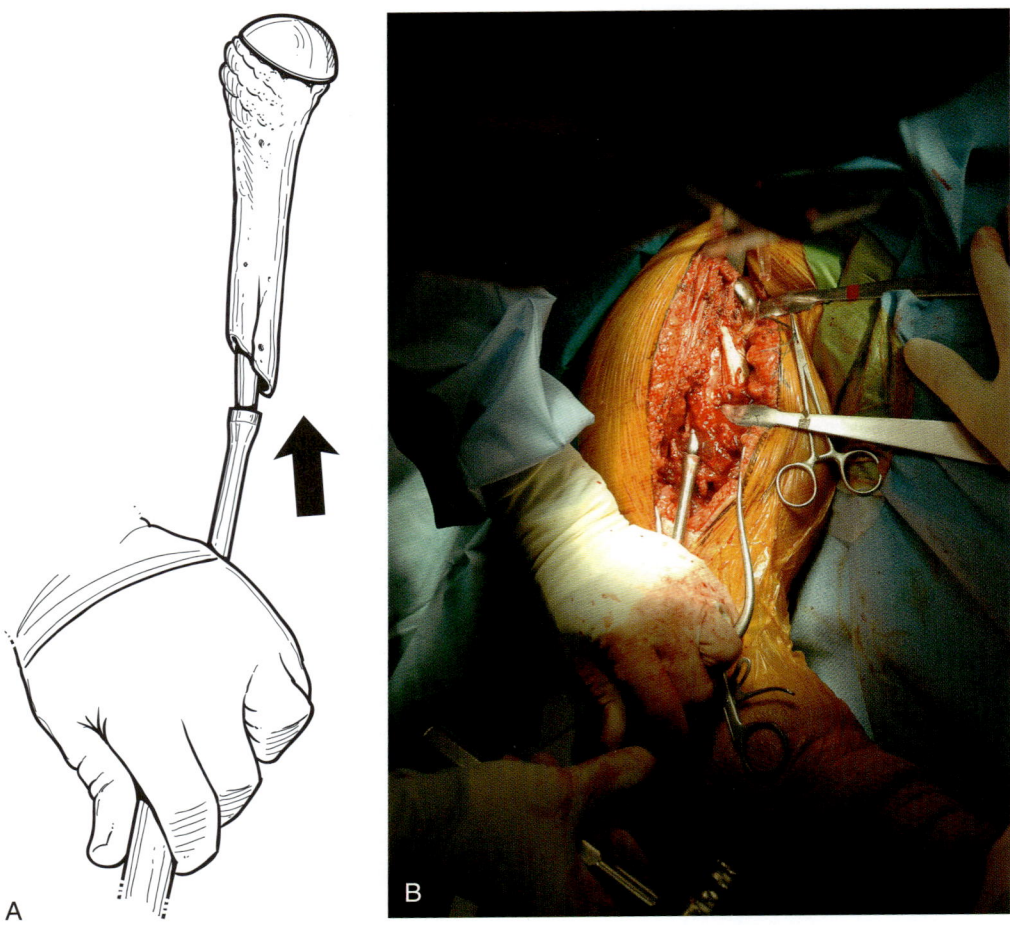

FIGURE 38.30 (A and B) Removal of the humeral stem through a periprosthetic fracture site.

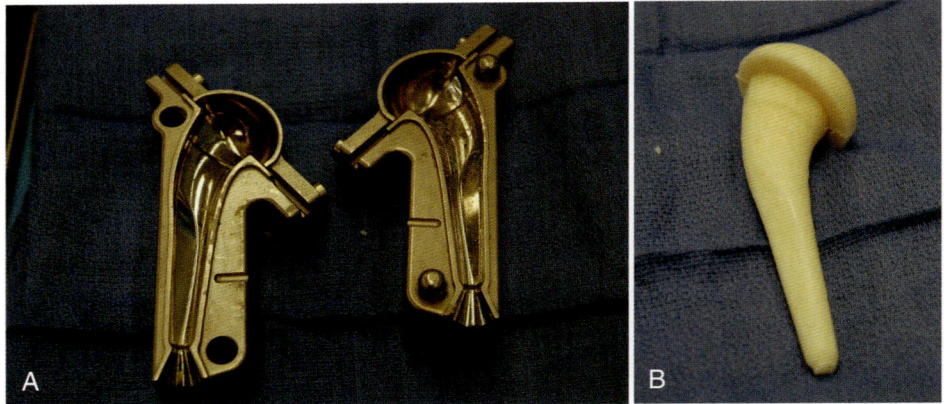

FIGURE 38.31 (A) Mold used for fabrication of antibiotic cement spacer. (B) Antibiotic cement spacer used in staged revision arthroplasty after infection.

the cultures are held for 21 days to allow for detection of *Propionibacterium acnes* and *Staphylococcus epidermidis*. We routinely send fluid and soft tissue specimen for analysis. After these samples are taken for culture, standard perioperative antibiotics are administered.

In cases of possible or suspected infection (preoperative aspiration negative, but other indicators of infection present), multiple synovial biopsy samples are submitted for intraoperative frozen section evaluation. While the pathologist is evaluating the tissue, the procedure continues with removal of the primary components. If findings on frozen section are indicative of infection (more than five polymorphonuclear leukocytes per high-power field in five consecutive fields) or in the case of confirmed infection (positive culture on preoperative aspirates), the components are removed and a custom-molded antibiotic-impregnated polymethylmethacrylate cement spacer is inserted as the first stage of a two-stage revision (Fig. 38.31).[2] We are more aggressive in cement removal from the proximal humerus in cases of infection and remove as much cement from the primary arthroplasty as possible without severely damaging the proximal humerus. In addition, in all cases of suspected infection, thorough irrigation is performed with at least 9 L of antibiotic-impregnated sterile saline (50,000 units bacitracin per liter sterile normal saline) introduced with a pulse lavage irrigator. Any necrotic-appearing tissue is sharply débrided.

The cement spacer is created with fast-setting bone cement (DePuy CMW 2, DePuy, Inc., Warsaw, Indiana). Two grams of vancomycin powder is mixed into each bag of cement. Two bags of cement are usually required for an average-size patient. In patients allergic to vancomycin, 2.4 g of tobramycin powder is mixed into each bag of cement. In cases with a preoperative culture positive infection, the antibiotic sensitivities can indicate the appropriate antibiotic to use in the antibiotic cement. As the cement becomes doughy, it is introduced into the cement spacer mold and allowed to polymerize.

Occasionally, we treat a patient with a chronically infected shoulder arthroplasty who is not a candidate for staged revision arthroplasty. In this case, we treat the patient by removing the prosthetic implants, performing irrigation and débridement, and implanting antibiotic-impregnated absorbable calcium sulfate pellets (Stimulan, Biocomposites, Ltd., Wilmington, North Carolina). A 10-mL package of pellets is mixed with 1 g of vancomycin or with 1.2 g of tobramycin for a vancomycin-allergic patient. Two 10-mL packages are usually sufficient to fill to the defect left by removal of the implant (Fig. 38.32).

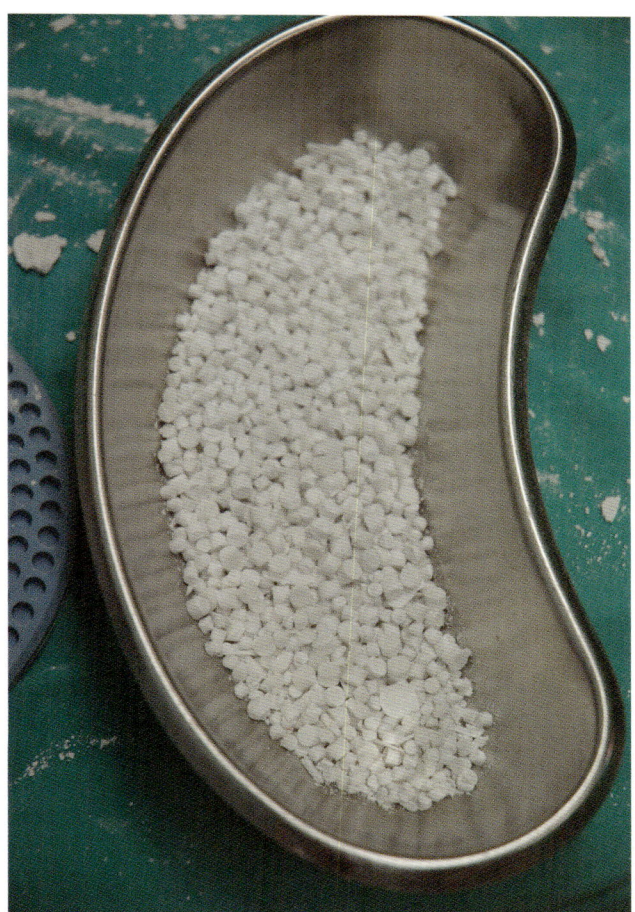

FIGURE 38.32 Absorbable antibiotic-impregnated pellets used for the treatment of an infected arthroplasty in a patient who is not a candidate for a staged revision arthroplasty.

REFERENCES

1. Walch G, Edwards TB, Boulahia A: Revision of the humeral stem: technical problems and complications. In Walch G, Boileau P, Molé D, editors: *2000 Prosthèses d'Epaule…Recul de 2 à 10 Ans*, Paris, 2001, Sauramps Medical, pp 443–454.
2. Feldman DS, Lonner JH, Desai P, et al: The role of intraoperative frozen sections in revision total joint arthroplasty, *J Bone Joint Surg Am* 77:1807–1813, 1995.

CHAPTER 39

Humeral component

Reconstruction of the proximal humerus can be a very difficult aspect of revision shoulder arthroplasty. During extraction of the previous humeral stem, every effort should be made to preserve as much native proximal humeral bone as possible (see Chapter 38). The overall condition of the proximal humerus and rotator cuff plays a significant role in determining the type of implant to be used in revision surgery (unconstrained vs. semiconstrained). In cases in which the rotator cuff is largely functional, preservation of the greater and lesser tuberosities helps to dictate which type of revision implant to use during revision surgery. After the type of revision implant to be used is selected, preparation of the proximal humerus and implantation of the humeral component proceed just as for primary arthroplasty. This chapter details our techniques for reconstruction and preparation of the proximal humerus and implantation of the humeral component in revision shoulder arthroplasty.

TECHNIQUE FOR PREPARATION OF THE PROXIMAL HUMERUS

Preparation of the proximal humerus is largely dependent on the residual osseous anatomy of the proximal humerus after the previously placed humeral stem has been extracted. In cases in which extraction of the previous humeral stem was relatively uncomplicated, with minimal compromise of the proximal humeral metaphysis and tuberosities, preparation of the proximal humerus can be straightforward and similar to proximal humeral preparation for primary shoulder arthroplasty. In cases in which the proximal humeral osseous anatomy has been compromised either before or during extraction of the humeral stem, preparation of the proximal humerus becomes substantially more complicated.

When proximal humeral osseous anatomy is well preserved, proximal humeral preparation for either an unconstrained stem or a reverse stem is performed similar to cases of primary arthroplasty.

Unconstrained Humeral Stem

In revision cases in which we are going to implant an unconstrained proximal humeral stem, we prefer to implant a cementless short stem whenever possible. If fixation into the metaphysis seems compromised, we will opt for a slightly longer stem (Fig. 39.1). Only in cases of periprosthetic fracture or when we have to bypass a humeral diaphyseal osteotomy used for stem extraction do we opt for a long-stem humeral component (Fig. 39.2). Only if press fit of the humeral component is deemed inadequate do we consider cementing the humeral component.

When using a short stem for revision, the humeral diaphysis is sounded just as in primary unconstrained arthroplasty (Fig. 39.3; see Chapter 11). The proximal humerus is then prepared using broaches for the standard short stem or the slightly longer stem, depending on the quality of the proximal humeral bone (Fig. 39.4).

After a humeral stem of appropriate size is selected, the proximal humerus can be planed, if necessary, to match the inclination of the humeral implant (Fig. 39.5). The appropriate size trial humeral head is then placed on the final humeral broach. The prosthetic head should provide adequate coverage of the proximal humeral metaphysis but not overhang the humerus at any portion. The system that we use allows variable medial-to-lateral and anterior-to-posterior offset. The prosthetic humeral head is placed on the trial humeral stem at the various offset positions to allow selection of the best offset index (Fig. 39.6). After the proper index has been selected, the glenohumeral joint is reduced and humeral version is judged. With the arm in neutral rotation, the center of the prosthetic humeral head should align with the center of the glenoid, provided that osseous glenoid morphology is intact and does not demonstrate a nonconcentric wear pattern (Fig. 39.7). In cases with nonconcentric glenoid morphology or cases in which the osseous glenoid is compromised, we judge humeral version by placing the prosthesis in approximately 30 degrees of retroversion relative to the long axis of the forearm (Fig. 39.8). The humeral stem retroversion can also be determined by using the version rod on the insertion handle relative to the forearm. If the version of the trial humeral stem is unacceptable, the humeral trial is removed and humeral version changed by revising the original plane of humeral head resection by way of a revision humeral cut to introduce more retroversion or anteversion, as deemed appropriate by the trial glenohumeral reduction. The trial humeral implant is reinserted and the trial reduction repeated to ensure that humeral version has been corrected acceptably.

Reverse-Design Humeral Stem

In cases in which a reverse-design humeral implant is to be used as the revision humeral stem and the osseous proximal humerus is relatively preserved, the proximal humerus is prepared in much the same way as for insertion of a reverse prosthesis as a primary implant (see Chapter 21). For revision

Text continued on p. 385

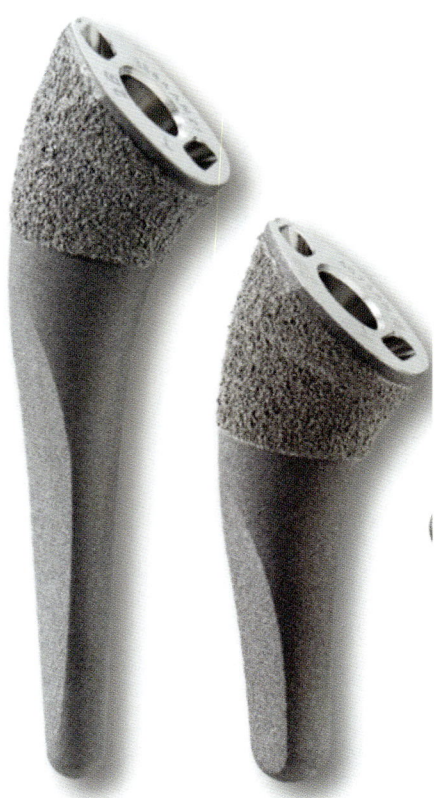

FIGURE 39.1 Unconstrained stems used in revision shoulder arthroplasty.

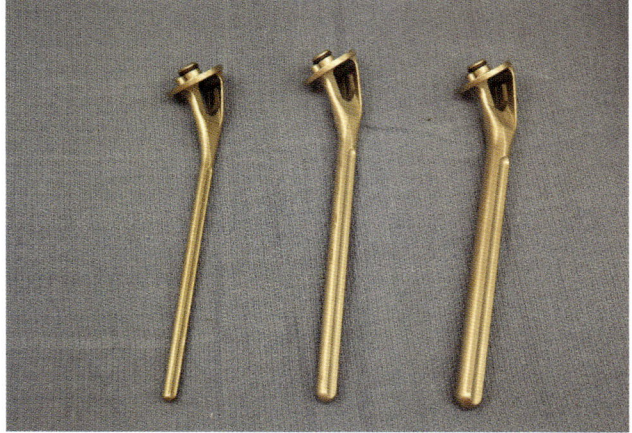

FIGURE 39.2 Long-stem unconstrained humeral implants used in the treatment of a periprosthetic fracture or when a diaphyseal humeral osteotomy has been required for stem removal.

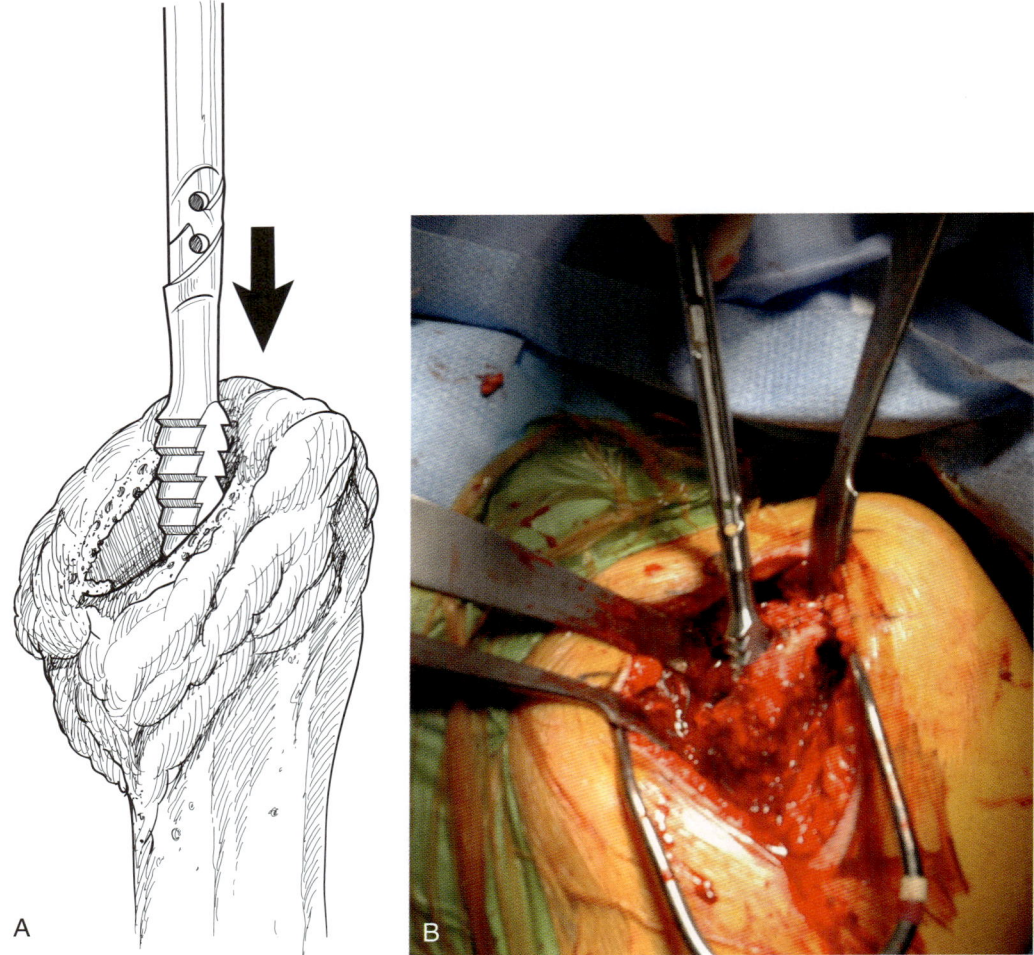

FIGURE 39.3 (A and B) The humeral canal is sounded to determine appropriate size of the humeral component.

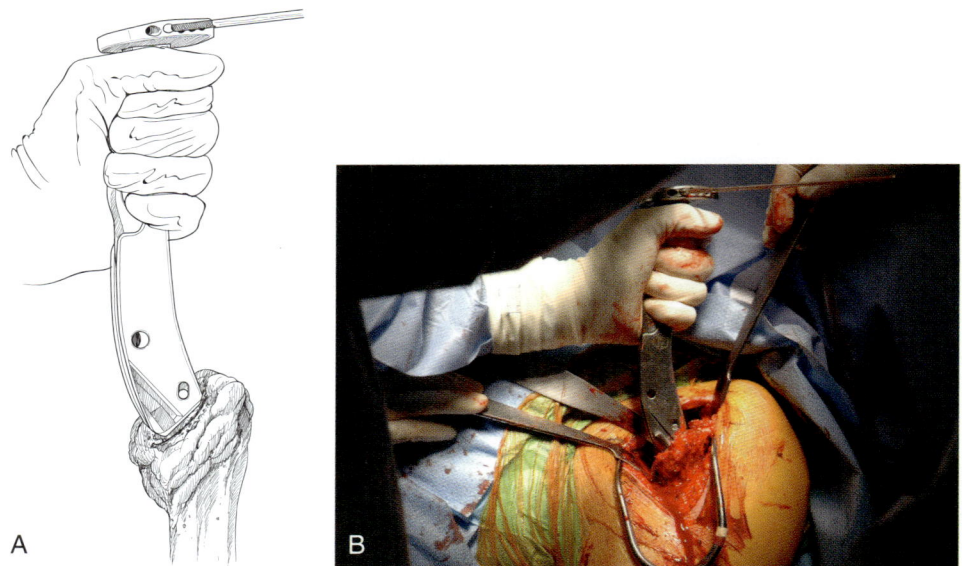

FIGURE 39.4 (A and B) Broaching of the proximal humerus.

CHAPTER 39 ■ Humeral Component

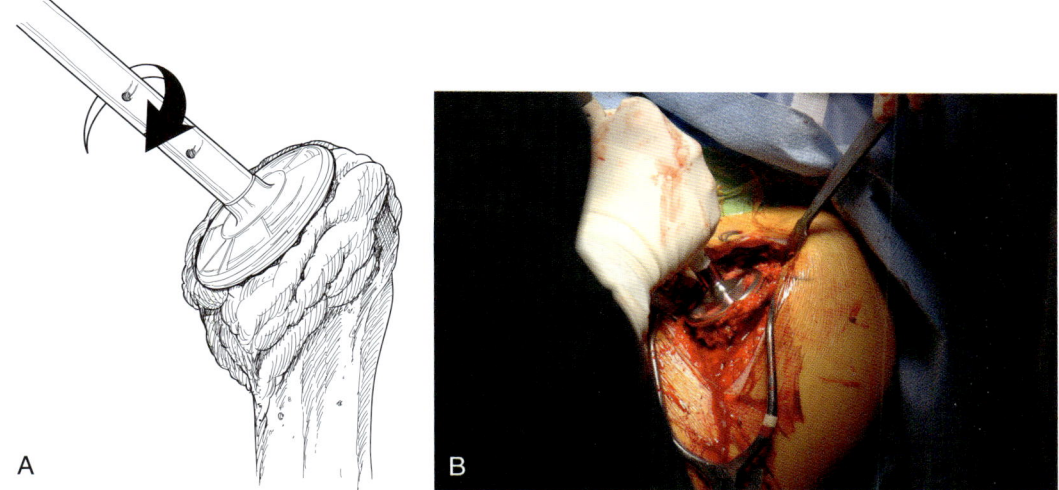

FIGURE 39.5 (A and B) The proximal humerus can be planed if necessary to match the inclination of the humeral implant.

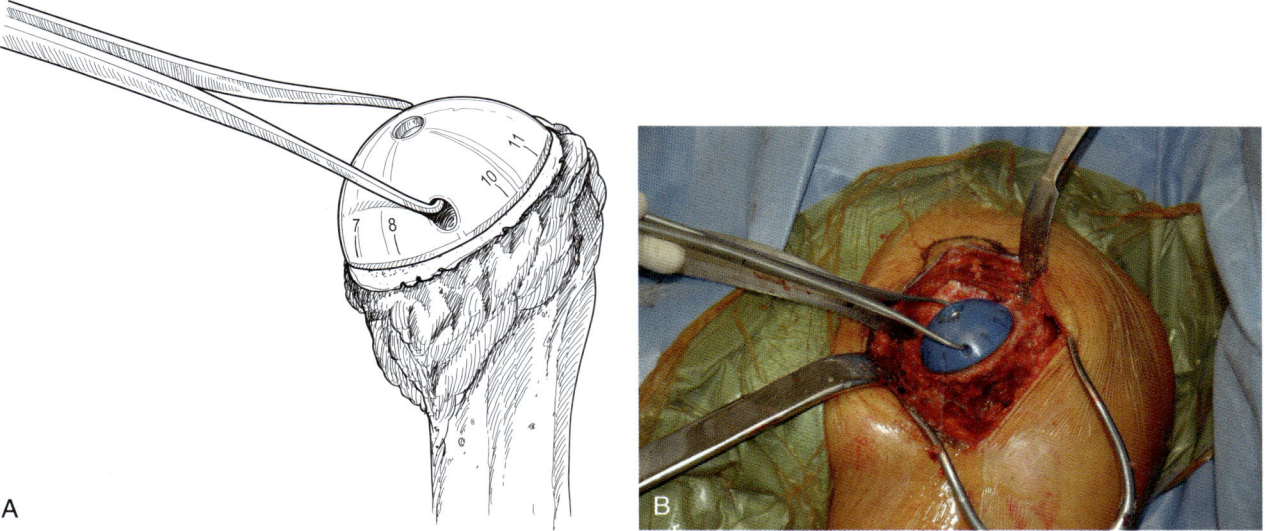

FIGURE 39.6 (A and B) The appropriate size trial humeral head is then placed on the final humeral broach.

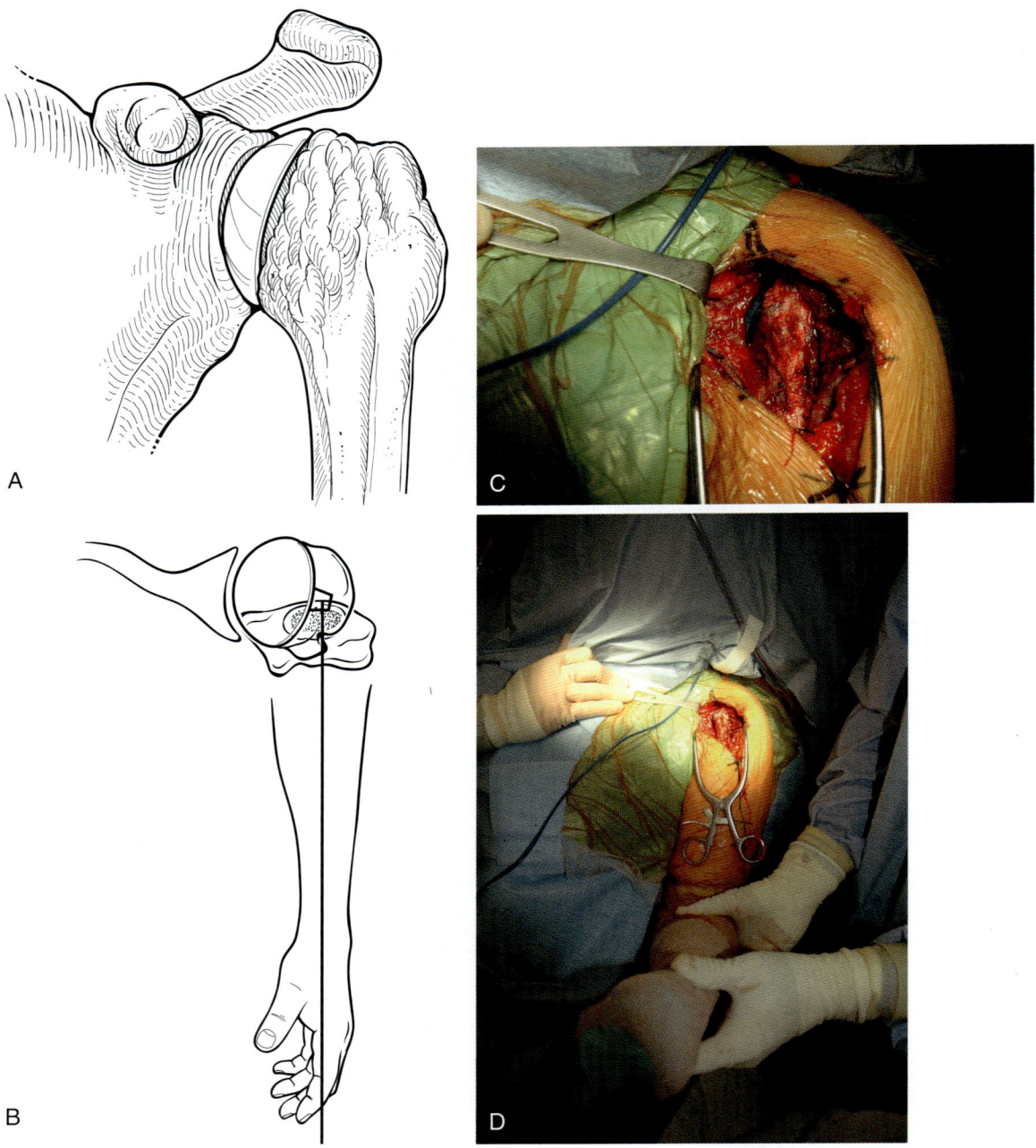

FIGURE 39.7 (A to D) Judgment of humeral version during revision shoulder arthroplasty by ensuring that the prosthetic head is centered in the glenoid with the arm in neutral rotation.

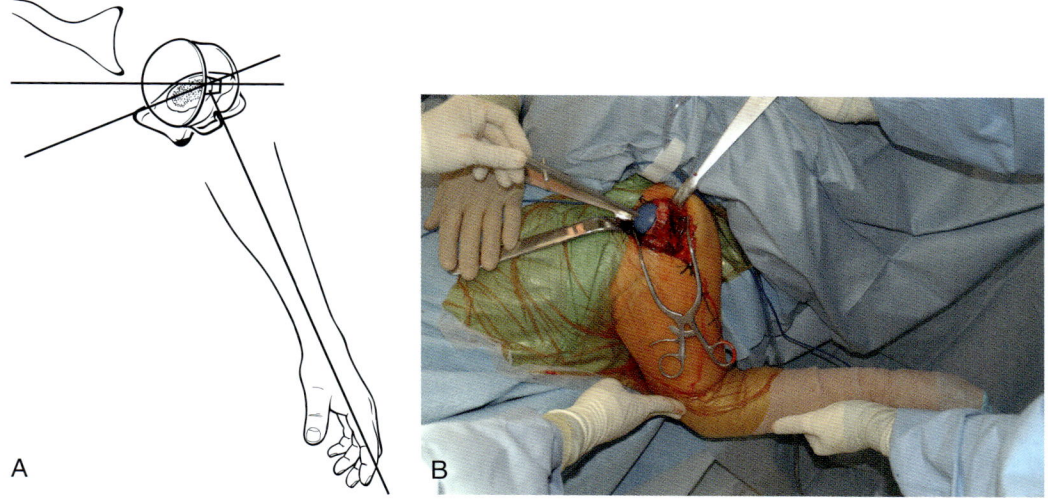

FIGURE 39.8 (A and B) Judgment of humeral version during revision shoulder arthroplasty by placing the humeral stem in 30 degrees of retroversion relative to the long axis of the forearm. This technique is used in patients with nonconcentric glenoid wear or in those with glenoid osseous deficiency.

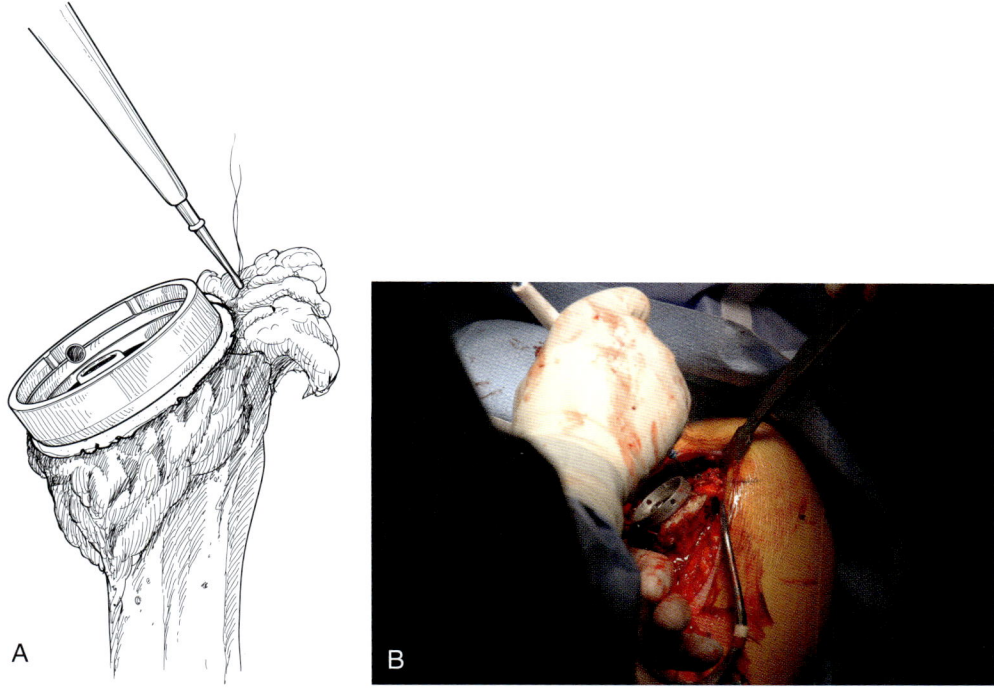

FIGURE 39.9 (A and B) Marking retroversion of the humeral component during revision shoulder arthroplasty with a reverse prosthesis.

using the reverse short stem, the diaphyseal and metaphyseal preparation is identical to revision using an unconstrained short stem (see Figs. 39.3 to 39.5). In cases in which identifiable anatomic landmarks that would normally guide prosthetic version are absent (i.e., the posterior rotator cuff), humeral broach is placed in approximately 30 degrees of humeral retroversion by using the forearm referencing insertion instrument. The position of the lateral aspect of the humeral implant is marked on the proximal humerus with the electrocautery (Fig. 39.9).

Revision cases with proximal humeral insufficiency may require proximal humeral osseous reconstruction with a bone graft. In general, in any case in which the rotator cuff insertion is compromised and glenoid bone stock allows, we will use a reverse prosthesis for revision arthroplasty. In cases of proximal humeral insufficiency limited to the proximal humeral metaphysis, no bone graft is indicated because the reverse prosthesis can be implanted into a proximal humerus that is partially compromised (Fig. 39.10). In cases in which proximal humeral bone loss includes the entire proximal humeral metaphysis and extends into proximal humeral diaphysis, bone graft reconstruction of the proximal humeral diaphysis is indicated (Fig. 39.11). In some cases, only a portion of the proximal humeral diaphysis is deficient

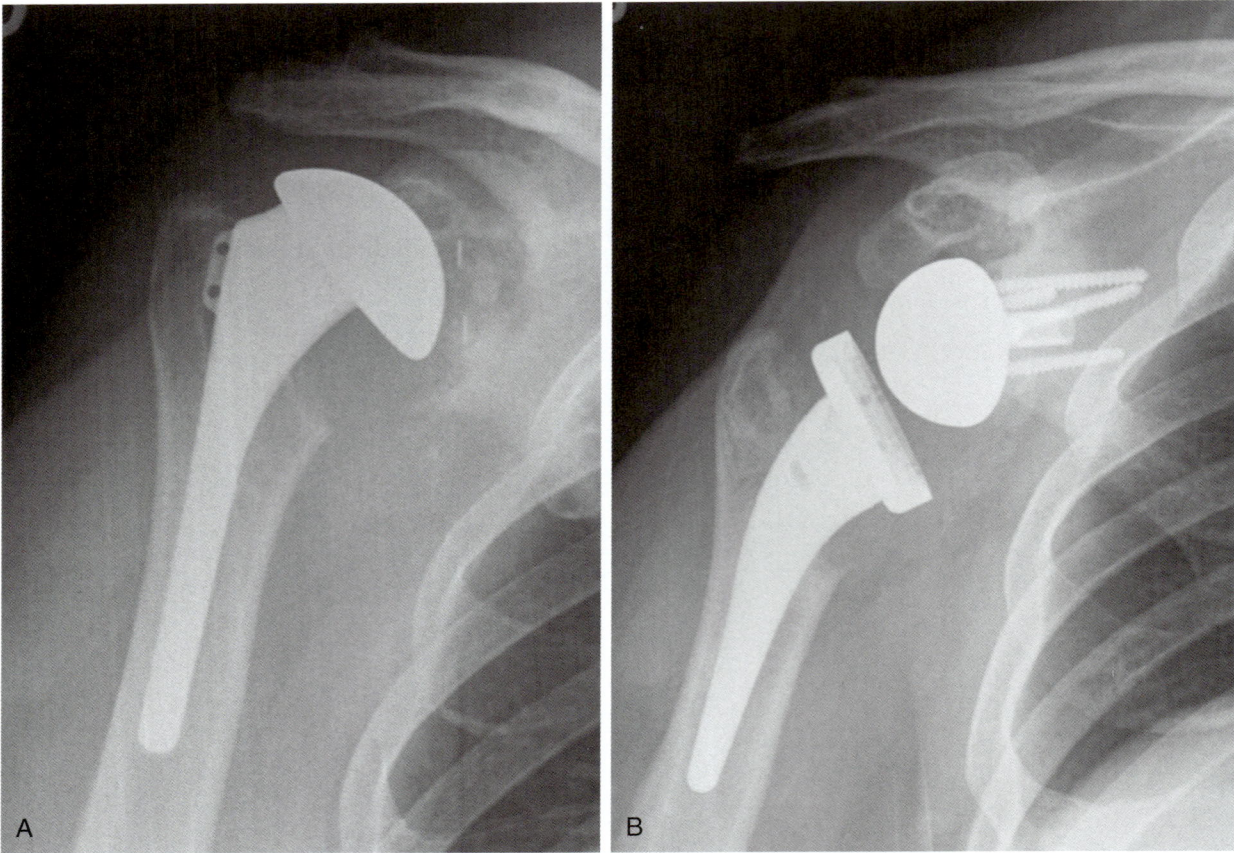

FIGURE 39.10 Patient with proximal humeral bone loss that did not require proximal humeral bone graft reconstruction before (A) and after (B) revision arthroplasty with a reverse prosthesis.

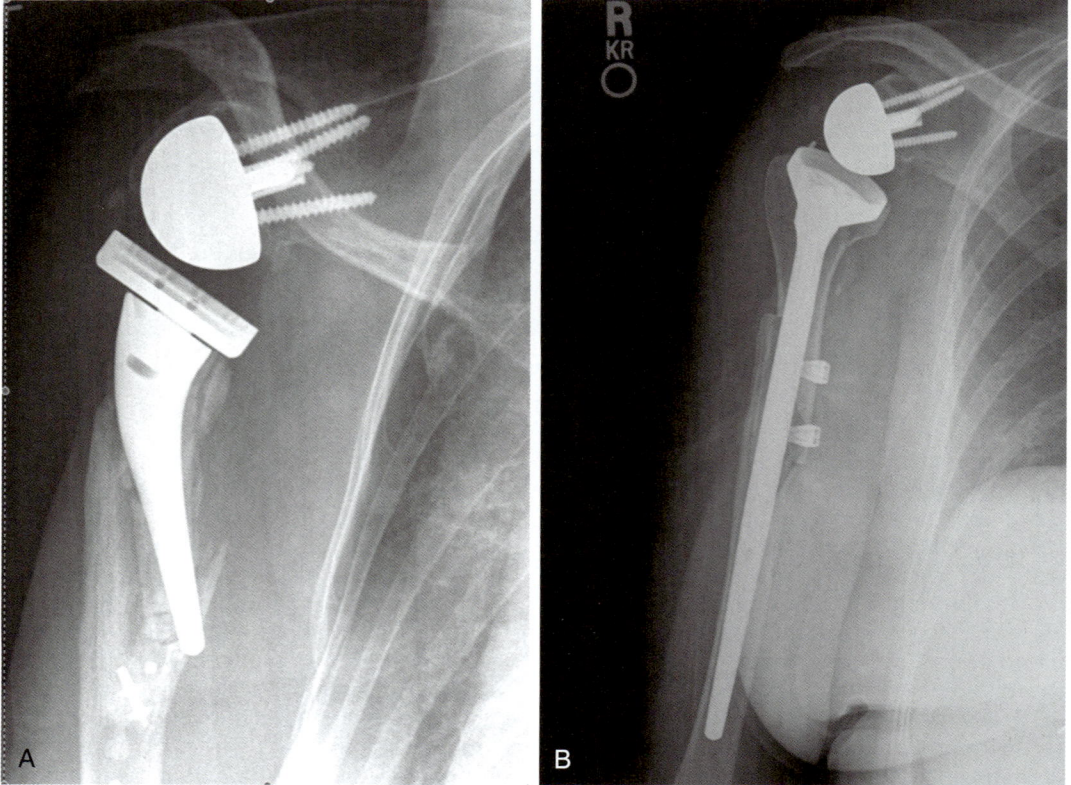

FIGURE 39.11 Patient with severe proximal humeral bone loss that required proximal humeral bone graft reconstruction before (A) and after (B) revision arthroplasty with a reverse prosthesis.

(anterior or posterior). For this reason, we prefer to reconstruct only the portion that is deficient and leave any native bone intact. Fresh frozen cortical strips of allograft tibia are used for the reconstruction (Fig. 39.12).

In cases in which an allograft proximal humeral reconstruction is anticipated or a proximal humeral osteotomy has been performed for removal of the humeral stem, we place two or three cables composed of a nylon monofilament core wrapped in a braided ultrahigh-molecular-weight polyethylene (Kinamed, Inc., Camarillo, CA) subperiosteally around the residual native humerus with the cable-passing instrumentation provided (Fig. 39.13). The cerclage cables are secured before removal of the trial humeral stem (see Chapter 38). In humeral osteotomy cases in which the native humeral cortex is excessively thin, fresh frozen allograft cortical struts are placed around the native humerus beneath the cables before tightening them to provide additional support for the proximal humerus, as shown in Chapter 38. The trial humeral stem is removed, and attention is turned to the glenoid, if indicated.

ALLOGRAFT RECONSTRUCTION OF THE PROXIMAL HUMERUS

Severe humeral metaphyseal bone loss in the revision setting clearly remains a challenge, and newer implants have been introduced to address the growing volume of revision reverse shoulder arthroplasty. Revision adjustable humeral implants are now available with press fit fixation. These adjustable humeral implants allow increased length options for severe humeral defects and are fixed within the native humeral diaphysis to improve deltoid tensioning. These implants are nearly always inserted with proximal humeral allografts in our practice.

Based on preoperative planning (see Chapter 36), an allograft is obtained of appropriate size. The humeral allograft is then prepared on the back table. Resection of the humeral head is performed using an intramedullary cutting guide in anatomic humeral version (Fig. 39.14). Epiphyseal preparation is performed with a 36-mm-diameter acetabular-type reamer while keeping the reamer's orientation perpendicular to the cut humeral surface (Fig. 39.15). Progressive diaphyseal reaming is performed until the appropriate diaphyseal diameter is attained, as evidenced by the diaphyseal reamer's reaching the inner humeral cortex (Fig. 39.16). The allograft is then cut to the appropriate length based on the preoperative

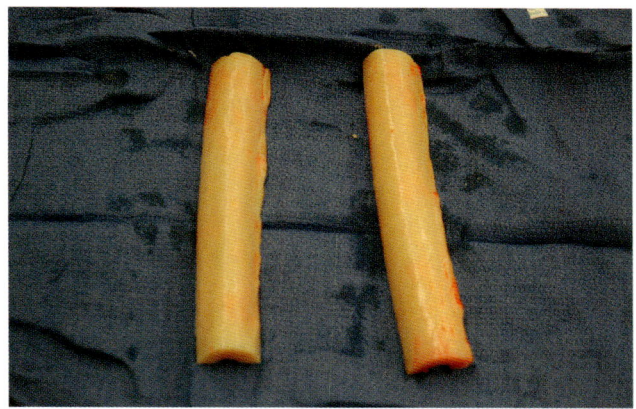

FIGURE 39.12 Fresh frozen allograft tibial strips used in proximal humeral reconstruction.

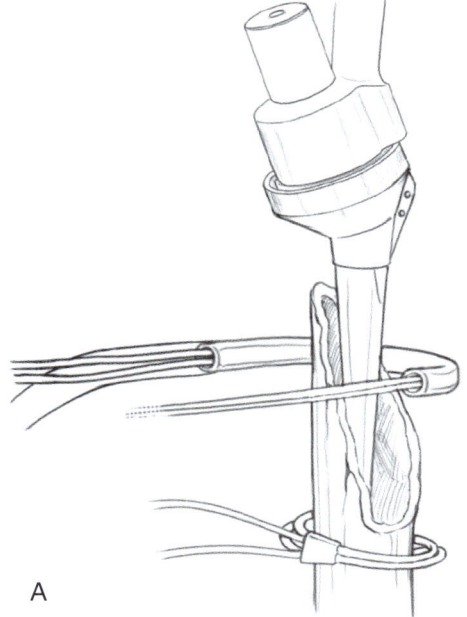
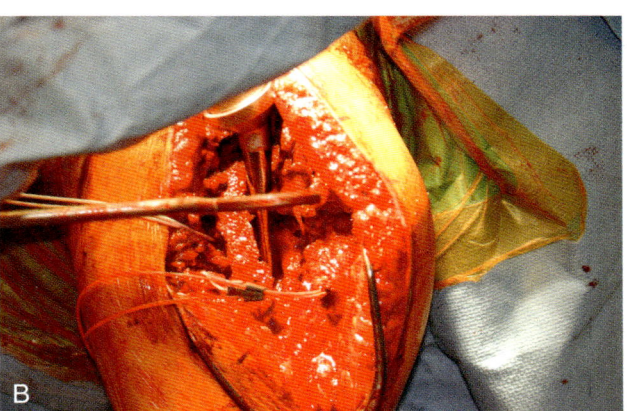

FIGURE 39.13 (A and B) Passage of fixation cables to secure the allograft during proximal humeral reconstruction.

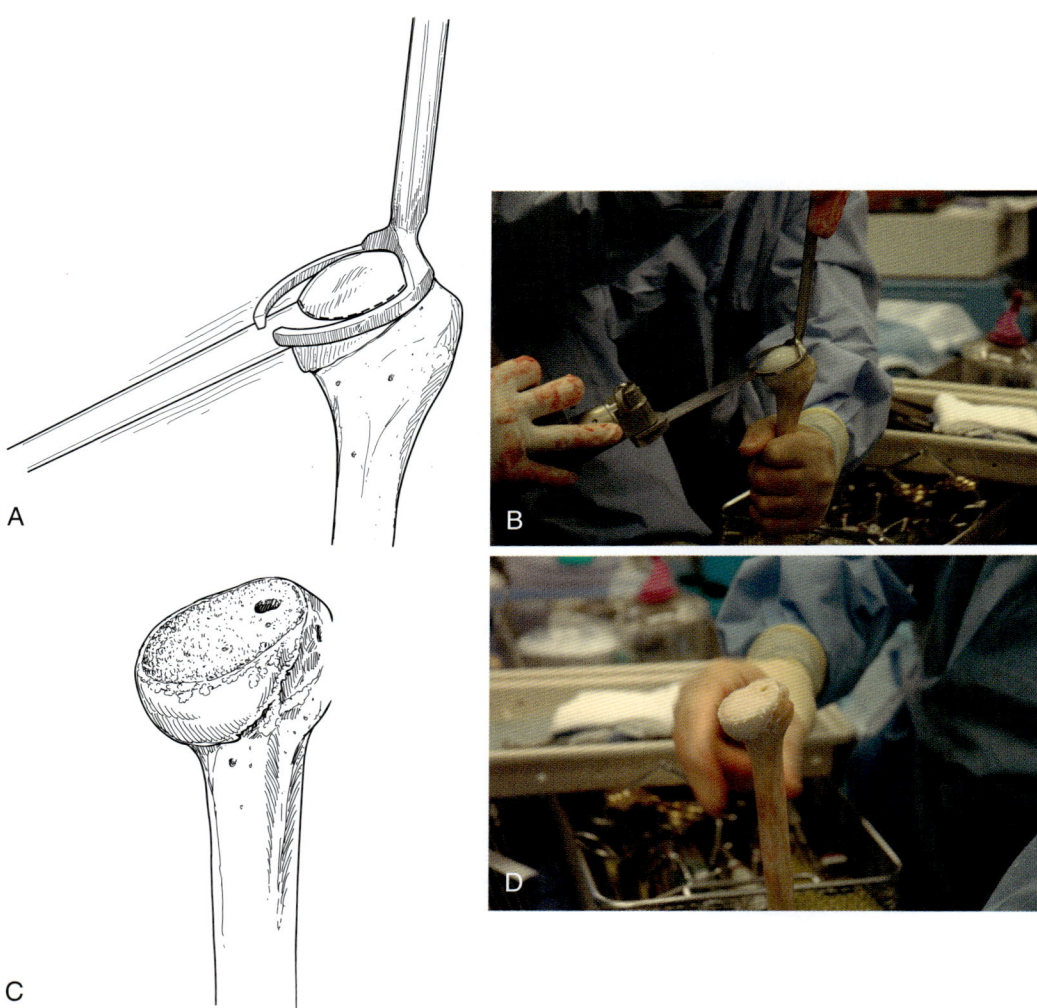

FIGURE 39.14 (A to D) Resection of the humeral head of a proximal humeral allograft to be used in a patient with severe proximal humeral bone loss.

CHAPTER 39 ■ Humeral Component

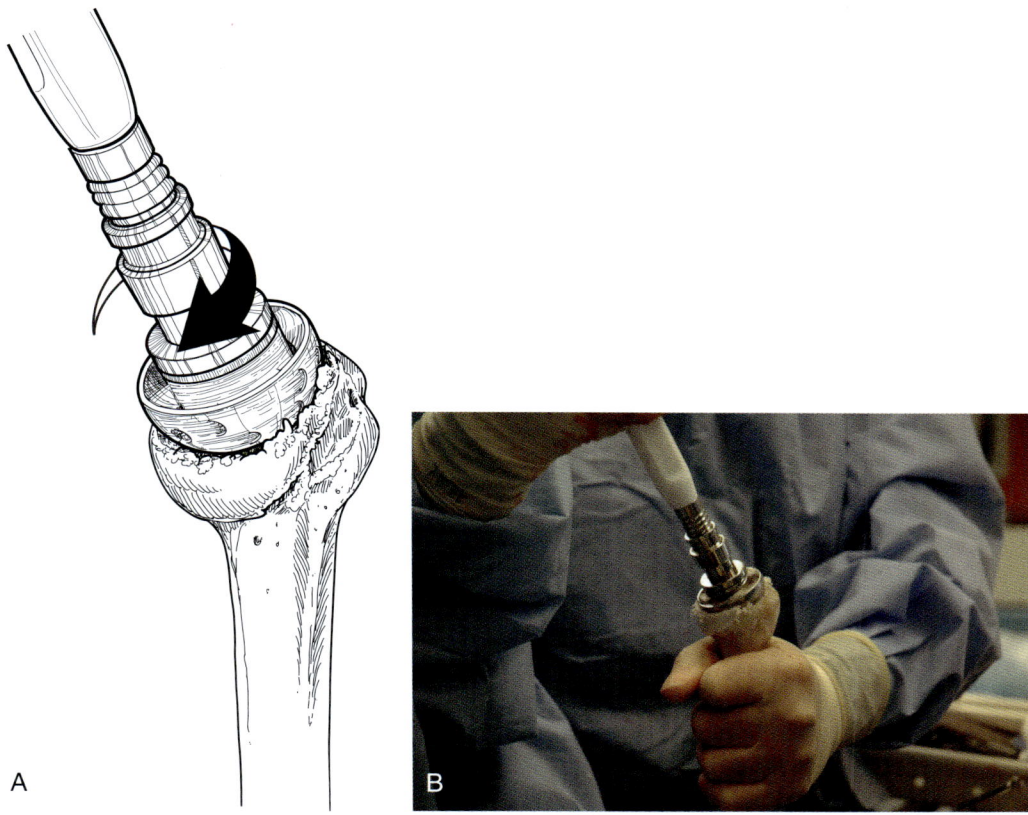

FIGURE 39.15 (A and B) Epiphyseal reaming of a proximal humeral allograft to be used in a patient with severe proximal humeral bone loss.

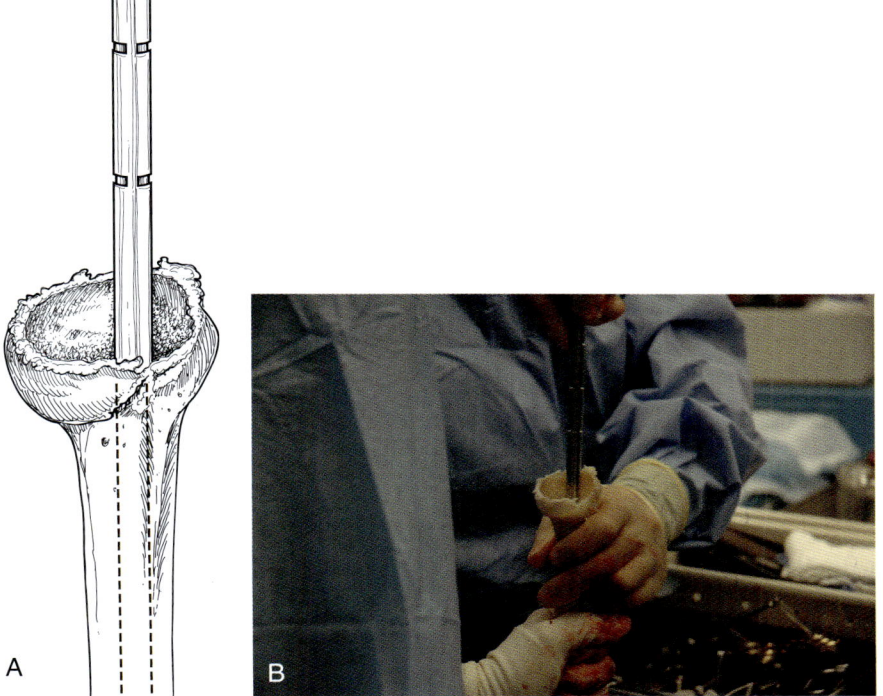

FIGURE 39.16 (A and B) Diaphyseal reaming of a proximal humeral allograft to be used in a patient with severe proximal humeral bone loss.

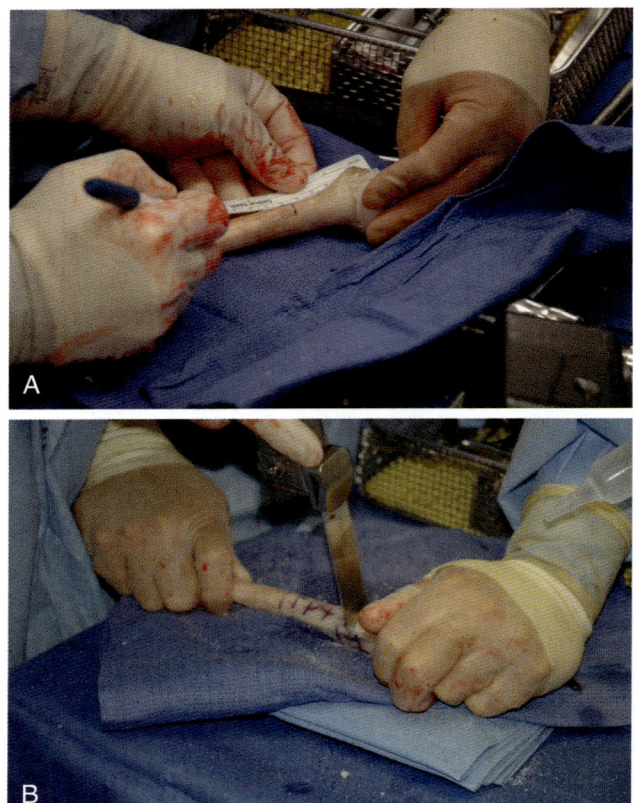

FIGURE 39.17 (A and B) The allograft is cut to the appropriate length based on the preoperative plan.

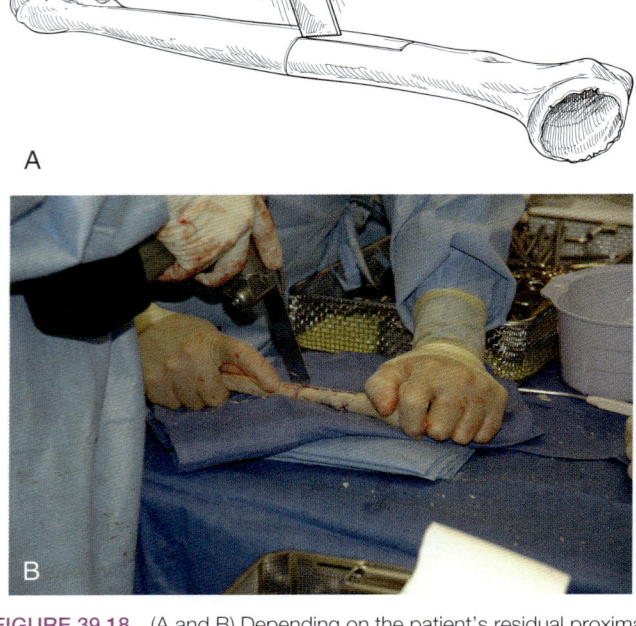

FIGURE 39.18 (A and B) Depending on the patient's residual proximal humeral morphology, a step cut may be used to facilitate graft fixation.

plan (Fig. 39.17). Depending on the patient's residual proximal humeral morphology, a step cut may be used to facilitate graft fixation (Fig. 39.18).

The residual native humerus is sized for the diaphyseal portion of the humeral implant (Fig. 39.19). The diaphyseal portion of the humeral implant is then placed (Fig. 39.20). The allograft is then placed (Fig. 39.21). The allograft is then fixed to the native humerus using cerclage cables at a step cut junction or with bridging allograft struts (Fig. 39.22).

TECHNIQUE FOR INSERTION OF A REVISION HUMERAL STEM

After any glenoid pathology has been addressed, the humeral stem may be implanted. We press-fit the humeral stem whenever possible. In cases in which an unconstrained shoulder arthroplasty is to be implanted, the trial humeral head is replaced after any glenoid procedure is completed and glenohumeral stability is evaluated. With the arm externally rotated approximately 30 degrees, force is applied in a posterior direction to the proximal humerus, as with primary unconstrained shoulder arthroplasty. The prosthetic humeral head should subluxate posteriorly approximately 30% to 50% of its diameter and spontaneously reduce on release of the posteriorly directed force. If spontaneous reduction does not occur, posterior capsulorrhaphy may be necessary, as described in Chapter 13. Conversely, if posterior translation of at least 30% of the diameter of the humeral head is not possible, posterior capsular release may be necessary.

After the shoulder is properly balanced, the final humeral implant is placed. Cement is used only in cases in which secure press fit fixation is not possible. Three no. 2 nonabsorbable braided sutures are placed first through the humeral stump of the subscapularis tendon, into the lesser tuberosity, and out through the intramedullary canal of the humerus for later use in reattachment of the subscapularis, as in cases of primary unconstrained shoulder arthroplasty (Fig. 39.23). These sutures are tagged with three different types of hemostats to identify the sutures as superior, middle, and inferior (we use a curved Kelly hemostat superiorly, a mosquito hemostat on the middle suture, and a regular hemostat inferiorly). The humeral canal is irrigated with sterile saline and dried with suction and gauze sponges. The final humeral implant is impacted into place (Fig. 39.24). The subscapularis is repaired with the previously placed transosseous sutures, as in cases of primary shoulder arthroplasty.

When implanting a reverse prosthesis during revision shoulder arthroplasty without significant proximal humeral bone loss, insertion of the humeral stem is performed nearly identically to primary reverse cases. We insert the trial humeral tray with the 6-mm polyethylene insert after

Text continued on p. 398

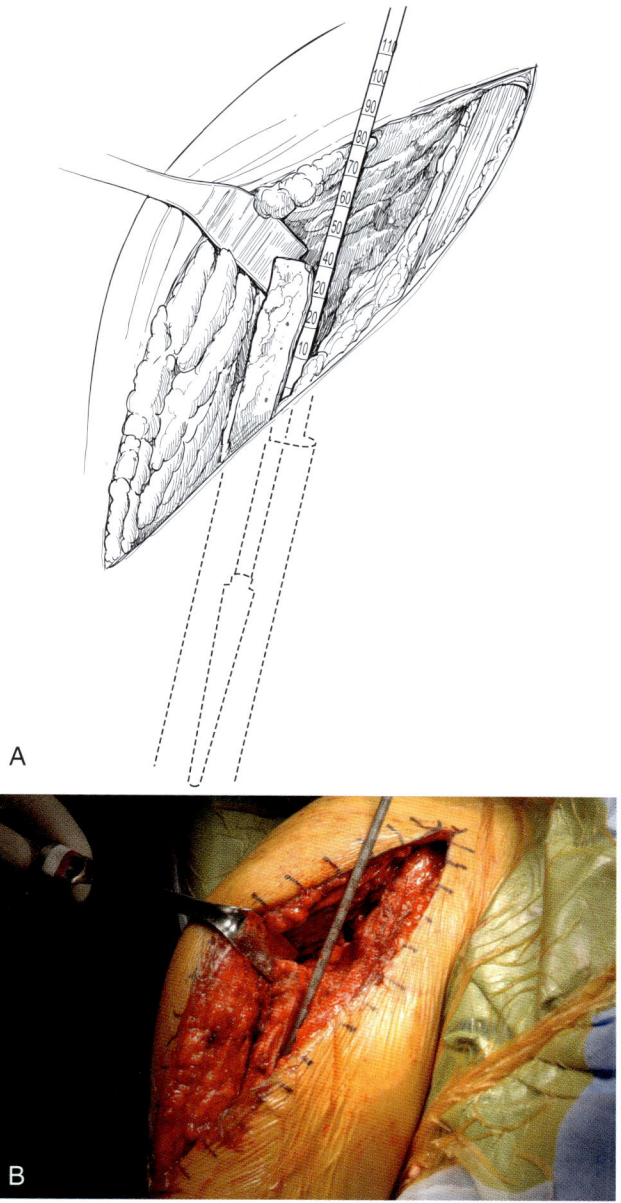

FIGURE 39.19 (A and B) The residual native humerus is sized for the diaphyseal portion of the humeral implant.

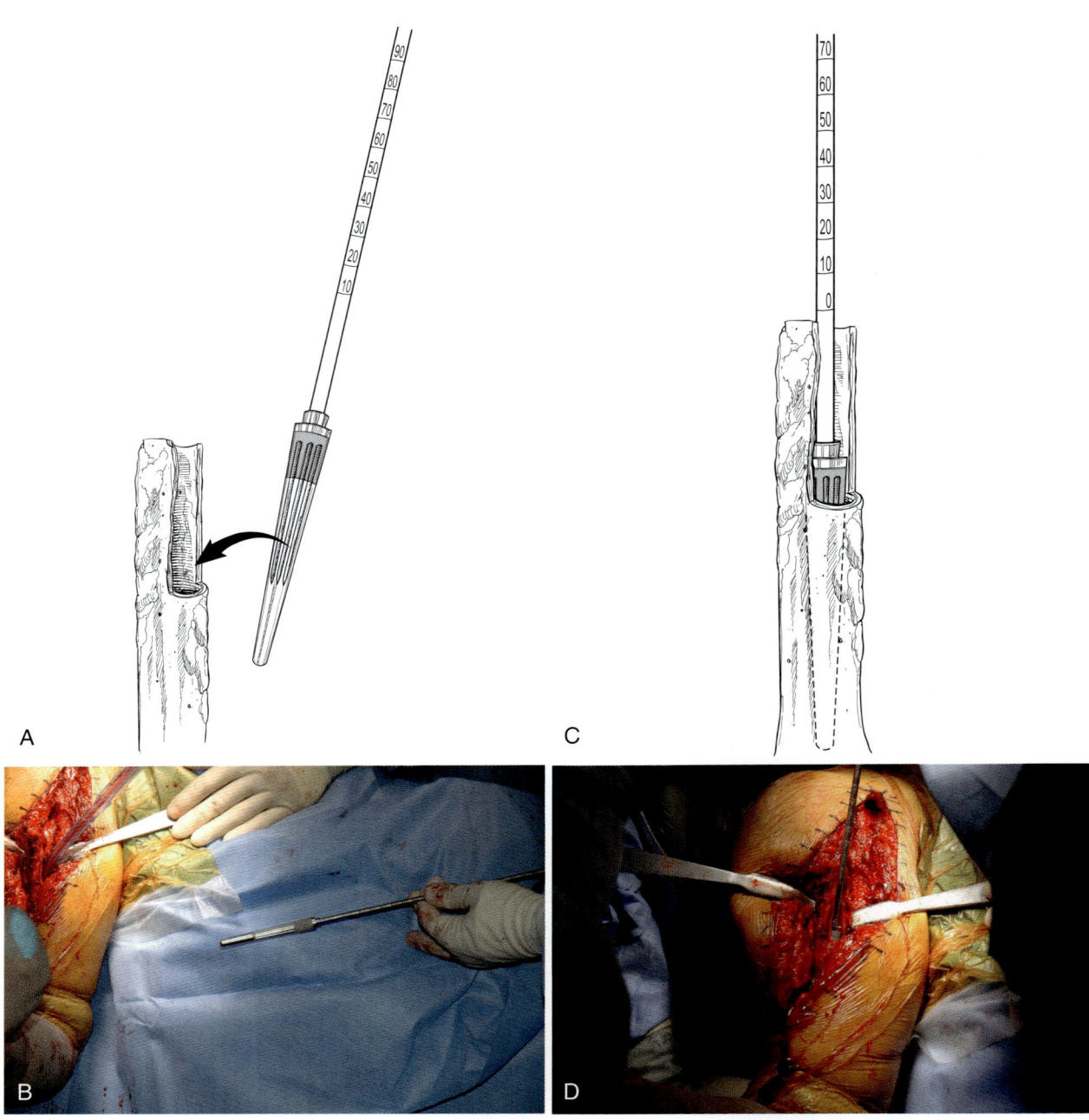

FIGURE 39.20 (A to F) Placement of the distal aspect of the prosthesis.

CHAPTER 39 ■ Humeral Component

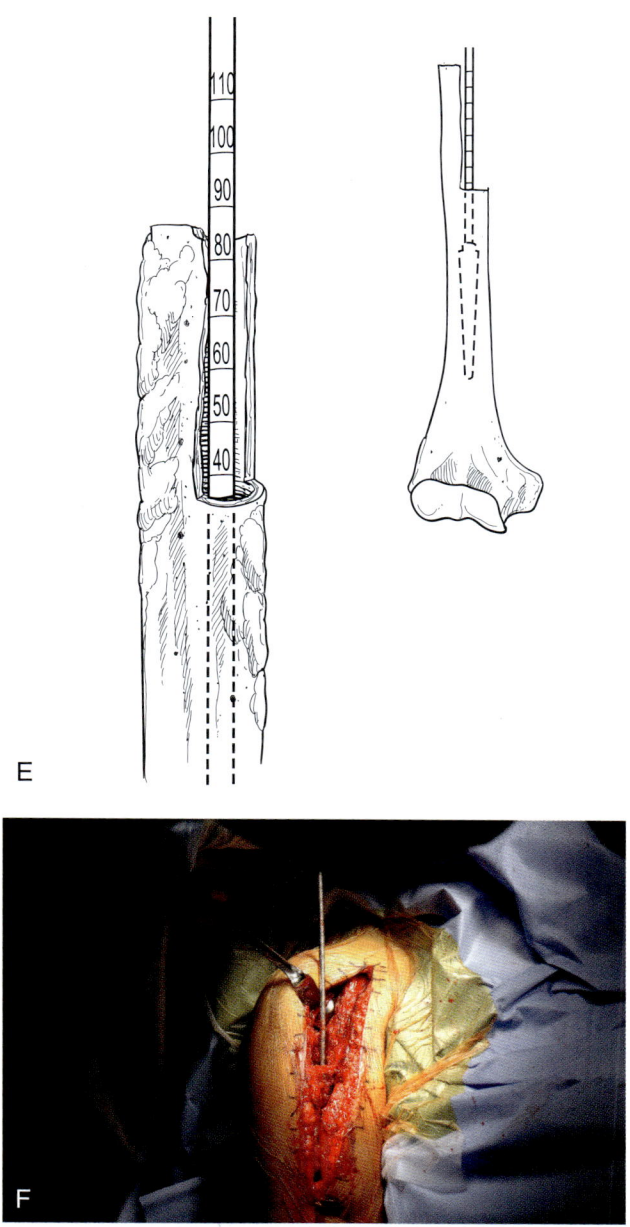

FIGURE 39.20, cont'd

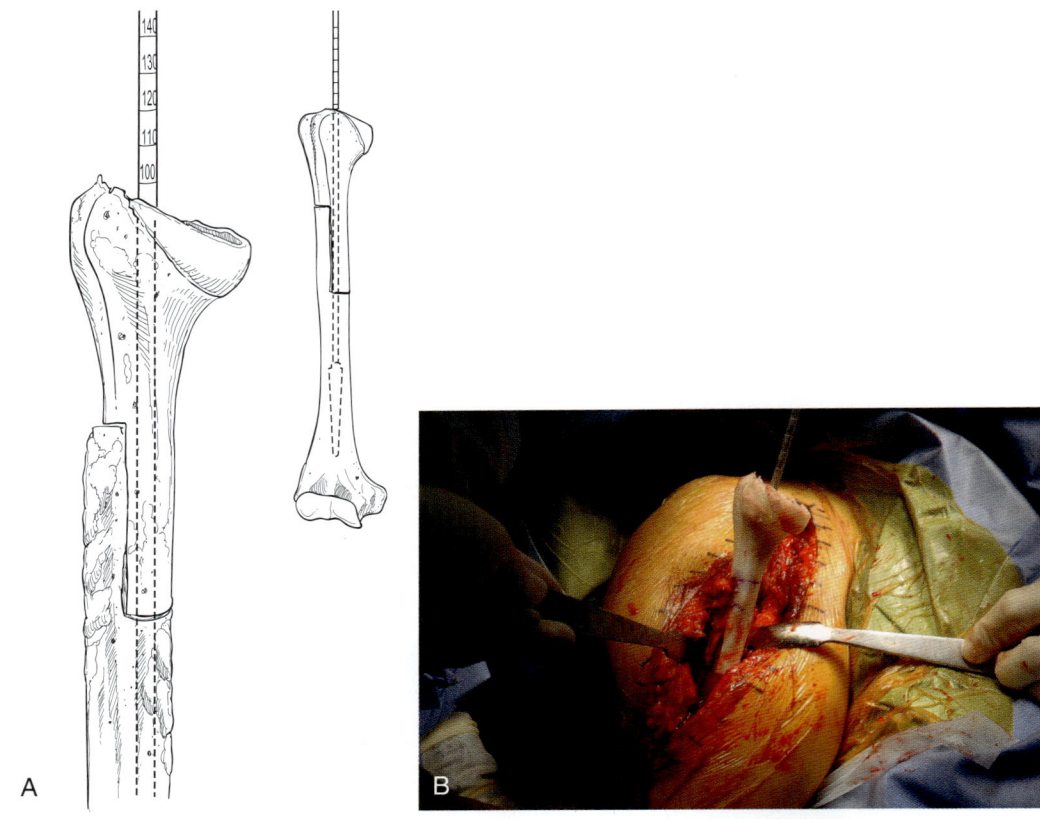

FIGURE 39.21 (A and B) Placement of the proximal humeral allograft.

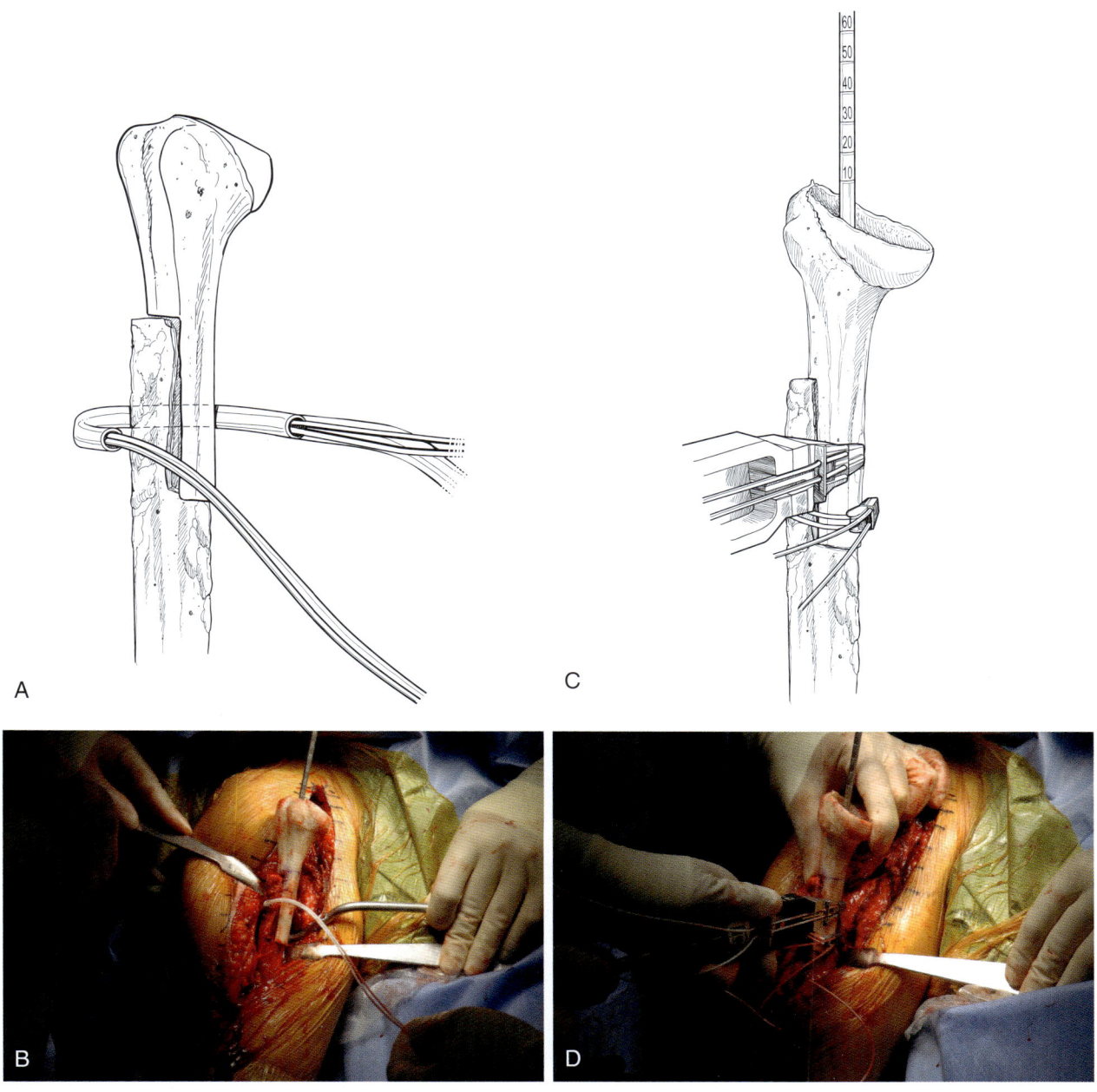

FIGURE 39.22 Fixation of the allograft to the native humerus using a step cut (A to F) or bridging allograft struts (G and H).

Continued

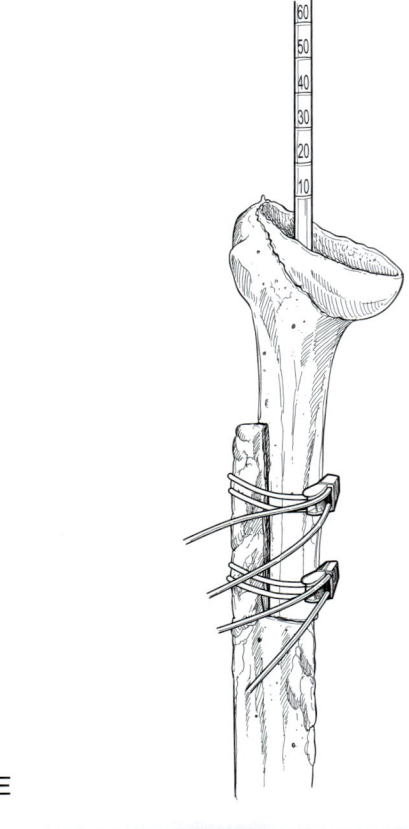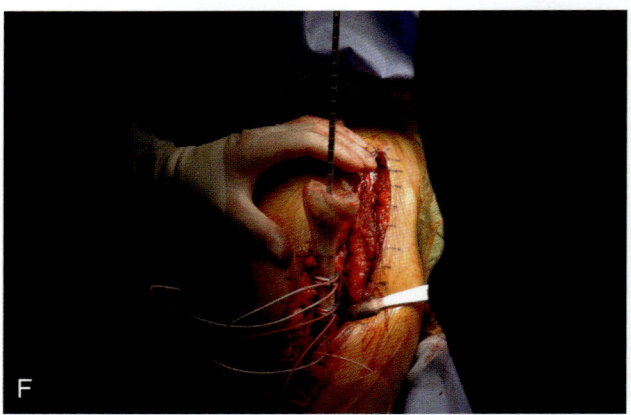

FIGURE 39.22, cont'd

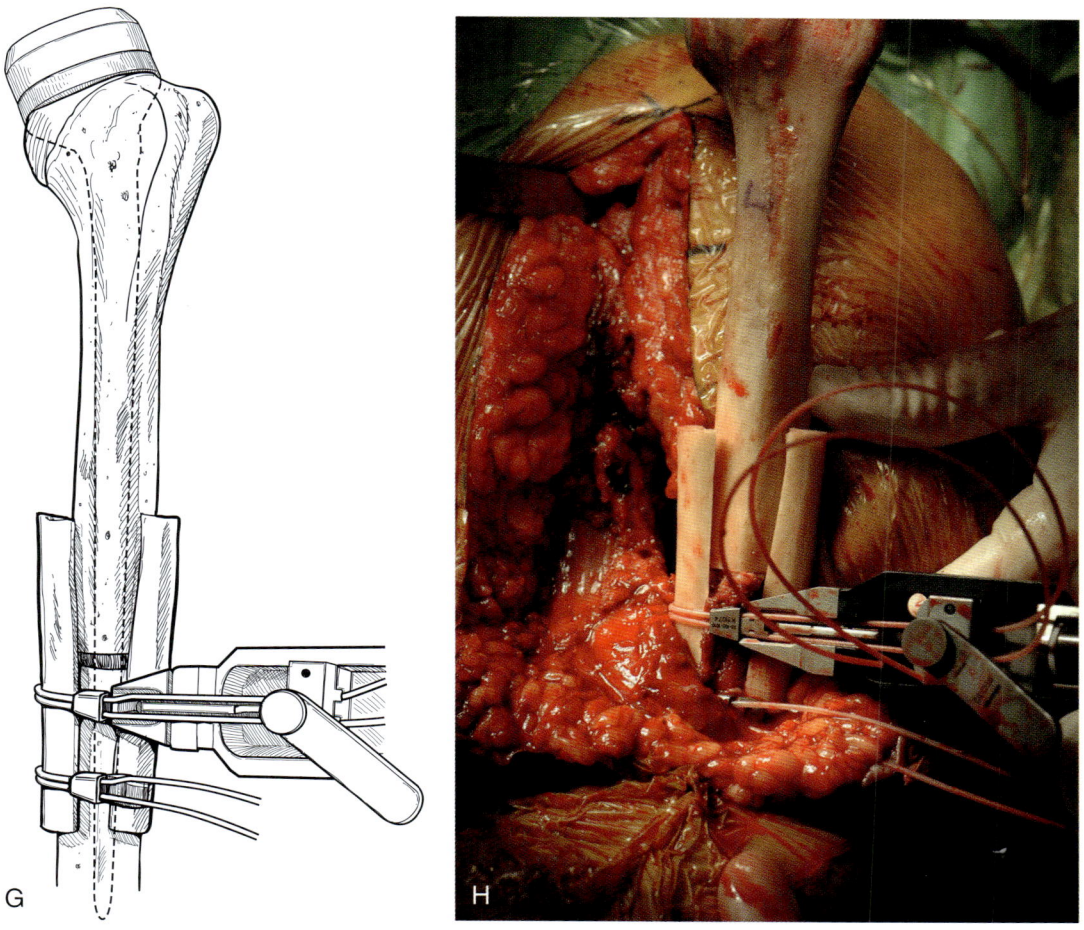

FIGURE 39.22, cont'd

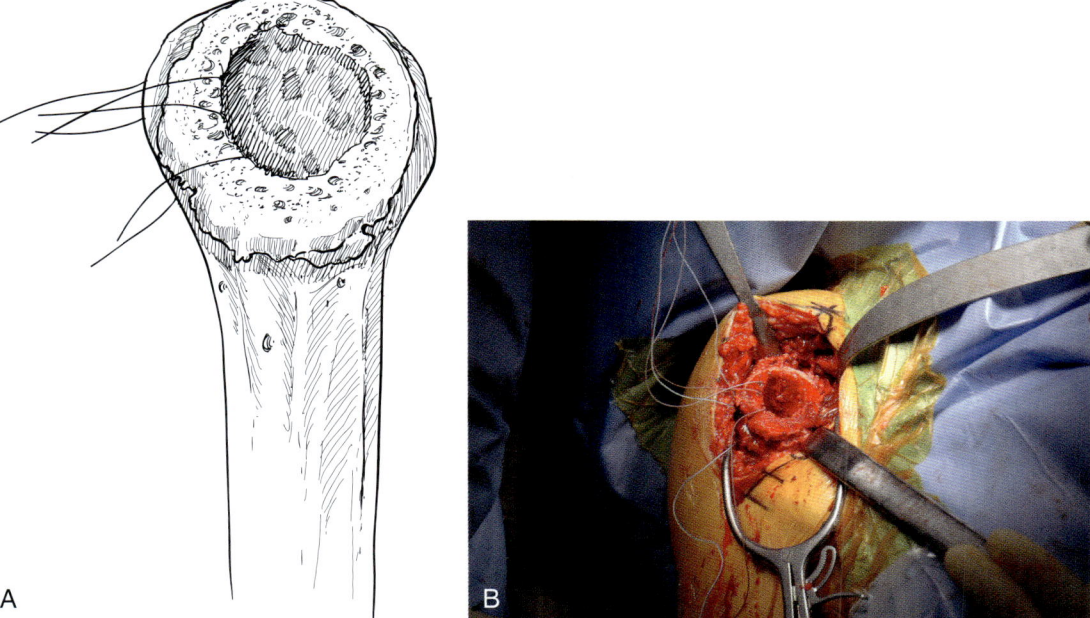

FIGURE 39.23 (A and B) Transosseous sutures placed before insertion of the humeral stem for later use in reattachment of the subscapularis.

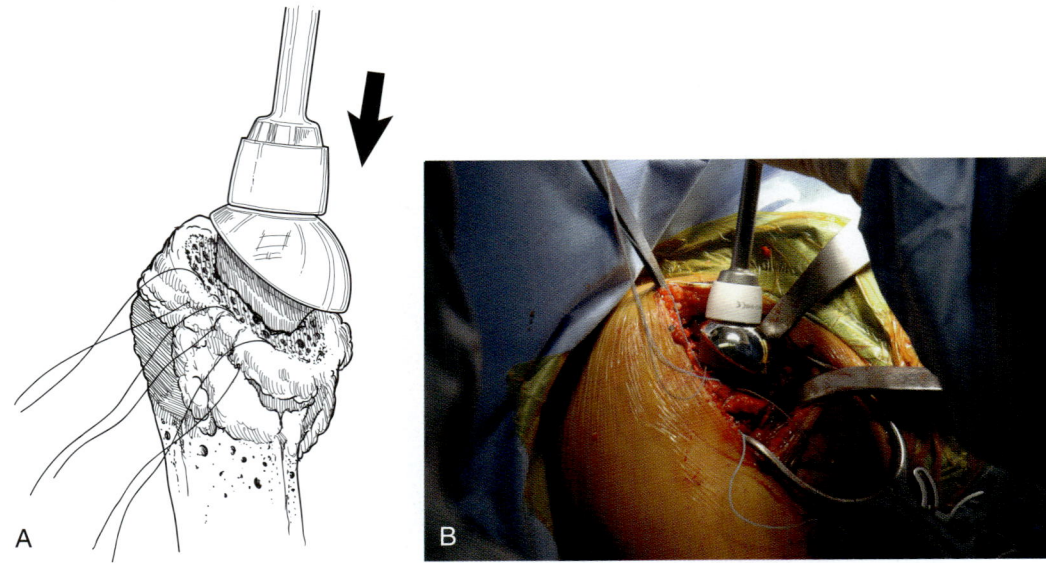

FIGURE 39.24 (A and B) The final humeral implant is impacted into place.

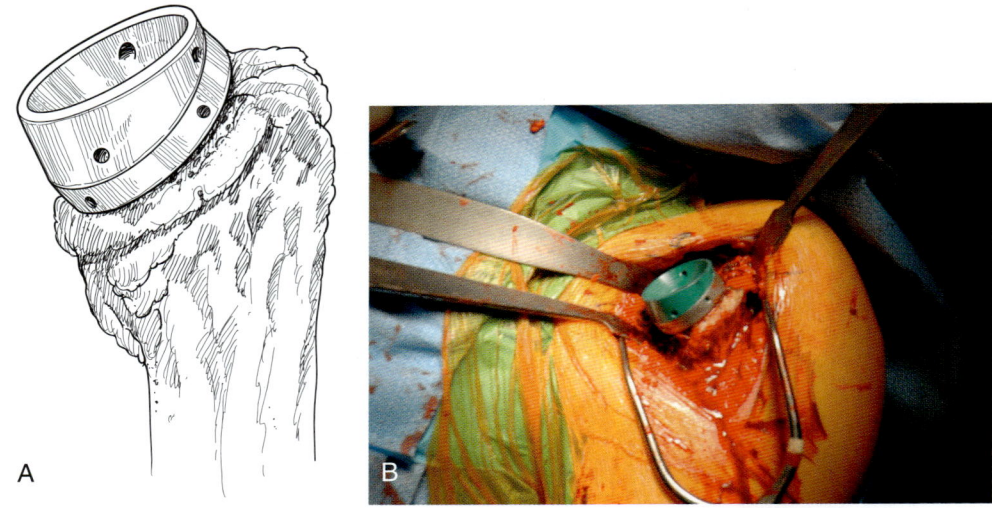

FIGURE 39.25 (A and B) Trialing of the humeral stem with various size polyethylene spacers.

completing implantation of the glenoid component and reduce the prosthetic glenohumeral joint (Fig. 39.25). Stability and mobility of the joint is assessed and adjustments are made to the thickness of the tray and polyethylene just as in primary reverse shoulder arthroplasty (see Chapter 23). Constrained polyethylene liners are available for additional stability when needed. After the appropriate tray and polyethylene liner are selected, the trial humeral component is removed and the final humeral component is placed (Figs. 39.26 and 39.27). If the subscapularis tendon is present and reparable, three no. 2 nonabsorbable braided sutures are placed through the humeral stump of the subscapularis tendon, into the lesser tuberosity, and out through the intramedullary canal of the humerus for later use in reattachment of the subscapularis, as in cases of primary and revision unconstrained shoulder arthroplasty, prior to placing the final implant.

In cases with significant proximal humeral bone loss requiring allograft reconstruction as described in the previous section, the adjustable humeral implant is inserted and assembled progressively through the allograft. The distal tip of the implant is inserted as described in the previous section using the calibrated rod (see Fig. 39.20). The appropriate length diaphyseal segment is introduced over the calibrated rod and advanced through the allograft and into the native humeral diaphysis until it rests in contact with the tip segment of the implant (Fig. 39.28). The metaphyseal portion of the implant is then introduced and advanced over the calibrated insertion rod (Fig. 39.29). An appropriate length linking screw is placed to assemble the segments of the implant (Fig. 39.30). The linking screw is further secured by placement of a locking cap (Fig. 39.31). Trialing of the various

Text continued on p. 406

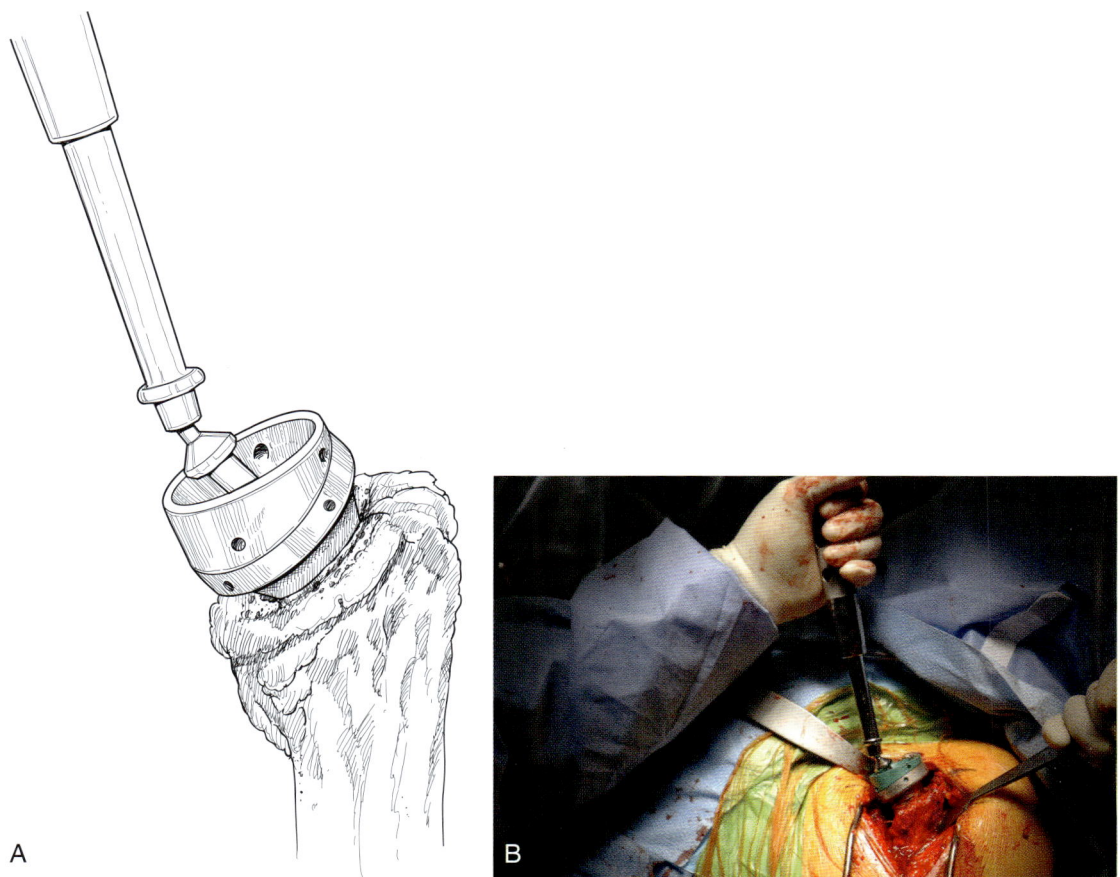

FIGURE 39.26 (A and B) Removal of the trial humeral stem.

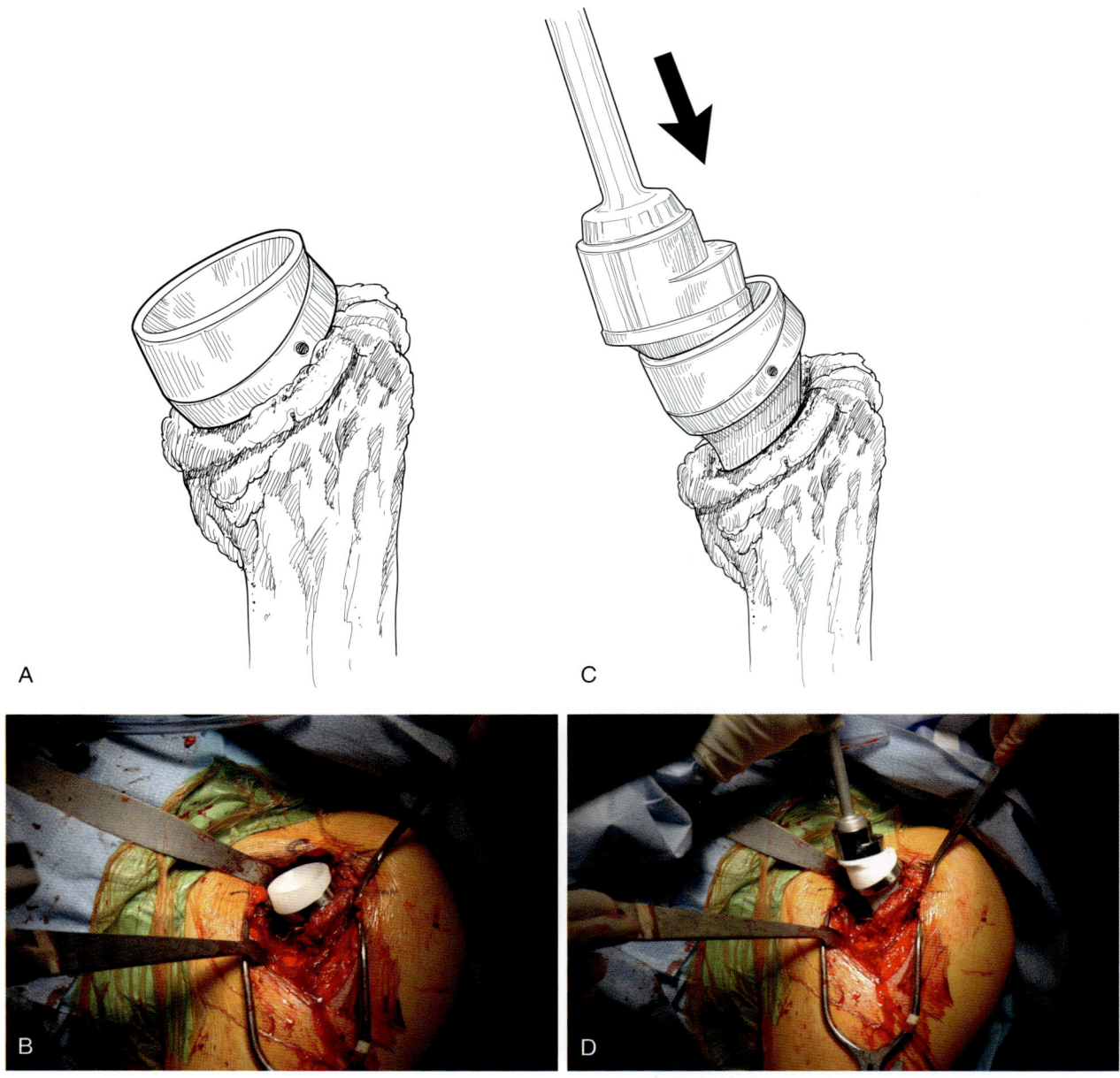

FIGURE 39.27 (A to D) Impaction of the final humeral stem of a reverse shoulder arthroplasty for revision.

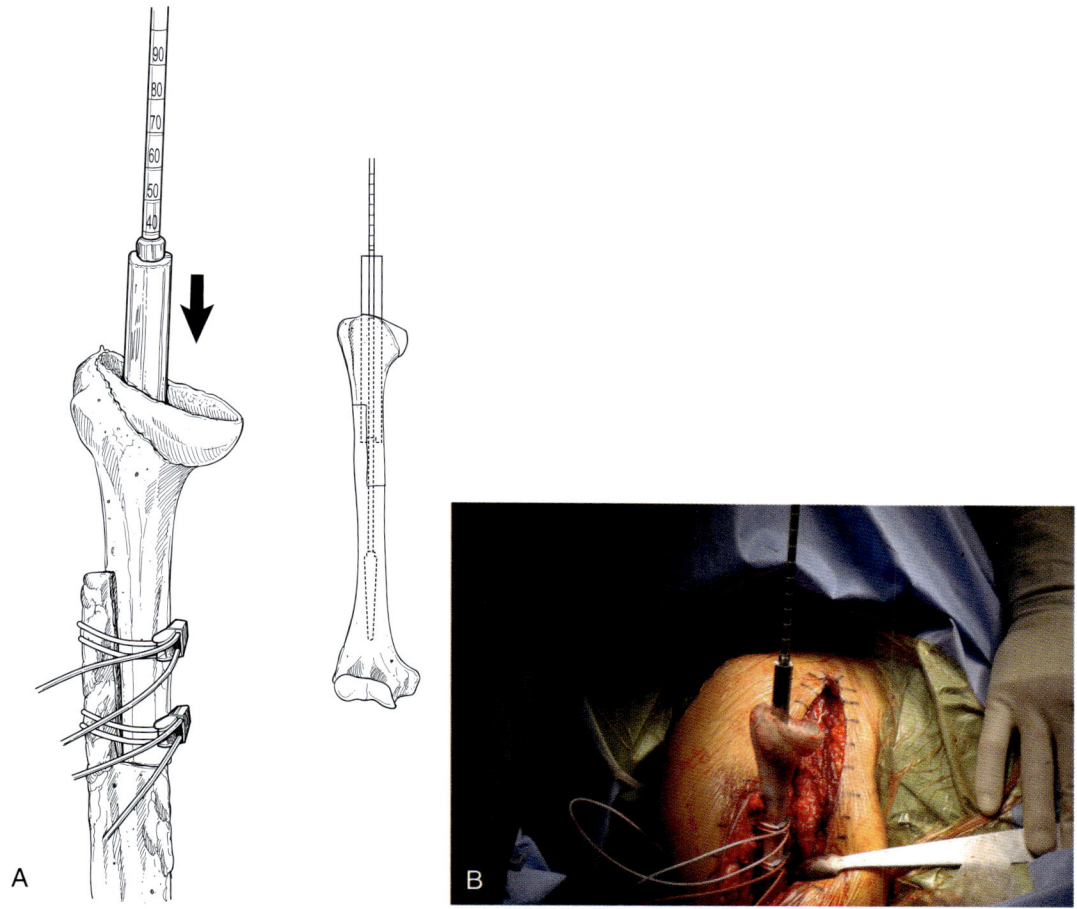

FIGURE 39.28 (A and B) The appropriate length diaphyseal segment is introduced over the calibrated rod and advanced through the allograft and into the native humeral diaphysis until it rests in contact with the tip segment of the implant.

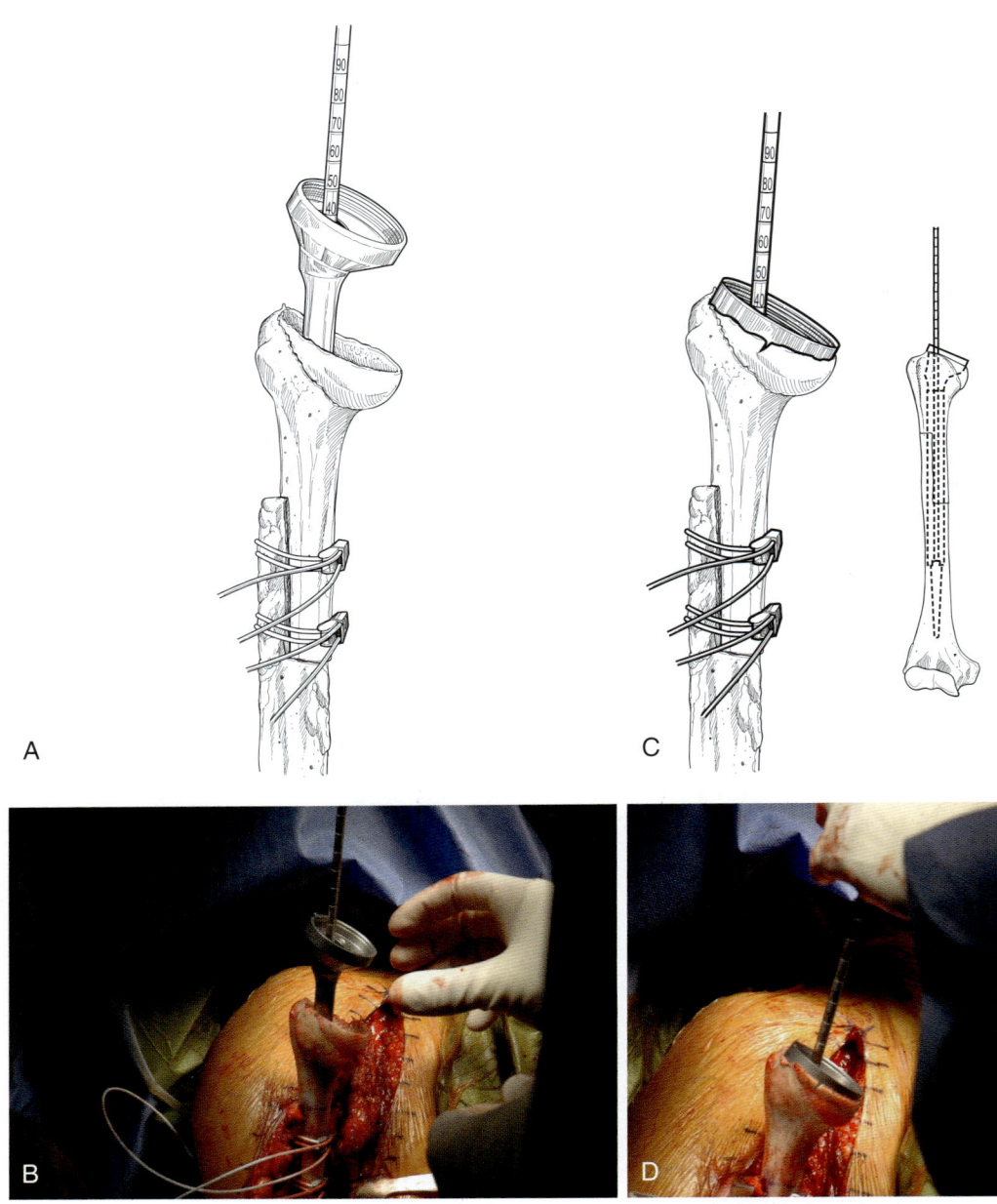

FIGURE 39.29 (A to D) The metaphyseal portion of the implant is then introduced and advanced over the calibrated insertion rod.

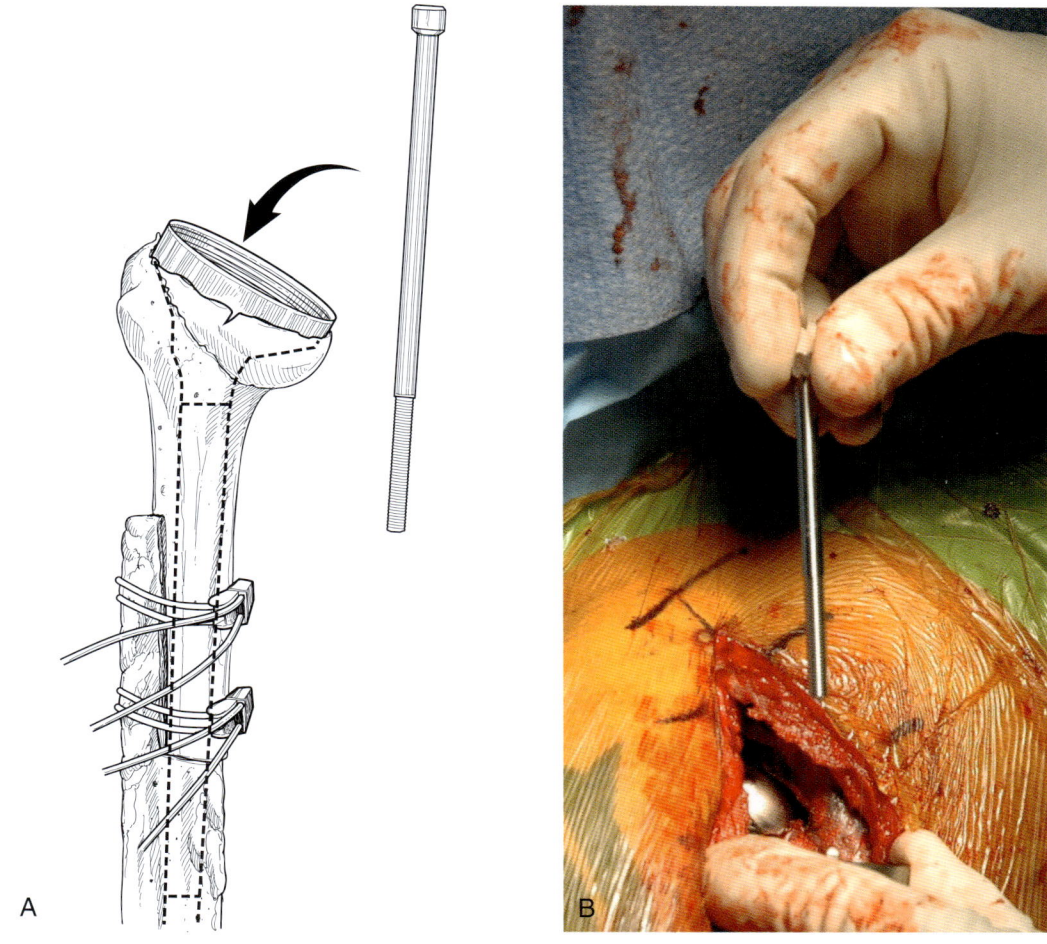

FIGURE 39.30 (A to D) An appropriate length linking screw is placed to assemble the segments of the implant.

Continued

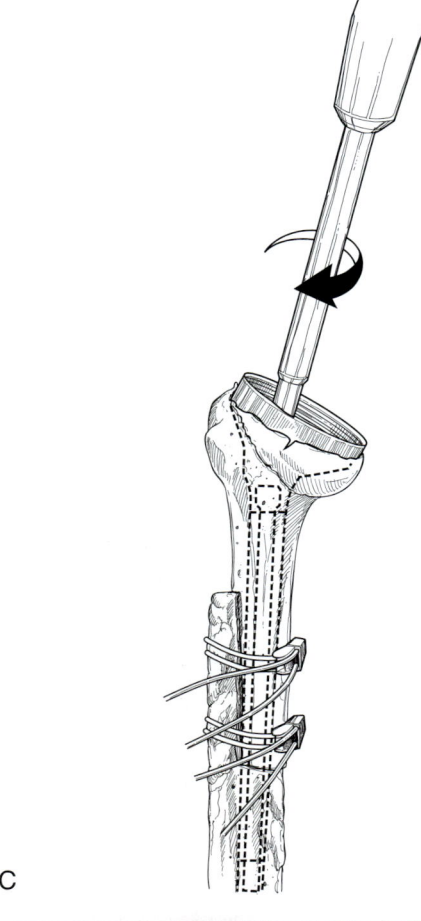
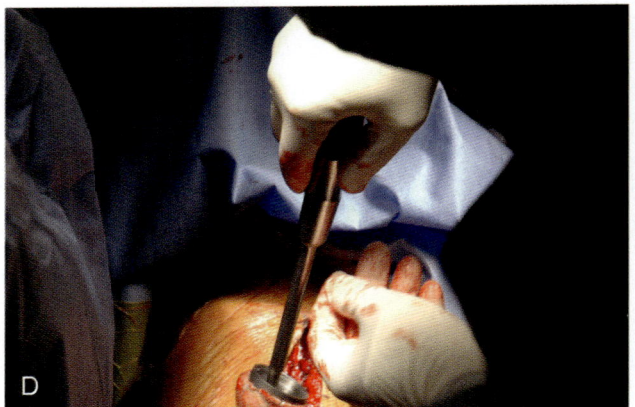

FIGURE 39.30, cont'd

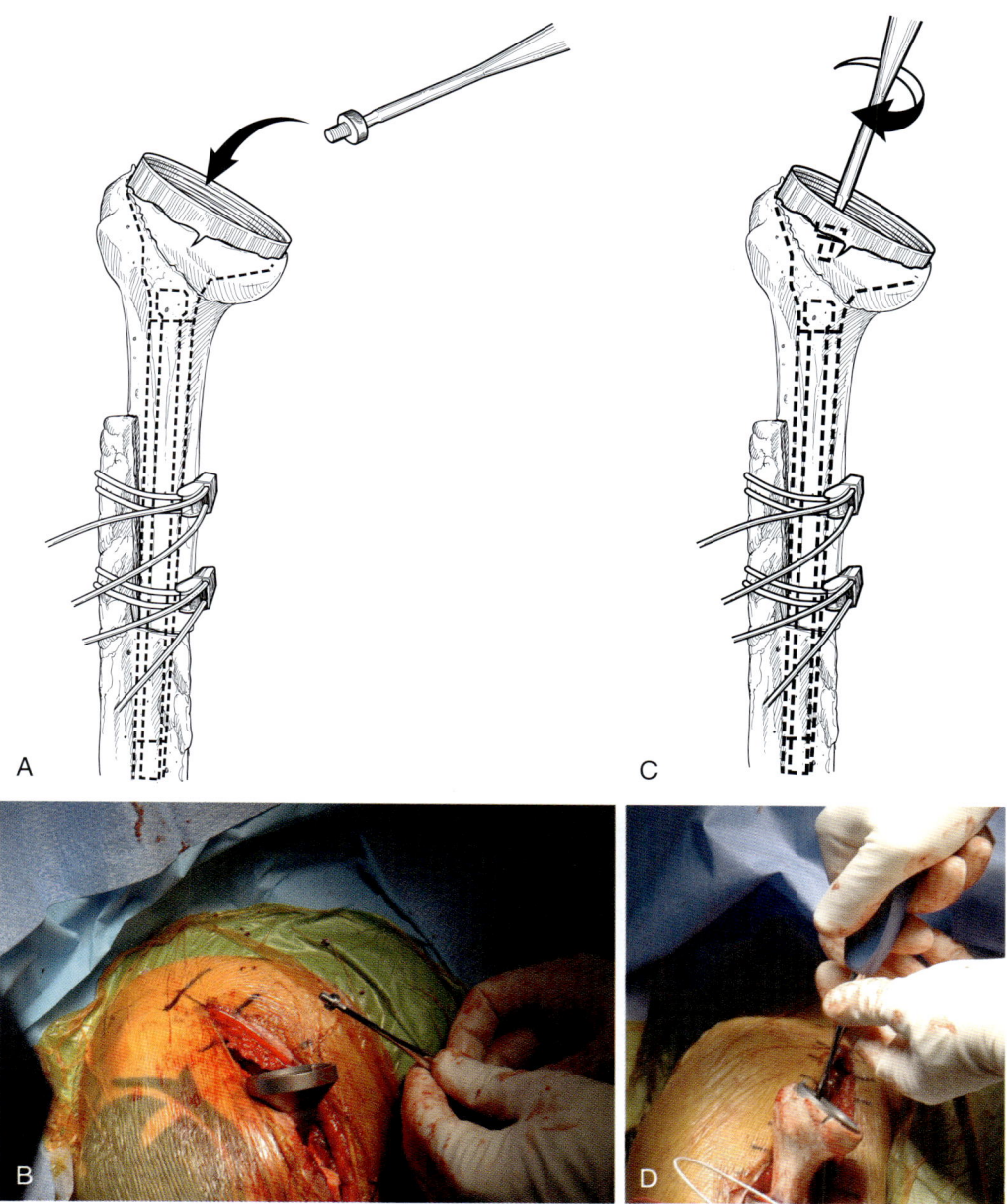

FIGURE 39.31 (A to D) The linking screw is further secured by placement of a locking cap.

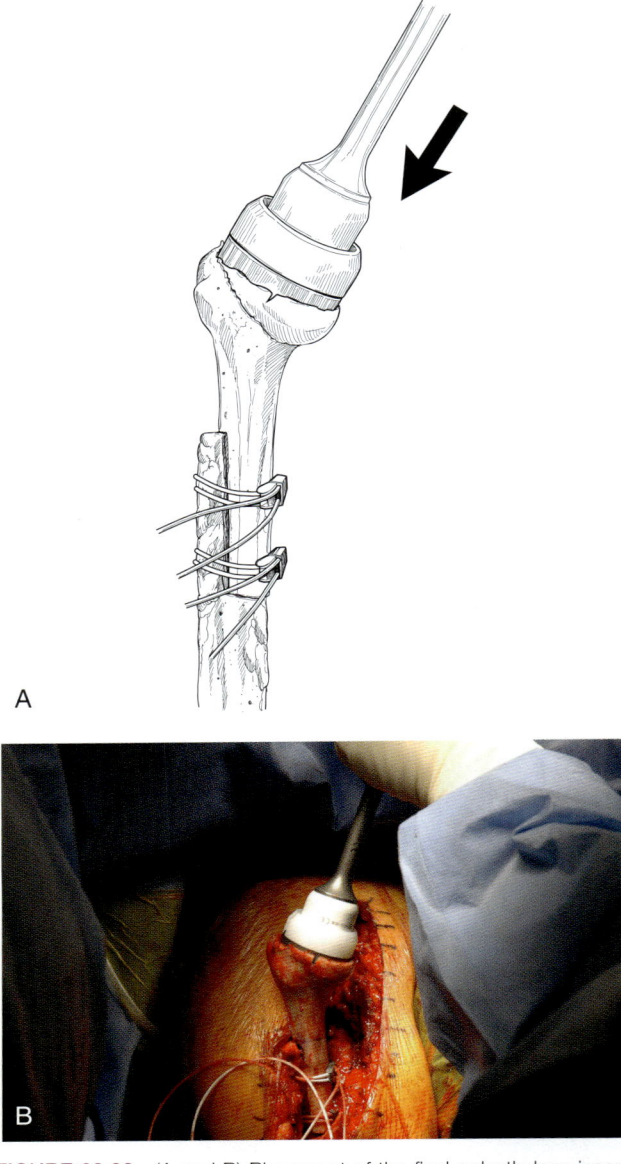

FIGURE 39.32 (A and B) Placement of the final polyethylene insert.

polyethylene spacers commences, as described in Chapter 23. Once appropriate tension has been obtained, the final polyethylene insert is placed (Fig. 39.32).

SPECIAL SITUATIONS

Periprosthetic Fracture

In cases of periprosthetic fracture, the fracture must be reduced before placement of the revision humeral stem. The fracture and associated structures (i.e., the radial nerve) are exposed as detailed in Chapter 37. The humerus distal to the fracture site is reamed with the diaphyseal reamers introduced at the fracture site (Fig. 39.33). The humerus proximal to the fracture site is prepared with the instrumentation provided for the selected humeral stem. It is often helpful to stabilize the proximal humeral fragment with a bone clamp during preparation of the proximal humerus (Fig. 39.34).

After the proximal humerus has been prepared, the fracture is reduced and the humeral stem is placed (Fig. 39.35). A humeral stem that bypasses the distal extent of the fracture by a minimum of two cortical diameters is selected (Fig. 39.36).[1] Fresh frozen cortical strips of allograft tibia are used on each side of the humerus and centered at the fracture site. We place two or four cables composed of a nylon monofilament core wrapped in a braided ultrahigh-molecular-weight polyethylene (Kinamed Inc., Camarillo, CA) subperiosteally around the residual native humerus with the cable-passing instrumentation provided while taking care to avoid the radial nerve posteriorly. The cables are tightened with the tensioning device (Fig. 39.37). The final humeral head or reverse polyethylene implant is placed completing the humeral reconstruction (Fig. 39.38).

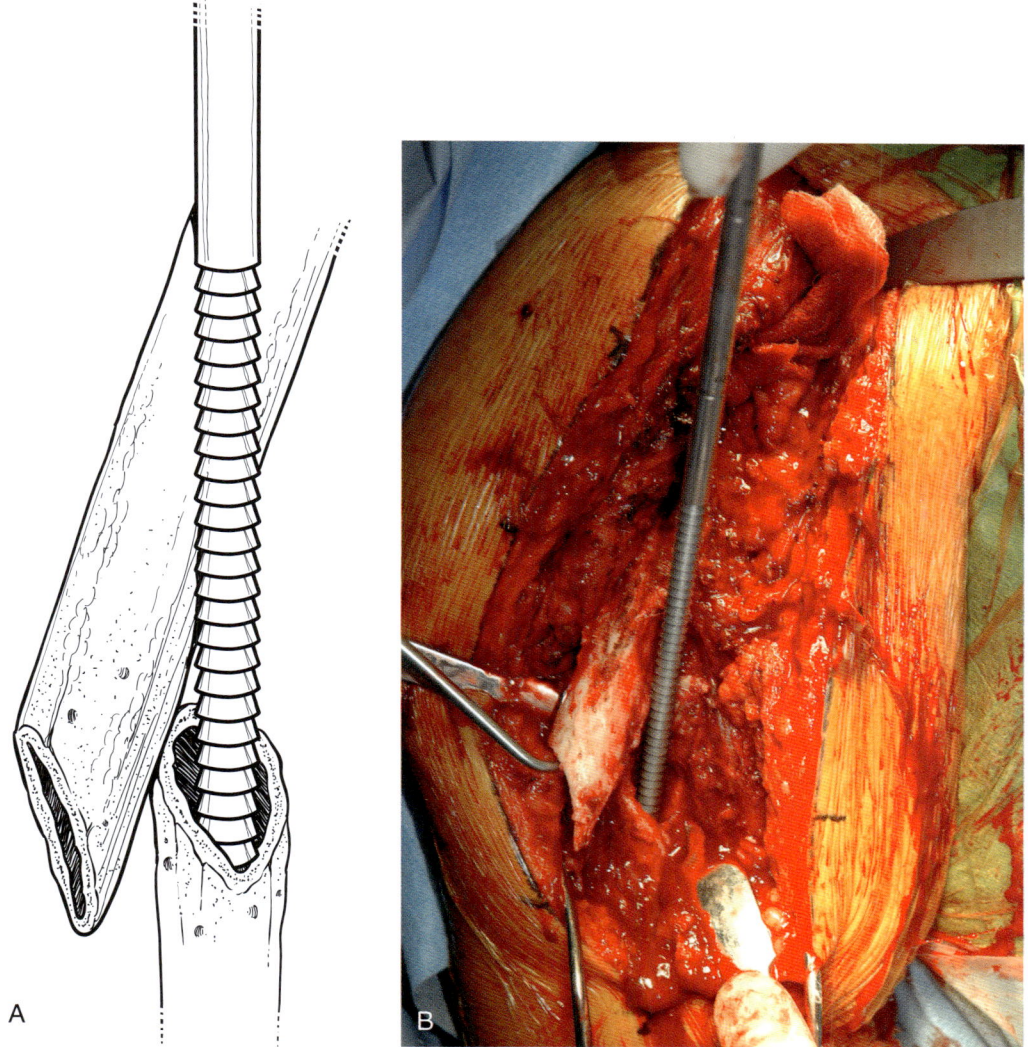

FIGURE 39.33 (A and B) The humerus distal to the fracture site is reamed with the diaphyseal reamers introduced at the fracture site.

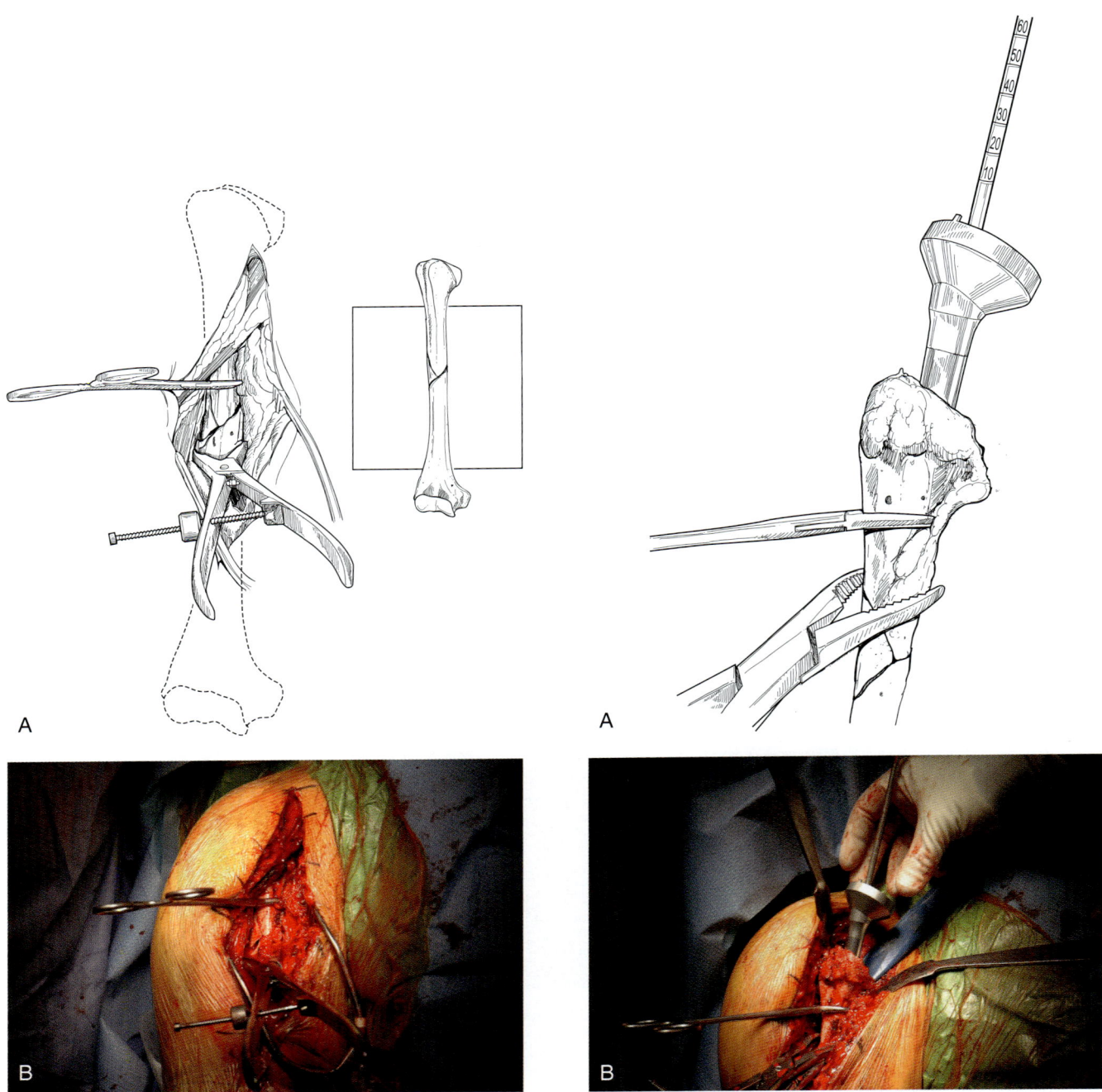

FIGURE 39.34 (A and B) The fracture is reduced and held with reduction clamps.

FIGURE 39.35 (A and B) The humeral implant is placed while the fracture is held reduced.

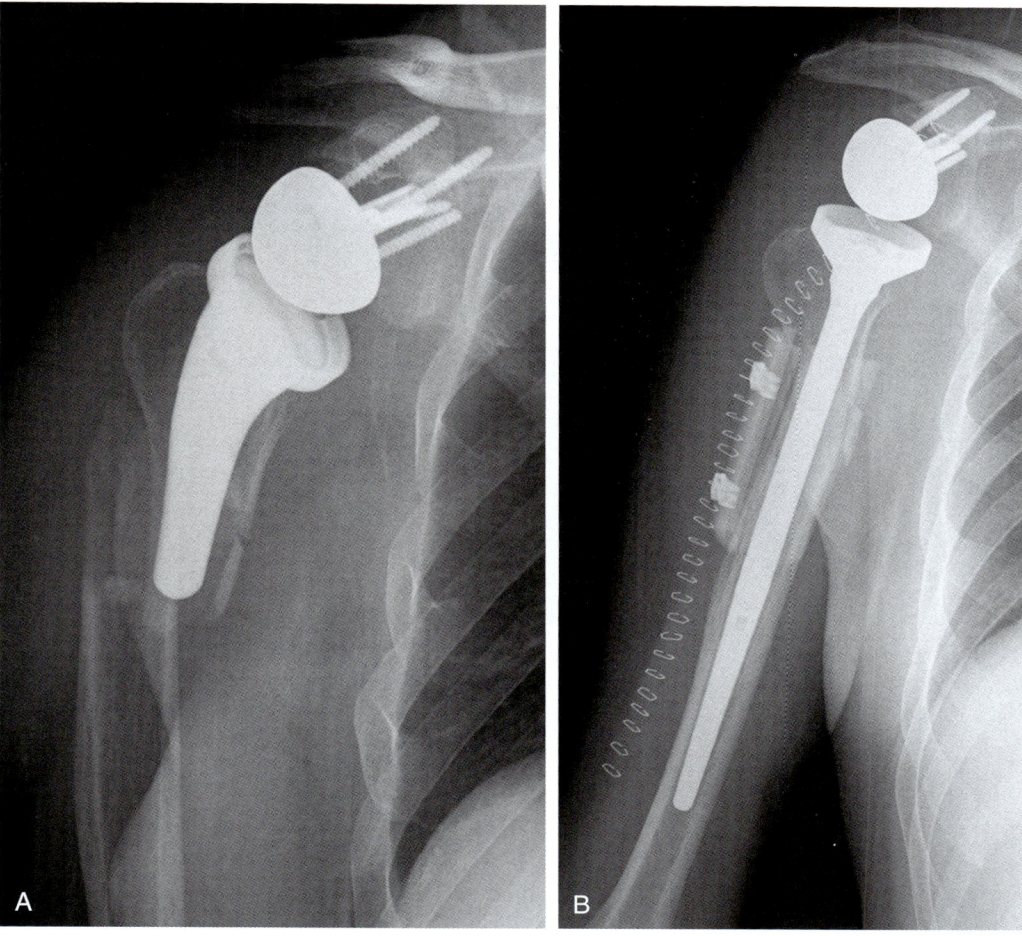

FIGURE 39.36 A humeral stem that bypasses the distal extent of the fracture by a minimum of two cortical diameters is selected. Preoperative radiograph (A) and postoperative radiograph (B).

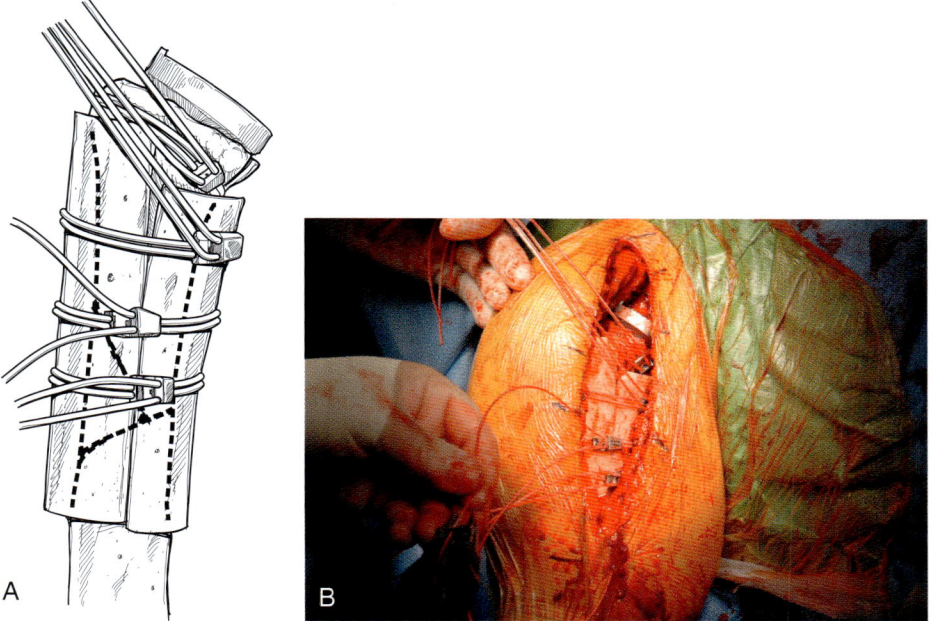

FIGURE 39.37 (A and B) Cables placed for fixation of a cortical strip allograft during treatment of a periprosthetic humeral fracture by revision arthroplasty.

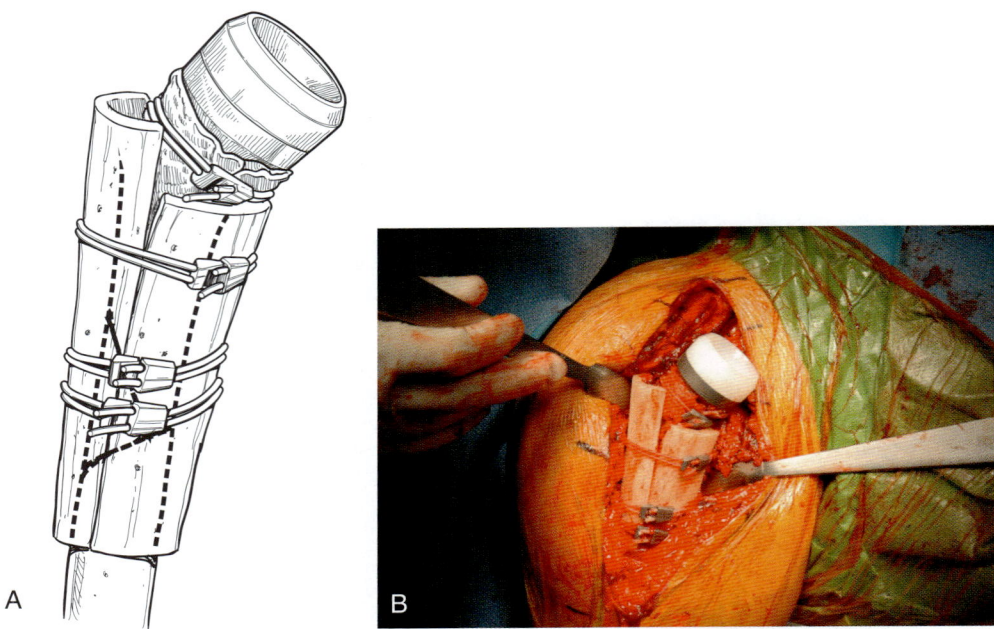

FIGURE 39.38 (A and B) The final polyethylene insert is placed completing the humeral reconstruction.

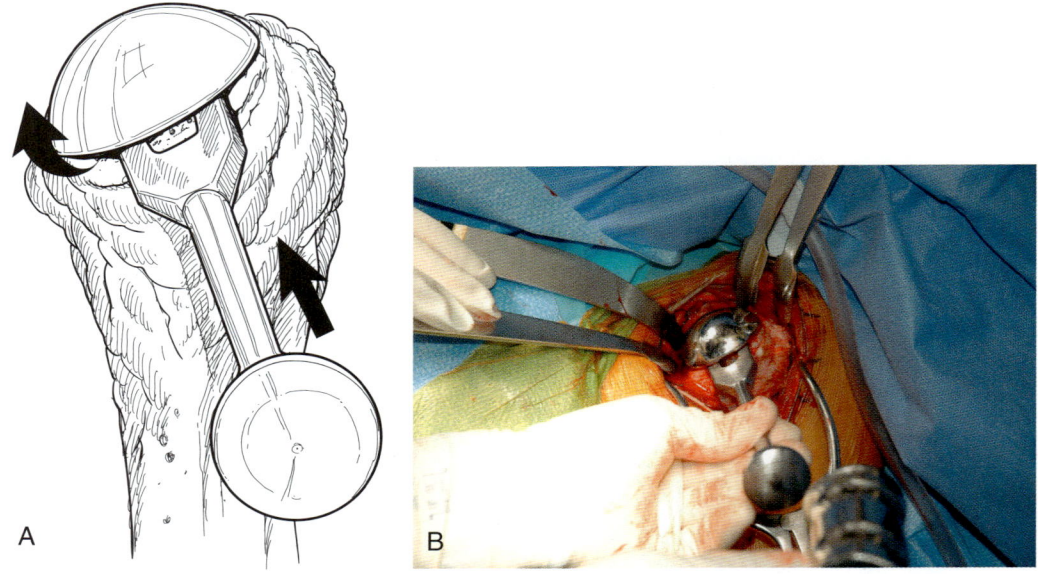

FIGURE 39.39 (A and B) When performing a conversion, the humeral head prosthesis is removed from the humeral stem with a tuning fork instrument.

Convertible Humeral Stems (Video 39.1)

Several companies now manufacture humeral stems that allow conversion from an unconstrained shoulder arthroplasty to a reverse shoulder arthroplasty and vice versa. In a revision case in which an unconstrained shoulder arthroplasty is being revised to a reverse shoulder arthroplasty such as rotator cuff failure, retention of the original stem and conversion of the arthroplasty design can be considered provided a convertible type stem had been primarily implanted.

When performing a conversion, the humeral head prosthesis is removed from the humeral stem with a tuning fork instrument (Fig. 39.39). All fibrous tissue is removed from the surface of the stem, and the stem is checked for

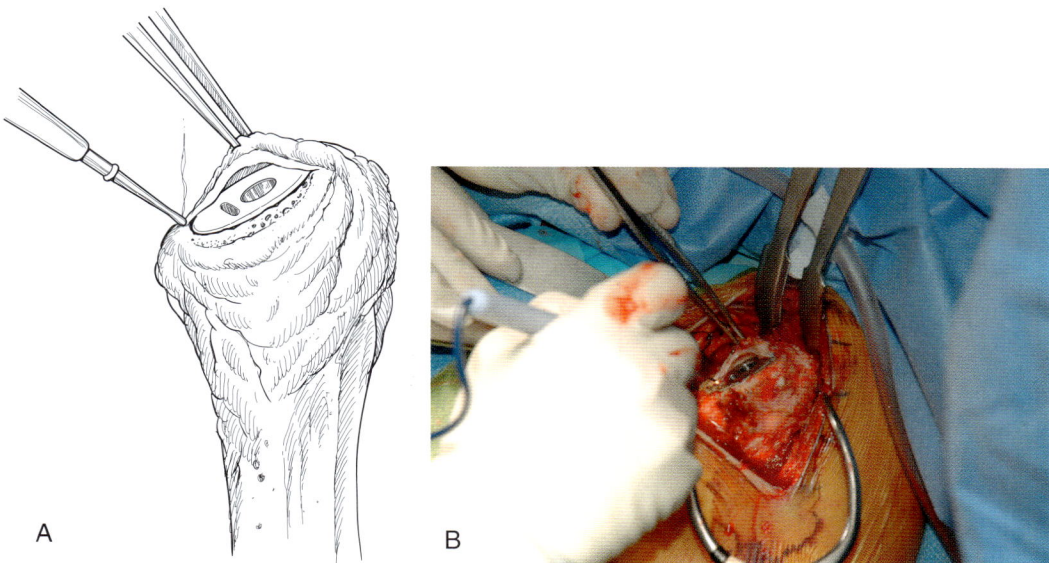

FIGURE 39.40 (A and B) All fibrous tissue is removed from the surface of the stem.

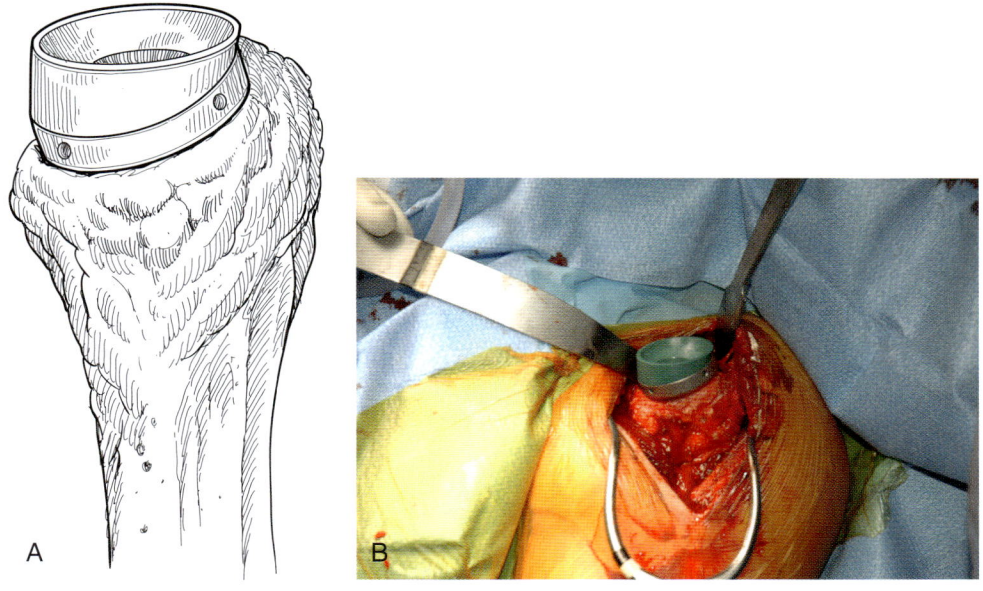

FIGURE 39.41 (A and B) A trial humeral tray and polyethylene insert are selected, placed, and adjusted.

stability (Fig. 39.40). At this point, any revision work on the glenoid is performed. The proximal humerus is dislocated and trialing of the reverse convertible components ensues. The system that we use allows restoration of a 145-degree neck inclination angle. It is important to know the inclination of the primarily placed humeral stem to allow selection of the proper revision components. A trial humeral tray and polyethylene insert are selected, placed, and adjusted as described in Chapter 21 (Fig. 39.41). Assessment of the trial components by reducing the prosthesis ensues to confirm the proper selection of components (see Chapter 23). After the proper component selection is confirmed, the final implants are placed, ensuring to clean and dry any Morse taper (Fig. 39.42).

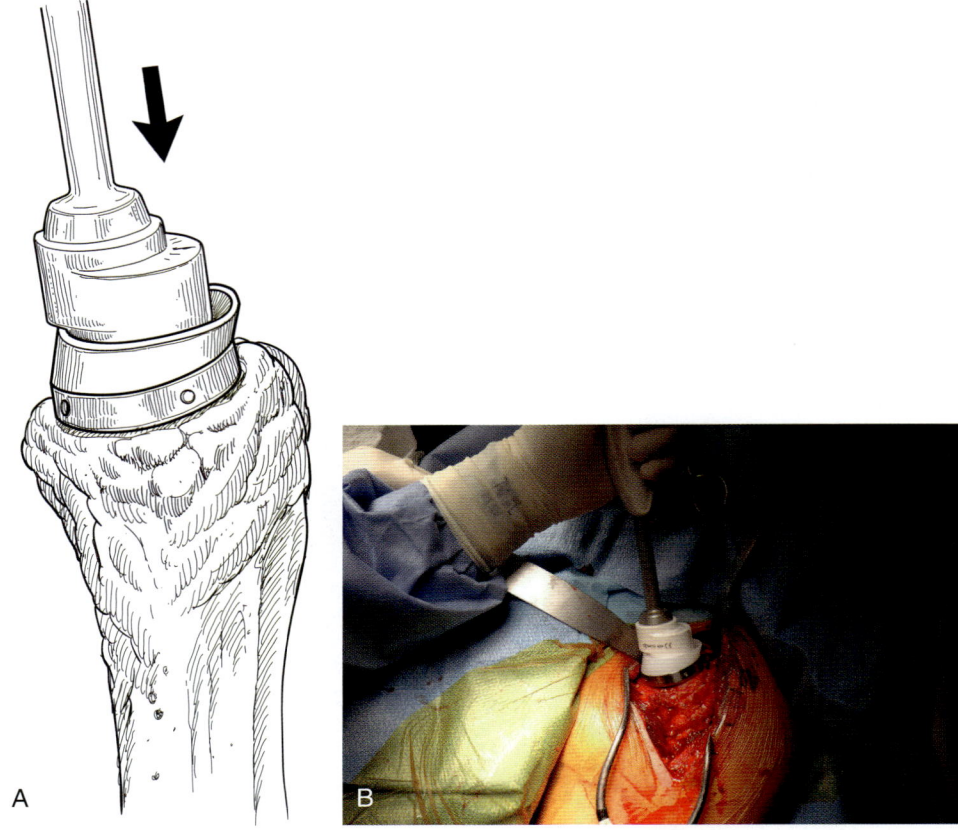

FIGURE 39.42 (A and B) The final implants are placed, ensuring to clean and dry any Morse taper.

REFERENCE

1. Johansson JE, McBroom R, Barrington TW, et al: Fractures of the ipsilateral femur in patients with total hip replacement, *J Bone Joint Surg Am* 61:1435–1442, 1981.

Glenoid component

CHAPTER 40

Problems with the glenoid are a common indication for revision arthroplasty. Such problems include failure of previously implanted glenoid components from total shoulder arthroplasty and osseous glenoid erosion after hemiarthroplasty. Frequently, glenoid problems involve substantial osseous compromise and require complex reconstruction. The ability to deal with these glenoid problems is necessary to successfully treat many cases of failed shoulder arthroplasty. Treatment of the various types of glenoid problems is addressed in detail in this chapter.

GLENOID REVISION NOT REQUIRING A BONE GRAFT

Glenoid erosion after hemiarthroplasty is a common indication for revision arthroplasty and occurs in two situations: (1) in patients with rotator cuff deficiency and superior glenoid erosion coupled with static superior (or anterior superior) humeral migration (Fig. 40.1) and (2) in patients with an intact rotator cuff and painful symptomatic humeral erosion that is central, anterior, or posterior (Fig. 40.2). Usually, the erosion is not severe enough to require a bone graft, but the surgeon should first determine the severity of the osseous glenoid defect with a preoperative computed tomography scan (Fig. 40.3).

Unconstrained Shoulder Arthroplasty Cases Not Requiring a Glenoid Bone Graft

In patients with glenoid erosion after hemiarthroplasty and a functional rotator cuff, revision surgery from hemiarthroplasty to total shoulder arthroplasty is performed similar to cases of primary unconstrained shoulder arthroplasty. In such cases, if the humeral component is properly sized and positioned, the surgeon may be able to retain the humeral stem while performing revision surgery. This almost always necessitates changing the humeral head of the modular implant. It is important to know preoperatively the type of implant that the patient had and the radius of curvature of the various head sizes of this implant. A different brand of glenoid component can be coupled with the previous humeral head component if prosthetic mismatch can be calculated and respected during revision arthroplasty (see Chapter 12 for discussion of prosthetic mismatch and its implications in unconstrained shoulder arthroplasty). In general, radial mismatch of greater than 5.5 mm and less than 10 mm should be respected and the glenoid component size selected accordingly.[1] If the humeral component is not properly sized or positioned or if adequate glenoid exposure cannot be obtained because of the humeral stem, the humeral component should be removed as described in Chapter 38.

After glenoid exposure is achieved, implantation of a glenoid component proceeds as in cases of primary unconstrained arthroplasty with either a keeled or pegged glenoid component (Fig. 40.4). The technique for insertion of an unconstrained glenoid component is detailed in Chapter 12.

Reverse Shoulder Arthroplasty Cases Not Requiring a Glenoid Bone Graft

In patients with glenoid erosion after hemiarthroplasty and a nonfunctional rotator cuff, revision surgery from hemiarthroplasty to reverse shoulder arthroplasty is performed similar to cases of primary reverse shoulder arthroplasty. In such cases the hemiarthroplasty component is removed and the glenoid exposed as described in Chapter 38. If a convertible implant had been placed primarily, removal of only the prosthetic humeral head may be necessary, leaving a well-fixed humeral stem (see Chapter 39). Implantation of a reverse glenoid component proceeds as in cases of primary reverse arthroplasty, as described later in this chapter and in detail in Chapter 22.

Occasionally, revision of an unconstrained total shoulder arthroplasty to a reverse shoulder arthroplasty in a patient with minimal glenoid bone loss is indicated (i.e., late rotator cuff insufficiency). Most of these patients have a pegged glenoid that is well fixed or minimally loose. After the glenoid component is removed, the previously created central hole can be used for placement of a reverse glenoid component (Fig. 40.5). The previously placed peripheral holes from the pegged unconstrained glenoid component may be ignored. The residual glenoid is reamed to a flat surface (Fig. 40.6). We prefer the use of a revision-type base plate with a central screw in this scenario (Fig. 40.7). The base plate is placed as described in Chapter 22. Because using the previously placed hole in the glenoid places the reverse base plate more superior than desired, an inferior offset glenosphere is used (Fig. 40.8). Fig. 40.9 shows the final construct.

GLENOID REVISION REQUIRING A BONE GRAFT

In cases of hemiarthroplasty with moderate to severe glenoid osseous erosion and in cases of failure of a primary glenoid

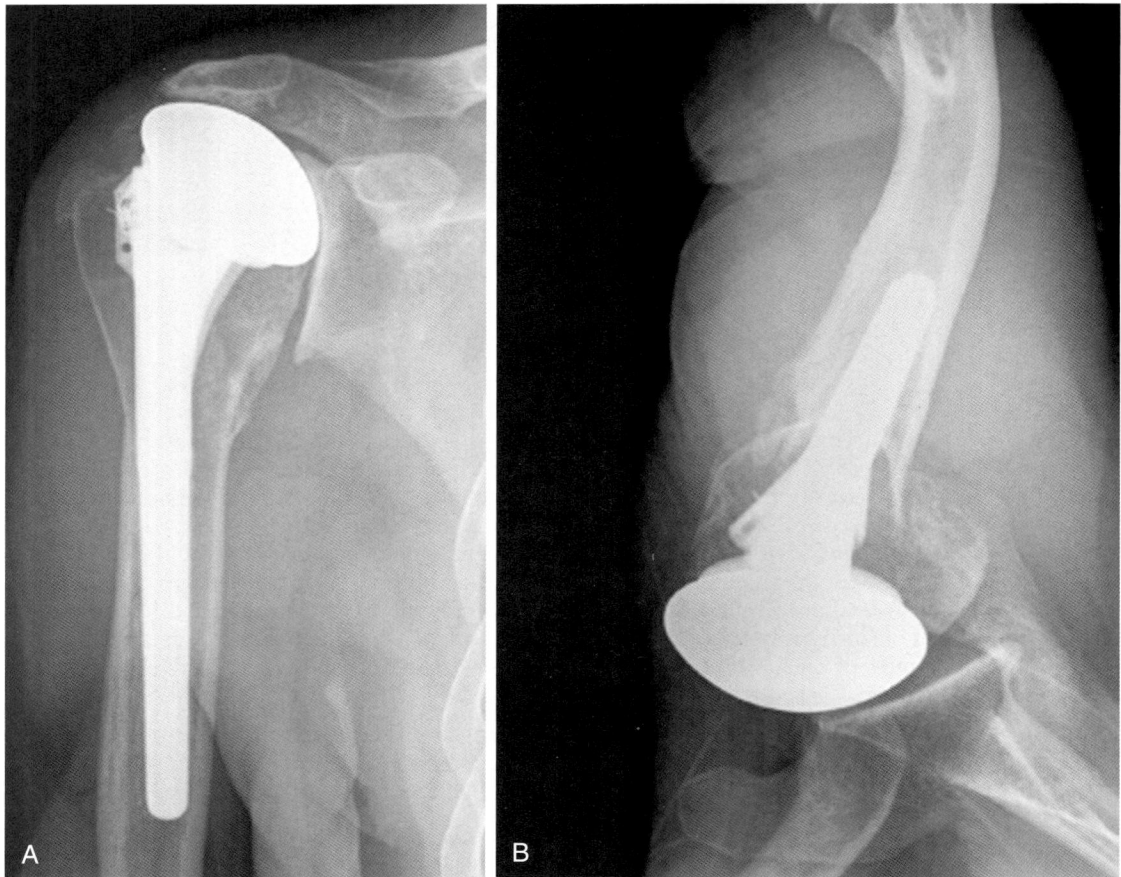

FIGURE 40.1 (A and B) Anterior superior escape of a hemiarthroplasty without significant glenoid bone loss.

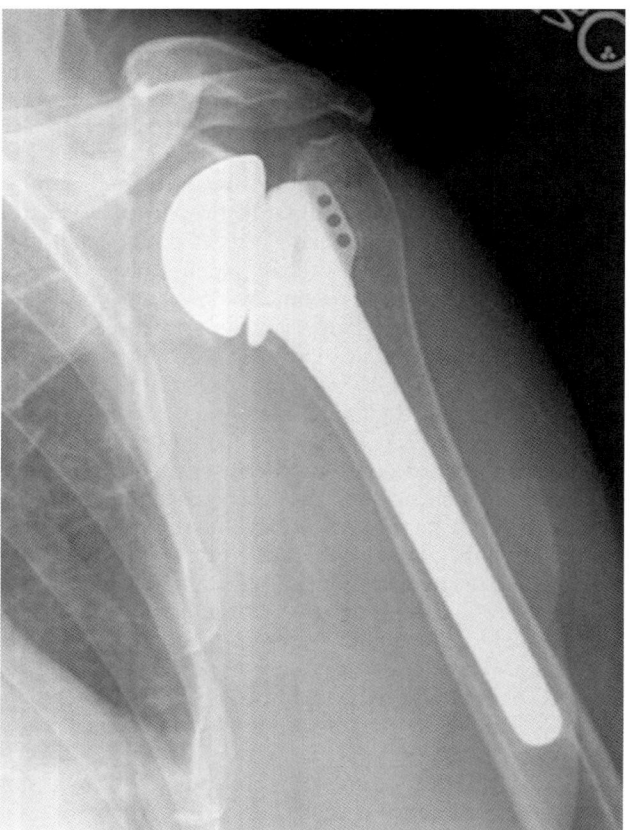

FIGURE 40.2 Painful central glenoid erosion after hemiarthroplasty.

FIGURE 40.3 Preoperative computed tomography scan of a patient after hemiarthroplasty demonstrating central erosion of the glenoid but with sufficient glenoid bone stock remaining to allow placement of a glenoid component without bone grafting of the glenoid.

CHAPTER 40 ■ Glenoid Component   415

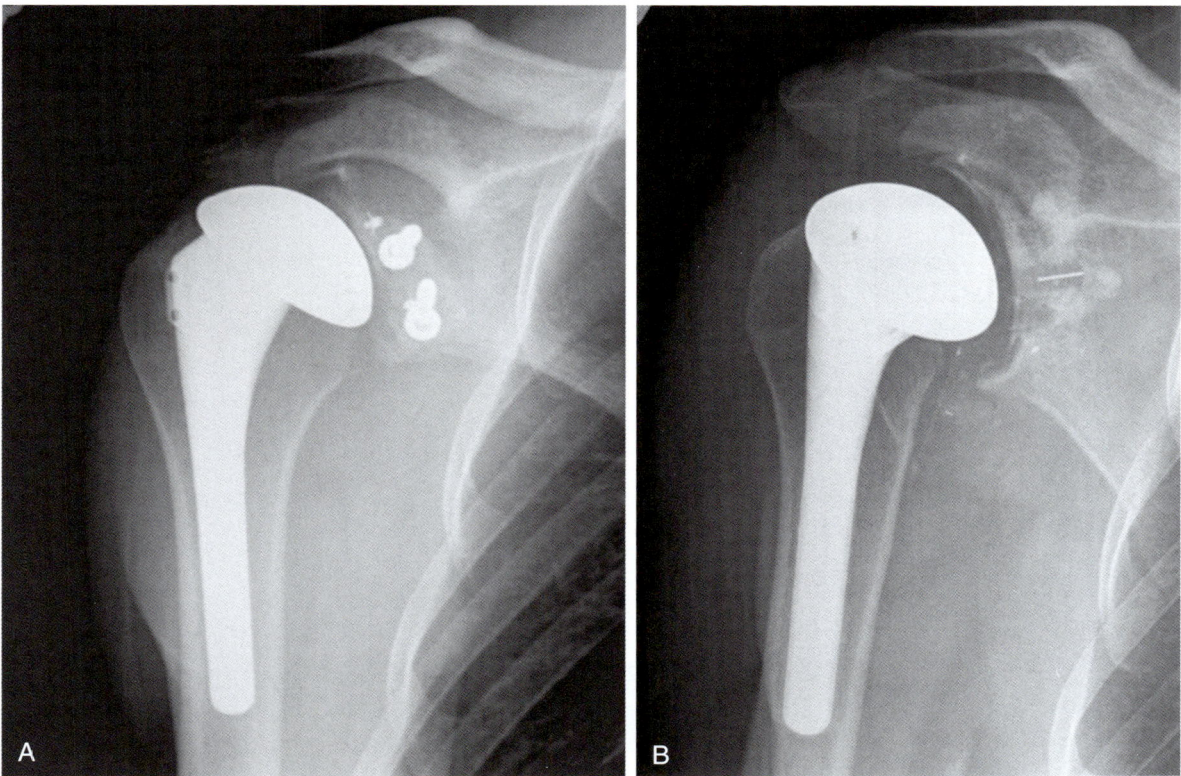

FIGURE 40.4 Prerevision (A) and postrevision (B) radiographs of a patient with conversion of a hemiarthroplasty to a total shoulder arthroplasty.

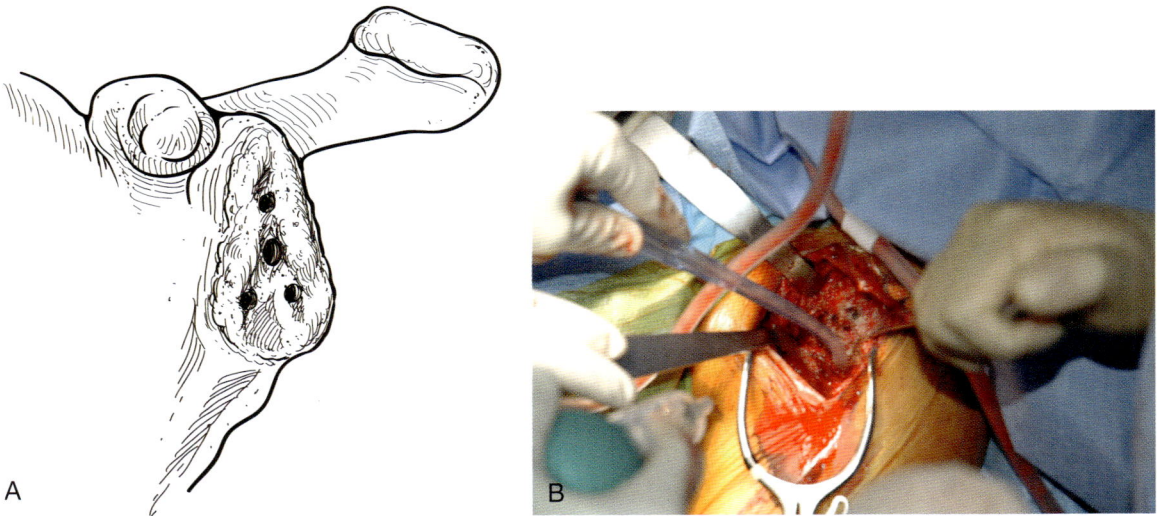

FIGURE 40.5 (A and B) The previously created central hole of a pegged anatomic glenoid component can be used for placement of a reverse glenoid component.

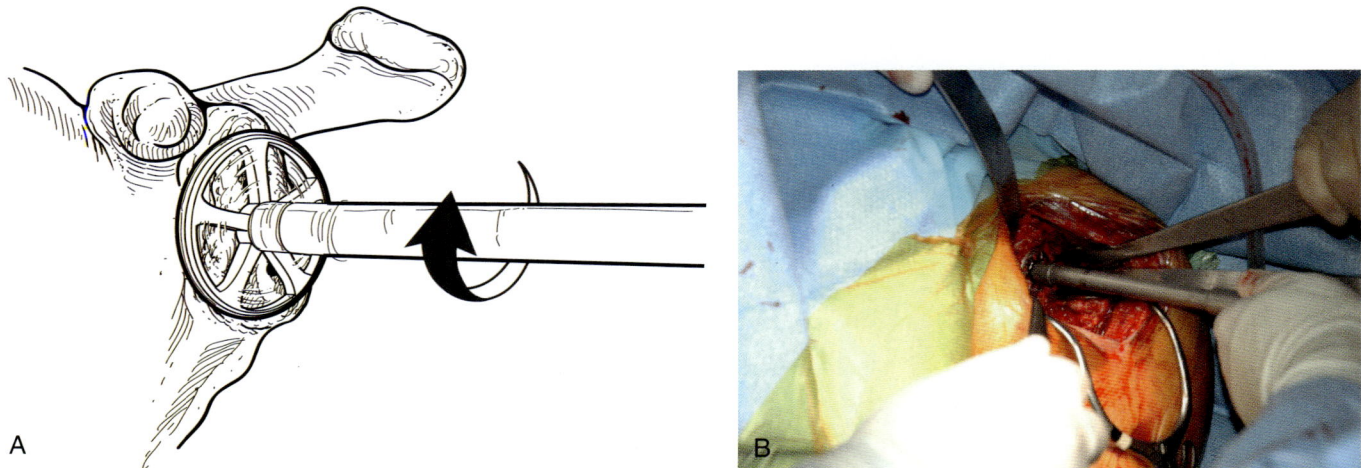

FIGURE 40.6 (A and B) The residual glenoid is reamed to a flat surface using the previously placed central hole.

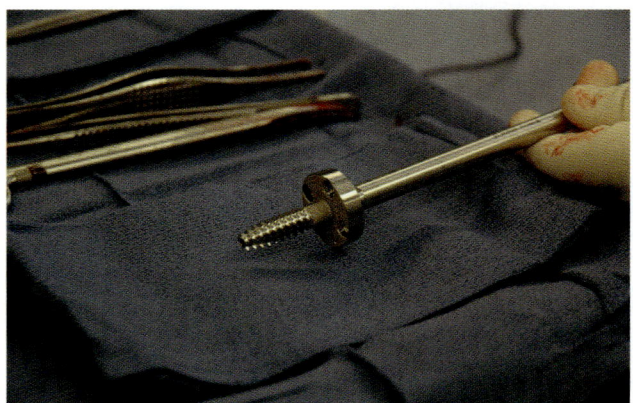

FIGURE 40.7 Revision-type base plate with a central screw.

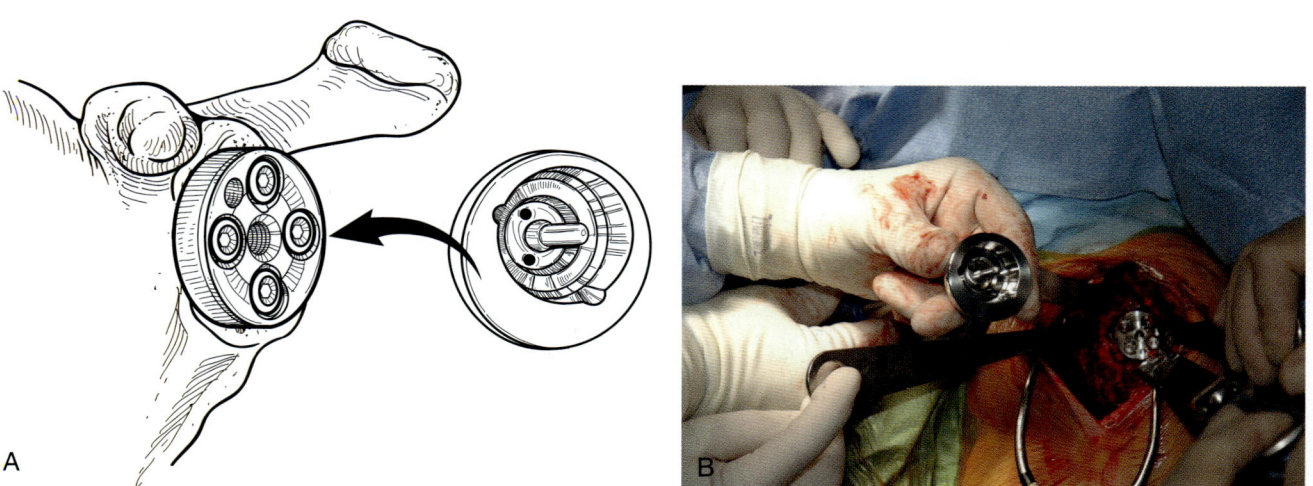

FIGURE 40.8 (A and B) Because using the previously placed hole in the glenoid places the reverse base plate more superior than desired, an inferior offset glenosphere is used.

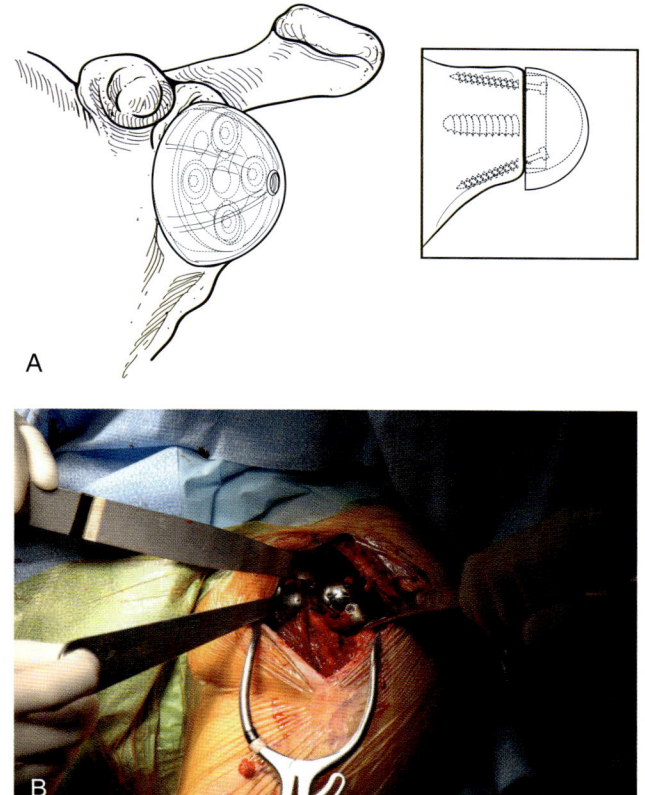

FIGURE 40.9 (A and B) The final glenoid construct using an inferior offset glenosphere.

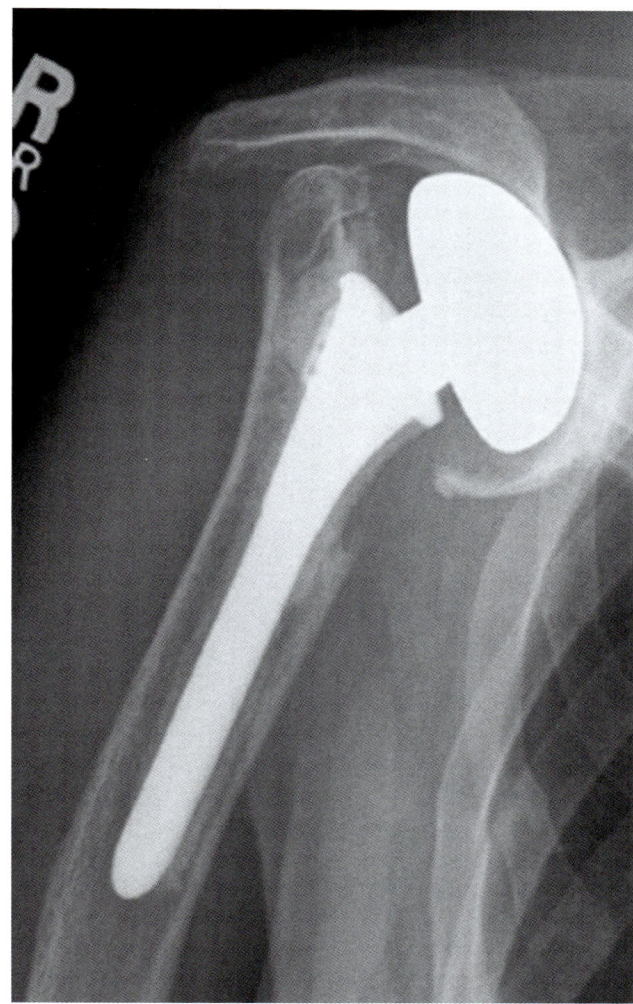

FIGURE 40.10 Patient with severe glenoid erosion after hemiarthroplasty prohibiting simple insertion of a glenoid component.

component, reconstruction of the glenoid with an autogenous iliac crest structural bone graft is indicated.[2] Our previous experience with cancellous bone grafts, allografts, and bone graft substitutes resulted in a high rate of graft resorption and led us to the technique that we now use.

Unconstrained Shoulder Arthroplasty Cases Requiring a Glenoid Bone Graft

Rarely, moderate to severe osseous insufficiency of the glenoid occurs after hemiarthroplasty of the shoulder, and poor glenoid bone stock prohibits insertion of an unconstrained glenoid component (Fig. 40.10). In these cases, two options exist: (1) conversion to resection arthroplasty by simple removal of the humeral component or (2) glenoid reconstruction with an iliac crest bone graft. Similarly, in patients with a failed glenoid component (loosening, component fracture), options include resection arthroplasty, removal of the glenoid component with retention of the humeral component, or glenoid reconstruction with an iliac crest bone graft (Fig. 40.11). We tell patients selected for glenoid reconstruction in unconstrained shoulder arthroplasty that we anticipate a second-stage operation for insertion of a polyethylene glenoid component after it is confirmed with computed tomography that the bone graft has been incorporated (Fig. 40.12), which occurs approximately 6 months after bone graft reconstruction. In patients who desire conversion to resection arthroplasty or removal of the glenoid component (usually elderly patients seeking only pain relief), this is easily accomplished by removing the humeral stem or glenoid component, or both, as described in Chapter 38 (Fig. 40.13).

For glenoid reconstruction, an autogenous iliac crest bone graft is first harvested, as described later in this chapter. The glenoid is exposed, as previously described. Any soft tissue covering the remaining osseous glenoid is removed to define the limits of the glenoid osseous margins (Fig. 40.14). The area of deficiency is identified. If the deficiency is central, it may be possible to fashion the bone graft to fit the defect via an interference fit and eliminate the need for internal fixation (Fig. 40.15). For peripheral deficits, it is necessary to secure the bone graft with internal fixation to avoid migration. In anterior or posterior osseous insufficiency, we usually opt for cannulated, partially threaded 4.0-mm-diameter screws with washers placed through the bone graft and into the intact osseous glenoid. In central glenoid osseous insufficiency (not amenable to interference fit of the bone graft) and superior glenoid osseous insufficiency, we opt for graft fixation with 1.5 × 60-mm bioabsorbable fixation pins (SmartPin, Linvtec, Inc., Largo, FL).

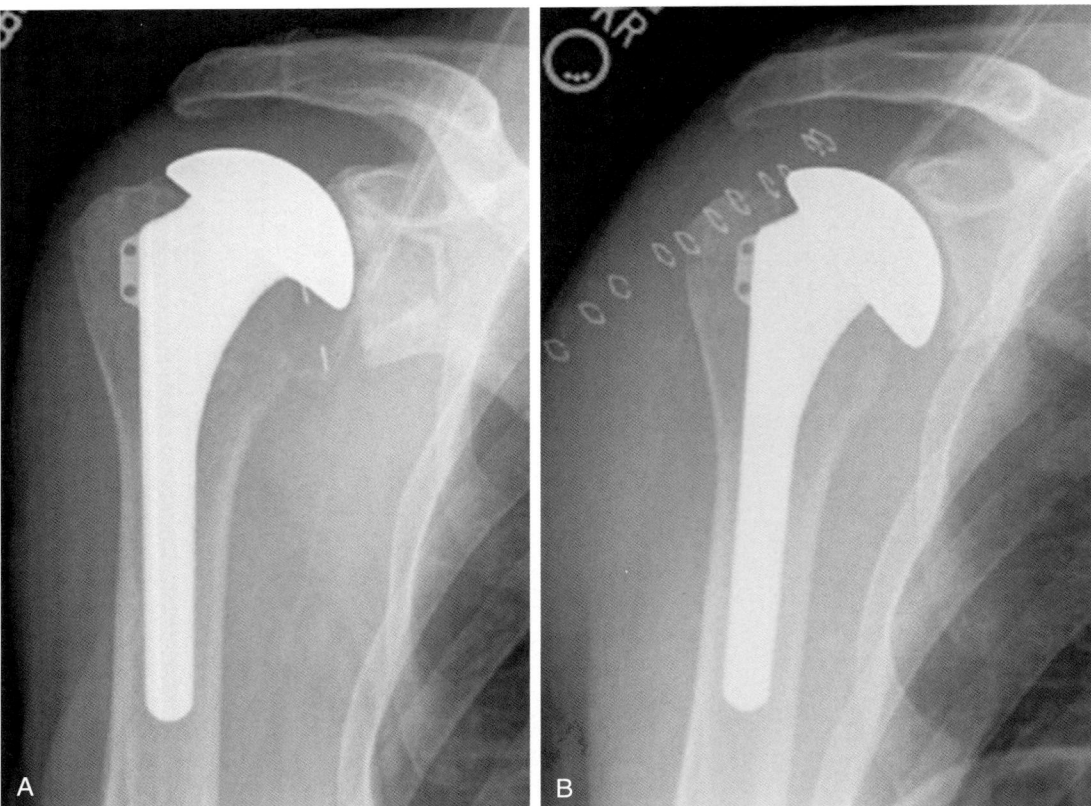

FIGURE 40.11 When considering revision using unconstrained arthroplasty in patients with a failed glenoid component (loosening, component fracture) (A), options include resection arthroplasty, removal of the glenoid component with retention of the humeral component, or glenoid reconstruction with an iliac crest bone graft (B).

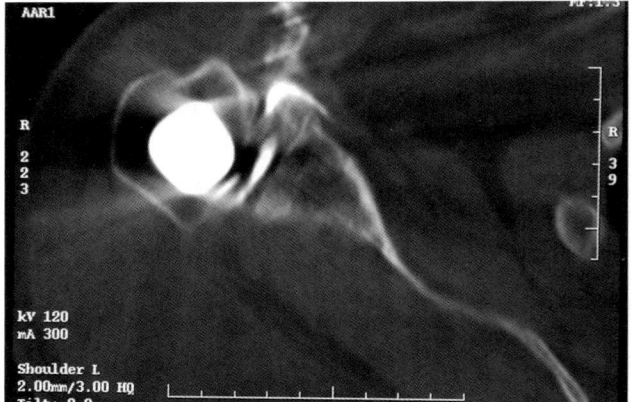

FIGURE 40.12 Computed tomography scan showing incorporation of an iliac crest bone graft used for reconstruction of the glenoid.

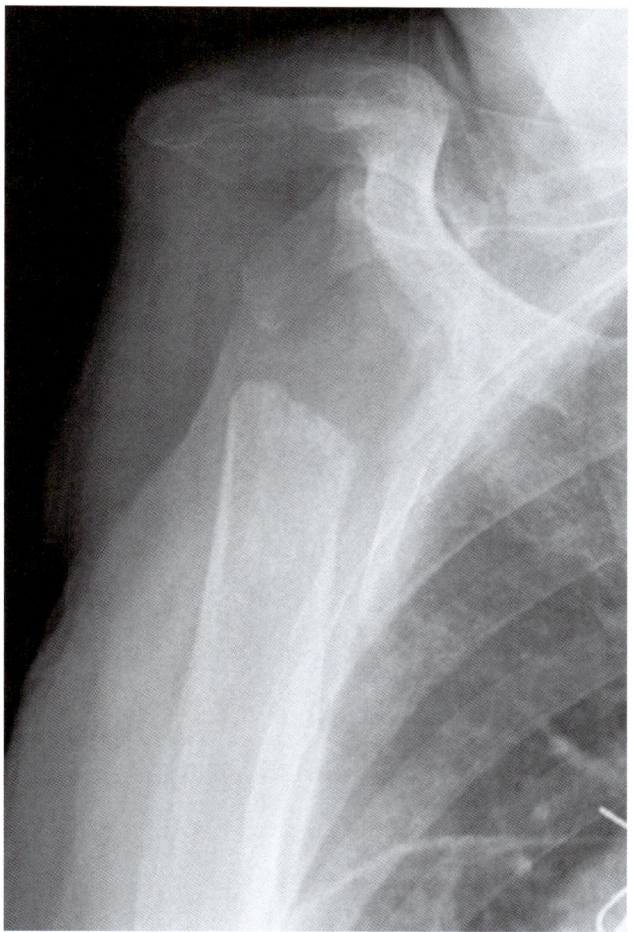

FIGURE 40.13 Patient undergoing resection arthroplasty for pain relief after failed shoulder arthroplasty.

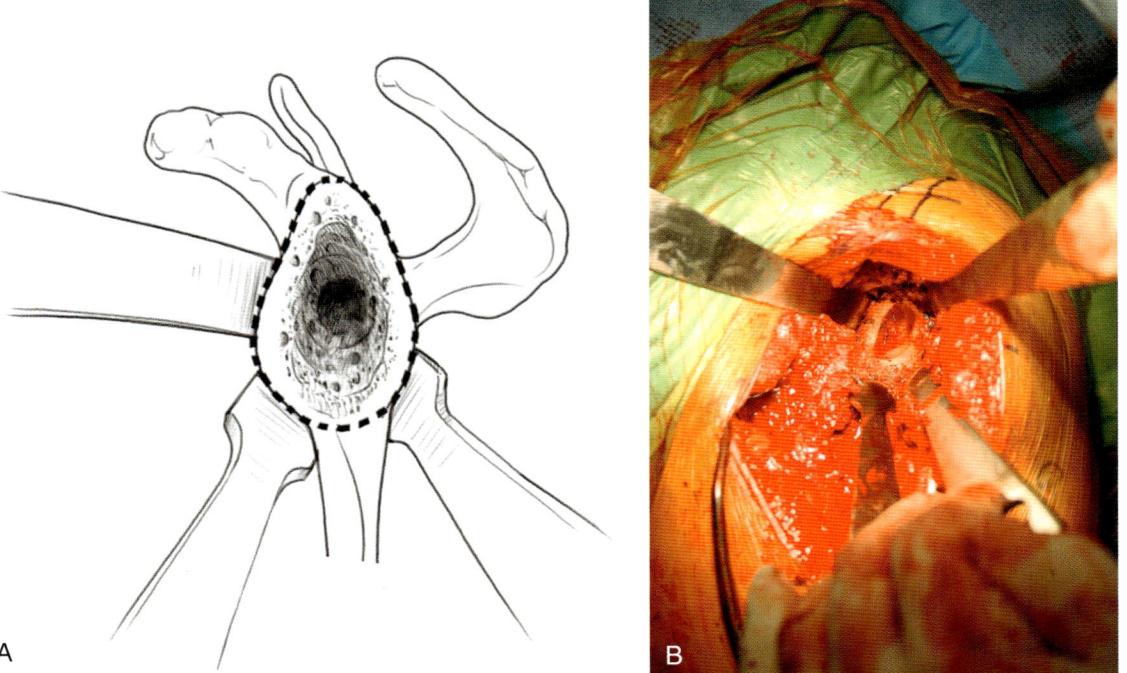

FIGURE 40.14 (A and B) The margins of the osseous glenoid are defined before reconstruction of the glenoid.

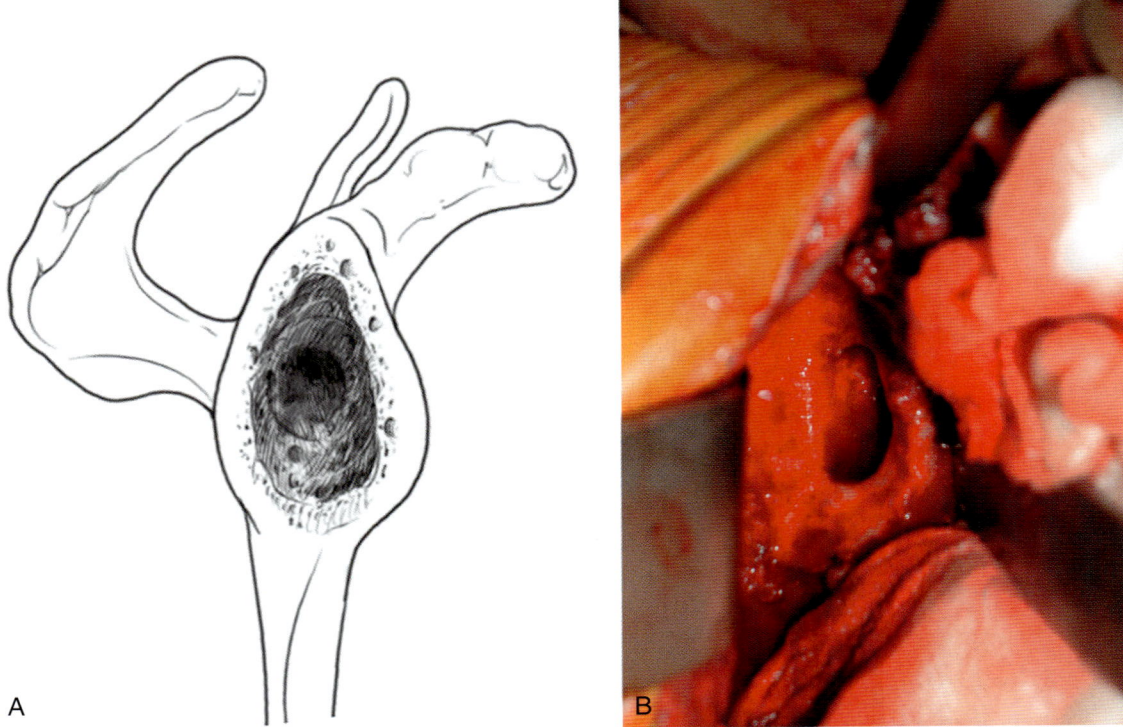

FIGURE 40.15 (A and B) Central glenoid deficiency that can be treated by bone graft reconstruction with interference-fit fixation.

Contained Osseous Deficit

For interference-fit fixation of a central osseous deficit, the defect is prepared by lightly abrading the glenoid surface with a 5-mm round burr (Fig. 40.16). The tricortical iliac crest bone graft is trimmed with a cutting rongeur or saw to a shape similar to the defect and slightly larger (Fig. 40.17). Cancellous bone is placed in the central defect, and the tricortical segment of the bone graft is placed in the defect and impacted into place with a large bone tamp until it is flush with the intact glenoid surface (Fig. 40.18). Care is taken to orient the tricortical graft so that a cortical surface faces laterally (Fig. 40.19).

Uncontained (Anterior or Posterior) Osseous Deficit

In cases of anterior or posterior glenoid insufficiency requiring bone graft reconstruction, the tricortical iliac crest bone graft is contoured to fit the defect with a cutting rongeur so that a cortical surface faces laterally (Fig. 40.20). Two guidewires for 4.0-mm screws are placed across the graft and the glenoid vault and into the opposite cortex of the native glenoid (Fig. 40.21). Care is taken to direct the guidewires so that they do not violate the central portion of the glenoid vault and thereby prohibit later placement of a glenoid component (Fig. 40.22). For anterior glenoid insufficiency, these guidewires can be placed through the deltopectoral approach. For posterior glenoid insufficiency, the guidewires are placed percutaneously from the posterior aspect of the shoulder (Fig. 40.23). Screw lengths are measured from the guidewire (Fig. 40.24). The drill provided is used over the guidewire (Fig. 40.25). The proper size screw with washer is placed over the guidewire and advanced until fully seated (Fig. 40.26).

When performing bone graft reconstruction of the glenoid, we avoid simultaneous implantation of an unconstrained glenoid component. Single-stage implantation of a glenoid component after reconstruction of the glenoid with a bone graft has resulted in an unacceptably high rate of failure of the glenoid component (Fig. 40.27). In this scenario, we will offer the patient implantation of a glenoid component 6 months after glenoid reconstruction if a computed tomography scan confirms incorporation of the bone graft and sufficient glenoid bone stock to allow insertion of a glenoid component (Fig. 40.28). In this situation, placement of the revision glenoid component is performed as in cases of primary glenoid resurfacing (see Chapter 12). Occasionally in young patients, we will perform fascia lata glenoid resurfacing at the time of glenoid reconstruction (Fig. 40.29; see Chapter 34).

Uncontained Combined (Anterior and Posterior) Osseous Deficit

For osseous glenoid defects that involve the anterior and posterior glenoid wall, bioabsorbable fixation pins are used to prevent migration of the bone graft (Fig. 40.30). This is done by first fixing the graft with two 0.062-inch Kirschner wires placed through the bone graft and into the native glenoid medially. These wires are intentionally placed so that they are not parallel to one another (Fig. 40.31). One

Text continued on p. 428

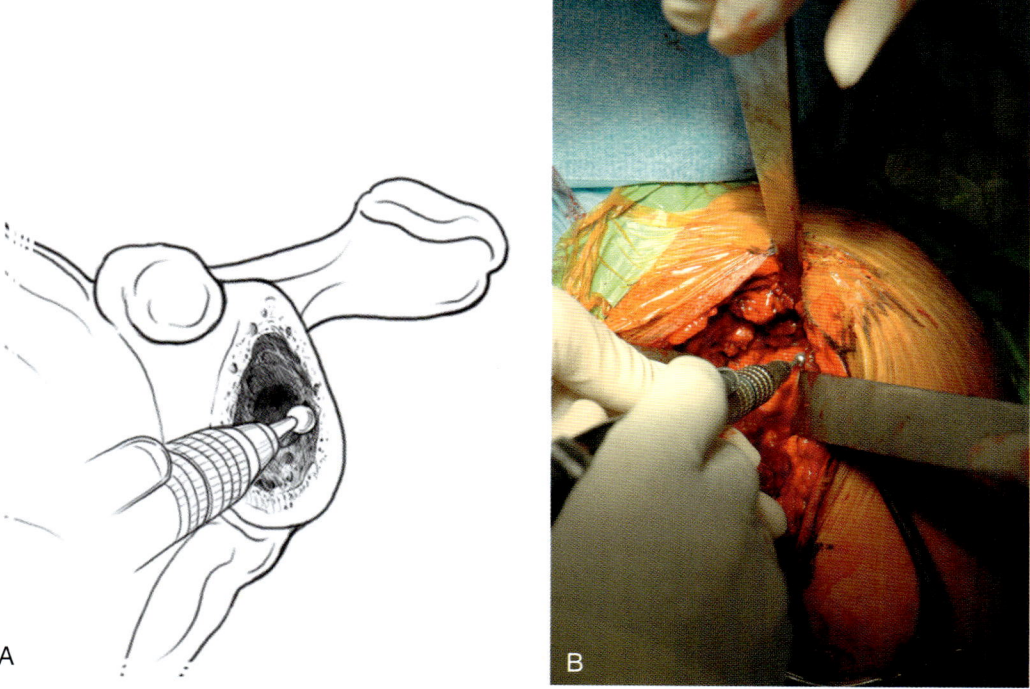

FIGURE 40.16 (A and B) Preparation of the glenoid with a 5-mm round burr.

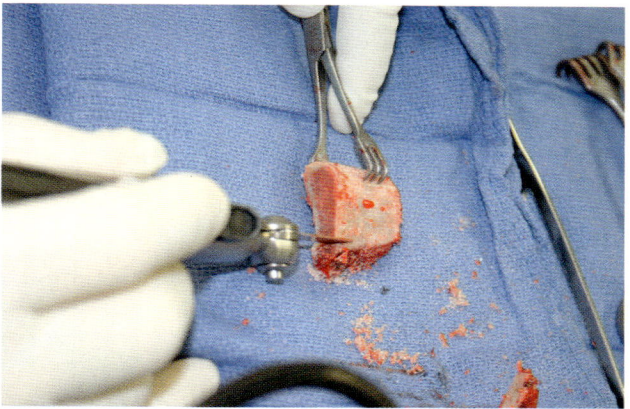

FIGURE 40.17 Contouring of the iliac crest bone graft before insertion into the glenoid cavity.

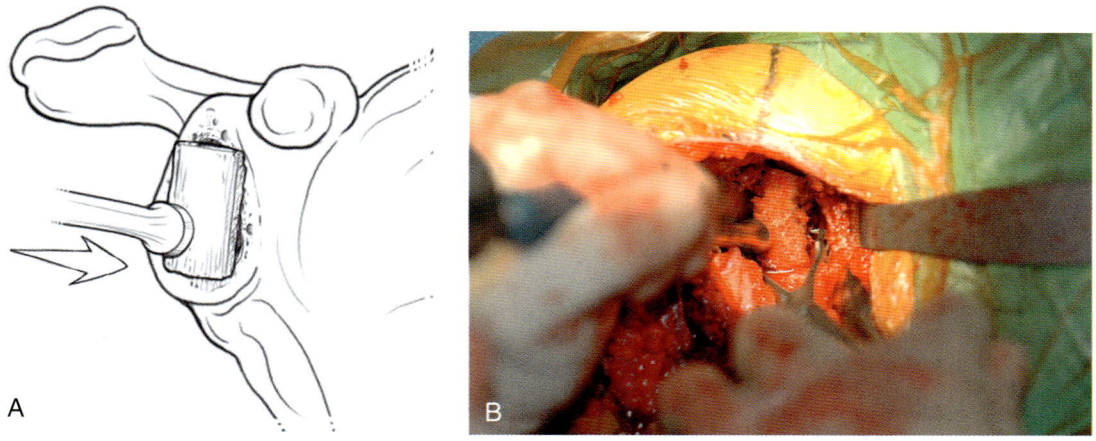

FIGURE 40.18 (A and B) Impaction of the glenoid bone graft.

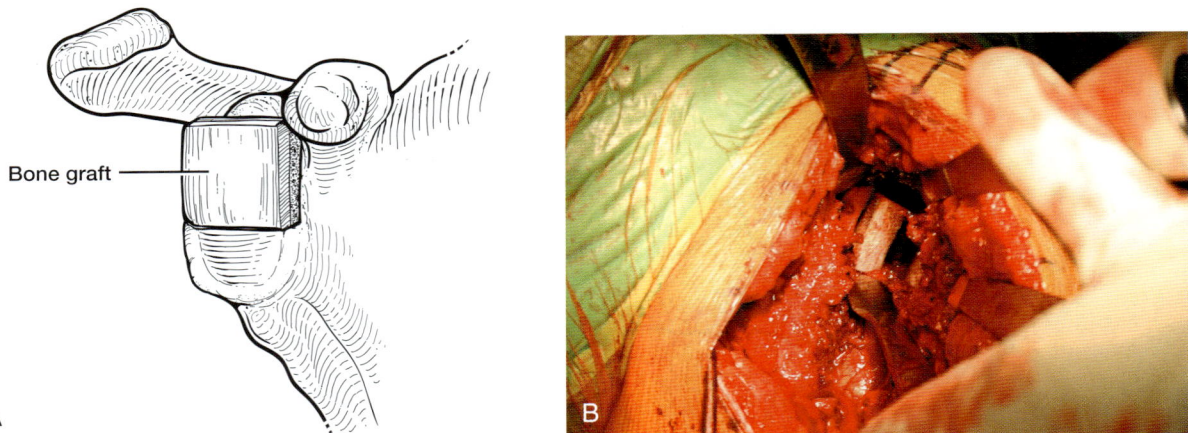

FIGURE 40.19 (A and B) The glenoid bone graft is inserted with a cortical surface facing laterally to resist medialization of the humeral head.

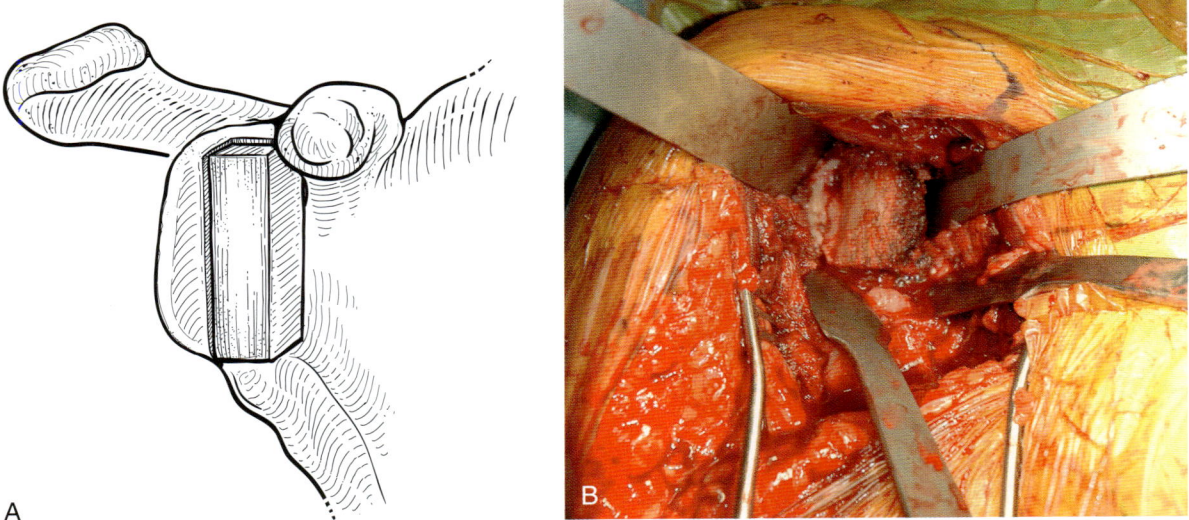

FIGURE 40.20 (A and B) Placement of a glenoid bone graft to fill an anterior glenoid defect.

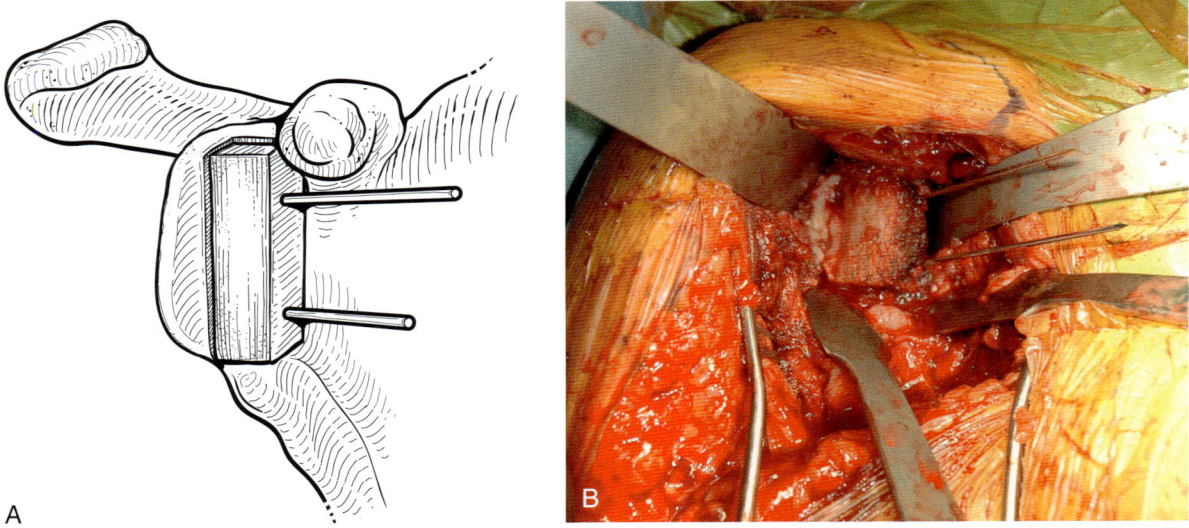

FIGURE 40.21 (A and B) Placement of guidewires for the 4.0-mm cannulated screws used for bone graft reconstruction of an anterior glenoid defect.

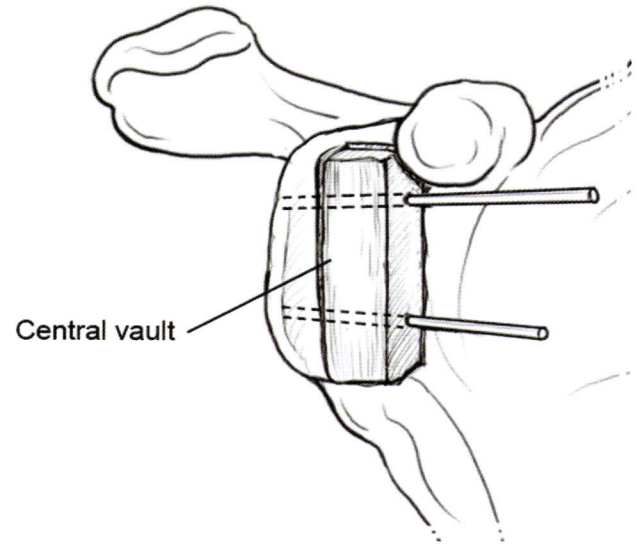

FIGURE 40.22 Guidewires are placed so that the central portion of the glenoid vault is not violated and later placement of the glenoid component prohibited.

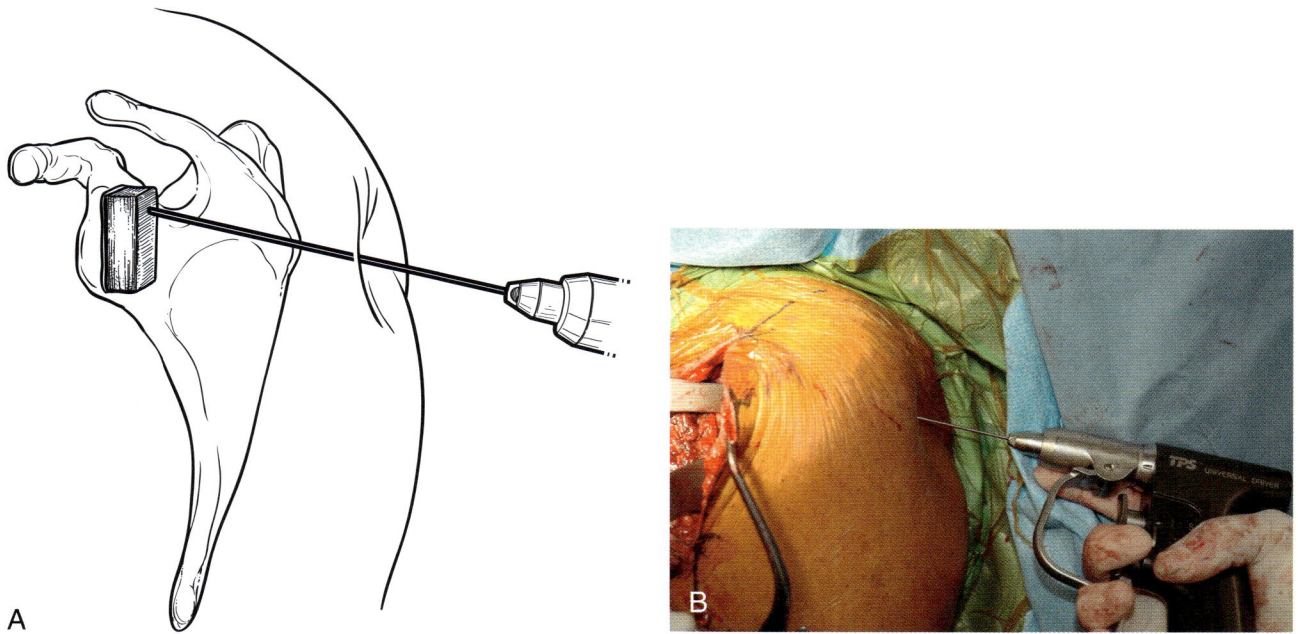

FIGURE 40.23 (A and B) Percutaneous placement for a posterior glenoid defect.

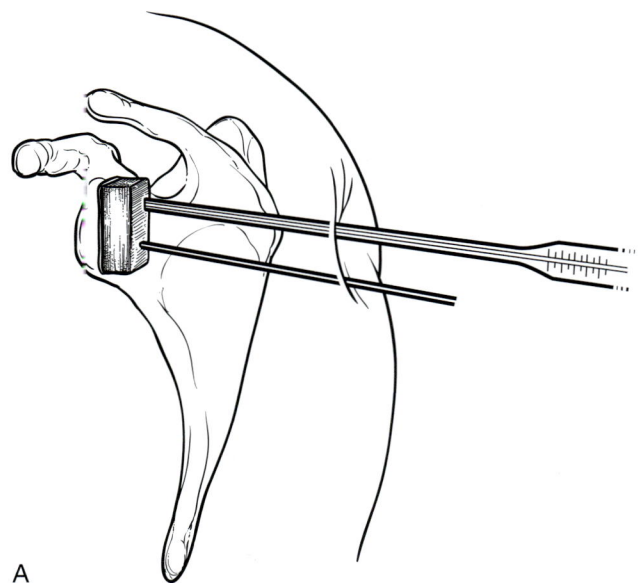
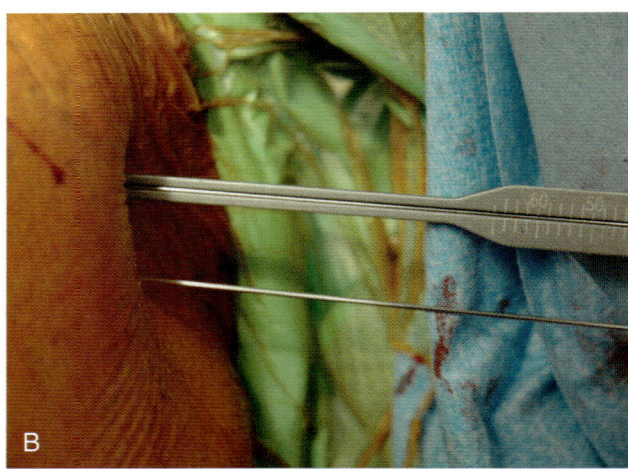

FIGURE 40.24 (A and B) Measurement of screw length from the guidewires.

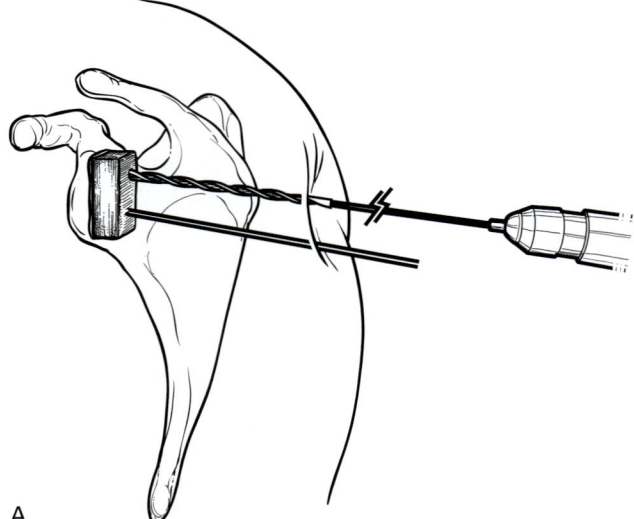
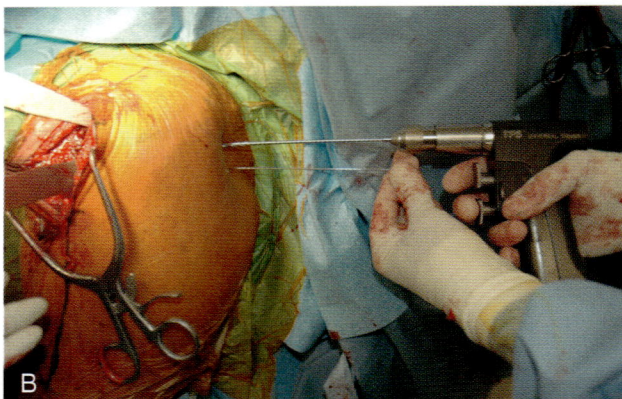

FIGURE 40.25 (A and B) Drilling the holes for the cannulated screws over the guidewires.

CHAPTER 40 ■ Glenoid Component

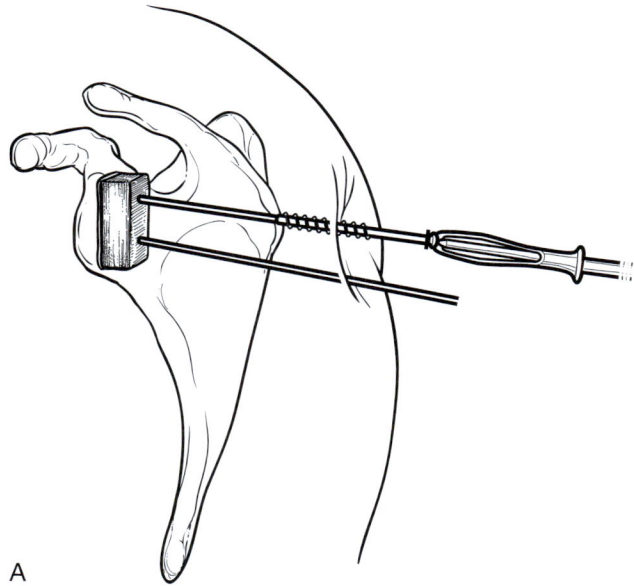

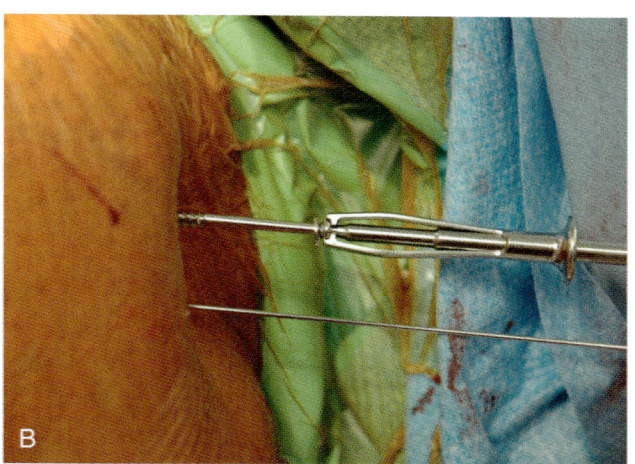

FIGURE 40.26 (A and B) Fixation of the bone graft with screws and washers.

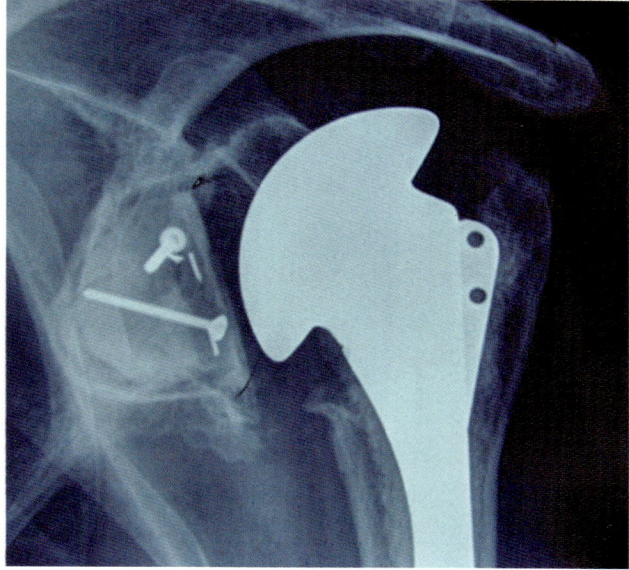

FIGURE 40.27 Failure of the glenoid component after attempted single-stage reconstruction of the glenoid with an iliac crest bone graft and placement of an unconstrained shoulder arthroplasty.

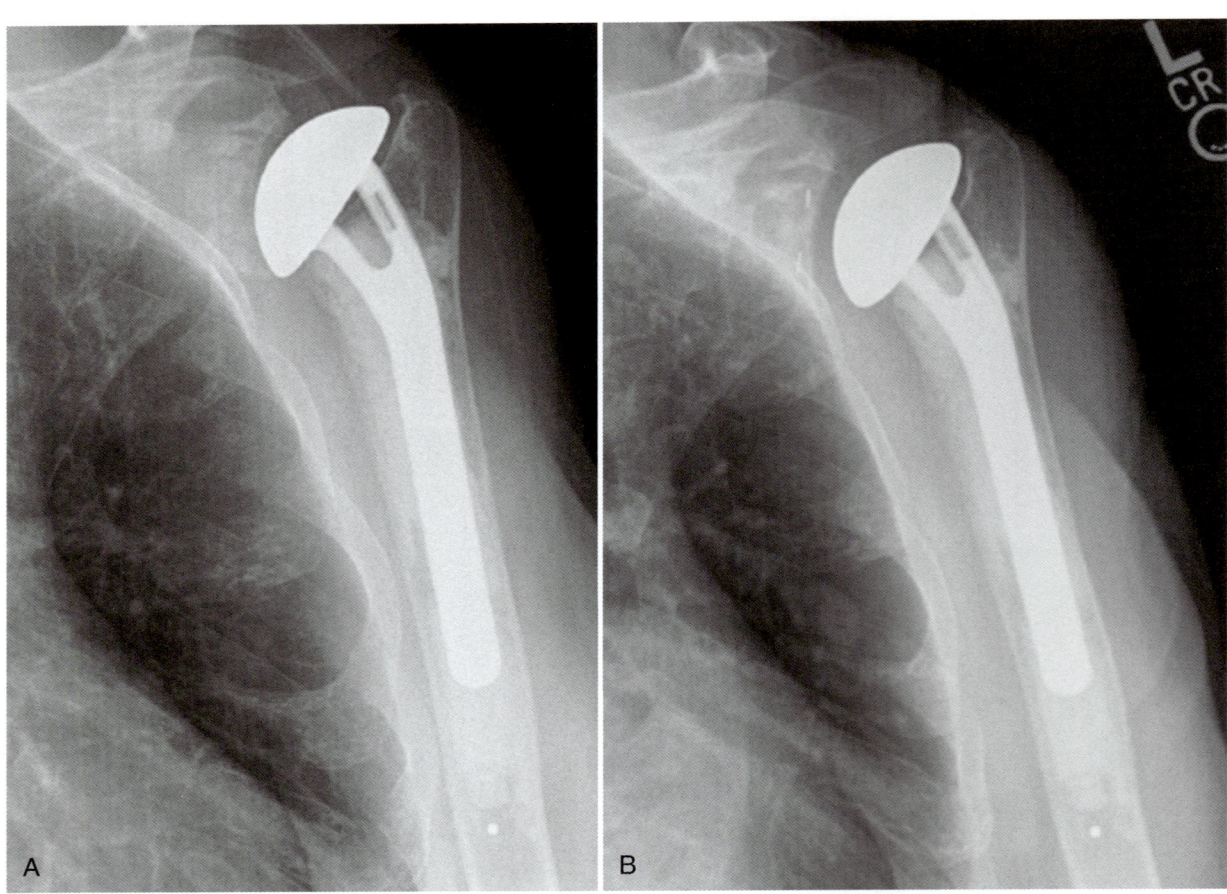

FIGURE 40.28 Revision total shoulder arthroplasty performed in two stages. The first stage consisted of glenoid reconstruction with a bone graft (A). The second stage involved implantation of a glenoid component 6 months after reconstruction of the osseous glenoid (B).

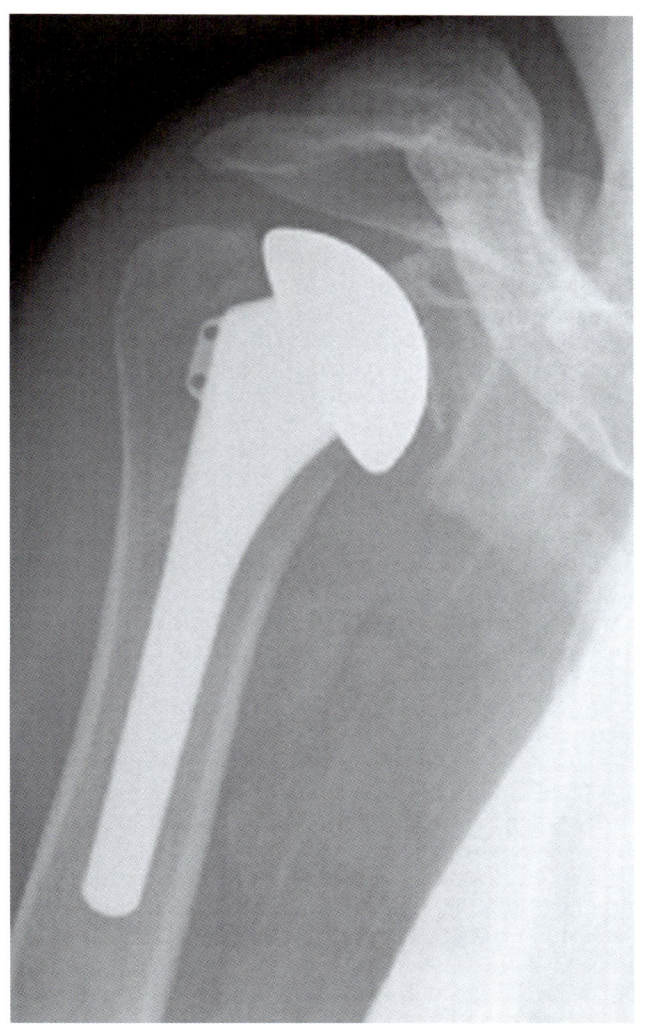

FIGURE 40.29 Biologic resurfacing of the glenoid after reconstruction of the osseous glenoid with a bone graft. It was performed as a single-stage procedure.

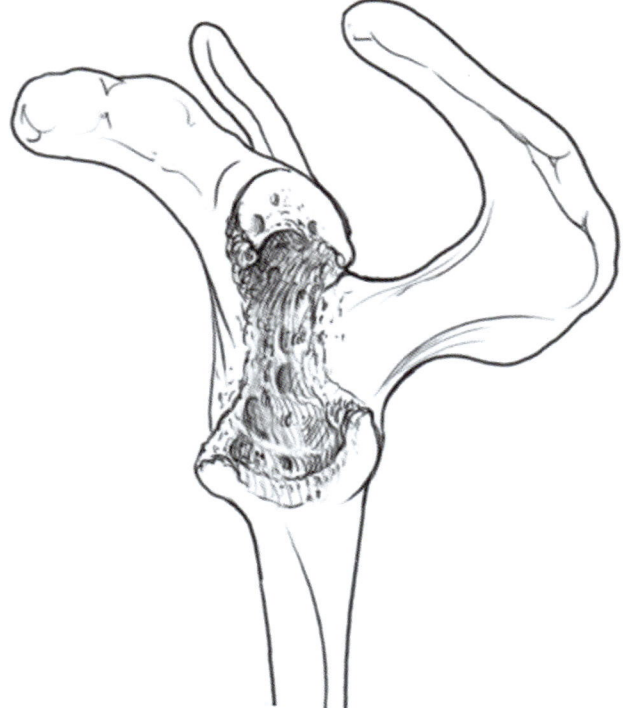

FIGURE 40.30 Uncontained combined anterior and posterior glenoid defect.

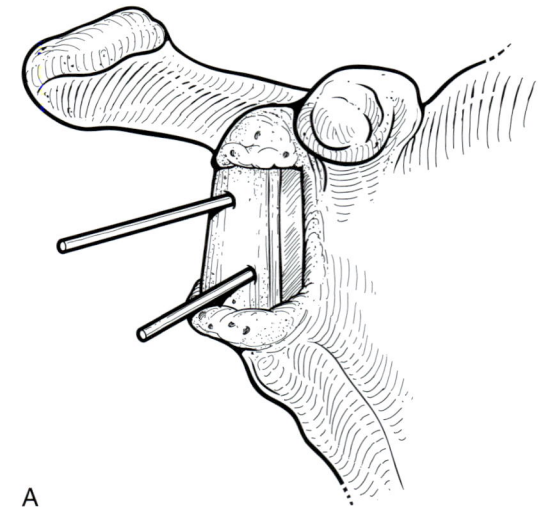

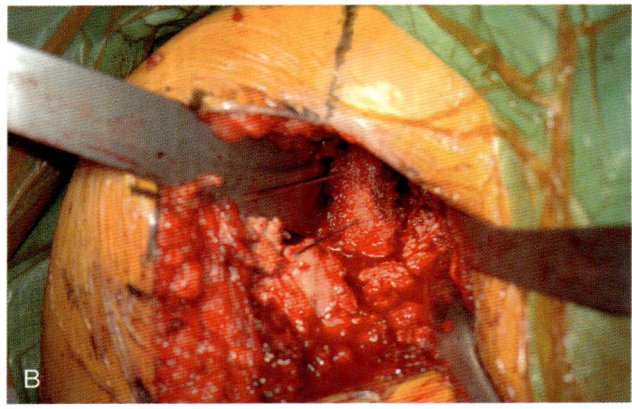

FIGURE 40.31 (A and B) Kirschner wires placed before insertion of bioabsorbable pins for bone graft fixation.

of the wires is removed, and a bioabsorbable pin is advanced into the hole left by the Kirschner wire with the insertion device (Fig. 40.32). Another wire is used to create another hole in a direction and orientation different from that of the previous two holes, and another bioabsorbable pin is placed (Fig. 40.33). This process is repeated until a minimum of four pins have been placed. To enhance fixation, we avoid placing any of the pins parallel to one another. The residual pin tips are clipped flush with the bone graft with a large rongeur to complete fixation of the bone graft (Fig. 40.34). This same technique is used for superior defects. After contouring the bone graft to fit the defect and preparation of the base of the defect, the graft is fixated with multiple bioabsorbable pins (Fig. 40.35).

Reverse Shoulder Arthroplasty Cases Requiring a Glenoid Bone Graft

Cases in which a primary hemiarthroplasty is to be revised to a reverse prosthesis occasionally require bone grafting of the glenoid. The defect is usually superior in cases of rotator cuff deficiency but may be anterior or posterior in cases of prosthetic instability after hemiarthroplasty (Fig. 40.36).

Similarly, cases with a failed glenoid component and rotator cuff insufficiency are an indication for glenoid reconstruction and placement of a reverse prosthesis (Fig. 40.37). The same techniques used for glenoid reconstruction with an autogenous iliac crest bone graft for unconstrained shoulder arthroplasty are performed. The main difference between revision with a reverse prosthesis and revision with an unconstrained prosthesis in this scenario is the potential ability to perform a single-stage procedure when using the reverse prosthesis. If the majority of the central post or screw of the reverse prosthesis base plate can be implanted into native glenoid bone, the reverse prosthesis can be implanted as a single-stage procedure (Fig. 40.38). An alternative base plate designed for revision surgery is available. This base plate has a central post or screw that is longer than the standard base plate. This extra length allows seating of the central post of the base plate into native glenoid bone with the use of a reconstructive bone graft (Fig. 40.39).

Pascal Boileau and colleagues described the bony increased-offset reversed shoulder arthroplasty technique (BIO-RSA) using a bone graft from the humeral head initially for use in lateralizing the glenoid in primary reverse shoulder arthroplasty (see Chapter 22).[3] In revision cases in which bone grafting is needed and the native humeral head is not available, the BIO-RSA technique is completed with harvest of iliac crest bone grafting using a modification of the original technique described by Tom Norris and colleagues.[4]

The technique for exposure to harvest autogenous iliac crest bone graft is described later. Once exposure of the anterior iliac crest is achieved, the technique for BIO-RSA graft harvesting is similar to the technique for BIO-RSA graft harvesting from the native humeral head (see Chapter 22).

The guide pin is placed into the center (from medial to lateral) of the iliac crest (Fig. 40.40), while ensuring the guide pin is parallel to the inner and outer tables. The BIO-RSA graft reamer is used to ream the iliac crest until a flat surface is created (Fig. 40.41). The central hole is drilled using a cannulated drill for the central hole of the base plate (Fig. 40.42). The guide pin is removed and the reverse glenoid base plate (long post or long screw) is inserted into the central hole created in the iliac crest (Fig. 40.43). A 1-inch curved osteotome is used to complete the osteotomy in the iliac crest created by the BIO-RSA reamer and free the tricortical bone graft (Fig. 40.44). The base plate, along with the attached bone graft, is then extracted (Fig. 40.45). The graft can be fashioned using a saw, burr, or rongeur as needed to match the defect on the glenoid (Fig. 40.46).

After preparation of the BIO-RSA bone graft on the long post or screw base plate, glenoid exposure is reestablished. As with primary reverse shoulder arthroplasty, we avoid using a Fukuda glenohumeral retractor during implantation of the reverse prosthesis because the base plate fixation screws may incarcerate the retractor. A guide pin is placed in the vault of the glenoid for placement of the central post or screw (Fig. 40.47). We attempt to place this pin in the area of maximal bone stock based on preoperative imaging and intraoperative observations. The guide pin is then overdrilled, penetrating the medial cortex of the scapula (Fig. 40.48). The base plate/bone graft construct is then placed in the central hole by either impaction with a mallet (posted base plate) or advancing via screw mechanism (threaded base

Text continued on p. 437

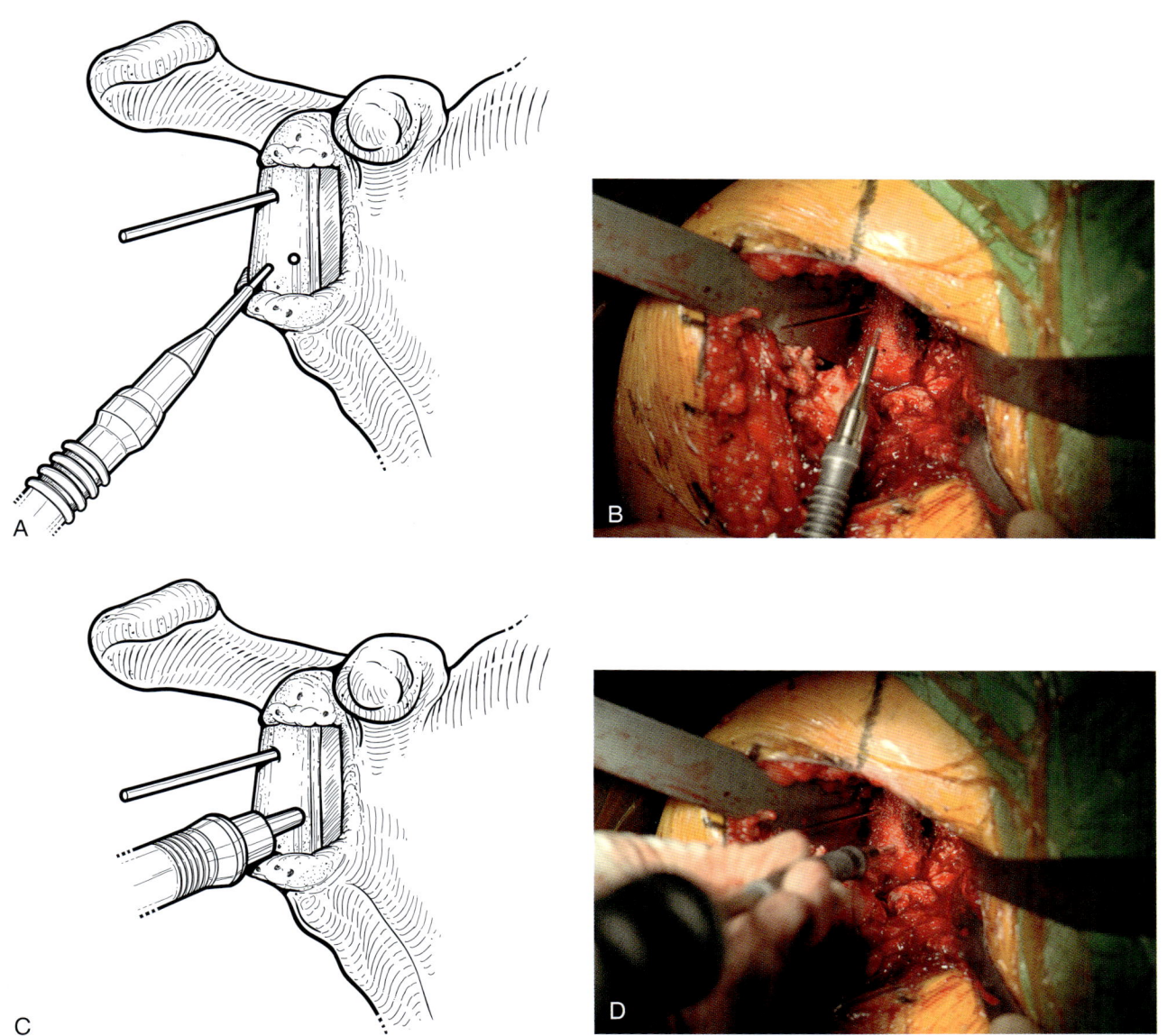

FIGURE 40.32 (A to D) Placement of a bioabsorbable pin for bone graft fixation.

430 SECTION VI ■ Revision Shoulder Arthroplasty

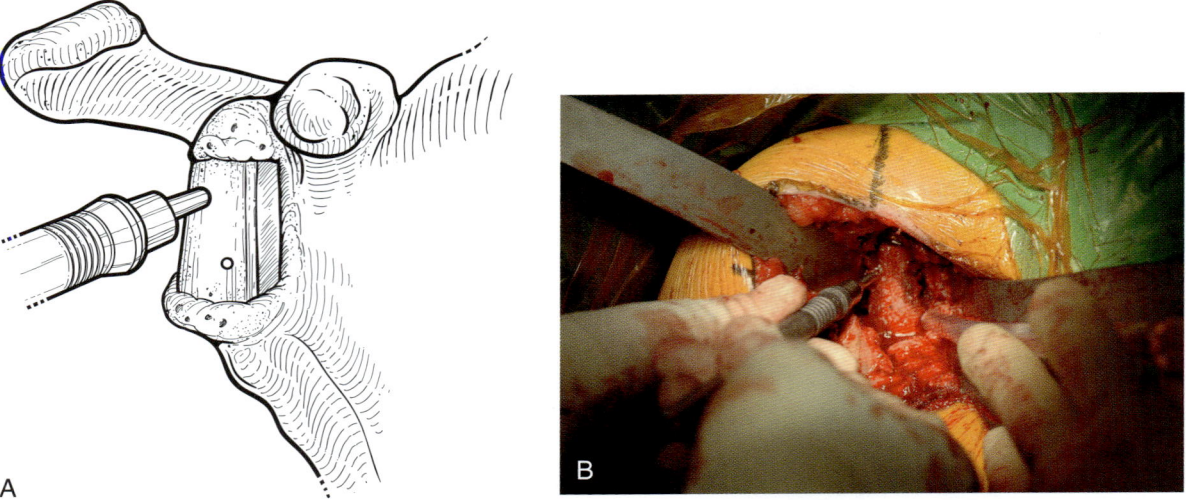

FIGURE 40.33 (A and B) Placement of a second bioabsorbable pin for bone graft fixation. The pin is not placed parallel to the initial pin.

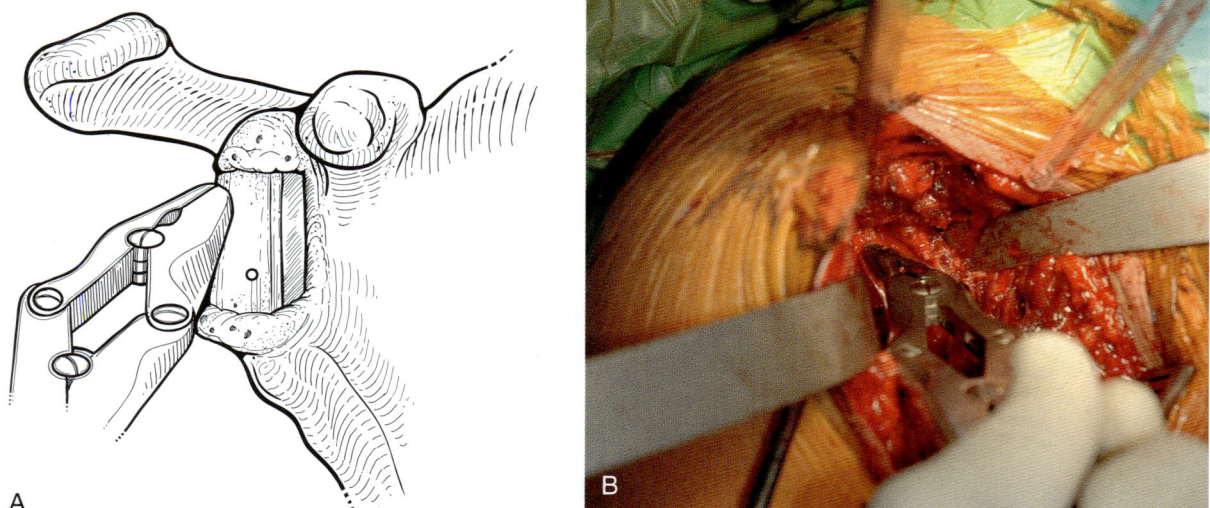

FIGURE 40.34 (A and B) The bioabsorbable pins are clipped flush to the surface of the bone graft with a rongeur.

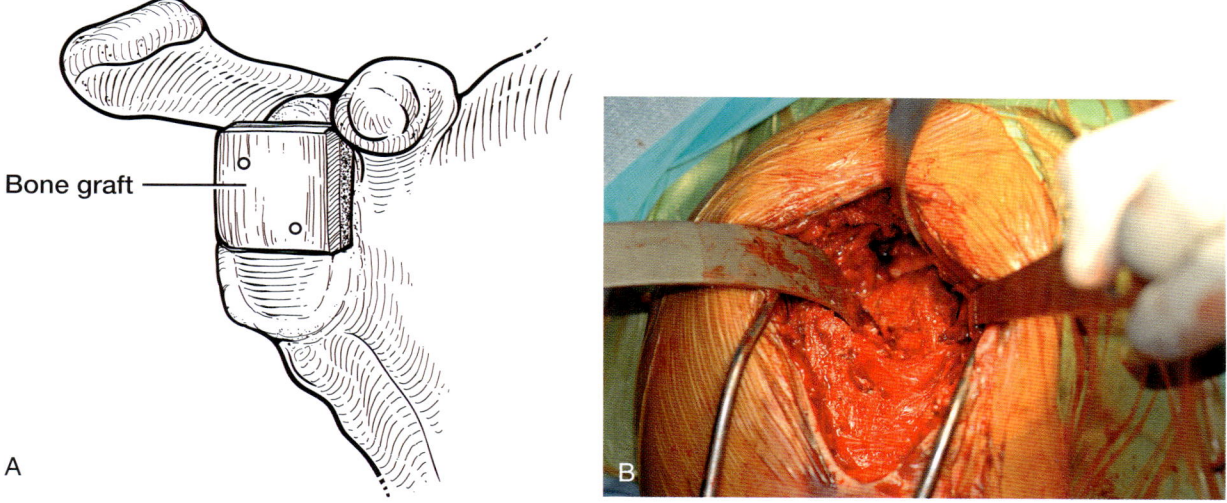

FIGURE 40.35 (A and B) After contouring the bone graft to fit the superior defect and preparation of the base of the defect, the graft is fixated with multiple bioabsorbable pins.

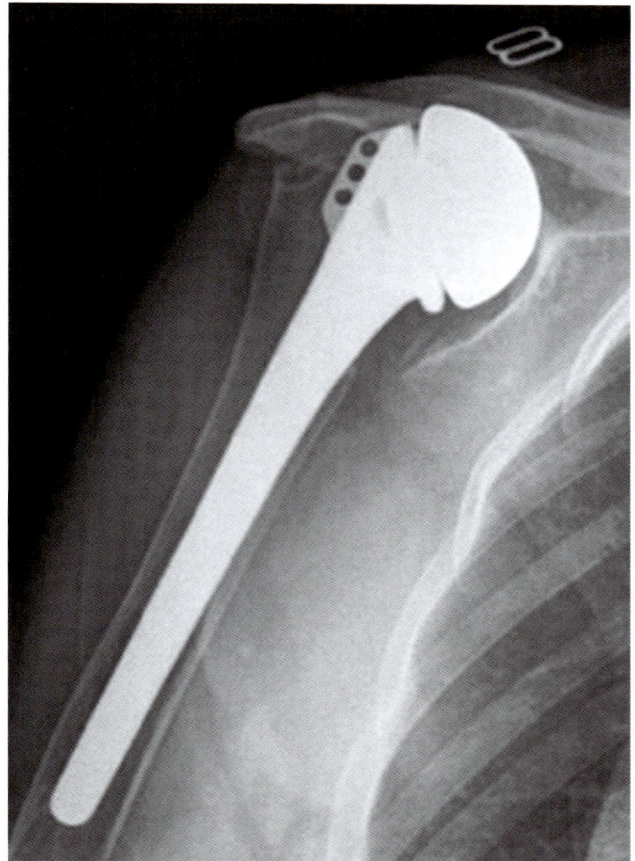

FIGURE 40.36 Failed hemiarthroplasty evaluated for conversion to a reverse prosthesis. The superior glenoid bone erosion necessitates osseous glenoid reconstruction with an iliac crest bone graft.

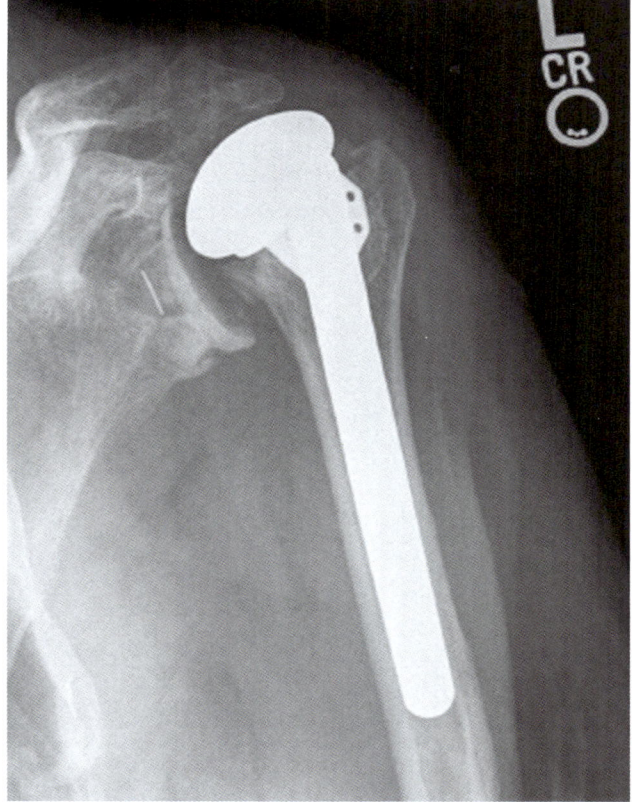

FIGURE 40.37 Case of failed total shoulder arthroplasty with rotator cuff insufficiency.

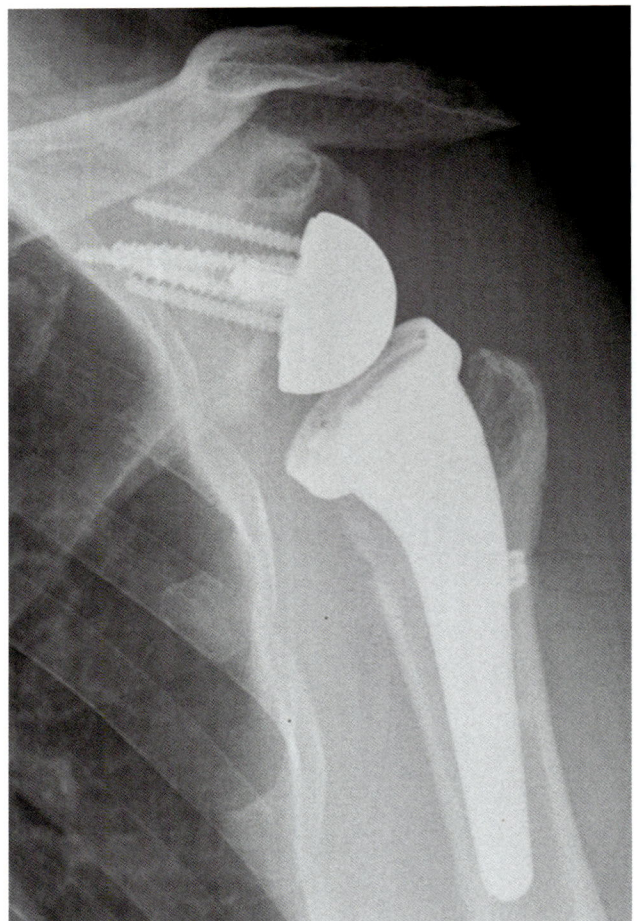

FIGURE 40.38 Case in which the majority of the central post of the reverse prosthesis base plate can be seated into native glenoid bone and allow single-stage revision.

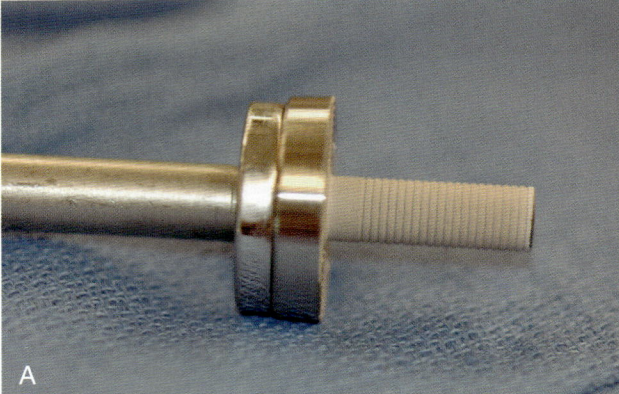
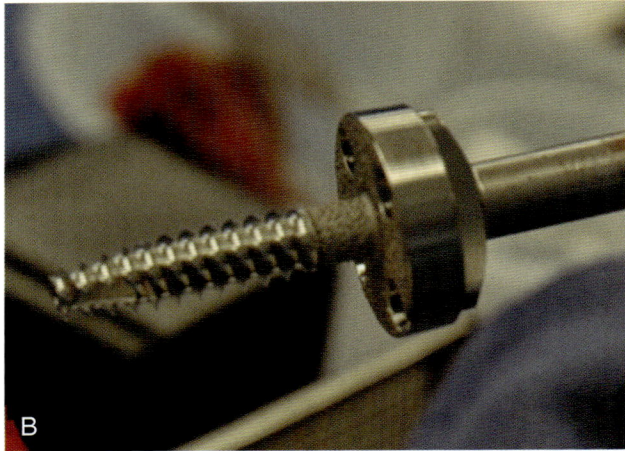

FIGURE 40.39 (A and B) Revision base plates with a central post or screw that is longer than the standard base plate allowing seating of the central post of the base plate into native glenoid bone with the use of a reconstructive bone graft.

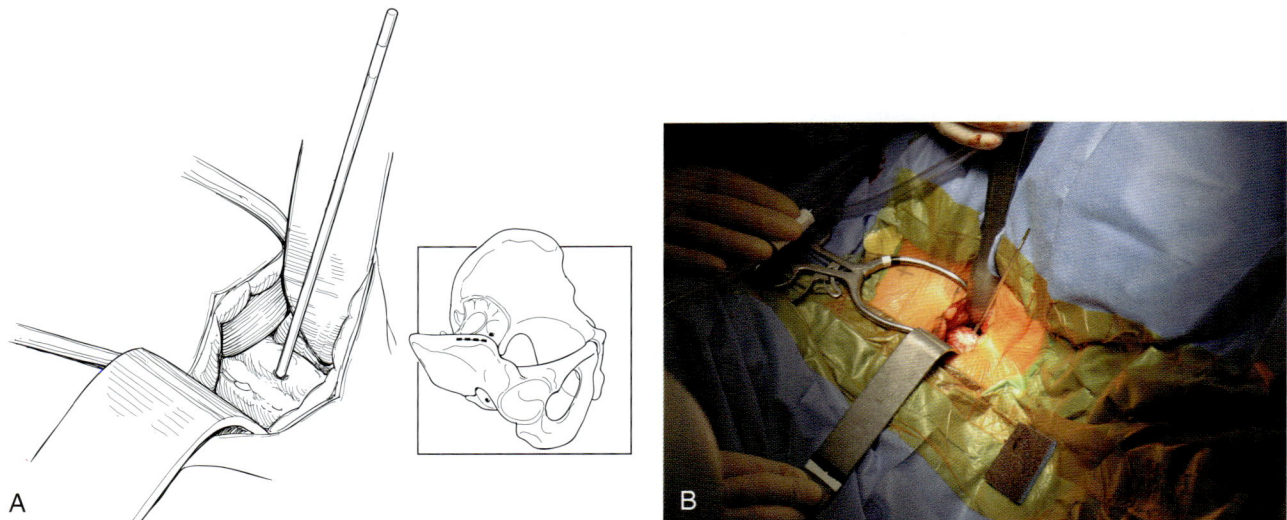

FIGURE 40.40 (A and B) The guide pin is placed into the center (from medial to lateral) of the iliac crest while ensuring the guide pin is parallel to the inner and outer tables.

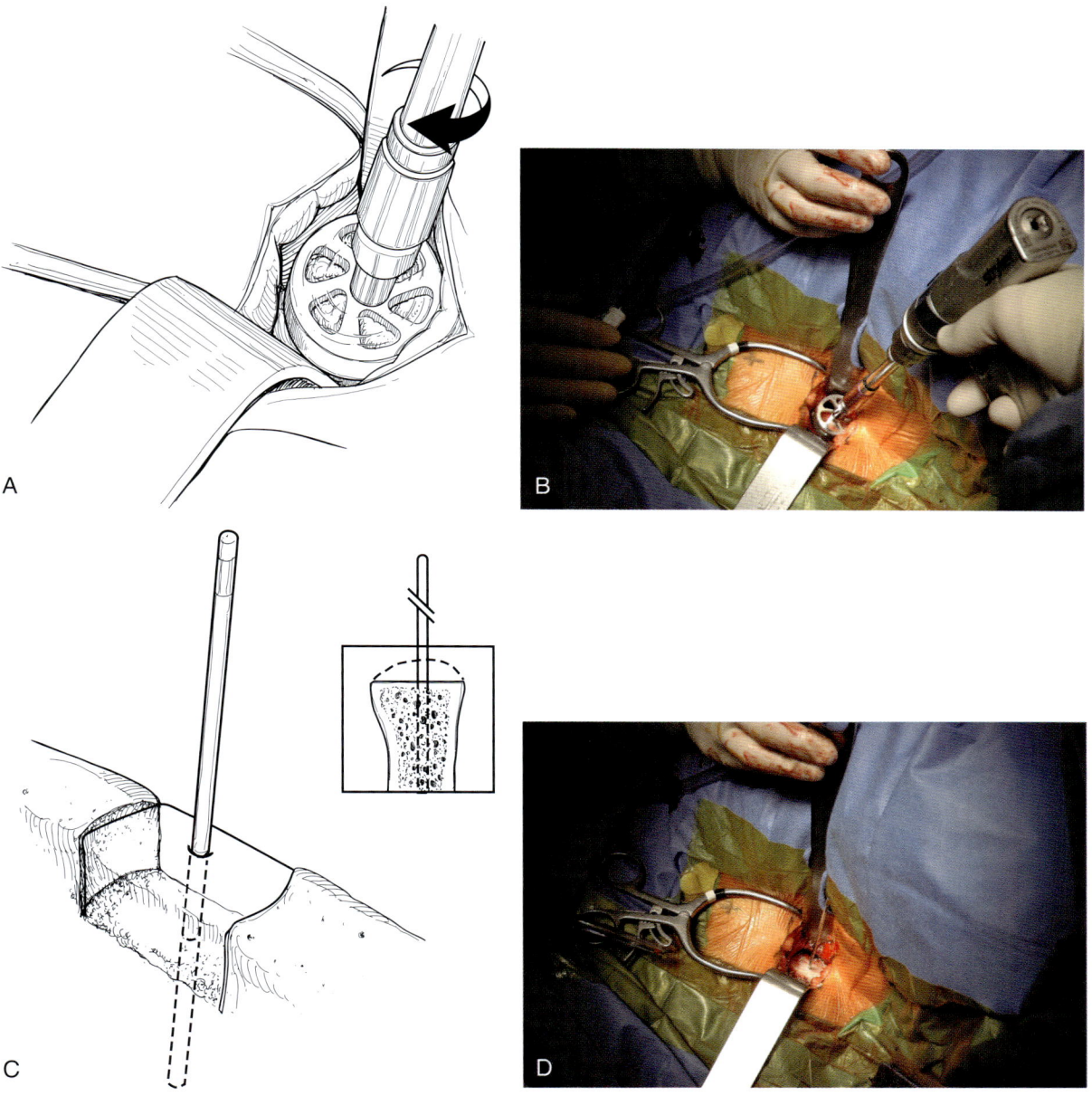

FIGURE 40.41 (A to D) The bony increased-offset reversed shoulder arthroplasty technique (BIO-RSA) graft reamer is used to ream the iliac crest until a flat surface is created.

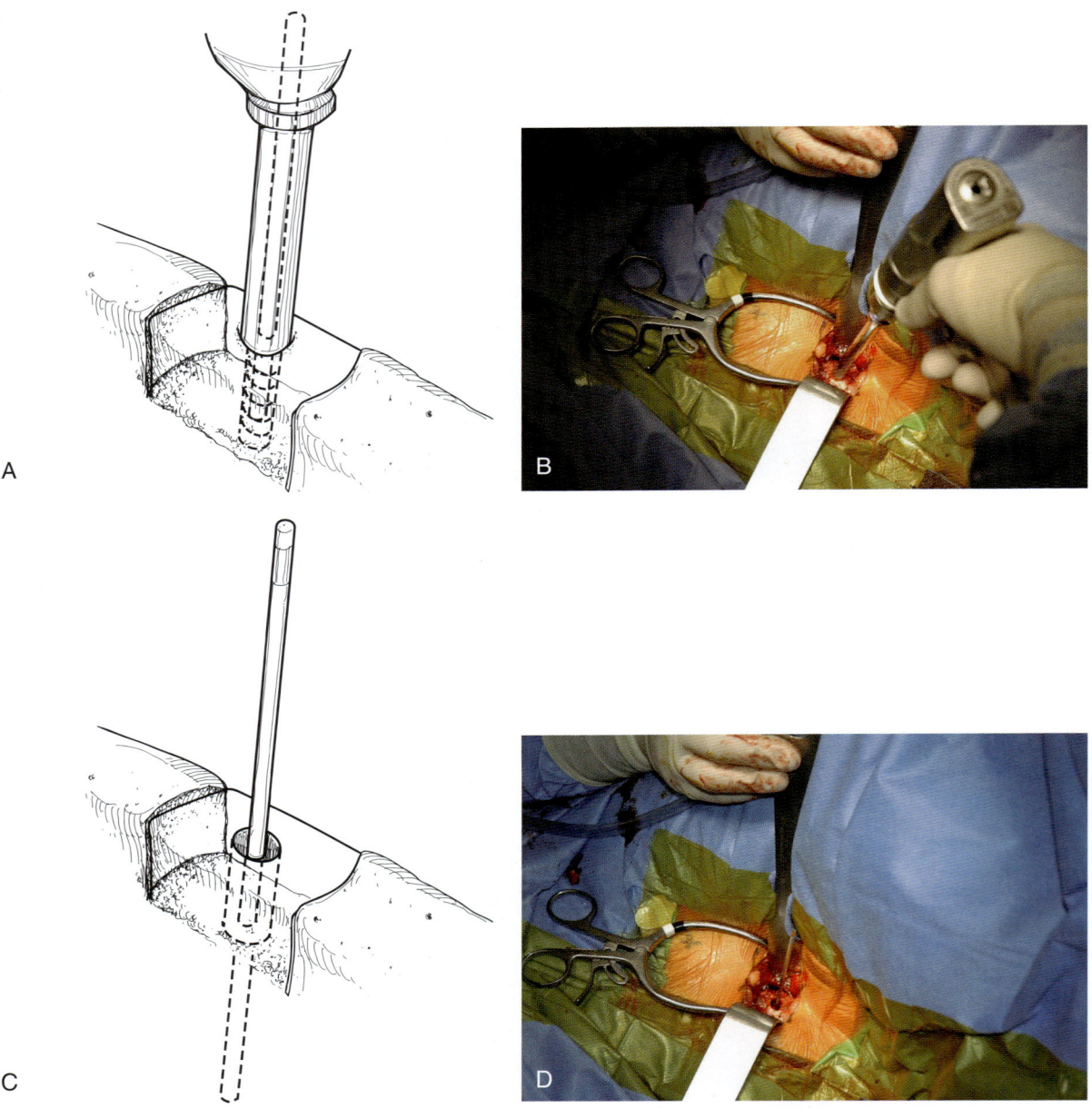

FIGURE 40.42 (A to D) The central hole is drilled using a cannulated drill for the central hole of the base plate.

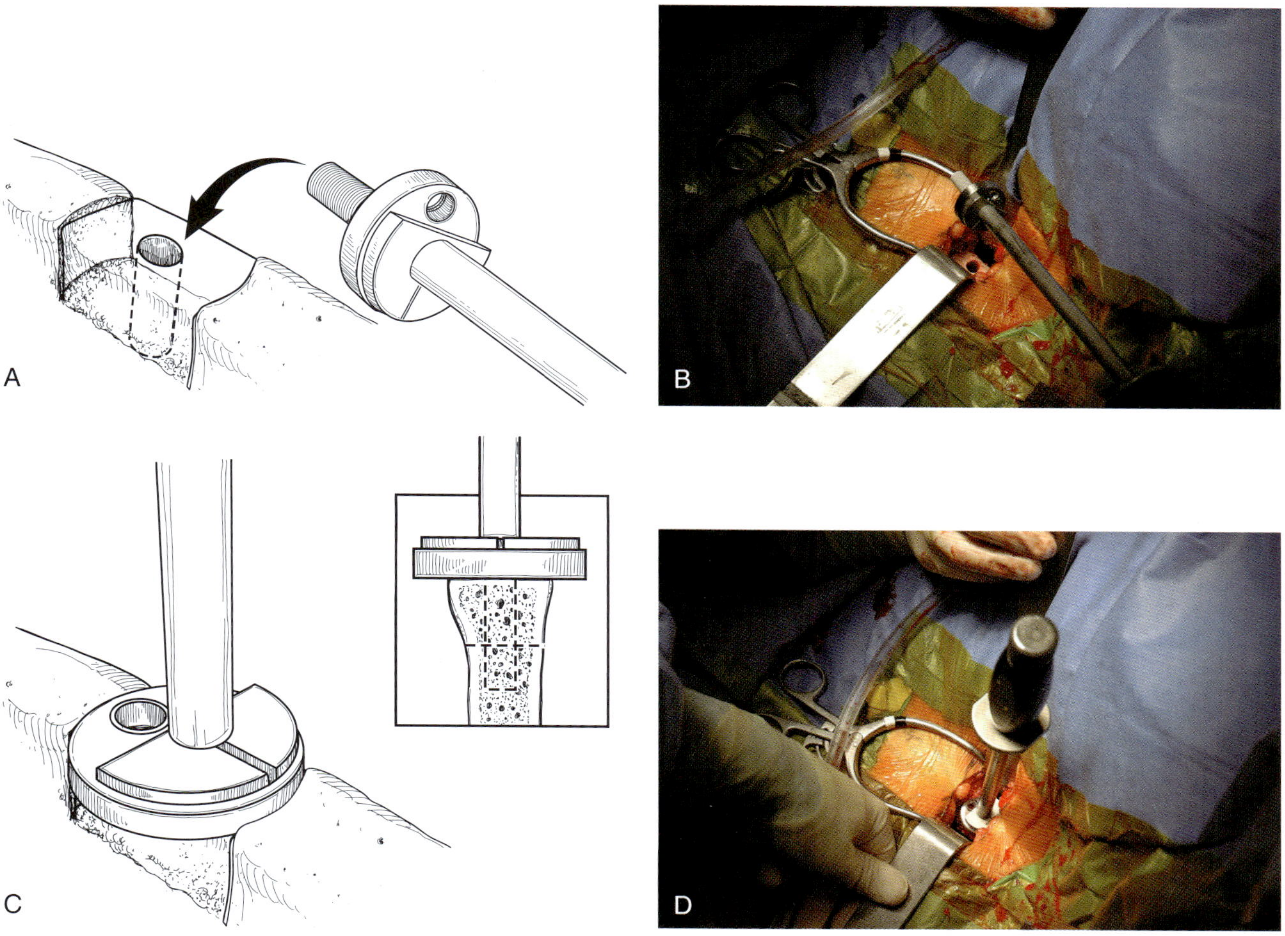

CHAPTER 40 ■ Glenoid Component

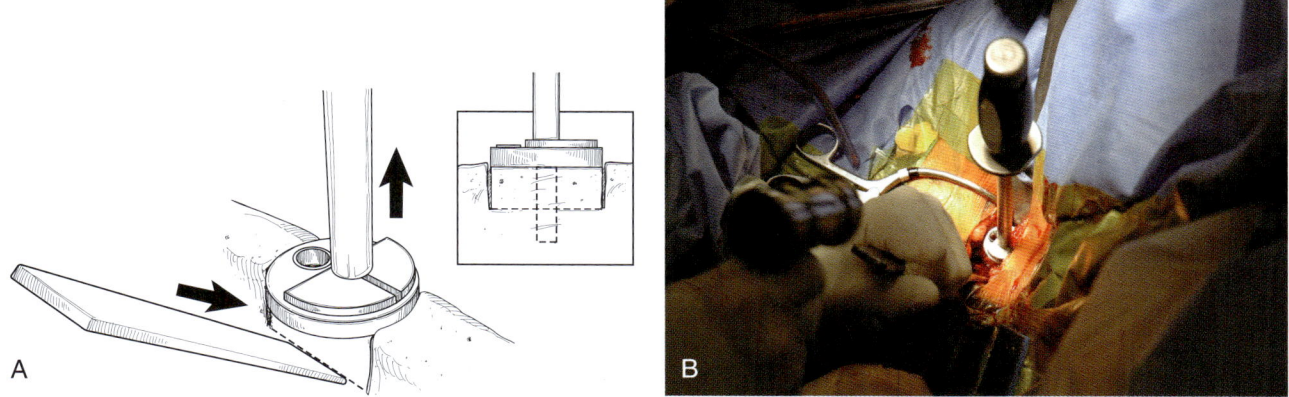

FIGURE 40.43 (A to D) The reverse glenoid base plate is inserted into the central hole created in the iliac crest.

FIGURE 40.44 (A and B) A 1-inch curved osteotome is used to complete the osteotomy in the iliac crest created by the bony increased-offset reversed shoulder arthroplasty technique (BIO-RSA) reamer and free the tricortical bone graft.

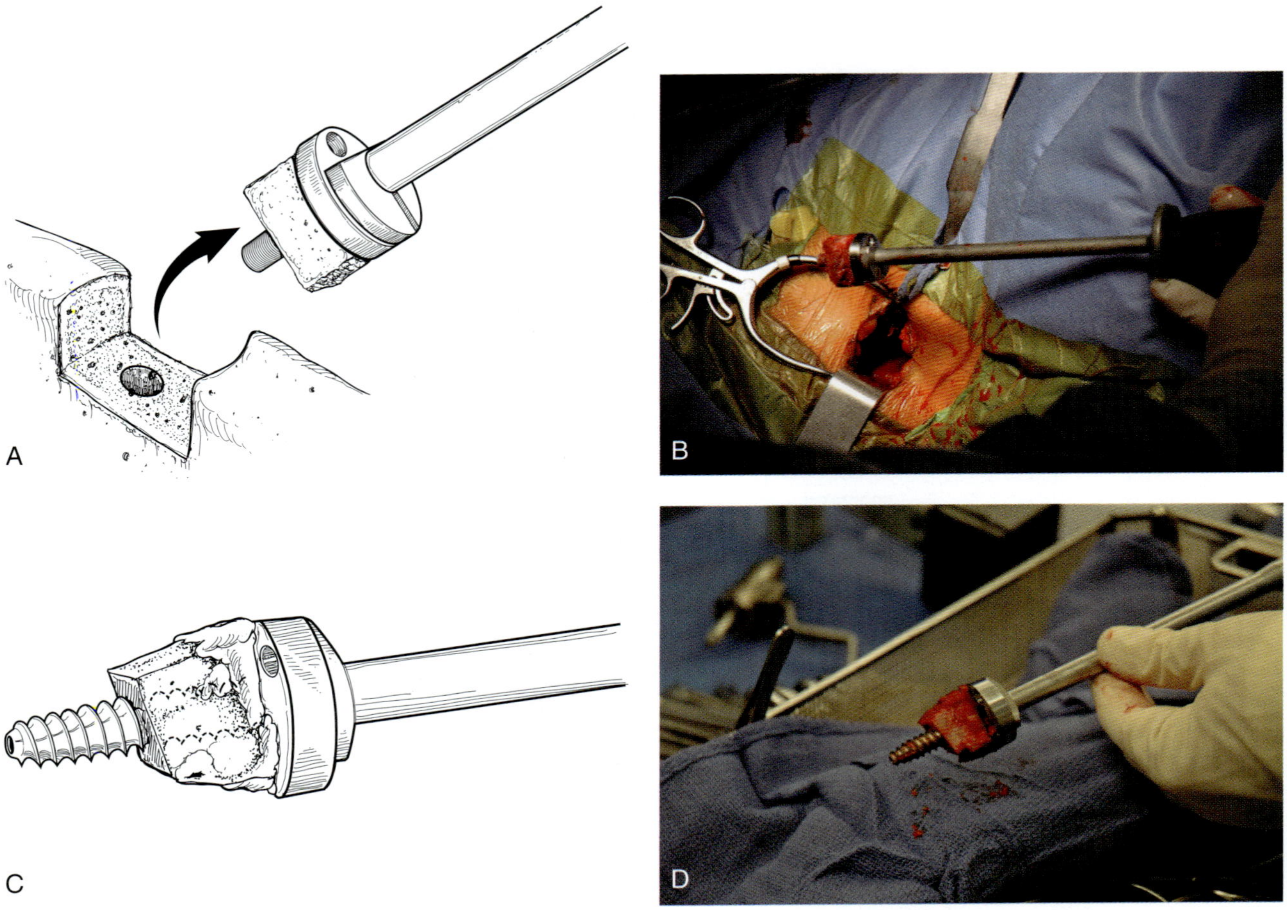

436 SECTION VI ■ Revision Shoulder Arthroplasty

FIGURE 40.45 The base plate along with the attached bone graft is then extracted. Either a long post base plate (A and B) or long screw (C and D) can be used.

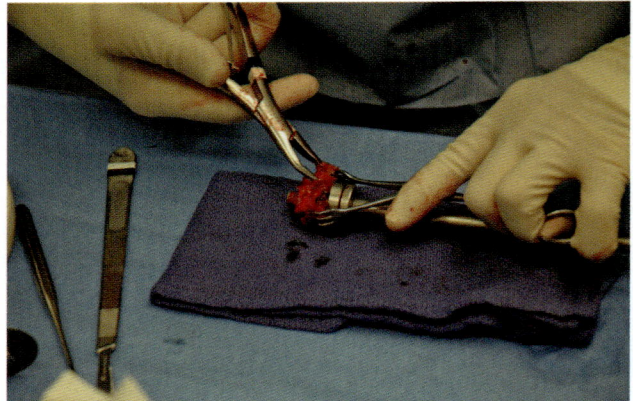

FIGURE 40.46 The graft is fashioned using a saw, burr, or rongeur as needed to match the defect on the glenoid.

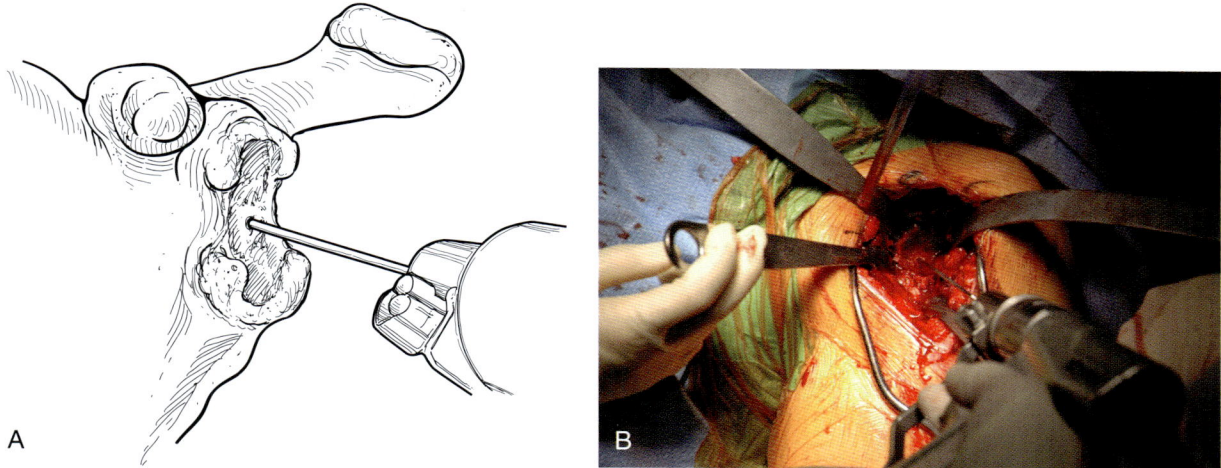

FIGURE 40.47 (A and B) A guide pin is placed in the vault of the glenoid for placement of the central post or screw.

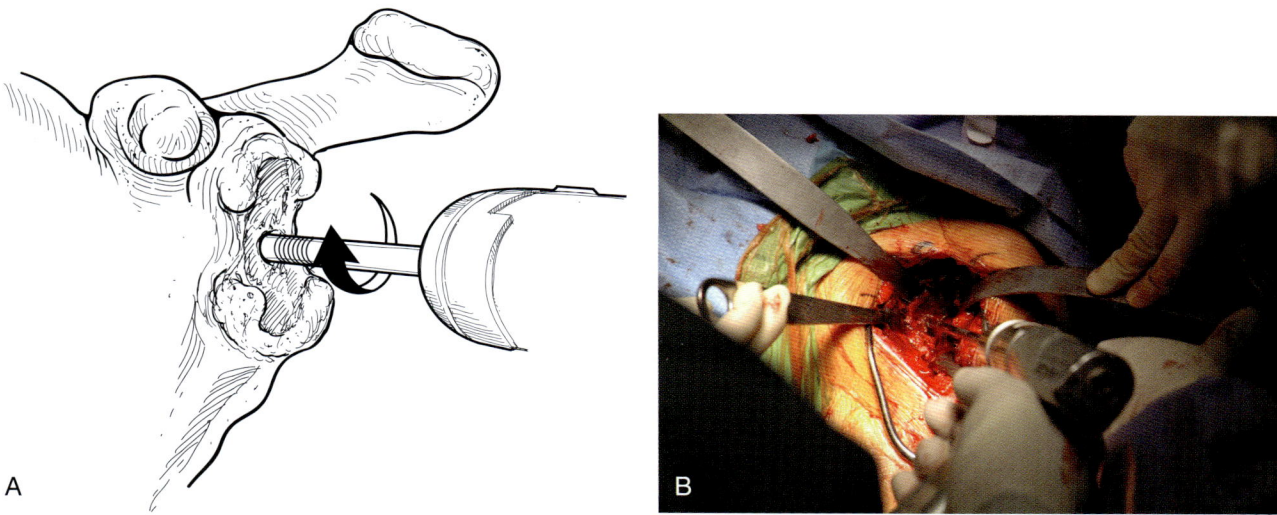

FIGURE 40.48 (A and B) The guide pin is then overdrilled penetrating the medial cortex of the scapula.

plate) (Fig. 40.49). If a threaded base plate is used, a special "tong clamp" is used to control rotation of the bone graft as the screw is advanced (Fig. 40.50).

After the base plate has been placed, peripheral screw fixation ensues via the same technique used during primary reverse shoulder arthroplasty (see Chapter 22). The inferior screw is placed first to ensure maintenance of inferior tilt of the glenoid component. A drill guide is placed in the inferior hole of the base plate. A drill (3.0-mm bit) is used through the guide to create a bicortical hole (Fig. 40.51). The direction of the drill should be chosen to maximize screw length so that the strongest fixation possible is provided. This is usually done by directing the drill halfway between the perpendicular and the maximal inferior direction allowed by the mechanical constraints of the base plate. After the second cortex is penetrated with the drill, a depth gauge is used or the calibrated drill bit can be read to determine the length. If a post base plate is used, a 4.5-mm screw is introduced and tightened until just before the threaded screw head engages the washer of the base plate. If the threaded head of the inferior screw engages the base plate washer, no further compression between the base plate and glenoid bone can be obtained. The drilling trajectory for the superior locking screw is directed toward the base of the coracoid process. The process of using the depth gauge is repeated for the superior locking screw. The superior screw is then inserted, once again making sure to not engage the base plate when the screw is advanced. For the anterior and posterior screws, the drill is typically angled toward the central peg of the glenoid base plate and passes just superior or inferior to the central peg to perforate the opposite cortex (i.e., the anterior drill hole passes just superior to the central peg and perforates the posterior cortex deep within the glenoid vault, and the posterior drill hole passes just inferior to the central peg and perforates the anterior cortex deep within the glenoid vault). The depth gauge or the calibrated drill bit is used for selection of screw length, and the anterior and posterior screws are inserted and fully tightened to

SECTION VI ■ Revision Shoulder Arthroplasty

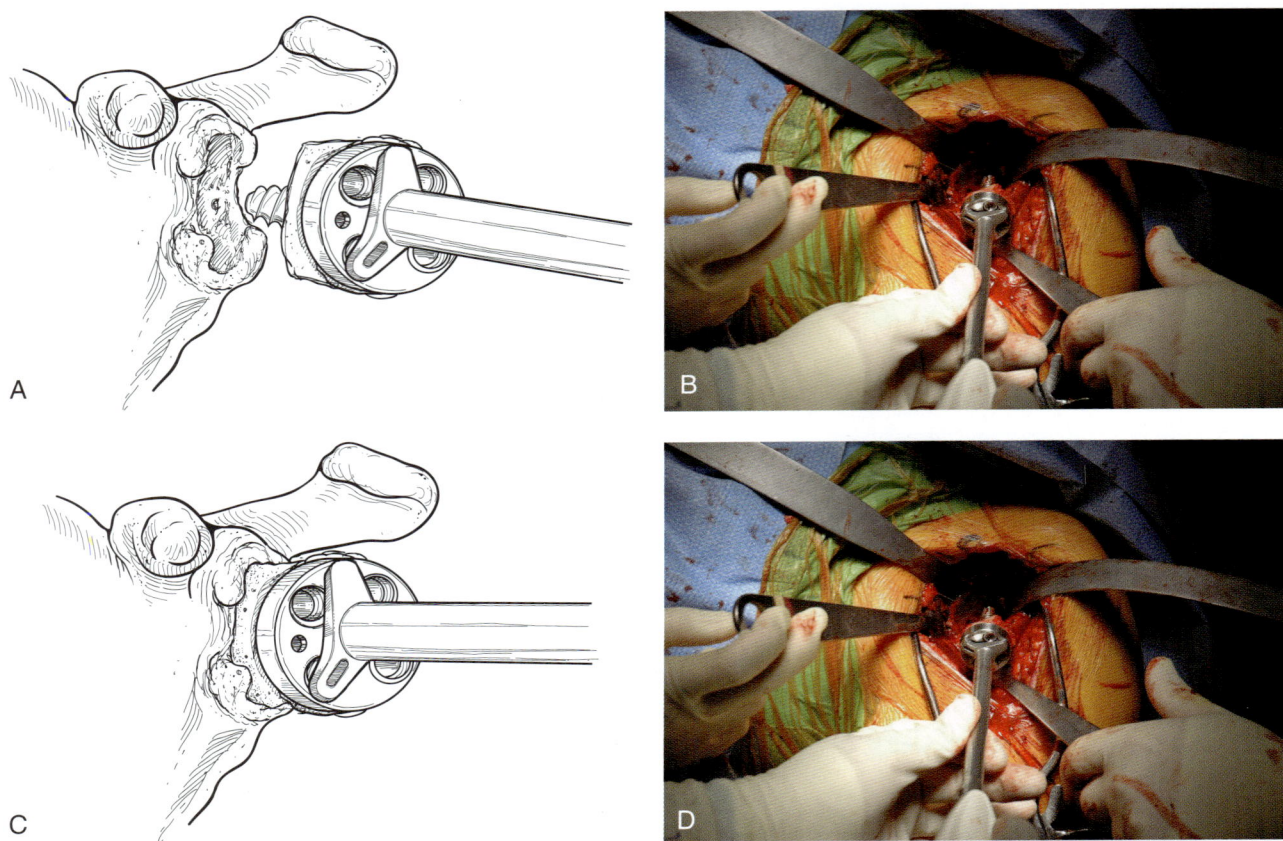

FIGURE 40.49 (A to D) The base plate/bone graft construct is then placed in the central hole.

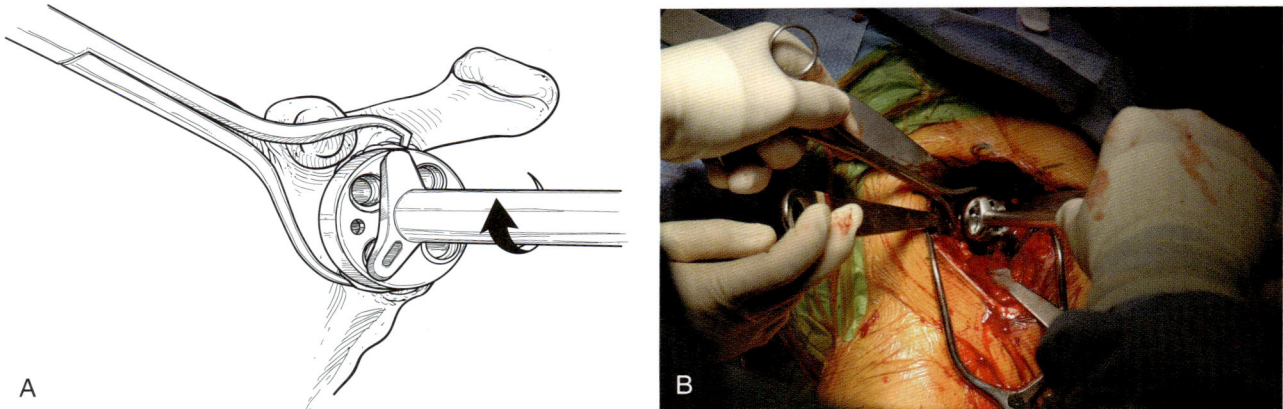

FIGURE 40.50 (A and B) When using a threaded base plate is used, a special "tong clamp" is used to control rotation of the bone graft as the screw is advanced.

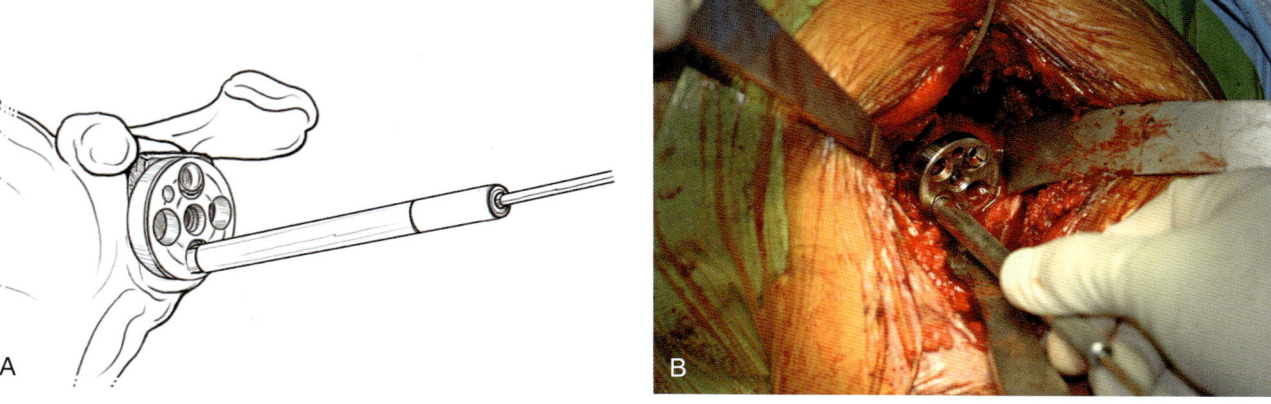

FIGURE 40.51 (A and B) Drilling of the peripheral screw holes.

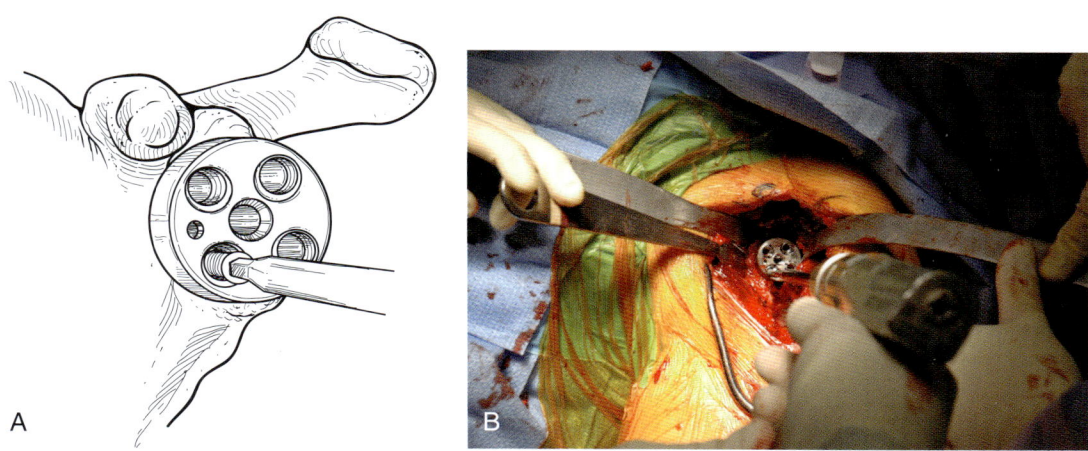

FIGURE 40.52 (A and B) Placement of the peripheral locking screws when using a threaded base plate.

provide compression between the base plate and the glenoid bone. After the anterior and posterior screws are fully seated, the inferior and then superior screws are fully tightened so that they engage and complete fixation of the base plate. Occasionally, the anterior or posterior screw will not obtain satisfactory osseous purchase because of underlying osteopenia. In this case the screw is left in place to provide interference-type resistance to loosening of the glenoid component. If using a threaded base plate, the screws are completely advanced, engaging the locking washer for all four peripheral screws (Fig. 40.52).

The periphery and central hole of the base plate are cleared of soft tissue and blood, and the glenosphere component is positioned on the base plate with a screwdriver used as an insertion device. The glenosphere attaches to the base plate via a peripheral rim Morse taper and is further secured with a central safety screw. The glenosphere is impacted into place with the impaction device, and the safety fixation screw is advanced to complete insertion of the glenoid component (Fig. 40.53).

After insertion of the glenoid component is complete, consideration can be given to performing a single-stage procedure. If the majority of the central post or screw of the reverse prosthesis base plate is implanted into native glenoid bone, the reverse prosthesis can be implanted as a single-stage procedure and attention directed toward insertion of the humeral component (Fig. 40.54). If the central post of the base plate is not well seated in native glenoid bone, a staged procedure should be performed. In this scenario the humeral implant is not inserted. Six months after the first stage, the humeral component is implanted at the second stage (Fig. 40.55).

TECHNIQUE FOR HARVEST OF AUTOGENOUS ILIAC CREST BONE GRAFT

In cases requiring reconstruction of the osseous glenoid, we use an autogenous anterior iliac crest tricortical bone graft. The iliac crest contralateral to the operative shoulder is selected in most cases. This allows easier surgical preparation and draping and, more importantly, permits more than one surgical team (if available) to work simultaneously. In our institution, one surgeon will frequently harvest the bone graft while the other surgeon performs the surgical approach on the operative shoulder. Exceptions occur when the patient has previously had an anterior bone graft harvested on the

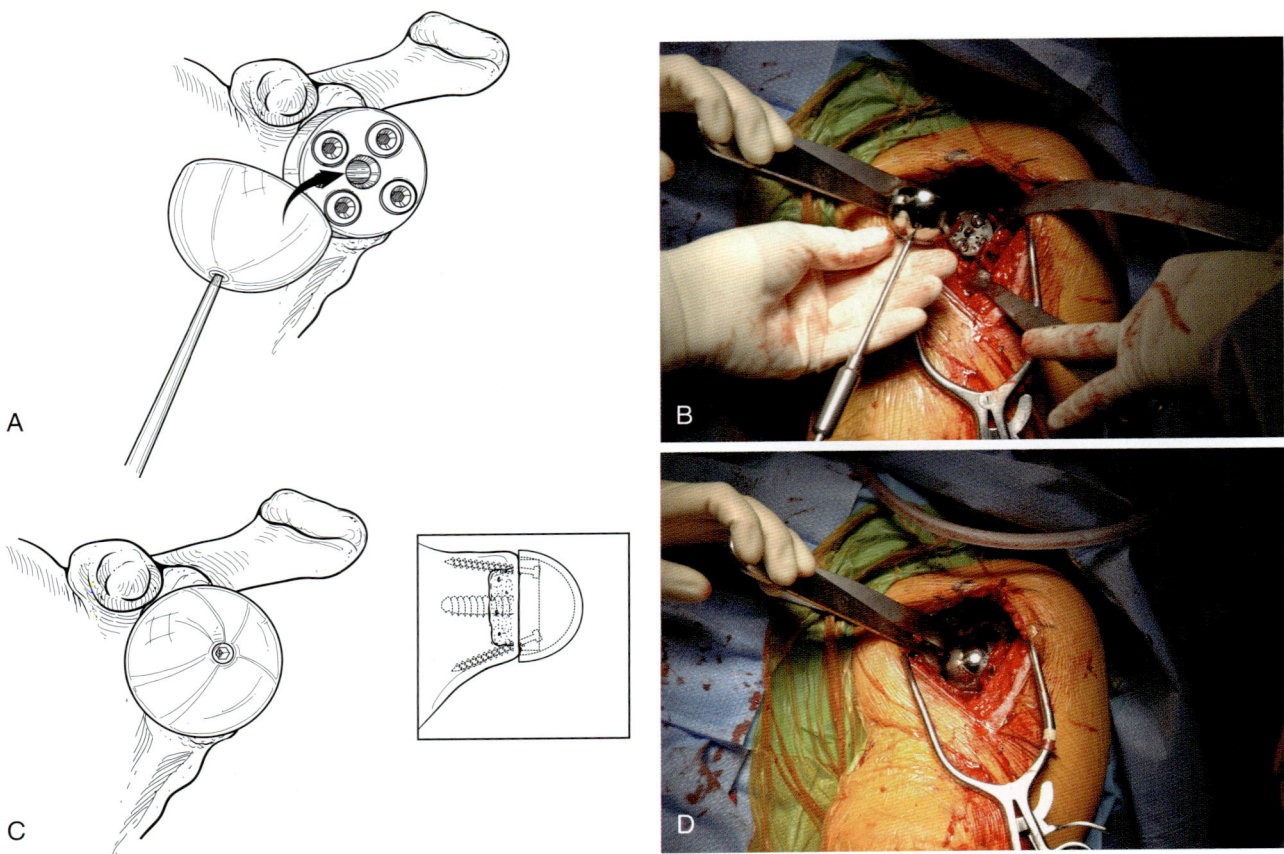

FIGURE 40.53 Final placement of the glenosphere (A and B) and completed glenoid reconstruction (C and D).

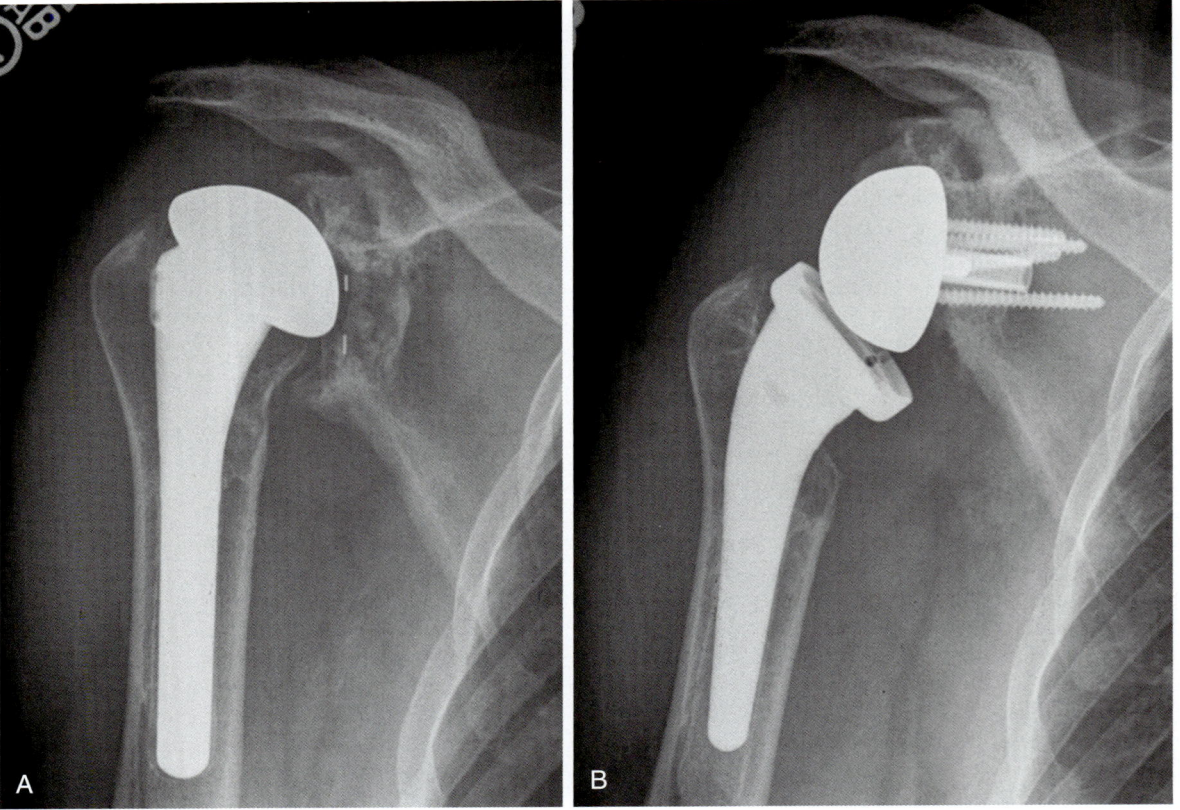

FIGURE 40.54 Case in which revision to a reverse prosthesis with bone graft reconstruction of the glenoid was performed as a single stage. (A) Prerevision. (B) Postrevision.

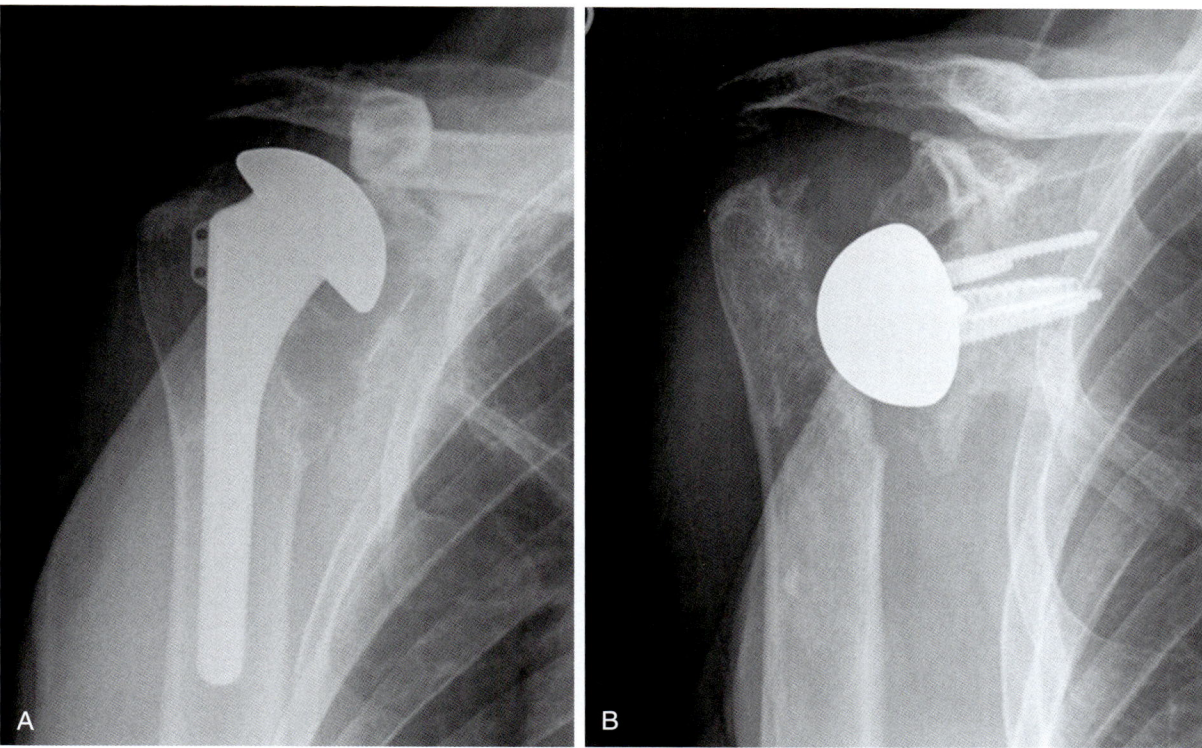

FIGURE 40.55 Case in which revision to a reverse prosthesis with bone graft reconstruction of the glenoid was performed as a two stage. (A) Prerevision. (B) Following the first stage of the revision.

contralateral side (although this does not represent an absolute contraindication if harvesting took place longer than 1 year previously and radiographs show reconstitution of the anterior iliac crest bone stock) or when the patient specifically requests that we use bone from the iliac crest ipsilateral to the operative shoulder.

The operative shoulder is prepared as described in Chapter 4. The area of the entire contralateral iliac crest is prepared. The skin is initially cleaned with isopropyl alcohol, after which a povidone-iodine (Betadine) scrub is performed. The surgical area is then dried with towels and painted with a Betadine preparative solution (Fig. 40.56). In patients with allergy or hypersensitivity to Betadine, the scrub is performed with a 4% chlorhexidine gluconate solution (Betasept). The solution is removed with sterile water and an isopropyl alcohol preparation is applied. The area is draped with sterile towels secured to the skin with skin staples (Fig. 40.57). The contralateral shoulder is routinely draped as described in Chapter 4. The anterior iliac crest is palpated through the drapes and a hole is cut in the drapes with bandage scissors (Fig. 40.58). Any residual Betadine is dried at the surgical site. An occlusive adhesive drape is applied to the surgical site. We prefer the occlusive drape to be impregnated with Betadine; however, in patients with Betadine allergy or hypersensitivity, we use a non–Betadine-impregnated version of the same drape. Completed draping of the iliac crest harvest site is shown in Fig. 40.59.

An incision is made with a no. 10 scalpel blade centered over the iliac crest, starting 4 cm posterior to the palpated anterior superior iliac spine and extending 8 cm posteriorly

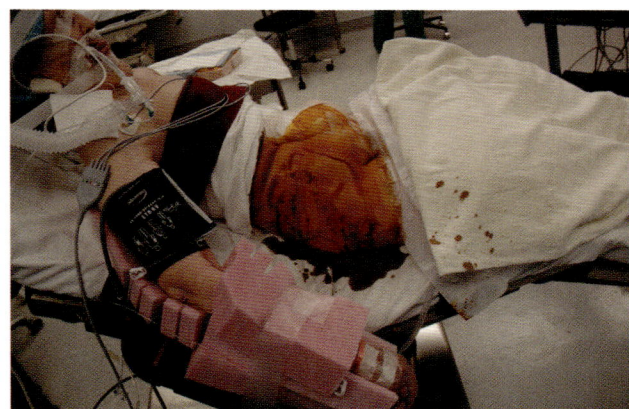

FIGURE 40.56 Skin preparation of the iliac crest bone graft harvest site.

along the iliac crest (Fig. 40.60). It is important not to extend the incision anteriorly, to avoid injury to the lateral femoral cutaneous nerve. A needle tip electrocautery is used to dissect through the subcutaneous tissue down to the periosteum of the iliac crest (Fig. 40.61). Exposure is maintained with a self-retaining retractor. The periosteum of the iliac crest is divided along the longitudinal axis of the iliac crest with the electrocautery and progressively elevated (Fig. 40.62). A Cobb elevator is used to expose the inner and outer tables of the iliac crest (Fig. 40.63). Hohmann-type retractors are

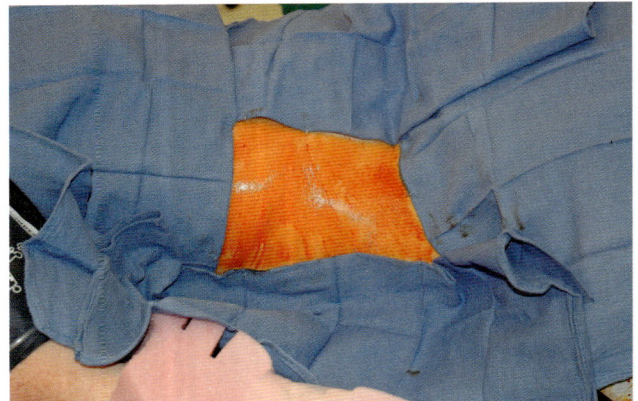

FIGURE 40.57 Draping of the iliac crest with sterile towels held with skin staples

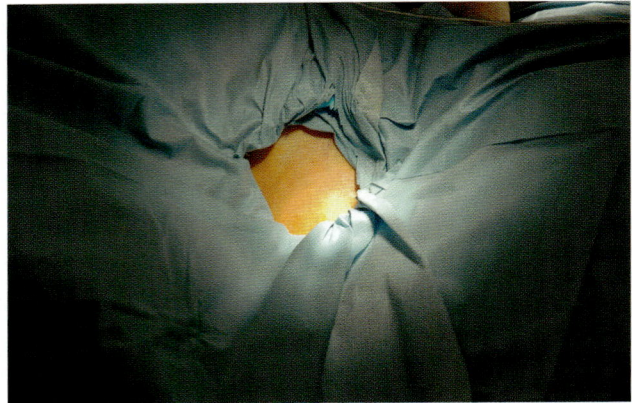

FIGURE 40.58 A hole is cut through the drapes over the iliac crest to allow exposure of the harvest site.

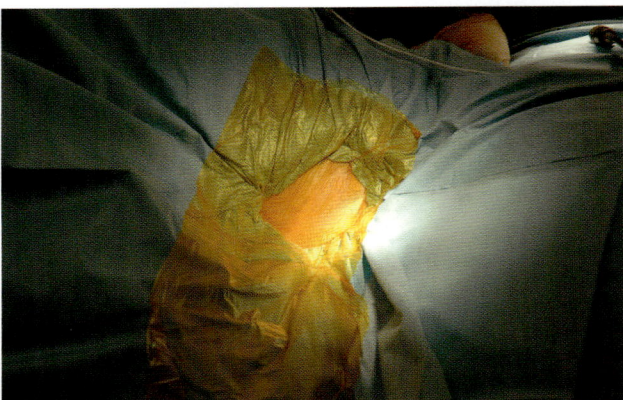

FIGURE 40.59 Completed skin preparation and draping of the iliac crest harvest site.

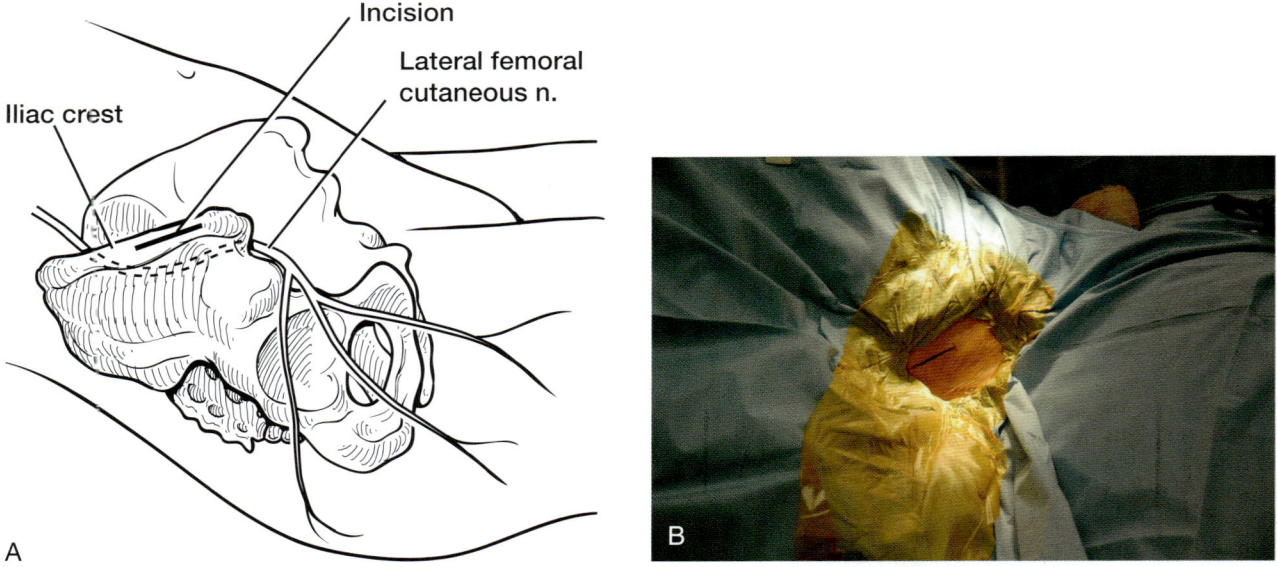

FIGURE 40.60 (A and B) Skin incision for harvesting the anterior iliac crest.

CHAPTER 40 ■ Glenoid Component   443

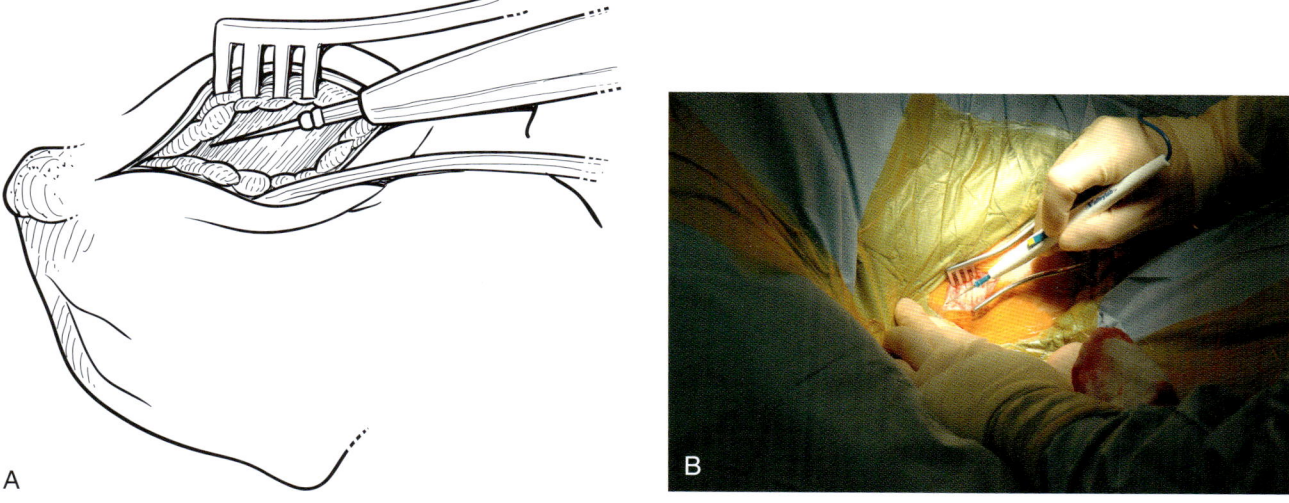

FIGURE 40.61   (A and B) Dissection through subcutaneous tissue with the needle tip electrocautery.

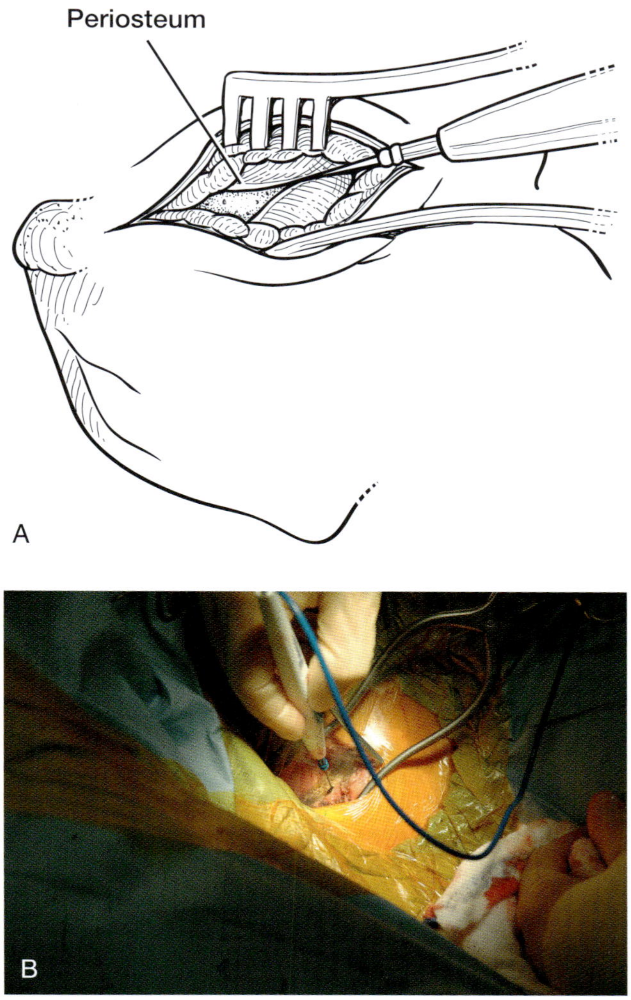

FIGURE 40.62   (A and B) The periosteum of the iliac crest is divided with the electrocautery.

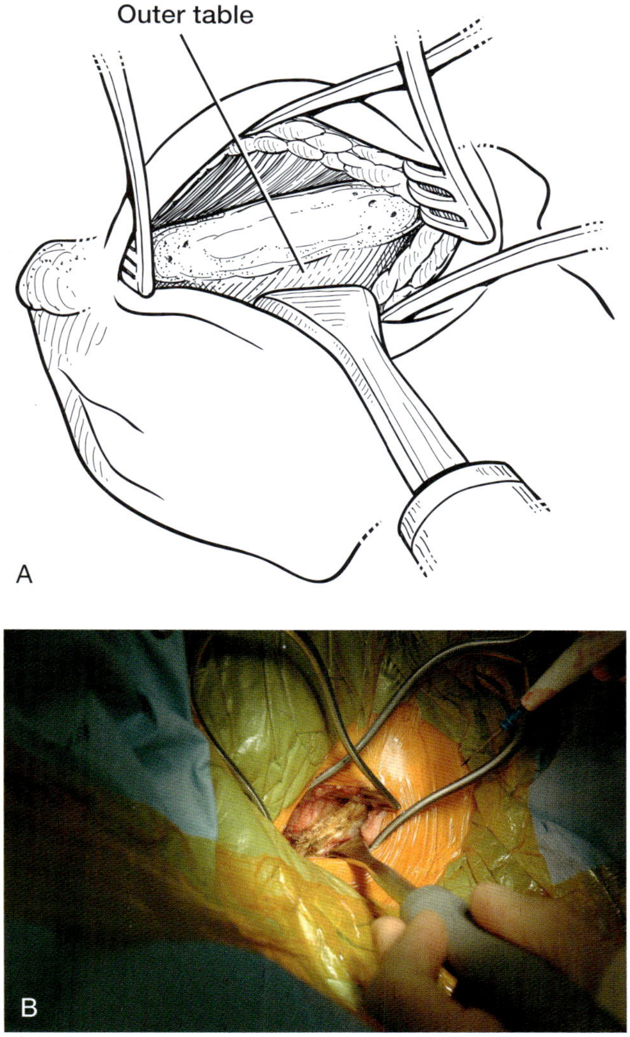

FIGURE 40.63   (A and B) A Cobb elevator is used to expose the inner and outer tables of the iliac crest.

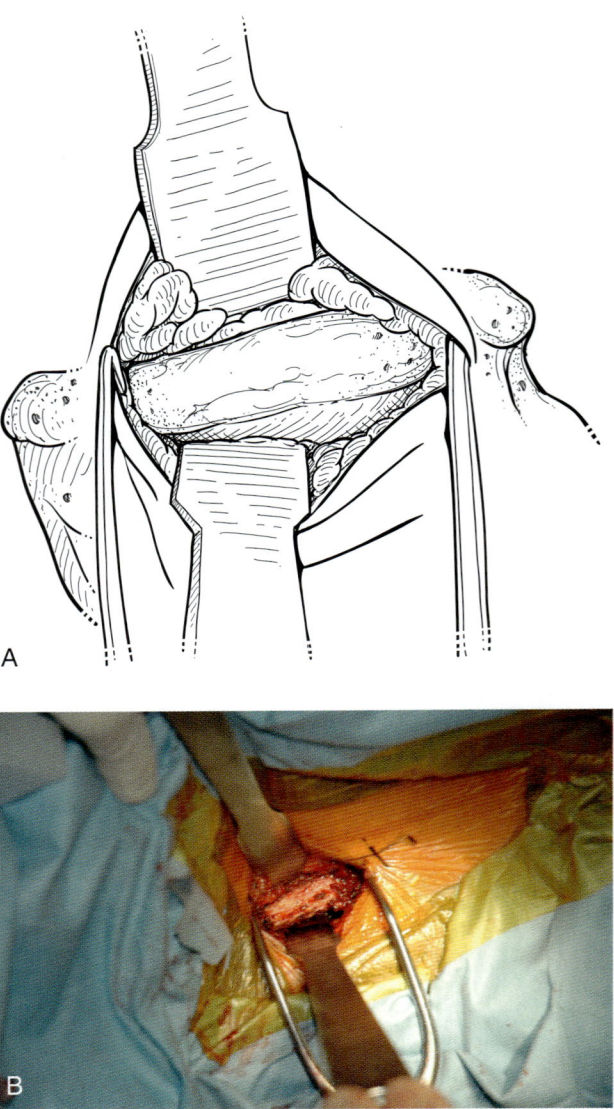

FIGURE 40.64 (A and B) Hohmann-type retractors are used to maintain exposure of the iliac crest.

placed on each side of the iliac crest to maintain exposure (Fig. 40.64). At this point the Norris modification of the BIO-RSA technique can be performed as described previously in this chapter.

If a bone graft is required that is not amenable to the Norris BIO-RSA technique, a 1-inch straight osteotome or small microsagittal saw is used to cut the iliac crest transversely in two places with a 3-cm-long intervening segment (Fig. 40.65). The osteotome or saw is advanced to a depth of at least 2 cm in each location (Fig. 40.66). A 1-inch curved osteotome is used to connect the two vertical cuts in the iliac crest and free the tricortical bone graft (Fig. 40.67). The bone graft is held with a Lahey-type clamp before its final removal to avoid inadvertent contamination.

The tricortical bone graft is placed on the back table and the underlying cancellous bone graft is removed from the pelvis with curettes of various size and shape (Fig. 40.68). The bone graft site is irrigated with antibiotic-impregnated sterile saline (50,000 units bacitracin per liter sterile normal saline) via a bulb syringe. Gelfoam (Pfizer, New York, NY) soaked in thrombin can be temporarily packed to obtain hemostasis. If the bone at the iliac crest harvest site continues to bleed, a medium closed suction drain is placed and maintained until the first postoperative day (Fig. 40.69). The periosteum is closed with no. 0 braided absorbable sutures in an interrupted technique. Local anesthetic can be infiltrated to help with postoperative pain relief. Subcutaneous tissue is closed with 2-0 braided absorbable sutures in an interrupted technique. The skin is closed with 3-0 monofilament absorbable sutures in a running subcuticular technique. Steri-Strips and a sterile dressing are applied (Fig. 40.70).

CHAPTER 40 ■ Glenoid Component 445

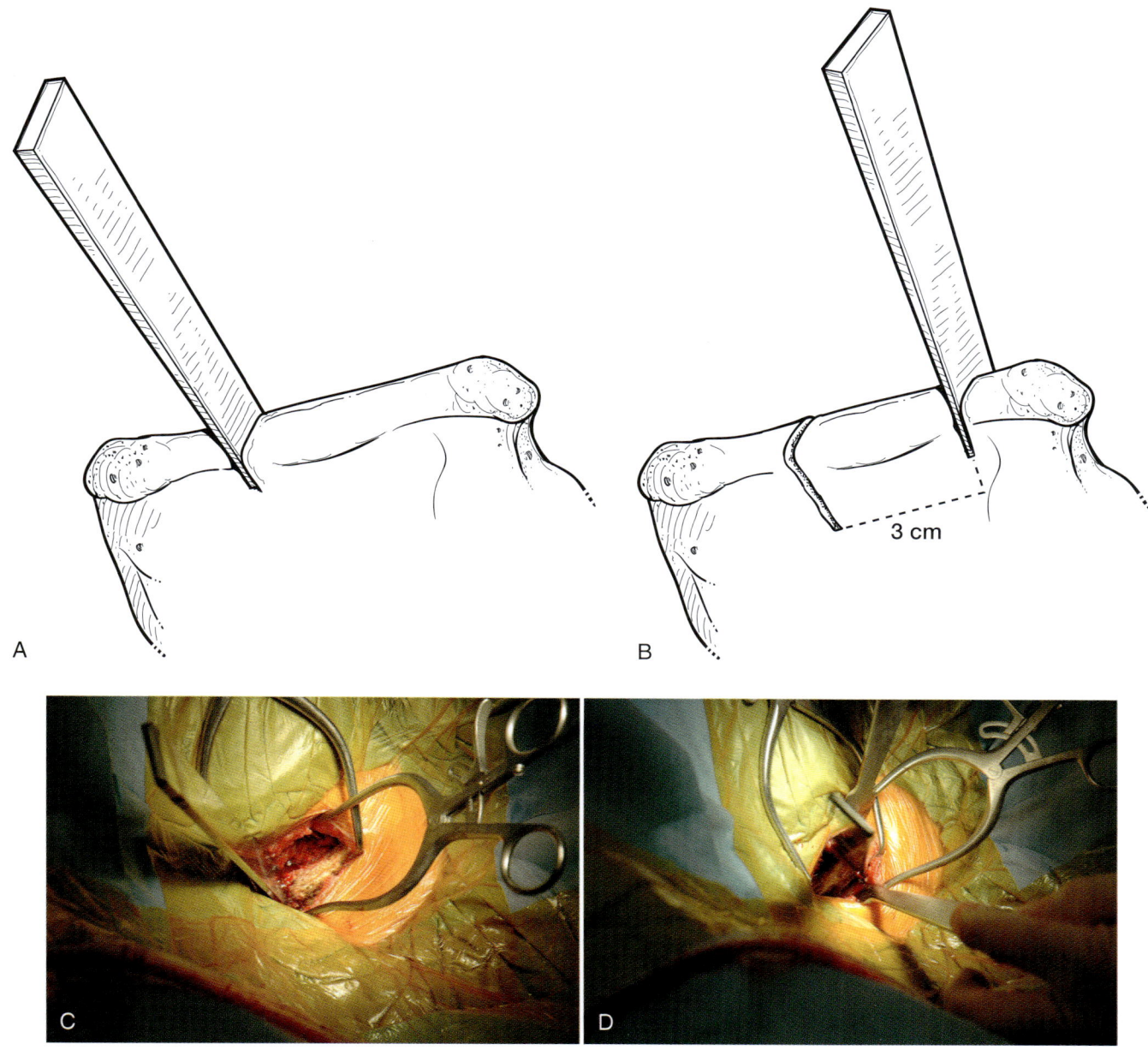

FIGURE 40.65 (A to D) Vertical cuts are made in the iliac crest 3 cm apart with a 1-inch osteotome.

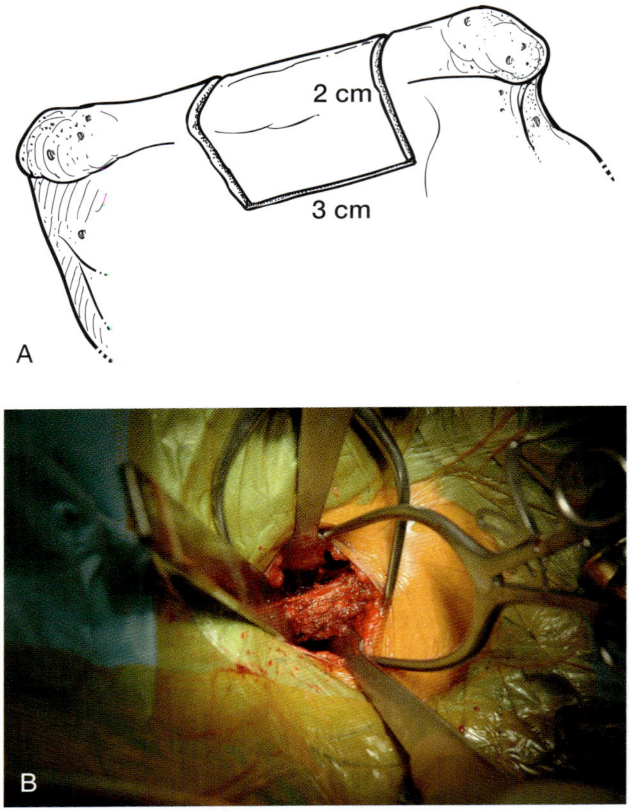

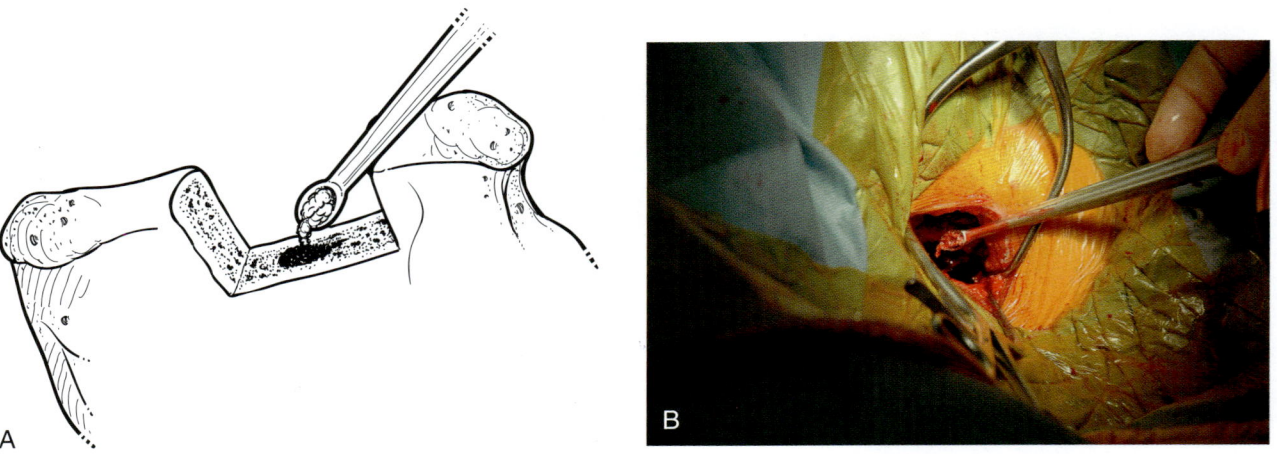

FIGURE 40.66 (A and B) The vertical cuts continue until they are 2 cm in depth.

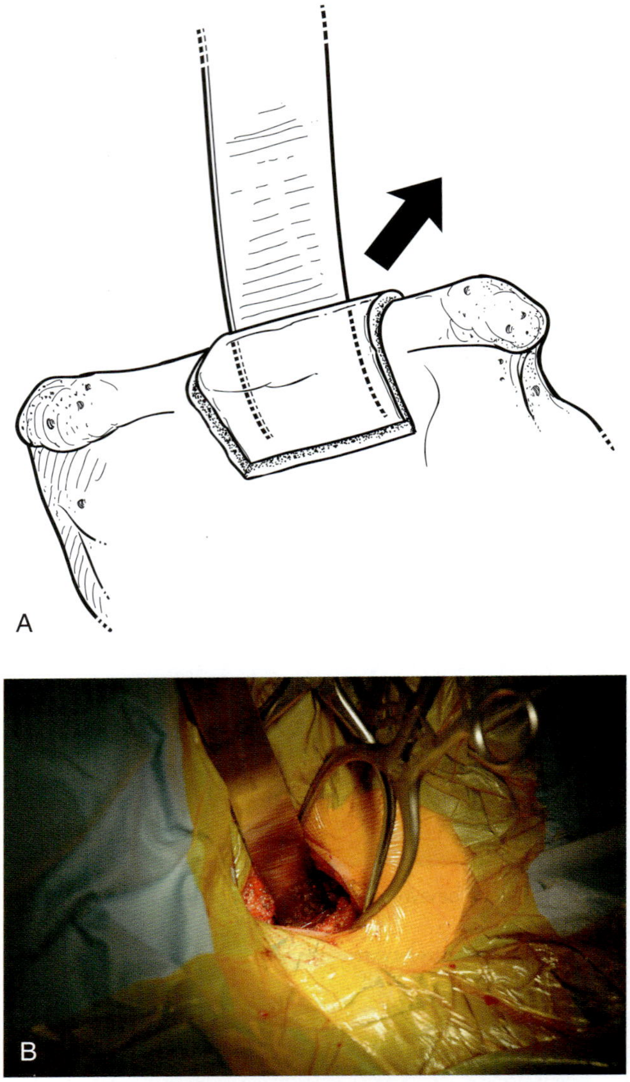

FIGURE 40.67 (A and B) A 1-inch curved osteotome is used to connect the two vertical cuts in the iliac crest and free the tricortical bone graft.

FIGURE 40.68 (A and B) Removal of cancellous bone with a curette.

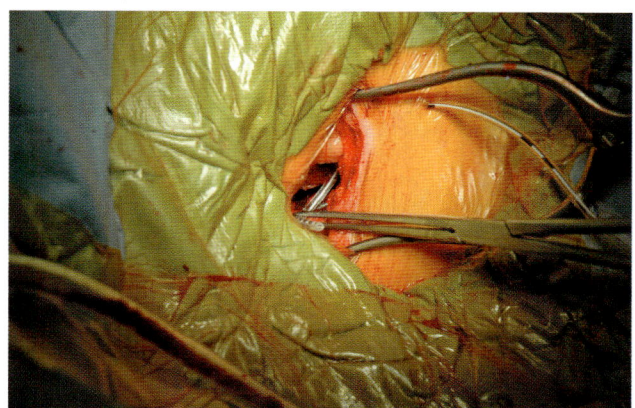

FIGURE 40.69 Placement of a medium closed suction drain in the iliac crest harvest site.

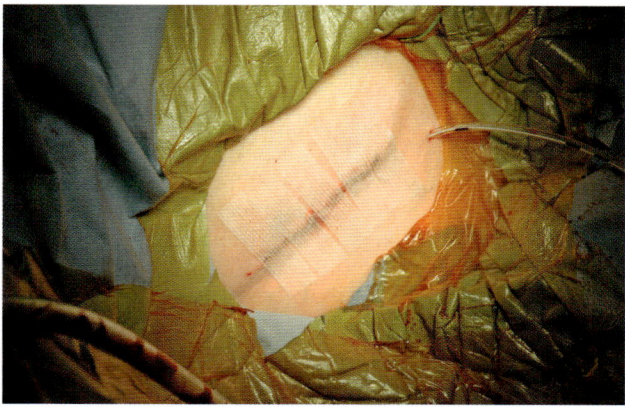

FIGURE 40.70 Final closure of the iliac crest harvest site.

REFERENCES

1. Walch G, Edwards TB, Boulahia A, et al: Adenleine P. The influence of glenohumeral prosthetic mismatch on glenoid radiolucent lines results of a multicenter study, *J Bone Joint Surg* 84-A(12):2186–2191, 2002.
2. Neyton L, Walch G, Nové-Josserand L, et al: Glenoid corticocancellous bone grafting after glenoid component removal in the treatment of glenoid loosening, *J Shoulder Elbow Surg* 15:173–179, 2006.
3. Boileau P, Moineau G, Roussanne Y, et al: Bony increased-offset reversed shoulder arthroplasty minimizing scapular impingement while maximizing glenoid fixation, *Clin Orthop Relat Res* 469:2558–2567, 2011.
4. Norris TR, Kelly JD, Humphrey CS: Management of glenoid bone defects in revision shoulder arthroplasty: a new application of the reverse total shoulder prosthesis, *Tech Should Elbow Surg* 8(1):37–46, 2007.

CHAPTER 41

Wound closure and postoperative orthosis

The final steps in revision arthroplasty are wound closure and placement of the postoperative orthosis. Wound closure after revision arthroplasty is performed similar to that for other arthroplasty cases. Revision shoulder arthroplasty often involves larger skin incisions, which can make wound closure an arduous task. The type of revision arthroplasty performed dictates the type of postoperative orthosis used and the duration of its use.

TECHNIQUE FOR WOUND CLOSURE

After reduction of the implant and closure of the subscapularis, if present, the wound is irrigated with 800 mL of antibiotic-impregnated sterile saline (50,000 units bacitracin per liter sterile normal saline) via a bulb syringe. The wound is checked to ensure that adequate hemostasis has been achieved. The electrocautery is used as necessary to minimize any residual hemorrhage. A medium-size closed suction drain is placed to help prevent postoperative hematoma formation in all cases in which a reverse prosthesis has been used, as described in Chapter 24.

Wound closure is initiated by reapproximation of the deep fascial layer with no. 0 braided absorbable suture in an interrupted figure-of-eight technique. As in cases of primary shoulder arthroplasty, we do not close the deltopectoral interval. The subcutaneous fascia is reapproximated with 2-0 braided absorbable suture in an interrupted figure-of-eight technique. The skin is reapproximated with skin staples (Fig. 41.1). We use skin staples in most revision cases because closure with subcuticular suture can be difficult in the presence of dermal scarring from a previous incision. In addition, the incision for revision shoulder arthroplasty can be large, especially if an extended approach is required. Use of skin staples facilitates closure of these large incisions (Fig. 41.2).

After skin closure is completed, the drain, if used, is checked to ensure that its position has been maintained. The occlusive draping is carefully removed from the site at which the drain tubing exits the skin. The skin in this area is cleaned and dried. Half-inch Steri-Strips are wrapped around the drain tubing to fix the drain to the skin and prevent inadvertent removal of the drain; we use two or three Steri-Strips (Fig. 41.3).

More of the occlusive draping is removed adjacent to the incision, and the skin is cleansed of blood with a saline-soaked sponge and then dried. Sterile gauze is placed over the incision, and a sterile absorbent pad is placed over the gauze. The dressing is secured with 3-inch foam tape. If applicable, the remainder of the surgical drain is connected to the drainage tube, and the suction function of the drain is activated. The remaining surgical drapes are then removed.

When used, the surgical drain is removed the day after surgery regardless of the amount of drainage recorded. The dressing is maintained in place until postoperative day 3, at which time it is removed. After removal of the dressing, the patient is allowed to shower, but submerging the incision in a bathtub is prohibited until 2 weeks postoperatively. The skin staples are removed 2 weeks postoperatively in the outpatient clinic.

POSTOPERATIVE ORTHOSIS

The postoperative orthosis is placed immediately after the dressing in the operating room. For unconstrained revision arthroplasty without a posterior capsulorrhaphy, we use a simple sling that the patient can discontinue as comfort allows within 2 to 4 weeks. For revision arthroplasty with a reverse prosthesis and unconstrained revision arthroplasty requiring an associated posterior capsulorrhaphy, we use a neutral-rotation sling (Ultrasling, Donjoy, Inc., Vista, California; Fig. 41.4). The patient is allowed to remove the sling for performance of hand, wrist, and elbow mobility exercises and for hygiene.

For revision with a reverse prosthesis, the duration for which the orthosis is maintained is determined by the presence or absence of humeral metaphyseal bone loss. In uncomplicated cases with sufficient metaphyseal bone, the sling is discontinued and physical therapy initiated 3 weeks postoperatively. In cases of humeral metaphyseal bone loss, the sling is maintained for an additional week, and physical therapy is initiated 4 weeks postoperatively.

In unconstrained revision arthroplasty requiring an associated posterior capsulorrhaphy, the neutral-rotation sling is maintained for 4 weeks to protect the posterior capsulorrhaphy. Patients are allowed to remove the sling only for hygiene and rehabilitation exercises. Details of the postoperative rehabilitation regimen are provided in Chapter 43.

CHAPTER 41 ■ Wound Closure and Postoperative Orthosis

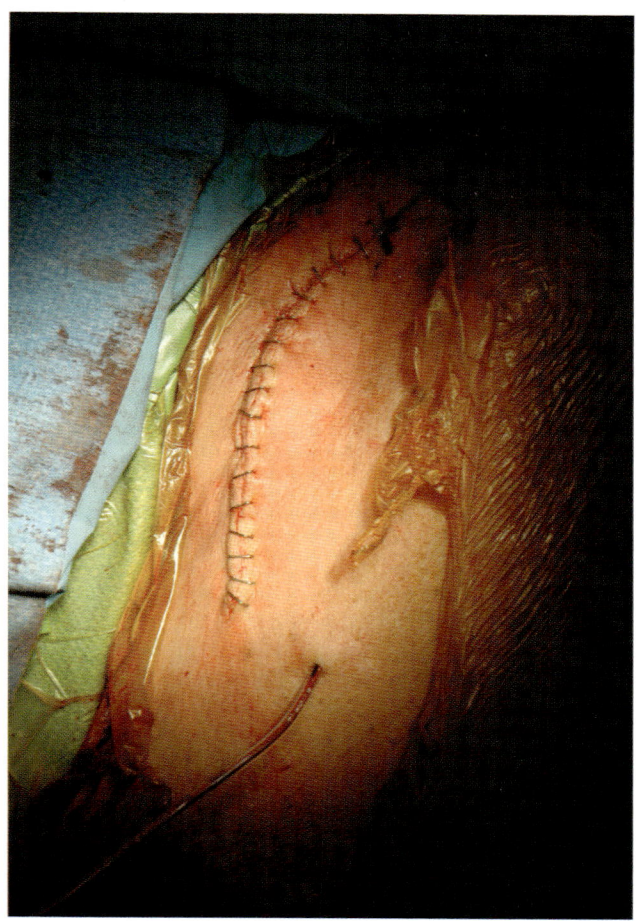

FIGURE 41.1 Skin closure with staples.

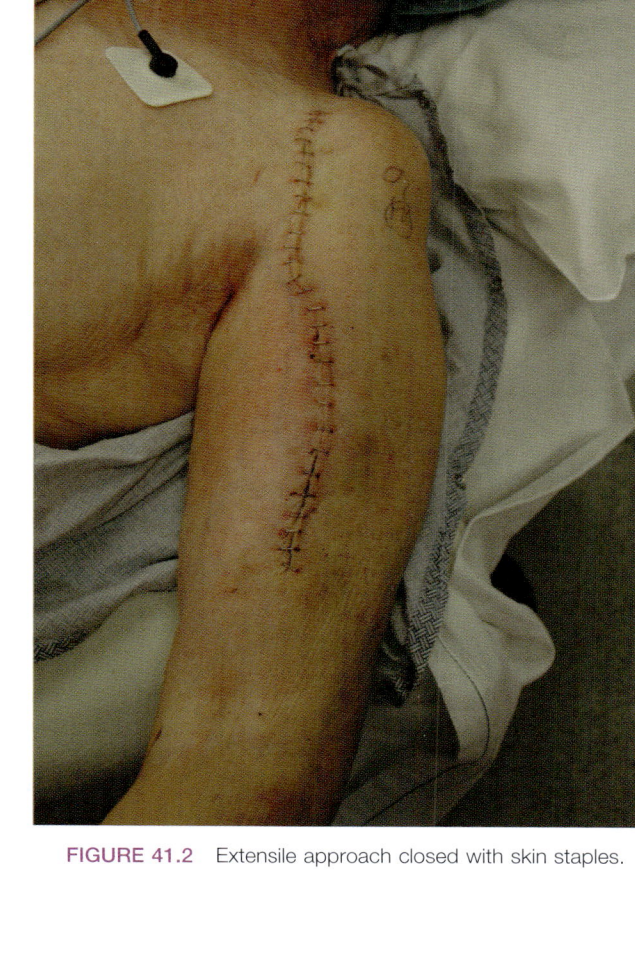

FIGURE 41.2 Extensile approach closed with skin staples.

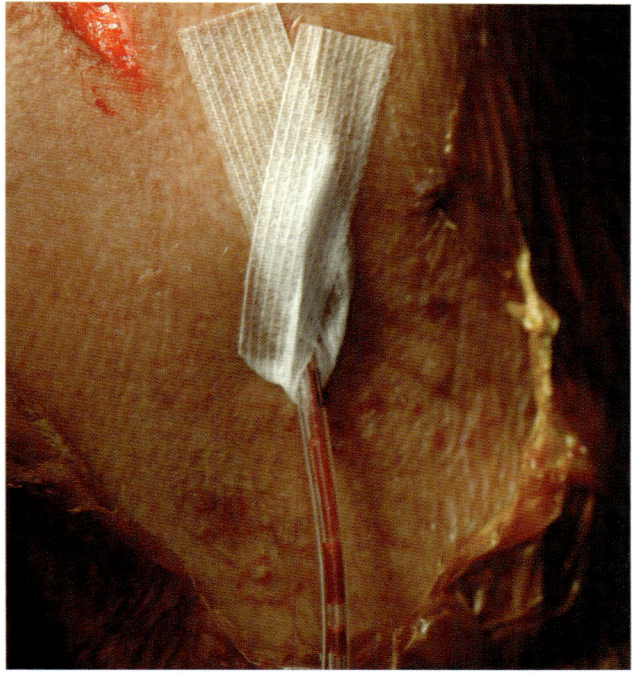

FIGURE 41.3 Steri-Strips hold the drain tube in place to prevent premature removal.

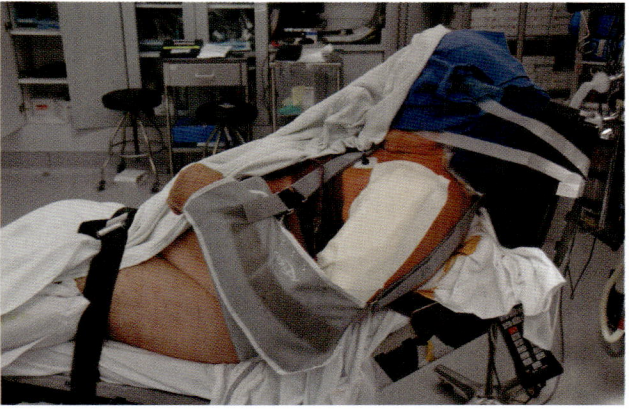

FIGURE 41.4 Neutral-rotation brace used after selected cases of revision shoulder arthroplasty.

CHAPTER 42

Results and complications

The results of revision shoulder arthroplasty are as variable as the indications for which it is performed. In general, outcomes after revision shoulder arthroplasty are less satisfactory than those after primary shoulder arthroplasty. Because of the paucity of results of revision shoulder arthroplasty reported in the literature, this chapter reports the results of revision shoulder arthroplasty by drawing from our own experience. In addition, the most frequent complications and their treatment are outlined.

RESULTS

The results of revision shoulder arthroplasty are hard to examine because of the diversity of indications for which revision is performed. A simple indication such as converting a hemiarthroplasty to a total shoulder arthroplasty for symptomatic glenoid erosion would logically yield a better outcome than would implantation of a revision shoulder arthroplasty for a chronic infection after multiple irrigation and débridement sessions. Unfortunately, the relative rarity of revision shoulder arthroplasty prevents definitive conclusions regarding outcomes. Table 42.1 details the results of revision shoulder arthroplasty from our prospective database initiated in 2003. This table expresses the results in terms of active mobility; patient satisfaction; the Constant score, a shoulder-specific outcomes device incorporating pain, mobility, activity, and strength; and the age- and gender-adjusted Constant score.[1,2]

INTRAOPERATIVE COMPLICATIONS

Intraoperative complications are common during revision shoulder arthroplasty and may be divided into complications involving the humerus, glenoid, musculotendinous soft tissues (rotator cuff), and neurovascular structures.

Humerus

Intraoperative complications involving the humerus are common. The most frequent humeral complication is iatrogenic fracture, which usually occurs during an overly aggressive dislocation maneuver without previous adequate soft tissue release or during extraction of a well-fixed humeral stem. Patients with osteopenia and those with severe preoperative stiffness are most at risk for this complication. These fractures may occur at the humeral diaphysis or proximally and involve the tuberosities. Fractures involving the diaphysis should be reduced and a long-stem humeral implant placed. Allograft struts and cerclage cables may be added in patients with severe osteopenia (Fig. 42.1).

Intraoperative fractures involving the greater or lesser tuberosities (or both) usually occur during removal of the humeral stem. Many of these fractures can be successfully stabilized by suture fixation. If a tuberosity fracture is not satisfactorily stable despite suture fixation, use of a reverse prosthesis is considered as the revision implant.

Glenoid

Intraoperative glenoid fractures at the time of revision shoulder arthroplasty occur during extraction of the glenoid component or during preparation (reaming) of the glenoid. Patients with osteopenia are most at risk. Fractures may involve only the peripheral glenoid rim or may extend significantly into the articular surface. Adequate capsular release helps to minimize the risk for glenoid fracture. In addition, a motorized reamer (not a drill) should be used for preparation of the glenoid surface. The reamer should be started before the surgeon applies force to engage the reamer onto the glenoid face. This avoids having the reamer "catch" an edge of the glenoid, which may cause a fracture.

When implanting an unconstrained glenoid component, fractures that involve only a small portion of the peripheral rim generally require no treatment and the glenoid component can be inserted as planned. Glenoid fractures that extend into the central portion of the glenoid (keel slot or peg holes) should be bone-grafted with autogenous iliac crest bone graft and placement of a glenoid component avoided. Placement of a glenoid component in the face of a fracture involving the central portion of the glenoid can result in early glenoid failure.

When implanting a reverse glenoid component, fractures that involve only a small portion of the peripheral rim generally require no treatment, and the glenoid component can be inserted as planned. Glenoid fractures that extend into the central portion of the glenoid should be bone-grafted with autogenous iliac crest bone graft. The reverse glenoid component can be placed to help secure the bone graft and internally fix the fracture. If the central post or screw of the reverse component (a long-post/screw revision base plate can be used) is firmly seated within native glenoid bone,

TABLE 42.1	Results of Revision Shoulder Arthroplasty Classified by the Type of Revision Implant Selected in the Authors' Prospective Database From 2003 to 2014								
	Absolute Constant Score (Points)		Adjusted Constant Score (%)		Active Forward Flexion (Degrees)		Active External Rotation (Degrees)		Excellent/Good Subjective Results (%)
Type of Revision Prosthesis	Preoperative	Postoperative	Preoperative	Postoperative	Preoperative	Postoperative	Preoperative	Postoperative	
Reverse prosthesis (n = 94)	18	49	24	66	38	115	13	19	72
Total shoulder arthroplasty (n = 8)	33	45	40	56	100	103	28	40	80
Hemiarthroplasty (n = 13)	25	54	30	66	65	127	13	36	76

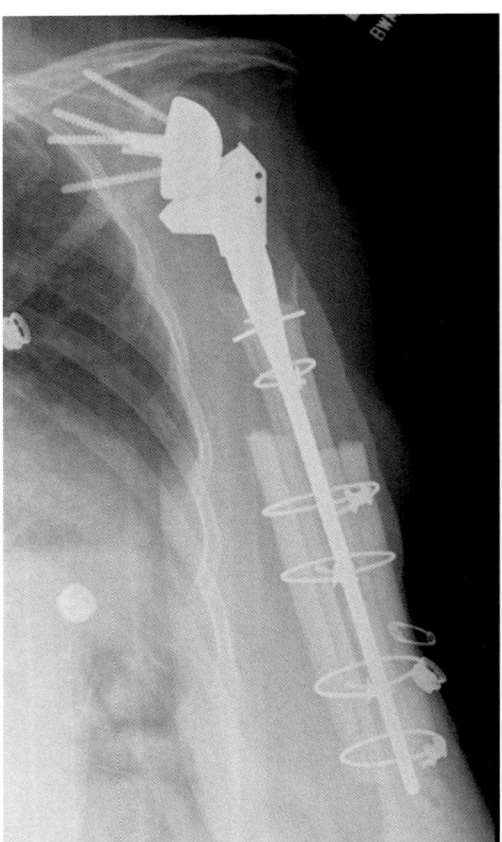

FIGURE 42.1 Radiograph of a patient with an intraoperative humeral shaft fracture incurred during revision arthroplasty that was treated with a long-stem humeral implant and allograft struts fixated with cerclage cables.

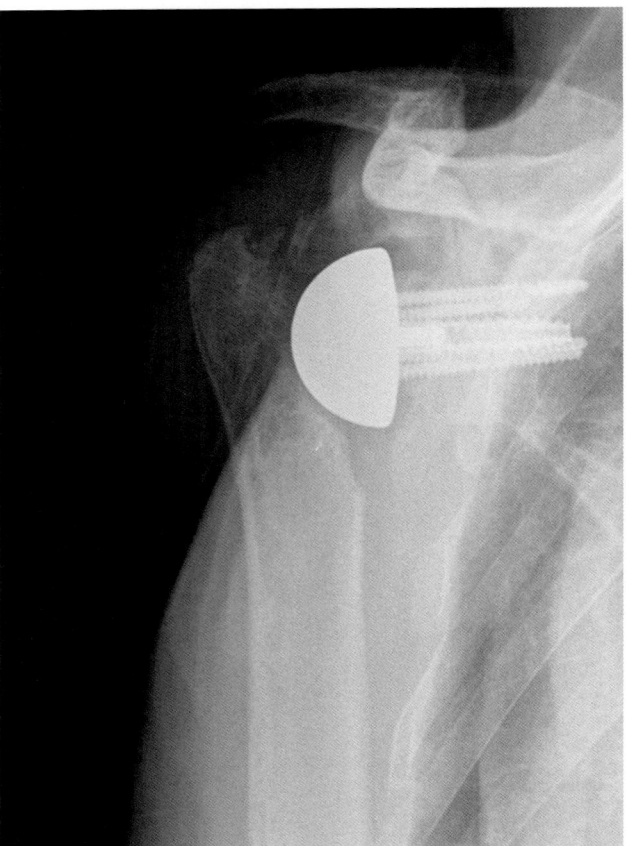

FIGURE 42.2 Revision arthroplasty during which the glenoid fractured and the glenoid component does not seem to be secure as the central screw of the glenoid base plate is not firmly seated in unfractured native glenoid bone. Insertion of the humeral component should be delayed for 6 months to allow the fracture to heal.

consideration can be given to placing the humeral component during the same surgical setting. If the glenoid component does not seem to be secure or the central post or screw of the glenoid base plate is not firmly seated in unfractured native glenoid bone, insertion of the humeral component should be delayed for 6 months to allow the fracture to heal (Fig. 42.2). After 6 months, a humeral component can be placed as the second part of a two-stage procedure. Alternatively, if an intraoperative glenoid fracture occurs, the fracture can be bone-grafted, and the humeral stem with a hemiarthroplasty adapter can be placed. After the fracture has healed and remodeled (approximately 6 months after the index attempt at reverse shoulder arthroplasty), the second stage of the procedure consisting of implantation of the glenoid component may be performed.

Rotator Cuff

Damage to the rotator cuff during revision shoulder arthroplasty usually occurs during the surgical approach and glenohumeral exposure. The anatomy is commonly distorted by the primary arthroplasty. Dissection should be slow and meticulous to avoid inadvertent damage to the rotator cuff. In the event that the rotator cuff is substantially compromised during the surgical procedure, consideration is given to implantation of a reverse prosthesis as the revision implant.

Neurovascular Structures

Catastrophic injury to the neurovascular structures around the shoulder is rare during revision shoulder arthroplasty. The neural structures most at risk during revision shoulder arthroplasty are the axillary and musculocutaneous nerves. If a humeral osteotomy is performed or if revision surgery is performed for a periprosthetic fracture, the radial nerve is also at risk. Nerve injury during revision shoulder arthroplasty can occur as a neuropraxic stretch injury or as a transection injury. Neuropraxic injury caused by stretch most commonly involves the axillary nerve but can involve any nerves within the brachial plexus. Care should be taken when positioning the patient to maintain the cervical spine in neutral alignment to avoid a stretch injury to the brachial plexus. When treating a periprosthetic fracture with revision arthroplasty or when a humeral osteotomy is anticipated for extraction of the humeral stem, the radial nerve should be carefully exposed to ensure its protection. Careful exposure of the radial nerve often results in transient neuropraxia. Patient education preoperatively is of paramount importance in dealing with neuropraxia inasmuch as patients are much more accepting if they have heard about the possibility of this complication before surgery. Axillary and radial nerve neuropraxia is treated by observation, with most patients recovering by 3 to 4 months postoperatively.

Neural transection injury is rare in revision shoulder arthroplasty. Careful identification of nerves at risk (axillary nerve and, in certain situations as outlined earlier, the radial nerve) is the best way to prevent this complication. If a transection injury does occur, the ends of the nerve are identified and consultation with a microvascular surgeon obtained.

Although tearing of the cephalic vein is common and largely without consequence, significant arterial and venous injuries do occur, although rarely, during revision reverse shoulder arthroplasty. The brachial artery is most at risk during revision surgery requiring an extensile exposure (periprosthetic fracture, humeral osteotomy). Should one of these injuries occur, after cross-clamping of the injured structure, emergency intraoperative consultation with a vascular surgeon is required.

POSTOPERATIVE COMPLICATIONS

Postoperative complications are more common after revision shoulder arthroplasty than after primary shoulder arthroplasty. The most frequent postoperative complications include wound problems (dehiscence, hematoma), glenoid problems, humeral problems, instability, rotator cuff problems, stiffness, infection, and when a reverse prosthesis is used as the revision implant, acromial problems and radiographic scapular notching.

Wound Problems

Wound problems occur early after revision shoulder arthroplasty. Hematoma is most easily avoided by extensive use of electrocautery during shoulder arthroplasty. When a reverse shoulder prosthesis is used for revision shoulder arthroplasty, closed suction drainage is maintained for 24 hours after surgery. When a hematoma occurs, it is managed by symptomatic nonoperative treatment (warm compresses, pain medication). Operative drainage is reserved for situations in which drainage persists beyond 1 week or infection is suspected (see later) but is rarely necessary.

In most revision cases the skin is closed with stainless steel skin staples. Problems with skin staples are extremely infrequent. Rarely, susceptible patients have a reaction to dissolving subcutaneous sutures. The presence of minimal serous drainage distinguishes this complication from the more serious deep infection. Superficial wound dehiscence is treated by local wound care, including removal of any residual dissolving suture material and chemical cauterization of any granulating tissue with silver nitrate applicators.

Glenoid Problems

Glenoid complications after revision arthroplasty are related to the type of revision arthroplasty performed—hemiarthroplasty, unconstrained total shoulder arthroplasty, or reverse shoulder arthroplasty. As with primary hemiarthroplasty, erosion of the remaining glenoid articular cartilage and osseous glenoid can occur. Successful treatment of glenoid erosion usually requires further revision surgery during which the glenoid is resurfaced.

Glenoid component failure after revision to unconstrained total shoulder arthroplasty can occur as a result of loosening

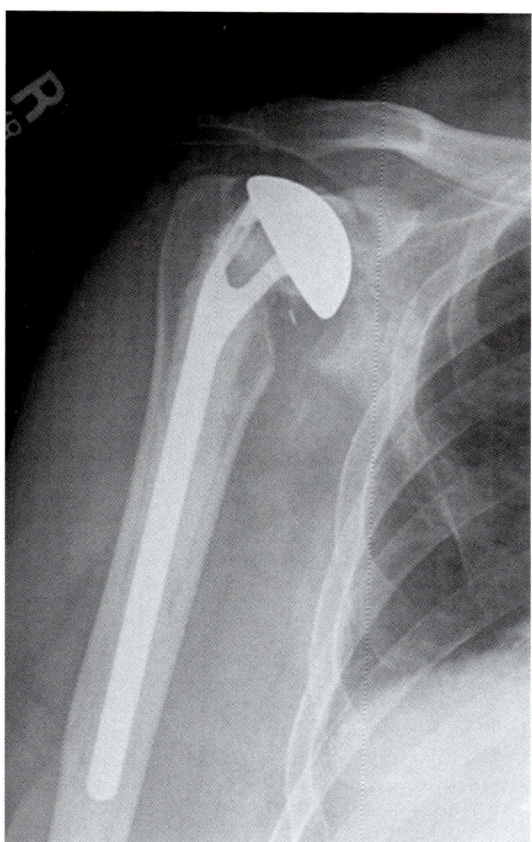

FIGURE 42.3 Unconstrained glenoid component loosening occurring 3 years after revision shoulder arthroplasty.

of the glenoid component from the host bone or mechanical breakage of the glenoid implant (Fig. 42.3). Glenoid component problems, when symptomatic, generally require further revision surgery.

Glenoid component failure after revision to reverse shoulder arthroplasty, as with primary reverse shoulder arthroplasty, has been associated in most cases of which we are aware with initial placement of the glenoid component in a superiorly oriented direction, implantation of the prosthesis in the presence of an intraoperative glenoid fracture, or insertion of the glenoid component with the central post anchored only in grafted bone. These complications are best avoided. As with primary reverse shoulder arthroplasty, we implant the reverse prosthesis for revision arthroplasty through a deltopectoral approach to avoid inadvertent placement of the glenoid component in a superiorly oriented position, which can occur with use of the superior lateral approach. If an intraoperative glenoid fracture occurs, we treat it as described previously in this chapter. When glenoid failure occurs, further revision surgery consisting of glenoid reconstruction and conversion to a hemiarthroplasty is required.

Humeral Problems

Humeral problems after revision shoulder arthroplasty are rare and can be divided into loosening of the humeral component and periprosthetic humeral fracture. Whenever possible, we use uncemented humeral stems in revision shoulder arthroplasty. Aseptic loosening of these stems is rare. Whenever loosening of a humeral stem occurs, infection must be ruled out (see later). In the rare instance of symptomatic aseptic loosening of an unconstrained humeral component, treatment is further revision of the humeral stem.

Loosening of a reverse humeral stem after revision surgery is uncommon. The predominant risk factor for aseptic loosening of a revision reverse humeral stem is proximal humeral bone loss (Fig. 42.4). Whenever loosening of a revision reverse humeral stem occurs, infection must be ruled out, as with loosening of an unconstrained revision humeral stem (see later). In the rare instance of symptomatic aseptic loosening of a revision reverse humeral component, treatment is further revision of the humeral stem, usually combined with allograft reconstruction of the proximal humerus to provide osseous support of the proximal portion of the revision stem.

Mechanical problems of a revision reverse humeral component are exceedingly rare and usually related to the polyethylene liner. Incomplete seating of the polyethylene component at the revision arthroplasty can be responsible for dissociation of the polyethylene liner from the humeral stem (Fig. 42.5). In this scenario, further revision surgery with replacement of the polyethylene liner is indicated. Polyethylene wear occurs medially on the rim of the polyethylene liner in many patients, as seen at the time of retrieval during revision surgery. It occurs as a result of scapular notching, as discussed later.

Periprosthetic humeral fractures after revision arthroplasty are more common than loosening of the humeral component and are almost always the result of a fall or similar low-energy

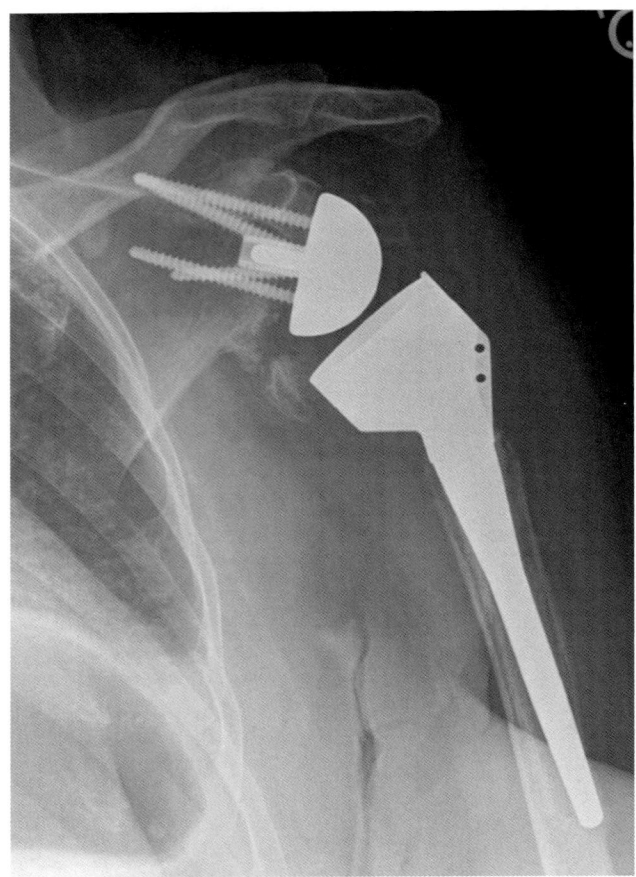

FIGURE 42.4 Aseptic loosening of a reverse humeral stem.

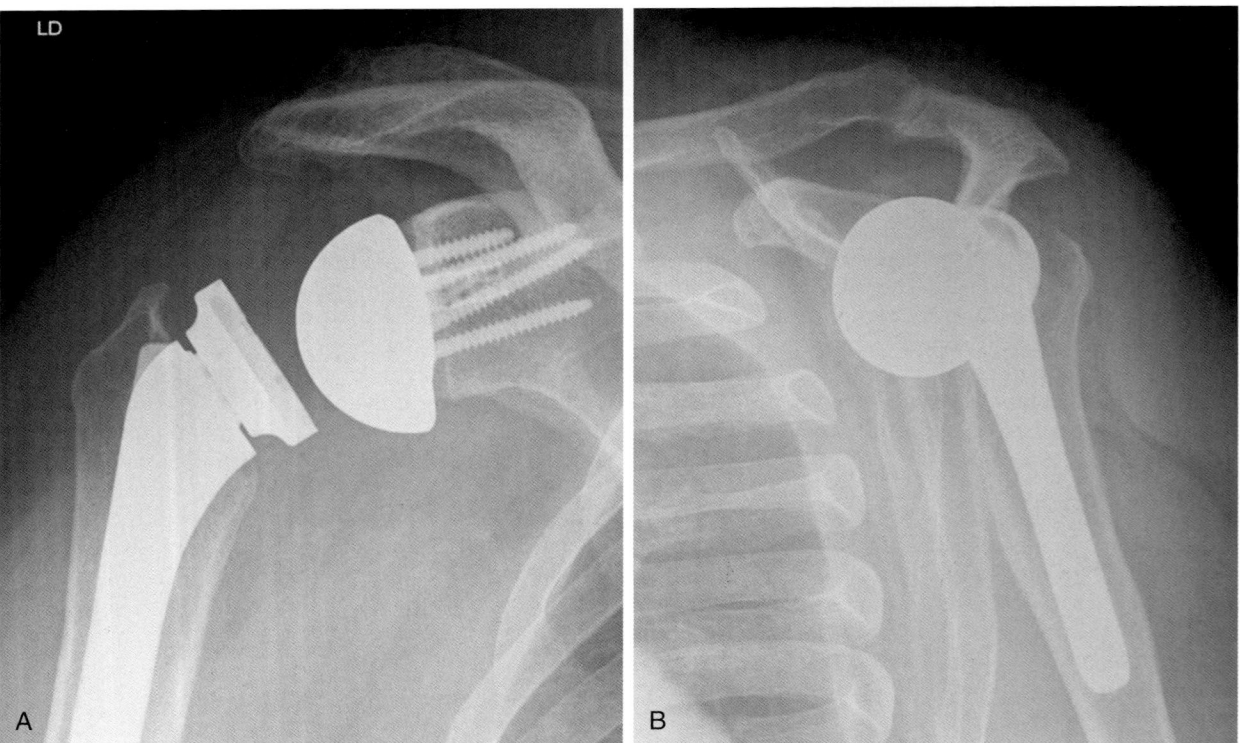

FIGURE 42.5 (A and B) Radiographs demonstrating dissociation of the polyethylene liner of a reverse shoulder arthroplasty. Note the subtle incongruence of the glenohumeral prosthetic articulation.

trauma. The majority of these fractures occur just distal to the tip of the humeral stem, and most can be treated nonoperatively. Nonoperative treatment consists of fracture bracing, activity modification, pain medication, and frequent radiographic monitoring. If the fracture has not healed within 3 months, we will incorporate the use of an external bone stimulator (OL 1000 Bone Growth Stimulator, Donjoy Orthopedics, Vista, CA). Despite these measures, periprosthetic humeral fractures treated nonoperatively may take longer than 9 months to heal.[3] Our criteria for recommending operative treatment of periprosthetic fractures include complete displacement, angulation greater than 30 degrees, loosening of the humeral component, or failure of nonoperative treatment.

Instability

Instability After Unconstrained Revision Shoulder Arthroplasty

Instability after unconstrained revision shoulder arthroplasty is usually related to one or more of three factors, including the prosthesis (alignment, size), the capsule, and the rotator cuff. Cases in which prosthetic problems have led to dynamic or static shoulder instability require correction to resolve the instability. Prosthetic problems may be related to the humeral side (excessive retroversion, causing posterior instability; excessive anteversion, causing anterior instability; too small a prosthetic head, causing global instability) or the glenoid side (failure to correct posterior glenoid wear, causing posterior instability). Further revision arthroplasty is the treatment of instability related to a prosthetic problem.

Capsular problems resulting in instability occur very infrequently after unconstrained revision shoulder arthroplasty. In this rare situation, soft tissue procedures do not reliably restore stability to the glenohumeral joint, and we perform further revision surgery with a reverse prosthesis.

Rotator cuff problems can cause static and dynamic instability after unconstrained revision shoulder arthroplasty. Unconstrained revision arthroplasty in patients with a compromised rotator cuff often results in static instability. These patients should undergo further revision with a reverse-design prosthesis to resolve the complication. Rarely, in a patient with a previously intact rotator cuff who has undergone unconstrained revision shoulder arthroplasty, a massive rotator cuff tear will develop and contribute to static instability. These patients, when symptomatic, are best treated by further revision surgery with a reverse-design prosthesis.

Dynamic instability after unconstrained revision shoulder arthroplasty most commonly occurs as anterior instability resulting from failure of the subscapularis repair. It occurs more commonly after revision arthroplasty because the subscapularis has been violated on multiple occasions. In the revision scenario, if the patient is symptomatic, we opt for revision to a reverse-design prosthesis and do not attempt isolated repair of the compromised subscapularis.

Instability After Revision Surgery With a Reverse Shoulder Prosthesis

Instability after revision surgery with a reverse shoulder prosthesis is twice as common as that observed in the primary reverse arthroplasty scenario. Dislocations after revision arthroplasty with a reverse prosthesis usually occur early (within 6 weeks of revision surgery). Instability of a reverse prosthesis can be related to various factors. In revision cases, proximal humeral bone loss seems to be the greatest risk factor for dislocation of a reverse prosthesis. In this scenario, deltoid muscle tension is often solely responsible for the stability of the implant because no rotator cuff or joint capsule exists to provide stability. Even if the deltoid is properly tensioned initially, it can gradually lose its tension and result in dislocation. A second major risk factor for dislocation of a Grammont-style reverse prosthesis is subscapularis insufficiency, a common condition encountered when performing revision shoulder arthroplasty with a reverse prosthesis. Instability associated with subscapularis insufficiency appears to be less problematic with newer designed reverse shoulder arthroplasty components; however, additional data will be needed to confirm our empiric results.

A less common factor contributing to dislocation of a reverse prosthesis is mechanical impingement causing the prosthetic socket to be levered away from the glenoid component. This impingement usually occurs inferiorly as the arm is adducted and is often related to too superior positioning of the glenoid component on the glenoid face, as detailed schematically in Chapter 25. Finally, in the revision situation, the integrity and function of the axillary nerve should be ensured before performing revision arthroplasty with a reverse prosthesis because this neural deficit can result in prosthetic dislocation.

In most cases, as with dislocation of a primary reverse prosthesis, treatment initially consists of closed reduction and a period of bracing. Closed reduction is performed in the operating room with the patient either heavily sedated or under general anesthesia. An attempt is made to reduce the dislocation under fluoroscopic guidance. If the prosthesis is successfully reduced, fluoroscopic examination is performed to ensure that mechanical impingement is not responsible for the instability. If the problem is not related to mechanical impingement and the prosthesis is successfully reduced, a brace is applied to maintain the arm with the humeral component centered on the glenoid component, usually in approximately 90 degrees of abduction and 30 degrees of forward flexion (Fig. 42.6). The patient maintains this brace

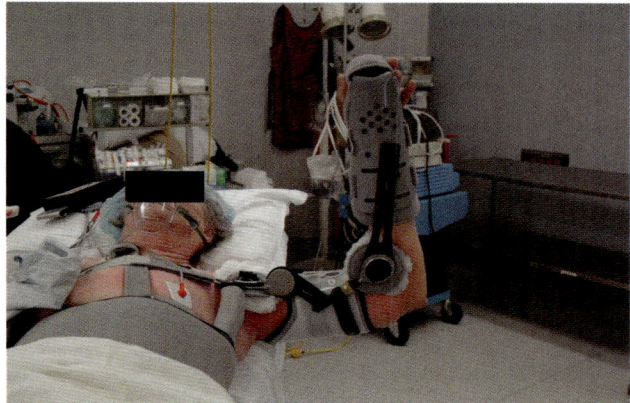

FIGURE 42.6 Placement of a brace used for the treatment of a dislocated revision reverse prosthesis after closed reduction.

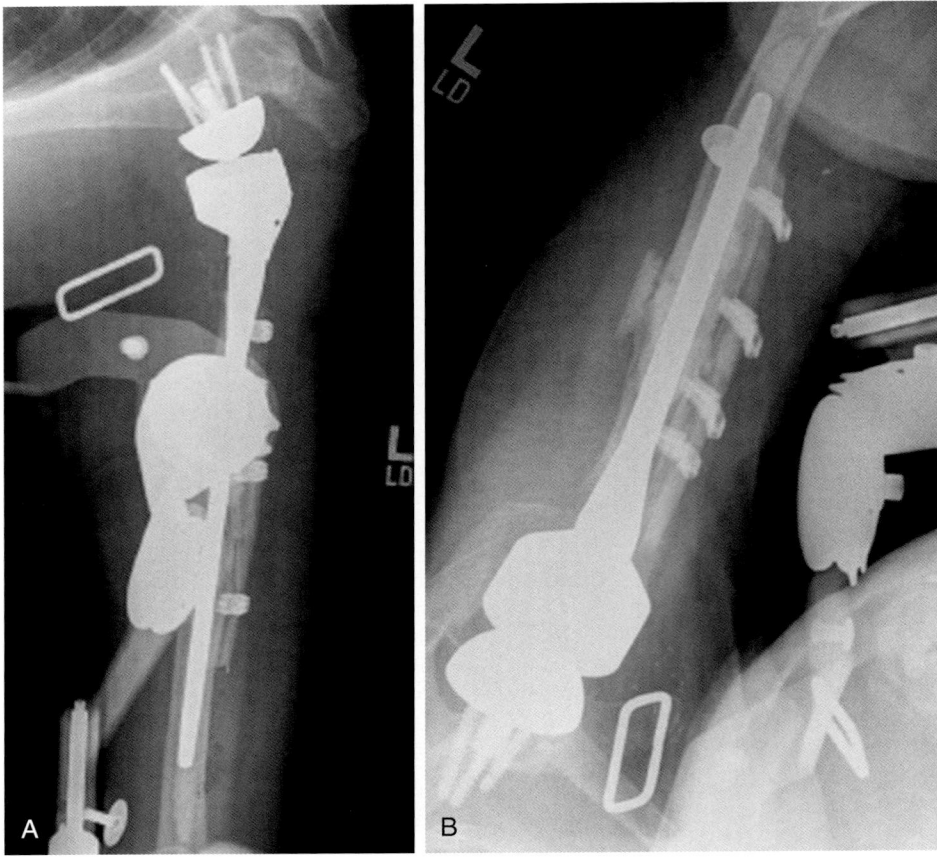

FIGURE 42.7 (A and B) Radiographs obtained in the brace confirming maintenance of prosthetic reduction.

at all times for 6 weeks, and radiographs are taken in the brace every 7 to 10 days to confirm that the prosthesis has remained located (Fig. 42.7). After 6 weeks the brace is discontinued and a normal rehabilitation regimen ensues.

If the prosthesis is not reducible by closed means, mechanical impingement causing dislocation exists, or closed reduction plus bracing has failed, open reduction with insertion of a thicker more constrained polyethylene spacer and/or larger diameter glenosphere is performed (Fig. 42.8). Any mechanical impingement can simultaneously be addressed by careful removal of bone at the lateral aspect of the scapula just inferior to the glenoid component, if necessary. Postoperatively, the patient is treated with the same bracing protocol used after closed reduction of a dislocated reverse prosthesis.

Rotator Cuff Problems

Symptomatic problems of the rotator cuff after unconstrained revision shoulder arthroplasty often result in instability and were described earlier. Failure of the subscapularis repair is the most common postoperative rotator cuff problem that we observe. When subscapularis failure is minimally symptomatic or asymptomatic, no treatment is indicated. When symptomatic, treatment is indicated as described previously in the "Instability" section of this chapter.

Isolated internal rotation weakness is not diagnostic of subscapularis failure after unconstrained revision shoulder arthroplasty. It is common for individuals to lose internal rotation strength after tenotomy and repair of the subscapularis during primary shoulder arthroplasty, and this finding becomes more pronounced after revision surgery. Subscapularis failure should be documented by computed tomography arthrography before considering operative treatment of this complication.

Stiffness

Glenohumeral stiffness after revision shoulder arthroplasty is related to capsular contracture or the prosthesis, or both. It is much more commonly observed when using an unconstrained revision implant than when using a reverse revision implant. Prosthetic problems resulting in stiffness are generally the result of implantation of too large an unconstrained humeral component or malpositioning of the revision component (Fig. 42.9). Rehabilitation with capsular stretching can be attempted in an effort to improve mobility. If this fails (no improvement over a 6-month period), revision surgery is indicated and consists of downsizing of the humeral head with open release of any capsular contractures that are present.

Stiffness related to capsular contracture almost always responds to nonoperative management involving aquatic-based rehabilitation (see Chapter 43). If the patient shows no improvement in mobility over a 6-month course of rehabilitation and has no obvious prosthetic problem, we will consider the patient a candidate for arthroscopic capsular

CHAPTER 42 ■ Results and Complications 457

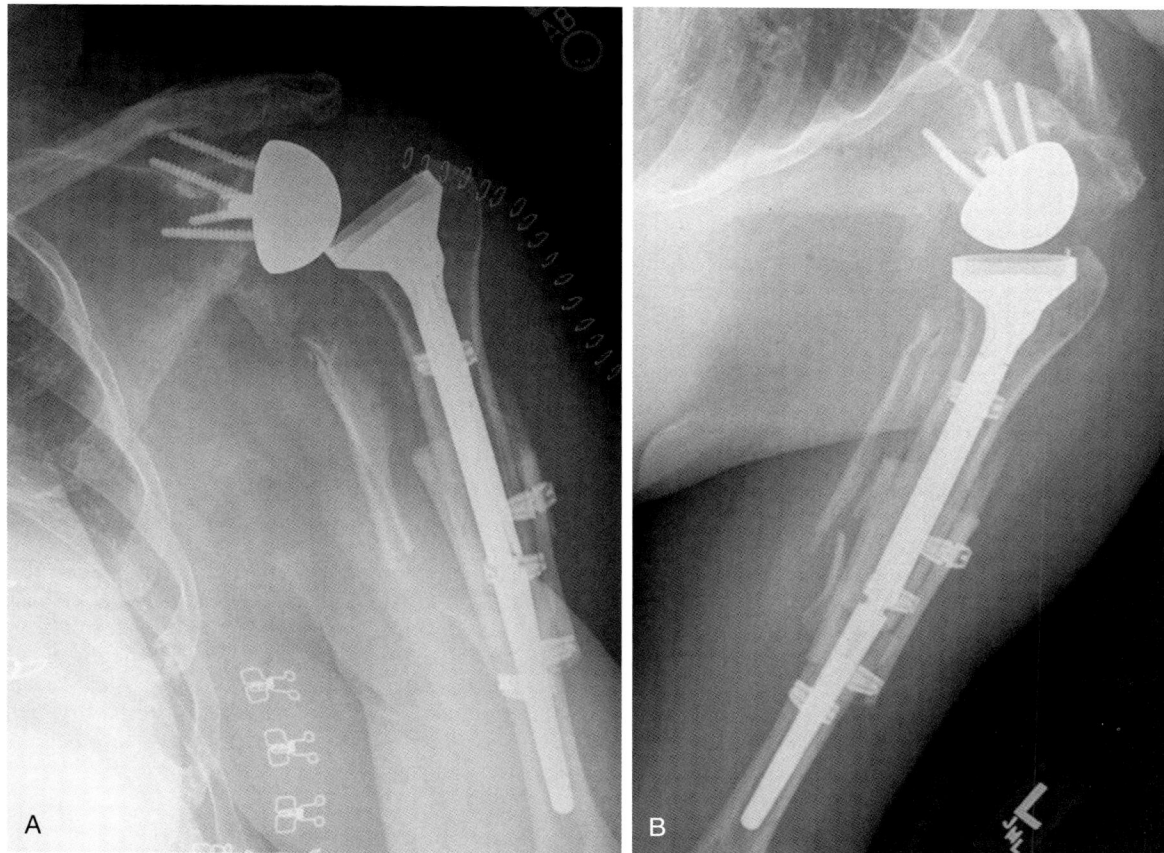

FIGURE 42.8 Treatment of a dislocated revision reverse prosthesis (A) with insertion of a thicker, more constrained polyethylene spacer and a larger diameter glenosphere (B).

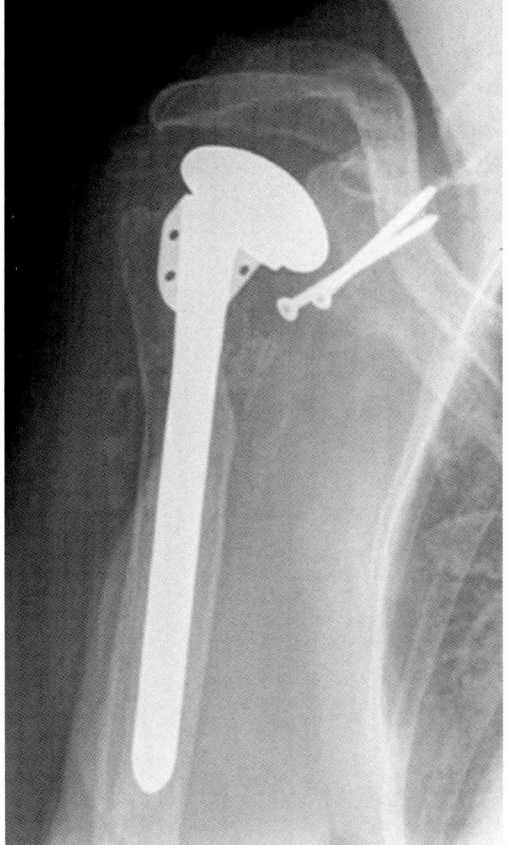

FIGURE 42.9 Malpositioned revision humeral stem contributing to glenohumeral stiffness.

contracture release if an unconstrained revision implant was used. We have no experience dealing with capsular contracture in a patient who has undergone revision shoulder arthroplasty with a reverse prosthesis.

Infection

Infection after revision shoulder arthroplasty is expectedly more common than infection after primary shoulder arthroplasty. Patients undergoing reverse shoulder arthroplasty for failed prior arthroplasty have been shown to be at a significantly increased risk for infection.[4] In addition, patients with systemic illness (diabetes mellitus), those with compromised soft tissues (radiation-induced osteonecrosis, posttraumatic arthritis), and those with inflammatory arthropathy (rheumatoid arthritis) are at increased risk for infection. These infections are most commonly caused by *Staphylococcus aureus* or *Propionibacterium acnes*. Infections after revision shoulder arthroplasty can be divided into perioperative (within 6 weeks of surgery) and late (hematogenous) infections.

Early perioperative infections are initially treated with two or three irrigation and débridement procedures and retention of the fixed components. With each irrigation and débridement procedure, the polyethylene liner of the humeral component is removed and the prosthesis is thoroughly cleaned. The original polyethylene liner is replaced after being cleaned during the initial one or two irrigation and débridement procedures. At the last planned irrigation and débridement procedure, absorbable antibiotic-impregnated beads (Stimulan, Biocomposites, Inc., Staffordshire, England) are placed in the soft tissues around the shoulder, and the polyethylene liner is replaced. Consultation with an infectious disease specialist is obtained, and a minimum of 6 weeks of intravenous antibiotics tailored to the specific organism causing the infection (or covering the most likely offending organisms, if cultures remain negative despite obvious infection) is usually recommended. If this regimen fails, prosthetic removal ensues.

Late-appearing infections are treated by removal of the prosthesis, placement of antibiotic spacer, and intravenous administration of antibiotics. The decision whether to place a revision shoulder arthroplasty or continue with a resection arthroplasty is patient specific.

Acromial Fractures

Occasionally, acromial stress fractures are seen after revision reverse shoulder arthroplasty, just as with primary reverse shoulder arthroplasty. These fractures result from deltoid tension applied to osteopenic bone. Frequently, these fractures exist preoperatively as a result of chronic superior migration of the humeral head with persistent acromiohumeral articulation (Fig. 42.10). Postoperatively, deltoid tension may cause the fracture fragment to tilt inferiorly.

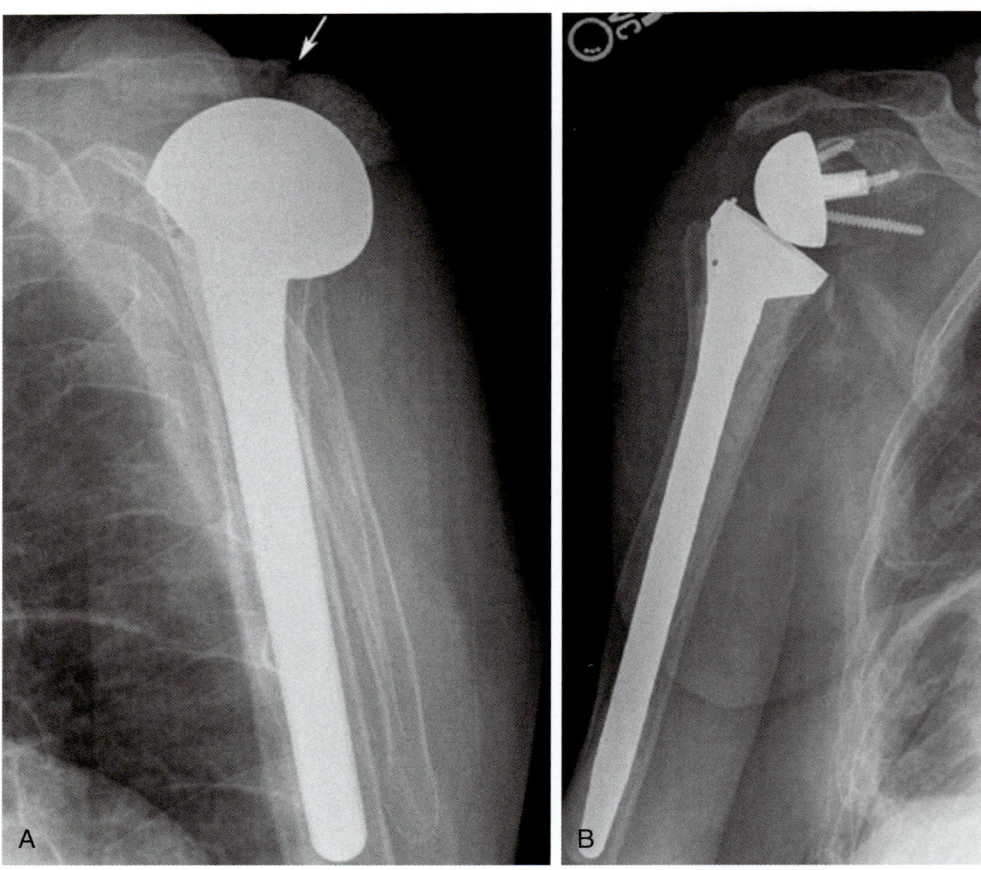

FIGURE 42.10 (A) Acromial stress fracture *(arrow)* occurring after hemiarthroplasty for rotator cuff tear arthropathy. (B) This patient underwent revision to a reverse prosthesis, with the stress fracture requiring no additional treatment.

Acromial fractures are likely more common than initially suspected, with a reported incidence of up to 3% in one series.[5] We tend to see these fractures approximately 2 to 3 months postoperatively, with the reported series noting an average of approximately 8 months postoperatively.[5] Acromial stress fractures are diagnosed with tenderness to palpation at the acromion and can sometimes be seen on radiographs. The diagnosis and treatment of acromial fractures are highlighted in Chapter 25. Reported outcomes for reverse shoulder arthroplasty after acromial stress fracture note significant improvements for preoperative to postoperative pain relief and function; however, these patients achieve decreased range of motion and decreased functional outcomes relative to controls.[5]

Scapular Body and Scapular Spine Fractures

Occasionally, scapular body and scapular spine fractures are seen after revision reverse shoulder arthroplasty, just as with primary reverse shoulder arthroplasty (Fig. 42.11). Scapular body and scapular spine fractures are not common after reverse shoulder arthroplasty. One series reported an incidence of 1% of scapular spine fractures (classified as "type III" fractures) after reverse shoulder arthroplasty.[6] Similar to acromial stress fractures, scapular fractures are thought to be secondary to osteopenic bone and deltoid tension and can potentially propagate through the superior screw of the baseplate. The superior screw has been noted to be a potential stress riser for scapular fracture propagation, with some advocating avoiding placing the superior screw when possible.[6] The diagnosis and treatment of scapular body and scapular spine fractures is highlighted in Chapter 25.

Scapular Notching

Although debatable whether it should be considered a complication, notching of the scapula occurs within 2 years of surgery in half the patients who have undergone reverse shoulder arthroplasty, both in the primary and in the revision situation (Fig. 42.12). This radiographic finding most likely occurs as a result of mechanical impingement of the medial aspect of the humeral component and the lateral aspect of the scapula just inferior to the glenoid. As the patient internally rotates the shoulder, the impingement is exacerbated. This mechanical impingement theory is further supported by the observation that patients' internal rotation seems to improve as the scapular notch progresses, thus suggesting that the prosthesis must "carve out" a portion of the scapula to maximize postoperative internal rotation. Another theory of the cause of scapular notching is polyethylene wear causing osteolysis, although this theory currently has less support than the mechanical impingement theory.

Scapular notching is commonly accompanied by a scapular osteophyte just medial to the notch. The degree of scapular notching has also been graded by severity.[7] The best way to avoid scapular notching was thought to be by placing the glenoid component inferiorly on the glenoid face and by introducing slight inferior tilt during glenoid reaming; however, we did not find a difference in scapular notching

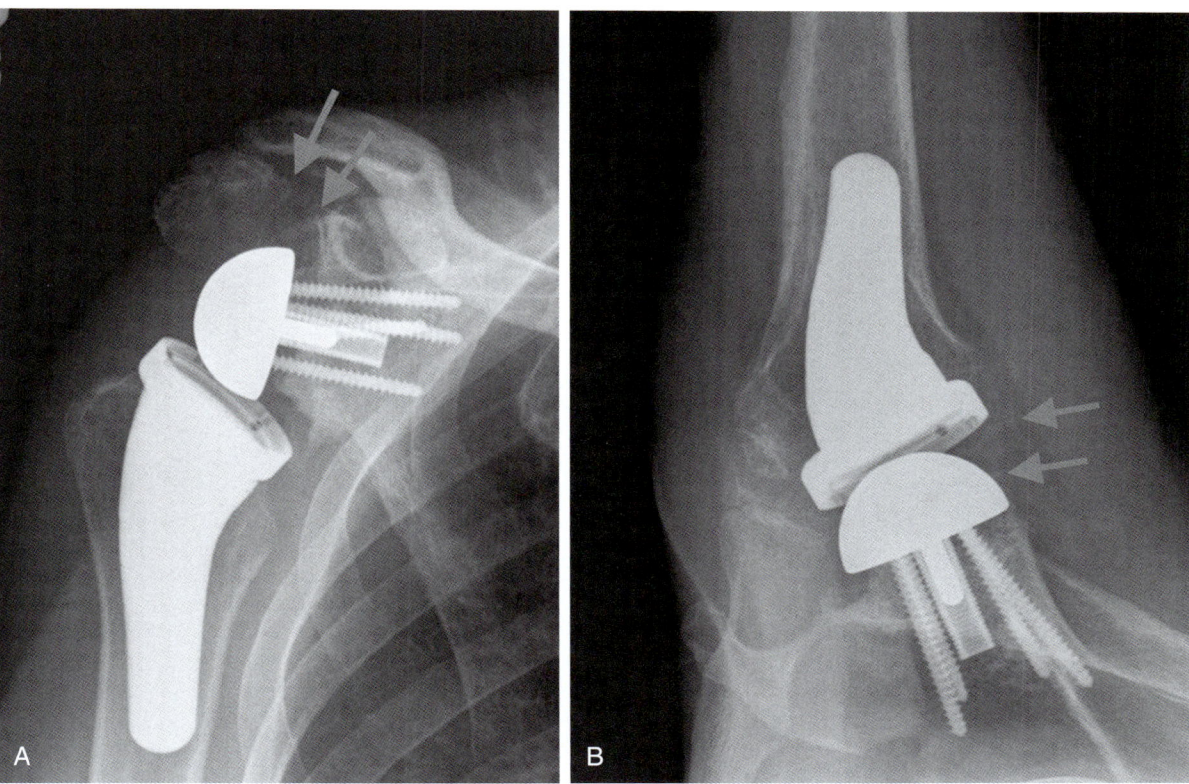

FIGURE 42.11 (A and B) Radiographs demonstrating scapular spine stress fracture *(arrows)* occurring 6 months following revision arthroplasty with a reverse prosthesis.

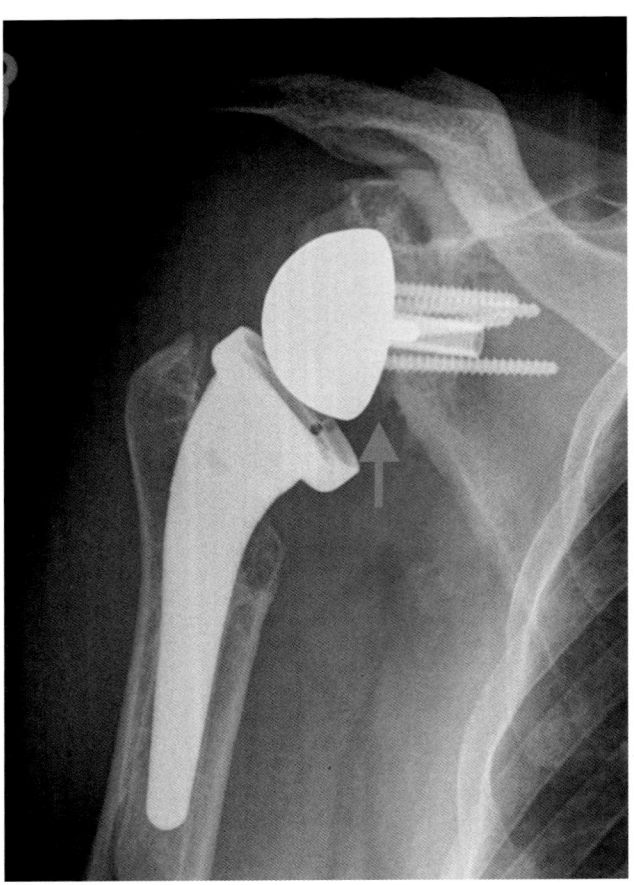

FIGURE 42.12 Scapular notching *(arrow)* occurring after revision arthroplasty with a reverse prosthesis.

when comparing neutral versus 10 degrees of inferior tilt in a prospective randomized trial.[8]

Despite the concerning appearance of this scapular notch, its clinical implications are unclear, with most of the evidence suggesting no adverse consequence. As long as the glenoid component remains stable, no treatment of an asymptomatic scapular notch is indicated.

REFERENCES

1. Constant CR, Murley AH: A clinical method of functional assessment of the shoulder, *Clin Orthop Relat Res* 214:160–164, 1987.
2. Constant CR: Assessment of shoulder function. In Gazielly D, Gleyze P, Thomas T, editors: *The cuff*, New York, 1997, Elsevier, pp 39–44.
3. Kumar S, Sperling JW, Haidukewych GH, et al: Periprosthetic humeral fractures after shoulder arthroplasty, *J Bone Joint Surg Am* 86:680–689, 2004.
4. Morris BJ, O'Connor DP, Torres D, et al: Risk factors for periprosthetic infection after reverse shoulder arthroplasty, *J Shoulder Elbow Surg* 24:161–166, 2015.
5. Teusink MJ, Otto RJ, Cottrell BJ, et al: What is the effect of postoperative scapular fracture on outcomes of reverse shoulder arthroplasty?, *J Shoulder Elbow Surg* 23:782–790, 2014.
6. Crosby LA, Hamilton A, Twiss T: Scapula fractures after reverse total shoulder arthroplasty: classification and treatment, *Clin Orthop Relat Res* 469:2544–2549, 2011.
7. Valenti P, Boutens D, Nerot C: Delta 3 reversed prosthesis for osteoarthritis with massive rotator cuff tear: long term results (>5 years). In Walch G, Boileau P, Molé D, editors: *2000 Prosthèses d'Epaule … Recul de 2 à 10 Ans*, Paris, 2001, Sauramps Medical, pp 253–259.
8. Edwards TB, Trappey GJ, Riley C, et al: Inferior tilt of the glenoid component does not decrease scapular notching in reverse shoulder arthroplasty: results of a prospective randomized study, *J Shoulder Elbow Surg* 21(5):641–646, 2012.

SECTION VII

POSTOPERATIVE REHABILITATION

CHAPTER 43

Rehabilitation after shoulder arthroplasty

The goal of rehabilitation after shoulder arthroplasty is restoration of functional shoulder mobility in a timely fashion. Biologic factors impose limitations in achieving mobility after shoulder arthroplasty. Histologically, collagenous connective tissues in the shoulder (tendons, ligaments, capsule) contract after shoulder arthroplasty. These connective tissues are subject to the biomechanical properties and limitations of collagen, including plasticity, stretching, and temperature sensitivity. The plasticity of collagen allows connective tissues to adapt to physiologic and pathologic conditions. Rehabilitation is designed to maximize these adaptations and provide functional recovery of mobility after shoulder arthroplasty. We use a hydrotherapy-based rehabilitation regimen after shoulder arthroplasty to regain shoulder mobility.[1]

PRINCIPLES OF HYDROTHERAPY

Rehabilitation in a warm-water pool facilitates gain of mobility after shoulder arthroplasty. Rehabilitation with the shoulder submerged or partially submerged in warm water provides a "weightless" environment. This "weightlessness" allows the arm to find the best path to achieve a specific movement. Additionally, a warm-water environment provides comfort and improves proprioception while minimizing pain. Whereas thermal neutrality is obtained with water heated to 34°C (93.2°F), a water temperature of 35°C (95°F) increases skin comfort while raising body temperature less than 1°C, thus minimizing the risk of a heat-induced inflammatory response.

REHABILITATION PROTOCOL

Rehabilitation starts with choosing the type of postoperative orthosis and its duration of use. This is largely based on the type of arthroplasty performed (unconstrained, fracture, reverse) and the performance of any associated procedures (posterior capsulorrhaphy). Table 43.1 summarizes the types of orthoses used and the duration of their use based on the procedure performed. All patients are instructed in hand, wrist, and elbow mobility exercises and scapular exercises on postoperative day 1. Patients undergoing unconstrained shoulder arthroplasty for chronic conditions without performance of an associated posterior capsulorrhaphy are also instructed in pendulum exercises on postoperative day 1. These exercises are performed three to five times per day for approximately 15 minutes each time and are continued throughout the rehabilitative program. The time of initiation of hydrotherapy depends on the type of arthroplasty performed. Table 43.2 summarizes the time at which hydrotherapy is instituted based on the procedure performed.

Hydrotherapy is performed in a warm (35°C, 95°F) rehabilitation pool that is approximately 1.3 m in depth at its deepest point. The pool is fitted with supports that can accommodate the straps and harnesses used in the rehabilitation process. The surgical wound is covered with a waterproof, air-permeable hypoallergenic adhesive dressing. Patients are equipped with a mask and snorkel if needed during hydrotherapy.

Hydrotherapy takes place daily (5 to 7 days per week, depending on availability) in a single 30- to 45-minute session. An abbreviated land-based verification session follows to affirm gains in mobility achieved in the pool. Various exercises designed to gain elevation, extension, horizontal adduction, internal rotation, and external rotation are performed in sets of 10 repetitions (Figs. 43.1 through 43.4). The unaffected extremity is used to help power the movement. Active mobility of the operated extremity is allowed in the form of a slow, gentle breaststroke motion with the palms placed horizontally (to avoid invoking resistance from the water), which is performed with the patient supported by a harness and the shoulders submerged (Fig. 43.5). In patients who have undergone unconstrained shoulder arthroplasty, external rotation beyond neutral is not allowed until 4 weeks postoperatively in patients with primary osteoarthritis or osteonecrosis and 6 weeks in patients with compromised soft tissues (inflammatory arthropathies, revision surgery) to protect the subscapularis repair. In patients who have undergone an associated posterior capsulorrhaphy, internal rotation and horizontal adduction are avoided until 4 weeks postoperatively. With the exception of these cases, no limitations on mobility are imposed.

Mobility exercises with total body immersion are advised for all patients; however, it is at the discretion of each

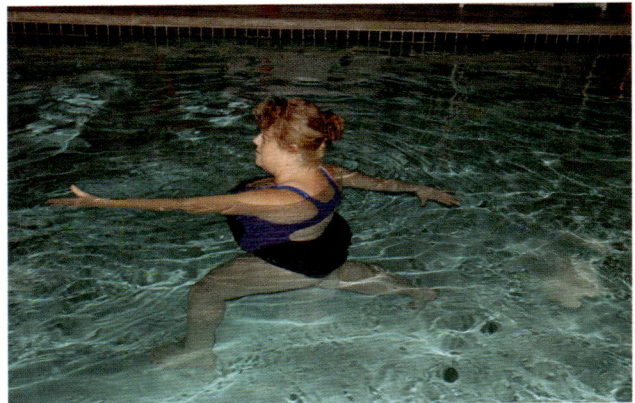

FIGURE 43.1 Shoulder flexion and extension exercises.

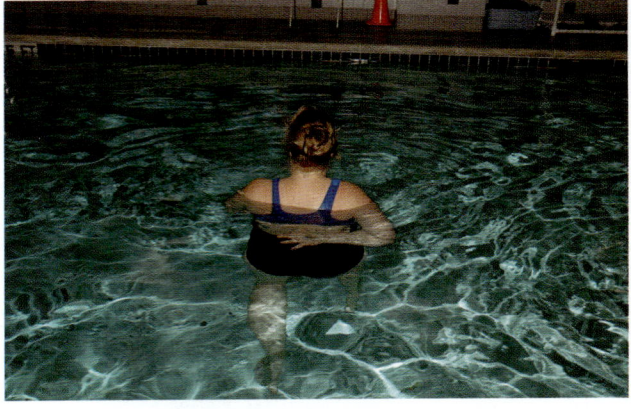

FIGURE 43.2 Internal rotation exercises.

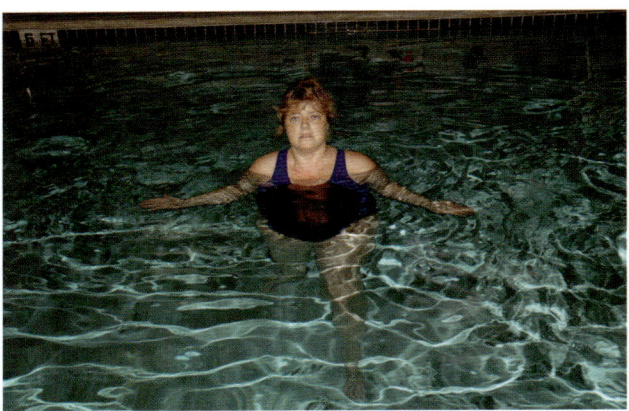

FIGURE 43.3 External rotation exercises.

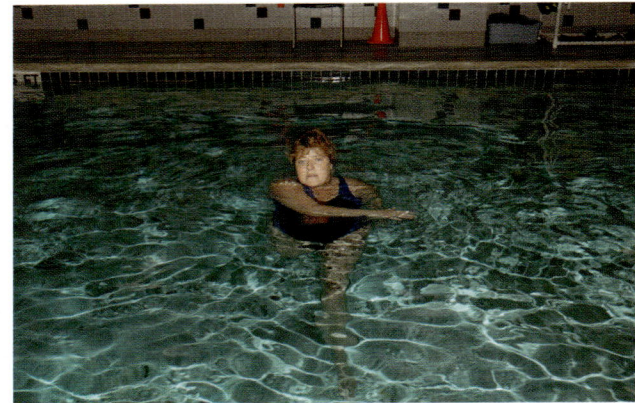

FIGURE 43.4 Horizontal adduction exercises.

TABLE 43.1	Type of Postoperative Orthosis Used and Duration of Use	
Procedure	Type	Duration (weeks)
Unconstrained arthroplasty	Simple sling	1–2
Unconstrained arthroplasty plus posterior capsulorrhaphy	Neutral rotation sling	4
Fracture prosthesis (unconstrained or reverse)	Neutral rotation sling	4–6
Reverse prosthesis	Neutral rotation sling	3–4

TABLE 43.2	Time for Initiation of Hydrotherapy
Procedure	Hydrotherapy Initiated (Postoperative Week)
Unconstrained arthroplasty	1
Unconstrained arthroplasty plus posterior capsulorrhaphy	1
Fracture prosthesis (unconstrained or reverse)	4–6
Reverse prosthesis	3–4

individual patient. Patients who wish to try such exercises are fitted with a weighted belt and instructed to hold their breath as they kneel or recline supine on the bottom of the pool (Fig. 43.6). The same mobility exercises are then performed in the more insulated underwater environment. This technique is very helpful in accelerating gains in mobility.

As soon as the patient has achieved 140 degrees of elevation, the hands can be clasped behind the head in the "siesta" position (Fig. 43.7). Additional stretching exercises for the anterior (Fig. 43.8) and posterior capsules (Fig. 43.9) can be performed in this position. From this position, motion is advanced until the "triple locking" position is achieved, which stretches the inferior capsule (Fig. 43.10). Both the siesta and triple-locking positions are used extensively in a self-rehabilitation program implemented after discharge from formal physical therapy.

An abbreviated session of land-based rehabilitation is used after the hydrotherapy session. The land-based session is performed principally to affirm the gains that the patient has made during the hydrotherapy session. The same exercises are used, but with fewer repetitions. Modality treatment (i.e., cryotherapy) is used on an as-needed basis. Analgesic medication is provided to patients for the first 6 postoperative weeks to alleviate the discomfort associated with surgery and subsequent rehabilitation.

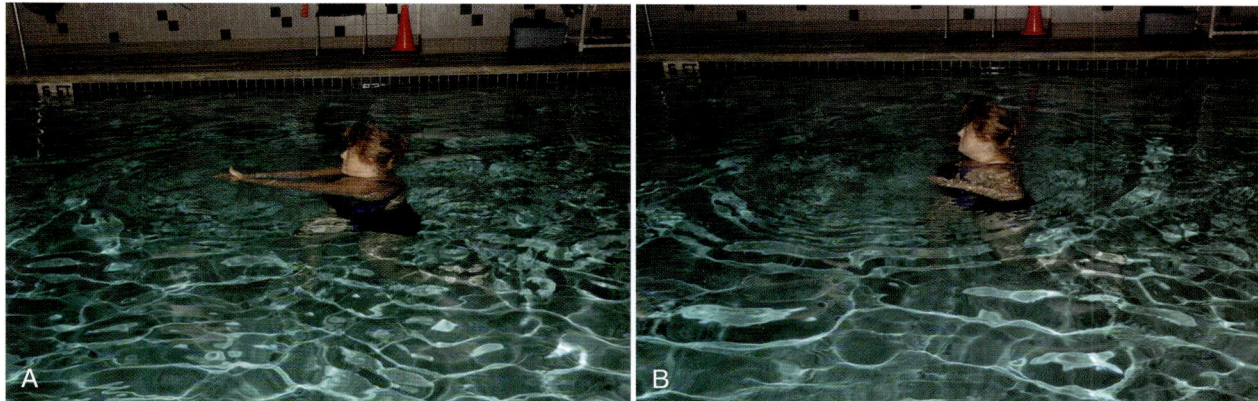

FIGURE 43.5 (A and B) Breaststroke exercise.

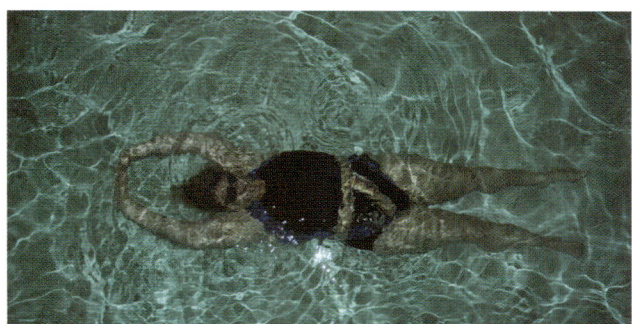

FIGURE 43.6 Total body immersion exercises.

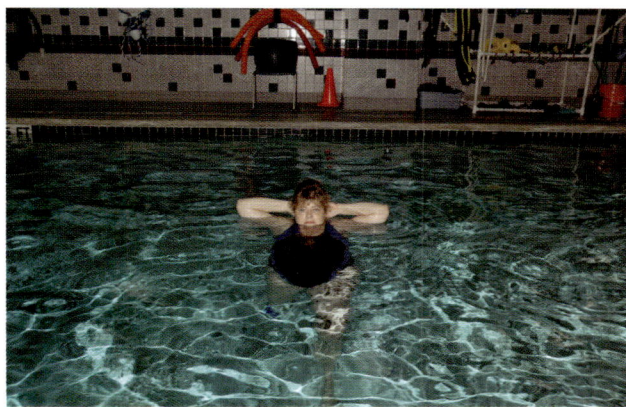

FIGURE 43.7 "Siesta" position.

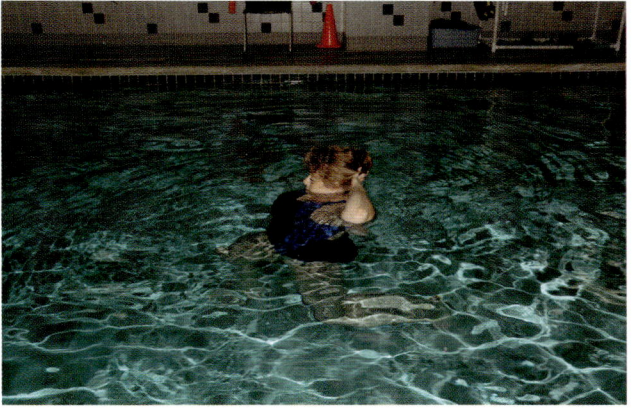

FIGURE 43.8 Anterior capsule stretching from the siesta position.

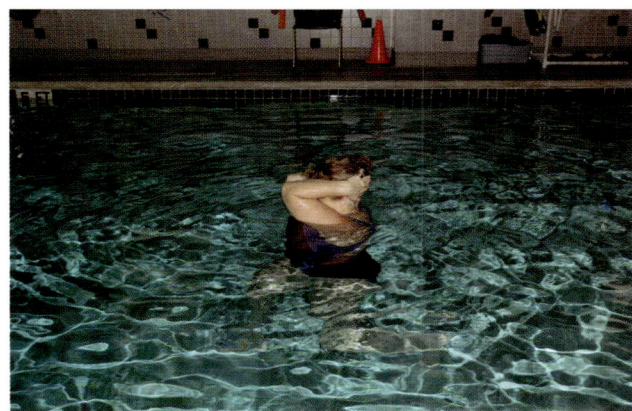

FIGURE 43.9 Posterior capsule stretching from the siesta position.

All patients participate in at least 5 weeks of hydrotherapy, after which they are reevaluated. If acceptable active mobility has been achieved, hydrotherapy is discontinued and the patient is graduated to a land-based self-rehabilitation regimen incorporating the siesta and triple-locking stretches performed several times per day indefinitely. If it is determined that the patient would benefit from continued hydrotherapy, 6 additional weeks of hydrotherapy are prescribed. Most patients are able to discontinue hydrotherapy and graduate to the self-rehabilitation program by 3 months postoperatively.

Some patients, particularly those living in rural areas, do not have access to a physical therapist with a rehabilitation pool. In these circumstances, patients learn the program from an experienced therapist in a more urban location and perform the program on their own in any public or private pool that they may have available. Additionally, any patients who prove adept at performing the exercises in the hydrotherapy program are allowed to complete the program independently with periodic monitoring by a physical therapist.

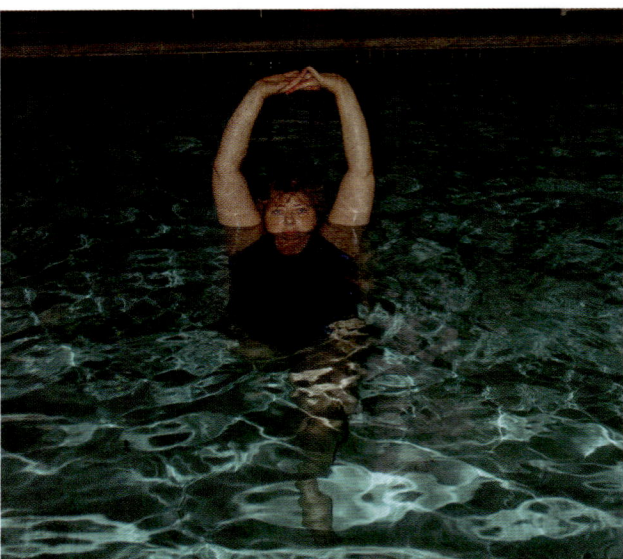

FIGURE 43.10 The triple-locking position.

Rarely, we encounter a patient with a true fear of water. Although an inability to swim is not a contraindication to hydrotherapy rehabilitation, anxiety or fearfulness at the prospect of aquatic-based rehabilitation is a contraindication. In these patients, we prescribe a land-based program incorporating the same exercises that are used in the rehabilitation pool. In general, the land-based program is effective in obtaining an end result similar to that achieved with hydrotherapy, but it usually takes longer to achieve this result and patients tend to have more pain during rehabilitation.

RETURN TO ACTIVITY

With this protocol, patients can be expected to resume activities of daily living on a normal basis before 3 months postoperatively. No specific strengthening exercises are performed in this protocol with the exception of scapular strengthening, which is permitted. Gradual resumption of normal activities is all that is required to regain strength, and it poses minimal risk to the patient.

We allow our patients to pursue most activities and sports after shoulder arthroplasty. We do limit patients to noncontact sports. The majority of our arthroplasty patients with athletic interests participate in golf and tennis. Restrictions placed on golfers and tennis players are designed to protect the subscapularis repair. Putting is allowed as soon as the patient can tolerate it postoperatively, usually within 6 weeks. At 3 months, half swings with a seven iron off a tee are allowed. This is advanced until the patient is allowed to hit a full swing with all clubs off a tee 4 to 5 months postoperatively. At 6 months after surgery, unrestricted golf is allowed. Tennis players are permitted to begin gentle ground strokes 3 months postoperatively. The intensity of the ground strokes is increased 4 to 5 months after surgery. Unrestricted tennis, including serves and overhead shots, is allowed 6 months postoperatively.

Although we do not recommend any specific strengthening exercises as part of the rehabilitation program, some of our younger patients enjoy weightlifting as part of their fitness regimen. Upper-extremity weightlifting is allowed starting 6 months postoperatively. Patients are encouraged to use weightlifting for muscle toning only and not to engage in any type of power-lifting exercises. We have had patients participate in sports such as trap shooting, water skiing, snow skiing, and mountain climbing 6 months after undergoing shoulder arthroplasty.

REFERENCE

1. Liotard JP, Edwards TB, Padey A, et al: Hydrotherapy rehabilitation after shoulder surgery, *Tech Shoulder Elbow Surg* 4:44–49, 2003.

SECTION VIII

THE FUTURE

CHAPTER 44

Future directions in shoulder arthroplasty

Shoulder arthroplasty has advanced immeasurably since the first shoulder replacement was implanted by Péan in 1893.[1] Implant designs continue to evolve and improve, as do the materials from which these designs are constructed. The reverse prosthesis has gained widespread use in the United States since 2004 and continues to evolve, with design changes introduced by many companies that manufacture a version of this semiconstrained device.

One of our personal interests in the future of shoulder arthroplasty focuses on patient-specific virtual surgery and the dynamic role of the scapula in shoulder arthroplasty.

PATIENT-SPECIFIC VIRTUAL SURGERY AND PATIENT-SPECIFIC INSTRUMENTATION

Preoperative planning software enables surgeons to plan surgery virtually, including humeral and glenoid implantation. The software is typically formatted off nonarthrogram computed tomography scans to create three-dimensional reconstructions that allow glenoid morphology to be evaluated, including degrees of retroversion and percentage of humeral head subluxation (Fig. 44.1). The surgeon can implant the glenoid component virtually to determine the appropriate size of the glenoid component, the backside radius of curvature, and the desired location to ensure appropriate version, seating, depth of reaming as well as to minimize glenoid perforation for anatomic shoulder arthroplasty and to find maximal bone purchase for reverse shoulder arthroplasty (Figs. 44.2 and 44.3). A patient-specific guide can be created to provide reproducibility of guide-pin placement for instrumentation of the glenoid (see Fig. 44.3). Multiple preoperative planning software programs and patient-specific guides have been shown to improve the reproducibility of guide-pin placement for glenoid instrumentation.[2-4] More clinical data are needed to show an advantage in glenoid component survival or patient outcomes with or without a patient-specific guide. The future role of virtual surgery and patient-specific instrumentation will be to determine implant size and placement for each patient to optimize individual outcomes.

RECOGNITION OF THE DYNAMIC ROLE OF THE SCAPULA IN SHOULDER ARTHROPLASTY

A greater understanding and application of the dynamic role of the scapula in shoulder arthroplasty is needed to improve outcomes and maximize implant survivability. Altered scapular motion or "scapular dyskinesis" is considered an impairment of normal scapular motion and has long been recognized as a finding in patients with shoulder pain.[5] Although little has been reported on scapular dyskinesis and shoulder arthritis, we know that up to 67% to 100%[6-8] of patients with shoulder injuries exhibit scapular dyskinesis. We have noted scapular dyskinesis preoperatively nearly universally in our shoulder arthroplasty patients. Scapular dyskinesis is associated with scapular protraction and a decrease in posterior scapular tilt.[9] Scapular protraction along with posterior humeral subluxation may contribute to the exacerbation of posterior glenoid wear. More work is needed to formalize the incidence and implications of preoperative and postoperative scapular dyskinesis in patients undergoing shoulder arthroplasty.

Newer implants and surgical experience have appeared to improve outcomes and instability rates after reverse shoulder arthroplasty; however, the incidence of acromial and scapular body fractures has been more readily identified. We postulate that poor scapular motion may contribute to both acromial stress fractures as well as scapular spine fractures. Patients exhibit increased scapulothoracic motion and less glenohumeral joint motion after reverse shoulder arthroplasty, as noted by significantly lower scapulohumeral rhythm after reverse shoulder arthroplasty compared with normal shoulders.[10] Optimization of scapular function with targeted preoperative and postoperative scapular rehabilitation may improve implant longevity and patient function. Further studies will be needed to address scapular motion as a potential key to the better understanding and prevention of acromial and scapular spine fractures after reverse shoulder arthroplasty.

Furthermore, for the purposes of preoperative planning software and virtual surgery, the scapula is currently considered a static structure. The scapula is clearly a dynamic structure

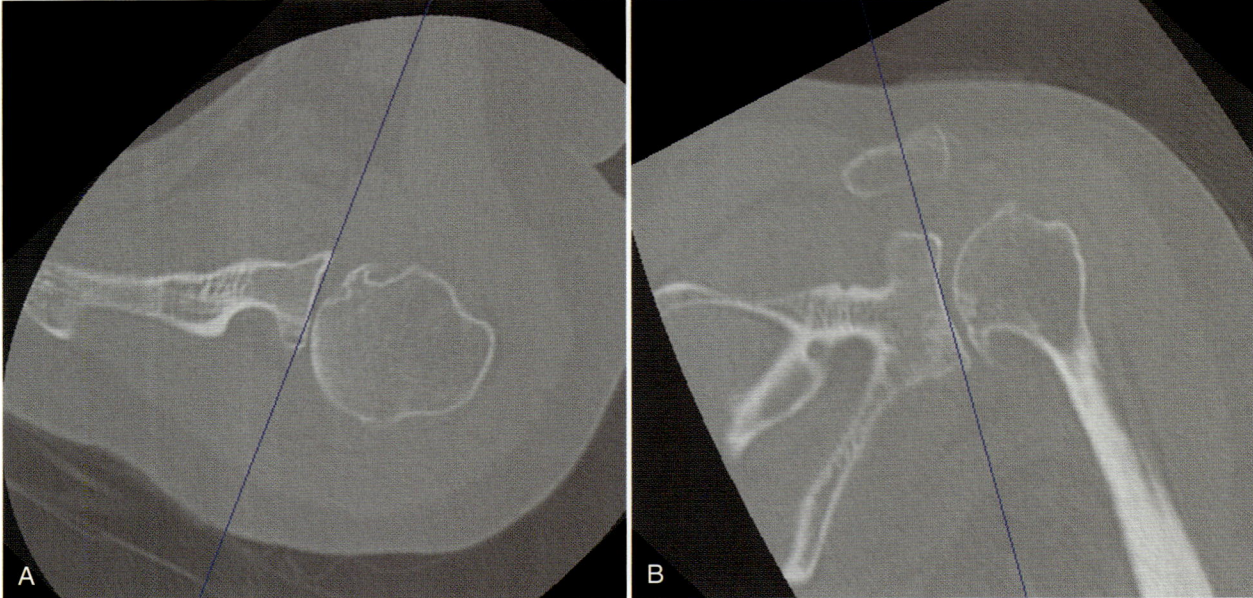

FIGURE 44.1 Preoperative planning software using computed tomography to determine retroversion (18 degrees; A) and superior inclination (12 degrees; B).

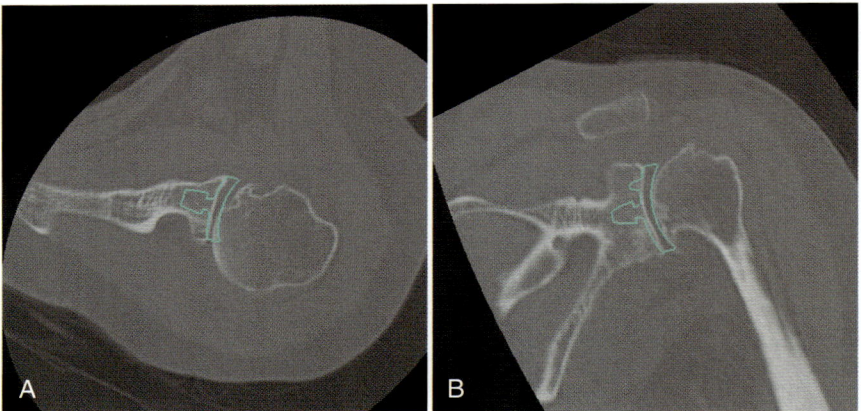

FIGURE 44.2 Preoperative planning software using computed tomography to determine axial (A) and coronal (B) virtual placement of the glenoid component. The *green-highlighted* glenoid component implies that there is no glenoid perforation, which would alternatively display as red with any glenoid perforation involving the peg(s) or keel.

and provides the foundation for rotator cuff function and shoulder motion. Scapular motion during shoulder elevation includes an average of 50 degrees upward rotation, 30 degrees posterior tilt, and 24 degrees external rotation.[11] Preoperative planning and virtual surgery with determination of native glenoid version is important; however, wide variations in scapular motion throughout the shoulder range of motion must also be considered. In the future, dynamic scapular modeling will allow preoperative planning with component placement based on dynamic scapular motion. Application of scapular principles for preoperative and postoperative rehabilitation and dynamic scapular modeling to improve component positioning will optimize outcomes.

ALTERNATIVE BEARING SURFACES

Long-term clinical outcomes after total shoulder arthroplasty have been superior to outcomes after hemiarthroplasty, likely secondary to glenoid erosion after hemiarthroplasty causing increased pain over time. However, there are some populations, especially comprising younger patients, regarding whom concerns exist for long-term implant survivability after total shoulder arthroplasty and the potential need for revision surgery. Furthermore, the glenoid component remains the weak link for long-term implant survival following total shoulder arthroplasty regardless of age. A hemiarthroplasty with a durable biocompatible material that generates minimal

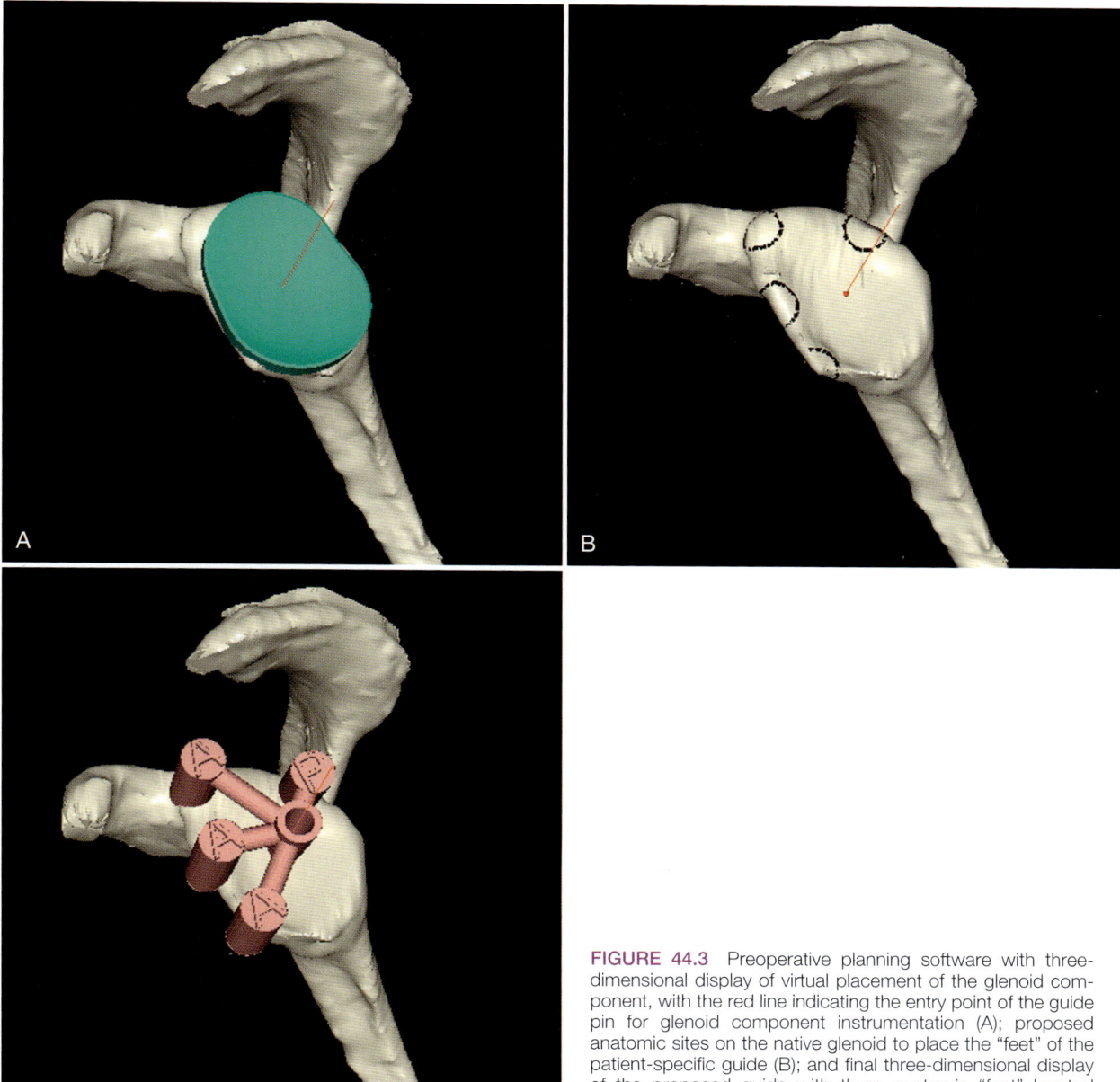

FIGURE 44.3 Preoperative planning software with three-dimensional display of virtual placement of the glenoid component, with the red line indicating the entry point of the guide pin for glenoid component instrumentation (A); proposed anatomic sites on the native glenoid to place the "feet" of the patient-specific guide (B); and final three-dimensional display of the proposed guide with three anatomic "feet" located anteriorly on the guide and a single foot posteriorly on the guide (C).

glenoid wear would be the ideal humeral head component. An alternative humeral head surface like this may decrease the need for the placement of a glenoid component.

One proposed alternative bearing surface has been pyrolytic carbon (pyrocarbon). Pyrocarbon has been identified as a durable biocompatible material that generates little wear and is felt to provide significant longevity.[12] Pyrocarbon has been used as an interposition shoulder arthroplasty implant.[12] The implant consisted of a graphite sphere with a pyrocarbon coating. Recent results were published with 2-year minimum follow-up in 67 patients with an average age of 49 years.[12] Seven patients (10.4%) had revision surgery. Overall, 6 patients out the 55 patients with complete data had glenoid erosion (10.9%) and 3 patients (5.5%) had thinning of the tuberosities. Complications were reported in nine patients. The authors acknowledged the uncertainties of pyrocarbon as an interposition arthroplasty and noted that "until long-term results are available, this type of innovative implant should remain to be tested in a few specialized shoulder centers."[12] It is important to note that these results were for interposition arthroplasty with pyrocarbon and not for a traditional hemiarthroplasty with pyrocarbon. It remains to be seen whether pyrocarbon in a traditional hemiarthroplasty will offer a promising humeral head bearing surface, and there are currently ongoing studies in the United States.

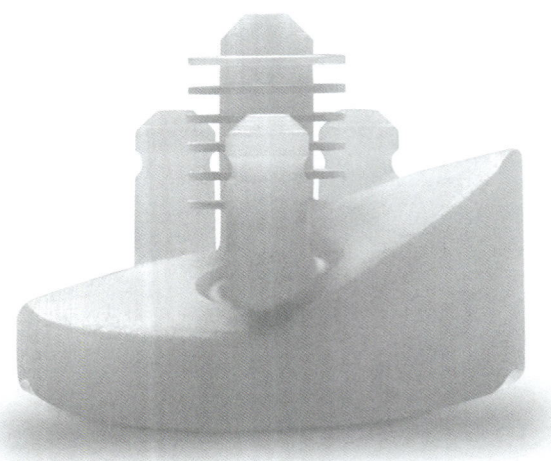

FIGURE 44.4 Posteriorly augmented all-polyethylene glenoid component. (Used with permission from Wright Medical N.V.)

TOTAL SHOULDER ARTHROPLASTY TECHNOLOGY ON THE HORIZON—GLENOID DESIGN AND CONVERTIBILITY

The glenoid has long been known as the limiting factor of anatomic shoulder arthroplasty. Metal-backed glenoid components have recently been resurrected with the goal of allowing bony ingrowth and for possible convertibility to a reverse shoulder arthroplasty. Some emerging glenoid components include a complete metal-backed component, while others have a metallic central post. Historically, metal-backed glenoid components have been fraught with significant polyethylene wear and osteolysis, causing glenoid loosening and a high revision rate (33% to 40%) at long-term follow-up.[13,14] It remains to be seen whether the newer metal-backed or hybrid glenoid components have offered good long-term solutions.

Additionally, posteriorly augmented all-polyethylene components are now available in multiple sizes and with various specifications (Fig. 44.4). Posteriorly augmented glenoid components have been proposed for glenoids with posterior wear (B2 or B2 glenoids) or potentially for glenoids with congenital retroversion without posterior wear (C glenoids). It is unclear whether posteriorly augmented glenoid components will offer a good long-term option. Short- and long-term data on posteriorly augmented all-polyethylene components are lacking at this time.

REVERSE SHOULDER ARTHROPLASTY TECHNOLOGY ON THE HORIZON

Much work is ongoing in reverse shoulder arthroplasty technology. Stemless reverse shoulder arthroplasty has been introduced to allow primary stemless reverse shoulder arthroplasty, or potentially conversion of a stemless anatomic total shoulder to a stemless reverse shoulder arthroplasty. Only very early data are available at this time regarding

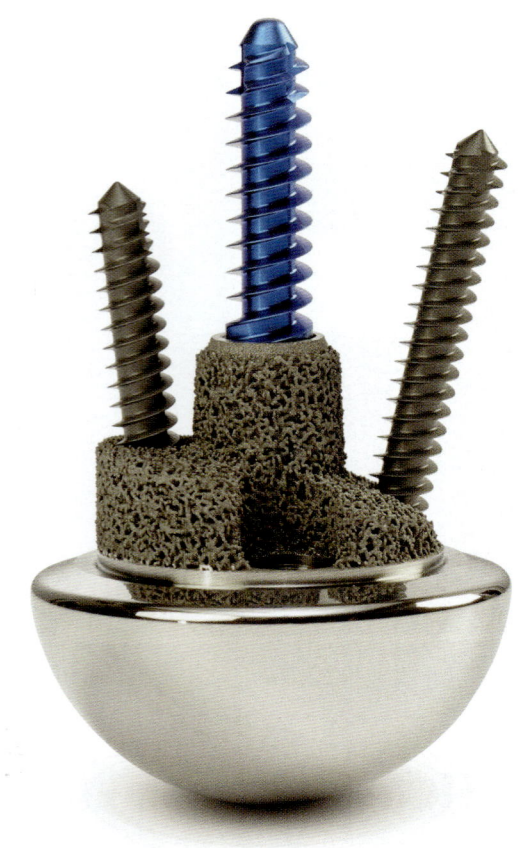

FIGURE 44.5 Reverse shoulder arthroplasty glenoid base plate with metal-augmented wedge. (Used with permission from Wright Medical N.V.)

primary stemless reverse shoulder arthroplasty; additional data and follow-up are needed.

An increase in shoulder arthroplasty cases being performed has led to a greater need for solutions in revision arthroplasty with bone loss. Autograft or allograft augmentation for bone loss has long been the only available option; however, newer technology offers metal augmentation for glenoid bone defects in reverse shoulder arthoplasty. Glenoid base-plate options with various metal augments now allow treatment of bone loss with metal augmentation rather that bone graft augmentation (Fig. 44.5). Preoperative planning software can now allow determination of the bone loss and appropriate sizing of the metal augment to treat the defect (Fig. 44.6).

Continuing studies are needed to determine the optimal humeral neck-shaft angle and location of the glenosphere. Some implants rely on relative lateralization compared with the original Grammont design. There may be an optimal humeral neck-shaft angle and glenosphere location for each patient for better function and longevity. Currently there are some proposed advantages of lateralized design versus a more traditional, Grammont-style implant; however, there is no definitive advantage of one design over the other. Preoperative modeling may be possible in the future to plan the ideal implant combination that will optimize results and longevity for each individual patient.

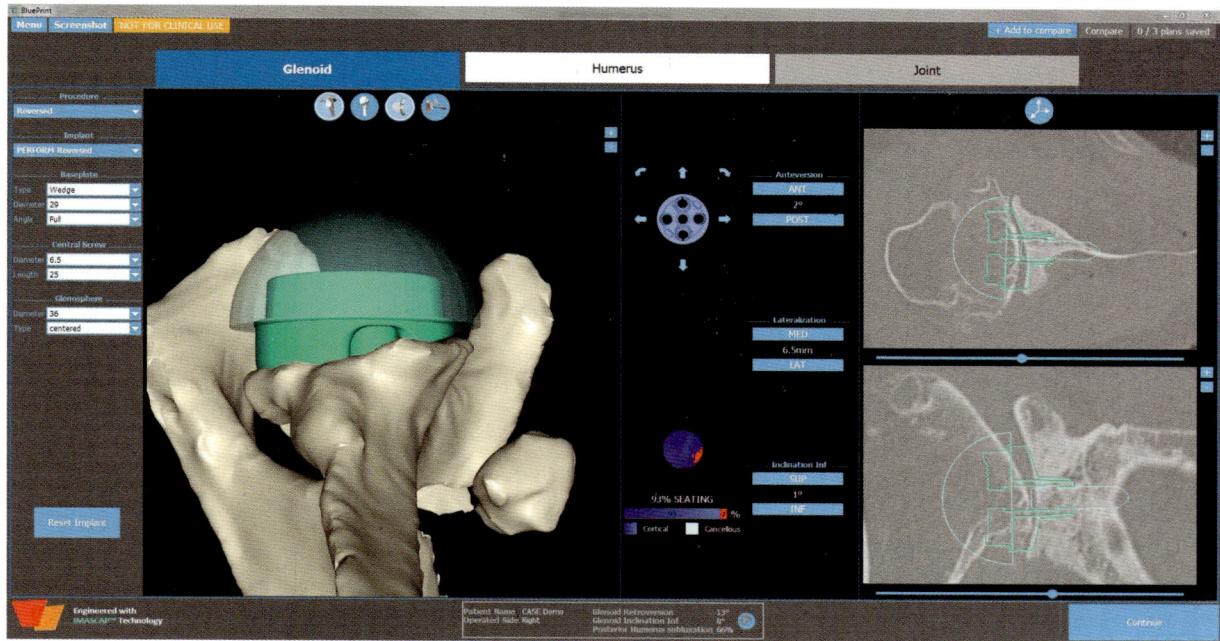

FIGURE 44.6 Preoperative surgical plan for a case with posterior glenoid bone loss and a base plate with a metal-augmented wedge. (Used with permission from Wright Medical N.V.)

REFERENCES

1. Lugli T: Artificial shoulder joint by Péan (1893). The facts of an exceptional intervention and the prosthetic method, *Clin Orthop* 133:215–218, 1978.
2. Hendel MD, Bryan JA, Barsoum WK, et al: Comparison of patient-specific instruments with standard surgical instruments in determining glenoid component position: a randomized prospective clinical trial, *J Bone Joint Surg Am* 94:2167–2175, 2012.
3. Throckmorton TW, Gulotta LV, Bonnarens FO, et al: Patient-specific targeting guides compared with traditional instrumentation for glenoid component placement in shoulder arthroplasty: a multi-surgeon study in 70 arthritic cadaver specimens, *J Shoulder Elbow Surg* 24(6):965–971, 2015, doi:10.1016/j.jse.2014.10.013. [Epub 2014 Dec 19].
4. Walch G, Vezeridis PS, Boileau P, et al: Three-dimensional planning and use of patient-specific guides improve glenoid component position: an in vitro study, *J Shoulder Elbow Surg* 24:302–309, 2015.
5. Kibler WB, McMullen J: Scapular dyskinesis and its relation to shoulder pain, *J Am Acad Orthop Surg* 11:142–151, 2003.
6. Warner JJP, Micheli LJ, Arslanian LE, et al: Scapulothoracic motion in normal shoulders and shoulders with glenohumeral instability and impingement syndrome, *Clin Orthop Relat Res* 285(191):199, 1992.
7. Gumina S, Carbone S, Postacchini F: Scapular dyskinesis and SICK scapula syndrome in patients with chronic type III acromioclavicular dislocation, *Arthroscopy* 25(1):40–45, 2009.
8. Paletta GA, Warner JJP, Warren RF, et al: Shoulder kinematics with two-plane x-ray evaluation in patients with anterior instability or rotator cuff tears, *J Shoulder Elbow Surg* 6:516–527, 1997.
9. Kibler WB, Sciascia A, Wilkes T: Scapular dyskinesis and its relation to shoulder injury, *J Am Acad Orthop Surg* 20(6):364–372, 2012.
10. Walker D, Matsuki K, Struk AM, et al: Scapulohumeral rhythm in shoulders with reverse shoulder arthroplasty, *J Shoulder Elbow Surg* 24:1129–1134, 2015.
11. McClure PW, Michener LA, Sennett BJ, et al: Direct 3-dimensional measurement of scapular kinematics during dynamic movements in vivo, *J Shoulder Elbow Surg* 10:269–277, 2001.
12. Garret J, Godeneche A, Boileau P, et al: Pyrocarbon interposition shoulder arthroplasty: preliminary results from a prospective multicenter study at 2 years of follow-up, *J Shoulder Elbow Surg* 2017; article in press. http://dx.doi.org/10.1016/j.jse.2017.01.002.
13. Boileau P, Moineau G, Morin-Salvo N, et al: Metal-backed glenoid implant with polyethylene insert is not a viable long-term therapeutic option, *J Shoulder Elbow Surg* 24:1534–1543, 2015.
14. Fox TJ, Cil A, Sperling JW, et al: Survival of the glenoid component in shoulder arthroplasty, *J Shoulder Elbow Surg* 18:859–863, 2009. http://dx.doi.org/10.1016/j.jse.2008.11.020.

Index

Page numbers followed by "f" indicate figures, and "t" indicate tables.

A

Abduction, 54f
Acromion
  anatomy of, 8, 15f
  stress fractures of
    after reverse shoulder arthroplasty, 229–231, 230f–231f
    after revision arthroplasty, 458–459, 458f
Activities of daily living, resumption of, 464
Adaptable glenoid implants, 4, 4f
Adduction exercises, horizontal, 462f
Adhesions
  release of, in subscapularis tenotomy, 73–82, 84f
  subdeltoid, release of, 351f
Allograft. *see also* Autograft; Bone graft
  cortical strips, in reverse-design humeral stem, 385–387, 387f
    passage of fixation cables, securing, 387, 387f
  plug, 308–312, 312f–313f
  proximal humeral, 308–312, 311f
Ancillary instrumentation, prosthetic positioning for, reverse shoulder arthroplasty for fracture, 244
Anesthesia, 29
Anterior capsule stretching, from siesta position, 463f
Anterior superior approach, to reverse arthroplasty, technique of, 170–174, 172f–174f
Antibiotic cement spacer, in staged revision arthroplasty, after infection, 378–379, 378f
Antibiotic-impregnated pellets, for infected arthroplasty, 379, 379f
Arthritis
  glenohumeral
    associated with neurologic pathology, 50
    associated with previous radiation therapy, 50, 50f
    associated with skeletal dysplasia, 50, 51f
    unconstrained arthroplasty for, 44–46

Arthritis (*Continued*)
  osteo-. *see* Osteoarthritis
  posttraumatic. *see* Posttraumatic arthritis
  rheumatoid. *see* Rheumatoid arthritis
Arthroscopic punch, for synovial biopsy, 49, 49f
Arthrotomy, glenohumeral, in subscapularis tenotomy, 73, 75f–76f
Articular cartilage lesion, 308
  exposure of, 308, 309f
  guide pin in, placement of, 308, 310f
  measurement of, 308, 309f
  scoring of, 308, 310f
Aseptic loosening
  of glenoid component, 138–140, 140f
  humeral stem, 138–140, 140f, 228, 228f, 289, 454, 454f
Aspiration, shoulder, fluoroscopically guided, 344
Authors' Prospective Database (2003–2014) results
  of reverse shoulder arthroplasty, 225t
  of revision arthroplasty, 451t
  of unconstrained arthroplasty, 136t
Autograft. *see also* Allograft; Bone graft
  fascia lata of, in biologic glenoid resurfacing, 312
  harvesting of, 313, 314f–316f
  implantation of, 313–321, 317f–321f
Awl, use of
  in reverse arthroplasty, 178–184, 181f
  in uncemented unconstrained arthroplasty, 89–94, 93f
Axillary nerve
  identification of
    in revision arthroplasty, 350–354
    in unconstrained arthroplasty, 72f
  injury to
    in revision arthroplasty, 452
    in unconstrained arthroplasty, 137–138
  surgical anatomy of, 8, 12f

B

Base plate
  in glenoid component
    inferior, screw insertion of, 194, 197f

Base plate (*Continued*)
    screw introduction and fixation in, 189–194, 194f–195f, 198f
    screw length in, determination of, 189–194, 196f–197f
    screw tightening in, 189–199, 194f, 199f
  in reverse shoulder arthroplasty cases requiring a glenoid bone graft, 428, 432f
    fixation of, 428–437
    introduction of, 428, 432f
    seating of, 428
Belly press test, for subscapularis insufficiency, 54, 57f
Biceps brachii
  dissection of, in extending deltopectoral approach into anterolateral approach to humeral diaphysis, 355, 356f
  surgical anatomy of, 8
Biceps tendon
  long head of, 35–38
    abnormalities of, 35, 36t
    technique for handling, 35, 36f–38f
  tenodesis of, 301, 305f
  tenotomy of, 301, 305f
Bioabsorbable fixation pins, for osseous glenoid defects, 420–428, 427f–428f
Biologic glenoid resurfacing, 312. *see also* Glenoid resurfacing, biologic
Biologic humeral resurfacing, 308. *see also* Humeral resurfacing, biologic
Biopsy, synovial, for postinfectious arthropathy, 49, 49f
Body fracture, scapular, after revision arthroplasty, 459
Bone graft. *see also* Allograft; Autograft
  glenoid revision with, 413–439
    iliac crest graft harvest in, 439–444, 441f–447f
    reverse shoulder arthroplasty cases requiring, 428–439, 431f–441f
    unconstrained shoulder arthroplasty requiring, 417–428, 417f–420f
    contained osseous deficit in, 420, 421f–422f

Bone graft (*Continued*)
   uncontained combined (anterior and posterior) osseous deficit in, 420–428, 427f–431f
   uncontained (anterior or posterior) osseous deficit in, 420, 422f–427f
   glenoid revision without, 413, 414f–417f
   preparation of
      for reverse shoulder arthroplasty, 264
      for unconstrained humeral head replacement for fracture, 260–261, 261f–262f
      reconstruction prior to, reverse-design humeral stem, in revision arthroplasty, 385–387, 386f
      for tuberosity fixation, 268, 271f
      placement of, 268
Bone loss
   glenoid
      with primary reverse prosthesis, 199–207, 203f–207f
      metaphyseal, in reverse arthroplasty, special considerations in, 209–218, 215f–218f
      new humeral implants for, 218, 219f
Bony glenoid deficiency, classification of, 339–344, 345f
Bony increased offset reverse shoulder arthroplasty (BIO-RSA), 199
Brachialis, splitting of, in extending deltopectoral approach into anterolateral approach to humeral diaphysis, 355, 357f
Bracing, of reverse prosthesis, after revision surgery, 455–456, 455f
Braided permanent sutures
   in implantation of fascia lata autograft, 316, 317f–320f
   for reattachment of subscapularis, 185–186, 186f
Breaststroke exercise, in rehabilitation, 463f
Bulb syringe, 26f

C

Calcium sulfate pellets, for infected arthroplasty, 379, 379f
Canal-sparing humeral components, 293
Cancellous bone, removal of, in iliac crest graft harvest, 444, 446f
Cannulated core drill, 299f

Capsular release, posterior, in soft tissue balancing, 118, 122f
Capsulorrhaphy, posterior, in soft tissue balancing, 118, 119f–121f
Catheter tip syringe, 26f
   for application of cement into canal, 186, 188f
Cement
   application of, into humeral canal, 103, 104f
   extravasation after unrecognized diaphyseal perforation, 287f, 289
Cement removal, in humeral stem removal, 373
   with Moreland osteotomes, 373, 375f–376f
   with pituitary-type forceps, 373, 375f
Cement removal osteotomes, 375f
Cement restrictor
   in cemented unconstrained arthroplasty, 103, 104f
   placement of, in reverse arthroplasty, 186, 187f
Cementation, of glenoid component, in unconstrained arthroplasty, 111–113, 116f–117f
Cephalic vein
   in deltopectoral interval, 8, 10f
   identification of, 66, 68f
      in revision arthroplasty, 346, 349f
   intraoperative tearing of
      in reverse arthroplasty, 227
      in revision arthroplasty, 453
Cerclage cables, placement of, in humeral osteotomy, 367
Chondrolysis, glenohumeral, in biologic glenoid resurfacing, 312, 313f
Clamps, 19t, 22f
Clavicle, anatomy of, 8, 11f
Clinical history
   preoperative
      in reverse arthroplasty, 160–161
      in shoulder arthroplasty, for fracture, 242
      in unconstrained arthroplasty, 53–54
   for revision shoulder arthroplasty, 337, 338f
Cobb elevator, in humeral stem removal, 360, 364f, 367, 368f
Computed tomography
   of osteoarthritis, 40f
   of posttraumatic arthritis, 46f
   preoperative
      in reverse arthroplasty, 165, 168f
      in revision shoulder arthroplasty, 339–344, 343f

Computed tomography (*Continued*)
   of rheumatoid arthritis, 41f
      with massive rotator cuff tear, 151, 154f
   of rotator cuff tear arthropathy, 149–151, 150f–152f
   in shoulder arthroplasty, for proximal humeral fractures, 242, 244f
Conjoined tendon
   identification of
      in revision arthroplasty, 346–350
      in unconstrained arthroplasty, 66
   release of, in revision arthroplasty, 350, 354f
   surgical anatomy of, 8, 11f
Convertible humeral stems, for revision arthroplasty, 410–411, 410f–412f
Convertible shoulder arthroplasty, 6–7, 7f
Copeland, Stephen, 293
Coracoacromial ligament, identification of, in deltopectoral approach, 66, 70f
Coracoid process
   identification of, in revision arthroplasty, 346–350, 352f
   surgical anatomy of, 8, 11f
Cortical allograft struts, in humeral osteotomy, 373, 374f
Crescent sign, in osteonecrosis of humeral head, 42

D

Dehiscence, wound, postoperative, 138, 138f, 227, 288, 453
Deltoid
   atrophy of, 337, 338f
   surgical anatomy of, 8, 11f
Deltoid tension
   with reverse prosthesis, 209–218
      in humeral component trialing, 209, 210f–214f
      metaphyseal bone loss, special considerations in, 209–218, 215f–218f
      polyethylene insert placement and, 209, 213f–214f
   restoration of, 147, 148f
   revision shoulder arthroplasty for, 329, 330f
Deltopectoral approach
   to reverse arthroplasty, technique of, 169–170, 171f
   to revision arthroplasty, 346–354
      axillary nerve identification in, 350–354
      conjoined tendon in
         identification of, 346–350
         release of, 350, 354f

Deltopectoral approach (Continued)
  coracoid process identification in, 346–350, 352f
  deltopectoral interval in, 346–350, 350f
  draping in, 346, 347f
  extension of, into anterolateral approach to humeral diaphysis, 354–355
    biceps brachii dissection in, 355, 356f
    brachialis splitting in, 355, 357f
    complete humeral shaft exposure in, 355, 357f
    deltoid humeral insertion in, 355, 358f
    radial nerve visualization in, 355, 359f
    skin incision in, 355, 355f–356f
  hypertrophic scar excision in, 346, 348f
  pectoralis major release, 346–350, 353f
  permanent sutures in, 354, 355f
  previous skin incisions for, 346, 347f
  subscapularis tenotomy in, 354, 355f
  to shoulder arthroplasty, 249
  skin incision for, 8, 9f
  to unconstrained arthroplasty
    anterior humeral circumflex vessel ligation in, 71f
    axillary nerve identification in, 66, 72f
    conjoined tendon retraction in, 66, 71f
    pectoralis major release in, 69f
    skin incision for, 67f
    steps in, 72t
Deltopectoral interval
  cephalic vein in, 8, 10f
  identification of, 66, 68f
  in revision arthroplasty, 346–350, 350f
Dislocation. see also Fracture-dislocation
  of glenohumeral joint
    reverse arthroplasty for, 156–157, 157f–158f
    unconstrained shoulder arthroplasty for, 46, 47f
  of proximal humerus, in humeral stem removal, 360, 363f
  of reverse prosthesis, revision shoulder arthroplasty for, 329, 330f

Drains, surgical
  after iliac crest graft harvesting, 444, 447f
  placement of, 283, 284f
  proximal extent of, 284f
  removal of, 283, 284f
Draping, surgical, 29–34, 31f–34f
  for autogenous fascia lata harvest, 313, 314f
  for iliac crest graft harvesting, 439–441, 442f
  in revision arthroplasty, 346, 347f
Dressings, sterile, after arthroplasty, 130, 133f, 283

E
Elderly, osteopenia in, proximal humeral fracture and, 238–239, 240f–241f
Electrocautery, 130
Electromyography, in revision shoulder arthroplasty, 344
Erosion, glenoid, after hemiarthroplasty, revision shoulder arthroplasty for, 323, 324f–325f
Extension exercises, in hydrotherapy, 462f
External rotation
  of arm, 55f
  lag sign, for infraspinatus integrity, 54, 56f
  passive, after subscapularis repair, 123, 128f
Extraction device, attachment of, in humeral stem removal, 360, 366f

F
Fascia lata autograft, in biologic glenoid resurfacing, 312
  harvesting of, 313, 314f–316f
  implantation of, 313–321, 317f–321f
Fibrous tissue, removal, of, in humeral stem removal, 360, 363f–365f
Figure-of-eight technique, of wound closure, 130, 131f
Fin blazer, in stemless unconstrained total shoulder arthroplasty, 297, 301f
First-generation shoulder arthroplasty, 1
Flexion exercises, in hydrotherapy, 462f
Fluoroscopically guided shoulder aspiration, 344
Forceps, 19t, 20f
Four-part proximal humeral fractures, 237, 238f–239f. see also Humeral fractures

Fracture(s)
  glenoid, 286
  intraoperative
    in reverse shoulder arthroplasty, 224–226, 226f–227f
    in unconstrained arthroplasty, 134, 137f
  humeral. see Humeral fractures
  periprosthetic, revision shoulder arthroplasty for, 334–336, 335f–336f
  stress, acromial
    after reverse shoulder arthroplasty, 229–231, 230f
    after revision arthroplasty, 458–459, 458f
  unconstrained arthroplasty. see Unconstrained arthroplasty, for fractures
Fracture-dislocation. see also Dislocation
  of humeral head, 238, 240f

G
Glenohumeral joint. see also Shoulder
  arthritis of
    associated with neurologic pathology, 50
    associated with previous radiation therapy, 50, 50f
    associated with skeletal dysplasia, 50, 51f
  arthrotomy of, 73, 75f–76f
  chondrolysis of, in biologic glenoid resurfacing, 312, 313f
  fixed dislocation of, 46, 47f
  instability, revision shoulder arthroplasty for, 332, 333f–334f
  osteoarthritis of
    with massive rotator cuff tear
      imaging findings in, 149–151, 149f–151f
      reverse arthroplasty for, 147–151
    primary, 40, 40f–41f
  other inflammatory arthropathies affecting, 42
  posttraumatic arthritis of, 44–46, 45f
  radiography of, 54–60
  rheumatoid arthritis of, 41–42, 41f
  stiffness of
    after reverse shoulder arthroplasty, 236
    after revision arthroplasty, 456–458, 457f
    after unconstrained arthroplasty, 144, 144f, 289
  tumor of, 50–51

Glenohumeral ligaments
　release of, in subscapularis tenotomy, 73–82, 81f–83f
　surgical anatomy of, 13, 14f
Glenohumeral prosthetic mismatch
　definition of, 3–4, 111
　values and recommendations, for Aequalis ascend flex/perform shoulder arthroplasty system, 112t
Glenoid
　anatomy of, 13, 15f
　biconcavity of, in osteoarthritis, 40
　bony deficiency, classification of, 339–344, 345f. see also Glenoid erosion
　exposure
　　during arthroplasty, 175
　　　technique for, 175, 176f–177f
　　in reverse arthroplasty, 169
　　in revision arthroplasty, 373–374, 376f–377f
　　in unconstrained arthroplasty, 86
　　　anterior release for, 86, 87f
　　　inferior release for, 86, 87f
　　　posterior release for, 86, 88f
　intraoperative complications involving, after revision arthroplasty, 450–452, 452f
　issues on, shoulder arthroplasty and, 239
　morphology, 60–61, 62f
　postoperative complications involving
　　after reverse shoulder arthroplasty, 227, 227f–228f
　　after revision arthroplasty, 453, 453f
　　after unconstrained arthroplasty, 138, 139f, 288–289
　preparation of, for implantation of keeled component, 113, 114f–115f
　reaming of, 107f–109f, 110–111, 111f–112f
　to produce inferior tilt, 189, 191f
　resurfacing of. see Glenoid resurfacing
　wear of. see Glenoid wear
Glenoid base plate, with metal-augmented wedge, 468, 468f
Glenoid bone loss, with primary reverse prosthesis, 199–207, 203f–207f
Glenoid component
　failure of
　　resection arthroplasty for, 417, 419f
　　revision shoulder arthroplasty for, 323–326, 326f–327f

Glenoid component (Continued)
　in unconstrained arthroplasty, 106–117
　　early, 134, 137f
　　final implantation in, 113, 116f–117f
　　preparation of glenoid bone in, 113, 114f–115f
　　reaming of glenoid surface in, 109f–110f, 110–111, 112f
　　selection of component size in, 111, 112t
　　type of, 111–113, 113f
　posteriorly augmented all-polyethylene, 468, 468f
　postoperative complications of, 227, 227f–228f
　reverse, revision shoulder arthroplasty for, 326–328, 328f–329f
　reverse prosthesis, primary, bone loss with, 199–207, 203f–207f
　in reverse shoulder arthroplasty, 189–208
　　glenoid base-plate selection-post, or threaded post, 199, 201f–202f
　　preparation and implantation of, 189–199, 190f, 192f–193f, 197f–198f
　revision of
　　with bone graft, 413–439
　　　harvest of autogenous iliac crest bone graft in, 439–444, 441f–447f
　　　reverse cases requiring, 428–439, 431f–441f
　　　unconstrained cases requiring, 413–439, 417f–420f
　　　contained osseous deficit in, 420, 421f–422f
　　　uncontained combined (anterior and posterior) osseous deficit in, 420–428, 427f–431f
　　　uncontained (anterior or posterior) osseous deficit in, 420, 422f–427f
　　without bone graft, 413, 414f–417f
　　stemless unconstrained total shoulder arthroplasty of, 297–301
　in unconstrained cases, revision of
　　with bone graft, 413–439, 417f–420f
　　　contained osseous deficit in, 420, 421f–422f
　　　uncontained combined (anterior and posterior) osseous deficit in, 420–428, 427f–431f

Glenoid component (Continued)
　　　uncontained (anterior or posterior) osseous deficit in, 420, 422f–427f
　　without bone graft, 413, 416f–417f
Glenoid erosion
　after hemiarthroplasty
　　biologic glenoid resurfacing in, 312–313, 314f
　　revision arthroplasty for, 323, 324f–325f
　　reverse shoulder arthroplasty for, 428, 431f
　　without bone graft, 413
　　unconstrained, 288
　after reverse arthroplasty, 199–203, 203f
　after unconstrained hemiarthroplasty, 239
Glenoid fracture, 286
　intraoperative
　　in reverse shoulder arthroplasty, 224–226, 226f–227f
　　in unconstrained arthroplasty, 134, 137f
Glenoid implant, 63f
Glenoid peg hole, enlargement of, in reverse arthroplasty, 189, 192f
Glenoid resurfacing
　advances in, 2–4
　biologic, 312
　　contraindications to, 312–313, 313f–314f
　　indications for, 312–313, 313f–314f
　　technique for, 313–321
　　　autogenous fascia lata harvest in, 313, 314f–316f
　　　fascia lata autograft, implantation of, 313–321, 317f–321f
　indications for, 39
　in unconstrained arthroplasty, 106, 109f–111f
Glenoid wear
　asymmetric, 110–111, 111f–112f
　osseous, 54–59, 59f
　superior, classification of, 151, 152f
Glenosphere, placement and fixation of, in reverse arthroplasty, 199, 200f–201f
Goutallier classification, of fatty infiltration of infraspinatus, 63f
Graft. see Allograft; Autograft; Bone graft
Grammont prosthesis, 6, 6f. see also Reverse-design prosthesis

Grammont-designed reverse prosthesis, 147, 148f
Greater tuberosity. *see also* Tuberosity(ies)
   Lahey forceps, 268, 274f
   migration of, after unconstrained arthroplasty for fracture, 287f–288f
   suture fixation technique for, 269f
   sutures controlling, 268, 275f, 279f–280f
   two looped sutures passing around the inferior aspect of, 268, 272f
Guide pin placement, in biologic humeral resurfacing, 308, 310f

H

Half-inch Steri-Strips, 130, 132f
Harvesting
   of autogenous fascia lata, 313, 314f–316f
   of autologous iliac crest bone graft, 439–444
     drains in, 444, 447f
     draping in, 439–441, 442f
     exposure and cutting of crest in, 441–444, 444f
     incisions in, 441–444, 442f–443f
     skin preparation in, 441, 441f–442f
   of osteochondral allograft plug, 308–312, 312f
Head-splitting humeral fracture, 238, 240f
Hematoma, postoperative, 138, 288, 453
Hemiarthroplasty
   glenoid erosion after
     biologic glenoid resurfacing in, 312–313, 314f
     reverse shoulder arthroplasty for, 428, 431f
     revision arthroplasty for, without bone graft, 413, 414f–417f
     revision shoulder arthroplasty for, 323, 324f–325f
   unconstrained, 239
   total shoulder arthroplasty *versus*, 39
History, for revision shoulder arthroplasty, 337, 338f
Hohmann retractor, 294
Horn blower's sign, in evaluation of teres minor, 54, 56f
Humeral allograft. *see also* Allograft
   proximal, 308–312, 311f
Humeral-based inferior capsular release, in humeral stem removal, 360, 362f

Humeral canal
   cement application into
     in reverse arthroplasty, 186, 188f
     in unconstrained arthroplasty, 103, 104f
   loose cement within, 373, 375f
   opening of
     in reverse arthroplasty, 178–184, 181f
     in uncemented unconstrained arthroplasty, 89–94, 93f
Humeral circumflex vessels
   anterior, ligation of, in deltopectoral approach, 66, 71f
   surgical anatomy of, 8, 12f
Humeral compactors, in uncemented unconstrained arthroplasty, 89–94, 96f
Humeral component, 178–186
   canal-sparing, 293
   in design for fracture cases, 4, 5f
   implantation of
     for reverse shoulder arthroplasty, 264, 266f–267f
     for unconstrained humeral head replacement for fracture, 261–263, 262f–264f
   postoperative complications of, 228, 229f–230f
   reverse-prosthesis
     insertion of, technique for, 178–186
       cement restrictor placement in, 186, 187f
       final implant assembly in, 185–186, 186f
       humeral preparation/exposure in, 178, 179f
       osteophyte removal in, 178, 180f
       resection with humeral cutting guide resection in, 178–184, 180f–185f
       suturing of subscapularis in, 185–186, 186f
       trial in, 178–184, 184f–185f
       use of starter awl in, 178–184, 181f
   trialing of, 209, 210f–214f
     metaphyseal bone loss, special considerations in, 209–218, 215f–218f
     new humeral implants for, 218, 219f
     polyethylene insert placement and, 209, 213f–214f
   in revision arthroplasty, 380–412
     allograft reconstruction, of proximal humerus, 387–390, 388f–397f
     insertion of stem in, technique for, 390–406, 397f–406f

Humeral component (*Continued*)
     preparation of, proximal humerus in, 380–387
     reverse-design, 329, 330f–331f
       humeral stem, 380–387, 385f–387f, 390–398
       special situations in, 406–411, 407f–412f
     unconstrained, 328, 329f
       humeral stem, 380, 381f–385f, 390
   short-stem, for metaphyseal press-fit fixation, 3f
   in unconstrained arthroplasty, 89–105
     cemented, 89, 90f
       indication of, 89, 91f
       technique for insertion of, 103, 104f–105f
     correct height and version of, ancillary instrumentation for, 4, 5f
     technique for insertion of, 89–103
     uncemented, 89, 90f
       technique for insertion of, 89–103
       humeral canal location and opening in, 89–94, 93f
       humeral cut protector placement in, 99–103, 100f
       humeral diaphysis reaming in, 89–94, 93f–94f
       humeral head resection in, 93f, 94–99, 99f
       humeral preparation/exposure in, 89, 90f–91f
       infraspinatus insertion identification in, 89, 92f
       neck inclination angle selection in, 89–94, 96f
       osteophyte removal in, 89, 91f–92f
       progressive metaphyseal broaching in, 89–94, 95f
       prosthetic assembly and placement in, 99–103, 101f, 103f
       suture placement for reattachment of subscapularis in, 99–103, 102f
       trial stem assembly and placement in, 94–99, 97f–99f
Humeral cut protector, 302f
   placement of, in reverse arthroplasty, 184–185, 185f
   in uncemented unconstrained arthroplasty, 94–99, 100f
Humeral cutting guide, resection with, 178–184, 180f–185f

Humeral diaphysis
　deltopectoral approach, extending into anterolateral approach, 354–355
　　biceps brachii dissection in, 355, 356f
　　brachialis splitting in, 355, 357f
　　complete humeral shaft exposure in, 355, 357f
　　deltoid humeral insertion in, 355, 358f
　　radial nerve visualization in, 355, 359f
　　skin incision in, 355, 355f–356f
　fractures of, intraoperative, 224, 226f
　identification and preparation of
　　for reverse shoulder arthroplasty for fracture, 263, 265f
　　for unconstrained humeral head replacement for fracture, 254, 256f–257f
　postoperative complications involving, 289
　reaming of
　　in revision arthroplasty, 380, 382f, 398–406, 401f
　　in uncemented unconstrained arthroplasty, 89–94, 94f
Humeral epiphysis, reaming of, in revision arthroplasty, 387–390, 389f
Humeral fractures
　intraoperative, in unconstrained arthroplasty, 134, 137f
　migration of, with massive rotator cuff tear, 155, 156f
　periprosthetic, 374, 378f
　　after revision arthroplasty, 454–455
　　with reverse prosthesis, 228, 229f–230f
　　treatment of, by revision arthroplasty, 380–385, 406, 409f
　　with unconstrained prosthesis, 140, 140f
　proximal, 286
　　dislocation with, 238, 240f
　　four-part, 237, 238f–239f
　　head-splitting, 238, 240f
　　malunion of, 154–155, 155f
　　nonunion of, 154, 154f
　　results of, 287t
　　shoulder arthroplasty for
　　　identification and handling of the tuberosity in, 249, 250f–253f
　　　preoperative planning and imaging of, 242–248

Humeral fractures (*Continued*)
　　　prosthetic positioning for, with ancillary instrumentation, 244
　　　surgical approach to, 249, 250f
　　three-part, 237–238, 239f–240f
　　tuberosity reduction and fixation in, 268
　　unconstrained arthroplasty for, 240–241
　　　complications of, 286
　　　postoperative orthosis in, 283
　shaft, results of, 286, 287f
　shoulder arthroplasty for, indications for, 237–241
Humeral head
　articular cartilage lesions, size of, 308, 309f
　completed exposure of, 308
　dislocation of, maneuver for, 89, 91f
　fracture-dislocation of, 238, 240f
　impactor, 301
　osteonecrosis of, unconstrained arthroplasty for, 42–43, 42f
　prosthesis, 306f
　reaming of, with triflange reamer, 308, 311f
　resection of
　　in reverse arthroplasty, 178–184, 180f–185f
　　in uncemented unconstrained arthroplasty, 93f, 94–99
　retractor, 294
　subluxation of, 54–59, 59f–60f
　trial, placement of, in uncemented unconstrained arthroplasty, 94–99, 97f, 99f
　unconstrained replacement for, fracture of, 254–263
　　humeral component for, implantation of, 261–263, 262f–264f
　　humeral diaphysis for, identification and preparation of, 254, 256f–257f
　　humeral implant for, selection of, 254, 258f
　　preparation of bone graft for, 260–261, 261f–262f
　　prosthetic positioning for (Gothic arch technique), 254–260, 258f–260f
Humeral implant, 301, 304f
Humeral insertion, deltoid, in extending deltopectoral approach into anterolateral approach to humeral diaphysis, 355, 358f

Humeral metaphysis
　bone loss of, in reverse arthroplasty, special considerations in, 209–218, 215f–218f
　new humeral implants for, 218, 219f
　progressive broaching of, in uncemented unconstrained arthroplasty, 89–94, 95f
　reaming of, in revision arthroplasty, 398–406, 402f
Humeral neck, selection of inclination angle of, in uncemented unconstrained arthroplasty, 89–94, 96f
Humeral osteophytes, peripheral, 295f
Humeral prosthetic positioning, 254–267, 255f
Humeral resurfacing, biologic, 308
　allograft plug in, 308–312, 312f–313f
　in articular cartilage lesion, 308
　exposure of, 308, 309f
　guide pin in, placement of, 308, 310f
　measurement of, 308, 309f
　scoring of, 308, 310f
　humeral head, reaming of, 308, 311f
　preparation for, 308, 311f
　proximal humeral allograft in, 308–312, 311f
　technique for, 308–312, 309f–313f
Humeral retroversion, 4, 5f
Humeral shaft
　completed exposure of, in extending deltopectoral approach to diaphysis, 355, 357f
　greater and lesser tuberosities to, 268, 271f
　intraoperative fracture of, 286
Humeral stem
　malposition of, glenohumeral stiffness due to, 456, 457f
　removal of, in revision arthroplasty, 360–373
　　cable placement in, 367, 370f
　　cement removal in, 373, 375f–376f
　　Cobb elevator in, 360, 364f, 367, 368f
　　dislocation maneuver in, 360, 363f
　　extraction device attachment in, 360, 366f
　　fibrous tissue removal in, 360, 363f–365f
　　humeral-based inferior capsular release in, 360, 362f
　　humeral osteotomy in, 360, 367–373, 367f, 369f–374f
　　implant exposure in, 360, 361f

Humeral stem (Continued)
  modular humeral implant, with Morse taper in, 360, 364f
  proximal humerus retraction in, 360, 362f
  rotator cuff inspection before, 360, 366f
  specialized instruments for, 361f
  in revision arthroplasty
    convertible, 410–411, 410f–412f
    postoperative complications of, 454, 454f
    reverse-design, 380–387, 385f–387f, 390–398
      allograft cortical strips in, 385–387, 387f
        passage of, fixation cables, securing, 387, 387f
      bone graft reconstruction prior to, 385–387, 386f
      diaphyseal reaming for, 387–390, 389f
      epiphyseal reaming for, 387–390, 389f
      markings for, 380–385, 385f
      metaphyseal portion of implant for, 398–406, 402f
      trial component removal in, 390–398, 399f–400f
      technique for insertion of, 390–406, 397f–406f
      transosseous sutures in, 390, 397f
    unconstrained, 380, 381f–383f, 390
      anterior-to-posterior offset of, 380, 383f
      in diaphyseal osteotomy, 380, 381f
      judgment of humeral version in, 380, 384f–385f
    in treatment of periprosthetic fracture, 380–385, 406, 409f
  trial
    in revision arthroplasty, impaction in, 390, 398f, 400f
    in uncemented unconstrained arthroplasty, assembly and placement of, 94–99, 97f–99f
Humerus
  intraoperative complications involving
    after revision arthroplasty, 450, 452f
    in reverse shoulder arthroplasty, 224, 226f
    in unconstrained arthroplasty, 134, 137f

Humerus (Continued)
  postoperative complications involving
    after revision arthroplasty, 453–455, 454f
    in reverse shoulder arthroplasty, 228, 228f–229f
    in unconstrained arthroplasty, 138–140, 140f
  proximal
    anatomy of, 13, 15f
      variability in, 2t
    preparation/exposure of
      in reverse arthroplasty, 178, 179f
      in uncemented unconstrained arthroplasty, 89, 90f–91f, 97f
    preparation of, in revision arthroplasty, 380–387
    revealing peripheral osteophytes, 295f
Hydrotherapy
  fear of water and, 464
  initiation of, time for, 462t
  land-based rehabilitation after, 462
  postoperative, 461–464, 462f–464f
  principles of, 461
Hypertrophic scar, excision of, in revision arthroplasty, 346, 348f

I
Iliac crest bone graft. see also Bone graft
  harvesting of, 439–444
    draping in, 439–441, 442f
    exposure and cutting of crest in, 441–444, 444f
    incisions in, 441–444, 442f–443f
    skin preparation in, 441, 441f–442f
Immersion exercises, total body, 463f
Implant(s). see Prosthesis; specific components
Incision
  for autogenous fascia lata harvest, 313, 315f
  in deltopectoral approach to arthroplasty, 67f
  in iliac crest graft harvest, 441–444, 442f–443f
  previous
    in primary shoulder arthroplasty, 337, 338f
    in revision arthroplasty, 346, 347f
Inclination angle, measurement of, for cemented humeral stem, 98f, 99–103, 100f

Infection
  after humeral stem removal, 374–379, 378f–379f
  after reverse shoulder arthroplasty, 236
  after revision arthroplasty, 332–334, 334f, 458
  after unconstrained arthroplasty, 145, 289–291
  history of, 53
  workup for, 54t
Infraspinatus
  atrophy of, 337, 338f
  identification of insertion of, in uncemented unconstrained arthroplasty, 89, 92f
  integrity of, external rotation lag sign for, 54, 56f
Instability
  after reverse shoulder arthroplasty, 231–236, 233f–235f
  after revision arthroplasty
    with reverse prosthesis, 455–456, 455f–457f
    unconstrained, 455
  after unconstrained arthroplasty, 140–144, 141f–144f, 289, 290f–291f
  arthropathy, of shoulder, unconstrained arthroplasty for, 43–44, 45f
  glenohumeral, revision shoulder arthroplasty for, 332, 333f–334f
Instruments
  disposable, 25t
  miscellaneous, 22f–25f, 25t
  specific set of, 26t, 27f–28f
  surgical, 16, 18f, 19t, 20f
Internal rotation, of arm, 55f

J
Jobe's test, for supraspinatus integrity, 54, 55f
Joint capsule
  release of, in subscapularis tenotomy, 73, 79f
  surgical anatomy of, 13, 14f
Juvenile-onset rheumatoid arthritis, 42

L
Lag sign, external rotation, for infraspinatus integrity, 54, 56f
Lesser tuberosity. see also Tuberosity(ies)
  identification and handling of, in shoulder arthroplasty, 249, 253f
  intraoperative fractures of, 224
  suture fixation technique for, 269f

Lift-off test, for subscapularis insufficiency, 54, 57f
Ligation of the anterior humeral circumflex vessels, 71f
Lighting, overhead, in operating room, 16, 18f
Looped suture, second, reduction and fixation of tuberosity, 268, 282f
Loose bodies, in subscapularis recess, 40, 40f, 54–59, 59f, 73–82, 84f
Loose cement, within humeral canal, 373, 375f

M

Malunion
　of proximal humeral fracture, 154–155, 155f
　tuberosity
　　after unconstrained arthroplasty for fracture, 287–288
　　revision shoulder arthroplasty for, 334, 335f
Mechanical impingement
　in dislocated revision of reverse prosthesis, 456
　in dislocation of a reverse prosthesis, 233
Medium skin rake, 20f
Metaphyseal bone, three-finned blazer in, 300f
Metaphyseal fin tracts, 297
Modern-day shoulder arthroplasty design, 293
Modified Hohmann retractor, 294
Modular humeral implant, with Morse taper, in humeral stem removal, 360, 364f
Moreland osteotomes, in cement removal, 373, 375f–376f
Morse taper, modular humeral implant with, in humeral stem removal, 360, 364f
Morselized bone graft, 268
Musculocutaneous nerve, surgical anatomy of, 8, 13f

N

Nerve conduction studies, in revision shoulder arthroplasty, 344
Neural injury, with humeral fracture, 239
Neurovascular structures
　in intraoperative complications, 286
　intraoperative complications involving, in revision arthroplasty, 452–453
　in reverse shoulder arthroplasty, 226–227
　unconstrained arthroplasty, 137–138

Neutral-rotation sling, 130, 133f, 220, 223f, 283, 285f, 448, 449f
Nice Multicenter Study results, of unconstrained arthroplasty, 135t
Nonunion
　of proximal humeral fracture, 154, 154f
　tuberosity
　　after unconstrained arthroplasty for fracture, 287–288
　　revision shoulder arthroplasty for, 334, 335f
Notching, scapular
　after reverse shoulder arthroplasty, 231, 232f
　after revision arthroplasty, 459–460, 460f
　avoidance of, 231, 233f

O

Operating room
　layout of, 16, 17f
　overhead lighting in, 16, 18f
　staff positioning in, 16, 17f
　surgical instrumentation in, 16, 18f, 19t
Orthosis, postoperative, 130, 133f, 220, 223f, 283, 285f, 448
　type of, 461, 462t
Osseous deficit
　of glenoid, after component removal, 374, 377f
　in glenoid revision with bone graft
　　contained, 420, 421f–422f
　　uncontained (anterior or posterior), 420, 422f–427f
　　uncontained combined (anterior and posterior), 420–428, 427f–431f
Osteoarthritis
　glenohumeral, with massive rotator cuff tear
　　imaging findings in, 149–151, 149f–151f
　　reverse arthroplasty for, 147–151
　primary
　　clinical findings in, 39
　　imaging findings in, 40, 40f–41f
　　unconstrained arthroplasty for, 39–41
Osteonecrosis, of humeral head, unconstrained arthroplasty for, 42–43, 42f
Osteopenia, severe, proximal humeral fracture and, 238–239, 240f–241f

Osteophytes
　peripheral, humeral, 295f
　removal of
　　in reverse arthroplasty, 178, 180f
　　in uncemented unconstrained arthroplasty, 89, 91f–92f
　　scapular notching accompanied by, 231, 231f
Osteotomes, for humeral stem removal, 367, 367f, 371f
Osteotomy, in humeral stem removal, 367–373, 369f–370f
　cable placement in, 373, 373f–374f
　by plastic deformation, 367, 372f
　unicortical, 367, 371f
Overhead lighting, in operating room, 16, 18f

P

Pain relief, resection arthroplasty for, 417, 419f
Passing sutures, in subscapularis repair, 123, 125f
Patient positioning, for arthroplasty, 29, 30f–31f
Pectoralis major
　release of, in revision arthroplasty, 346–350, 353f
　surgical anatomy of, 8, 11f
　in unconstrained arthroplasty, 66, 69f
Peripheral humeral osteophytes, 295f
Peripheral osteophytes, humerus, 295f
Periprosthetic fracture, revision shoulder arthroplasty for, 334–336, 335f–336f
Periprosthetic humeral fractures, 374, 378f
　after revision arthroplasty, 454–455
　with reverse prosthesis, 228, 229f–230f
　treatment of, by revision arthroplasty, 380–385, 406, 409f
　with unconstrained prosthesis, 140, 140f, 289
Physical examination
　preoperative, 53, 54f
　in reverse arthroplasty, 160–161, 161f
　for revision shoulder arthroplasty, 337, 338f
　in shoulder arthroplasty, for fractures, 242
Pins, bioabsorbable, for osseous glenoid defects, 420–428, 427f–430f

Polyethylene glenoid components. *see also* Glenoid component
 convex-back
  implantation of, 113, 116f–117f
  selection of, 111–113, 113f
 posteriorly augmented, 468, 468f
Polyethylene inserts, in reverse-prosthesis humeral component trialing, 209, 213f, 215f
Polyethylene wear, of humeral component, 228, 229f
Posterior capsule stretching, from siesta position, 463f
Postinfectious arthropathy
 imaging findings of, 48, 48f
 unconstrained arthroplasty for, 47–49
Posttraumatic arthritis
 glenohumeral, unconstrained arthroplasty for, 45f
 with proximal humeral malunion, 155f
 with severe proximal humeral malunion., 44, 45f
Power equipment, 19t, 22f
Preoperative planning
 for reverse arthroplasty
  clinical history and examination in, 160–163, 161f
  radiography in, 161–163, 162f–166f
  secondary imaging, 163–168, 166f–168f
 for revision shoulder arthroplasty, 337–345
  clinical history in, 337, 338f
  physical examination in, 337, 338f
  radiography in, 337–339, 339f–343f
  secondary imaging in, 339–344, 343f–345f
  special tests in, 344
 for shoulder arthroplasty
  clinical history and examination in, 242
  prosthetic positioning, with ancillary instrumentation, 244
  radiography in, 242, 243f
  secondary imaging in, 242, 244f
 software, 168
  in reverse shoulder arthroplasty, 468, 469f
  in shoulder arthroplasty, 465, 466f–467f
 for unconstrained arthroplasty
  clinical history and examination in, 53–65
  computed tomography for, 64f
  radiography in, 54–60
  results of, 54

Preoperative planning (*Continued*)
  secondary imaging in, 60–61
  software and patient-specific, 61–63, 64f
Prosthesis. *see also specific component*
 dislocation of, 233f
 humeral, positioning, 254–267, 255f
  head replacement for fracture, 254–260, 258f–260f
 humeral head, 306f
  placement of, Gothic arch technique in, 242–244, 244f–248f
 reverse-design, 2f, 6, 6f, 148f
 instability of, 233, 234f–235f
Pseudoparalysis, chronic, massive rotator cuff tear with, reverse arthroplasty for, 155–156, 156f
Pyrocarbon implant, in shoulder arthroplasty, 467

R
"Racking hitch" technique, 268, 276f–278f
Radial nerve
 injury to, in revision arthroplasty, 452
 visualization, in extending deltopectoral approach into anterolateral diaphysis, 355, 359f
Radiography
 of osteoarthritis, 40, 40f–41f
 of osteonecrosis of humeral head, 42, 42f–44f
 of postinfectious arthropathy, 48f
 of posttraumatic arthritis, 45f, 46
 preoperative
  for proximal humeral fractures, 242, 243f–244f
  in reverse arthroplasty, 161–163, 162f–166f
 templates for, 163, 164f
 for revision shoulder arthroplasty, 337–339, 339f–343f
 of rheumatoid arthritis, 41, 41f
 with massive rotator cuff tear, 151, 153f
 of rotator cuff tear arthropathy, 46–47, 47f, 149–151, 149f–151f
 in unconstrained arthroplasty, 54–60, 57f–58f
 templates for, 60, 60f–61f
Reamer, insertion of, in stiff shoulder, 106–110, 108f, 110f
Reaming
 of glenoid surface, 107f–112f, 110–111
  to produce inferior tilt, 189, 191f
 of humeral diaphysis, 89–94, 95f, 387–390, 389f, 407f

Reaming (*Continued*)
 of humeral epiphysis, 387–390, 389f
 of humeral head, with triflange reamer, 308, 311f
 of humeral metaphysis, 398–406, 402f
Rehabilitation, after shoulder arthroplasty, 461–464
 hydrotherapy in
  principles of, 461
  protocol for, 461–464, 462f–464f, 462t
 return to activity following, 464
Resection arthroplasty, for pain relief, 417, 419f
Retractors, 19t, 20f–21f
 deltopectoral approach, 66, 70f
 humeral head, 294
 modified Hohmann, 294
Reverse arthroplasty
 complications of
  intraoperative, 224–227, 226f
  postoperative, 227–236, 227f–235f
 contraindications to, 147–159, 158t
 deltoid violation, 169
 extensile exposure, 169
 familiarity, 169
 for fracture, 263–264
  bone graft for, preparation of, 264
  humeral component for, implantation of, 264, 266f–267f
  humeral diaphysis for, identification and preparation of, 263, 265f
  humeral implant for, selection of, 263–264, 265f–266f
  prosthetic positioning for, 263–264
 glenoid component in, 189–208
  glenoid base-plate selection-post, or threaded post, 199, 201f–202f
  positioning in, 169, 170f
  preparation and implantation of, 189–199, 190f, 192f–193f, 197f–198f
   anterior and posterior screws, placement of, 194–199, 199f
   base plate screw introduction and fixation in, 189–194, 194f–195f, 198f
   base plate screw length in, determination of, 189–194, 196f–197f
   base plate screw tightening in, 189–199, 194f, 199f
   enlargement of peg hole in, 189, 192f
   glenosphere placement and fixation in, 199, 200f–201f

Reverse arthroplasty (Continued)
    inferior base-plate screw, insertion of, 194, 197f
    optimal inferior screw placement in, 189–194, 196f
    reaming to produce inferior tilt in, 189, 191f
    primary reverse prosthesis, glenoid bone loss with, 199–207, 203f–207f
  glenoid exposure during, 169, 175
    technique for, 175, 176f–177f
  glenoid problems after, 288–289
  humeral component in, 178–186
  humeral resection, level of, 169
  indications for, 147–159
    acute proximal humeral fracture as, 156, 156f
    fixed glenohumeral dislocation, 156–157, 157f–158f
    humeral malunion as, 155, 155f
    massive rotator cuff tear with chronic pseudoparalysis as, 155–156, 156f
    postinfectious arthropathy, 157–158, 158f
    rheumatoid arthritis with massive rotator cuff tear as, 151–154, 153f–154f
    rotator cuff tear arthropathy as, 147–151, 149f–151f
    tumor, 158, 159f
  preoperative planning for
    clinical history and examination in, 160–161, 161f
    radiography in, 161–163, 162f–166f
    secondary imaging, 163–168, 166f–168f
  reduction and deltoid tensioning in, 209–218
  results of, 224–236, 225t
  surgical approach to, 169–174, 170f–174f
  technology in, 468, 468f–469f
Reverse-design prosthesis, 6, 6f
  early, forces acting on, 148f
  Grammont-designed, 147, 148f
  instability of, 233, 234f–235f
Reverse glenoid component, revision shoulder arthroplasty for, 326–328, 328f–329f
Reverse humeral component, revision shoulder arthroplasty for, 329, 330f–331f
Revision arthroplasty
  clinical history for, 337, 338f
  complications in
    intraoperative, 450–453, 452f
    postoperative, 453–460, 453f–460f
  contraindications to, 336, 336t

Revision arthroplasty (Continued)
  deltopectoral approach to, 346–354
    axillary nerve identification in, 350–354
    conjoined tendon in
      identification of, 346–350
      release of, 350, 354f
    coracoid process identification in, 346–350, 352f
    deltopectoral interval in, 346–350, 350f
    draping in, 346, 347f
    extension of, into anterolateral approach to humeral diaphysis, 354–355
      biceps brachii dissection in, 355, 356f
      brachialis splitting in, 355, 357f
      complete humeral shaft exposure in, 355, 357f
      deltoid humeral insertion in, 355, 358f
      radial nerve visualization in, 355, 359f
      skin incision in, 355, 355f–356f
    hypertrophic scar excision in, 346, 348f
    pectoralis major release, 346–350, 353f
    permanent sutures in, 354, 355f
    previous skin incisions for, 346, 347f
    subscapularis tenotomy in, 354, 355f
  glenoid exposure in, 373–374, 376f–377f
  humeral component in, 380–412
    allograft reconstruction, of proximal humerus, 387–390, 388f–397f
    insertion of stem in, technique for, 390–406, 397f–406f
    preparation of, proximal humerus in, 380–387
    reverse-design humeral stem implant as, 380–387, 385f–387f, 390–398
    special situations in, 406–411, 407f–412f
    unconstrained humeral stem implant as, 380, 381f–385f, 390
  humeral stem removal in, 360–373
    cable placement in, 367, 370f
    cement removal in, 373, 375f–376f
    Cobb elevator in, 360, 364f, 367, 368f
    dislocation maneuver in, 360, 363f
    extraction device attachment in, 360, 366f

Revision arthroplasty (Continued)
    fibrous tissue removal in, 360, 363f–365f
    humeral-based inferior capsular release in, 360, 362f
    humeral osteotomy in, 360, 367–373, 367f, 369f–374f
    implant exposure in, 360, 361f
    modular humeral implant, with Morse taper in, 360, 364f
    proximal humerus retraction in, 360, 362f
    rotator cuff inspection before, 360, 366f
    specialized instruments for, 361f
  imaging for, 337–345
    secondary, 339–344, 343f–345f
  indications for, 323–336
    glenoid problems as, 323–328
    humeral problems as, 328–329
    infection in, 332–334
    periprosthetic fracture as, 334–336, 335f–336f
    soft tissue problems as, 329–332
    tuberosity problems in, 334, 335f
  physical examination for, 337, 338f
  preoperative planning for, 337–345
  radiography for, 337–339, 339f–343f
  results of, 450–460, 451t
  with reverse prosthesis, instability after, 455–456, 455f–457f
  special tests for, 344
  surgical approach to, 346–355
  unconstrained, instability after, 455
Rheumatoid arthritis
  imaging findings of, 41, 41f
  juvenile-onset, 42
  with massive rotator cuff tear
    imaging findings in, 151–154, 153f–154f
    reverse arthroplasty for, 151–154
  unconstrained arthroplasty for, 41–42
Rotation exercises, in hydrotherapy, 462f
Rotator cuff
  inspection of, before humeral stem removal, 360, 366f
  instability after unconstrained revision arthroplasty, 455
  insufficiency, in glenoid revision with bone graft, 428, 431f
  intraoperative complications involving, in revision arthroplasty, 452
  postoperative injury to, in revision arthroplasty, 456
  problems, revision shoulder arthroplasty for, 332, 333f
  surgical anatomy of, 13, 14f

Rotator cuff (Continued)
  in unconstrained arthroplasty
    intraoperative injury to, 134–137
    postoperative injury to, 144, 144f
Rotator cuff tear
  after unconstrained arthroplasty, 140, 143f
  arthropathy, after unconstrained shoulder arthroplasty, 46–47, 47f
  massive
    with chronic pseudoparalysis, 155–156, 156f
    with glenohumeral osteoarthritis
      imaging findings in, 149–151, 149f–151f
      reverse arthroplasty for, 147–151
    with rheumatoid arthritis, 151–154
Rotator interval
  glenohumeral arthrotomy through, in subscapularis tenotomy, 73, 75f–76f
  repair of, technique of, 123, 124f–128f
  surgical anatomy of, 13, 14f

S
Scapula
  anatomy of, 15f
  body and spine fractures of, after revision arthroplasty, 459, 459f
  in shoulder arthroplasty, recognition of dynamic role of, 465–466
Scapular notching
  after reverse shoulder arthroplasty, 231, 231f–233f
    avoidance of, 231, 233f
    classification of, 232f
  after revision arthroplasty, 459–460, 460f
  after unconstrained arthroplasty, 289
Scissors, 19t, 20f
Screw holes, for glenoid base plate, 189–194, 194f
Second-generation shoulder arthroplasty, 1
Second looped suture, reduction and fixation of tuberosity, 268, 282f
Secondary imaging, for revision shoulder arthroplasty, 339–344, 343f–345f
"Shoehorn" technique, of reduction, of reverse arthroplasty, 218, 218f
Short-stem arthroplasty, 2

Shoulder. see also Glenohumeral joint
  instability arthropathy of, 43–44, 45f
  surgical anatomy of, 8–13, 9f, 15f
  tumor of, 50–51, 158, 159f
Shoulder arthroplasty
  alternative bearing surfaces for, 466–467
  biologic alternatives to, 308–321
  constrained and semiconstrained, 6, 6f
  convertible, 6–7, 7f
  evolution of, 1–7
  first-generation, 1
  future directions in, 465–469
  hemiarthroplasty versus, 39
  implants and techniques of, 13–15
  intraoperative complications of, 286
  rehabilitation after, 461–464
  resources for, 15
  reverse. see Reverse arthroplasty
  revision. see Revision arthroplasty
  scapula in, recognition of dynamic role of, 465–466
  second-generation, 1
  short-stem, 2
  Simpliciti stemless, 294f
  stemless, 2
  surgical approach to, 249
  third-generation, 1–2, 2t, 3f
  unconstrained. see Unconstrained arthroplasty
Shoulder aspiration, fluoroscopically guided, 344
Siesta position
  anterior capsule stretching from, 463f
  posterior capsule stretching from, 463f
  in rehabilitation, 463f
Simpliciti stemless shoulder arthroplasty, 294f
Skeletal dysplasia, glenohumeral arthritis associated with, 50, 51f
Skin closure. see Wound closure
Skin incision. see Incision
Skin preparation, 29, 31f–34f
  for iliac crest bone graft harvesting, 441, 441f–442f
Skin staples, for wound closure, 448, 449f
Sling(s)
  neutral-rotation, 130, 133f, 220, 223f, 283, 285f, 448, 449f
  simple, 130, 133f
Soft tissue, revision shoulder arthroplasty for, 329–332

Soft tissue balancing, in unconstrained arthroplasty, 118
  need for, 118
  posterior capsular release in, 118, 122f
  posterior capsulorrhaphy in, 118, 119f–121f
Soft tissue removal, in glenoid exposure, 374, 376f
Software, preoperative planning
  in reverse shoulder arthroplasty, 468, 469f
  in shoulder arthroplasty, 465, 466f–467f
Spine fracture, scapular, after revision arthroplasty, 459, 459f
Staff positioning, in operating room, 16, 17f
Stay sutures
  control of subscapularis with, 123, 125f
  placement of, before subscapularis tenotomy, 73, 74f
Stemless humeral implant, 2, 3f
Stemless shoulder arthroplasty, 293–307
  Simpliciti, 294f
Stemless unconstrained total shoulder arthroplasty
  contraindications to, 294
  indications for, 294
  technique for, 294–301, 296f–298f
Steri-Strips, in wound closure, 220, 223f, 283, 285f, 448, 449f
Sterile dressings, after arthroplasty, 130, 133f, 283
Stiffness, glenohumeral
  after reverse shoulder arthroplasty, 236
  after revision arthroplasty, 456–458, 457f
  after unconstrained arthroplasty, 144–145, 144f
Stress fractures, acromial
  after reverse shoulder arthroplasty, 229–231, 230f
  after revision arthroplasty, 458–459, 458f
Subcuticular running closure, 130, 132f
Subdeltoid adhesions, release of, 351f
Subluxation, of humeral head, 54–59, 59f–60f
Subscapularis, 73–82
  placement of stay sutures in, 73, 74f
  problems, revision shoulder arthroplasty for, 332, 332f
  visualization of, 73
Subscapularis insufficiency
  belly press test for, 57f
  lift-off test for, 54, 57f
  in reverse prosthesis, 233

Subscapularis recess, loose bodies in, 40, 40f, 73–82, 84f
Subscapularis repair
  failure of, 144, 144f
  technique of, 123, 124f–128f
Subscapularis tendon, surgical anatomy of, 13f
Subscapularis tenotomy, 360
  glenohumeral arthrotomy in, 73, 75f–76f
  glenohumeral ligaments in
    release of, 73–82, 81f–83f
    visualization of, 73–82, 80f
  identification of loose bodies in, 73–82, 84f
  placement of stay suture before, 73, 74f
  release of extra-articular adhesions in, 73–82, 84f
  release of humeral joint capsule in, 73–82, 79f
  in revision arthroplasty, 354, 355f
  technique of, 73–82, 74f–85f
  transection of tendon in, 73, 77f–78f, 82f
  tucking of subscapularis into subscapularis fossa in, 73–82, 85f
Suction tip with tubing, 26f
Supraspinatus
  atrophy of, 337, 338f
  computed tomography of, 63f
  integrity of, Jobe's test for, 54, 55f–56f
Surface planar, 297, 297f
Surgical approach, to unconstrained arthroplasty, 66
  completed retractor placement in, 70f
  conjoined tendon retraction in, 70f
  coracoacromial ligament in, 70f
  deltopectoral interval identification in, 66, 68f
  skin incision for, 66, 67f
  topographic anatomy identification in, 66, 67f
Surgical drains
  after iliac crest graft harvesting, 444, 447f
  placement of, 283, 284f
  proximal extent of, 284f
  removal of, 283, 284f
Surgical draping, 29–34, 31f–34f
  for autogenous fascia lata harvest, 313, 314f
  for iliac crest graft harvesting, 439–441, 442f
  in revision arthroplasty, 346, 347f
Surgical instrumentation, 16, 18f, 19t

Suture(s), 25f, 25t. *see also specific types*
  dissolving, reaction to, 453
  permanent, in revision arthroplasty, 354, 355f
Suture anchor placement, for biologic glenoid resurfacing, 316, 320f
Suture fixation technique, of tuberosity reduction and fixation, 268, 269f
Synovial biopsy, for postinfectious arthropathy, 49, 49f

T
Teaching resources, for shoulder arthroplasty, 15
Tenotomy, subscapularis. *see Subscapularis tenotomy*
Teres minor, evaluation of, horn blower's sign in, 54, 56f
Texas Orthopedic Hospital, shoulder arthroplasty performed at, long head of biceps tendon abnormalities in, 35, 36t
Third-generation shoulder arthroplasty, 1–2, 2t, 3f
Three-part proximal humeral fractures, 237–238, 239f
"Thumb test", 296
Total shoulder arthroplasty
  stemless unconstrained
    contraindications to, 294
    indications for, 294
    technique for, 294–301, 296f–298f
  technology in, 468, 468f
Transosseous sutures
  in insertion, of humeral stem, in revision arthroplasty, 390, 397f
  placement of
    for reattachment of subscapularis, in uncemented unconstrained arthroplasty, 99–103, 102f
    in subscapularis repair, 123, 126f
Trial prosthetic humeral head, 301, 302f
  placement of, 303f
Trial stem. *see Humeral stem, trial*
Triple-locking position, in rehabilitation, 464f
Tuberosity(ies). *see also Greater tuberosity; Lesser tuberosity*
  complications of, after unconstrained arthroplasty for fracture, 287–288, 287f
  malunion and nonunion, revision shoulder arthroplasty for, 334, 335f
  reduction and fixation of, 268–282

Tuberosity(ies) (*Continued*)
  bone graft plug in, 268, 271f
  placement of, 268
  suture fixation technique of, 268, 269f
  technique for, 268, 269f–282f
  vertical fixation, 268, 281f–282f
Tumors, about shoulder girdle
  reverse arthroplasty for, 158, 159f
  unconstrained arthroplasty for, 50–51
Twist test, for reverse-prosthesis humeral component, 178–184, 184f

U
Unconstrained arthroplasty
  for chronic conditions. *see also specific chronic conditions*
    complications of
      intraoperative, 134–138, 137f
      postoperative, 138–145, 138f–144f
      results of, 134, 135t–136t, 143f
    glenoid component in, 106–117
    glenoid exposure in, 86, 87f–88f
    humeral components in
      cemented, 89, 90f
        indication for, 89, 91f
        technique for insertion of, 103, 104f–105f
      uncemented, 89
    soft tissue balancing in, 118, 119f–122f
  for fractures, 4–6, 5f
    complications
      intraoperative, 286
      postoperative, 287–291
    contraindications to, 239, 241t
    identification and handling of the tuberosity in, 249, 250f–253f
    indications for, 237–241
      four-part proximal humeral fractures as, 237, 238f–239f
      fracture-dislocation as, 238, 240f
      glenoid issues as, 239
      head-splitting fracture as, 238, 240f
      neural injury as, 239
      rotator cuff pathology as, 239
      severe osteopenia as, 238–239, 240f–241f
      three-part proximal humeral fractures as, 237–238, 239f
    results of, 286
    in special situations, 238–239, 241f
    surgical approach to, 249, 250f
    wound closure in, 283
    greater and lesser tuberosities, 269f

Unconstrained arthroplasty (Continued)
  indications for, 39–52
    contraindications to, 51, 51t
    fixed glenohumeral dislocation as, 46, 47f
    glenohumeral chondrolysis as, 49–50, 49f–50f
    humeral head osteonecrosis as, 42–43, 42f
    instability arthropathy as, 43–44
    postinfectious arthropathy as, 47–49
    posttraumatic arthritis as, 44–46, 46f
    primary osteoarthritis as, 39–41, 40f
    rheumatoid arthritis as, 41–42, 41f
    rotator cuff tear arthropathy as, 46–47, 47f
  postoperative orthosis in, 130, 133f, 220
  preoperative planning for clinical history and examination in, 53–65, 54f
  results of, 54
  subscapularis and rotator interval repair in, technique of, 123, 124f–128f

Unconstrained arthroplasty (Continued)
  total, stemless
    contraindications to, 294
    indications for, 294
    technique for, 294–301, 296f–298f
  tuberosity reduction and fixation in bone graft plug in, 268, 270f–271f
  suture fixation technique of, 272f–275f, 279f–282f
  wound closure in, 130, 220, 222f
Unconstrained humeral component, revision shoulder arthroplasty for, 328, 329f
Unconstrained humeral head replacement, for fracture, 254–263
  humeral component for, implantation of, 261–263, 262f–264f
  humeral diaphysis for, identification and preparation of, 254, 256f–257f
  humeral implant for, selection of, 254, 258f
  preparation of bone graft for, 260–261, 261f–262f
  prosthetic positioning for (Gothic arch technique), 254–260, 258f–260f

V
Vascular injuries, intraoperative, during shoulder arthroplasty, 286
Vertical tuberosity fixation, 268, 281f–282f
Virtual surgery, of shoulder arthroplasty, 465, 466f–467f

W
Wound closure
  in iliac crest graft harvest, 444, 447f
  in reverse arthroplasty, 220, 221f–223f
  in revision arthroplasty, 448, 449f
  in unconstrained arthroplasty, 130, 133f
    for fracture, 283, 284f–285f
Wound dehiscence, postoperative, 138, 138f, 227, 288, 453
Wound problems
  after reverse shoulder arthroplasty, 227
  after revision arthroplasty, 453
  after unconstrained arthroplasty, 138, 138f